OSCES IN
Obstetrics and Maternal-Fetal Medicine

An Evidence-Based Approach

EDITED BY

Amira El-Messidi
McGill University

Alan D. Cameron
University of Glasgow

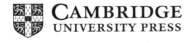 CAMBRIDGE
UNIVERSITY PRESS

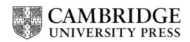

Shaftesbury Road, Cambridge CB2 8EA, United Kingdom

One Liberty Plaza, 20th Floor, New York, NY 10006, USA

477 Williamstown Road, Port Melbourne, VIC 3207, Australia

314–321, 3rd Floor, Plot 3, Splendor Forum, Jasola District Centre, New Delhi – 110025, India

103 Penang Road, #05–06/07, Visioncrest Commercial, Singapore 238467

Cambridge University Press is part of Cambridge University Press & Assessment, a department of the University of Cambridge.

We share the University's mission to contribute to society through the pursuit of education, learning and research at the highest international levels of excellence.

www.cambridge.org
Information on this title: www.cambridge.org/9781108972185

DOI: 10.1017/9781108975780

First published 2023

Printed in the United Kingdom by TJ Books Limited, Padstow Cornwall

A catalogue record for this publication is available from the British Library

ISBN 978-1-108-97218-5 Paperback

Additional resources for this publication at www.cambridge.org/9781108972185

Cambridge University Press & Assessment has no responsibility for the persistence or accuracy of URLs for external or third-party internet websites referred to in this publication and does not guarantee that any content on such websites is, or will remain, accurate or appropriate.

....

To my parents – thank you for your untiring encouragement, unwavering affection, and experienced advice. Thank you for always providing me your all. Words fall short in expressing my gratefulness to you.

To my teachers – thank you for grounding me as a clinician and for inspiring me to explore my talent to maintain your legacy.

To the array of clinical trainees, the '*brothers and sisters*' who have put themselves through and reaped the benefits of hours of teaching and learning with me, not to forget all without breaks, accommodating what has evolved as '*Dr. El-Messidi's guidelines*: food is permitted, but she won't be impressed if you waste time for *urological* breaks, so have your coffee at least two hours before her sessions!'

To Professor Alan Cameron, my coeditor and mentor, and Ms. Anna Whiting, our Senior Commissioning Editor at Cambridge University Press, who saw my vision and believed in my *labor of love*.

Amira El-Messidi

Contents

SECTION 3: Placental Complications

SECTION 4: Neurological Disorders in Pregnancy

SECTION 5: Psychiatric Disorders in Pregnancy

SECTION 6: Cardiopulmonary Conditions in Pregnancy

SECTION 7: Hepato-Renal and Gastrointestinal Conditions in Pregnancy

SECTION 8: Connective Tissue Disorders in Pregnancy

SECTION 9: Hematologic Conditions in Pregnancy

SECTION 13: Miscellaneous Conditions

Preface

> He who studies medicine without books sails an unchartered sea, but he who studies medicine without patients does not go to sea at all.
>
> Sir William Osler (1849–1919)

Traditionally, the crux of factual knowledge in obstetrics is presented within a myriad of formats that include textbooks, handbooks, point-of-care resources, and diverse nations' practice guidelines, while didactic simulations using simulated patients, manikins, or virtual patients assess different dimensions of clinical performance. Given the daily activities of obstetric care providers in an era of continuously evolving practice standards, intertwined with the responsibility of transmission of knowledge and skill to learners, this innovative resource was envisioned to blend evidence-based practice standards in obstetrics and medical complications of pregnancy with academic fundamentals into a patient-centered approach using standardized objective structured clinical examination (OSCE)-type scenarios.

Introduced in 1975 in response to criticisms regarding the reliability and validity of traditional clinical examinations, OSCEs have been adopted worldwide and are now recognized as gold standard for assessment of clinical competence [1]. Each of the 77 OSCE chapters starts with a brief case scenario and guides obstetric practitioners and trainees to focused history taking, which implies the extrapolation of essential patient information, to then offer evidence-based counseling and management from preconception or early pregnancy to the postpartum period. With reference to contemporary British, American, Canadian, Australian, and other international clinical policy makers, the intent of the book is to provide an evidence-based approach to clinical care, synchronizing practice recommendations where possible and otherwise allowing international readers to appreciate diverse evidence-based practices. Developed from the selected 'Suggested Readings,' with a maximum of 10 per chapter, where possible, each scenario assumes the reader is the obstetric care provider, accompanied by a clinical trainee, providing comprehensive coverage of the obstetric patient, thereby helping trainees prepare for high-stakes certification examinations or health care workers in providing care. The pedagogical approach also serves to stress important elements of basic science and physiology required to appreciate clinical practice.

The marking mechanism is intended as a simple and schematic tool to objectify progress in self-assessment or peer review, with the total points per OSCE chapter in multiples of 5 for homogeneity of structure throughout the book. The weight of allotted points is open to modification according to the level of the learner, as is the content presented throughout any chapter. For example, the objectives of a junior obstetric trainee may be solely to extrapolate a patient's medical history and initiate necessary investigations, while a senior trainee may be expected to provide counseling, analyze laboratory results, structure clinical care, and manage complications in pregnancy or postpartum. Unlike real-time settings, where OSCEs are intended to be completed within the specified time frame, this book offers teachers and learners flexibility according to individual needs. Readers are encouraged to recognize that clinical blurbs depicting the progress of an OSCE scenario often contain clinically relevant academic information presented partly for learning purposes. To interconnect clinical content while avoiding overlap of concepts addressed elsewhere in the book, readers will find selected 'Special notes' directing them to complementary content addressed in other OSCE chapters or otherwise providing adjunctive literary reference or highlighting learning points.

This textbook is intended for all obstetric care providers and learners as a stimulus for excellence in modern evidence-based clinical and academic dimensions of obstetrics. We hope you enjoy the art of teaching and the lifelong journey of learning, amid providing medical care to the mother and fetus, as much as we enjoyed crafting these innovative OSCE chapters.

REFERENCE

1. Harden RM, Laidlaw JM. Clinical and Performance-Based Assessment. Chapter 30 in: *Essential Skills for a Medical Teacher: An Introduction to Teaching and Learning in Medicine.* New York: Elsevier; 2012.

Amira El-Messidi and Alan D. Cameron

Acknowledgments

Fundamental to the sculpting of this textbook are pillars of countless supporters to whom I remain indebted. Thank you to all my clinical 'brothers and sisters,' including physicians, nurses, and allied health professionals, who were instrumental in different dimensions throughout the journey of my endeavor.

Consistent with the metaphor 'as an arrow can only be shot by pulling it backward, just focus and you'll be launched forward,' I value the challenges that propelled me to continue aiming for this book's construction.

Professor Cameron and I are appreciative of the collaboration and expertise of all contributors, who were fundamental to the construction of a tome of this breadth. We are also grateful to our entire team at Cambridge University Press, in particular, Ms. Beth Pollard, our Content Manager, and Ms. Camille Lee-Own, our Senior Editorial Assistant. We appreciate Mr. Nicholas Dunton, who committed to launching the early creation of this production shortly prior to his well-deserved retirement, and we remain indebted to Ms. Anna Whiting, who continued as our Senior Commissioning Editor; thank you, Anna, for your executive managerial skills, which you lace with an unwavering presence and experienced insight.

Amira El-Messidi

As a part of the University of Cambridge, Cambridge University Press's mission is to unlock people's potential with the best learning and research solutions. It is a privilege for me to work on the medical books list, and particularly on our obstetrics and gynecology books, which directly assist clinicians in what is a varied role that offers no typical days – helping them to improve outcomes for women and babies. Never more has a book exemplified these aims than this one, on which the editors and contributors have worked tirelessly to ensure that this book innovatively provides a valuable resource for clinicians at all levels. It's been a joy to work with a team that is so committed to making change by sharing their knowledge.

Anna Whiting

List of Abbreviations

A	ACEi	Angiotensin-converting enzyme inhibitor
	A&E	Accident & Emergency
	ADR	Autonomic dysreflexia
	AED	Antiepileptic drug
	AFE	Amniotic fluid embolism
	AFLP	Acute fatty liver of pregnancy
	AFV	Amniotic fluid volume
	AMA	Advanced maternal age
	ANA	Antinuclear antibody
	aPTT	Activated partial thromboplastin time
	AREDF	Absent (or reversed) end diastolic flow
	ART / cART	Antiretroviral therapy /combined antiretroviral therapy
	ALT, AST	Alanine aminotransferase, aspartate aminotransferase
B	BCG	Bacillus Calmette-Guerin (vaccine)
	ß-hCG	Beta human chorionic gonadotropin
	BMI	Body mass index
	BNP	Brain natriuretic peptide
	BPP	Biophysical profile
C	CBC or FBC	Complete blood count, or full blood count
	CD	Crohn's disease
	CF	Cystic fibrosis
	cfDNA	Cell-free DNA
	CFTR	Cystic fibrosis transmembrane conductance regulator
	ChEI	Cholinesterase inhibitors
	CKD	Chronic kidney disease
	CMA	Chromosomal microarray analysis

	CMV	Cytomegalovirus
	CNV	Copy number variants
	CPAP	Continuous positive airway pressure
	CPR	Cerebroplacental ratio
	CRL	Crown-rump length
	CTG	Cardiotocography
	CVS	Chorionic villus sampling
D	DIC	Disseminated intravascular coagulation
	DID	Delayed interval delivery
	DKA	Diabetic ketoacidosis
	DMD	Disease-modifying drugs
	DMPA	Depot medroxyprogesterone acetate
	dsDNA	Double-stranded DNA
	DV	Ductus venosus
	DVP	Deep vertical pocket (*of amniotic fluid*)
	DVT	Deep vein thrombosis
E	ECG	Electrocardiogram
	ECMO	Extracorporeal membrane oxygenation
	EFW	Estimated fetal weight
	ELISA	Enzyme-linked immunoassay
	EMB	Ethambutol
	EPDS	Edinburgh Postnatal Depression Scale
	ERCP	Endoscopic retrograde cholangiopancreatogram
	E.R.	Emergency Room
F	FAST	Focused abdominal sonography for trauma
	FEV1	Forced expiratory volume in the first second of expiration
	FISH	Fluorescent in-situ hybridization
	fFN	Fetal fibronectin
	FGFR	Fibroblast growth factor receptor
	FGR	Fetal growth restriction
	FRC	Functional residual capacity
	FVC	Forced vital capacity

G	GBS	Group B Streptococcus
	GCT	Glucose challenge test
	GDM	Gestational diabetes mellitus
	GGT	Gamma-glutamyl transferase
H	HbA1c	Glycosylated hemoglobin
	HAV	Hepatitis A virus
	HBV	Hepatitis B virus
	hCG	Human chorionic gonadotropin
	HCV	Hepatitis C virus
	HELLP	Hemolysis, elevated liver enzymes, low platelets
	HIG	Hyperimmunoglobulin
	HIV	Human immunodeficiency virus
	HLA	Human leukocyte antigen
	HPEP	Hemoglobin protein electrophoresis
	HPV	Human papilloma virus
	HSV	Herpes simplex virus
I	ICP	Intrahepatic cholestasis of pregnancy
	ICU/ITU	Intensive care unit/ intensive treatment unit
	IGF	Insulin-like growth factor
	IGFBP	Insulin growth factor binding protein
	IM	Intramuscular
	INH	Isoniazid
	INR	International normalized ratio
	IPS	Integrated prenatal screening
	ITP	Immune thrombocytopenic purpura
	IUD	Intrauterine device
	IUFD	Intrauterine fetal demise/death
	IV	Intravenous
	IVH	Intraventricular hemorrhage
	IVIG	Intravenous immunoglobulin
	IOL	Induction of labor
J	....	
K	....	

L	LCHAD	Long-chain- 3-hydroxyacyl CoA dehydrogenase
	LDASA	Low-dose acetylsalicylic acid (aspirin)
	LDH	Lactate dehydrogenase
	LMWH	Low molecular weight heparin
	LNG-IUS	Levonorgestrel intrauterine system
	LVEF	Left ventricular ejection fraction
M	MCA	Middle cerebral artery
	MCDA	Monochorionic diamniotic
	MG	Myesthenia gravis
	MMF	Mycophenolate mofetil
	MMR(V)	Measles, mumps, rubella, varicella
	MoM	Multiples of the median
	MRCP	Magnetic resonance cholangiopancreatogram
	MRI	Magnetic resonance imaging
	MS	Multiple sclerosis
	MSAFP	Maternal serum alpha-fetoprotein
	MTCT	Mother-to-child transmission
N	NAAT	Nucleic acid amplification test
	NASH	Nonalcoholic steatohepatitis
	NICU	Neonatal intensive care unit
	NPH (insulin)	Neutral protamine Hagedorn
	NPV	Negative predictive value
	NSAIDs	Nonsteroidal anti-inflammatory drugs
	NST	Nonstress test
	NT	Nuchal translucency
	NTD	Neural tube defect
	NVP	Nausea/vomiting of pregnancy
	NYHA	New York Heart Association classification
O	OASIS	Obstetric anal sphincter injuries
	OGTT	Oral glucose tolerance test
	OSA	Obstructive sleep apnea
	OUD	Opioid use disorder

P	PAPP-A	Pregnancy-associated plasma protein-A
	PCI	Percutaneous coronary intervention
	PCR	Polymerase chain reaction
	PE	Pulmonary embolism
	PEFR	Peak expiratory flow rate
	PEP	Positive expiratory pressure
	PFT	Pulmonary function tests
	PI	Pulsatility index
	PlGF	Placental growth factor
	PO	Per os (oral)
	PPCM	Peripartum cardiomyopathy
	PPH	Postpartum hemorrhage
	PPROM	Preterm prelabor rupture of membranes
	PPV	Positive predictive value
	PTB	Preterm birth
	PTL	Preterm labor
	PT	Prothrombin time
	PV	Per vaginal
	PZA	Pyrazinamide
Q	QF-PCR	Quantitative fluorescence polymerase chain reaction
R	RIF	Rifampin
S	SCA	Sickle cell anemia
	SCI	Spinal cord injury
	sFGR	Selective fetal growth restriction
	sFlt-1	Soluble fms-like tyrosine kinase-1
	SLE	Systemic lupus erythematosus
	SSRI	Selective serotonin reuptake inhibitor
	STI	Sexually transmitted infection
T	T1DM, T2DM	Type 1 diabetes mellitus, type 2 diabetes mellitus
	TB	Tuberculosis
	TCP	Thrombocytopenia
	TEE/ TTE	Transesophageal echocardiography/ transthoracic echocardiography

	TIPS	Transjugular intrahepatic portosystemic shunt
	tPA	Tissue plasminogen activator
	TRAb, anti-TPO	Thyroid receptor antibody, thyroid peroxidase antibody
	TSH, T_3, T_4	Thyroid stimulating hormone, triiodothyronine, thyroxine
	TST	Tuberculin skin test
	TTN	Transient tachypnea of the newborn
	TTP	Thrombotic thrombocytopenic purpura
	TTTS	Twin–twin transfusion syndrome
	TORCH	Toxoplasmosis, others (e.g., syphilis, parvovirus B19, Listeria monocytogenes, Zika), rubella, cytomegalovirus, herpes, HIV
U	UA	Umbilical artery
	UAE	Uterine artery embolization
	UC	Ulcerative colitis
	UFH	Unfractionated heparin
	UPCR	Urine protein/creatinine ratio
	UtAD	Uterine artery Doppler
V	VBAC	Vaginal birth after Cesarean section
	VDRL, RPR test	Venereal disease research laboratory, rapid plasma reagin test
	V/Q scan	Ventilation/perfusion scan
	VTE	Venous thromboembolism
	VWD, VWF	Von Willebrand disease, Von Willebrand factor
	VZIG	Varicella zoster immunoglobulin
W - Z	....	

Contributors

Nimrah Abbasi MD MSc FRCSC
Assistant Professor, Department of Obstetrics and Gynecology, Ontario Fetal Centre, Mount Sinai Hospital, Toronto, Ontario, Canada

Rasha Abouelmagd DipA MSc PhD MD FRCA
Consultant Anaesthetist, Department of Anaesthesia, King's College Hospital, London, UK

Alfred Abuhamad, MD
President, Provost and Dean, Eastern Virginia Medical School, Norfolk, Virginia, USA

Neha Agrawal MD
Assistant Professor, Department of Gastroenterology & Hepatology, University of Florida, Jacksonville, Florida, USA

Waseem Ahmed MD
Postgraduate Fellow, Department of Medicine, Division of Gastroenterology & Hepatology, Weill Cornell Medicine, New York, NY, USA

Noor Amily MD, FRCSC
Assistant Professor, Department of Obstetrics, Gynecology and Newborn Care, Division of Maternal-Fetal Medicine, The Ottawa Hospital, Ottawa, Ontario, Canada

Anita Banerjee FHEA FRCP
Obstetric Physician, Internal Medicine Physician, Division of Women's Health, Guy's and St Thomas' Hospitals, NHS Foundation Trust, London, UK

Robert Battat MDCM, FRCPC
Assistant Professor, Department of Medicine, Division of Gastroenterology & Hepatology, Weill Cornell Medicine, New York, NY, USA

Nicolas Beaulieu, MD, FRCPC, M.A. Philosophy
Assistant Professor, Department of Psychiatry Université Laval, Québec Canada

Talat Bessissow MDCM MSc FRCPC
Associate Professor, Department of Medicine, Faculty of Medicine and Health Sciences, McGill University Division of Gastroenterology and Hepatology, McGill University Health Center, Montreal, Quebec, Canada

Nathaniel Bouganim MDCM FRCPC
Assistant Professor, Department of Medical Oncology, Faculty of Medicine and Health Sciences, McGill University, Montreal, Quebec, Canada

Richard Brown MBBS FRCOG FACOG
Associate Professor, Department of Obstetrics and Gynecology, Faculty of Medicine and Health Sciences, McGill University Director of Obstetrics and Maternal-Fetal Medicine, McGill University Health Centre, Montreal, Quebec, Canada

William M. Buckett MD FRCOG
Associate Professor, Department of Obstetrics and Gynecology, Faculty of Medicine and Health Sciences, McGill University Medical Director and Chief, Division of Reproductive Endocrinology and Infertility, McGill University Health Center, Montreal, Quebec, Canada

Alan D Cameron MD FRCP(Glas) FRCOG
Honorary Professor of Fetal Medicine, University of Glasgow, UK

Victoria E. Canelos MD
Postgraduate Resident, Department of Psychiatry, Massachusetts General Hospital, Boston, Massachusetts, USA

Elyce H. Cardonick MD
Professor of Obstetrics & Gynecology, Division of Maternal-Fetal Medicine, Director of the Cancer and Pregnancy Registry, Cooper University Hospital, MD Anderson at Cooper, Camden, New Jersey, USA

Andrea Carlson MD
Attending Physician and Director of Toxicology, Department of Emergency Medicine, Associate Program Director, Emergency Medicine Residency, Advocate Christ Medical Center, Chicago, Illinois, USA

Gabrielle Cassir MD FRCSC
Assistant Professor, Department of Obstetrics and Gynecology, Faculty of Medicine and Health Sciences, McGill University Division of Maternal-Fetal Medicine, St Mary's Hospital, Montreal, Quebec, Canada

Stella S. Daskalopoulou MD MSc DIC PhD
Associate Professor, Department of Medicine, Faculty of Medicine and Health Sciences, McGill University Director, Vascular Health Unit, Division of Internal Medicine, Montreal General Hospital, Montreal, Quebec, Canada

Bruno De Souza Ribeiro MD
Assistant Professor, Department of Gastroenterology & Hepatology, University of Florida, Jacksonville, Florida, USA

Hannah Douglas MRCP PhD
Consultant Cardiologist, Department of Cardiology, St Thomas' Hospital, London, UK

Rohan D'Souza MD PhD FRCOG
Associate Professor, Department of Obstetrics & Gynecology and Department of Health Research Methods, Evidence and Impact, McMaster University, Ontario, Canada

Genevieve Eastabrook, MD, FRCSC
Associate Professor, Department of Obstetrics & Gynaecology; Scientist, Division of Maternal, Fetal & Newborn Health, Children's Health Research Institute, and Director of Maternal-Fetal Medicine Subspecialty Training Program, Schulich School of Medicine and Dentistry, Western University, Ontario, Canada

Alexa Eberle MD
Postgraduate Resident, Department of Obstetrics and Gynecology, Faculty of Medicine and Health Sciences, McGill University, Montreal, Quebec, Canada

Maria Loren Eberle MD
Postgraduate Resident, Department of Emergency Medicine, Advocate Christ Medical Center, Chicago, Illinois, USA

Amira El-Messidi MDCM FRCSC RDMS
Associate Professor, Department of Obstetrics and Gynecology, Faculty of Medicine and Health Sciences, McGill University Consultant, Maternal-Fetal Medicine, McGill University Health Centre, Montreal, Quebec, Canada

Oseme Etomi MRCP
Specialty Registrar, Department of Rheumatology, Royal Free Hospital, London, UK

Majed S. Faden MBBS FRCSC
Consultant, Department of Obstetrics and Gynecology, Division of Maternal-Fetal Medicine, Women's Specialized Hospital, King Fahad Medical City, Riyadh, Saudi Arabia

Nader Fahmy MD PhD FRCSC
Assistant Professor, Department of Surgery, Faculty of Medicine and Health Sciences, McGill University Division of Urology, McGill University Health Center, Montreal, Quebec, Canada

Karen Fung-Kee-Fung MD FRCSC MHPE
Professor, Department of Obstetrics & Gynecology, Division of Maternal-Fetal Medicine, The Ottawa Hospital, Ontario, Canada

Robert Gagnon MD, FRCSC
Professor, Department of Obstetrics & Gynecology, Postgraduate Residency Program Director, Faculty of Medicine and Health Sciences, McGill University Division of Maternal-Fetal Medicine, McGill University Health Center, Montreal, Quebec, Canada

Natasha Garfield MDCM FRCPC
Assistant Professor, Department of Medicine, Faculty of Medicine and Health Sciences, McGill University Division of Endocrinology and Metabolism, McGill University Health Centre, Montreal, Quebec, Canada

Laura M. Gaudet MSc MD FRCSC
Associate Professor of Obstetrics & Gynecology, and of Radiology, Queen's University Division Head of Maternal Fetal Medicine, Kingston Health Science Center, Kingston, Ontario, Canada Adjunct Professor, School of Epidemiology and Public Health, University of Ottawa, and Affiliate Scientist, Ottawa Hospital Research Institute, Ottawa, Ontario Canada

Maged Peter Ghali MDCM MSc(epid) FRCPC
Professor, Department of Medicine, Chief of Gastroenterology & Hepatology; Program director, Gastroenterology Fellowship, University of Florida, Jacksonville, Florida, USA

Lucy Gilbert MD MSc FRCOG
Robert Kinch Chair in Women's Health, Professor, Department of Obstetrics & Gynecology, Department of Oncology, McGill University Director, Gynecologic Cancer Service, McGill University Health Center, Carole Epstein Leadership Award, Cedars Cancer Centre, Montreal, Quebec, Canada

Walter H. Gotlieb, MD, PhD
Professor of Obstetrics, Gynecology & Oncology, Director of Surgical Oncology, McGill University Chief, Department of Obstetrics & Gynecology, and Division of Gynecologic Oncology, Jewish General Hospital McGill University, Montreal, Quebec, Canada

Erica Hardy MD MMSc
Assistant Professor of Medicine, Divisions of Obstetric Medicine and Infectious Disease, The Warren Alpert Medical School of Brown University, Providence, Rhode Island, USA

Roupen Hatzakorzian MD
Assistant Professor, Departments of Anesthesia and Intensive Care, Faculty of Medicine and Health Sciences, McGill University, Montreal, Quebec, Canada

Michelle Hladunewich MD MSc
Chief of Medicine and Nephrologist, Sunnybrook Health Science Centre Professor of Medicine, University of Toronto, Toronto, Ontario, Canada Medical Lead, Glomerulonephritis and Specialty Clinics, Ontario Renal Network

Charlotte S. Hogan MD ABPN
Psychiatrist, Massachusetts General Hospital Instructor of Psychiatry, Harvard Medical School, Boston, Massachusetts, USA

Neel S. Iyer, DO, MPH
Postgraduate Fellow, Division of Maternal Fetal Medicine, Department of Obstetrics and Gynecology Thomas Jefferson University Hospital, Philadelphia, Pennsylvania, USA

Paula D. James MD
Professor, Department of Internal Medicine, Division of Hematology, Queen's University, Kingston, Ontario, Canada

Meena Khandelwal MD
Professor, Department of Obstetrics & Gynecology, Division of Maternal-Fetal Medicine, Cooper Medical School of Rowan University, Camden, New Jersey, USA

Srinivasan Krishnamurthy FRCS(Ed) FRCOG
Associate Professor, Vice-Chair of Education, Faculty of Medicine and Health Sciences, Department of Obstetrics and Gynecology, McGill University, Montreal, Quebec, Canada

Audrey-Ann Labrecque MDCM FRCSC
Postgraduate Fellow, Department of Obstetrics and Gynecology, Division of Maternal-Fetal Medicine, University of Calgary Cumming School of Medicine, Calgary, Alberta, Canada

Marie-France Lachapelle MDCM, FRCSC
Assistant Professor, Department of Obstetrics and Gynecology, Faculty of Medicine and Health Sciences, McGill University Division of Maternal-Fetal Medicine, Jewish General Hospital, McGill University, Montreal, Quebec, Canada

Jennifer Landry MD MSc FRCPC
Associate Professor, Department of Medicine, Faculty of Medicine and Health Sciences, McGill University Division of Respiratory Medicine, McGill University Health Centre, Montreal, Quebec, Canada

Catherine Legault, MD, FRCPC
Assistant Professor, Department of Neurology and Neurosurgery, Faculty of Medicine and Health Sciences, McGill University Stroke Neurologist, Montreal Neurological Institute and Hospital, Montreal, Quebec, Canada

Isabelle Malhamé, MD, MSc FRCPC

Assistant Professor, Department of Medicine, Faculty of Medicine and Health Sciences, McGill University McGill University Health Centre, Montreal, Quebec, Canada

Amanda Malik MD MPH

Clinical Instructor, Cooper Medical School of Rowan University, Camden, New Jersey, USA

Juliana Martins MD

Assistant Professor, Department of Obstetrics and Gynecology, Division of Maternal-Fetal Medicine, Eastern Virginia Medical School, Norfolk, Virginia, USA

Cynthia Maxwell MD FRCSC RDMS DABOG

Professor, Department of Obstetrics and Gynaecology, University of Toronto Maternal Fetal Medicine and Obesity Medicine Specialist Medical Lead, Women and Infants Ambulatory Health, Division Head, Maternal Fetal Medicine, Sinai Health Equity, Diversity and Inclusion Officer Toronto, Ontario, Canada

Anne-Maude Morency MD FRCSC

Assistant Professor, Postgraduate Fellowship Program Director Department of Obstetrics and Gynecology, Faculty of Medicine and Health Sciences, McGill University Division of Maternal-Fetal Medicine, Director of Obstetric Ultrasound, McGill University Health Center, McGill University, Montreal, Quebec, Canada

Ahmed Nazer MBBS FRCSC

Gynecologic Oncologist, Department of Obstetrics and Gynecology, King Faisal Specialist Hospital and Research Center, Riyadh, Saudi Arabia

Catherine Nelson-Piercy MA FRCP FRCOG

Professor of Obstetric Medicine and Consultant Obstetric Physician, Guy's and St. Thomas' Hospitals Trust, London, UK

Raluca Pana MD FRCPC CSCN(EEG)

Assistant Professor, Department of Neurology and Neurosurgery, Faculty of Medicine and Health Sciences, McGill University Neurologist and Epileptologist, Montreal Neurological Institute and Hospital, Montreal, Quebec, Canada

Jessica Papillon-Smith MD, FRCSC, MEHP

Assistant Professor, Department of Obstetrics and Gynecology, Faculty of Medicine and Health Sciences, McGill University Division of Minimally Invasive Gynecologic Surgery, McGill University Health Centre, Montreal, Quebec, Canada

Andrea S. Parks BSc MD FRCPC

Postgraduate Fellow in Neuromuscular Disorders, Division of Neurology, University of Toronto, Toronto, Ontario, Canada

Melissa-Rosina Pasqua MD FRCPC

Department of Medicine, Division of Endocrinology, McGill University Health Centre, Montreal, Quebec, Canada

Tiina Podymow MD FRCPC

Associate Professor, Department of Medicine, Faculty of Medicine and Health Sciences, McGill University Division of Nephrology, McGill University Health Centre, Montreal, Quebec, Canada

Vincent Ponette BSc (MIT), MD MBA FRCSC
Assistant Professor, Department of Obstetrics and Gynecology, Faculty of Medicine and Health Sciences, McGill University Division of Maternal-Fetal Medicine, McGill University Health Center, Montreal, Quebec, Canada

Glenn D. Posner MDCM MEd FRCSC
Professor, Department of Obstetrics, Gynecology and Newborn Care, University of Ottawa, Ottawa, Ontario, Canada

Oded Raban MD
Postgraduate Fellow, Department of Obstetrics and Gynecology, Faculty of Medicine and Health Sciences, McGill University Division of Gynecologic Oncology, McGill University Health Centre, Montreal, Quebec, Canada

Michelle Rougerie MD FRCSC
Postgraduate Fellow, Division of Maternal-Fetal Medicine, Department of Obstetrics and Gynecology, Monash Health, Melbourne, Victoria, Australia

Greg Ryan MD
Professor, Fetal Medicine Unit, Ontario Fetal Center, Mount Sinai Hospital, and Division of Maternal-Fetal Medicine, Department of Obstetrics and Gynaecology, University of Toronto, Toronto, Ontario, Canada

Marwa Salman MBBCh FRCA LLM MSc EDRA
Consultant anaesthetist, Guy's and St. Thomas' NHS Foundation Trust, London, UK

Megan Schneiderman BSc MDCM FRCSC
Assistant Professor and Assistant Program Director, Department of Obstetrics & Gynecology, McGill University, St Mary's Hospital, Pediatric and Adolescent Gynecologist, Montreal Children's Hospital, Montreal, Quebec, Canada

Cynthia H. Seow MBBS (Hons), MSc, FRACP
Professor, Division of Gastroenterology and Hepatology, Departments of Medicine and Community Health Sciences, University of Calgary, Canada

Samantha So MD
Postgraduate Resident, Department of Obstetrics and Gynecology, Cooper Medical School of Rowan University, Camden, New Jersey, USA

Bianca Stortini MD FRCSC
Assistant Professor, Department of Obstetrics and Gynecology, Pediatric and Adolescent Gynecologist, Sherbrooke University, Sherbrooke, Quebec, Canada

Eva Suarthana MD PhD
Adjunct Professor, Department of Obstetrics and Gynecology, Faculty of Medicine and Health Sciences McGill University Associate Investigator at the Research Institute of McGill University Health Center, Montreal Quebec, Canada

Marie-Julie Trahan MD, MSc
Postgraduate Resident, Department of Obstetrics and Gynecology, Faculty of Medicine and Health Sciences, McGill University, Montreal, Quebec, Canada

Michael A. Tsoukas MD FRCPC
Assistant Professor, Department of Medicine, Faculty of Medicine and Health Sciences, McGill University Division of Endocrinology, McGill University Health Center, Montreal, Quebec, Canada

Karen Wou MDCM FRCSC FACMG
Department of Obstetrics and Gynecology, Faculty of Medicine and Health Sciences, McGill University Division of Maternal-Fetal Medicine, McGill University Health Center, Montreal, Quebec, Canada

Tricia E. Wright MD MS FACOG DFASAM
Professor, Department of Obstetrics, Gynecology and Reproductive Sciences, University of California, San Francisco, SF, California, USA

Ji Wei Yang MD FRCPC
Assistant Professor, Department of Medicine, Faculty of Medicine and Health Sciences, McGill University Division of Endocrinology, McGill University Health Center, Montreal, Quebec, Canada

Andrew Zakhari MDCM, MGSC, FRCSC
Assistant Professor, Department of Obstetrics and Gynecology, Faculty of Medicine and Health Sciences, McGill University Division of Minimally Invasive Gynecologic Surgery, McGill University Health Centre, Montreal, Quebec, Canada

Cleve Ziegler MD FRCSC
Assistant Professor, Department of Obstetrics and Gynecology, Faculty of Medicine and Health Sciences, McGill University Jewish General Hospital, McGill University, Montreal, Quebec, Canada

SECTION 1

Obstetric Aspects of Antenatal Care

CHAPTER 1

Routine Prenatal Care

Megan Schneiderman and Amira El-Messidi

A 27-year-old primigravida at 11^{+1} weeks' gestation by menstrual dating presents for her first visit for routine prenatal care, accompanied by her husband. While discussing the comprehensive medical history with you before you meet the couple, your obstetric trainee mentions that the patient is allergic to penicillin.

LEARNING OBJECTIVES

1. Take a comprehensive prenatal history, demonstrating the ability to appropriately assign a gestational age based on clinical and sonographic parameters
2. Appreciate defining features for a severe penicillin allergy and provide safe alternative intrapartum pharmacologic treatment where clinically indicated
3. Address common aspects of prenatal care for a low-risk patient, including, but not limited to, routine prenatal investigations and pharmacologic treatments, vaccinations, nutritional intake, chemical exposure, umbilical cord blood banking, and potential for air travel during pregnancy
4. Appreciate the importance of maintaining a low threshold for multidisciplinary collaboration where unexpected events occur among low-risk singleton pregnancies
5. Recognize important elements of the routine postpartum visit

SUGGESTED READINGS

Antenatal Care
1. National Institute for Health and Care Excellence. Antenatal care; NICE guideline NG201, August 2021. Available at www.nice.org.uk/guidance/ng201. Accessed October 11, 2021.

Chemical Exposure during Pregnancy
2. Royal College of Obstetricians and Gynaecologists. Chemical exposures during pregnancy: dealing with potential but unproven risks to child health; Scientific Impact Paper No. 37. May 2013. Available at www.rcog.org.uk/en/guidelines-research-services/guidelines/sip37/. Accessed October 11, 2021.

Gestational Age Assignment
3. Butt K, Lim KI. Guideline No. 388 – determination of gestational age by ultrasound. *J Obstet Gynaecol Can.* 2019;41(10):1497–1507.

4. Committee Opinion No. 700: Methods for estimating the due date. *Obstet Gynecol.* 2017;129(5):e150–e154.
5. Van den Hof MC, Smithies M, Nevo O, et al. No. 375 – clinical practice guideline on the use of first trimester ultrasound. *J Obstet Gynaecol Can.* 2019;41(3):388–395.

Immunizations

6. ACOG Committee Opinion No. 718: Update on immunization and pregnancy: tetanus, diphtheria, and pertussis vaccination. *Obstet Gynecol.* 2017;130(3):e153–e157.
7. ACOG Committee Opinion No. 732: Influenza vaccination during pregnancy. *Obstet Gynecol.* 2018;131(4):e109–e114.
8. Castillo E, Poliquin V. ACOG Committee Opinion No. 357 – Immunization in pregnancy. *J Obstet Gynaecol Can.* 2018;40(4):478–489.

Iron-Deficiency Anemia and Rh Immunoglobulin

9. ACOG Committee on Practice Bulletins – Obstetrics. Anemia in pregnancy: ACOG Practice Bulletin, No. 233. *Obstet Gynecol.* 2021;138(2):e55–e64.
10. Fung KFK, Eason E. ACOG Committee Opinion No. 133 – Prevention of Rh alloimmunization. *J Obstet Gynaecol Can.* 2018;40(1):e1–e10.
11. Pavord S, Daru J, Prasannan N, et al. UK guidelines on the management of iron deficiency in pregnancy. *Br J Haematol.* 2020;188(6):819–830.
12. Practice Bulletin No. 181: Prevention of Rh D alloimmunization. *Obstet Gynecol.* 2017;130(2): e57–e70.
13. Qureshi H, Massey E, Kirwan D, et al. BCSH guideline for the use of anti-D immunoglobulin for the prevention of haemolytic disease of the fetus and newborn. *Transfus Med.* 2014;24(1):8–20.

Physical Activity

14. Mottola MF, Davenport MH, Ruchat SM, et al. No. 367 – 2019 Canadian guideline for physical activity throughout pregnancy. *J Obstet Gynaecol Can.* 2018;40(11):1528–1537. [Correction in *J Obstet Gynaecol Can.* 2019 Jul;41(7):1067]
15. Physical activity and exercise during pregnancy and the postpartum period: ACOG Committee Opinion, No. 804. *Obstet Gynecol.* 2020;135(4):e178–e188.

Travel during Pregnancy

16. ACOG Committee Opinion No. 746: Air travel during pregnancy. *Obstet Gynecol.* 2018;132(2):e64–e66.
17. Antony KM, Ehrenthal D, Evensen A, et al. Travel during pregnancy: considerations for the obstetric provider. *Obstet Gynecol Surv.* 2017;72(2):97–115.
18. Royal College of Obstetricians and Gynaecologists. Air travel and pregnancy; Scientific Impact Paper No. 1. May 2013. Available at www.rcog.org.uk/en/guidelines-research-services/guidelines/sip1/. Accessed October 11, 2021.
19. Van de Venne M, Mahmood T. EBCOG position statement – travelling when pregnant. *Eur J Obstet Gynecol Reprod Biol.* 2019;233:158–159.

Umbilical Cord Blood Banking

20. ACOG Committee Opinion No. 771: Umbilical cord blood banking. *Obstet Gynecol.* 2019;133(3):e249–e253.
21. Armson BA, Allan DS, Casper RF. Umbilical cord blood: counselling, collection, and banking. *J Obstet Gynaecol Can.* 2015;37(9):832–844.

Universal Cervical Length Screening in Low-Risk Singleton Pregnancies

22. AIUM-ACR-ACOG-SMFM-SRU Practice parameter for the performance of standard diagnostic obstetrical ultrasound examinations. 2018. Available at https://onlinelibrary.wiley.com/doi/full/10.1002/jum.14831. Accessed October 14, 2021.
23. Butt K, Crane J, Hutcheon J, et al. No. 374 – universal cervical length screening. *J Obstet Gynaecol Can.* 2019;41(3):363–374.
24. Committee on Practice Bulletins – Obstetrics and the American Institute of Ultrasound in Medicine. Practice Bulletin No. 175: Ultrasound in pregnancy. *Obstet Gynecol.* 2016;128(6):e241–e256.
25. FIGO Working Group on Best Practice in Maternal-Fetal Medicine, International Federation of Gynecology and Obstetrics. Best practice in maternal-fetal medicine. *Int J Gynaecol Obstet.* 2015;128(1):80–82. [Correction in *Int J Gynaecol Obstet.* 2015 Apr;129(1):89]
26. McIntosh J, Feltovich H, Berghella V, et al. The role of routine cervical length screening in selected high- and low-risk women for preterm birth prevention. *Am J Obstet Gynecol.* 2016;215(3):B2–B7.

POINTS

1. Elaborate on defining features for high risk of anaphylaxis or a severe reaction to penicillin, appreciating that *one* feature is satisfactory. *(1 point each)* — Max 5

High risk for IgE-mediated reactions:
- ☐ Pruritic rash
- ☐ Urticaria (hives)
- ☐ Immediate flushing
- ☐ Hypotension
- ☐ Angioedema
- ☐ Respiratory distress (*e.g.*, wheezing, stridor, dyspnea, throat/chest tightness, repetitive dry cough)

High risk for severe non-IgE-mediated reactions:
- ☐ Eosinophilia and drug-induced hypersensitivity syndrome
- ☐ Stevens–Johnson syndrome
- ☐ Toxic epidermal necrolysis

Other:
- ☐ Positive penicillin allergy test
- ☐ Reaction to multiple beta-lactam antibiotics
- ☐ Recurrent reactions

Special note:
Refer to Prevention of Group B Streptococcal Early-Onset Disease in Newborns: ACOG Committee Opinion No. 797. *Obstet Gynecol.* 2020;135(2):e51–e72. [Correction in *Obstet Gynecol.* 2020 Apr;135(4):978–979]

2. In the absence of drug or environmental allergies, outline aspects of the comprehensive patient history elicited by your obstetric trainee at this patient's first prenatal visit. *(1 point each)*

Max 30

Current/recent pregnancy-related features and management, *if any*:
☐ Nausea and/or vomiting (*i.e.*, duration, frequency, quantity); effect of symptoms on daily living
☐ Vaginal bleeding
☐ Pelvic cramping, especially that prevents or awakens from sleep
☐ Determine whether a dating sonography or other investigations were performed

Gynecologic history:
☐ First day of the last menstrual period
☐ Cycle regularity
☐ Recent contraceptive use and whether pregnancy was planned
☐ Determine if and when prenatal vitamins have been initiated
☐ History of sexually transmitted infections (STIs); specifically, inquire about history of genital herpes simplex virus (in the patient or her partner)
☐ Duration since last cervical cytology test (*i.e.*, Papanicolaou test) and history of abnormal results
☐ Inquire about spontaneous or therapeutic undisclosed early pregnancy losses *in confidence with the patient* (individualized timing and setting)

Medical and surgical history:
☐ Determine if the patient accepts transfusion of blood products (*e.g.*, enquire whether patient is a Jehovah's Witness) and prior receipt of blood transfusions
☐ Chronic active or dormant medical or psychological conditions, including treatments
☐ Prior surgeries (*e.g.*, cerebral, cardiothoracic, abdominal-pelvic)

Social history and routine health maintenance:
☐ Ethnicity of the patient and partner
☐ Occupation (*e.g.*, exposure to daycare children, toxic chemicals, radiation, prolonged standing, physical activity, or risk of injury) and socioeconomic status (including food and housing security and potential barriers to accessing medical care)
☐ Dietary restrictions (*i.e.*, assess adequacy of calcium and iron intake)
☐ Vaccination status, namely, to COVID-19, hepatitis B, and annual *H. influenza*, and history of varicella disease or prior vaccination
☐ Exercise patterns (*i.e.*, type, frequency, and duration per week)
☐ Cigarette smoking, including quantity (*i.e.*, type [cigarette, cigar, water pipe/hookah, vape], quantity, and duration of use)
☐ Alcohol consumption (*i.e.*, type, quantity, and duration of use)
☐ Illicit drug use (*i.e.*, source, type, quantity, and duration of use)

☐ Nonmedical use of medications

☐ Recent travel, or intended trips, to areas endemic for infectious diseases (*e.g.*, Zika virus, tuberculosis, malaria, Lyme disease)

☐ Past, present, and future risk of abuse (*e.g.*, intimate partner violence or other forms of physical, sexual, psychological, or emotional trauma)

☐ Pets at home, specifically cats (*refer to Chapter 66, 'Toxoplasmosis in Pregnancy'*)

Family history:

☐ *e.g.*, Cardiovascular, autoimmune, or pregnancy-associated complications

☐ Congenital anomalies or aneuploidies

☐ *e.g.*, Mental or developmental delays, autism spectrum disorders

Male partner:

☐ Consanguinity

☐ Personal history of neural tube defect (NTD)

☐ History of STIs, specifically genital herpes simplex virus (HSV)

☐ Smoking (with regard to the gravida's exposure to second-hand smoke)

You learn that the patient continues to practice as an attorney, as she has not experienced any obstetric complications to date. Sonographic pregnancy dating has not been performed, although the patient is confident of her menstrual dates. Medical and surgical histories are unremarkable; she confirms having remotely had varicella infection. She practices noncontact aerobic as well as strength-conditioning exercise as 30-minute sessions four times weekly and consumes a Mediterranean diet, as consistent with her ethnicity. Neither of the couple smokes cigarettes or uses illicit substances; they do not have pets. As the couple planned conception two months prior to pregnancy, she discontinued her two-year use of combined oral contraception, initiated folic acid-containing prenatal vitamins, received the COVID-19 and flu vaccines, and has abstained from twice-weekly glasses of wine with dinner. Although she has never received blood products, the patient is not against receipt for medical indications. In confidence, the patient ascertained to your obstetric trainee that there are no undisclosed pregnancies; neither she nor her husband has had STIs. A routine cervical smear performed eight months ago was normal, as per her usual. Family history is noncontributory.

She elaborates that her penicillin allergy entails onset of hives and a generalized pruritic rash shortly after exposure; the patient does not have any other drug or environmental allergies.

Having met the couple and reviewed the clinical history, you confirm that she is normotensive and that her prepregnancy body mass index is 23.5 kg/m^2, and remaining maternal findings on physical examination are unremarkable. You inform the patient that in addition to routine prenatal investigations discussed earlier by your obstetric trainee, you advise an obstetric ultrasound scan at this time.

3. Indicate advantages of first-trimester sonography for consideration in counseling this patient. *(1 point each)*

10

☐ Determine pregnancy location

☐ Confirm viability

☐ Improved accuracy for determining gestational age compared to menstrual dating among spontaneously conceived pregnancies, regardless of menstrual cycle regularity

☐ Ascertain fetal number, and ascertain chorionicity and amnionicity in the case of multiples

☐ Highlight that her recent discontinuation of oral contraceptives may contribute to inaccurate menstrual dating

☐ Inform the patient that bleeding in early pregnancy may have been misperceived as menses

☐ Allow early detection of embryo-fetal malformations

☐ Contribute to fetal aneuploidy risk assessment, improving performance of prenatal screening

☐ Contribute to preeclampsia risk assessment

☐ Decreased maternal anxiety about pregnancy[†]

Special note:

[†] *Refer to* Crowther CA, Kornman L, O'Callaghan S, et al. Is an Ultrasound Assessment of Gestational Age at the First Antenatal Visit of Value? A Randomised Clinical Trial. *Br J Obstet Gynaecol.* 1999;106(12):1273–1279.

The patient appreciates your counseling and understands that ultrasound is a nonionizing form of radiant energy where the risk of bioeffects is minimal when performed in accordance with sonographic principles. As such, ultrasound performed during this clinical visit by your colleague with sonographic expertise reveals a viable intrauterine singleton at 12^{+2} weeks' gestation with normal early morphology and no markers of aneuploidy. To optimize aneuploidy risk assessment, the patient agrees to complement first-trimester sonographic findings with noninvasive tests available in your jurisdiction.[†]

Special note:

[†] Refer to Chapter 5.

4. Among the reported fetal crown–rump length (CRL) and mean diameters of gestational sac and yolk sac, inform your obstetric trainee how the sonographic estimated due date was established.

2

☐ Direct measurement of the CRL is the most accurate indicator of dating spontaneous conceptions when the embryo is clearly seen, where the narrowest confidence interval appears to be between 7 and 60 mm for CRL *(SOGC[3])*.

5. Based on clinical and sonographic estimated due dates, <u>rationalize</u> your chosen assigned gestational age for this patient. *(1 point each)*   Max 2

Superiority of ultrasound redating:

☐ There is a greater than seven-day discrepancy between clinical and ultrasound dating at gestational age between 9^{+0} and 13^{+6} weeks *(ACOG[4])*;[†] accepted practice also favors selecting first-trimester CRL dating, when appropriate, irrespective of discrepancy from clinical dating *(SOGC[3,5])*.

☐ Improved performance of prenatal screening programs (*i.e.*, increase the sensitivity for Down syndrome and/or decrease false-positive rates).

☐ Reduced rates of postdate pregnancy, related labor inductions, or iatrogenic prematurity.

Special note:

† At $\leq 8^{+6}$ weeks' gestation, the CRL-based dating is accurate within five days of the birthdate.

You explain that guidance for an optimal frequency of prenatal visits is limited: among nulliparous women with uncomplicated pregnancies, this may involve 10 visits per pregnancy *(NICE[1])*,[†] or scheduled to accommodate a minimum of 8 visits, which would entail 1 visit in the first trimester, 2 in the second trimester, and 5 thereafter, regardless of parity *(WHO)*,[§] or prenatal visits arranged at monthly intervals until ~28 weeks' gestation, followed by bimonthly visits until 36 weeks and weekly visits thereafter until delivery.[†‡]

Special notes:

† Parous women with uncomplicated pregnancies may have less frequent prenatal visits.

‡ For postdate pregnancies, increased fetal surveillance is recommended according to local protocols.

§ WHO Recommendations on Antenatal Care for a Positive Pregnancy Experience. November 2016. Available at www.who.int/publications/i/item/9789241549912, accessed October 12, 2021.

6. Outline your recommended routine prenatal investigations for *this* patient and provide her with an overview of subsequent routine investigations until the estimated due date. *(1 point each)*

Max 15

Initial prenatal visit:§
☐ Full/complete blood count (FBC/CBC)
☐ Ferritin
☐ Blood type and antibody screen
☐ Hepatitis B surface antigen (HBsAg) and antibody (HBsAb)
☐ Hepatitis C antibody
☐ Human immunodeficiency virus (HIV) conventional third-generation enzyme-linked immunoassay (ELISA) or fourth-generation antigen/antibody assay *(using the 'opt-out' approach)*
☐ Rubella IgG antibodies
☐ Syphilis nontreponemal or treponemal test†
☐ Hemoglobin protein electrophoresis (HPEP) [*i.e., Mediterranean ethnicity*]
☐ Fetal aneuploidy screening by either the first component of integrated prenatal screening (IPS) test or cell-free DNA (cfDNA) [*the second component of the IPS test is performed in the second trimester, if indicated*]
☐ Urinalysis and culture
☐ Urine chlamydia nucleic acid amplification test (NAAT); a vaginal or endocervical swab demonstrates similar sensitivity to urine testing

Second trimester:
☐ Sonographic fetal morphology survey at 18–22 weeks' gestation
☐ Screening for gestational diabetes at 24–28 weeks' gestation
☐ Repeat a CBC between 24^{+0} and 28^{+6} weeks' gestation to screen for anemia

Third trimester:
☐ Vaginal-rectal group B *Streptococcus* swab (GBS) at 36–37 weeks' gestation, unless known positive GBS bacteriuria at any time during pregnancy or a positive vaginal-rectal swab resulted during investigations for preterm labor# [*screening all women for GBS colonization is not routinely offered in the United Kingdom; refer to the clinical description after Question 19*]‡

Special notes:
† Refer to Chapter 65, 'Syphilis in Pregnancy'
§ Given self-reported history of infection, varicella serology is unnecessary for this patient; *refer to* Question 2 in Chapter 67, 'Varicella in Pregnancy.' There are no specified high-risk features in this case scenario to suggest routine toxoplasmosis, cytomegalovirus (CMV), or parvovirus serologies, although international practice variations exist.
# A positive vaginal-rectal GBS swab may also be repeated if more than five weeks have elapsed since the at-risk episode for preterm labor; *refer to* Question 1 in Chapter 15, 'Labor at Term.'
‡ *Refer to* **(a)** UK National Screening Committee. UK NSC Group B Streptococcus (GBS) Recommendation. London: UK NSC; 2017; **(b)** Hughes RG, Brocklehurst P, Steer PJ, et al. Prevention of early-onset neonatal group B streptococcal disease. Green-Top Guideline No. 36. *BJOG*. 2017;124:e280–e305.

You inform her that she will complete a short, validated screening tool for depression and anxiety at least once during the antenatal and/or postpartum period, which she is pleased to complete today. You explain that the *routine* physical examination components of each prenatal visit will entail measurement of her blood pressure (BP), weight, and auscultation of the fetal heart rate, while fundal height assessments will commence at ~24 weeks' gestation.

7. Address a patient inquiry regarding <u>routine</u> antenatal pharmacologic treatments, apart from vitamin and mineral supplementation. *(1 point per main bullet)* ... 3

☐ Flu vaccine in any trimester if the patient is pregnant in the fall or winter
☐ Pertussis vaccine, ideally at 27–32 weeks' gestation; administration outside this gestational window, including while breastfeeding, is also possible
☐ Single-dose Rh immunoglobulin at 28–30 weeks' gestation or two-dose regimen given at around 28 and 34 weeks, respectively, if D-negative and nonsensitized; repeat antibody screen is necessary prior to drug administration[†]
   ○ Where cell-free DNA (cfDNA) is available for fetal blood group genotyping, maternal prophylactic anti-D immunoglobulin may be obviated, particularly among male fetuses

<u>Special note:</u>
[†] Selection of single- or two-dose regimen may depend on cost and local practice.

8. Highlight the contraindicated vaccinations during pregnancy, which you intend to teach your obstetric trainee after this consultation. *(1 point each)* ... Max 5

Live-attenuated bacterial vaccines	Live-attenuated viral vaccines	Inactivated viral vaccines
☐ Oral typhoid	☐ Measles, mumps, rubella (MMR)	☐ Human papilloma virus (HPV)
☐ Bacillus Calmette–Guérin	☐ Varicella	
	☐ Zoster	
	☐ Rotavirus	
	☐ Yellow fever[†]	
	☐ Japanese encephalitis	
	☐ Live-attenuated influenza	
	☐ Smallpox (vaccinia)	

<u>Special note:</u>
[†] Pregnancy is a *precaution* for receipt of the yellow fever vaccine by the Advisory Committee on Immunization Practices (ACIP) as risk of exposure to yellow fever virus may outweigh risks of vaccination; *refer to* www.cdc.gov/vaccines/pregnancy/hcp/guidelines.html, accessed August 26, 2022.

Keen to maintain a healthy lifestyle, the patient inquires about optimal gestational weight gain and foods to avoid in pregnancy. You take the opportunity to offer her your local 'nutrition in pregnancy' resource manuals as well as consultation with a perinatal dietitian, if preferred.

9. With reference to the patient's BMI, inform her of the advised overall gestational weight gain, and summarize nutritional intake to be avoided during pregnancy. *(1 point each)*

6

☐ Based on a BMI of 23.5 kg/m^2, the ideal gestational weight gain is 11.5–16 kg (25–35 lb)

Food and beverages to avoid in pregnancy: *(max 5)*
☐ Alcohol
☐ Caffeine >250–300 mg/d
☐ Soy protein or isoflavone supplements
☐ Raw or undercooked fish, meat, eggs, poultry
☐ Cold deli meat
☐ Cold smoked salmon
☐ Fish with high levels of methylmercury (*e.g.*, fresh/frozen tuna, shark, swordfish, escolar, martin, orange roughly)
☐ Fish considered to have had high exposure to pollutants
☐ Unpasteurized dairy products
☐ Unpasteurized juices
☐ Unwashed fruits and vegetables

In response to a concern, you advise that she remain in well-ventilated areas or minimize use of scent-producing hair and nail chemicals. You explain that despite the lack of high-quality evidence, avoidance of ammonia- or formaldehyde-containing hair products and nail polishes containing toluene, formaldehyde, and dibutyl phthalate is prudent, as inhaled products may trigger asthma or allergic reactions during pregnancy or pose theoretical risks due to absorption through the scalp or nail bed.

You later receive results of prenatal genetic screening, showing low risks of trisomies 13, 18, and 21 and of sex chromosome aneuploidies. Her blood group is B-negative without atypical antibodies. First-trimester maternal investigations are only significant for the following:

Hemoglobin concentration	99 g/L (9.9 g/dL)
Mean corpuscular volume	78 fL
Hematocrit	30% (*i.e.*, <33%)
Ferritin	10 ng/ml (10 ug/L)[†]
HPEP	HbA, 96.5%
	HbA2, 2.5%
	HbF, 1%
	HbS, HbC, absent

Special note:
† Serum ferritin <30 ug/L confirms iron-deficiency anemia.

10. What is the most specific diagnosis?													2

☐ Iron-deficiency anemia[†] with a normal hemoglobin pattern

Special note:
† Anemia is defined as hemoglobin concentration <110 g/L (11.0 g/dL) in the first and <105 g/L (10.5 g/dL) in the second trimester, respectively (*Suggested Readings 9 and 11*); hemoglobin concentration <110 g/L (11.0 g/dL) or <105 g/L (10.5 g/dL) defines abnormal values in the third trimester (*Suggested Readings 9 and 11, respectively*).

11. In preparation for patient counseling, teach your trainee the recommended initial			10
management and identify perinatal risks that have been associated with iron-deficiency anemia. *(1 point each; max points specified per section)*

Initial management: *(3)*
☐ Explain the diagnosis and advise a trial of oral iron supplementation
☐ Plan reassessment of hemoglobin to monitor response to oral therapy (*e.g.*, in two to three weeks [*Suggested Reading 11*] after commencing treatment)
☐ Inform the patient of associated perinatal complications with iron-deficiency anemia

Maternal risks: *(max 6)*
☐ Fatigue
☐ Thyroid dysfunction or altered metabolism
☐ Preterm birth
☐ Preeclampsia
☐ Need for parenteral iron or blood transfusion
☐ Postpartum hemorrhage (PPH)[†]
☐ Peripartum hysterectomy[‡]
☐ Postpartum depression
☐ Mortality, in low- and middle-income countries

Fetal-infant risks: *(max 1)*
☐ Low birthweight or small-for-gestational-age newborn
☐ Low Apgar score, <5 at one minute
☐ Perinatal and neonatal mortality
☐ Mental and psychomotor delays

Special notes:
† Possibly due to suboptimal uterine contractility with decreased availability of oxygen; consideration for active management of the third stage of labor for women with iron-deficiency anemia at time of delivery
‡ After adjustment for confounding factors, such as PPH

You communicate with the patient in advance of the subsequent prenatal visit; she appreciates your counseling and agrees to initiate oral supplemental iron while continuing routine prenatal vitamins. In response to her query, you inform her that neither extended release nor enteric coated formulations are recommended, as absorption of iron from these preparations is limited.[§] As she is concerned about not tolerating or responding to oral iron supplements, you reassure her of the availability of intravenous iron therapy.[#] Further to your discussion, she has confirmed that brands of prenatal vitamins she uses contain vitamin D 400[†]–600[‡] IU (10–15 mcg) per day, consistent with recommendations for pregnancy and lactation.

Special notes:

§ Refer to *Suggested Readings 9, 11* and Tapiero H, Gaté L, Tew KD. Iron: Deficiencies and Requirements. *Biomed Pharmacother.* 2001;55(6):324–332.

\# Intravenous iron therapy is also indicated for noncompliance to oral treatment or women presenting at >34 weeks' gestation with confirmed iron-deficiency anemia and hemoglobin concentration <100 g/L *(Suggested Reading 11).*

† *Refer to* National Institute for Health and Care Excellence. Vitamin D: Supplement Use in Specific Population Groups. Public Health Guideline [PH56]. Last updated August 2017. Available at www.nice.org.uk/guidance/ph56, accessed October 14, 2021.

‡ *Refer to* **(a)** Institute of Medicine. Dietary Reference Intakes for Calcium and Vitamin D. Washington, DC: National Academy Press; 2010; **(b)** Health Canada website, available at www.canada.ca/en/health-canada/services/food-nutrition/healthy-eating/vitamins-minerals/vitamin-calcium-updated-dietary-reference-intakes-nutrition.html, accessed October 14, 2021.

---

12. Instruct the patient how to ingest oral iron supplements. *(1 point each)*   3

☐ Take iron supplements on an empty stomach, with water or a source of vitamin C to maximize absorption

☐ Avoid simultaneous ingestion of other medications, such as multivitamins and antacids

☐ Consideration for alternate-day dosing to optimize absorption relative to consecutive daily dosing[†]

Special note:

† *Refer to* Stoffel NU, Cercamondi CI, Brittenham G, et al. Iron Absorption from Oral Iron Supplements Given on Consecutive versus Alternate Days and as Single Morning Doses versus Twice-Daily Split Dosing in Iron-Depleted Women: Two Open-Label, Randomised Controlled Trials. *Lancet Haematol.* 2017;4(11):e524–e533.

---

13. Facilitate your trainee's learning of contraindications for intravenous iron therapy, as requested after your telecommunication with the patient. *(1 point each)*   Max 3

☐ First trimester of pregnancy

☐ Active acute or chronic bacteremia

☐ Decompensated liver disease

☐ Anaphylactic reactions

The patient tolerates oral ferrous iron well, and serial laboratory assessments demonstrate a positive response to supplementation. Second-trimester ultrasound shows appropriate fetal biometry and amniotic fluid volume and normal fetal–placental morphology; assessment of maternal cervical length was feasible and is normal.[†]

Glucose screening test and anti-D immunoglobulin are planned simultaneously at 28 weeks' gestation. Routine repeat antibody screen at 28 weeks remains negative.

Special note:

† Practice variations exist with regard to routine cervical length screening at second-trimester morphology ultrasound; as examples:

1. AIUM[22] recommends transvaginal or transperineal sonographic imaging if the cervix appears shortened or funneled or is not adequately visualized during transabdominal ultrasound examination.
2. SOGC[23] does not fully recommend stand-alone universal cervical length screening across Canada at this time.
3. ACOG[24] recommends assessment of the maternal cervix when clinically appropriate and when technically feasible.
4. FIGO[25] recommends transvaginal sonographic cervical length in all women at 19^{+0}–23^{+6} weeks' gestation.
5. Although SMFM[26] does not mandate universal cervical length screening in singleton gestations without history of preterm birth, it may be reasonable for individual practitioners' consideration.
6. NICE, RCOG, and ISUOG do not address routine cervical length screening at the second-trimester morphology ultrasound.

---

14. Based on your proposed treatment, outline aspects to discuss in the informed consent process for routine administration of anti-D immunoglobulin in this D-negative, nonsensitized patient. *(1 point each)*

Max 4

Benefit/efficacy:
☐ The risk of RhD alloimmunization after two deliveries of D-positive ABO-compatible infants would decrease from ~16% to 0.17%–0.28% through routine third-trimester prophylaxis

Risks:
☐ Provide reassurance that only negative plasma for antibodies to hepatitis B and C viruses, human immunodeficiency viruses (HIV), and parvovirus B19 is used to make anti-D immunoglobulin; viral inactivation steps (viral clearance ultrafiltration) further reduce risks of infection
☐ Allergic reactions are very rare; the risk of severe hypersensitivity and anaphylaxis is increased if the patient has IgA antibodies due to trace amounts of IgA in the drug preparation
☐ *Theoretical* risk of transmitting variant Creutzfeldt–Jakob disease

Alternatives:
☐ The only alternative is not to administer prophylactic anti-D immunoglobulin

---

The glucose screening test is negative, and the patient tolerated anti-D immunoglobulin† well. She has also received routine pertussis vaccination, as recommended in each pregnancy. All aspects of routine prenatal care are unremarkable.

At 28^{+6} weeks' gestation, the patient calls your office requesting a timely visit, as she needs to travel for an urgent family matter to a destination five hours away by air for one week. Accommodating the patient, you ensure absence of medical contraindications to air travel and document normal maternal-fetal assessment. As she may be exposed to a forested area, you inform her on ways to prevent insect bites.[‡] She will obtain travel insurance. You will provide a copy of her medical records and a letter confirming the due date and fitness to travel.

Special notes:
† Dosing varies by international jurisdiction and brand name.
‡ Refer to Question 23 in Chapter 68.

---

15. Prior to her travels, review with the patient clinical features requiring immediate medical care; she recalls this discussion earlier in pregnancy as well. *(1 point each)*   7

- ☐ Pelvic or abdominal pain
- ☐ Vaginal bleeding
- ☐ Potential rupture of chorioamniotic membranes
- ☐ Uterine contractions or other features of preterm labor
- ☐ Signs or symptoms of preeclampsia (*e.g.,* headache unrelieved by acetaminophen or paracetamol, nausea and/or vomiting, visual changes, epigastric or right upper quadrant pain)
- ☐ Severe vomiting, diarrhea, or signs of dehydration
- ☐ Signs or symptoms of possible deep vein thrombosis (DVT) or pulmonary embolism (PE) (*e.g.,* unusual swelling of leg with pain in calf or thigh, unusual shortness of breath)

Special note:
Refer to Centers for Disease Control and Prevention. Yellow Book; Chapter 7. Available at wwwnc.cdc.gov/travel/yellowbook/2020/family-travel/pregnant-travelers, accessed October 15, 2021.

---

16. Address an inquiry about maternal-fetal risks of radiation exposure from airport body scanners and cosmic radiation with air travel. *(1 point each)*   2

Body scanners:
- ☐ Reassure the patient that the total radiation dose from airport body scanners (*e.g.,* two to three scans) is less than that from two minutes flying at cruising altitude or from one hour at ground level; negligible radiation doses are absorbed into the body, therefore fetal dose is much lower than maternal dose

Cosmic radiation:
- ☐ Based on the recommended maximum of 1 millisievert (mSv) radiation exposure over the course of a 40-week pregnancy,[†] fetal risks from cosmic radiation are negligible; the longest available intercontinental flights would expose passengers to no more than 15% of this limit for *occasional* flyers (*restrictions are entailed for aircrew or frequent flyers who may exceed these limits*)

Special note:

† *Refer to* **(a)** ACOG[16] and **(b)** Barish RJ. In-Flight Radiation Exposure during Pregnancy. *Obstet Gynecol.* 2004;103(6):1326–1330.

17. Provide the patient with practical considerations and advice in preparation for and during air travel, particularly a medium- to long-haul flight of more than four hours' duration. *(1 point each)*

Max 8

Pretravel:

☐ Avoid gas-producing foods and beverages before the flight due to expansion of entrapped gases at altitudes

☐ Consider having prophylactic antiemetic medication for travel-associated maternal discomfort

☐ Avoid restrictive clothing

☐ Wear properly fitted graduated elastic compression stockings (DVT prevention)

General in-flight safety:

☐ Encourage wearing the seatbelt continuously while seated, belted below the abdomen and onto the thighs

In-flight measures for DVT prevention:†

☐ Have an aisle seat to facilitate ease of movement

☐ Walk regularly in the cabin

☐ Perform in-seat exercises approximately every 30 minutes

☐ Maintain adequate hydration, and avoid caffeinated drinks due to risk of dehydration

Special note:

† For patients at increased risk of thrombosis, pharmacologic prophylaxis with low molecular weight heparin (LMWH) should be considered; low-dose aspirin alone is not recommended for thromboprophylaxis associated with air travel.

During a weeknight† hospital call duty, your patient calls the obstetric emergency assessment unit as she panicked after her husband just removed a tick with tweezers from the back of her knee. She was in a forested area yesterday morning,† and although she used insect repellants, she forgot to wear long pants or shower within two hours of being outside, as you had advised. The couple kept the insect for laboratory analysis. Having seen the insect by a photograph she sent you, there is a high suspicion for a blacklegged tick bite. The patient has no systemic or obstetric complaints; fetal activity is normal. You consult with a maternal-fetal medicine/infectious disease expert(s) to assist in counseling and management of your patient.

Special note:

† Clinical scenario implies at least 24 hours have passed since attachment of the blacklegged tick.

18. In collaboration with the maternal-fetal medicine/infectious disease expert, indicate aspects to discuss with the patient after removal of the tick attached for over 24 hours. *(1 point per main and subbullet)*

☐ Reassure the patient that the risk of vertical transmission appears to be very low; transplacental transmission is *theoretical*, without a defined congenital syndrome

☐ Pregnancy does not affect the manifestations or severity of Lyme disease, if it develops

☐ Encourage preserving the tick as the laboratory can determine the length of time it was embedded based on its engorgement

☐ Offer single-dose prophylactic **doxycycline 200 mg** to be taken within 72 hours of tick removal to decrease the risk of developing Lyme disease by 10-fold (*i.e.*, 2.2%–0.2%), based on reassuring drug-related literature and clinical experience:[§]

    ○ No doxycycline-associated teratogenicity in pregnancy

    ○ No permanent tooth staining from in utero exposure or use by children under eight years old

    ○ No hepatotoxicity

    ○ No permanent inhibitory effects on bone growth

☐ Advise the patient to report signs and/or symptoms of Lyme disease that may manifest within the next 30 days (*e.g.*, single, localized, painless, nonpruritic skin lesion that slowly increases in size from >5 to ~60 cm [erythema migrans], fever, arthralgia, myalgia, headache), regardless of doxycycline prophylaxis

☐ Breastfeeding will not be contraindicated, even if she does develop Lyme disease

Special note:

Refer to **(a)** National Institute for Health and Care Excellence (NICE). Lyme disease (NG95). London, United Kingdom: NICE; 2018 Available at www.nice.org.uk/guidance/ng95, accessed October 15, 2021.

(b) Smith GN, Moore KM, Hatchette TF, et al. Committee Opinion Number 399: Management of Tick Bites and Lyme Disease During Pregnancy. *J Obstet Gynaecol Can.* 2020;42(5):644–653.

§ *Refer to* Cross R, Ling C, Day NP, McGready R, Paris DH. Revisiting doxycycline in pregnancy and early childhood–time to rebuild its reputation? *Expert Opin Drug Saf.* 2016;15(3):367–382.

The patient returns from her trip and remains asymptomatic after the tick bite, as the insect was confirmed in the local infectious disease laboratory. She was reassured by your evidence-based counseling on doxycycline prophylaxis.

At a 32-week routine prenatal visit, you address patient inquiries on umbilical cord blood banking, after having provided her with patient-focused references earlier in gestation. She recalls that the chance for a future sibling to be a full human leukocyte antigen (HLA) match is 25%.

19. Review with the patient the advantages and disadvantages of hematopoietic stem cell collection from umbilical cord blood. *(1 point each; max points specified per section)* 4

Advantages: *(max 2)*
☐ Potential use in numerous conditions (*e.g.,* correction of inborn errors of metabolism, treatment of certain hematopoietic malignancies or genetic disorders of the hematologic and immune systems)
☐ Relative to bone marrow or peripheral stem cell collection, umbilical cord blood collection is easier, with negligible collection-related risks to the donor
☐ Relative to receipt of bone marrow or peripheral stem cells, umbilical cord blood hematopoietic stem cells have a low risk of acute graft-vs-host reaction
☐ The recipient of hematopoietic stem cells from umbilical cord blood should tolerate greater mismatch or disparity in human leukocyte antigen (HLA) relative to receipt of bone marrow or peripheral stem cells

Disadvantages: *(max 2)*
☐ Limited amounts of hematopoietic stem cells are available in umbilical cord blood units
☐ Slow engraftment rates
☐ Potential genetic transfer of abnormal or premalignant cells to the recipient

(Continuation of scenario for countries where <u>universal</u> bacteriological screening for GBS is practiced):

At the 36-week visit, you collect the vaginal-rectal GBS swab, recalling that if positive, routine first-line intrapartum penicillin therapy would have to be substituted by a safe alternative.

(Continuation of scenario for countries where <u>risk factor-based</u> screening for early-onset GBS disease is practiced):

You learn that an international visiting obstetric trainee incidentally performs vaginal-rectal GBS screening, unknowing of risk factor-based screening in your local jurisdiction; the swab has already been sent to the laboratory. You take this opportunity to inform your trainee of numerous reasons for risk factor-based screening, among which are that offspring of many women who carry the bacteria do not develop an infection and universal screening in late pregnancy cannot accurately predict which neonates will develop GBS infection; in addition, between 17% and 25% of women who have a positive swab will be GBS-negative at delivery, while 5%–7% of women who are GBS-negative in late pregnancy will be GBS-positive at delivery.‡

‡ *Refer to* UK National Screening Committee. UK NSC Group B Streptococcus (GBS) Recommendation. London: UK NSC; 2017 and Hughes RG, Brocklehurst P, Steer PJ, Heath P, Stenson BM on behalf of the Royal College of Obstetricians and Gynaecologists. Prevention of early-onset neonatal group B streptococcal disease. Green-Top Guideline No. 36. *BJOG* 2017;124:e280–e305

20. Review with your trainee the particularities related to completion of *this* patient's laboratory requisition for vaginal-rectal GBS swab.   2

☐ Highlight the importance of documenting the high-risk penicillin allergy on the laboratory requisition to ensure that GBS isolates are tested for clindamycin sensitivity

21. Where the GBS bacteria are <u>resistant</u> to clindamycin, state the intrapartum prophylactic regimen.   4

☐ Intravenous vancomycin 20 mg/kg every eight hours, with a maximum of 2 g per single dose and minimum infusion time of one hour

The patient presents in spontaneous labor at 38^{+4} weeks' gestation with rupture of chorioamniotic membranes; intravenous clindamycin is commenced, based on susceptibility of GBS isolates.

22. State the regimen for prophylactic intrapartum clindamycin   4

☐ Intravenous clindamycin 900 mg every eight hours until delivery

A healthy neonate delivers spontaneously after an uncomplicated labor and delivery. The patient receives guidance with breastfeeding and is discharged from hospital with planned postpartum follow-up with you in approximately six weeks, as routine.

23. Identify important elements of <u>maternal care</u> to discuss at the routine postpartum visit for this healthy patient after a generally uncomplicated pregnancy and spontaneous vaginal delivery. *(1 point each)*   Max 7

☐ Breastfeeding status
☐ Continued use of prenatal vitamins, preferably at least until end of breastfeeding
☐ Resumption of exercise and a healthy diet for healthy living and to facilitate gestational weight loss
☐ Screen for postpartum depression using a validated questionnaire
☐ Availability of social support systems (*e.g.,* family, community resources)
☐ Quantity and quality of lochia, or possible resumption of menses
☐ Symptoms of urinary incontinence or anal incontinence to flatus or stool
☐ Sexual function and resumption of sexual activity
☐ Contraception and subsequent resumption of fertility and ovulation

Special note:
As this patient had a normal cervical smear within the past two years, repeat testing is not presently required.

You learn from comprehensive discussion that the postpartum period has been well; she continues to exclusively breastfeed, resumed exercise and sexual function, and scored 3/30 on the Edinburgh

Postnatal Depression Scale (EPDS).[†] She has not yet resumed menses. The patient is interested in learning of her options for postpartum contraception.

Special note:
† Refer to Question 1 in Chapter 29.

---

24. Summarize the available options for postpartum contraception[§] for this healthy patient who continues to breastfeed. *(1 point each)* — 4

☐ Systemic progestin-only contraceptives, namely progestin-only pill, intramuscular Depo-Provera, or progestin implants can be safely used without restrictions (Category 1), reassuring the patient of no impact on quantity or quality of breast milk

☐ Intrauterine contraceptives, namely copper intrauterine device (IUD) or levonorgesterel intrauterine system (LNG-IUS) can be safely used without restrictions as of four weeks postpartum (Category 1)
  ○ *Beware of the higher risk of perforation within the first year postpartum among breastfeeding women*

☐ Systemic combined hormonal contraceptives, namely pill, patch, or vaginal ring can be used when the patient is primarily breastfeeding and is at least six weeks to six months postpartum as the advantages outweigh theoretical or proven risks (Category 2)[†]; reassuringly, estrogen-containing agents should not have an impact once breastfeeding is well established *(combined hormonal contraceptives are safe while breastfeeding once the patient is greater than or equal to six weeks postpartum)*

☐ Barrier methods can be used without restriction (Category 1)

Special notes:
§ *Refer to* UK and US Medical Eligibility Criteria (MEC) for Contraceptive Use, 2016; UK-MEC revised September 2019, US-MEC amended 2020
† If not breastfeeding, the patient may use combined hormonal contraceptives as of ≥6 weeks postpartum without restriction (Category 1)

While exclusively breastfeeding, she inquires about its reliability as a contraceptive method until she decides upon a long-term reliable method.

---

25. Refer to the required criteria that must be met for lactational amenorrhea to be considered an effective contraceptive method. *(1 point each)* — 3

☐ The patient must be within six months of delivery

and

☐ Exclusively, or near-exclusively (*i.e.,* at least ¾ of feeds) breastfeeding

and

☐ Amenorrheic

TOTAL: 155

CHAPTER 2

Advanced Maternal Age

Amira El-Messidi and William M. Buckett

A 43-year-old G1P1 is referred by her primary care provider to your hospital center's high-risk obstetrics unit for preconception counseling for advanced maternal age (AMA). She started folic-containing prenatal vitamins and has recently discontinued five-year use of a copper intrauterine contraceptive device. They wish to attempt spontaneous conception prior to considering fertility evaluation.

Special note: Although social and medical comorbidities are often present or detected in preconception counseling for women of advanced age, the case scenario is presented as such for academic purposes and to avoid content overlap. The reader is encouraged to complement this subject matter with chapters in which respective comorbidities or pregnancy complications are addressed.

LEARNING OBJECTIVES

1. Appreciate the importance of referral to the high-risk obstetrics unit for preconception counseling for AMA-associated maternal-fetal risks, including formulation of surveillance strategies during potential pregnancy
2. Recognize that preconceptional investigations for AMA-associated perinatal morbidities are largely tailored to individually identified risk factors for pregnancy complications
3. Advise on mode and timing of delivery in relation to the relative and absolute risks of stillbirth based on AMA
4. Recognize that women referred for preconception counseling for AMA may have partners of advanced *paternal* age, which implicates discussion of potential paternal age related effects

SUGGESTED READINGS

1. Attali E, Yogev Y. The impact of advanced maternal age on pregnancy outcome. *Best Pract Res Clin Obstet Gynaecol.* 2020;S1521–6934(20):30096-1.
2. Chronopoulou E, Raperport C, Serhal P, et al. Preconception tests at advanced maternal age. *Best Pract Res Clin Obstet Gynaecol.* 2021;70:28.
3. Frick AP. Advanced maternal age and adverse pregnancy outcomes. *Best Pract Res Clin Obstet Gynaecol.* 2020;S1521–6934(20):30112-7.
4. Kawwass JF, Badell ML. Maternal and fetal risk associated with assisted reproductive technology. *Obstet Gynecol.* 2018;132(3):763–772.
5. Liu KE, Case A. No. 346 – advanced reproductive age and fertility. *J Obstet Gynaecol Can.* 2017;39(8):685–695.
6. Walker KF, Thornton JG. Timing and mode of delivery with advancing maternal age. *Best Pract Res Clin Obstet Gynaecol.* 2020;S1521–6934(20):30095-X.

1. With regard to AMA and referral of early consultation for fertility evaluation, which aspects of a focused history would you want to know? *(1 point per main bullet unless indicated)*

Max 15

Medical AMA-associated comorbidities:
☐ Chronic hypertension including micro/macrovascular complications
☐ Diabetes, including micro/macrovascular complications
☐ Psychological conditions

Reproductive history:
☐ Determine if patient had prior, *undisclosed,* ectopic pregnancy, spontaneous/therapeutic pregnancy losses, or fetal/neonatal deaths
☐ Details of prior pregnancy (*i.e.*, maternal and gestational age at delivery, mode of conception, maternal-fetal-neonatal complications)

Social habits and lifestyle assessment:
☐ Smoking, alcohol, recreational drug use
  ○ *Smoking is associated with decreased ovarian follicular pool, earlier menopause, perinatal morbidity and mortality*
☐ Amount of caffeine intake
  ○ *Women seeking fertility should limit caffeine intake per day to 200 mg (European Food Safety Authority) or 300 mg/d (WHO) (Suggested Reading 2)*
☐ Exercise habits and nutrition
☐ Current/prior teratogenic medications
☐ Coital frequency and any difficulties (*e.g., pain for either partner, or erectile/ejaculatory dysfunction*)

Gynecological history *(as relevant to AMA or fertility status)*:
☐ Conditions associated with ovarian injury or surgery: *(1 point per subbullet)*
  ○ Leiomyomas[§]
  ○ Tubal disease[§]/pelvic inflammatory disease
  ○ Endometriosis[§]
  ○ Medical treatment with gonadotoxic therapy, or prior pelvic radiation
☐ Menstrual cycle details (patient may have experienced common side effects of copper IUD)

Family history: *(ideally, a three-generation pedigree)*
☐ Early menopause
☐ Genetic disorders related to ethnicity or where prenatal genetic diagnosis may be offered/mitochondrial mutations/familial diseases with a major genetic component

Male partner:
☐ Age
☐ Paternity history
☐ Chronic medical/genetic conditions affecting fertility, livebirth rates or offspring genetic risk
☐ History of mumps infection
☐ Current/recent use of teratogenic or sperm-toxic agents

Special note:
§ Aging has cumulative effects

You learn that the patient is healthy, has a well-balanced diet, and performs moderate-intensity exercise routinely. She does not consume alcohol, smoke cigarettes, or use recreational drugs. Nine years ago, she conceived spontaneously and had an unremarkable pregnancy and vaginal delivery at 41 weeks' gestation. The patient has not had any undisclosed pregnancies. Family history is noncontributory. While completing postgraduate studies, she and her husband of 10 years chose to delay conception, for which she relied on intrauterine contraception. Over the past two years, her menstrual cycles have become nearly a week shorter than her mean throughout her reproductive years.

Her husband, present at this encounter, is a 51-year-old court judge. He does not take teratogenic medications and has not had children with other partners. As he has to return to work shortly, you take the opportunity to address the impact of advanced paternal age[†] on fertility and obstetric outcomes prior to counseling the patient.

Special note:
† Advanced paternal age is generally defined as >40 years, based on age-related spermatogenic changes

2. Detail your counseling of the couple regarding the impact of advanced paternal age, particularly above 50 years, on fertility and adverse obstetric outcome. *(1 point per main bullet)*   9

☐ Inform the couple that although advanced paternal age has been associated with fetal genetic conditions, the excess risk is very small
☐ Provide reassurance that medical evidence does not justify dissuading older men from attempting to achieve spontaneous conception
☐ Mention that sperm banking is not recommended based on age alone

Potential fetal/offspring risks and obstetric features of advanced paternal age: *(max 6 points)*
☐ Increased interval to conception/decreased conception rates
☐ Early pregnancy loss *(even when controlling for maternal age)*
☐ Preeclampsia
☐ Low birthweight
☐ Congenital anomalies *(weak association)*
  ○ Paternal age may play a small role; associations have been made with neural tube defects, facial clefts, trachea-esophageal fistula, atrial-ventricular septal defects
☐ Klinefelter syndrome (47, XXY)
  ○ *Half of cases are related to a male X etiology*
☐ Spontaneous mutations in X-linked genes can lead to the 'grandfather effect' (carrier daughters of this father transmit mutations to affected grandsons)
  ○ *e.g.,* hemophilia A, Duchenne muscular dystrophy

□ Down syndrome, although to a much lesser extent than advancing maternal age
  ○ *In up to 10% of nondisjunction trisomy 21, the extra chromosome is of paternal origin*
□ Neurocognitive disorders
  ○ Paternal age may play a small role; associations have been made with neurological tumors, epilepsy, autism spectrum disorders, schizophrenia
□ Autosomal dominant genetic mutations in offspring
  ○ *e.g.*, achondroplasia, neurofibromatosis type 1, osteogenesis imperfecta, retinoblastoma, thanatophoric dysplasia, genetic syndromes such as Marfan, Apert, Crouzon, Pfeiffer, and Waardenburg
□ Childhood leukemia (paternal age may play a small role)

The couple understand that although there is an exponential increase in incidence of autosomal dominant conditions in offspring of older men, the actual risk is ≤0.5%. You indicate that neither chromosomal microarray nor karyotype analysis screen for autosomal dominant diseases and that prenatal genetic diagnosis (PGD) is only useful when testing is done for targeted genes. Prior to his return to work, the patient's husband is interested in the biological foundation for male age-related genetic aberrations or disorders in offspring.

3. Identify four pathogenic mechanisms in sperm biology of older fathers that may account for increases in autosomal dominant conditions in offspring. *(1 point each)*   4

Spermatic changes with advanced age:
□ Altered integrity of DNA/decreased function of DNA repair mechanisms
□ Altered telomere lengths
□ Point mutations
□ De novo mutations
□ Epigenetic factors
□ Apoptosis

The patient's blood pressure is 130/78 mmHg, heart rate 73 bpm, and BMI 23.8 kg/m². You inform her that similar to the cutoff for defining advanced paternal age, there is international variation in defining AMA based on age at the time of delivery, varying from >35 years to >40 years, and the term 'very advanced maternal age' (vAMA) has been introduced with similarly varying cutoffs at ≥45 years, ≥48 years, or ≥50 years. Her primary care provider indicated that despite a prior low-risk gestation, AMA incurs risk of maternal-fetal complications. Prior to addressing complications by stage of pregnancy and outlining a gestational management plan, you highlight that most pregnancy outcomes are reassuring, and AMA patients cope well with the emotional and physical challenges of pregnancies and parenting.

4. Discuss <u>first-trimester</u> AMA-associated features or complications, offer possible biologic causations and prenatal management recommendations, where possible.
(1 point per main bullet)

Max 6

Ectopic pregnancy: [**four- to eightfold risk compared to younger women**]
☐ Causation involves cumulative features including decreased tubal function and delayed oocyte transport, multiple partners, pelvic infections[†]
☐ *Plan* for early sonography to identify pregnancy location

Spontaneous abortion of both euploid and aneuploid viable embryos (*independent* **of parity or previous pregnancy loss**)
☐ Biological causes involve poor oocyte quality and hormonal changes
☐ Potential plan involves oocyte donation, as pregnancy rates are based on donor's age, not the recipient

Aneuploidy (**contributes to spontaneous abortion**)
☐ Biological causes include less discriminating oocyte selection leading to a poorer dominant follicle, cumulative oxidative stress, and inherent diffuse spindle arrangement predisposing to meiotic error
Plan:
☐ First-trimester sonography for markers of aneuploidy and detection of malformations
☐ Offer noninvasive cell-free DNA (cfDNA) screening or integrated prenatal screening *(international practices may vary)*
☐ Diagnostic testing by amniocentesis or chorionic villous sampling is offered as needed

Multiple pregnancy (*refer to Chapter 11*)

Special note:
† Risk factors may not be specific to this patient, and are presented for academic purpose

You inform her that the chance of spontaneous conception of a multiple gestation is increased among women of advanced age, which entails increased maternal-fetal complications.

As fertility decreases with age, she wonders whether lifestyle behaviors may boost her natural fertility potential, positively influencing obstetric outcome. With natural conception among older women, the patient is curious to know approximate risks of aneuploidy after age 40.

5. Although part of general counseling for all women, address important <u>modifiable lifestyle</u> factors for optimal fertility rates and obstetric outcomes in consultation for AMA.
(1 point each)

Max 4

☐ Mediterranean diet and folic acid supplementation
☐ Smoking cessation or continued abstinence
☐ Avoid alcohol (no safe amount)
☐ Stop/seek professional help for illicit drug use
☐ Weight optimization and regular, moderate intensity exercise
☐ Screen for, and take appropriate action against domestic violence *(Suggested Reading 2)*

6. Among <u>spontaneously</u> conceived pregnancies in women aged 40 and 45, elaborate on the age-related risk of Down syndrome and all chromosomal abnormalities at term, respectively. *(1 point each)*

4

Approximate risks at age 40:
☐ 1/85 (Down syndrome)
☐ 1/39 (all chromosomal abnormalities)

Approximate risks at age 45:
☐ 1/34 (Down syndrome)
☐ 1/2 (all chromosomal abnormalities)

Special note:
Fetal risk of aneuploidy improves with oocyte donation

The patient appreciates your knowledge and communication. She intends to pursue aneuploidy screening upon natural conception. She wishes to prepare for potential later pregnancy risks, should the first trimester progress unremarkably.

7. Provide a structured outline of <u>antenatal</u> risks in the second and third trimesters for AMA gravidas with spontaneous conceptions. *(1 point per main bullet)*

8

Maternal: *(max 4)*
☐ Gestational diabetes
☐ Hypertensive syndromes of pregnancy
☐ Mid-trimester pregnancy loss
☐ Preterm birth (spontaneous or medically indicated)
  ○ Preterm neonates are not at increased risk of morbidity due to maternal age alone
☐ Hospitalizations, due to co-existing or new-onset pregnancy complications
☐ Cesarean delivery
☐ Mortality *(not limited to second/third trimesters: international variations in risk)*

Fetal-placental: *(max 4)*
☐ Fetal growth restriction (FGR)/suboptimal growth velocity
  ○ *Exact mechanisms for FGR are incompletely understood; likely related to placental vascular dysfunction with AMA and associated comorbidities*
☐ Placenta previa
  ○ The only placental condition strongly and independently linked to AMA; absolute risk is low
☐ Placental abruption[§]
☐ Intrauterine fetal demise (IUFD), despite nonanomalous fetuses and absence of maternal comorbidities *(small absolute risk; international variations in risk)*

Special note:
§ Placental abruption is mostly associated with multiparity and hypertensive conditions

You explain that evidence for the association between AMA and congenital anomalies among *euploid* fetuses is controversial, as recent literature[‡] suggests absence of an independent risk for major congenital anomalies due to AMA.

Special note:
‡ Refer to: **(a)** Marozio L et al. *J Matern Neonatal Med* 2019; 32:1602e8.; **(b)** Frederiksen LE et al. *Obstet Gynecol* 2018;131:457e63; **(c)** Goetzinger KR et al. *Am J Perinatol* 2017;34:217e22.

8. Discuss your plan for screening and preconceptional advice for AMA-associated maternal-fetal morbidities with spontaneous conception <u>or</u> in vitro fertilization. *(1 point per main bullet or subbullet)*

        Max 8

☐ Recommend care and delivery in a center with adequate maternal-fetal support services *(e.g., maternal-fetal medicine, neonatal intensive care, anesthesia, intensive care unit, accessibility to blood products)*

☐ Preconceptional screening for occult type 2 diabetes mellitus is reasonable, although no universal recommendations exist for routine screening

☐ Consider early screening for diabetes at 16–18 weeks' gestation, in addition to screening for gestational diabetes at 24–28 weeks *(preferably early in the window)*

☐ Preeclampsia prophylaxis: *(3 points for primary subbullet)*
  ○ Initiation of nightly low dose aspirin (LDASA) 75–162 mg,[†] started <16 weeks' gestation; AMA ≥35 or 40 years *(varies by jurisdiction)* is considered a <u>strong</u> risk factor for preeclampsia [Refer to Chapter 38]
  ○ Calcium supplementation 1.2–2.5 g elemental calcium/d in women with low calcium intake is recommended by the ISSHP* and SOGC**, however ACOG*** does not endorse calcium supplementation for preeclampsia prevention [Refer to Chapter 38]

☐ Serial monitoring for hypertension and associated clinical manifestations

☐ Second-trimester fetal morphology scan with attention to placental location, suggestions of accreta spectrum,[‡] velomentous cord insertion,[‡] and vasa previa[‡]

☐ Serial sonographic fetal growth assessment (risk stratification is recommended for frequency of follow-up)

☐ Consideration for antenatal anesthetic consultation, particularly for women of very advanced maternal age (vAMA), or based on comorbidities in AMA gravidas

Special notes:
Universal *preconception* screening for thyroid dysfunction is not currently recommended; individualized approach is advised
† Dosing varies by jurisdiction
* ISSHP: International Society for the Study of Hypertension in Pregnancy
** SOGC: Society of Obstetricians and Gynaecologists of Canada
*** ACOG: American College of Obstetricians and Gynecologists
‡ Particularly with invasive procedures for assisted reproduction

The patient recalls you mentioning that older women, particularly >40, have a greater risk of stillbirth earlier in the term period than do younger women, although the absolute risk remains small and is likely influenced by factors other than maternal age alone. She is curious whether mechanisms for fetal monitoring and timing of delivery can mitigate this risk. She asks about practice recommendations for mode of delivery among AMA gravidas, reflecting on your mention of the potential need for Cesarean delivery.

---

9. With focus on risks of stillbirth with AMA, counsel the patient on the value or limitations of antenatal monitoring and provide evidence-based recommendations for delivery planning. *(1 point each)*   4

☐ Advise the patient that **no** fetal surveillance protocol (ultrasound, cardiotocography, kick counting) prevents stillbirth; additional risk of stillbirth with AMA is insufficient on its own to recommend any additional routine monitoring

☐ Although no universal consensus exists for *exact* timing of delivery in AMA gravidas, induction of labor at 39 weeks' gestation may be considered to mitigate the risk of stillbirth, without increasing risks of Cesarean section

☐ Provide the patient with an explanation for your recommended timing of delivery, such as the similar risk of stillbirth at 39 weeks in women 40–44 years as at 41 weeks among women 25–29 years[†]

☐ Trial of vaginal delivery is advised for AMA gravidas; elective Cesarean delivery solely for AMA is not advocated

Special note:

[†] *Refer to* (1) Royal College of Obstetricians and Gynaecologists, Scientific Impact Paper No. 34, Induction of labor at term in older mothers, February 2013; (2) Reddy Uma M *et al. Am J Obstet Gynecol* 2006; 195(3):764–770. Other statistical presentations may be shared with the patient to support safe practice recommendations

---

10. Facilitate your obstetric trainee's understanding as to why AMA gravidas have a greater risk of elective or emergent Cesarean delivery. *(1 point each)*   Max 3

☐ Medical or obstetrical complications
☐ Maternal request
☐ Greater risk of second-stage labor dystocia *(particularly among primiparous women)*
☐ Lower physician threshold

11. Inform the patient of immediate and long-term postpartum risks associated with AMA, which may be associated with related comorbidities. *(1 point each)*   Max 5

☐ Postpartum depression† *(Offer continued psychological and social support services)*
☐ Venous thromboembolism
☐ Peripartum hysterectomy
☐ Postpartum hemorrhage and need for blood transfusion
   ○ *Consider blood product availability and encourage active management of the third stage of labor*
☐ Fever/infection morbidity
☐ Prolonged hospitalization
☐ Future cardiovascular morbidity, especially after hypertensive diseases of pregnancy
☐ Future hemorrhagic stroke

Special note:
† *Refer to* Muraca GM, Joseph KS. The association between maternal age and depression. *J Obstet Gynaecol Can.* 2014;36(9):803–810.

At the end of your encounter, the patient provides constructive feedback in appreciation for your comprehensive information and well-structured approach. She understands a consultation note will be reported to her physician and that perinatal risks discussed in association with AMA may be compounded by in vitro fertilization, even though age appears to be a primary independent predictor of adverse perinatal outcomes.

TOTAL: **70**

CHAPTER 3

Teenage Pregnancy

Amira El-Messidi and Bianca Stortini

A 16-year-old primigravida at 16^{+5} weeks' gestation, confirmed two days earlier by dating sonography, is sent by her school nurse to your tertiary center's teen-pregnancy clinic. She presents accompanied by her mother, whom she prefers to be present during your encounter. Early fetal anatomy appeared normal without sonographic markers suggestive of aneuploidy. Urine pregnancy testing was initiated by her school nurse, who was concerned when the patient recently complained of increasing bloating and nausea over the past two months. The nurse assures you she had addressed the possibility of pregnancy with the teenager *prior* to urine testing.

Special note: *Although adolescents have increased rates of comorbidities, including alcohol consumption, smoking, illicit substance use, and psychiatric illness, the case scenario is presented as such for academic interest and to avoid content overlap of material addressed in respective chapters; readers are encouraged to complement subject matter where required.*

LEARNING OBJECTIVES

1. Take a focused history from a pregnant adolescent, appreciating the importance of screening questions for domestic violence and assessing for social determinants of health
2. Recognize causes for delayed prenatal care among pregnant teenagers amd provide counseling in a respectful, nonjudgmental manner
3. Demonstrate a structured approach to the identification of maternal-fetal-neonatal complications among pregnant adolescents, formulating an adolescent-focused multidisciplinary antenatal and postnatal care plan, consistent with the gold standard of care
4. Provide prenatal counseling for an active urogenital *C. trachomatis* infection, including comprehensive discussion on social health measures pre- and post effective treatment

SUGGESTED READINGS

1. ACOG Committee Opinion No. 735: Adolescents and long-acting reversible contraception: implants and intrauterine devices. *Obstet Gynecol.* 2018;131(5):e130–e139.
2. Apter D. International perspectives: IUDs and adolescents. *J Pediatr Adolesc Gynecol.* 2019;32(5S):S36–S42.
3. Workowski KA, Bachmann LH, Chan PA, et al. Sexually Transmitted Infections Treatment Guidelines, 2021. *MMWR Recomm Rep.* 2021;70(4):1–187. Accessed August 12, 2022.

4. Faculty of Sexual and Reproductive Healthcare of the Royal College of Obstetricians and Gynaecologists (FRSH) Clinical Guideline: contraceptive choices for young people (March 2010, amended May 2019). Available at www.fsrh.org/standards-and-guidance/documents/cec-ceu-guidance-young-people-mar-2010/. Accessed February 8, 2021.
5. Fleming N, O'Driscoll T, Becker G, et al. Canadian Paediatric and Adolescent Gynaecology and Obstetricians (CANPAGO) Committee: adolescent pregnancy guidelines. *J Obstet Gynaecol Can.* 2015;37(8):740–756.
6. Lanjouw E, Ouburg S, de Vries HJ, et al. 2015 European guideline on the management of chlamydia trachomatis infections. *Int J STD AIDS.* 2016;27(5):333–348.
7. Leftwich HK, Alves MV. Adolescent pregnancy. *Pediatr Clin North Am.* 2017;64(2):381–388.
8. McCarthy FP, O'Brien U, Kenny LC. The management of teenage pregnancy. *BMJ.* 2014;349: g5887.
9. Peterson SF, Goldthwaite LM. Postabortion and postpartum intrauterine device provision for adolescents and young adults. *J Pediatr Adolesc Gynecol.* 2019;32(5S):S30–S35.
10. Public Health England. Collection on teenage pregnancy. Available at www.gov.uk/government/collections/teenage-pregnancy. Accessed February 8, 2021.

POINTS

1. Before you meet the patient, alert your obstetric trainee to the significance for pretest counseling appropriately performed by the school nurse prior to urine pregnancy testing. *(1 point each)*

2

Positive pregnancy test:
☐ Asking the teenager to consider potential pregnancy prior to confirmation provided opportunity to ensure her safety, in case of dangerous behavior including suicidality/homicidality

Negative pregnancy test:
☐ Encouraging the teenager to entertain possible pregnancy may provide strategic opportunities for contraception education (long-term and emergency contraception as well as providing sex education)

2. With regard to a teenage pregnancy, what aspects of a focused history would you want to know? *(1 point per main bullet; max points specified per section)*

30

Pregnancy: (9)
☐ Ensure pregnancy is not due to sexual violence (*e.g.*; sex trafficking, rape, coercion) *[i.e., a form of 'structural conflict'*[$]*
☐ Age and involvement of the fetus' father and her current partner, if not the father
　○ *Recognize that sociomedical comorbidities may prohibit the pregnant teen from identifying the father (e.g., mental handicap, was under drug/alcohol influence, multiple partners)*
☐ Assess her attitude toward pregnancy
☐ Assess for possible mood disorders, including past or present depressive symptoms, and possibly suicidal ideation or prior suicidal tendencies, anxiety
☐ Current vaginal bleeding, or within past months when she was unknowingly pregnant
☐ Current or recent lower abdominal cramps/pains
☐ Symptoms suggestive of genitourinary infections (*e.g.*, abnormal vaginal discharge, pruritis, dysuria)

☐ Current/recent vomiting, with her concurrent nausea

☐ Determine if patient had prior, *undisclosed,* spontaneous or therapeutic pregnancy losses

Socio-sexual history: *(3)*

☐ History of sexually transmitted infections (STI) or need for hospitalization/surgery for pelvic inflammatory disease

☐ Assess whether patient is in a consensual relationship or experiences peer pressure to have sex *(i.e., a form of 'structural conflict'§)*

☐ Current/prior multiple sexual partners

Medical comorbidities most relevant to pregnancy in teenagers: *(4)*

☐ Known history of iron-deficiency anemia

☐ Mood disorder *(e.g.,* history of depression and/or anxiety conditions)

   ○ *Obtain name/contact of treating physician*

☐ History of eating disorders (anorexia or bulimia nervosa); assess self-esteem

☐ Presence of neurodevelopmental delay/mental disability

Socioeconomic features: *(max 5)*

☐ Living situation and basic house amenities§; receipt of public financial benefits

☐ Food security§

☐ Access and financial coverage of transportation costs for prenatal visits, vitamins, or other treatments that may not be covered by the local health care system

   ○ *(i.e., 'access to affordable health services of decent quality'§)*

☐ Social supports§ *(i.e., family, community support, social worker)*

☐ Education§ – patient's progress, access to a supportive system, and future plans

☐ Ethnicity and cultural attitude toward extramarital pregnancy

Social habits: *(3)*

☐ Cigarette smoking and amount

☐ Alcohol consumption and amount

☐ Use of illicit substances, including type, frequency, supply source, mode of use *(e.g., IV, inhaled, smoked, snorted, oral),* and enrollment in treatment programs

Health maintenance: *(2)*

☐ Assess if was on contraceptive method that led to inadvertent pregnancy/prior use of other contraceptives

☐ Vaccination status *(e.g., MMR, influenza, hepatitis A and B, tetanus)*

Medications and allergies: *(2)*

☐ Prescribed or over-the-counter agents, particularly assess for use of psychotropic agents

☐ Allergies *(particularly important as pregnant teenagers have increased rates of STIs in pregnancy)*

Family history: *(max 2)*

☐ Parental separation in early childhood *(i.e., a form of 'structural conflict'§)*

☐ Exposure to family violence in early childhood *(i.e., a form of 'structural conflict'§)*

☐ Family history of teenage pregnancy

Special note:

§ Items are among the 'social determinants of health' delineated by the World Health Organization; readers are encouraged to refer to www.who.int/health-topics/social-determinants-of-health#tab=tab_1, accessed February 9, 2021.

3. In conversation with the patient, demonstrate how you may phrase questions addressing the risk of <u>domestic violence</u> using a <u>validated screening approach</u>. You inform the patient she may decline to answer. *[the following provides five questions from one validated system; other approaches may be accepted]* (1 point each)

☐ 1) Do you *feel safe* in your relationship with your partner or family?

☐ 2) Are there situations in the past six months when you have *felt afraid* of your partner or a family member?

☐ 3) In the past six months, have you ever been a *victim of domestic violence* from your partner or family member?

☐ 4) In the past six months, have you ever been hit, kicked, punched, or *physically hurt* by a partner or a family member?

☐ 5) In the past six months, have you ever been *forced* to have sex or do sexual things that you did not want to do by a partner or family member?

Special note:

Refer to Quinlivan JA, Evans SF. A prospective cohort study of the impact of domestic violence on young teenage pregnancy outcomes. *J Pediatr Adolesc Gynecol.* 2001; 14(1):17–23.

You learn that the patient lives with her 33-year-old mother and her younger sister in a small two-bedroom home in a poor socioeconomic sector of town. They have been unaware of the father's whereabouts for numerous years. The mother works as a part-time cashier and the family receives monthly governmental financial aid, which helps supply basic necessities of living. Until nine months ago, her mother's boyfriend was living with them for two years, during which the patient endured his verbal aggression. During that time, the school psychologist provided close care for the teen's resultant depressed mood, though she has never required antidepressant or other prescribed medications; she reports emotional stability since his departure. There is no history of smoking, alcohol intake, or use of illicit substances. Although one year behind her peers in schooling due to social disadvantages, her performance has been satisfactory.

The patient is generally healthy. With irregular menses and continued sporadic bleeding over the past few months, she did not suspect pregnancy. She has been taking a combined oral contraceptive pill, although she forgets at least once weekly. She assures you her sexual encounters have been consensual. Two months ago, she broke up with her 'long-term' partner of one year, whom she is certain is the father of her child. Over the past few months, she has been feeling unwell from bouts of vomiting and increased somnolence. She has had prior vaginal infections in the past, although is unable to confirm the etiologies; the patient was reportedly cured after short courses of medical treatment. She ascertains the last infection was over one year ago and is currently asymptomatic.

You sketch contributing factors for late prenatal care among adolescents, intending to teach your trainee after this clinical visit.

4. Discuss your sketched notes regarding why adolescents may delay prenatal care.   Max 5
(1 point each)

☐ Limited knowledge about the importance of prenatal care
☐ Limited understanding of consequences from lack of prenatal care
☐ Fear of apprehension of the newborn by youth protection authorities
☐ Fear of violence
☐ Contemplating termination of pregnancy (abortion)
☐ Fear of lack of confidentiality from the health care professional
☐ Fear of being judged by the treating team
☐ Financial implications

5. Cognizant of being respectful and nonjudgmental, identify three pregnancy management   3
options for the patient's consideration, assuming jurisdictional laws allow women to make
informed choices on early pregnancy management. *(1 point each)*

☐ Continuation of pregnancy and parenting
☐ Arranging for child adoption or kinship care
☐ Termination of pregnancy

The patient and her mother appreciate your professional approach: the patient has indeed considered her options and plans to continue pregnancy and care for the child within her family home. With support from the social worker, the patient intends to notify her former partner, should he wish to participate in the care of his child.

You explain that this adolescent-focused multidisciplinary clinic is structured to provide **gold standard** comprehensive antenatal care with delivery planned in the affiliated hospital center with appropriate access to maternal-fetal and neonatal support services.

6. In addition to a welcoming environment for the pregnant adolescent, identify a <u>key</u>   1
characteristic of adolescent-focused multidisciplinary care units.

☐ Different dimensions of prenatal care are provided in one place at one time (*i.e.*, one-stop
shopping: nutritionist, social worker, public health worker, nurse/midwife, pediatric
gynecologist or obstetrician, psychologist/psychiatrist, expert in addiction medicine)
   ○ *Ease of access to prenatal services improves compliance with care*
   ○ *Nonjudgmental approach by the health professionals*
   ○ *Adolescent-focused multidisciplinary clinics have been shown to result in better outcomes
     relative to standard prenatal care units, potentially leading to significant reductions in
     health care costs*

Before you prepare an outline for the antenatal management most particular to this pregnant adolescent, you think of potential perinatal complications more common in this population.

7. Verbalize your structured thinking of maternal-fetal complications more common in the pregnant adolescent, upon which you will base the framework for prenatal care.[†]
(1 point each; max points per section specified)

                                                          9

Maternal: *(max 6)*
- ☐ Iron-deficiency anemia
- ☐ Urinary tract infections
- ☐ STIs
- ☐ Preeclampsia/eclampsia *(controversial)*
- ☐ Preterm prelabor rupture of membranes
- ☐ Preterm labor/preterm birth
- ☐ Depression (antepartum and postpartum)
- ☐ Suicidality
- ☐ Increased rates of instrumental vaginal delivery
  - ○ *Possibly associated with less maternal cooperation in the second stage or 'uterine immaturity' of young mothers*
  - ○ *Note that teenagers are less likely to have a Cesarean delivery than older patients*

Fetal/neonatal: *(max 3)*
- ☐ Certain congenital anomalies are more common in this population *(see Question 15)*
- ☐ FGR, suboptimal growth velocity; low birthweight
- ☐ IUFD
- ☐ NICU admissions
- ☐ Neonatal death/sudden infant death syndrome

Special note:
† In the clinical setting, risks of morbidity and mortality would not be presented in this fashion to the (perhaps) vulnerable pregnant adolescent; the above represents your *thinking* process for academic purposes of this exercise

8. Recognizing that sociodemographic factors partly account for adverse perinatal outcomes, pinpoint the most likely <u>biologic mechanism</u> for the 'high-risk' nature of adolescent pregnancies.

                                                           1

- ☐ Biologic immaturity of the adolescent (uterine immaturity)

9. In collaboration with multidisciplinary professionals, present a model for your <u>antepartum</u> management most relevant to the care of this pregnant adolescent.
(1 point per main bullet)

                                                         13

Maternal:
- ☐ Initiate treatment of her nausea to maintain/improve nutritional support
- ☐ Anticipate frequent antenatal follow-up *(e.g., every two to three weeks in the second and early third trimester, or individualized interval)*
- ☐ Educate for daily intake of 0.4 mg folic acid-containing multivitamins
- ☐ Consideration for providing samples/free access to prenatal vitamins or at reduced cost
- ☐ Screening and treatment of iron-deficiency anemia (free access or reduced cost)

☐ Early nutritional referral
  o *Increased risk of nutritional deficiencies and higher needs due to pubertal change*
  o *Assess for adequate intake of vitamins and nutrients important in pregnancy, such as folic acid, iron, calcium, and vitamin D*
  o *Consideration for arranging food donation services, if required*
☐ Careful monitoring of gestational weight gain
☐ Routine screening for gestational diabetes, as per local recommendations
☐ Ensure testing for STIs and bacterial vaginosis at this initial prenatal visit and in the third trimester; further testing is dependent upon symptoms
  o *Vaginal swab specimens self-collected by the patient improve patient acceptance over pelvic examination*
  o *Prioritize the adolescent's right to privacy and confidentiality and consider her preference regarding her mother's presence*
☐ Screen for urinary tract infections at the first prenatal visit and with symptoms
☐ Serial prenatal screening to assess for domestic violence, mental health, and social habits

Fetal:
☐ Second-trimester detailed morphology scan *(more frequent rates of congenital anomalies)*
☐ Serial growth scans *(individualized frequency in the second and third trimesters with minimum one third-trimester growth ultrasound)*
☐ Consideration for early neonatology consultation, where clinical concern exists

Special note:
Routine monitoring for risk of hypertensive syndromes of pregnancy is practiced in adolescents; there is no evidence to support prophylaxis as in high- and moderate-risk populations (refer to Chapter 38)

Having provided adequate time to counsel the patient, discuss her prenatal care plan, and allow the patient to meet allied professionals who will be involved in her care, you proceed to assess her vital signs, which are unremarkable. Ascertaining fetal viability has evidently reassured the patient and her mother. Sensitive to the patient's privacy, you offer her self-collection of vaginal swabs for chlamydia,[§] gonorrhea,[§] and bacterial vaginosis, which she indeed prefers relative to pelvic examination.

Three days later, the patient attends to this specialized obstetric adolescent unit upon your request. Transportation costs have been facilitated. You intend to counsel and manage the *C. trachomatis*[†] infection detected on vaginal swab[‡§] at the initial prenatal visit. There is no concomitant gonococcal infection. You will also reassure the patient that all other routine prenatal investigations are normal. The fetal morphology sonogram is arranged for next week. The patient appears to be doing well and has no obstetric or other socio-medical complaints.

Special notes:
§ Urogenital *C. trachomatis* and *N. gonorrhea* infections can also be diagnosed with NAATs on first-catch urine specimen
† *C. trachomatis* infection has been found in up to 30% of pregnant adolescents presenting for the first prenatal visit
‡ Optimal, first choice, specimens for diagnosis of urogenital chlamydial infections using nucleic acid amplification tests (NAATs) are vaginal or vulvo-vaginal swabs *(2015 CDC[3] and 2015 European Guidelines[6], respectively)*

10. Address your obstetric trainee's inquiry about the technical procedure performed by the microbiology laboratory for detection of *C. trachomatis* infection.

2

☐ Nucleic acid amplification tests (NAATs)
  ○ *(2015 European Guidelines[6])* Where *C. trachomatis* NAAT is unavailable or not affordable, cell culture or direct fluorescent assays can be used for diagnosis

11. Indicate important aspects you would discuss in counseling the patient on social health measures with *C. trachomatis* infection. *(1 point per main bullet)*

3

☐ Discuss partner notification within the past 60 days (interpersonally or via partner services programs)
  ○ *Note that the recommended exposure interval for identification of at-risk sex partners is based on limited evidence; as such, the most recent sex partner should be evaluated and treated, even if the last sexual contact was >60 days before the patient's diagnosis, or symptom-onset (CDC[3])*
☐ Inform the patient that public health reporting of *C. trachomatis* infections may be required by jurisdictional policies *(consult local legal counsel, if necessary)*
  ○ Always reassure the patient of confidential proceedings
☐ Recommend systematic future condom use during sexual intercourse to decrease risk of STIs

The patient appreciates your sensitive approach to counseling; she prefers a professional service program to contact her former boyfriend, in case he stigmatizes her. Incidentally, the patient informs you the father of her unborn child is aware of the pregnancy but has chosen to 'move on' in life; he does not intend to play a role in his unborn child's life.

As you confirm the patient does not have drug allergies, she agrees to comply with recommended treatment and required follow-up for *C. trachomatis*. Treatment will be provided for the teenager and directly observed therapy will be assured at this visit. The patient confirms she is asymptomatic.

12. In the absence of drug allergies, provide the recommended regimen for *C. trachomatis* infection in pregnancy and specify the management course posttreatment. *(1 point per main bullet)*

Max 4

☐ Azithromycin 1 g as a single oral dose
☐ Encourage the patient (and sexual partner, if any) to abstain from sexual intercourse for seven days until after *initiating* treatment (*i.e.*, seven days after single-dose therapy, or after completing a seven-day regimen)
  ○ *Abstinence would also be advised until resolution of symptoms, where present*
☐ Test of cure is recommended at three to four weeks after *completion* of treatment
☐ Retesting for infection in ~12 weeks after treatment
☐ Serial testing every trimester is planned for this adolescent with documented infection in pregnancy, as would be *considered* in routine prenatal care of an adolescent

Special note:
Amoxicillin is an alternative therapy for *C. trachomatis* for pregnant women; erythromycin is no longer recommended because of the frequency of gastrointestinal side effects that can result in therapy nonadherence.

13-A. Concerned about bacterial eradication after taking azithromycin, the patient inquires whether you may perform the diagnostic test of cure at the next prenatal visit in two weeks' time. Justify your advisory.

□ Test of cure is <u>not</u> advised before three weeks after completion of treatment as nucleic acid amplification tests may detect persistent dead organisms, leading to false-positive results

13-B. Should the test of cure demonstrate a persistent infection, address the patient's question regarding subsequent treatment.

□ Repeat the standard preferred azithromycin regimen, as *C. trachomatis* resistance to this agent has not been demonstrated

14. Inform the patient of the two principal <u>neonatal infections</u> that may occur consequent to exposure to *C. trachomatis* pathogens harboring an untreated/inadequately treated genital tract at delivery. *(1 point each)*

□ Ophthalmia neonatorum (presenting as conjunctivitis)
□ Chlamydia pneumonia

Special note:
Vertical transmission risk for newborn ranges from 30%–50% *(Suggested Reading 5)* to 50%–75% *(Suggested Reading 6)*

You later find your obstetric trainee surfing the internet for therapeutic agents used outside the context of pregnancy for treatment of *C. trachomatis* infection.

15. Facilitate your trainee's learning by identifying three antibiotic <u>agents</u> that would treat *C. trachomatis* infection but are generally contraindicated in pregnancy and during breastfeeding. *(1 point each)*

□ Doxycycline[§]
□ Ofloxacin/levofloxacin[†]
□ Erythromycin estolate *(drug-associated hepatotoxicity)*

Special notes:
§ Refer to Question 18 in Chapter 1 for discussion on updated drug-related literature and clinical experience with use of doxycycline in pregnancy
† Human data show low risk to the fetus during pregnancy, yet animal studies raise concern about neonatal cartilage damage; use of alternative agents in pregnancy is wise

The patient is looking forward to the second-trimester fetal morphology sonogram arranged next week, where her mother will be able to accompany her.

After this clinical visit, your obstetric trainee takes note of congenital malformations more common among adolescent populations, as you had alluded to during initial consultation. He or she recognizes that lifestyle-related factors, such as smoking, alcohol consumption, illicit drug use, and insufficient periconceptional folic acid supplementation may play a role in risk of congenital anomalies, although independent associations with teenager status have been shown. You hereby reinforce that adequate counseling and support for the teenage patient is an opportunity for prevention and may positively impact public health.

---

16. Identify <u>congenital fetal malformations</u> that may be more common in teenage pregnancies.   Max 4
    (1 point each)

- ☐ Gastroschisis
- ☐ Omphalocele
- ☐ Facial clefts (lip and/or palate)
- ☐ Polydactyly, syndactyly/adactyly
- ☐ Central nervous system anomalies <u>other than</u> anencephalus, spina bifida/meningocele, hydrocephalus, and microcephalus

Special note:
Refer to Chen XK, Wen SW, Fleming N, Yang Q, Walker MC. Teenage pregnancy and congenital anomalies: which system is vulnerable? *Hum Reprod.* 2007;22(6):1730–1735.

The fetal morphology scan is normal and serial growth biometric assessments remain on the 13th–15th percentile with normal amniotic fluid volume. Test of cure for *C. trachomatis* infection is negative, with normal results thereafter. The patient's socio-medical progress is appropriate, and she remains compliant with multidisciplinary care.

She presents to the obstetrics emergency assessment unit at 36^{+2} weeks' gestation in spontaneous preterm labor and has an uneventful vaginal delivery. Her GBS (group B streptococcus) vaginal-rectal swab, which you had just performed two days ago, was negative. Although you had discussed essential elements of postpartum management well in advance of delivery, you visit the patient and her newborn on postpartum day 1 and review aspects of care.

---

17. Provide essential elements of <u>postpartum</u> management with regard to a teenage pregnancy.   9
    (1 point per main bullet)

Mental well-being and health maintenance:
- ☐ Screen for postpartum depression and continue to ensure hospital-based psychosocial support services with simultaneous engagement in community care programs for young postpartum women/families
- ☐ Arrange for a clinic visit early in the postpartum period (*e.g.*, two weeks) and at six weeks postpartum
- ☐ Plan for repeat STI screening postpartum

Breastfeeding:
- ☐ Encourage breastfeeding by proving extensive education and support (*e.g.*, lactation expert) as teenagers have high discontinuation rates

o *Ensure no concurrent maternal substance use or medications that may incur risk to the breastfed infant*

Contraception:

☐ Engage the patient in comprehensive sexuality educational services

☐ Reassure the patient that contraceptive counseling and prevention of rapid repeat pregnancy *(i.e., variably defined as pregnancy within 18–24 months of a previous pregnancy)* serves to avoid unplanned and unwanted pregnancy, while also empowering her to achieve the desired interpregnancy interval and allow her socio-economic stability

☐ Advocate long-acting reversible contraception *[i.e., intrauterine devices (IUDs) or subdermal implants]* **as soon as possible after delivery**

   o Although copper or levonorgesterol IUD may be inserted immediately (<10 minutes postplacental) or early postpartum (10 minutes up to 48 hours) after vaginal or Cesarean delivery, rates of expulsion are greater than with interval placement (at least four weeks postpartum)

   o Multiple organizations[†] endorse long-acting reversible contraception as safe contraceptive methods for adolescents

      ▪ American Academy of Pediatrics (AAP)[†] and Canadian Pediatric Society (CPS)[†] endorse long-acting reversible contraception as *first-line* for adolescents seeking contraception

☐ Encourage male condom use for dual contraception and prevention of STIs

Primary care:

☐ Communicate with her primary physician/pediatrician for ongoing care after the approximately six weeks postpartum period

Special note:

† Including the Faculty of Sexual and Reproductive Healthcare (FRSH)-2019, American College of Obstetricians and Gynecologists (ACOG)-2018, American Academy of Pediatrics (AAP)-2014, Society of Obstetricians and Gynaecologists of Canada (SOGC)-2018, and Canadian Pediatric Society (CPS)-2018

TOTAL: **100**

CHAPTER 4

Hyperemesis Gravidarum

William M. Buckett and Amira El-Messidi

A 25-year-old G2P1 presents for prenatal care at 8^{+2} weeks' gestation by menstrual dates with complaints of nausea and vomiting for the past two weeks. Your clinical nurse reassures you the patient is not in acute distress and converses well. There is no history of vaginal bleeding.

Although your obstetric trainee tells you she recently learned about nausea and vomiting of pregnancy (NVP) and will be comfortable initiating patient care, you highlight that this is a diagnosis of exclusion.

LEARNING OBJECTIVES

1. Elicit risk factors for, and clinical manifestations of, first-trimester nausea and vomiting of pregnancy (NVP) to determine severity and set management goals
2. Counsel on diet, lifestyle changes, and pharmacologic interventions to improve symptoms and quality of life of patients with NVP
3. Recognize the importance of interprofessional collaboration to optimize management and prevent serious maternal complications of hyperemesis gravidarum
4. Understand that variations exist in the line of pharmacologic treatments among national guidelines, with mostly similar drug regimens

SUGGESTED READINGS

1. Austin K, Wilson K, Saha S. Hyperemesis gravidarum. *Nutr Clin Pract*. 2019;34(2):226–241.
2. Boelig RC, Barton SJ, Saccone G, et al. Interventions for treating hyperemesis gravidarum: a Cochrane systematic review and meta-analysis. *J Matern Fetal Neonatal Med*. 2018;31(18):2492–2505.
3. Bustos M, Venkataramanan R, Caritis S. Nausea and vomiting of pregnancy – what's new? *Auton Neurosci*. 2017;202:62–72.
4. Campbell K, Rowe H, Azzam H, et al. The management of nausea and vomiting of pregnancy. *J Obstet Gynaecol Can*. 2016;38(12):1127–1137.
5. Committee on Practice Bulletins – Obstetrics. ACOG Practice Bulletin No. 189: nausea and vomiting of pregnancy. *Obstet Gynecol*. 2018;131(1):e15–e30.
6. Dean CR, Shemar M, Ostrowski GAU, et al. Management of severe pregnancy sickness and hyperemesis gravidarum. *BMJ*. 2018;363:k5000.

7. Jennings LK, Krywko DM. Hyperemesis gravidarum. In: *StatPearls*. Treasure Island, FL: StatPearls; 2020.

8. London V, Grube S, Sherer DM, et al. Hyperemesis gravidarum: a review of recent literature. *Pharmacology*. 2017;100(3–4):161–171.

9. Royal College of Obstetricians and Gynaecologists. The management of nausea and vomiting of pregnancy and hyperemesis gravidarum. Green-Top Guideline No. 69, 2016. Available at www.rcog.org.uk/en/guidelines-research-services/guidelines/gtg69/. Accessed February 27, 2021.

10. Tsakiridis I, Mamopoulos A, Athanasiadis A, et al. The management of nausea and vomiting of pregnancy: synthesis of national guidelines. *Obstet Gynecol Surv*. 2019;74(3)161–169.

POINTS

1. Regarding nausea and vomiting, what aspects of a focused history would you want to know? *(1 point per main bullet, unless specified; max points indicated per section)*   Max 30

General aspects of the clinical complaints:
- ☐ Determine the ability to tolerate food and liquids
- ☐ Changes in frequency and severity of symptoms since onset
- ☐ Attempted interventions and their effects on symptom-control
- ☐ Identify whether sensory stimuli or time of day trigger symptoms
- ☐ Effect on her quality of life
- ☐ Clinical manifestations:
  - ○ Retching/dry heaves
  - ○ Hypersalivation (ptyalism), spitting
  - ○ Hematemesis
  - ○ Weight loss

Tool to measure the severity of NVP: *(1 point for each component of the PUQE score; total 3)*
- ☐ Pregnancy-Unique Quantification of Emesis [PUQE score][$] *(or other validated, standardized tool)*
  - ○ 3 questions regarding nausea, vomiting, and retching during previous 12 h *(original version)* or 24 hours *(most commonly used version)*
    - ▪ Total score is the sum to each of the three questions: mild ≤6; moderate 7–12; severe 13–15

Features related to differential diagnoses: *(max 5)*
- ☐ Recent travel or sick contacts
- ☐ Possible contaminated food ingestion
- ☐ Fever
- ☐ History of migraines or neurologic illness
- ☐ Abdominal pain
- ☐ Change in bowel habits
- ☐ Symptoms of urinary tract infections

Obstetric and medical risk factors or associations with NVP: *(max 4)*
- ☐ NVP or hyperemesis gravidarum in prior pregnancy, severity, and effective treatments
- ☐ History of *H. pylori* infection, gastroesophageal reflux disease, esophagitis, or gastritis

□ Known endocrinologic condition, such as diabetes or hyperthyroidism
□ *Current* features of depression and/or anxiety disorder
    ○ *poor mental health is a result of the suffering from NVP rather than being causal; prior history of depression is not a determinant*

Social history: *(2)*
□ Occupation
□ Alcohol consumption, illicit drug use, cigarette smoking[†]

Medications and allergies: *(4)*
□ Current medications
□ Preconception use of vitamin supplements[†]
□ Prior adverse reactions to antiemetics
□ Food or drug allergies

Family history: *(2)*
□ NVP or hyperemesis gravidarum in her mother and/or sisters
□ Arrhythmias or prolonged QT interval (for the patient or family members)

Special notes:
§ Refer to (a) Koren G et al. *Am J Obstet Gynecol.* 2002; 186: S228; (b) Koren G et al. *Obstet Gynecol* 2005; 25:241; (c) Lacasse A et al. *Am J Obstet Gynecol.* 2008; 198: 71.e1–7; (d) Ebrahimi N et al. *J Obstet Gynaecol Can.* 2009;31:803–7
† Vitamins for one month prior to conception and smoking are protective against NVP

You learn the patient immigrated two years ago with her husband and then one-year-old daughter[†] to pursue studies in pharmacology. Although her obstetrical chart from her homeland is unavailable, she vividly recalls having nausea and vomiting in pregnancy, requiring outpatient therapy until mid-second trimester, and a brief hospitalization for hydration in early pregnancy. Unfortunately, the patient does not know which medicines provided her with symptomatic relief. She is grateful that her experience with NVP did not require enteral nutrition, as did her older sister's pregnancy.

Her current pregnancy is a pleasant surprise after failed barrier contraception. Urine pregnancy testing six weeks after her last menses validated her morning sickness. Her only medications include prenatal vitamins which she recently started, although they aggravate her symptoms. The patient is generally healthy, does not drink alcohol or use illicit substances. She has no food or drug allergies.

Over the past two weeks, nausea has progressed to include vomiting and spitting. In the last 24 hours, she has been nauseous for 1 hour, vomited twice, and had two episodes of dry heaves.[‡] She tolerates mid-day meals yet vomits in the morning and when she lays down after supper. The patient continues to attend activities related to her studies yet is often disturbed by aromatic compounds in the laboratory; reassuringly, all compounds are nontoxic. No therapeutic modalities for symptomatic relief have been tried to date. Review of systems is unremarkable for other possible causations to explain her symptoms. Although she has not weighed herself, her average weight is quoted to be 73 kg (160.0 lb), which you confirm. Physical examination is unremarkable, with no evidence of dehydration; the patient retched once during your encounter and complains of mild nausea.

Special notes:

† Female fetuses may be associated with greater risk of hyperemesis gravidarum *(Basso, O et al. Epidemiology 2001;12:747–749)*

‡ PUQE score is 6, consistent for mild NVP

2. In addition to baseline prenatal tests, indicate the <u>next</u> most appropriate investigation and justify your plan. *(1 point per main and subbullet)*		Max 3

☐ Obstetric ultrasound:
  o Confirm viable intrauterine pregnancy
  o Exclude multiple pregnancy
  o Exclude trophoblastic disease

Obstetric ultrasound at this first visit confirms an intrauterine singleton consistent with menstrual dates. While the patient is at the imaging unit, you take this opportunity to address your trainee's inquiry about the causes of NVP syndromes and make arrangements for the obstetric dietician to subsequently counsel the patient with you at this initial visit.

3. Although multifactorial and largely unknown, discuss three possible etiologies in the pathogenesis[$] of NVP. *(1 point per main bullet)*	3

☐ <u>Genetic predisposition:</u> *(one or more prevailing theories)*
  o Increased incidence in mothers, sisters, particularly monozygotic twins, or other relatives of women with NVP/hyperemesis gravidarum
  o Ethnic variations – *NVP appears more common in Asian, Indian, Pakistani, and New Zealanders compared to European, American Indian and Inuit populations*
☐ <u>Endocrine aspects:</u>[†]
  o High levels of human chorionic gonadotropin (hCG) *(correlation may relate to isoforms of hCG; causality is not proven)*
  o High estradiol and progesterone levels *(not a strong association)*
  o Other placental-mediated hormones
☐ <u>Evolutionary adaptation:</u>
  o Aversion to foods and smell in early pregnancy may protect the mother and fetus from potentially harmful foods
☐ <u>Infectious:</u>
  o *H. pylori* has been positively correlated, yet unlikely a main mechanism, in hyperemesis gravidarum

Special notes:

§ Psychogenic etiologies are erroneous, despite the common belief of health care professionals

† Hyperthyroidism itself rarely causes vomiting; attention is focused on hCG and estrogen

4. In collaboration with the obstetric nutritionist, provide <u>dietary and lifestyle</u> strategies to manage nausea and vomiting in early pregnancy. *(1 point per main bullet)*

Max 8

Recommended interventions:
- ☐ Rest periods, as required, to alleviate symptoms *(RCOG[9])*
  - ○ Laying on the left side may aggravate symptoms [delays gastric emptying]
- ☐ Small, frequent meals every one to two hours to avoid an empty or a full stomach that aggravate nausea
  - ○ *(SOGC[4] and ACOG[5])*
- ☐ Protein-dominant, salty, starchy, bland and/or dry foods
  - ○ *e.g., BRAT diet (banana, rice, applesauce, toast), tea-cookies, butter, mashed potato, noodles, cheese, egg, turkey slices, soft fruits/vegetables, nuts*
- ☐ Delay liquid intake by 30–60 minutes before or after tolerated food
- ☐ Clear, cold, carbonated/sour liquids drunk slowly or with a straw
- ☐ Consumption of ginger-containing foods, or oral capsules of 250 mg four times daily
  - ○ *(SOGC, ACOG, RCOG recommendation)*
- ☐ Peppermint tea/candy may reduce postprandial nausea
- ☐ Brush teeth after meals or frequent mouth-washing
- ☐ Acustimulation of the pericardium-6 point [P6] located on the distal forearm, three fingerbreadths above the wrist
  - ○ *(SOGC, ACOG, RCOG recommendation)*
- ☐ Consideration for behavioral interventions such as mindfulness-based cognitive therapy
  - ○ *(SOGC recommendation)*

Avoid or minimize:
- ☐ Environmental triggers (*e.g.*, odors, noise, visual stimuli, driving, heat, humidity)
- ☐ Iron-containing supplements in the first trimester; substitute with folic acid or noniron vitamin supplements instead
  - ○ *(SOGC, ACOG, RCOG recommendation)*
- ☐ Fatty, spicy, sweet, odorous, fried, or acidic foods, milk, cream soups, tomato sauce, coffee

The patient appreciates this counseling session; she is an avid eater of ginger-containing foods and is reassured about its fetal safety. She wonders, however, about maternal side effects.

5. Discuss potential maternal adverse effects from ginger ingestion or supplementation. *(1 point each)*

Max 2

- ☐ Gastric irritation
- ☐ Anticoagulant effects
- ☐ Drug interactions with benzodiazepines and beta-blockers

You explain that NVP is associated with lower rates of miscarriage and does not increase perinatal or neonatal mortality. Fetal risks of low birthweight and prematurity are controversial and may vary by severity of disease.

At this visit, you counsel the patient on the safety and effectiveness of pharmacologic treatment of NVP and inform her that early treatment may improve her quality of life, which may be impaired even with mild manifestations. As no antiemetic has demonstrated clear superiority over another for symptomatic relief, choice is largely based on side-effect profile, safety, and cost.

Noting differences exist in the line of pharmacologic patterns between North America and the United Kingdom, you highlight to your trainee that regimens are largely similar. You are confident with names of drug therapies, although require your trainee to validate prescription regimens.

---

6. Detail two first-line pharmacologic regimens for NVP, recognizing that international practice variations exist in drug selection.   Max 4

   (any two comprehensive regimens for 2 points each; alternative antihistamines and phenothiazines may be accepted; practice variations exist)

ACOG/SOGC:
- ☐ Pyridoxine (vitamin B6) 10–25 mg PO, three to four times daily
- ☐ Pyridoxamine 10–25 mg/doxylamine 12.5 mg PO, three to four times daily
- ☐ Pyridoxamine 10 mg/doxylamine 10 mg PO, up to four times daily
- ☐ Pyridoxamine 20 mg/doxylamine 20 mg PO, up to twice daily

RCOG:[†]
- ☐ Antihistamines (H1-receptor antagonists):
  - ○ Cyclizine 50 mg PO/IM/IV every eight hours
  - ○ Diphenhydramine or dimenhydrate 25–50 mg PO every four to six hours *(SOGC, ACOG; second line)*
  - ○ Diphenhydramine 10–50 mg IV every four to six hours
  - ○ Dimenhydrinate 50–100 mg PR every four to six hours
  - ○ Dimenhydrinate 50 mg IV over 20 minutes
- ☐ Phenothiazines (a type of dopamine antagonists):
  - ○ Prochlorperazine 5–10 mg PO every six to eight hours
  - ○ Prochlorperazine 12.5 mg IM/IV every eight hours
  - ○ Prochlorperazine 25 mg PR one to two times daily
  - ○ Chlorpromazine 10–25 mg PO/IV/IM every four to six hours
  - ○ Chlorpromazine 50–100 mg PR every six to eight hours
  - ○ Promethazine 12.5–25 mg PO/PR/IM/IV[‡] every four to eight hours

Special notes:
† RCOG does not recommend pyridoxine based on limited evidence supporting its use (Matthews A, et al. *Cochrane Database Syst Rev.* 2015;2015(9):CD007575); subsequent studies showed mild improvement and decreased hospitalizations
‡ IV is last resort due to risk of gangrene in affected extremity and severe extravasation injury PO. = per os; IM = intramuscular; IV = intravenous; PR = per rectum

---

As pyridoxine regimens are not recommended in the United Kingdom, you inform your trainee that the treatment line of therapy results in a four-tier system in Canada and the United States and a three-tier system in the United Kingdom, resorting to PO/IV corticosteroids[†] when standard therapies fail.

The patient will practice the discussed lifestyle and dietary strategies, resorting to antihistaminic support if necessary. Follow-up with the nutritionist has been arranged and the patient will contact you within one week if current management is nonrelieving. She understands a drug from a *different* class may be added to her antihistaminic, if needed. Attendance at your ambulatory care unit for daily parenteral therapy is also practiced provided hospitalization is not required.

Special note:
† *Refer to Chapter 45 for **fetal** effects, and Chapter 46 for **maternal** effects, of maternal corticosteroids*

7. Detail two drug regimens from two different classes for treatment of NVP after failed response to initial therapy. You are reserving corticosteroids as a last resort. *(2 points per drug regimen)*   4

   ☐ Dopamine antagonists:
     ○ Metoclopramide 5–10 mg PO/IM/IV every eight hours[†]
     ○ Domperidone 10 mg PO every eight hours
     ○ Domperidone 30–60 mg PR every eight hours
   ☐ Serotonin 5-hydroxytryptamine type 3 receptor antagonists:
     ○ Ondansetron 4–8 mg PO every six to eight hours
     ○ Ondansetron 8 mg IV, over 15 minutes, every 12 hours

Special note:
† Consideration for limiting metoclopramide treatment to five days with maximum of 30 mg/24 hours or 0.5 mg/kg/d due to extrapyramidal effects, tardive dyskinesia, and oculogyric crisis

The following week, the patient notifies you she is now nauseous five hours per day, vomits three to four times per day, and still retches twice daily.[‡] She is able to tolerate some oral intake; you do not detect indications for hospitalization. You decide to add metoclopramide to her diphenhydramine regimen. The patient is reassured that metoclopramide is not associated with risks of congenital malformations, prematurity, low birthweight, or perinatal mortality.

Special note:
‡ PUQE score is now 9, consistent for moderate NVP

8-A. Indicate two adverse effects to mention in counseling requiring prompt cessation of metoclopramide. *(2 points each)*   4

   ☐ Extrapyramidal symptoms – *prompt cessation of treatment is indicated*
   ☐ Oculogyric crisis– *prompt cessation of treatment is indicated*

8-B. Indicate three other side effects of metoclopramide you would mention to the patient. *(1 point each)*   3

   ☐ Restlessness, irritability
   ☐ Insomnia
   ☐ Dry mouth
   ☐ Drowsiness
   ☐ Diarrhea
   ☐ Rash

The patient recalls reading about ondansetron upon a friend's request when she required it for treatment of hyperemesis gravidarum; she remembers conflicting information on risks of fetal malformations. Prior to addressing her inquiry, you mention that lack of an opportunity for patients with hyperemesis gravidarum to discuss risks and benefits of treatment and ask questions, increases distress.[†] You address the patient's inquiry about common side effects with ondansetron. Interestingly, you note an ongoing randomized trial investigating the effect of ondansetron and mirtazapine *(appetite stimulating and antiemetic antidepressant)* in hyperemesis gravidarum.[‡]

Special notes:
† Dean C, Marsden J. *MIDIRS Midwifery Digest* 2017;27:177–86.
‡ Ostenfeld A, Petersen TS, Futtrup TB, et al. Validating the effect of Ondansetron and Mirtazapine In Treating hyperemesis gravidarum (VOMIT): protocol for a randomised placebo-controlled trial. *BMJ Open.* 2020;10(3): e034712.

9. Address the patient's concerns regarding <u>fetal safety</u> with first-trimester use of ondansetron.   1

☐ Inform the patient that available data suggest a possibly small absolute risk increase in cleft palate (0.03% above baseline) and septal cardiac defects (0.3% above baseline); some large studies did not show associations
  ○ Route of administration does not appear to affect obstetric risk, if any

Special note: *Refer to*
(a) Huybrechts KF, et al. *JAMA.* 2018;320(23):2429–2437.
(b) Huybrechts KF, et al. *JAMA.* 2020;323(4):372–374.
(c) Picot C, et al. *Birth Defects Res.* 2020;112(13):996–1013.
(d) Andrade C. et al. *J Clin Psychiatry.* 2020;81(3):20f13472.

Although combinations of different drugs are advocated with suboptimal response to a single antiemetic, you inform your trainee that guidance is dictated by risks, benefits, adverse effects, and cost: as an example, you mention that various phenothiazines warrant caution when used in parallel with some antiemetics.

10. Specify two drug-classes and resulting adverse events when combined with certain   4
    phenothiazines for treatment of NVP/hyperemesis gravidarum. *(2 points each)*

	Drug classes	Adverse events in combination with certain phenothiazines
☐	Dopamine antagonists (*e.g.,* metoclopramide)	- Extrapyramidal effects - Neuroleptic malignant syndrome
☐	Serotonin 5-hydroxytryptamine type 3 receptor antagonist (*e.g.,* ondansetron)	Prolonged QT interval

Despite lifestyle modifications and a trial of combined diphenhydramine and metoclopramide, the patient returns at 10 weeks' gestation weighing 68 kg (149.6 lb), compatible with a 6.8% loss from her prepregnancy weight and clinical symptoms consistent with a PUQE score of 13. Together with physical examination findings, you advise laboratory investigations and hospitalization for parenteral therapy, to which she concurs. Fetal viability is ascertained.

11. Identify three indications for hospitalization of patients for NVP or hyperemesis gravidarum. *(1 point each)*   3

☐ Signs of dehydration, change in mental status, change in vital signs, or continued weight loss
☐ Refractory response to outpatient treatment and inability to tolerate oral intake without vomiting
☐ Confirmed or suspected comorbidity (*e.g.*, urinary tract infection, with inability to tolerate oral antibiotics)

12. Specify aspects of your physical examination <u>focused</u> to assessment of her volume status. *(1 point each)*   Max 6

☐ General appearance, alertness, lethargy
☐ Orthostatic blood pressure
☐ Pulse
☐ Weight
☐ Capillary refill
☐ Dry skin and mucous membranes (eyes, mouth)
☐ Decreased skin turgor
☐ Low jugular venous pressure

Special note:
Urine output would also be a marker of volume status, although not relevant to *physical examination* of this patient.

13. Although no universally accepted definition exists, highlight four <u>most commonly</u> cited criteria for hyperemesis gravidarum. *(1 point each)*   4

☐ Protracted NVP, unrelated to other causes
☐ Greater than 5% of prepregnancy weight
☐ Electrolyte imbalance
☐ Dehydration, ketonuria

14. Indicate <u>laboratory investigations</u> you would/may include in the initial clinical work-up upon her admission. *(1 point each)*   Max 5

☐ Urinalysis for ketonuria and specific gravity
☐ Urine culture and sensitivity
☐ CBC *(to assess for leukocyte concentration hemoglobin, and hematocrit)*
☐ Serum creatinine and electrolytes (sodium, potassium, chloride, calcium, phosphate, urea)
☐ Random serum glucose

☐ Liver transaminases (AST, ALT) and function tests
☐ Thyroid stimulating hormone (TSH)
☐ Serum amylase *(exclude pancreatitis)*
☐ Consideration for arterial blood gas *(exclude metabolic disturbances and monitor severity)*
☐ Consideration for *H. pylori* testing, particularly if hyperemesis gravidarum is refractory to treatment

Special note:
Serum β-hCG would be ordered in the absence of earlier sonographic assessment for molar pregnancy; otherwise, not indicated in this context

15. Identify three features that distinguish hyperemesis-associated biochemical thyrotoxicosis from underlying thyroid gland-induced dysfunction. *(1 point each)*   3

Features common to biochemical thyrotoxicosis:
☐ Vomiting *(rare with primary thyroid diseases)*
☐ Absence of common symptoms and signs of thyroid disease *(e.g., sweating, heat intolerance, tremor)*
☐ Absence of features of hyperthyroidism on physical examination *(e.g., opthalmopathy, goiter)*
☐ Absence of antithyroid hormone receptor antibodies or antithyroid peroxidase antibodies
☐ Absence of symptomatic improvement with antithyroid drugs

16. While awaiting results of her investigations, provide your trainee with 10 laboratory abnormalities that <u>may be</u> associated with hyperemesis gravidarum or protracted NVP. *(1 point each)*   10

Urinary:
☐ Ketonuria
☐ Increased urine specific gravity

Electrolyte and metabolic:
☐ Hyponatremia
☐ Hypokalemia or hyperkalemia
☐ Hypomagnesemia
☐ Hypocalcemia
☐ Hypouricemia
☐ Low preserum albumin *(poor protein nutrition)*
☐ Metabolic hypochloremic alkalosis (or metabolic acidosis if severe volume contraction)

Hematologic, hepatic, gastrointestinal, renal:
☐ Increased hematocrit *(hemoconcentration; plasma volume depletion)*
☐ Raised lymphocyte count
☐ Increased serum aminotransferases (ALT > AST; *most common liver abnormality*)
☐ Mild hyperbilirubinemia
☐ Increased serum creatinine *(severe hypovolemia affecting the glomerular filtration rate)*
☐ Increased serum amylase *(mostly salivary in origin)* and serum lipase

Endocrine:
☐ Increased free thyroxine levels with/without TSH suppression, absent antithyroid receptor and antithyroid peroxidase antibodies

Laboratory investigations confirm low serum electrolyte concentrations, volume contraction with mild secondary renal dysfunction.

---

17. Excluding antiemetic treatments, discuss important aspects of <u>inpatient</u> management given the patient's intolerance to liquids and clinical signs of dehydration. *(1 point per main bullet)*

Max 10

☐ Arrange for multidisciplinary care with the obstetrics medical/midwifery team
   ○ *e.g., nurses, nutritionists, pharmacists, endocrinologists, gastroenterologists, and psychotherapists/mental health experts*
☐ Daily weight
☐ Daily serum electrolytes and urea
☐ IV normal saline is the preferred solution, with added potassium chloride guided by serum levels *(RCOG)*
☐ *Hypomagnesemia:* use magnesium sulfate 2 g IV bolus over 10–20 minutes, followed by 1 g/hr in 100 mL IV solution; follow serum levels
☐ *Hypocalcemia:* When persistent despite correction of magnesium levels, consider calcium gluconate 1–2 g IV in 50 mL dextrose-solution over 10–20 minutes
☐ *Hypophosphatemia:* Consider IV sodium or potassium phosphate, or oral replacement where tolerated
☐ Administer thiamine (vitamin B1) <u>before</u> dextrose-containing solution or parenteral nutrition *(ACOG, RCOG)*
   ○ Thiamine 100 mg IV daily for each day IV dextrose-containing solution is used *(RCOG)*
   ○ Oral thiamine supplementation is a recommended follow-up measure after IV treatment
☐ Avoid dextrose-solution during correction of hypokalemia
   ○ Dextrose-induced insulin release drives potassium into cells, transiently reducing extracellular potassium
☐ Aim for urine output of ~100 mL/hr
☐ Administer IV multivitamin dose daily
☐ Thromboprophylaxis with low molecular weight heparin until discharge or clinical resolution *(RCOG)*
☐ Consideration for histamine H2 receptor antagonists or protein pump inhibitors where gastroesophageal reflux, gastritis, or esophagitis is present/suspected

---

You stress the importance of thiamine replacement, as deficiency may arise from a combination of excessive vomiting, poor dietary intake, and increased glucose demands (*shown in 60%[$] of pregnant women with hyperemesis gravidarum*); failure to do so may lead to neurological deficits or fatality.

[[$]*Suggested Reading 1*, and refer to: Van Stuijvenberg ME et al. *Am J Obstet Gynecol.* 1995;172(5): 1585–1591]

18. Elicit clinical manifestations of the syndrome associated with thiamine deficiency. *(1 point each)*   Max 4

Wernicke's encephalopathy:
- ☐ Confusion, drowsiness, memory loss
- ☐ Blurred vision
- ☐ Unsteady gait
- ☐ Finger-nose ataxia
- ☐ Oculomotor symptoms – nystagmus, ophthalmoplegia
- ☐ Hyporeflexia

Although the patient is reassured that hyperemis gravidarum most often portends well for pregnancy outcome, she recognizes its socioeconomic implications, including treatment expenses and loss of job productivity, in addition to adverse medical events.

19. Discuss seven other <u>maternal medical complications</u> of hyperemis gravidarum with your trainee. *(1 point each)*   Max 7

- ☐ Higher rates of depression, anxiety, or psychologic problems
- ☐ Complications from electrolyte abnormalities
- ☐ Vitamin deficiencies, dehydration, malnutrition
- ☐ Central pontine myelinolysis/osmotic demyelination syndrome *(due to rapid correction of sodium)*
- ☐ Retinal hemorrhage
- ☐ VTE (venous thromboembolism)
- ☐ Hamman syndrome (pneumomediastinum)
- ☐ Mallory–Weiss tears or Boerhaave syndrome *(i.e., esophageal rupture)*
- ☐ Diaphragmatic tear
- ☐ Rhabdomyolysis *(due to hypokalemia)*
- ☐ Splenic avulsion
- ☐ Acute tubular necrosis
- ☐ Pregnancy termination due to intractable hyperemis gravidarum
- ☐ Decreased likelihood to attempt repeat pregnancy
- ☐ Rarely, maternal mortality

By 72 hours of admission, the patient's symptoms improve with IV hydration and antiemetic therapy; her laboratory investigations have normalized and oral feeds and antiemetics are gradually introduced, to which she responds well and is ready for discharge after six days of admission. You reassure her that continuation of an oral antiemetic will help decrease relapse rate and readmission and inform her you will reassess the need for continued therapy at subsequent follow-up. A second antiemetic agent is provided for breakthrough symptom-control.

20. Indicate particular aspects in discharge management after treatment for hyperemis gravidarum. *(1 point per main bullet)*   Max 3

☐ Advise continuation of her antiemetics
☐ Ensure follow-up is arranged with nutritionist and obstetric provider (in approximately one to two weeks)
  ○ *RCOG[9]: specific recommendation for women suffering from hyperemis gravidarum*
☐ Provide the patient with easy access to care with recurrent symptoms and/or signs of NVP/ hyperemis gravidarum
  ○ Consideration for home ketonuria assessment if vomiting recurs
☐ Individualized consideration for psychosocial support services

The remainder of her pregnancy progresses well, and the patient has an uncomplicated vaginal delivery at term.

At the postpartum obstetric visit, you highlight the importance of future preconception care with regard to NVP and hyperemis gravidarum during the recent pregnancy.

21. Specify your evidence-based recommendations for the <u>preconception</u> care plan of a patient, focusing on prior NVP or hyperemis gravidarum.[†] *(1 point per main bullet)*   Max 4

☐ Encouraging the patient to time conception, where possible, may help reduce challenges in managing childcare, household duties, and financial obligations
☐ Achieving or maintaining a healthy prepregnancy weight may decrease the risk of NVP
  ○ *Low prepregnancy weight is associated with increased hospitalizations*
  ○ *Obesity increases the risk of NVP (possibly via endocrine etiology)*
☐ Adjusting meals (*e.g.*, frequency, food types) prepregnancy may facilitate maintenance once pregnant
☐ Commencing prenatal vitamins at least one month preconception decreases the risk of NVP
☐ Providing preemptive, or early prescription of, antiemetics that were priorly effective is encouraged (*may be preventative, or reduce symptom-duration and severity*)

Special note:
† *Refer to* Suggested Reading 6 (Box 4).

TOTAL: 125

CHAPTER 5

Prenatal Genetic Screening

Karen Wou and Amira El-Messidi

A 33-year-old primigravida with a sonographically confirmed spontaneous viable intrauterine singleton at 10^{+3} weeks' gestation presents for her first prenatal visit. She has been taking routine prenatal vitamins containing folic acid for the past four months. Her medical, surgical, social, and family histories are unremarkable. The patient does not have any obstetric complaints. She is normotensive with a body mass index (BMI) of 22.5 kg/m^2. A follow-up fetal sonography has been arranged between 11^{+0} and 13^{+6} weeks' gestation. Your obstetric trainee asks for your assistance to address the patient's options for prenatal genetic screening.

LEARNING OBJECTIVES

1. Appreciate the different options for prenatal genetic screening for a singleton pregnancy
2. Understand the biology of cfDNA and different maternal serum biomarkers
3. Discuss essential elements in pretest counseling for aneuploidy screening using cell-free DNA (cfDNA)
4. Provide posttest counseling of a 'no call' result with cfDNA testing and discuss evidence-based management considerations
5. Outline the prenatal management plan of a high-risk result for trisomy 21 on integrated prenatal screening (IPS), being cognizant of adverse obstetric outcomes associated with abnormal maternal serum biomarkers

SUGGESTED READINGS

1. American College of Obstetricians and Gynecologists' Committee on Practice Bulletins – Obstetrics; Committee on Genetics; Society for Maternal-Fetal Medicine. Screening for fetal chromosomal abnormalities: ACOG Practice Bulletin, No. 226. *Obstet Gynecol*. 2020;136(4): e48–e69.
2. Audibert F, De Bie I, Johnson JA, et al. No. 348 – Joint SOGC-CCMG guideline: update on prenatal screening for fetal aneuploidy, fetal anomalies, and adverse pregnancy outcomes. *J Obstet Gynaecol Can*. 2017;39(9):805–817. [Correction in *J Obstet Gynaecol Can*. 2018 Aug;40(8):1109]
3. Benn P, Borrell A, Chiu RW, et al. Position statement from the Chromosome Abnormality Screening Committee on behalf of the Board of the International Society for Prenatal Diagnosis. *Prenat Diagn*. 2015;35(8):725–734.

4. Chitayat D, Langlois S, Wilson RD. No. 261 – prenatal screening for fetal aneuploidy in singleton pregnancies. *J Obstet Gynaecol Can.* 2017;39(9):e380–e394.

5. Dugoff L. Cell-free DNA screening for fetal aneuploidy. *Topics Obstetr Gynecol.* 2017;37(1): 1–7.

6. Gil MM, Accurti V, Santacruz B, et al. Analysis of cell-free DNA in maternal blood in screening for aneuploidies: updated meta-analysis. *Ultrasound Obstet Gynecol.* 2017;50(3): 302–314.

7. Gregg AR, Skotko BG, Benkendorf JL, et al. Noninvasive prenatal screening for fetal aneuploidy, 2016 update: a position statement of the American College of Medical Genetics and Genomics. *Genet Med.* 2016;18(10):1056–1065.

8. Royal College of Obstetricians and Gynaecologists, Scientific Impact Paper No. 15. Non-invasive prenatal testing for chromosomal abnormality using maternal plasma DNA. March 2014. Available at https://obgyn.onlinelibrary.wiley.com/doi/10.1111/tog.12099. Accessed May 1, 2021.

9. Sachs A, Blanchard L, Buchanan A, et al. Recommended pre-test counseling points for noninvasive prenatal testing using cell-free DNA: a 2015 perspective. *Prenat Diagn.* 2015;35(10):968–971.

10. (a) Norton ME, Biggio JR, Kuller JA, et al. The role of ultrasound in women who undergo cell-free DNA screening. *Am J Obstet Gynecol.* 2017;216(3):B2–B7.

    (b) Society for Maternal-Fetal Medicine (SMFM) Publications Committee. Prenatal aneuploidy screening using cell-free DNA, SMFM Consult Series No. 36. *Am J Obstet Gynecol.* 2015;212(6):711–716.

POINTS

1. Highlight to your trainee the advantages of the patient's early obstetric imaging and planned sonogram between 11^{+0}- and 13^{+6}-weeks' gestation. *(1 point each)*	Max 5

☐ Confirm viability
☐ Provide accurate pregnancy dating of spontaneous conception
☐ Assess fetal number
☐ Determine chorionicity and amnionicity in multiple pregnancy
☐ Assess markers of aneuploidy (*e.g.*, nuchal translucency, intracranial translucency, presence of the nasal bone, tricuspid regurgitation, ductus venosus Doppler interrogation)
☐ Detection of major structural malformations

Knowing that all women should be offered aneuploidy screening in early pregnancy *(ACOG[1])*, you intend to provide comprehensive nondirective counseling on available options which is necessary for informed consent. There are no restrictions in availability of screening tests for Down syndrome (trisomy 21) in your jurisdiction.

2. Inform the patient on prenatal genetic screening options,[§] while simultaneously elaborating on specific test components to your trainee, where relevant. *(1 point per main and each subbullet)*

Max 10

☐ No screening
☐ Maternal plasma cell-free DNA (cfDNA)
☐ First-trimester screening at 11^{+0}-and 13^{+6}-weeks' gestation[†]
　○ Maternal age, NT measurement, pregnancy-associated plasma protein A (PAPP-A), free β-hCG
☐ Second-trimester/quadruple screening at 15–22 weeks' gestation[‡]
　○ Maternal age, free β-hCG, unconjugated estriol, dimeric inhibin-A, maternal serum α-fetoprotein (MSAFP)
☐ Serum IPS[‡]
　○ Provides a single test result after first-trimester PAPP-A followed by second-trimester quadruple serum screening; maternal age is <u>not</u> included in the risk assessment
☐ Integrated prenatal screening (IPS)
　○ Provides a <u>single</u> test result after first-trimester NT and PAPP-A, followed by second-trimester quadruple serum screening; maternal age <u>is</u> included in the risk assessment
☐ Sequential prenatal screening
　○ Women with a high-risk result on first-trimester screening (*e.g.*, ≥1/50) are offered invasive testing or cfDNA; all other women proceed to second-trimester screening
☐ Contingent prenatal screening
　○ Women with a high-risk result on first-trimester screening (>1/50) are offered invasive testing or cfDNA, while those at low risk (<1/1500) require no further testing; women at intermediate risk proceed to second-trimester testing and receive combined results

Special notes:
§ Maternal age and NT measurement alone is not recommended in singleton pregnancies, although accepted screening for twin gestations; refer to Chapter 11
† *Enhanced* first-trimester screening would include placental growth factor (PlGF)
‡ Performed in the event that specialized NT scan is missed or unavailable; accurate pregnancy dating is critical

SCENARIO A
Maternal plasma cell-free DNA (cfDNA)
The patient expresses a preference to receive results as early as possible while the pregnancy is still private, to allow for timely prenatal diagnosis. She inquires about your recommendations for the most accurate test to detect a trisomy 21-affected fetus with the lowest chance of a screen-positive result.

3. Which of the prenatal screening tests best suits the patient's values?

1

☐ Maternal plasma cfDNA screening

4. Elaborate on the <u>biology</u> of pregnancy-associated cfDNA. *(1 point per main bullet)*   Max 2

☐ After 9–10 weeks' gestation, ~5%–15% of the total cfDNA (maternal + fetal) in maternal plasma derives from apoptosis of syncytiotrophoblast (*i.e.*, fetal fraction)

☐ Entire fetal genome is represented in short cfDNA fragments (<200 base pairs) in maternal plasma

☐ Fetal fraction increases with advancing gestation and is rapidly cleared, by two days, postpartum *(pregnancy specific)*
  ○ *Increase of ~0.1% per week from 10–21 weeks, then 1.0% per week until term[§]*

Special note:
[§] Refer to Wang E, Batey A, Struble C, Musci T, Song K, Oliphant A. Gestational age and maternal weight effects on fetal cell-free DNA in maternal plasma. *Prenat Diagn.* 2013;33(7):662–666.

5. Indicate essential elements you would convey to this patient in <u>pretest counseling</u> for cfDNA aneuploidy screening. *(1 point per main and subbullet bullet)*   Max 12

☐ Screening is intended to classify the patient as high or low risk for the intended fetal aneuploidies; confirmation of high-risk screening test would require an invasive diagnostic test

☐ cfDNA screening appears to be the most accurate screening test for the most common fetal trisomies, performed after 10 weeks' gestation.
  ○ Detection rate for trisomy 21 is >99% with a false-positive rate <1%
  ○ Detection rates for trisomy 13 and 18 are 99% and 98%, respectively

☐ The positive predictive value (PPV) of a cfDNA result is affected by numerous variables including the aneuploidy studied, population prevalence, clinical features (*e.g.*, maternal age, ultrasound findings, obstetric history)
  ○ Positive result for trisomy 21 does *not* imply that the likelihood of an affected fetus is >99%
  ○ As trisomy 13 and 18 are less prevalent than trisomy 21, their PPV from a screen-positive test will be lower

☐ cfDNA does not screen for all chromosomal conditions

☐ False-positive and false-negative results do occur with cfDNA testing

☐ In the event of abnormal cfDNA test results, amniocentesis or chorionic villous sampling (CVS) would be offered for definitive diagnosis, prior to considering termination of pregnancy

☐ A negative cfDNA test result indicates a decreased risk of trisomy 21 or other chromosome conditions tested for but does not *confirm a normal* fetal karyotype
  ○ If a fetal structural abnormality is identified, invasive diagnostic testing *may be* indicated after counseling, regardless of a negative cfDNA screen result

☐ Screening may fail to provide a result

☐ Results may raise suspicion for conditions apart from the intended fetal aneuploidies

☐ Screening does not assess for fetal structural abnormalities or screen for neural tube defects; second-trimester fetal morphology sonogram remains fundamental to prenatal care

☐ Mention that serum biomarker screening in parallel with cfDNA testing is not recommended

☐ Potential cost implications

You alert your trainee that cfDNA testing may also be performed for a variety of genetic conditions, including blood type, single gene disorders, and fetal gender where inherent risk of X-linked diseases exist.

---

6. Apart from trisomy 21, address the patient's inquiry about additional fetal chromosomal abnormalities detected by cfDNA analysis.† *(1 point per main bullet unless specified)*

    Max 5

☐ Trisomy 13
☐ Trisomy 18
☐ Most common sex chromosome abnormalities *(any two subbullets for 1 point each)*
    ○ 47, XXX
    ○ 47, XXY (Klinefelter syndrome)
    ○ 47, XYY
    ○ 45, XO (Turner syndrome, monosomy X)
☐ Microdeletion/microduplication syndromes
☐ Triploidy *(only SNP-based method screens for triploidy)*

Special note:
† This list is not intended to be all-inclusive; testing for other aneuploidies is laboratory-dependent.
  Routine screening of trisomy 9, 16, 22, microdeletion syndromes, and screening for late copy-number changes is not recommended

---

After this consultation visit, you intend to explain to your obstetric trainee that as cfDNA in maternal plasma is a mixture of maternal and placental DNA, a number of biologic phenomena can cause discordant results from fetal karyotype.

---

7. Formulate a differential diagnosis for a positive cfDNA result where fetal karyotype is normal. Features *may or may not* apply to this patient. *(1 point each)*

    Max 5

☐ Statistical chance
☐ Vanishing twin
☐ Sample mix-up/laboratory error†
☐ Confined placental mosaicism†
☐ Maternal copy-number variants†
☐ Maternal sex chromosome abnormality (often in mosaic form)
☐ Maternal malignancy‡

Special notes:
† May also account for false-negative cfDNA results
‡ Although rare, maternal malignancies should be included in the differential diagnosis of unusual cell-free DNA patterns in pregnancy, such as multiple concurrent aneuploidies

---

Fetal sonogram at 11+5 weeks' gestation reveals normal early fetal morphology. You inform your obstetric trainee that although NT measurement does not add benefit in detecting aneuploidy when cfDNA screening has been performed in a singleton pregnancy (*ACOG[1]*, *SOGC[2]*), it may be valuable to assess risk of single gene disorders and malformations associated with thickened NT.[†] You have just received the patient's cfDNA laboratory report indicating a 'no-call result.'

You inform your obstetric trainee that the overall chance of test failure is 0.9%–8.1%, the magnitude of which varies, in part, by laboratory methodology. Upon your request, she presents to your office for timely counseling. Results of all routine maternal prenatal laboratory tests were unremarkable; her blood group is B-positive.

Special note:
† *Refer to* Chapter 13 for discussion of associations with thickened NT

---

8. Elaborate on cfDNA test failures according to the three laboratory platforms used and outline other causes for 'no call' results. Features *may or may not* apply to this patient. *(1 point each; points specified per section)*

10

'No-call result' by cfDNA methodologies: *(max 3)*
☐ Massive parallel shotgun sequencing *(lowest failure rates of 1.58%[†])*
☐ Chromosome-selective/targeted sequencing *(3.56% failure rate[†])*
☐ Single nucleotide polymorphism (SNP)-based approach *(highest failure rate of 6.39%[†])*
☐ Suboptimal sample collection and handling that leads to maternal leukocyte-associated reduction of fragmented fetal cfDNA

Other causes for a 'no-call result': *(max 7)*
☐ Low fetal fraction (<4%)
☐ Fetal aneuploidy, particularly trisomy 13, 18, monosomy X, and triploidy
☐ Testing prior to 10 weeks' gestation
☐ Obesity *(inverse relationship with free fraction)[‡]*
☐ Increasing maternal age
☐ Maternal chromosomal abnormalities
☐ Large chromosomal segments with homozygosity
☐ Anticoagulation with low molecular weight heparin (LMWH)[§]
☐ Twin gestations[#]
☐ In vitro fertilization
☐ South Asian and black women (more frequently than white women)

Special notes:
† Yaron Y. The implications of noninvasive prenatal testing failures: a review of an under-discussed phenomenon. *Prenat Diagn.* 2016;36(5):391–396.
‡ Laboratory cannot adjust for maternal weight as with serum biomarker screening; likely due to a dilutional effect and increased adipocyte turnover
§ Nakamura N, Sasaki A, Mikami M, et al. Nonreportable rates and cell-free DNA profiles in noninvasive prenatal testing among women with heparin treatment. *Prenat Diagn.* 2020;40 (7):838–845.
# Refer to Question 5 in Chapter 11 for cfDNA testing characteristics among multiple gestation

9. What are the principal, evidence-based management considerations for this patient after primary failed cfDNA fetal aneuploidy testing? *(1 point per main bullet unless specified)*

Max 3

☐ Referral for consultation with a maternal-fetal medicine expert, geneticist, or genetic counselor
☐ Offer invasive diagnostic testing without repeating the cfDNA test, as test failure due to low fetal fraction itself increases risk of fetal aneuploidy (up to 5%)
  ○ *i.e., chorionic villous sampling (CVS) or amniocentesis with molecular testing including karyotype, chromosomal microarray, fluorescent in-situ hybridization (FISH), or quantitative fluorescence polymerase chain reaction (QF-PCR)*
☐ Controversy exists regarding repeat maternal plasma cfDNA screening: *(1 point for either subbullet)*
  ○ Redraw is successful to report a result in 50%–80% of cases, at the expense of prolonging reporting time
  ○ ACMG[7]: Repeat blood draw is not recommended given the marginal rate of increase in cfDNA before 20 weeks' gestation (0.1% per week)
☐ Arrange for comprehensive fetal sonographic assessment

In collaboration with a genetic counselor, the implications and management options for the failed cfDNA result due to a fetal fraction of 3.4% were comprehensively discussed with the patient. Although a CVS[†] would provide earlier results, considerations for the potential for confined placental mosaicism was addressed, as both cfDNA and CVS are based on placental cells. An amniocentesis is thereby planned at ≥15 weeks' gestation to optimize fetal genotypic representation from tested amniocytes.

At the following prenatal visit, the patient asks for your advice regarding an early-amniocentesis and whether she may have obviated genetic screening.

Special note:
† *Refer to* Questions 10 and 11 in Chapter 64 for discussion on chorionic villous sampling (CVS)

10. Indicate the risks associated with amniocentesis performed before 14–15 weeks' gestation.[†] *(1 point each)*

Max 4

☐ Inadequate amniotic fluid sampling
☐ Failed cell culture
☐ Pregnancy loss
☐ Clubfoot (talipes equinovarus)
☐ Early preterm prelabor rupture of membranes (PPROM) with its related anomalies and complications

Special note:
† Refer to (a) Practice Bulletin No. 162: Prenatal Diagnostic Testing for Genetic Disorders. *Obstet Gynecol.* 2016;127(5):e108–e122, and (b) Wilson RD, Gagnon A, Audibert F, Campagnolo C, Carroll J; Genetics Committee. Prenatal Diagnosis Procedures and Techniques to Obtain a Diagnostic Fetal Specimen or Tissue: Maternal and Fetal Risks and Benefits. *J Obstet Gynaecol Can.* 2015;37(7):656–668.

11. Address the patient's inquiry by illustrating clinical situations where invasive diagnostic testing for cytogenetic analysis would be considered without initial prenatal screening. *(1 point each)*

Parental:
☐ Known carrier(s) of a chromosome rearrangement that increases the risk of having a fetus with a chromosomal abnormality
☐ Conception occurred by in vitro fertilization with intracytoplasmic sperm injection

Fetal/child:
☐ NT measurement >(or ≥) 3.5 mm regardless of gestational age
☐ Other sonographic markers that increase the risk of fetal aneuploidy, particularly in combination *(e.g., nasal bone hypoplasia, tricuspid regurgitation, ductus venosus waveform abnormalities)*
☐ Fetal malformations detected on first-trimester sonogram
☐ Previous fetus or child with a chromosomal abnormality

You later receive a call from a fetal medicine expert with regard to another patient of yours whose 20-week fetal morphology sonogram clearly demonstrates female external genitalia despite earlier cfDNA confirmed male gender, assessed for risk of an X-linked disorder.

12. In the absence of a laboratory error, summarize aspects on obstetric history to review in her medical chart to potentially explain the fetal gender discordance in genotype and phenotype. *(1 point each)*

Maternal factors:
☐ Organ-transplant or bone marrow transplant recipient from a 46, XY individual or donor of uncertain biologic gender
☐ Receipt of a blood transfusion from 46, XY individual or donor of uncertain biologic gender less than four weeks prior to the blood draw for cfDNA *(ACMG[7])*
☐ Malignancy [rarely] *(ACMG[7])*

Fetal-placental factors:
☐ Vanishing twin or multiple pregnancy
☐ Confined placental mosaicism *(ACMG[7])*

Special note:
Disorders of sexual development *(e.g., SRY-gene defects, androgen receptor defects)* may account for genotype–phenotype discordance.

SCENARIO B
(*This is a continuation of the clinical scenario after Question 2*)
Traditional biochemical screening
As cfDNA screening is unavailable in your jurisdiction, the patient inquires about your recommended prenatal screening test that would provide the most accurate detection of a trisomy 21-affected fetus. She would not consider early invasive diagnostic testing, if required.

13. Select the prenatal screening test that would best suits the patient's values and inform her of its test characteristics for trisomy 21. (*1 point for main and subbullet*)

   2

☐ Integrated prenatal screening (IPS)
  ○ Detection rate 96% with a screen-positive rate of 5% (*ACOG[1]*)

14. Outline principal aspects of the <u>biology</u> of each maternal serum biomarker included in the second-trimester component of the IPS test. You have previously discussed the first-trimester serum marker, PAPP-A,[†] with your trainee. (*1 point per main bullet; max specified per section*)

   Max 6

hCG: (*max 2*)
☐ Principally produced by syncytiotrophoblast and secreted into the intervillous space; cytotrophoblast also contributes to hCG formation
  ○ Initially, immature syncytiotrophoblast produce free β-hCG
  ○ Cytotrophoblast production of α-subunit lags by several days
☐ Peak concentrations reach ~100,000 mU/mL by ~10 weeks' gestation
☐ Major biologic role of hCG in early pregnancy is to *rescue* the corpus luteum from demise while maintaining progesterone production

Estriol:
☐ Synthesized in the placenta from the androgenic precursor, dehydroepiandrosterone sulfate made by the fetal adrenal cortex

Inhibin A:
☐ Initially synthesized by the corpus luteum, followed by the placenta

Alpha-fetoprotein (AFP): (*max 2*)
☐ Initially synthesized by the fetal yolk sac followed by the fetal liver and gastrointestinal tract
☐ Peak concentrations in amniotic fluid and fetal serum occur at ~13 weeks' gestation, followed by a rapid decline
☐ AFP enters maternal serum by diffusion and transport mechanisms, with peak concentrations by ~32 weeks' gestation

Special note:
† *Refer to* Question 6-C in Chapter 9 for biological function of PAPP-A

15. Indicate <u>maternal factors</u> that affect maternal serum AFP levels (MSAFP). *(1 point each)*   5

- ☐ Maternal weight
- ☐ Ethnicity
- ☐ Pregestational diabetes mellitus
- ☐ Gestational age
- ☐ Multifetal pregnancy

At 12^{+2} weeks' gestation, first-trimester sonogram reveals normal early fetal morphology with an NT of 1.3 mm. With a written reminder for the patient to present for the second serum testing component to avoid the risk of 'no result' without the second blood draw, the patient complied with screening requirements.

At 17^{+3} weeks' gestation, you receive results of her IPS indicating a trisomy 21 risk at 1/150 and notice the following derangements in serum biomarker values:

	Multiples of the median (MoM)	Normal MoM
PAPP-A	0.30	>0.40
MSAFP	3.0	0.25–2.5

Although maternal biochemical marker screening tests should not be repeated to avoid false reassurance, you emphasize to your trainee that verifying the accuracy of clinical characteristics documented in the laboratory report is paramount. You teach your trainee that although many of the associations between maternal serum markers and adverse obstetric outcomes are statistically significant, the sensitivity and PPVs for individual outcomes are too low to recommend maternal serum biomarker screening for risk of adverse pregnancy outcomes.

The patient is concerned about having a trisomy 21-affected fetus and is contemplating pregnancy termination.

16. Specify the patient's <u>clinical characteristics</u> that are most relevant to the performance of the aneuploidy screening report. *(1 point each)*

Max 6

☐ Accurate gestational age dating
☐ Maternal age
☐ Weight
☐ Spontaneous vs. in vitro fertilization
☐ Insulin-dependent diabetes mellitus *(lower MSAFP and unconjugated estriol only)*
☐ Past pregnancy with aneuploidy
☐ Ethnicity

17. Which adverse obstetric outcomes have been associated with decreased PAPP-A levels? *(1 point each)*

Max 6

☐ Fetal growth restriction (FGR)
☐ Gestational hypertension and preeclampsia
☐ Spontaneous preterm labor and preterm delivery
☐ Pregnancy loss <24 weeks
☐ Preterm prelabor rupture of membranes (PPROM)
☐ Placental abruption
☐ IUFD >24 weeks' gestation

18. Which adverse obstetric outcomes have been associated with <u>unexplained</u> increased MSAFP levels? *(1 point each)*

Max 6

☐ Fetal growth restriction (FGR)
☐ Gestational hypertension and preeclampsia before 32 weeks
☐ Oligohydramnios
☐ Spontaneous preterm labor and preterm delivery
☐ Placental abruption
☐ Placenta accreta spectrum
☐ IUFD >24 weeks' gestation

19. With focus on the IPS results, outline your prenatal management plan. *(1 point per main and subbullet)*   Max 6

☐ Offer amniocentesis for confirmation of fetal karyotype
☐ Inform the patient that cfDNA screening is an accepted alternative to invasive diagnostic testing for patients who screen-positive by traditional screening tests if she wishes to avoid an invasive diagnostic test
  ○ Inform the patient that cfDNA testing may delay definitive diagnosis and will not identify all chromosomal abnormalities
  ○ Inform the patient that if cfDNA screening reveals a low risk for the tested aneuploidies, after the abnormal traditional screening test (*i.e.*, IPS), the residual risk of a chromosomal abnormality is about **2%**
☐ Arrange for a detailed fetal morphology sonogram at 16–18 week's gestation to assess for (a) major malformations or other markers suggestive of trisomy 21, and (b) assess for fetal malformations or placental features associated with increased MSAFP levels
☐ Discuss the implications of abnormal serum biomarkers in contributing to adverse obstetric outcomes
☐ Consideration for close surveillance of signs/symptoms of adverse obstetric outcomes and serial fetal growth biometry, placenta and amniotic fluid assessments
☐ Consideration for referral to a genetic counselor, geneticist, or maternal-fetal medicine expert

Special note:
Although the option of *no further antepartum testing with planned postnatal testing* is valid after patient counseling of a screen-positive result, it would not be appropriate for this case scenario as the patient is contemplating pregnancy termination.

TOTAL: **100**

CHAPTER 6

Obesity in Pregnancy

Gabrielle Cassir, Amira El-Messidi, and Cynthia Maxwell

A 31-year-old nulligravida with a body mass index (BMI) of 42 kg/m^2 is referred by her primary care provider to your high-risk obstetrics clinic for preconception counseling. Prior to the consultation, you highlight to your obstetric trainee that motivational interviewing with nonstigmatizing terminology avoids negative influences on mood and self-esteem, promoting patient uptake of weight management strategies and a healthy lifestyle.

Special note: *Although pregnant women with obesity have increased rates of concomitant maternal-fetal morbidities including, but not limited to, hypertension, diabetes, mental health issues, and fetal growth aberrations, the case scenario is presented as such for academic purposes and to avoid overlap of content addressed in other chapters. Readers are encouraged to complement subject matter where clinically required.*

LEARNING OBJECTIVES

1. Take a focused preconception history and verbalize essentials of the physical examination of a patient with obesity, recognizing the importance of screening for, and managing, obstructive sleep apnea
2. Provide counseling on adverse perinatal outcomes related to obesity in pregnancy
3. Understand the unique aspects of prenatal care for a patient with obesity and the pregnancy-related challenges post bariatric surgery
4. Appreciate the importance of multidisciplinary collaboration for the obstetric care of patients with obesity
5. Recognize particularities for vaginal and Cesarean delivery of a parturient with obesity

SUGGESTED READINGS

1. (a) American College of Obstetricians and Gynecologists' Committee on Practice Bulletins – Obstetrics. Obesity in pregnancy: ACOG Practice Bulletin, No. 230. *Obstet Gynecol.* 2021;137(6):e128–e144.
   (b) ACOG Practice Bulletin no. 105: Bariatric surgery and pregnancy. *Obstet Gynecol.* 2009;113(6):1405–1413.
2. Benhalima K, Minschart C, Ceulemans D, et al. Screening and management of gestational diabetes mellitus after bariatric surgery. *Nutrients.* 2018;10(10):1479.
3. Ciangura C, Coupaye M, Deruelle P, et al. Clinical practice guidelines for childbearing female candidates for bariatric surgery, pregnancy, and post-partum management after

bariatric surgery. *Obes Surg.* 2019;29(11):3722–3734. [Correction in *Obes Surg.* 2020 Sep;30(9):3650–3651]

4. (a) Denison FC, Aedla NR, Keag O, et al. Care of women with obesity in pregnancy. Green-Top Guideline No. 72. *BJOG* 2018.

   (b) Royal College of Obstetricians and Gynaecologists. The role of bariatric surgery in improving reproductive health. Scientific Impact Paper No. 17. October 2015.

5. D'Souza R, Horyn I, Pavalagantharajah S, et al. Maternal body mass index and pregnancy outcomes: a systematic review and metaanalysis. *Am J Obstet Gynecol MFM.* 2019;1(4):100041.

6. (a) Maxwell C, Gaudet L, Cassir G, et al. Guideline No. 391 – Pregnancy and maternal obesity part 1: pre-conception and prenatal care. *J Obstet Gynaecol Can.* 2019;41(11):1623–1640.

   (b) Maxwell C, Gaudet L, Cassir G, et al. Guideline No. 392 – Pregnancy and maternal obesity part 2: team planning for delivery and postpartum care. *J Obstet Gynaecol Can.* 2019;41(11):1660–1675. [Correction in *J Obstet Gynaecol Can.* 2020 Mar;42(3):385]

7. McAuliffe FM, Killeen SL, Jacob CM, et al. Management of prepregnancy, pregnancy, and postpartum obesity from the FIGO Pregnancy and Non-Communicable Diseases Committee: A FIGO (International Federation of Gynecology and Obstetrics) guideline. *Int J Gynaecol Obstet.* 2020;151(Suppl 1):16–36.

8. Royal Australian and New Zealand College of Obstetricians and Gynaecologists. Management of obesity in pregnancy. C-Obs 49, March 2017.

9. Simon A, Pratt M, Hutton B, et al. Guidelines for the management of pregnant women with obesity: a systematic review. *Obes Rev.* 2020;21(3):e12972.

10. Vitner D, Harris K, Maxwell C, et al. Obesity in pregnancy: a comparison of four national guidelines. *J Matern Fetal Neonatal Med.* 2019;32(15):2580–2590.

POINTS

1. With regard to obesity, what aspects of a focused history would you like to know for preconception counseling? *(1 point per main bullet)* — Max 20

☐ Height and current body weight *(an aspect of history and physical examination)*

Clinical features related to body weight
☐ Detailed evolution of challenges with weight gain/loss
☐ Current/prior nutritional counseling
☐ Use of fad diets or fasting as means for weight loss
☐ Exercise regimens, if any
☐ History of bariatric surgical procedures *(e.g., sleeve gastrectomy, Roux-en-Y gastric bypass, adjustable gastric band, biliopancreatic diversion)*
☐ Current/prior use of adjunctive medical therapies *(e.g., orlistat,[†] liriglutide,[‡] lorcaserin hydrochloride*)*

Patient or familial medical comorbidities, including treatments where applicable

Respiratory:
☐ Obstructive sleep apnea (OSA)/use of a continuous positive airway pressure (CPAP) machine
  ○ If no prior evaluation for OSA, consider use of an evaluation tool[§] for OSA-risk evaluation *(e.g., STOP-Bang questionnaire, Berlin questionnaire, or other validated tools)*

Cardiovascular:
- ☐ Chronic hypertension/other cardiovascular diseases
- ☐ Arrhythmias
- ☐ Venous thromboembolism (VTE)

Hematologic:
- ☐ Iron, folate, vitamin B12-deficiency anemia

Neuro-psychiatric:
- ☐ Stroke
- ☐ Depression, anxiety, suicidality
- ☐ Eating disorders (*e.g.*, binge-purging)

Endocrine:
- ☐ Type 2 diabetes mellitus
- ☐ Dyslipidemia

Hepato-renal:
- ☐ Nonalcoholic steatohepatitis (NASH)
- ☐ Chronic renal insufficiency

Gynecologic:
- ☐ Patient's last menstrual period, cycle regularity, meno-metrorrhagia (*evaluate for risk of anovulation*)
- ☐ Prior attempts to conceive, if any
- ☐ Current/prior contraceptive mechanisms, if any

Musculoskeletal:
- ☐ Osteoarthritis

Allergies and contraindications to potential therapeutics in pregnancy
- ☐ Asthma (*potential contraindication to aspirin, labetalol*)
- ☐ Nasal polyps (*contraindication to aspirin*)

Social history:
- ☐ Occupation, smoking, alcohol consumption, and use of illicit substances
- ☐ Consider inquiring about ethnicity (*variations on BMI, body fat percentage, and risks of chronic disease*)
- ☐ Screening question(s) for intimate partner violence

Special notes:
† Provides reversible inhibition of pancreatic and gastric lipases, resulting in ~30% inhibition of dietary fat absorption; use is contraindicated in pregnancy

‡ Antidiabetic agent resulting in increased insulin and decreased glucagon section with slowed gastric emptying and less food intake; use is contraindicated in pregnancy

* Highly selective 5-HT$_{2c}$ serotonin receptor agonist that promotes satiety; use is contraindicated in pregnancy

§ *Refer to* (a) Chung F, Subramanyam R, Liao P, et al. High STOP-Bang score indicates a high probability of obstructive sleep apnoea. *Br J Anaesth* 2012; 108:768 and (b) Senaratna CV, Perret JL, Matheson MC, et al. Validity of the Berlin questionnaire in detecting obstructive sleep apnea: A systematic review and meta-analysis. *Sleep Med Rev.* 2017;36:116–124.

You learn that the patient is an administrative assistant of English ancestry, who has struggled with obesity for 10 years; her weight has been stable for the last five years during which a psychological support group for obese women has helped manage her weight-related anxiety. The patient has never experienced suicidality or required anxiolytics. At 5 ft 2 in (1.57 m), she weighed 103.5 kg this morning on her home scale. The patient last consulted a nutritionist several years ago; she has never used weight loss pharmaceutical agents. There are no known comorbidities; she was normotensive at her physician's office last week. Upon questioning, she describes nonrestorative sleep, often leading to daytime drowsiness and fatigue. Her husband has not voiced complaints related to her sleep behaviors, although she feels this may stem from his sensitivity toward her body weight. To date, the couple has not tried to conceive, consistently using the male condom. With irregular menstrual cycles, she is concerned about difficulty conceiving as planned in the next few months. She takes supplements for iron-deficiency anemia and practices yoga once weekly. Her social habits are unremarkable.

2. You inform your trainee that despite its effects on fecundity, most women with obesity have regular ovulation and normal fertility. Address your trainee's inquiry regarding the etiologies of reduced <u>fertility</u> among women with obesity. *(1 point each)*

Max 2

Note that features may be independent of polycystic ovarian syndrome
- ☐ Anovulation/oligo-ovulation
- ☐ Suboptimal oocyte maturation or embryo quality
- ☐ Abnormal endometrial development and implantation
- ☐ Insulin resistance

Special notes:
(a) No evidence that obesity results in decreased frequency of sexual intercourse
(b) Refer to Kominiarek MA, Jungheim ES, Hoeger KM, Rogers AM, Kahan S, Kim JJ. American Society for Metabolic and Bariatric Surgery position statement on the impact of obesity and obesity treatment on fertility and fertility therapy Endorsed by the American College of Obstetricians and Gynecologists and the Obesity Society. *Surg Obes Relat Dis.* 2017;13(5):750–757.

3. Discuss your recommendations to this patient for body weight management, indicating general benefits on prospective obstetric outcomes. *(1 point per main bullet)*

Max 4

Interventions:
- ☐ Augment her physical activity, adopting *moderate* intensity exercise regime for 150 minutes/week over at least four to five days/week
  - ○ *Consideration for professional advice to gradually build physical activity*
- ☐ Dietary revision and referral to a nutritionist
- ☐ Respirology assessment for OSA
- ☐ Consideration for consultation with an expert in bariatric medicine

General benefits:
- ☐ Even small amounts of prepregnancy weight loss with a booking BMI <30 mg/m^2 improves maternal-fetal outcomes
  - ○ A realistic target is 5%–10% loss of original body weight over six months *(FIGO)*

4. Highlight four maternal-fetal benefits of treating OSA. *(1 point each)*

4

Decreased risk of:
☐ Small for gestational age or fetal growth restriction (FGR)
☐ Hypertensive syndromes of pregnancy
☐ Cardiomyopathy
☐ Gestational diabetes mellitus (GDM)
☐ Pulmonary emboli
☐ In-hospital mortality *(particularly with postpartum use of the CPAP machine)*
☐ Iatrogenic preterm birth

5. Present a <u>structured</u> outline of obesity-related pregnancy complications <u>or</u> features you may discuss at this preconception consultation. *(1 point each)*

25

Maternal – antepartum: *(max 6)*
☐ Early pregnancy loss
☐ Dizygotic twin pregnancy *(due to increased follicle stimulating hormone levels)*
☐ Hypertensive syndromes of pregnancy *(e.g., gestational hypertension, preeclampsia)*
☐ VTE *[≥2-times increased risk]*
☐ GDM *[more than three times increased likelihood relative to normal BMI]*
☐ Iatrogenic preterm birth
☐ Prolonged pregnancy >41 weeks' gestation
☐ Mental health problems
☐ Mortality

Maternal – intrapartum: *(max 7)*
☐ Anesthetic-related complications *(e.g., higher epidural resite rate,[†] difficult airway management, postoperative atelectasis, postoperative ICU stay)*
☐ Induction of labor
☐ Prolonged first stage (but not second stage) of labor
☐ Instrumental delivery and failed instrumental delivery
☐ Atonic postpartum hemorrhage (PPH) after vaginal (but not Cesarean) birth
  ○ *Blood transfusion requirements are not clearly higher*
☐ Third-degree perinatal lacerations
☐ Elective and emergency Cesarean section
☐ Genital tract injury at Cesarean section
☐ Peripartum death

Maternal – postpartum: *(max 4)*
☐ Mental health problems
☐ VTE
☐ Delayed wound healing and infection *(regardless of mode of delivery or use of prophylactic antibiotics at Cesarean section)*
☐ Failure to initiate or maintain breastfeeding

Fetal-neonatal: *(max 8)*

☐ Major congenital malformations *(see Question 7-A)* and suboptimal antenatal sonographic diagnosis

☐ Large for gestational age fetal biometry/postnatal macrosomia *(independent of GDM)*

☐ Suboptimal fetal growth biometry/FGR

☐ Shoulder dystocia

☐ Meconium aspiration

☐ Difficulties with fetal heart rate monitoring

☐ Neonatal metabolic complications *(e.g., jaundice, hypoglycemia, metabolic acidemia)* and low Apgar scores

☐ NICU admission

☐ Stillbirth or neonatal death

☐ Long-term health risks *(see Question 18)*

Special note:

† Repeat epidural placement with overall similar success rates in *achieving* neuraxial analgesia compared to parturients with normal body weight

---

6. Based on obesity-related health risks, which screening <u>investigations</u> would you initiate at this preconception visit, unless recently performed? *(1 point each)*   Max 8

☐ Renal function tests *(i.e., proteinuria and serum creatinine)*

☐ Liver function tests *(i.e., INR, serum bilirubin, serum albumin)*

☐ Aminotransferases *(i.e., AST, ALT)* and LDH

☐ Lipid profile *(i.e., serum total cholesterol, triglycerides, low- and high-density lipoproteins)*

☐ Thyroid function tests *(e.g., serum TSH, total and free thyroxine [T4], total and free triiodothyronine [T3])*

☐ Fasting plasma glucose and HbA1c

☐ Electrocardiogram (ECG)

☐ CBC/iron studies *(known anemia)*

Special note:

Hormonal profile for menstrual irregularity is not a direct screening test to address obesity-related health risks

---

The patient appreciates evidence-based counseling and agrees to adhere to your professional recommendations for body weight optimization prior to conception. Attentive to your discussion, she requests elaboration on congenital malformations more commonly detected among pregnant women with obesity. In addressing her inquiry, you mention that recent literature shows that risks of major congenital malformations in offspring progressively increase with maternal spectrum of obesity.[§]

Special note:

§ *Refer to* Persson M, Cnattingius S, Villamor E, et al. Risk of major congenital malformations in relation to maternal overweight and obesity severity: cohort study of 1.2 million singletons. *BMJ.* 2017;357:j2563

7-A. Independent from diabetes, present four obesity-associated birth defects. *(1 point each)*   4

Congenital anomalies:‡
- ☐ Cardiac anomalies
- ☐ Neural tube defects (NTDs)
- ☐ Hydrocephaly
- ☐ Facial clefting
- ☐ Anorectal atresia
- ☐ Limb reduction anomalies

7-B. Counsel the patient on a <u>specific strategy</u> proven to modify baseline risk of certain congenital malformations.   1

Risk reduction: *(1 point based on local policy)*
- ☐ Folic acid supplementation for risks of NTDs *(international disparities on dose-recommendations for women with obesity)*:
  - ○ *RCOG[4]*: High dose folic acid 5 mg/d starting at least one month preconception with continuance through antenatal period
  - ○ *SOGC[6]*: Routine dose folic acid 0.4 mg/d starting three months preconception (consideration for up to 5 mg/d until the end of the first trimester)
  - ○ *FIGO[7]*: At least folic acid 0.4 mg/d and consider up to 5 mg/d for at least one to three months preconception
  - ○ *RANZCOG[8]*: High dose folic acid 5 mg/d preconception with continuation antenatally

Special note:
‡ Risk of gastroschisis appears to be *reduced* among offspring of women with obesity

8. Noting that mechanisms for fetal death and stillbirth among women with obesity are largely unclear, discuss biologically plausible theories for this featured risk. *(1 point each)*   Max 3

- ☐ Fetal hypoxic episodes during untreated OSA
- ☐ Congenital malformations
- ☐ Maternal confounding factors, such as smoking, cardiovascular, or diabetes-related morbidity
- ☐ Suboptimal ability to obtain fetal cardiotocography (CTG) tracings
- ☐ Increased decision-to-delivery interval for emergency Cesarean section

Special note:
Women with obesity *do not* have decreased perception of fetal movements relative to women of normal weight

The patient mentions she has been contemplating gastric bypass surgery as a timely means to improve her personal and gestational health outcomes. She realizes that bariatric surgery is <u>not</u> a primary treatment for infertility, if present.

---

9. In the event of a bariatric procedure, counsel the patient on the preferred surgery-to-conception interval and provide rationale for your recommendation. *(1 point each)*   6

☐ Although limited supporting evidence, a minimum wait-period of at least 12–18 months *(FIGO, RCOG)*, 12–24 months *(ACOG, RANZCOG)*, or 24 months *(SOGC)* are advocated

<u>**Maternal benefits:**</u> *(relative to conception at shorter intervals)*
☐ Body weight stabilization
☐ Identification and treatment of nutritional deficiencies

<u>**Fetal benefits:**</u> *(relative to conception at shorter intervals)*
☐ Lower risk of small-for-gestational-age biometry
☐ Decreased risk of prematurity
☐ Decreased NICU admissions

---

10. The patient appreciates the importance of a delayed pregnancy interval after a bariatric procedure. Discuss important aspects related to <u>hormonal contraceptives</u> after gastric bypass. *(1 point per main and subbullet)*   Max 4

☐ Long-acting reversible contraceptives, such as IUDs or progestin implants are preferred options
☐ Depot-medroxyprogesterone acetate (DMPA) is safe, but may not be ideal due to more prolonged ovulation suppression among women with obesity relative to normal weight women
   ○ DMPA is <u>not</u> associated with additional weight gain in adult women with obesity *(data is conflicting for teenagers with obesity)*
   ○ Consideration for deltoid injection or longer needles for appropriate intramuscular dose
☐ Nonoral combined hormonal contraception (*i.e.*, vaginal ring, transdermal patch) is safe
☐ Oral contraceptives (combined or progesterone-only) are not reliably absorbed after bariatric procedures and are not recommended

---

Two years later, you receive a request for transfer of the patient's prenatal care to your tertiary center's high-risk obstetric unit after sonographic dating confirmed an intrauterine singleton at 9^{+3} weeks' gestation. The combination of lifestyle modifications, diagnosis and management of OSA, as well as an uncomplicated Roux-en-Y gastric bypass 20 months ago, improved her prepregnancy BMI$^\$$ to 38.97 kg/m^2. As anticipated, weight loss led to menstrual regularity and improved anxiety. Maintaining use of a CPAP machine for persistent OSA, she credits you with her increased energy and concentration. Folic acid supplements were started several months preconception. There have not been other germane changes in her biopsychosocial dimensions of health since your consultation.

Special note:
§ This prepregnancy BMI serves to illustrate that obesity is still very common (>50%) among women of childbearing age after bariatric surgery

11. Use the World Health Organization (WHO) definition to classify the patient's prepregnancy BMI.

1

☐ Obesity class II *(i.e., BMI 35.00–39.99 kg/m²)*

Special notes:
(i) *Refer to* World Health Organization (WHO). BMI Classification. Geneva: WHO; 2006. Available at https://gateway.euro.who.int/en/indicators/mn_survey_46-recommendations-on-weight-gain-include-guidance-for-each-obese-class/, accessed March 30, 2021.
(ii) Obesity class I and III are defined as BMI 30.00–34.99 kg/m² and ≥40.00 kg/m², respectively

12. Relative to your counseling of obstetric risks prior to her gastric bypass, discuss <u>specific</u> maternal-fetal features following bariatric surgery. (*1 point each*)

Max 4

Decreased:
☐ Gestational diabetes
☐ Pregnancy-associated hypertensive disorders
☐ Large-for-gestational-age fetuses/macrosomic newborns
☐ Congenital defects *(controversial)*
☐ Preterm birth *(controversial)*
☐ Cesarean section *(controversial)*

Increased:
☐ Maternal anemia
☐ Nutritional deficiencies
☐ Cholelithiasis *(associated with both pregnancy and Roux-en-Y gastric bypass)*
☐ Small-for-gestational-age infants/FGR
  ○ *Possibly attributed to nutritional deficiencies and/or weight loss*

13. Outline aspects of your physical examination most focused on her body habitus. Fetal viability has been ascertained. (*1 point each, unless specified*)

☐ Vital signs (with appropriately sized blood pressure cuff) *(2 points)*
  ○ *Cuff size used at the earliest time point should be documented in her medical notes (FIGO)*
  ○ *Large cuff is used when mid/upper arm circumference >33 cm[†]*
☐ Cardiopulmonary examination
☐ Abdominal assessment : *(1 point per subbullet)*
  ○ Subcutaneous tissue distribution (*i.e.*, examine the panniculus)
  ○ Bariatric surgery incisions
  ○ Abdominal hernias
  ○ Intertriginous infections
☐ Pressure wounds
☐ Lower extremities signs of VTE

Special note:
[†] *Refer to* Pickering TG, Hall JE, Appel LJ, et al. Recommendations for blood pressure measurement in humans and experimental animals: part 1: blood pressure measurement in humans: a statement for professionals from the Subcommittee of Professional and Public Education of the American Heart Association Council on High Blood Pressure Research. *Circulation.* 2005;111(5):697–716.

14. Detail your counseling and <u>antenatal</u> management plan pertaining to maternal obesity and/or prior gastric bypass surgery. (*1 point per main bullet, unless specified*)

☐ Highlight the importance of multidisciplinary consultations and serial collaboration (*e.g., digestive surgery, obstetrics/maternal-fetal medicine, obstetric medicine, perinatal mental health, nutrition, anesthesia, neonatology, midwifery, nursing, lactation expert*)

Maternal management: *(max 10)*
☐ Inform the patient that international variations exist regarding recommended gestational weight gain *(1 point for any one subbullet)*
  ○ *SOGC[6], FIGO[7], Institute of Medicine[†]* (now, 'National Academy of Medicine') *and ACOG[†]* recommend 5.0–9.0 kg (11–20 lbs) for singleton pregnancies with BMI ≥ 30 kg/m^2
  ○ *RCOG[4]* advises a healthy diet may be more applicable than prescribed weight gain targets
☐ Advise against excess weight gain due to associated increased risks of adverse maternal-fetal outcomes, including postpartum weight retention
☐ Maintain high index of suspicion for complications of bariatric surgery (*e.g., bowel obstruction, intussusception, dumping syndrome*) which may present as common pregnancy complaints (*e.g, abdominal cramps, bloating, nausea/vomiting/diarrhea*)
☐ Encourage continued moderate intensity physical activity (*unless contraindicated*)

☐ Low-dose ASA 75–162 mg taken nightly as preeclampsia prophylaxis **is** recommended for this patient given two moderate risk factors (*i.e.*, primigravida and obesity),[‡] provided her risk of gastrointestinal hemorrhage post-ariatric surgery is low
  ○ *Evidence suggests a dose response prophylactic effect*
☐ Encourage early reporting of symptoms or signs suggestive of hypertensive diseases or VTE
☐ Ensure use of an appropriately sized blood pressure cuff both in the clinical setting and if home-monitoring is required
☐ Serum screening <u>every trimester</u> for micronutrient deficiencies, with supplementation as needed *(additional point for first subbullet)*
  ○ *i.e.*, ferritin, iron, folate, calcium, vitamins A, B1, B12, D, and K
  ○ *RCOG[4] recommends vitamin D 10 ug/d for BMI $\geq$30 kg/m^2*
  ○ *RAZCOG[8] recommends iodine 150 ug/d preconception*
☐ *Avoid* standard glucose tests for GDM after gastric bypass due to potential for dumping syndrome *(additional point for first subbullet)*
  ○ Use HbA1c, fasting plasma glucose, and home capillary-glucose monitoring**
  ○ *Dumping syndrome is not typical after gastric banding (i.e., restrictive-type surgery)*
☐ Offer perinatal psychosocial support services for increased risk of anxiety and depression among pregnant women with obesity
☐ Third-trimester assessment for tissue viability issues/risk of pressure sores by a qualified professional [where booking BMI is $\geq$40 kg/m^2] *(RCOG[4])*

Fetal management: *(max 6)*
☐ Counsel that fetal fraction of cfDNA at noninvasive prenatal genetic screening is decreased with maternal obesity, raising risks of test failure (~24%), irrespective of gestational age[#]
☐ Consideration for timing the second-trimester morphology[$] sonogram at a minimum of 20 weeks' gestation *(SOGC[6])*
☐ Inform the patient of, and arrange for, extra time to complete the morphology sonogram
☐ Inform the patient of suboptimal abdominal image quality and antenatal detection of anomalies; transvaginal scanning may improve image acquisition
☐ Arrange for serial sonographic fetal biometry in the third trimester ($\pm$ second trimester)
  ○ *Fetal growth aberrations and limitations in fundal height assessment*
☐ Provide greater fetal surveillance in the case of reduced fetal movements due to increased risks of stillbirth; for this patient with obesity class II, weekly antenatal fetal surveillance may be considered beginning by 37^{+0} weeks' gestation *(ACOG[1a])*
☐ Maintain a low threshold for sonographic confirmation of fetal presentation at ~36 weeks' gestation if palpation is inadequate, and at delivery hospitalization
☐ Individual discussion is warranted for timing of induction of labor: *(1 point for any one subbullet)*
  ○ *ACOG[1] and RCOG[4] advise against induction of labor for obesity alone; spontaneous labor is encouraged*
  ○ *SOGC[6] recommends delivery at 39–40 weeks' gestation for class III obesity*
  ○ *FIGO[7] recommends induction of labor at 41^{+0} weeks' gestation for class II, III obesity*

Special notes:

† Institute of Medicine (now, 'National Academy of Medicine'): Weight gain during pregnancy: reexamining the guidelines. National Academy of Sciences. 28 May 2009; endorsed by the American College of Obstetricians and Gynecologists. ACOG Committee opinion no. 548: weight gain during pregnancy. *Obstet Gynecol.* 2013;121(1):210–212.

‡ Refer to Chapter 38, Question 6

** Post-gastric bypass, GDM is defined if ≥20% of all capillary blood glucose exceed glycemic targets: premeals ≥95 mg/dL (5.3 mmol/L), one-hour postprandial ≥140 mg/dL (7.8 mmol/L), two-hour postprandial ≥120 mg/dL (6.7 mmol/L) *(Suggested Reading 3)*

Yared E, Dinsmoor MJ, Endres LK, et al. Obesity increases the risk of failure of noninvasive prenatal screening regardless of gestational age. *Am J Obstet Gynecol.* 2016;215(3):370. e1–370.e3706.

§ Fetal echocardiography is <u>not</u> indicated for maternal obesity alone; refer to <Donofrio MT, Moon-Grady AJ, Hornberger LK, et al. Diagnosis and treatment of fetal cardiac disease: a scientific statement from the American Heart Association [published correction appears in *Circulation.* 2014 May 27;129(21):e512]. *Circulation.* 2014;129(21): 2183–2242. >

By 36^{+2} weeks' gestation, maternal-fetal aspects of prenatal care have been uneventful; compliance was maintained and adherence to physical activity, dietary regimes, and micronutrient supplementations collectively resulted in 7 kg gestational weight gain and obviated pregnancy complications. *{The patient's BMI is now nearly 42 kg/m².}*

Fetal sonographic assessment today shows a cephalic presentation with growth velocity maintained on the 79th percentile and normal markers of fetal well-being. Although intrapartum management has been serially updated during the antepartum period, you review delivery plans with her at this visit. You have just performed the group B streptococcus (GBS) vaginal-rectal swab for which routine care is anticipated.

In discussion on timing of delivery, you inform the patient that although obesity alone is not an indication for induction of labor, elective induction at term in women with obesity may obviate the risk of stillbirth and reduce the risk of Cesarean section without increasing adverse outcomes.

15. In planning for vaginal delivery, outline pertinent treatment and management considerations with regard to maternal obesity. *(1 point per main and subbullet)*   Max 8

☐ Consideration for labor and delivery to proceed in an obstetric unit with adequate maternal-fetal support, particularly in this patient with OSA and bariatric bypass surgery

□ Early notification of the on-duty obstetric anesthesiologist upon patient admission
  o Consideration for early placement of an epidural catheter is advisable in case of emergency Cesarean delivery *(FIGO[7])*
  o Exercise caution with use of opioid analgesics given known OSA
□ Establishing venous access (>1 cannula) early in labor *(FIGO[7])*
□ Consideration for blood product availability

Labor:
□ Where induction of labor is planned, preferred use of mechanical cervical ripening over prostaglandins
□ Use BMI-adjusted labor curves
□ Anticipate increased oxytocin doses in the first stage of labor relative to nonobese women
□ Maintain continuous maternal pulse oximetry to identify hypoxemia *(i.e., patient has known OSA)*
□ Consideration for continuous electronic fetal monitoring in active labor with possible recourse to fetal scalp electrode if abdominal monitoring is inadequate
□ Active management of the third stage of labor is advised to reduce risks of PPH

Spontaneous amniorhexis of clear fluid, followed by oxytocin augmentation occurs at 39^{+2} weeks' gestation. The patient's GBS swab was negative. An early epidural was inserted. Despite increasing doses of oxytocin, the cervix has not dilated past 7 cm over several hours. Fetal CTG tracing has remained normal although detection of the contraction pattern is suboptimal.

16. What is your <u>next best step</u> in management of this patient?   1

□ Insertion of an intrauterine pressure catheter
  o *Although not recommended for <u>routine</u> use*

An adequate uterine contraction pattern and Montevideo unit measurement >200 units for at least four hours does not result in cervical change. Fetal tracing remains normal. The patient consents to Cesarean section for first stage arrest. Neuraxial anesthesia is adjusted for surgical delivery. Blood products remain available.

17. As a senior obstetric surgeon, detail your surgical delivery management of this patient. *(1 point per main bullet)*

Max 7

☐ Ensure availability of proper length surgical instruments and additional experienced surgical assistance

☐ Administer single-dose cefazolin IV at 15–60 minutes before the skin incision *(precluding allergies)* with additional intraoperative doses based on blood loss or surgical duration
  ○ Weight-adjusted dosage (*i.e.*, cefazolin 3 g for women ≥120 kg and 2 g for women <120 kg†) may be considered; conclusive recommendations are difficult to establish given the lack of evidence demonstrating different adipose tissue concentrations or decreased surgical site infections with higher dosage strategies in an obese cohort *(ACOG[1a])*

☐ Mechanical thromboprophylaxis (graduated compression stockings or sequential compression devices) is recommended before and after Cesarean section *(FIGO[7])*

☐ Individual variations in maternal habitus, surgical anatomy, and operator's experience preclude recommendations for a specific abdominal incision; options include: *(any one route)*
  ○ Transverse infrapanniculus/suprapubic (usually with maternal weight ≤180 kg)
  ○ Transverse suprapanniculus
  ○ Vertical suprapanniculus *(consideration for risk of surgical site infections)*

☐ Maintain meticulous hemostasis, minimize blood loss and tissue handling

☐ Close subcutaneous tissue in multiple layers, particularly when >2 cm in thickness

☐ Keep the subcutaneous layer dry to decrease wound complications

☐ Limited evidence to recommend staples or subcuticular sutures for skin closure at Cesarean section among women with obesity[‡]

☐ Consideration for LMWH thromboprophylaxis after Cesarean section at least until mobilization *(jurisdictional recommendations vary)*

Special notes:

† Bratzler DW, Dellinger EP, Olsen KM, et al. Clinical practice guidelines for antimicrobial prophylaxis in surgery. *Surg Infect (Larchmt).* 2013;14(1):73–156.

‡ Refer to (a) <Rodel RL, Gray KM, Quiner TE, et al. Cesarean wound closure in body mass index 40 or greater comparing suture to staples: a randomized clinical trial. *Am J Obstet Gynecol MFM.* 2021;3(1):100271 >and (b) <Zaki MN, Wing DA, McNulty JA. Comparison of staples vs subcuticular suture in class III obese women undergoing Cesarean: a randomized controlled trial. *Am J Obstet Gynecol.* 2018;218(4):451.e1–451. e8. >

(a) Subcutaneous drains are <u>not</u> *routinely* recommended due to increased risk of wound complications

(b) Routine use of negative pressure dressing therapy to the Cesarean wound is not recommended

An uncomplicated Cesarean delivery is performed under neuraxial anesthesia with a 90-minute operating time and estimated blood loss of 900 mL. A healthy male is delivered weighing 3300 grams; arterial pH is 7.25. Neonatology evaluation is in progress.

On postoperative day 1, the medical chart indicates normal vital signs. The patient reports adequate pain control, and you are reassured her abdominal incision is dry. Thromboprophylaxis has been initiated. The patient is tolerating meals. Her husband remains supportive at her bedside.

18. What are important short- and long-term postpartum considerations related to maternal obesity and prior gastric bypass? *(1 point per main bullet, unless specified)*   Max 15

Postoperative analgesic considerations:
- ☐ *Avoid* nonsteroidal anti-inflammatory drugs (NSAIDs) in patients with gastric bypass *(i.e., risk of gastric ulcers)*
- ☐ Continue to exercise caution with opioid analgesics in view of her OSA

Wound care monitoring:
- ☐ Encourage post–hospital discharge monitoring for wound complications
- ☐ Counsel on maintaining the surgical site dry, especially with suprapubic skin incisions

Physical and mental health monitoring:
- ☐ Encourage early ambulation
- ☐ Encourage adequate hydration
- ☐ Ensure continuation of CPAP treatment
- ☐ Continue to offer psychosocial support services and screen for postpartum depression and anxiety
  - ○ *Although crucial for all postpartum women with obesity, recall this patient's antecedent history of obesity-related anxiety*
- ☐ Encourage interpregnancy weight loss, regardless of appropriate gestational weight gain; even modest weight retention is associated with increased risk of adverse outcomes among women with obesity *(additional 1 point per subbullet)*
  - ○ Interpregnancy weight loss reduces risk of stillbirth, hypertensive complication, and macrosomia
  - ○ Improved prepregnancy BMI <u>may</u> be associated with improved VBAC success rates *(this has not been confirmed in all studies[†])*
- ☐ Continue to offer professional nutritional expert services to support postpartum weight reduction (including routine care post–bariatric surgery)
- ☐ Continue to encourage moderate intensity physical activity
- ☐ Arrange for postpartum obstetric and medical outpatient follow-up *(individual considerations based on clinical context)*
- ☐ Promote long-term follow-up with her primary care provider for risk of metabolic syndrome[§] *(i.e., hypertension, insulin resistance, hypertriglyceridemia, central obesity, low high-density lipoprotein cholesterol)*

Breastfeeding and contraception:
- ☐ Offer specialist support to promote breastfeeding initiation and maintenance, which are decreased with maternal obesity
  - ○ *Consideration for difficult positioning, nipple flattening with increased edema, individual perceptions, physiological delay in lactogenesis with obesity, and possibly impaired prolactin response to suckling*

- [ ] Reassure the patient that quality and quantity of breast milk is not negatively affected by her weight loss *(FIGO[7])*
- [ ] Advise her that breastfeeding, exclusively and mixed, is inversely related to postpartum weight retention and may be protective against childhood obesity
- [ ] *(For contraception, see Question 10)*

Encourage long-term pediatric follow-up for health risks:
- [ ] Child and adolescent obesity
- [ ] Asthma
- [ ] Neurodevelopmental problems
- [ ] Type 2 diabetes mellitus

Special notes:
† Mei JY, Havard AL, Mularz AJ, Maykin MM, Gaw SL. Impact of obesity class on trial of labor after cesarean success: does prepregnancy or at-delivery obesity status matter?. *J Perinatol.* 2019;39(8):1042–1049.

§ For diagnostic criteria, refer to National Institutes of Health: Third report of the National Cholesterol Education Program Expert Panel on detection, evaluation, and treatment of high blood cholesterol in adults (Adult Treatment Panel III), NIH Publication 01–3670. Bethesda, National Institutes of Health, 2001

TOTAL: **140**

CHAPTER 7

Preterm Labor

Jessica Papillon-Smith and Amira El-Messidi

During your obstetric call duty in a tertiary hospital center, you receive a telephone call from a colleague on call duty at a community hospital center where a 34-year-old G3P2 presented with uterine contractions at 27 weeks' gestation.

Special note: *For comprehensive presentation of resources, clinical, and academic subject matter addressed in this chapter, the 'Suggested Readings' list exceeds 10.*

LEARNING OBJECTIVES

1. Collaborate with an obstetric care provider for management of possible preterm labor, appreciating general and individual consideration for tocolysis
2. Provide counseling on the benefits of antenatal pulmonary corticosteroids and risks of repeat courses, and appreciate select situations where a rescue course may be considered
3. Understand the indications for magnesium sulfate administration for fetal neuroprotection and outline potential mechanisms for reductions in risk of cerebral palsy and gross motor dysfunction
4. Initiate recognized pharmacologic regimens for preterm prelabor rupture of membranes (PPROM) based on perinatal benefits
5. Recognize and manage select obstetric emergency complications of PPROM

SUGGESTED READINGS

1. American College of Obstetricians and Gynecologists' Committee on Practice Bulletins – Obstetrics. Prediction and prevention of spontaneous preterm birth: ACOG Practice Bulletin, No. 234. *Obstet Gynecol.* 2021;138(2):e65–e90.
2. Bachnas MA, Akbar MIA, Dachlan EG, et al. The role of magnesium sulfate (MgSO$_4$) in fetal neuroprotection. *J Matern Fetal Neonatal Med.* 2021;34(6):966–978.
3. Committee on Obstetric Practice. Committee Opinion No. 713: Antenatal corticosteroid therapy for fetal maturation. *Obstet Gynecol.* 2017;130(2):e102–e109.
4. Committee Opinion No. 455: Magnesium sulfate before anticipated preterm birth for neuroprotection. *Obstet Gynecol.* 2010;115(3):669–671.
5. Di Renzo GC, Cabero Roura L, Facchinetti F, et al. Preterm labor and birth management: recommendations from the European Association of Perinatal Medicine. *J Matern Fetal Neonatal Med.* 2017;30(17):2011–2030.

6. Jain V, McDonald SD, Mundle WR, et al. Guideline No. 398: Progesterone for prevention of spontaneous preterm birth. *J Obstet Gynaecol Can.* 2020;42(6):806–812.

7. Magee LA, De Silva DA, Sawchuck D, et al. No. 376 – magnesium sulphate for fetal neuroprotection. *J Obstet Gynaecol Can.* 2019;41(4):505–522.

8. McGoldrick E, Stewart F, Parker R, et al. Antenatal corticosteroids for accelerating fetal lung maturation for women at risk of preterm birth. *Cochrane Database Syst Rev.* 2020;12(12): CD004454.

9. Medley N, Poljak B, Mammarella S, et al. Clinical guidelines for prevention and management of preterm birth: a systematic review. *BJOG.* 2018;125(11):1361–1369.

10. (a) National Institute for Health and Care Excellence. Diagnostic guidance on biomarker tests to help diagnose preterm labour in women with intact membranes. NICE Guidance NG33, July 4, 2018. Available at www.nice.org.uk/guidance/dg33. Accessed July 19, 2021.

    (b) National Institute for Health and Care Excellence. Preterm labour and birth. NICE Guidance NG25, November 20, 2015, last updated August 2, 2019. Available at www.nice.org.uk/guidance/ng25?unlid=9291036072016213201257. Accessed July 10, 2021.

    (c) National Institute for Health and Care Excellence. Preterm labour and birth overview; NICE Pathways. Last updated April 20, 2021. Available at https://pathways.nice.org.uk/pathways/preterm-labour-and-birth. Accessed July 10, 2021.

11. Prelabor rupture of membranes: ACOG Practice Bulletin, No. 217. *Obstet Gynecol.* 2020;135(3):e80–e97.

12. Reddy UM, Deshmukh U, Dude A, et al. Society for Maternal-Fetal Medicine Consult Series No. 58: Use of antenatal corticosteroids for individuals at risk for late preterm delivery: replaces SMFM Statement No. 4, implementation of the use of antenatal corticosteroids in the late preterm birth period in women at risk for preterm delivery. *Am J Obstet Gynecol.* 2021; S0002–9378(21):00859–0.

13. Royal College of Obstetricians and Gynaecologists. Umbilical cord prolapse. Green-Top Guideline No. 50, November 2014. Available at www.rcog.org.uk/en/guidelines-research-services/guidelines/gtg50/. Accessed October 8, 2021.

14. SMFM preterm birth toolkit. Available at www.smfm.org/publications/231-smfm-preterm-birth-toolkit. Accessed July 10, 2021.

15. Skoll A, Boutin A, Bujold E, et al. No. 364 – antenatal corticosteroid therapy for improving neonatal outcomes. *J Obstet Gynaecol Can.* 2018;40(9):1219–1239.

16. Society for Maternal-Fetal Medicine (SMFM) Publications Committee. The choice of progestogen for the prevention of preterm birth in women with singleton pregnancy and prior preterm birth. *Am J Obstet Gynecol.* 2017;216(3):B11–B13.

17. Tchirikov M, Schlabritz-Loutsevitch N, Maher J, et al. Mid-trimester preterm premature rupture of membranes (PPROM): etiology, diagnosis, classification, international recommendations of treatment options and outcome. *J Perinat Med.* 2018;46(5): 465–488.

18. Thomson AJ; Royal College of Obstetricians and Gynaecologists. Care of women presenting with suspected preterm prelabour rupture of membranes from 24[+0] weeks of gestation: Green-Top Guideline No. 73. *BJOG.* 2019;126(9):e152–e166.

19. Tsakiridis I, Mamopoulos A, Athanasiadis A, et al. Antenatal corticosteroids and magnesium sulfate for improved preterm neonatal outcomes: a review of guidelines. *Obstet Gynecol Surv.* 2020;75(5):298–307.

20. Tsakiridis I, Mamopoulos A, Chalkia-Prapa EM, et al. Preterm premature rupture of membranes: a review of 3 national guidelines. *Obstet Gynecol Surv.* 2018;73(6): 368–375.

21. WHO recommendations on interventions to improve preterm birth outcomes, 2015. Available at www.who.int/reproductivehealth/publications/maternal_perinatal_health/preterm-birth-guideline/en/. Accessed October 5, 2021.
22. Yudin MH, van Schalkwyk J, Van Eyk N. No. 233 – antibiotic therapy in preterm premature rupture of the membranes. *J Obstet Gynaecol Can.* 2017;39(9):e207–e212.

	POINTS
1. What aspects of a focused history would you inquire about in <u>telephone conversation</u> with the obstetric provider? *(1 point each; max points indicated where required)*	Max 45

Demographic information:

Obstetric provider
☐ Name and contact information (*e.g.,* telephone, license number)

Hospital center
☐ Name, location, and distance of the community hospital center from the tertiary center by potential modes of transport

Patient and pregnancy
☐ Two patient identifiers (*e.g.,* name, health care number, date of birth)
☐ Singleton or multiple pregnancy
☐ Method used for pregnancy dating (*i.e.,* last menstrual period vs. ultrasound); calculate a more precise gestational age
☐ Prior similar presentation(s) or hospitalization(s)

Obstetric features of the clinical presentation:
☐ Duration of uterine contractions and changes in frequency and intensity over time
☐ Possibility of, or confirmed, rupture of chorioamniotic membranes
☐ Presence of vaginal bleeding (*i.e.,* unexplained, or secondary to known placenta previa or suspected placental abruption)
☐ Confirmation of fetal viability *(also a component of the physical examination)*
☐ Known fetal features associated with uterine overdistension (*e.g.,* polyhydramnios, space-occupying fetal malformation, multiple gestation)
☐ Inquire about the presence of a short cervix at 16–24 weeks' gestation and if the patient takes progesterone supplementation

Maternal features in this pregnancy related to the clinical presentation:

Medical and surgical aspects (max 4)
☐ Compliance with prenatal care
☐ Current/recent infection (*e.g.,* periodontal disease, genitourinary, gastrointestinal, systemic infection) and medical treatments
☐ Trauma, abuse, or recent sexual activity (*interval since last sexual activity relates to the interpretation of clinical investigations*)
☐ Pregnancy-associated medical complications (*e.g.,* anemia, poorly controlled gestational diabetes) and medical treatments

☐ Antecedent medical complications (*e.g.,* pregestational diabetes, chronic hypertension, collagen vascular disorder, uncontrolled thyroid disorder, mental illness) and medical treatments

☐ Emergency surgical procedures in pregnancy (*e.g.,* appendicitis, cholecystitis, cervical cerclage)

☐ Antecedent gynecologic features[†] (*e.g.,* Mullerian anomaly, uterine fibroids, cone biopsy, particularly undisclosed uterine evacuations [either induced termination or spontaneous pregnancy loss])

Social aspects (max 3)
☐ Cigarette smoking
☐ Alcohol abuse/heavy consumption
☐ Illicit drug use (especially cocaine and/or heroin)
☐ High-risk sexual practices

Obstetric history:
☐ Mode of deliveries
☐ Gestational age at deliveries; inquire about circumstances of past preterm deliveries *if any*
☐ Interval since last pregnancy (*i.e.,* primarily to assess for short interpregnancy interval <18 months)

Inquire on physical examination findings:
☐ General appearance (*e.g.,* body habitus, apparent distress from uterine contractions)
☐ Blood pressure, temperature, pulse rate, oxygen saturation, and respiratory rate
☐ Findings on cardiotocographic monitoring of the fetal heart and uterine activity
☐ Presence, duration, and frequency of palpable uterine contractions
☐ Fundal height
☐ Abdominal tenderness unrelated to uterine contractions
☐ Costovertebral angle tenderness
☐ Findings on sterile speculum examination (*i.e.,* cervical dilation, visualization of the chorioamniotic membranes and/or fetal parts, suggestion of cervico-vaginal infection)
☐ Bimanual pelvic examination, if clinically warranted (*i.e.,* characterize cervical dilation, effacement, station, position, consistency)

Investigations performed in relation to the presenting complaint:
☐ Sonography for fetal presentation, estimated fetal weight, amniotic fluid volume, suggestion of placental abruption, placental and umbilical cord localization (if not already known)
☐ Transvaginal sonography for cervical length, *if deemed complementary to clinical management*
☐ Full/complete blood count (FBC/CBC) with differential
☐ Vaginal cultures (*e.g.,* trichomonas vaginalis)
☐ Consideration for wet-prep evaluation for bacterial vaginosis
☐ Vaginal-rectal group B *Streptococcus* (GBS) swab, or known positive status based on GBS bacteriuria at any time during pregnancy or a positive vaginal-rectal swab resulted during investigations of preterm labor within the past five weeks
☐ Urinalysis and urine culture, including testing for chlamydia and gonorrhea
☐ Cervicovaginal fetal fibronectin (fFN), *if clinically indicated*

> ○ NICE[10a, 10b]: *fFN testing may be considered for women $\geq 30^{+0}$ weeks to determine the likelihood of birth within 48 hours*
> ○ *While NICE does not recommend combined fFN and transvaginal ultrasound for measurement of cervical length, other guidance allow use of two methods to improve diagnostic accuracy (European Association of Perinatal Medicine[5])*
>
> **Pharmacologic aspects related to current management:**
> ☐ Drug allergies
> ☐ Tocolysis
> ☐ Analgesia
> ☐ Antibiotics for positive or unknown GBS status
> ☐ Intravenous hydration
> ☐ Initiation of fetal pulmonary corticosteroids (*i.e.,* dexamethasone or betamethasone)
> ☐ Magnesium sulfate for fetal neuroprotection
>
> **Special note:**
> † *Refer to* Saccone G, Perriera L, Berghella V. Prior uterine evacuation of pregnancy as independent risk factor for preterm birth: a systematic review and metaanalysis. *Am J Obstet Gynecol.* 2016;214(5):572–591.

You learn the patient is healthy, at 27^{+4} weeks' gestation by early sonographic dating of a spontaneous singleton. She presented with a two-hour history of unprovoked contractions increasing in intensity, lasting ~45 seconds, and occurring at 15-minute intervals; there are no other obstetric complaints or associated symptoms.

There is a long-standing history of multiple uterine fibroids, the largest being 10 cm with intramural-submucosal components, distant from the cervix on ultrasound 10 days ago, at 26^{+1} weeks' gestation, when the patient was hospitalized for threatened preterm labor and a positive qualitative cervicovaginal fFN test; transvaginal cervical length was 26 mm. Investigations were otherwise unremarkable. The patient received fetal pulmonary corticosteroids, hydration, and a 48-hour course of indomethacin tocolysis. She was later discharged in stable condition.

As the patient had a spontaneous vaginal birth after Cesarean section (VBAC) at 33 weeks' gestation, seven months prior to the current pregnancy, she has thereby remained adherent to vaginal progesterone supplementation, based on local availability. She also takes oral iron for long-standing anemia. Planned serial sonographic cervical lengths until 24 weeks' gestation were stable at 27–29 mm. Fetal aneuploidy screening showed 46, XY chromosomes and routine morphology survey was normal. Routine prenatal serologies were unremarkable; GBS bacteriuria was detected on first-trimester urine culture. Asymptomatic candidiasis and bacterial vaginosis, detected on first-trimester screening, were treated accordingly. She does not engage in high-risk behaviors.

Eleven years ago, she had an uncomplicated first pregnancy where she delivered at term by Cesarean section in the second stage for fetal indications. Based on her medical chart, the physician learned of two remote uterine evacuations, consisting of one induced termination and one early spontaneous loss; in confidence, the patient requested her true gravidity remain undisclosed.

Your colleague indicates that vital signs and body habitus are normal. On continuous cardiotocography, fetal heart tracing remains appropriate for gestational age while contraction frequency increased to eight in the past hour. She is uncomfortable from the uterine contractions despite oral acetaminophen (paracetamol) and one 5-mg dose of subcutaneous morphine. Fetal presentation is cephalic and amniotic fluid volume appears normal on bedside sonography; assessment for sonographic evidence of placental abruption is beyond the physician's expertise. Over the past two hours, the cervix has dilated from 1 to 2 cm with softening consistency. Repeat cervicovaginal fFN was deferred. There is no vaginal bleeding or fluid loss. The physician confirms that routine cultures you suggested were collected at presentation. Intravenous hydration and GBS prophylactic antibiotics have been initiated. While you agree with the request for transfer to a tertiary center to optimize neonatal outcomes, particularly among women who may deliver prior to 30 weeks' gestation, you inform the physician that an optimal risk scoring system for preterm birth prediction remains unknown.[†]

Special note:

† *Refer to* Meertens LJE, van Montfort P, Scheepers HCJ, et al. Prediction models for the risk of spontaneous preterm birth based on maternal characteristics: a systematic review and independent external validation. *Acta Obstet Gynecol Scand.* 2018;97(8):907–920.

---

2. Elicit this patient's risk factors that <u>may contribute</u> to preterm labor and/or spontaneous preterm birth, as highlighted in your notes during the conversation with the physician. *(1 point each)*   Max 7

Patient-specific risk factors:
- ☐ Previous preterm birth *(most significant risk factor)*
- ☐ Short interpregnancy (<18 months[‡]) interval prior to the current pregnancy[§]
- ☐ Previous episode of threatened preterm labor in the incident pregnancy
- ☐ Second stage Cesarean section
- ☐ Bacterial vaginosis[†#]
- ☐ GBS bacteriuria
- ☐ Nondilutional anemia
- ☐ Male fetal gender
- ☐ Multiple uterine fibroids, including a large fibroma (*i.e.,* >6 cm)
- ☐ Previous uterine evacuations for an induced pregnancy termination and spontaneous loss

Special notes:

‡ *Refer to* Conde-Agudelo A, Rosas-Bermúdez A, Kafury-Goeta AC. Birth spacing and risk of adverse perinatal outcomes: a meta-analysis. *JAMA.* 2006;295(15):1809–1823.

§ The long interpregnancy interval (≥60 months[‡]) after the first delivery increased risk for preterm birth in the second pregnancy

† Antibiotic treatment has not been shown to consistently reduce the risk of preterm birth; *refer to* Brocklehurst P, Gordon A, Heatley E, Milan SJ. Antibiotics for treating bacterial vaginosis in pregnancy. *Cochrane Database Syst Rev.* 2013;(1):CD000262. Published 2013 Jan 31.

Asymptomatic vaginal candidiasis is *not* associated with preterm birth; *refer to* Schuster HJ, de Jonghe BA, Limpens J, Budding AE, Painter RC. Asymptomatic vaginal Candida colonization and adverse pregnancy outcomes including preterm birth: a systematic review and meta-analysis. *Am J Obstet Gynecol MFM.* 2020;2(3):100163.

3. Discuss important considerations prior to initiating patient transfer. *(1 point each)*   Max 6

Safety features: (*i.e.,* **ensure no contraindications to transport**)
- ☐ Maternal hemodynamic stability
- ☐ Fetal well-being
- ☐ Likelihood of delivery during transport
- ☐ Presence of skilled health care provider(s) for maternal and neonatal care during transport
- ☐ External factors, such as weather restrictions, distance, and availability of medical transport

Administrative features:
- ☐ Availability of maternal and neonatal hospital beds at the receiving hospital
- ☐ Availability of allied medical personnel (*e.g.,* nurses, midwives)
- ☐ Ensure that the receiving hospital provides necessary neonatal care for gestational age

4. Explore reasons why the referring physician may have deferred repeating the cervicovaginal fFN test performed 10 days prior. *(1 point each)*   Max 2

- ☐ Inherent risk of a false-positive[†] result due to administration of intravaginal medications (*i.e.,* vaginal progesterone)
- ☐ No change in patient management
- ☐ Cost

Special note:
† Other causes for a false-positive fFN test, not specific to this case scenario, include a grossly bloody specimen, sexual intercourse within the previous 24 hours, lubricants, and digital cervical assessment

Having confirmed your maternal-neonatal unit can accommodate transfer, the patient is estimated to arrive by ambulance within two hours based on distance of the referring center. All medical notes will be provided with the patient. If uterine contractions persist, you suggest cervical assessment just prior to departure. A midwife skilled in neonatal resuscitation will accompany the paramedics; the patient will remain in the left lateral decubitus position, fetal heart rate will be verified by intermittent auscultation, uterine contractions will be recorded by palpation and vital signs assessed, as routine. You take this opportunity to discuss initiation of tocolysis prior to transfer.

5. Address the referring physician's inquiry about a repeat course of indomethacin, providing other evidence-based options for tocolysis, where indicated. *(1 point each)*   3

☐ While indomethacin treatment may be repeated after a five-day interval at <32 weeks' gestation *(European Association of Perinatal Medicine[5])*, consideration for sonographic imaging of amniotic fluid volume, and blood flow in the pulmonary trunk and across the tricuspid valve

Other classes of drugs for tocolysis:[†] *(max 2)*
☐ Calcium-channel blocker (*i.e.*, oral nifedipine)
☐ Oxytocin-receptor antagonist (*i.e.*, intravenous atosiban)[‡]
☐ ß-adrenergic receptor agonists/betamimetics (*i.e.*, subcutaneous terbutaline)[§]

Special notes:
[†] Preferred choice of agent depends on patient factors and international practice recommendations; magnesium sulfate is not recommended for tocolysis because it is ineffective *(SOGC[7])*, and there is insufficient evidence to support use of the nitroglycerin transdermal patch for tocolysis
[‡] International variations exist regarding drug availability
[§] Not recommended by *NICE* [10b] due to risk of adverse events

Having agreed to a trial of a calcium-channel blocker, you inform the referring physician that while the optimal regimen of nifedipine for management of preterm labor remains to be determined, the optimal initial dose appears to be 10 mg orally or sublingually. If contractions persist, a repeat dose could be given every 15–20 minutes up to 40 mg in the first hour; continued regimen would entail 20 mg orally every 6–8 hours for 48–72 hours.[†]

Special note:
[†] *Refer to* Conde-Agudelo A, Romero R, Kusanovic JP. Nifedipine in the management of preterm labor: a systematic review and metaanalysis. *Am J Obstet Gynecol.* 2011;204(2):134.e1–134.20.

6. Review the maternal-fetal side effects of nifedipine with the referring physician as you advise monitoring thereof during patient transfer. *(1 point each)*   4

Maternal:
☐ Symptoms related to the effects of peripheral vasodilation include dizziness, nausea, headache, palpitations, flushing
☐ Compensatory sign includes reflex tachycardia *(among compensatory physiological changes to maintain normotension among women without cardiac dysfunction)*
☐ Severe hypotension *(described in case reports)*

Fetal:
☐ No known side effects from oral nifedipine tocolysis

Special note:
Refer to Cornette J, Duvekot JJ, Roos-Hesselink JW, Hop WC, Steegers EA. Maternal and fetal haemodynamic effects of nifedipine in normotensive pregnant women. *BJOG.* 2011;118(4): 510–540.

7-A. Address the referring physician's inquiry regarding general conditions that preclude tocolysis. *(1 point each)*

Max 5

General contraindications to tocolysis: *(max 5)*

Maternal
- ☐ Gestational age >34 weeks
- ☐ Bleeding with hemodynamic instability
- ☐ Chorioamnionitis
- ☐ Preterm prelabor rupture of membranes, except in absence of infection to support maternal transfer and fetal benefit of pulmonary corticosteroids
- ☐ Conditions, such as severe preeclampsia, eclampsia, HELLP syndrome, acute fatty liver of pregnancy

Fetal
- ☐ Demise
- ☐ Lethal fetal anomaly or aneuploidy
- ☐ Abnormal or nonreassuring fetal status
- ☐ Documented fetal maturity

7-B. Highlight the situations precluding use of nifedipine for treatment of preterm labor. *(1 point each)*

Max 3

Contraindications to nifedipine:
- ☐ Hypotension
- ☐ Preload-dependent cardiac lesions
- ☐ Heart failure with decreased ejection fraction
- ☐ Known hypersensitivity to the drug

As the physician inquires about a repeat or rescue course of antenatal corticosteroids, you highlight that although geographic practice patterns vary based on conflicting evidence, a repeat course should not be routinely offered, but *considered* based on gestational age, likelihood of delivery within 48 hours, and interval since the last course *(NICE [10b])*. Depending on jurisdictional practices, a single rescue course may either be considered as early as seven days from the initial course *(ACOG[3], WHO[21])* or after a time interval of more than 14 days *(ACOG[3], SOGC[15])*, up to 34 weeks' gestation. As such, administration of a rescue course for this patient merits multidisciplinary consultation and a discussion of risks and benefits with the patient.

8. Outline the risks of repeat courses of antenatal pulmonary corticosteroids for consideration in patient counseling. *(1 point each)*

Max 3

☐ Reduction in mean birthweight
☐ Smaller neonatal head circumference
☐ Neonatal death
☐ Childhood impairments in neuromotor (*i.e.*, nonambulatory cerebral palsy), neurocognitive (abnormal attention, memory, or behavior) or neurosensory (vision or hearing) skills at five years of age among children born at ≥37 weeks' gestation

9. Apart from the commonly disclosed benefits with regard to the risk of respiratory distress syndrome, address the physician's inquiry regarding other benefits of a primary course of antenatal pulmonary corticosteroids for consideration in future counseling of patients, where clinically indicated. *(1 point each)*

5

Benefits of a *primary course* of antenatal pulmonary corticosteroids:

Decreased rates of
☐ Intraventricular hemorrhage (IVH)
☐ Necrotizing enterocolitis (NEC)
☐ Systemic infections in the first 48 hours of life
☐ Perinatal and neonatal death

Decreased needs for
☐ Mechanical ventilation

In conversation with the physician, you mention your intent to determine whether intravenous magnesium sulfate, given for a maximum of 24 hours to achieve fetal neuroprotection, is indicated at this time. You highlight that although international guidance varies with regard to gestational age ranges,[†] dosing regimens,[‡] and aspects surrounding repeat treatments, this gravida at 27^{+4} weeks' gestation could benefit from mechanisms by which magnesium sulfate is theorized to reduce the risk of cerebral palsy and gross motor dysfunction.

Special notes:
† Refer to Question 18 in Chapter 9
‡ Refer to Question 29 in Chapter 38 indicating the intravenous loading and maintenance dose of magnesium sulfate

10. In the absence of contraindications,[†] elaborate on the indications for initiating magnesium sulfate for in utero neuroprotection.

2

☐ Intravenous magnesium sulfate for fetal neuroprotection is indicated when either cervical dilatation is ≥4 cm regardless of chorioamniotic membrane status, or preterm birth is planned for maternal or fetal indications within the next 24 hours (*i.e., imminent preterm birth*)

Special note:
† Refer to the Question 29 in Chapter 38 indicating contraindications to magnesium sulfate

11. Reflecting on your conversation with the referring physician, outline mechanisms that may explain how in utero exposure to magnesium sulfate provides neuroprotection for preterm newborns. *(1 point each)*

Max 3

☐ Antioxidants effects

☐ Correction of the balance between oxygen delivery versus consumption by lowering oxygen demand

☐ Cerebral vasodilatation

☐ Stabilization of neuronal membranes to prevent early abnormal neuronal cell apoptosis

☐ Promotion of neurogenesis in premature brain cell maturation by stimulating secretion of neurotrophic factors

☐ Protection against neuroinflammation

☐ Protection against injury from excitatory neurotransmitters, such as glutamate

☐ Decreasing cerebellar hemorrhage

Upon arrival two and a half hours later, maternal-fetal hemodynamic stability is ascertained while cervical dilatation has progressed to 4 cm since departure from the referring center, despite initiation of nifedipine tocolysis. Fetal viability is ascertained, and presentation remains cephalic by your bedside sonography. Intravenous penicillin G and subcutaneous morphine were last given three hours ago. The paramedic and accompanying obstetric personnel indicate the patient experienced mild side effects of nifedipine, which spontaneously resolved. The neonatology team will provide timely consultation and the patient concurs with your plan to commence magnesium sulfate neuroprotection; she appreciates knowledge of potential side effects in advance of treatment as disclosed in counseling.[†] You take this opportunity to reassure your obstetric trainee that no contraindication exists for co-administration of magnesium sulfate for neuroprotection and nifedipine, as the risk of neuromuscular blockade does not appear to be increased *(SOGC[7])*.

Over the next 12 hours, uterine contractions abate, the cervix remains unchanged, and labor is no longer considered imminent. Magnesium sulfate and antibiotics are thereby discontinued. Fetal heart tracing has been unremarkable and estimated fetal weight is consistent for gestational age.

At 28^{+0} weeks' gestation, the patient reports a sudden gush of clear vaginal fluid, for which you are promptly notified. In the absence of visual evidence, you proceed with diagnostic tests that confirm spontaneous rupture of chorioamniotic membranes.[‡] The patient is otherwise well, and electronic fetal heart tracing is appropriate; uterine quiescence is ascertained. Counseling and documentation have been completed; the neonatology team has been updated on the patient's clinical status.

Special notes:
† Refer to the Question 27 in Chapter 38 indicating side effects of magnesium sulfate
‡ Refer to Question 4 in Chapter 15 for discussion on noninvasive tests, their rationale, and caveats in diagnosis of spontaneous rupture of chorioamniotic membranes

12. Outline the perinatal benefits of antibiotics that you disclosed in patient counseling on management of preterm prelabor rupture of membranes (PPROM). *(1 point each)*

6

Increased:
☐ Latency period between PPROM and delivery *(i.e.,* decreased risk of delivery within 48 hours)

Decreased:
☐ Risk of chorioamnionitis
☐ Risk of neonatal infection
☐ Need for oxygen therapy
☐ Need for surfactant administration
☐ Abnormal cerebral ultrasound, including intraventricular hemorrhage (IVH)

You highlight to your obstetric trainee that while international practice patterns vary regarding antibiotic regimens in management of PPROM, antenatal use of amoxicillin-clavulanate (*i.e.,* co-amoxiclav) should be uniformly avoided.

13. Explain why antenatal use of amoxicillin-clavulanate is not recommended.

2

☐ Increased risk of necrotizing enterocolitis in the preterm neonate

Special note:
Refer to Kenyon S, Boulvain M, Neilson JP. Antibiotics for preterm rupture of membranes. *Cochrane Database Syst Rev.* 2013;(12):CD001058. Published 2013 Dec 2.

14. Having confirmed the patient has no drug allergies, provide one accepted antibiotic regimen for management of PPROM. *(4 points for either bullet; other regimens may be deemed appropriate based on international practice variations)*

4

Options may include:
☐ Intravenous ampicillin 2 g *plus* intravenous erythromycin 250 mg every 6 hours for 48 hours, followed by oral amoxicillin 250 mg *plus* oral erythromycin base 333 mg[†] every 8 hours for five days (ACOG[7]; *recognized by SOGC*[22])
☐ Oral erythromycin 250 mg every six hours for 10 days (RCOG[18], NICE[10b]; *recognized by SOGC*[22])

Special note:
† Oral erythromycin 250 mg every six hours for 10 days is optional

At 28[+3] weeks' gestation, the patient complains of bothersome pelvic cramping; moderate-intensity uterine contractions are palpated. Maternal vital signs are normal while the fetal heart rate is 100 bpm on auscultation. Promptly presenting to the antepartum unit, you auscultate the fetal heart rate at 90 bpm, ensuring to differentiate it from maternal pulse. On sterile digital examination, the cervix is 6 cm dilated, completely effaced with the cephalic presenting at the level of the ischial spines. Protruding beyond the fetal vertex is a soft, bulging pulsatile mass.

15. What is the most probable diagnosis?	1

☐ Umbilical cord prolapse

16. Discuss your clinical management of this obstetric emergency, noting that steps are often performed simultaneously and ensuring ongoing communication with the patient. *(1 point each)*	6

☐ Do not remove the hand inside the vagina; elevate the presenting part gently to remove pressure from the umbilical cord
☐ Activate the local obstetric emergency protocol (*i.e.,* notification of anesthesia, neonatology, operating room/theater personnel, obstetrical colleague to assist in emergency delivery, additional midwifery or nursing support, patient transport services)
☐ Continue fetal heart monitoring
☐ Consider placing the patient in Trendelenburg or knee-chest positions to alleviate cord compression
☐ Consider administration of a rapid-acting tocolytic agent to reduce pressure from the umbilical cord in the presence of uterine contractions
☐ In case of a delay to start emergency Cesarean delivery, consider filling the urinary bladder with 500–700 mL of saline to elevate the fetal presenting part and clamping the catheter; drain the bladder prior to Cesarean delivery

Emergent Cesarean delivery is uncomplicated, and the newborn cried upon delivery. In collaboration with the attending neonatology team, a 60-second delayed umbilical cord clamp (DCC) is performed. Postoperative debriefing among the medical team as well as the patient is planned. You now intend to complete your documentation, and plan to encourage the primary care provider to promote a healthy lifestyle given the long-term risk of cardiovascular morbidity and mortality after spontaneous preterm birth.

17. State the neonatal benefits of DCC, as discussed with your obstetric trainee assisting in the delivery of this patient. *(1 point each)*	Max 3

Decreased:
☐ Need for red blood cell transfusion (due to improved hemoglobin and hematocrit levels)
☐ Intraventricular hemorrhage (IVH)
☐ Necrotizing enterocolitis (NEC)
☐ In-hospital mortality[†]

Special note:
† *Refer to* Fogarty M, Osborn DA, Askie L, et al. Delayed vs early umbilical cord clamping for preterm infants: a systematic review and meta-analysis. *Am J Obstet Gynecol.* 2018;218(1):1–18.

TOTAL:	110

CHAPTER 8

Cervical Insufficiency

Marie-Julie Trahan, Amira El-Messidi,. and Richard Brown

A 30-year-old G6P2A4L1 is referred by her primary care provider to your high-risk obstetrics clinic for preconception counseling after a pregnancy loss at 21^{+4} weeks' gestation last year, shortly after incidental transvaginal cervical shortening was noted at second-trimester fetal morphology survey. After an uncomplicated first pregnancy and term delivery, she experienced four consecutive first-trimester losses for which comprehensive investigations were unremarkable.

Special note: The clinical and educational content in this case scenario relates to singleton pregnancies; readers are encouraged to refer to Question 11 in Chapter 11, 'Dichorionic Twin Pregnancy,' for evidence-based management of short cervix in twin pregnancies.

LEARNING OBJECTIVES

1. Elicit risk factors for cervical insufficiency in focused preconception history taking and provide evidence-based future prenatal management
2. Outline antenatal and intrapartum strategies that may contribute to prevention or progression of cervical insufficiency
3. Understand technical requirements in transvaginal sonographic image acquisition and cervical length assessment
4. Demonstrate the ability to counsel for transvaginal cerclage and manage postoperative care
5. Recognize indications for, timing of, and prenatal management considerations for transabdominal cerclage

SUGGESTED READINGS

1. ACOG Practice Bulletin No. 142: cerclage for the management of cervical insufficiency. *Obstet Gynecol.* 2014;123(2 Pt 1):372–379.
2. (a) Alfirevic Z, Stampalija T, Medley N. Cervical stitch (cerclage) for preventing preterm birth in singleton pregnancy. *Cochrane Database Syst Rev.* 2017;6(6):CD008991.
   (b) Eleje GU, Eke AC, Ikechebelu JI, et al. Cervical stitch (cerclage) in combination with other treatments for preventing spontaneous preterm birth in singleton pregnancies. *Cochrane Database Syst Rev.* 2020;9(9):CD012871.
3. Conde-Agudelo A, Romero R, Nicolaides KH. Cervical pessary to prevent preterm birth in asymptomatic high-risk women: a systematic review and meta-analysis. *Am J Obstet Gynecol.* 2020;223(1):42–65.

4. Gluck O, Mizrachi Y, Ginath S, et al. Obstetrical outcomes of emergency compared with elective cervical cerclage. *J Matern Fetal Neonatal Med.* 2017;30(14):1650–1654.

5. Pergialiotis V, Bellos I, Antsaklis A, et al. Presence of amniotic fluid sludge and pregnancy outcomes: a systematic review. *Acta Obstet Gynecol Scand.* 2020;99(11):1434–1443.

6. Preterm Labour and Birth. NICE Guideline NG25, November 20, 2015, last updated August 2, 2019. Available at www.nice.org.uk/guidance/ng25?unlid=9291036072016213201257. Accessed July 10, 2021.

7. Senarath S, Ades A, Nanayakkara P. Cervical cerclage: a review and rethinking of current practice. *Obstet Gynecol Surv.* 2020;75(12):757–765.

8. Shennan A, Chandiramani M, Bennett P, et al. MAVRIC: a multicenter randomized controlled trial of transabdominal vs transvaginal cervical cerclage. *Am J Obstet Gynecol.* 2020;222(3):261. e1–261.e9.

9. (a) Brown R, Gagnon R, Delisle MF. No. 373 – cervical insufficiency and cervical cerclage. *J Obstet Gynaecol Can.* 2019;41(2):233–247.

    (b) Lim KI, Butt K, Nevo O, et al. Guideline No. 401: sonographic cervical length in singleton pregnancies: techniques and clinical applications. *J Obstet Gynaecol Can.* 2020;42(11): 1394–1413.

10. Sperling JD, Dahlke JD, Gonzalez JM. Cerclage use: a review of 3 national guidelines. *Obstet Gynecol Surv.* 2017;72(4):235–241.

POINTS

1. What aspects of a focused history would you want to know? *(1 point each; max point specified per section)*

Max 10

Pregnancy-related risk factors for cervical insufficiency: *(max 6)*

General
☐ Determine whether any conceptions occurred by in vitro fertilization

First pregnancy
☐ Establish the mode of delivery
☐ Inquire whether an instrumental vaginal delivery was required, particularly if failed procedure resulted in a second-stage Cesarean section
☐ Consider obtaining delivery records to assess for intrapartum complications *(e.g., spontaneous or iatrogenic cervical tears at vaginal delivery or extensions of the surgical incisions at Cesarean section)*

Early pregnancy losses
☐ Need for dilatation and curettages in any of the pregnancy losses

Second-trimester pregnancy loss
☐ Determine whether there was a uterine overdistension-associated cause for cervical changes *(e.g., multiple gestation, polyhydramnios of any cause)*
☐ Inquire whether the patient recalls any mild abdominopelvic symptoms, changes in vaginal discharge, or symptoms of genitourinary infections prior to incidental detection of a short, dilated cervix in the mid-trimester

General medical/surgical risk factors for cervical insufficiency:[†] *(max 3)*
☐ Prior cervical surgery procedures *(e.g., loop electrocautery excision procedure [LEEP], cold knife conizaton)*

☐ Inquire about receipt of human papilloma virus vaccine *(promotes prevention of dysplasia-associated cervical surgery)*
☐ Prior hysteroscopy for any cause
☐ Polycystic ovarian syndrome *(SOGC[9a])*
☐ Mullerian anomaly *(either known to the patient or identified at her Cesarean section)*
☐ Collagen vascular disorder *(e.g., Marfan syndrome,[‡] Ehler Danlos syndrome)*

Social features:[§] *(max 1)*
☐ Cigarette smoking
☐ Illicit drug use *(e.g., cocaine)*

Special notes:
† Although in utero exposure of the patient to diethylstilbesterol increases risk of cervical insufficiency, its clinical relevance has diminished over the past decades
‡ Refer to Question 4 in Chapter 50
§ Risk factors for preterm labor may contribute to differentiation from cervical insufficiency

You learn that her first pregnancy, conceived via in vitro fertilization for sperm-related pathology, required an emergency Cesarean section after failed forceps delivery. The operative note in your center's electronic database indicates a unilateral extension of the uterine incision into the cervical mucosa which was repaired transvaginally. She subsequently had four spontaneous pregnancies, two of which required dilatation and curettages at 8 and 10 weeks' respectively; the remaining two intrauterine early pregnancy losses were managed expectantly. In vitro fertilization was performed for her latest pregnancy, which progressed well until the fetal morphology scan at 21^{+1} weeks' gestation when the cervix was noted to be 21 mm in length on transvaginal imaging, concurrent with 2 cm cervical dilatation on digital palpation. The patient had been asymptomatic. Clinical history and speculum examination did not reveal premature rupture of membranes. Fetal morphology appeared normal, without suspected uterine overdistension. Absence of genitourinary infections was confirmed within 48 hours, yet silent cervical dilatation progressed to 4 cm when uterine contractions commenced. Delivery ensued without the need for manual or surgical uterine revision.

The patient is healthy and has not required cervical procedures unrelated to pregnancies; there is no history of cervical dysplasia. Her social habits are unremarkable. As the couple are planning an in vitro procedure, the patient presents to seek your professional opinion on future antenatal management with regard to her obstetric history.

2. Identify clinical descriptors of the most recent pregnancy that raise suspicion for cervical insufficiency. *(1 point per main bullet)*

☐ History of second-trimester pregnancy loss associated with painless cervical dilatation
☐ Physical examination showed cervical dilatation at 16–23 weeks[†]
☐ Sonographic transvaginal cervical length ≤25 mm before 24 weeks' gestation, without alternative diagnoses

Special note:
† This emphasizes to the learner how findings on physical examination can define cervical insufficiency, even in the absence of pregnancy loss

3. Highlight the patient's risk factors for structural cervical weakness. *(1 point each)*   7

☐ In vitro fertilization procedures
☐ Second-stage Cesarean section
☐ Trial of instrumental vaginal delivery
☐ Cervical laceration and repair at her first delivery
☐ Recurrent pregnancy loss[†]
☐ Rapid mechanical cervical dilatation at prior dilatation and curettage procedures
☐ Prior second-trimester loss associated with asymptomatic[‡] cervical dilatation

Special notes:
† Associated with cervical insufficiency in ~8% of patients
‡ Minimal symptoms may have also been present

You inform your trainee that the incidence of cervical insufficiency is 0.5%–1% of the obstetric population, with acquired or congenital causes contributing to the individual risk assessment. Without a history to suggest congenital features, which remain rare, you take note of her multiple acquired risk factors and intend to discuss strategies that may decrease recognized contributors to cervical insufficiency.

The patient is aware that laboratory tests are not helpful in screening, diagnosis, or management of cervical insufficiency, yet inquires about the potential role of other investigations in ascertaining a diagnosis outside of pregnancy.

4. Indicate nonlaboratory investigations that have been studied as potential diagnostic tools   5
   for cervical insufficiency in the nonpregnant state, highlighting which have proven most
   useful, if any. *(1 point each, unless specified; max points indicated where relevant)*

Investigations: *(max 3)*

Radiologic modalities
☐ Magnetic resonance imaging (MRI)
☐ Ultrasound
☐ Hysterosalpingography

Mechanical techniques
☐ Cervical dilators
☐ Balloon traction
☐ Cervical resistance studies[†]

Surgical procedure[†]
☐ Hysteroscopy

Value: *(2)*
☐ None of the investigations are diagnostic, although imaging modalities (*i.e.*, MRI, ultrasound, and hysterosalpingography) contribute to determining utero-cervical anomalies

Special notes:

† *Refer to* Anthony GS, Walker RG, Robins JB, Cameron AD, Calder AA. Management of cervical weakness based on the measurement of cervical resistance index. *Eur J Obstet Gynecol Reprod Biol.* 2007;134(2):174–178.

5. Discuss <u>pregnancy-related strategies</u> that may contribute to prevention or progression of cervical insufficiency in this patient's future singleton pregnancy. *(1 point per main bullet)*

Max 5

Antepartum:

☐ Routine genitourinary culture screening at the first prenatal visit

☐ In case of early pregnancy failure or therapeutic termination, consider medical methods[†] and/or gentle cervical ripening (*e.g.*, laminaria) for uterine evacuation over a primary aspiration procedure

☐ Arrange for serial transvaginal cervical length assessments starting at 16 weeks until 24 weeks' gestation

　　○ *There is no consensus on optimal timing or frequency of serial cervical length assessments (SOGC[9b])*

☐ Prophylactic supplemental progesterone from 16 to 34 weeks, at least *(may continue to ~36^{+6} weeks' gestation)*

☐ *Consideration* for prophylactic cerclage in subsequent pregnancy

　　○ *International jurisdictions differ in required number of prior second-trimester losses for history-indicated cerclage*

　　○ *Ultrasound-based cerclage requires a short cervix ≤ 25 mm prior to 24 weeks in the next pregnancy in the context of her prior loss*

Intrapartum:

☐ Reinforce the importance of achieving complete cervical dilatation prior to starting the active second stage of labor

☐ Ensure proper technique/skilled provider at instrumental delivery, where required

Special note:

† As this patient had one prior Cesarean section, misoprostol may be administered for future first- or second-trimester pregnancy loss (*e.g.*, pregnancy failure, therapeutic termination, or fetal demise) in the absence of placenta previa or accreta spectrum

6. Counsel the patient on potential benefits of cerclage in a future singleton pregnancy with confirmed cervical insufficiency. *(1 point each)*

2

☐ Decreased likelihood of preterm delivery/pregnancy loss *(Cochrane review[2a])*

☐ No difference in serious neonatal morbidity *(Cochrane review[2a])*

☐ Presumptive prevention of intra-amniotic infection, preterm prelabor rupture of membranes (PPROM), and prolapsed amniotic membranes

You teach your trainee that while cerclage can improve obstetric outcome, its use <u>without</u> a clear history of cervical insufficiency may be detrimental to maternal-fetal outcome.

7. Highlight *potentially* negative consequences associated with elective cerclage for a patient whose clinical history of cervical insufficiency is *unclear*. *(1 point each)*	Max 2

Increased risks of:
- ☐ Preterm birth prior to 37 weeks' gestation
- ☐ Preterm prelabor rupture of membranes (PPROM)
- ☐ Perinatal morbidity and mortality

8. Apart from an inconsistent clinical history, list circumstances where you would <u>not</u> offer a cerclage procedure for cervical insufficiency. *(1 point each)*	Max 7

Contraindications to cerclage:[†]
- ☐ Active preterm labor, nonresponsive to tocolytic agents, where applicable
- ☐ Cervical dilatation >4 cm
- ☐ Clinical or sonographic signs of intrauterine infection
- ☐ Preterm prelabor rupture of membranes (PPROM)
- ☐ Active vaginal bleeding
- ☐ Evidence of fetal compromise (*e.g.*, demise, lethal anomaly)
- ☐ *Controversial* upper gestational age limit: the procedure is not generally considered at >24 weeks' gestation [*i.e.*, viability] *(ACOG[1], SOGC[9a])*, or >27[+6] weeks' gestation *(NICE[6])[‡]*
- ☐ Müllerian anomalies *(Controversial; limited evidence suggests consideration for high vaginal or transabdominal cerclage)*

Special notes:
- † Presence of placenta previa (without bleeding) does not prohibit cerclage placement
- ‡ Physical examination-indicated cerclage may be considered up to 27[+6] weeks' gestation with asymptomatic cervical dilation in the presence of exposed, unruptured amniotic membranes *(NICE[6])*

Within 18 months, planned repeat in vitro fertilization results in a viable singleton pregnancy. First-trimester fetal morphology is unremarkable, with a low risk of aneuploidy. No infections are detected on routine genitourinary screening; serial transvaginal cervical lengths are arranged, and vaginal progesterone commenced at 16 weeks' gestation. Extensive counseling was considered with regard to the potential for offering a cerclage.

9. In addition to the antenatal care plan, indicate important aspects of clinical counseling with regard to cervical incompetence at the principal prenatal visit. *(1 point per main and subbullet)*   5

☐ Reassure her that bed rest, activity restriction, or pelvic rest *(i.e., avoidance of sexual activity)* are not warranted, given unproven benefits on pregnancy outcomes as well as significant associated psychosocial stressors

☐ Encourage early reporting of symptoms potentially associated with cervical insufficiency:[†]
  ○ Lower abdominal cramps or contractions
  ○ Pelvic pressure
  ○ Increased amount, change in color, or thinning of vaginal discharge

Special note:

† On its own, this statement response provides suboptimal directive counseling; mention of specific symptoms to address in patient counseling is preferred

At 18 weeks' gestation, transvaginal cervical length is 30 mm; no change is noted with Valsalva maneuver. The routine fetal biometry and morphology sonogram at 20^{+2} weeks' gestation shows the following, where cervical length is now 15 mm at rest[†]; the patient remains asymptomatic and amniotic membranes are intact.

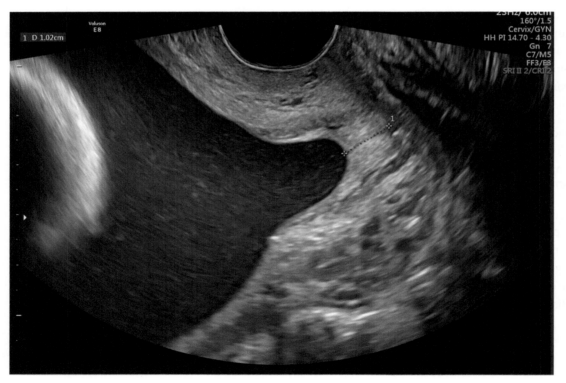

Figure 8.1

With permission: Courtesy of Dr R. Brown

There is no association between this case scenario and this patient's image. Image used for educational purposes only.

As the patient wishes to salvage the pregnancy, she chooses to undergo therapeutic cerclage procedure, with primary objective to support the internal os and prevent further opening.

You teach your trainee that had transvaginal cervical length ≤25 mm occurred in a patient *without* prior preterm birth, evidence would not support cerclage placement given absence of preterm birth reduction or improved neonatal outcomes *(ACOG[1], SOGC[9a], NICE[6])*, with limited evidence of benefit for transvaginal cervical length <10–15 mm. You also mention that cervical pessaries do not reduce preterm birth or improve perinatal outcome *(Suggested Reading 3)*.

Special note:
† There is no amniotic debris, sludge or biofilm to suggest intra-amniotic infection; application of Valsalva maneuver is not required in presence of a short or open cervix

10. You report the presence of funneling of the internal cervical os. Explain to your trainee why objective measurements including its width, length, and proportion within the cervix are not specified in your sonographic report.

2

☐ Quantifiable measurements of the cervical funneling vary during the examination and are not useful prognosticators

11. Using a clean covered probe, explain to your trainee the technical steps required to obtain this transvaginal cervical length assessment. *(1 point per main bullet)*

6

☐ Ensure the bladder is empty
☐ Gently insert the probe into the anterior vaginal fornix, while adjusting the probe to avoid excessive pressure; anterior and posterior cervical tissue should be of nearly equal thickness
☐ Obtain a sagittal long-axis image of the entire cervix to occupy 75% of the screen
☐ Ensure the internal os, external os, and endocervical mucosa are visible
☐ Measure the cervical length along the endocervical canal between the internal and external os
☐ Use the shortest-best measurement of three image sets/measurements taken over approximately three minutes
  ○ *Selecting the best image of the top three introduces variability and is not advised*

Special note: (a) The Society for Maternal-Fetal Medicine. CLEAR – Cervical Length Education and Review. 2018. Available at https://clear.perinatalquality.org/default.aspx; (b) Fetal Medicine Foundation. Cervical assessment. Available at https://fetalmedicine.org/fmf-certification-2/cervical-assessment-1, accessed July 18, 2021.

Using the patient's image, you show your trainee that the endocervical canal commonly appears straight when the cervix is short, contrary to an occasional curvilinear appearance with longer length. You mention that in the later circumstance, cervical length may be measured as a straight line between the internal and external os or as a sum of two straight lines formed along the curvature.

12. Address three reasons why tracing the endocervical canal in cervical length assessment is not preferred. *(1 point each)*   3

☐ Hypotenuse of a 'triangle' represents the shortest distance between two points
☐ Manual tracing method introduces variation in measurement
☐ Curvilinear endocervical canal commonly implies a longer cervix

13. Identify two of each hematologic, amniotic fluid biomarkers and sonographic features that may indicate an intra-amniotic inflammatory process or infection. *(1 point per main bullet)*   6

Hematologic:
☐ Leukocytosis *(above normal pregnancy range)*
☐ Increased C-reactive protein

Sonographic:
☐ Evidence of intra-amniotic debris *(i.e., 'sludge' or biofilm)*
  ○ *Majority of evidence demonstrates risk of preterm birth and possibly increased neonatal morbidity and mortality (Suggested Reading 5)*
☐ Hour-glassing or prolapsing membranes into the vaginal cavity

Amniotic fluid biomarkers:[†]
☐ Interleukin-6
☐ Lactate dehydrogenase
☐ Leukocyte count
☐ Glucose concentration

Special note:
† Gram stain is not considered a 'biomarker'

14. Indicate clinical management considerations for this patient prior to the cerclage procedure.[†] *(1 point each)*   Max 3

☐ Urinalysis and culture
☐ Vaginal culture for bacterial vaginosis
☐ Consideration for a short course of indomethacin therapy for amniotic fluid reduction and its anti-inflammatory benefit
☐ Consideration for screening for vaginal *Mycoplasma hominis* and *Ureaplasma* species *(where locally available)*

Special note:
† Routine screening for sexually transmitted infections does not improve outcomes after cerclage; screening is warranted for women at increased risk

15. Rationalize why genitourinary screening for *M. hominis* and *Ureaplasma* spp. infections is not uniformly practiced despite known associations with adverse obstetric outcome. *(1 point each)*

Max 2

☐ Difficulty in establishing causality between *Mycoplasma* species and infection as such pathogens are rarely found in isolation
☐ Pathogens are found in asymptomatic colonization of the genitourinary tract
☐ Limited explanations for biologic pathogenicity

You utilize the available simulation model to demonstrate to your obstetric trainee the technical aspects of the McDonald and Shirodkar approaches which may be performed using different suture materials, including braided Mersilene tape, prolene, delayed absorbable materials or mesh. You explain that available evidence does not favor a surgical technique or suture *(ACOG[1], SOGC[9a], NICE[6])*.

Your trainee recalls learning of the low cerclage-related complication rate, generally being <6%,[†] for *elective* procedures, increasing with advancing gestation and cervical change.

Special note:
† Final report of the Medical Research Council/Royal College of Obstetricians and Gynaecologists multicentre randomised trial of cervical cerclage. MRC/RCOG Working Party on Cervical Cerclage. *Br J Obstet Gynaecol.* 1993;100(6):516–523.

16. Indicate procedure-related risks of <u>transvaginal cerclage</u> you may discuss during the patient consent process. *(1 point each)*

Max 8

Intraoperative risks:
☐ Iatrogenic rupture of amniotic membranes
☐ Cervical laceration *(may occur postoperatively with cervical dilatation prior to cerclage removal)*
☐ Injury to the bladder or rectum (± vesicocervical, cervicovaginal, or rectovaginal fistula)
☐ Vaginal bleeding/hemorrhage *(lower risk with transvaginal than transabdominal cerclage)*

Postoperative risks:
☐ Uterine contractions/irritability ± preterm labor
☐ Infection *(e.g., cervicovaginal, chorioamnionitis, septicemia)*
☐ Suture migration
☐ Spontaneous preterm prelabor rupture of amniotic membranes *(controversial)*
☐ Uterine rupture
☐ Intrapartum pyrexia and endometritis
☐ Cervical dystocia and Cesarean delivery *(possibly due to cervical scarring or stenosis)*

Consent is obtained, absence of genitourinary infections confirmed, and fetal viability is ascertained just prior to the operative procedure. Following an uncomplicated cerclage, the patient will be discharged from hospital upon ambulation and voiding after regional anesthesia.[†] Paracetamol (acetaminophen) has been satisfactory for postoperative analgesia.

Special note:
† Hospitalization for clinical monitoring postcerclage may be warranted for cerclage-associated cervical dilation with/without bulging amniotic membranes

---

17. Outline your evidence-based clinical and sonographic management postcerclage.   6
    (1 point per main bullet)

☐ Inform the patient that she may have mild lower abdominal cramps, vaginal spotting, and dysuria for several days
  ○ *Lower abdominal cramps relate to transiently increased prostaglandin levels postcerclage*
  ○ *Dysuria relates to the effect of surgical retractors*
☐ Encourage reporting of vaginal fluid loss
☐ Evidence for combined surgical and nonsurgical (*e.g.*, continuation of the patient's progesterone) therapy is lacking (*Cochrane review[2b]*)
☐ Discuss the lack of evidence proving benefit from abstinence from sexual activity or decreased physical activity on obstetric outcome, while acknowledging individual provider practice variations exist
☐ While evidence does not show benefit from routine postcerclage sonographic monitoring, ultrasound assessment may be considered for patients at increased risk of preterm delivery to allow for timely administration of fetal pulmonary corticosteroids and consideration for neuroprotection with magnesium sulfate
☐ Plan elective removal of the cerclage at 36^{+0} to 37^{+0} weeks (*ACOG[1], NICE[6]*), or up to 38 weeks (*SOGC[9a]*); if this patient opts for a repeat Cesarean delivery, the cerclage may be removed at the time of surgery (*ACOG[1], NICE[6]*)

SCENARIO A
Pregnancy progresses well with the transvaginal cerclage. At 28 weeks' gestation, she presents with confirmed preterm prelabor rupture of membranes (PPROM) without contractions or vaginal bleeding; the patient is afebrile and serum laboratory investigations do not demonstrate an infectious process. The fetus is in the cephalic presentation; cardiotocography (CTG) is appropriate for gestational age.

---

18. What are your general management considerations with respect to timing of cerclage   2
    removal in the context of PPROM between 24- and 34-weeks' gestation? *(1 point each)*

☐ Serum C-reactive protein can assist with decision-making about immediate or delayed (48 hours) removal of the cerclage to benefit from fetal pulmonary corticosteroids (*SOGC[9]*)

OR

Cerclage removal or retention is reasonable, after consideration of risks of preterm delivery and infection, respectively (*ACOG[1]*)

Special note:
Latency antibiotics for longer than seven days is not recommended (*ACOG[1]*)

SCENARIO B

(This is a continuation of the clinical scenario after Question 17)

Pregnancy progresses well with the transvaginal cerclage. At 28 weeks' gestation, she presents with uterine contractions appearing as 250 Montevideo units on the CTG tracing; fetal cardiac tracing is appropriate for gestational age. Fetal presentation is cephalic, amniotic membranes are intact and there is no vaginal bleeding. The patient is afebrile and serum laboratory investigations do not demonstrate an infectious process.

19. Inform your trainee of maternal-fetal circumstances that may require emergency removal of the cerclage; clinical circumstances may or may not relate to this patient. *(1 point each)*

Max 4

☐ Uterine contractions associated with cervical dilatation or cerclage under tension
☐ Chorioamnionitis or sepsis
☐ Active vaginal bleeding
☐ PPROM
☐ Other complications requiring delivery *(e.g., fetal demise/termination for malformation, abnormal fetal CTG tracing, maternal medical/obstetric morbidities)*

SCENARIO C

(This is a continuation of the clinical scenario after either scenario A or B)

Shortly after removal of the cerclage, the patient progresses in labor and delivers a vigorous newborn appropriate for gestational age. Her postpartum course is unremarkable, and a postpartum visit is arranged.

You subsequently counsel her that transabdominal cerclage, preferably placed laparoscopically at the cervico-isthmic region, is offered after transvaginal cerclage resulted in second-trimester pregnancy loss[†] *(ACOG[1], SOGC[9a], NICE[6])* with associated reductions in preterm birth *(Suggested Reading 8)*.

Special note:

† Other indications include posttrachelectomy or in the presence of dense cervical scarring preventing transvaginal procedures

20. In general terms, inform your trainee of possible timing considerations for abdominal cerclage procedures. *(1 point each)*

4

☐ Prepregnancy
☐ First trimester
☐ Early second trimester *(i.e., 14–15 weeks' gestation)*
☐ At the time of trachelectomy

21. Counsel the patient on prenatal management considerations after transabdominal cerclage. *(1 point each)*   4

Early intrauterine pregnancy loss:
☐ Trans-cerclage uterine suction curettage or dilatation and extraction is possible prior to ~18 weeks' gestation

Therapeutic pregnancy termination:
☐ The cerclage can be cut via a posterior colpotomy *(NICE[6])*
☐ Delivery through a hysterotomy is required if dilatation and extraction is not feasible

Delivery planning:
☐ Elective Cesarean delivery is required, or at onset of labor *(i.e., to avoid risk of uterine rupture)*

Prior to leaving for vacation, a colleague later transfers care of a patient at 21[+6] weeks' gestation with incidental discovery of bulging amniotic membranes into the vaginal cavity at second-trimester morphology survey. Fetal assessment is unremarkable. Your colleague informs you the cervix is 2 cm dilated and genitourinary screening tests for infections have been performed. As the patient requests all measures to salvage the pregnancy, she has been extensively counseled about risks and complications associated with a rescue cerclage procedure and has consented to surgery.

22. Highlight essential aspects of your clinical management and surgical approach to cerclage placement with prolapsing amniotic membranes. *(1 point each)*   Max 4

☐ Preoperative indomethacin administration for up to 48 hours to benefit from its effect on fetal renal function in decreasing fluid production
☐ Preoperative and intraoperative Trendelenburg position to facilitate recession of bulging amniotic membranes
☐ Consideration for preoperative amnioreduction to reduce amniotic fluid volume *(ACOG[1], NICE[6])*, or amniocentesis to both reduce fluid volume and rule out infection *(SOGC[9a])*
☐ Consideration for use of nitroglycerin to promote uterine relaxation for membrane replacement into the cervix
☐ Gently support amniotic membranes into the cervix using ring forceps loaded with a surgical sponge, a bladder catheter balloon, sponge-filled condom, or operator's fingers

Special note:
The ongoing trial, Israfil-Bayli F, Morton VH, Hewitt CA, et al. C-STICH: Cerclage Suture Type for an Insufficient Cervix and its effect on Health outcomes-a multicentre randomised controlled trial. *Trials.* 2021;22(1):664, is expected to provide high-quality evidence on the selection of suture material

<u>**TOTAL:**</u>   **100**

CHAPTER 9

Fetal Growth Restriction

Amira El-Messidi, Juliana Martins, and Alfred Abuhamad

A 29-year-old G2P1 at seven weeks' gestation is referred to your tertiary center for consultation and prenatal care. Obstetric history is significant for fetal growth restriction (FGR) requiring preterm delivery at 33 weeks' gestation. Her son's birthweight was 1400 g. The patient's prenatal care and delivery were at another center, and her medical chart is unavailable at the time of initial consultation.

LEARNING OBJECTIVES

1. Take a focused history, recognizing maternal, fetal, and placental risk factors in a prenatal patient with prior FGR
2. Recognize maternal vascular malperfusion and structural abnormalities of the placental unit as possible etiologies for the early-onset FGR phenotype
3. Understand the potential roles of maternal sonographic parameters and serum analytes in screening for early FGR
4. Detail the contribution of arterial and venous Doppler assessments in the assessment and management of early-onset FGR
5. Establish an evidence-based management for early-onset FGR, appreciating international protocol variations

SUGGESTED READINGS

1. Fetal growth restriction: ACOG Practice Bulletin, No. 227. *Obstet Gynecol.* 2021;137(2): e16–e28.
2. Figueras F, Gratacos E. Stage-based approach to the management of fetal growth restriction. *Prenat Diagn.* 2014; 34(7):655–659.
3. Kingdom JC, Audette MC, Hobson SR, et al. A placenta clinic approach to the diagnosis and management of fetal growth restriction. *Am J Obstet Gynecol.* 2018;218(2S):S803–S817.
4. Khong TY, Mooney EE, Ariel I, et al. Sampling and definitions of placental lesions: Amsterdam placental workshop group consensus statement. *Arch Pathol Lab Med.* 2016;140(7): 698–713.
5. Lausman A, Kingdom J. Intrauterine growth restriction: screening, diagnosis, and management. *J Obstet Gynecol Can.* 2013;35(8):741–748.

6. Lees CC, Stampalija T, Baschat AA, et al. ISUOG Practice Guidelines: diagnosis and management of small-for-gestational-age fetus and fetal growth restriction. *Ultrasound Obstet Gynecol.* 2020; 56(2):298–312.

7. McCowan LM, Figueras F, Anderson NH. Evidence-based national guidelines for the management of suspected fetal growth restriction: comparison, consensus, and controversy. *Am J Obstet Gynecol.* 2018;218(2S): S855–S868.

8. Melamed N, Baschat A, Yinon Y, et al. FIGO (International Federation of Gynecology and Obstetrics) initiative on fetal growth: best practice advice for screening, diagnosis, and management of fetal growth restriction. *Int J Gynaecol Obstet.* 2021;152(Suppl 1):3–57.

9. Robson SC, Martin WL, Morris RK. The investigation and management of the small-for-gestational age fetus. Green Top Guideline No. 31, 2013. 2nd ed. Available at www.rcog.org.uk/globalassets/documents/guidelines/gtg_31.pdf. Accessed August 15, 2020.

10. Salomon LJ, Alfirevic Z, Da Silva Costa F, et al. ISUOG Practice Guidelines: ultrasound assessment of fetal biometry and growth. *Ultrasound Obstet Gynecol.* 2019;53(6):715–723.

11. Society for Maternal-Fetal Medicine, Martins JG, Biggio JR, et al. Society for Maternal-Fetal Medicine (SMFM) Consult Series No. 52: diagnosis and management of fetal growth restriction. *Am J Obstet Gynecol.* 2020;223(4):B2–B17.

POINTS

1. What aspects of a focused history would you want to know? *(1 point per main bullet, unless specified)*   Max 25

Current pregnancy:
☐ Establish whether artificial reproductive techniques were required
☐ Determine if gestational age is established by menstrual or ultrasound dating
☐ Interval since last pregnancy
☐ Establish whether preconceptional folic acid was taken *(ideally three months preconceptionally)*
☐ Presence of bleeding, cramping, nausea or vomiting
☐ Determine whether conception occurred with the same partner as prior pregnancy
☐ Inquire about prepregnancy weight

Obstetric and medical history:
☐ Antenatal chronology of FGR: early vs late onset, results of laboratory and sonographic investigations
☐ Fetal causes of FGR: *(2 points for indicating four fetal factors)*
  ○ *e.g* aneuploidy, major malformations, genetic syndromes, congenital infections, inborn errors of metabolism, multiple gestation
☐ Maternal causes of FGR: *(1 point per subbullet)*
  ○ Pregnancy-associated causes: heavy first-trimester bleeding, preeclampsia syndromes, placental abruption
  ○ Vascular disorders: *e.g.,* chronic hypertension, thromboembolic events
  ○ Autoimmune disorders: *e.g.,* lupus, antiphospholipid antibody syndrome
  ○ Hematologic conditions: sickle cell disease, severe chronic anemia
  ○ Endocrinopathies: *e.g.,* pregestational diabetes mellitus type 1 or 2, systemic lupus erythematosus

- ○ Cardiac disorders: *e.g.*, cyanotic congenital heart disease, cardiomyopathy, heart failure
- ○ Chronic pulmonary diseases
- ○ Renal insufficiency (primary or secondary)
- ○ Gastrointestinal: *e.g.*, inflammatory bowel diseases
- ○ Infectious diseases including maternal travel history to malaria-, tuberculosis-, or Zika-endemic areas
- ○ Nutritional disorders
- ○ Teratogenic exposures: *e.g.*, prepregnancy pelvic radiation, or therapeutic radiation during pregnancy, inadvertent use of teratogenic agents
- ○ Substance-use: cigarette smoking (or second-hand exposure), chronic alcohol use, or illicit drug use
- ○ Social factors: consanguinity, ethnicity, residing in high altitudes, stress
- ○ Psychiatric conditions
- ○ Structural factors: uterine cavity anomalies, uterine fibroids
- ☐ Placental factors: *(1 point per subbullet)*
- ○ Sonographic abnormalities: *e.g.*, implantation or cord aberrations, tumors *(chorioangioma)*, chronic abruption, bilobed placenta
- ○ Pathology report: low weight, abnormal histology or morphology, infections
- ☐ Delivery information: *(1 point per subbullet)*
- ○ Indications for timing of prior preterm delivery
- ○ Mode of delivery (ideally, obtain operative note if delivery was by Cesarean section)

Medications:
- ☐ Prescribed and nonprescribed pharmacologic agents *(may contribute to decreased fetal growth: e.g., atenolol)*

Surgical history:
- ☐ Prior surgeries, particularly uterine

Family history:
- ☐ Fetal or maternal causes of FGR

You learn that the patient is a healthy Caucasian and note she has a normal body habitus. This is a planned spontaneous pregnancy with the partner who is also the father of her son. Gestational age has been determined by menstrual dating based on regular menstrual cycles. She does not have obstetric complaints. Neither she nor her partner smoke cigarettes or use illicit substances; the patient does not drink alcohol while pregnant.

Two years ago, her pregnancy progressed unremarkably until 25 weeks' gestation when fundal height significantly lagged behind gestational age. Fetal growth restriction was confirmed, and her care was transferred to a high-risk center. The patient remained healthy antenatally and post-natally and recalls that maternal and fetal investigations for FGR were unremarkable. A Cesarean section was required at 33 weeks' gestation for static fetal growth and abnormal fetal Doppler velocimetry. Her son was admitted to the neonatal intensive care unit (NICU) for several weeks; he had no malformations, aneuploidy, or perinatal infections. Placental pathology and details of her operative delivery remain unavailable.

The patient agrees to a dating ultrasound which confirms a single viable intrauterine pregnancy with normal size and morphology of the yolk sac and gestational sac. Images are satisfactory: dating corresponds to 7^{+6} weeks by clinical dating and 7^{+1} weeks by crown–rump length (CRL).

2-A. Discuss your choice of gestational age estimate.   1

☐ Sonographic gestational age assignment by CRL is superior in dating of spontaneously conceived pregnancies compared to menstrual dating regardless of menstrual cycle regularity[†]

2-B. For a CRL corresponding to 7^{+1} weeks, approximate the embryonic size in millimeters.   1

☐ 7^{+1} weeks = 50 days; 50 − 42 = ~8 mm
  ○ *[where '42' is a constant; 'rule of thumb' CRL (mm) + 42 = gestation (days)]*

Special note:
† Refer to Questions 3 and 5 in Chapter 1 for general advantages of first-trimester sonography and superiority of ultrasound in redating pregnancy, respectively

3. With regard to prior early-onset FGR, which laboratory investigations <u>might</u> you test the patient for, in addition to the routine prenatal work-up?   3

☐ Antiphospholipid antibodies (*i.e.,* lupus anticoagulant, anticardiolipin antibodies, anti-β2-glycoprotein-I antibodies)
  ○ *This patient fulfills the criteria of at least one premature birth of a morphologically normal fetus before 34 weeks' gestation due to placental insufficiency*

Special note:
FIGO[8] does not recommend routine screening for antiphospholipid antibodies in women with a history of FGR, in the absence of a history of thromboembolism or pregnancy loss

Antiphospholipid antibodies are within normal limits and prenatal investigations are normal.

You have now received her medical chart indicating unremarkable antenatal and neonatal work-up for FGR. The operative delivery report indicates a bicornuate uterus and pathology was significant for infarcts in the circumvallate placenta, with histologic decidual vasculopathy and syncytial knotting.

4. Explain how the Mullerian anomaly may have contributed to FGR. *(1 point each)*   2

☐ Cavitary limitations
☐ Implantation of the placenta over suboptimally vascularized myometrium

5. In addition to infarction and circumvallate placenta, identify five _structural_ abnormalities   Max 5
    of the placental unit that may, _in part,_ contribute to FGR. _(1 point each)_

☐ Hemangioma
☐ Chorioangioma/teratoma
☐ Hydatidiform mole
☐ Bilobed placenta
☐ Velomentous cord insertion
☐ Marginal/eccentric cord insertion _(via attenuated vascular branching in the contralateral chorionic plate)_
☐ Placenta of multiple gestation
☐ Single umbilical artery
☐ Hypercoiled umbilical cord
☐ Increased length of the umbilical cord
☐ True knot in the umbilical cord

The patient progresses well and has the 12 weeks' routine first-trimester sonogram for anatomy and aneuploidy risk assessment.

Multiple algorithms in screening of FGR are currently being investigated, with controversial value to date.

6-A.   Discuss the Doppler parameter that may contribute to early identification of FGR in   1
       predefined pregnancies at-risk. _(1 point for main bullet and either subbullet, respectively)_

☐ Uterine artery Doppler[§]
   ○ Assesses flow impedance due to maternal vascular malperfusion of the placenta
   ○ Mean pulsatility index (PI) >2.35 has a sensitivity of 11.7% for isolated prediction of FGR _(Normal Doppler indices have a high negative predictive value in women with a baseline increased risk of FGR)_

Special note:
§ _SMFM suggests against the use of uterine artery Doppler in management of early- (or late-) onset FGR_

                                                                                               Max 2

6-B.   Which maternal serum analytes may be associated with FGR? _(1 point each)_

☐ Low PAPP-A (pregnancy-associated plasma protein-A)
☐ Low PlGF alone or high sFlt: PlGF ratio, which is a ratio of an anti-angiogenic: pro-angiogenic marker (placental growth factor; soluble fms-like tyrosine kinase-1)
☐ Low free ß-hCG (beta human chorionic gonadotropin)
☐ High MSAFP (maternal serum alpha-fetoprotein)

                                                                                               1

6-C.   What is the mechanism by which low PAPP-A _may_ contribute to FGR?

☐ PAPP-A normally cleaves IGFBP-4 (insulin growth factor binding protein-4), which is a potent inhibitor of insulin-like growth factors (IGF-1, IGF-2) that play a central role in fetal growth

Ultrasound shows an NT of 1.0 mm and fetal morphology is normal for 12 weeks' gestation. As she was scanned in your high-risk unit, uterine artery Dopplers were assessed: mean PI is 2.85. PAPP-A is <0.41 MoM and PlGF is <100 pg/mL.

7. Discuss your counseling and management of the patient's risk for FGR. *(1 point per main bullet)*	Max 6

☐ Inform the patient of the increased risk for recurrence based on her obstetric history and current prenatal screening parameters

☐ Suggest cell-free DNA (cfDNA) testing or sonographic and maternal serum prenatal screening (*e.g.,* sequential or contingent screening) for aneuploidy risk assessment, explaining to the patient that, in isolation, maternal age and nuchal translucency (NT) risk assessment are not recommended screening tests

☐ Consideration for nightly low-dose aspirin (controversial)
  ○ *Low-dose aspirin may be ineffective in reducing recurrence of normotensive FGR*
  ○ *While SOGC and RCOG recommend low-dose aspirin for prior FGR, ACOG recommends against low-dose aspirin for prevention of recurrent FGR in otherwise low-risk women, and FIGO indicates insufficient evidence for routine use of low-dose aspirin for women at high-risk of FGR*

☐ Plan the second-trimester fetal morphology scan, informing the patient that early FGR or malformations increase the risk of aneuploidy and adverse outcome

☐ Document fundal height measurements from 24 weeks' gestation, despite its low sensitivity of ~17% in detection of FGR

☐ Plan serial sonographic fetal growth monitoring starting from ~24 weeks' gestation

☐ Plan monitoring of gestational weight gain, providing information about target weight gain based on BMI

Special notes:
- Screening for inherited thrombophilias in the context of placental-mediated pregnancy complications is not indicated
- Treatment with sildenafil is not advised
- Anticoagulant treatment/prophylaxis is not advised
- Activity restriction for the purpose of improving fetal growth is not advised

Results of genetic screening reveal a low risk for trisomy 13, 18, and 21. Fetal biometry is on the 20th percentile at 20 weeks' gestation with normal morphology and no soft markers detected. Placental implantation is fundal, umbilical cord insertion is normal, and amniotic fluid volume appears appropriate.

At 26 weeks' gestation, suboptimal growth velocity is noted, with overall biometry falling to the 9th percentile with abdominal circumference being on the 8th percentile from the prior 17th percentile. Head circumference remains within normal limits on the 18th centile. Amniotic fluid volume is normal. Umbilical artery (UA) Doppler shows continuous forward flow with UA pulsatility index (UA-PI) >95th percentile.

The patient is clinically well and has no obstetric complaints. She remains normotensive with adequate weight gain.

8. Variations exist in defining early FGR. What are the most common definitions for <u>early FGR</u>, assuming absence of congenital anomalies? *(1 point each)*   4

☐ **(1)** Estimated fetal weight (EFW) below the 10th percentile for gestational age *(ISUOG: EFW below the third percentile; RCOG and SMFM: Severe FGR below the third percentile)*

OR

☐ Abdominal circumference below the 10th percentile for gestational age *(ISUOG: Abdominal circumference below the third percentile; RCOG also considers reduction in abdominal circumference growth velocity in defining FGR as a change of <5 mm over 14 days)*

☐ **(2)** EFW or abdominal circumference<10th percentile **and** uterine artery PI>95th percentile *(ISUOG)*

☐ **(3)** EFW or abdominal circumference<10th percentile **and** umbilical artery PI>95th percentile *(ISUOG)*

☐ **(4)** Gestational age <32 weeks with umbilical artery absent end-diastolic flow [UA-AEDF] *(ISUOG)*

9. What is the rationale for using '32 weeks' as a gestational cutoff in differentiating early versus late FGR?   Max 2

Normal fetal growth pattern: *(1 point for either bullet)*
☐ Increase in cell number and cell size until 32 weeks *(principally cellular hyperplasia until 16 weeks, followed by both hyperplasia and hypertrophy until 32 weeks)*
☐ Cellular hypertrophy is principally responsible for fetal growth after 32 weeks

Differences in fetal pathophysiological behavior: *(1 point for either bullet)*
☐ Early-onset FGR <32 weeks exhibits abnormal placental implantation that leads to increased uterine arterial resistance; fetal hypoxia ensues and requires cardiovascular adaptation
☐ Late-FGR ≥32 weeks exhibits slight deficiencies in placentation causing mild hypoxia and requiring little cardiovascular adaptation

10. Discuss the physiological bases for decreased abdominal circumference biometry among growth restricted fetuses. *(1 point each)*   2

☐ Depletion of adipose tissue
☐ Decreased hepatic size due to depleted glycogen stores

11. Assuming FGR was associated with periventricular calcifications or echogenic bowel, which perinatal infections might you consider testing for by maternal serology, based on proven causality for FGR? *(2 points per main bullet)*   4

- ☐ Cytomegalovirus (CMV)
  - ○ *Proposed mechanism via cytolysis and organ necrosis*
- ☐ Rubella
  - ○ *Proposed mechanism via necrotizing angiopathy and endothelial damage*
  - ○ *Rubella is no longer part of routine serology in the United Kingdom, although it may be considered in the work-up of FGR*

Special note:
Some jurisdictions support routine maternal serum TORCH testing in the context of FGR, despite unproven causation

She remains normotensive with no obstetrical complaints. Screening for gestational diabetes mellitus is normal. While you inform the patient that recurrent FGR is likely secondary to uteroplacental insufficiency, she is curious whether nonpathologic factors may be contributing to fetal weight.

12. Indicate nonpathological variables that affect fetal weight and growth potential. *(1 point each)*   Max 3

- ☐ Maternal age
- ☐ Parity
- ☐ Ethnicity
- ☐ Height and weight, for calculation of the body mass index
- ☐ Fetal gender

13. Attentive to your counseling whereby invasive genetic testing is not indicated based on current clinical and sonographic findings, your obstetric trainee inquires about situations where fetal karyotyping, including chromosomal microarray, would be recommended for comprehensive assessment of FGR. *(1 point each)*   4

- ☐ Presence of structural anomalies associated with genetic etiologies
- ☐ Sonographic soft markers for aneuploidy
- ☐ Early-onset FGR prior to 24 weeks' gestation, particularly in the absence of obvious signs of placental dysfunction
- ☐ Unexplained polyhydramnios

14. Given a low risk of aneuploidy and absence of suggested congenital infection, identify the   2
fetal risks of growth restriction in this case scenario. *(1 point each)*

☐ Stillbirth (~1.5% with biometry <10th percentile, and 2.5% with biometry <5th percentile)
☐ Prematurity

You intend to teach your trainee the differentiation between FGR and constitutional growth delay after this patient encounter.

15. Elaborate on the differences between pathological FGR and constitutional fetal growth   Max 3
delay *(1 point each)*

Supporting features for constitutional growth delay:
☐ Maintenance of growth velocity[†]
☐ Moderately decreased growth biometry (between 5th and 10th percentiles)[§]
☐ Appropriate fetal growth in relation to maternal factors (habitus, ethnicity)[‡]
☐ Normal sonographic markers of well-being (*i.e.,* amniotic fluid volume and Doppler velocimetry)

Special notes:
† *Refer to* Dubinsky TJ, Sonneborn R. Trouble With the Curve: Pearls and Pitfalls in the Evaluation of Fetal Growth [published correction appears in *J Ultrasound Med.* 2020 Dec;39(12):2491]. *J Ultrasound Med.* 2020;39(9):1839–1846.
§ *Refer to* Mlynarczyk M, Chauhan SP, Baydoun HA, et al. The clinical significance of an estimated fetal weight below the 10th percentile: a comparison of outcomes of <5th vs 5th–9th percentile. *Am J Obstet Gynecol.* 2017;217(2):198.e1–198.e11
‡ *Refer to* Buck Louis GM, Grewal J, Albert PS, et al. Racial/ethnic standards for fetal growth: the NICHD Fetal Growth Studies. *Am J Obstet Gynecol.* 2015;213(4):449.e1–449.e41.

The patient is compliant with medical care and lives within reasonable distance of the tertiary hospital center.

16. Discuss your management plan for this new-onset FGR at 26 weeks' gestation with increased UA resistance. *(1 point each)*

4

☐ Continue outpatient management at this time
☐ Arrange for weekly sonography for fetal Doppler and fluid assessment
  ○ *UA is the principal Doppler index; variations exist regarding assessment of other arterial indices (e.g., middle cerebral artery [MCA]) and/or venous Doppler (e.g., umbilical vein [UV] or ductus venosus [DV])*
☐ Consideration for twice weekly cardiotocographic (CTG) monitoring
☐ Plan assessment of fetal growth biometry at two-week intervals
☐ Advise early reporting of decreased fetal activity, or other obstetric complaints

Special note:
There is no consensus on the ideal frequency of monitoring in idiopathic FGR; international variations exist

Your obstetric trainee asks you about the physiological basis of the UA Doppler and its interpretation.

17. Outline the physiology and prognostic value of the UA Doppler in monitoring growth restricted fetuses. *(1 point each)*

Max 2

☐ UA Doppler reflects downstream placental resistance to the flow of deoxygenated blood returning to the uteroplacental unit
☐ All UA Doppler indices (systolic/diastolic ratio, resistive index, pulsatility index) should normally decrease progressively in the third trimester
☐ UA resistance is increased when ~30% of the villous vasculature is nonfunctional *(decreased end-diastolic flow)*
☐ Once 60%–70% of villous vasculature is obliterated, UA Doppler shows absent or reversed end-diastolic flow (UA-AEDF or UA-REDF)

At 28^{+0} weeks' gestation, UA Doppler shows AEDF. Amniotic fluid volume has decreased to the 10th percentile for gestational age. Appropriate interval fetal growth is noted. Fetal behavior, as assessed by movement and tone, is normal.

The patient remains normotensive with no history suggestive of chorioamniotic membrane rupture; fetal activity is unchanged.

18. With respect to the fetal sonographic findings, discuss your counseling and management plan at this time. *(1 point per main bullet)*   Max 7

☐ Recommend hospitalization

☐ CTG monitoring at least once to twice daily

☐ Ultrasound Doppler assessment two to three times weekly
  ○ UA-AEDF coincides with increased perinatal morbidity and mortality and changes in acid-base balance

☐ Considerations for fetal pulmonary corticosteroids if high risk of delivery is anticipated within seven days, where treatment options include either betamethasone 12 mg intramuscularly, repeated once in 24 hours, **or** dexamethasone 6 mg intramuscularly for four doses at 12-hour intervals

	NICE guideline (NG25)[†]	WHO, 2015[‡]	ACOG No. 713[#]	SOGC No. 364[§]
General timing of administration	24^{+0}–33^{+6}	24^{+0}–34^{+0}	24^{+0}–36^{+6}	24^{+0}–34^{+6}
Periviable period	23^{+0}–23^{+6} should be considered	Not mentioned	23^{+0}–24^{+0} should be considered	22^{+0}–23^{+6} should be considered
Late preterm period	34^{+0}–35^{+6} should be considered	Not mentioned	34^{+0}–36^{+6} may be considered for risk of preterm birth within seven days if no prior course was given	35^{+0}–36^{+6} may be considered

Table provided for clinical and academic interest

☐ Neonatology consultation *(assuming patient is under the care of maternal-fetal medicine)*

☐ Offer psychosocial support services

☐ If premature delivery is anticipated, fetal neuroprotection by intravenous magnesium sulfate should be given for a maximum duration of 24 hours

NICE guideline (NG25)[†]	WHO, 2015[‡]	ACOG No. 455[##]	SOGC No. 376[§§]
23^{+0}–23^{+6} (consider administration), 24^{+0}–29^{+6} (recommend administration) 30^{+0}–33^{+6} (consider administration)	Viability to 31^{+6} weeks	Viability to 31^{+6} weeks	24^{+0}–33^{+6}

Table provided for clinical and academic interest

☐ Plan to repeat sonographic fetal growth biometry in two weeks, unless earlier delivery indicated

Special notes:

† *Refer to* National Institute for Health and Care Excellence. Preterm labor and birth (2015); NICE guidance NG25. London, UK; November 20, 2015, last updated August 2, 2019. Available at www.nice.org.uk/guidance/ng25?unlid=9291036072016213201257, accessed July 10, 2021.

‡ WHO recommendations on interventions to improve preterm birth outcomes, 2015. Available at www.who.int/reproductivehealth/publications/maternal_perinatal_health/ preterm-birth-guideline/en/, accessed October 5, 2021.

Refer to Committee on Obstetric Practice. Committee Opinion No. 713: Antenatal Corticosteroid Therapy for Fetal Maturation. *Obstet Gynecol.* 2017;130(2):e102-e109. Reaffirmed 2020.

§ *Refer to* Skoll A, Boutin A, Bujold E, et al. No. 364-Antenatal Corticosteroid Therapy for Improving Neonatal Outcomes. *J Obstet Gynaecol Can.* 2018;40(9):1219–1239.

Refer to Committee Opinion No. 455: Magnesium sulfate before anticipated preterm birth for neuroprotection. *Obstet Gynecol.* 2010;115(3):669–671. Reaffirmed 2020.

§§ *Refer to* Magee LA, De Silva DA, Sawchuck D, Synnes A, von Dadelszen P. No. 376-Magnesium Sulphate for Fetal Neuroprotection. *J Obstet Gynaecol Can.* 2019;41(4): 505–522.

Follow-up sonogram in 48 hours demonstrates *'improved'* UA Doppler with continuous forward flow, although downstream resistance is increased. There are no other sonographic changes noted.

---

19. While mechanisms for the brief and transitory (7–10 days) improvements in UA Doppler in response to fetal pulmonary corticosteroids are not well established, highlight two possible explanations for this phenomenon. *(1 point each)*   2

☐ Increased blood pressure due to corticosteroid administration
☐ Increased placental corticotropin releasing hormone (CRH) mediates an increase in nitric oxide-associated vasodilation

---

20. What is the proposed pathophysiology for the idiopathic decrease in amniotic fluid volume in FGR?   1

☐ Decreased fetal urination due to hypoxia-induced redistribution of blood flow to vital organs *(i.e., brain, heart, adrenals)*

Over the following week of admission, CTG monitoring remains normal. Sonography at 29 weeks' gestation shows episodic reversed flow in the UA. Amniotic fluid volume is unchanged relative to the prior week and fetal behavioral state is normal.

During the patient's scan, your trainee seems anxious to make delivery arrangements in view of the current UA Doppler waveform.

21. Based on a current gestational age of 29 weeks with FGR and reversed UA flow, provide your evidence-based recommendation for timing of delivery.　　2

☐ Anticipate delivery planning for 30^{+0} to 32^{+0} weeks' gestation *(FIGO[8], [ACOG and SMFM][§])*

Special note:
§ *Refer to* American College of Obstetricians and Gynecologists' Committee on Obstetric Practice, Society for Maternal-Fetal Medicine. Medically Indicated Late-Preterm and Early-Term Deliveries: ACOG Committee Opinion, No. 831. *Obstet Gynecol.* 2021;138(1): e35–e39.

22. Albeit controversial, discuss the role of venous Doppler in the management of this FGR, given gestational age is below 32 weeks with UA flow reversal and otherwise stable findings. *(1 point each)*　　3

Ductus venosus Doppler:[§]
☐ May play an important role in delaying centralization by redirecting a significant amount of fetal blood from the liver to the heart to support the brain
☐ Single, strongest predictor of short-term risk of stillbirth in early FGR *(Absent/reversed a-wave doubles the daily odds of stillbirth)*

Umbilical venous Doppler:
☐ Biphasic or triphasic pulsatility reflects hemodynamic instability *(normal flow is nonpulsatile due to a high capacitance vessel)*

Special note:
§ SMFM suggests against the use of ductus venosus Doppler in management of early- (or late-) onset FGR

Your trainee recalls middle cerebral artery (MCA) Doppler being assessed in growth restricted fetuses, although is uncertain of its adjunctive value for clinical decision-making.

23. Explain to your trainee the physiological changes in the MCA, outlining its value and limitations in clinical management of FGR. *(1 point per main bullet)*   Max 3

☐ Cerebral vasodilation occurs in compensation to hypoxemia (brain-sparing), resulting in a decrease in MCA-PI

☐ Low CPR, defined by the ratio of MCA-PI/UA-PI reflects brain sparing, resulting in possible adverse perinatal outcomes, neonatal intensive care admission, decreased fetal growth velocity, intrapartum abnormal fetal heart tracings, and lower Apgar scores
  ○ Variable thresholds exist in defining abnormal CPR *(e.g., <1, <1.08, <fifth percentile, MoM<0.6765)*
  ○ Umbilico-cerebral ratio, the reverse of CPR, has been proposed to better detect abnormalities in early-FGR *(there is no strong evidence in favor of either ratio)*
  ○ Ratios are more sensitive to fetal hypoxia and more strongly associated with adverse perinatal outcome than individual Doppler components

☐ Once redistribution is present, a seemingly improved fetal state by normalization of the CPR reflects a loss of autoregulation and worsening of hemodynamic status

☐ There is no evidence-based value for use of MCA Doppler in timing delivery

Special note:
SMFM suggests against the use of MCA Doppler in management of early- (or late-) onset FGR

By 30^{+1} weeks, the UA shows unchanged velocimetry with normal flow in the DV and low MCA-PI. The umbilical vein Doppler is nonpulsatile. Amniotic fluid volume is stable on the 10th percentile for gestational age. Several echogenic foci are noted in the placental plate. The biophysical profile (BPP) score is 8/8.

The patient inquires about the discrepancy between fetal Doppler and the BPP score.

24. Interpret the relationship between fetal cardiovascular parameters and behavioral states in FGR.   1

☐ Doppler and BPP changes may occur independently *(abnormal DV may precede BPP by 48–72 hours)*
  ○ Sequence of change in BPP follows a reverse order of embryological development *(i.e., fetal heart rate is the first parameter to deteriorate, followed by breathing, movements, and lastly, tone)*

Special note:
International protocols differ regarding utility of the BPP in high-risk pregnancies
- *ISUOG, ACOG, SOGC: surveillance accepted*
- *SMFM, RCOG: surveillance disfavored*

By 30^{+3} weeks, the patient remains normotensive and continues to report fetal activity. Fetal growth velocity has plateaued, and amniotic fluid volume has further decreased. Large echogenic lesions are imaged near the fetal plate of the placenta. Doppler interrogation reveals the following:

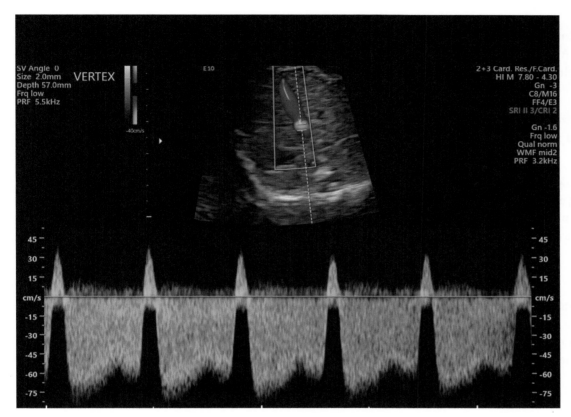

Figure 9.1

Courtesy of Professor A. Abduhamad

There is no association between this case scenario and this patient's image. Image used for educational purposes only.

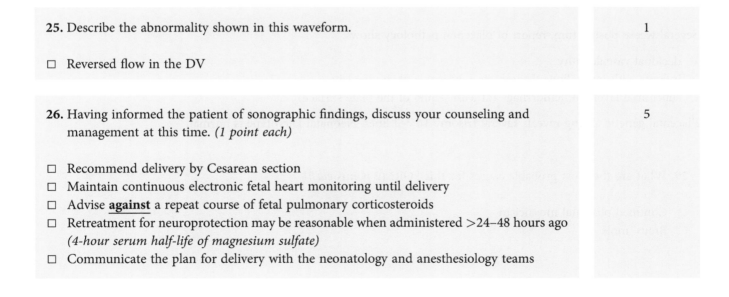

25. Describe the abnormality shown in this waveform.   1

☐ Reversed flow in the DV

26. Having informed the patient of sonographic findings, discuss your counseling and   5
management at this time. *(1 point each)*

☐ Recommend delivery by Cesarean section
☐ Maintain continuous electronic fetal heart monitoring until delivery
☐ Advise **against** a repeat course of fetal pulmonary corticosteroids
☐ Retreatment for neuroprotection may be reasonable when administered >24–48 hours ago
   (4-hour serum half-life of magnesium sulfate)
☐ Communicate the plan for delivery with the neonatology and anesthesiology teams

27. Elaborate on the mode of delivery for a growth restricted singleton in the cephalic presentation, in the absence of maternal-placental indications for Cesarean section. *(1 point each)*

2

☐ Cesarean section is recommended for spontaneous decelerations on CTG, abnormal DV Doppler, UA-AREDF, or abnormal BPP[†]; induction of labor and vaginal delivery may otherwise be clinically accepted

Special note:
† Societal organizations differ regarding assessment of the BPP score (refer to the 'special note' indicated in Question 24)

The patient has a low-transverse Cesarean section at 30^{+3} weeks. The 940-gram male neonate is vigorous and crying at birth. One-minute delayed cord-clamp is performed. Scant, clear amniotic fluid is noted. The placenta appears small and heavily calcified; histopathological assessment is planned. The uterine cavity is indeed bicornuate. Umbilical cord arterial pH is 7.20 and base excess is −9.

28. List the neonatal <u>metabolic</u> aberrations associated with FGR. *(1 point each)*

Max 6

☐ Hypoglycemia or hyperglycemia
☐ Hyperbilirubinemia
☐ Polycythemia
☐ Jaundice
☐ Hypothermia
☐ Hypocalcemia
☐ Metabolic acidemia

Several weeks postpartum, report of placental pathology shows:

- decidual vasculopathy
- infarcts with intervillous thrombi and extensive fibrin deposits
- subchorial layers of hemorrhage (at least ≥50% of the plate surface)

Placental genetic testing reveals several trisomy 16 cell lines. Neonatal karyotype is normal.

29. What are the most probable causes for this FGR? *(2 points each)*

4

☐ Confined placental mosaicism
☐ Breus' mole

At a six-week postpartum visit, you use this opportunity to discuss future health risks as both the patient's pregnancies were affected by FGR.

30-A. Explain the Barker hypothesis.	1

☐ Adverse nutrition early in life (*i.e.,* birthweight) increases the risk of metabolic syndrome

30-B. State the long-term morbidities of FGR. *(1 point each)*	Max 4

☐ Obesity
☐ Hypertension
☐ Coronary artery disease/stroke
☐ Hyperlipidemia
☐ Chronic pulmonary insufficiency and reactive airways
☐ Chronic kidney disease
☐ Neurodevelopmental impairment
☐ Non-insulin-dependent diabetes mellitus
☐ Osteoporosis

30-C. With reference to two *different* organ system manifestations in FGR, discuss the fetal pathophysiological changes that result in long-term adverse health outcomes. *(1 point per organ system)*	2

Cardiovascular
☐ Altered vascular tone starting in fetal life
☐ Increased myocardial performance index from greater afterload causes wall stress and hypertrophy

Pulmonary
☐ Abnormal pulmonary vascular development from chronic hypoxia
☐ Disruption in alveolarization from decreased fetal breathing activity, in response to a lower metabolic rate with placental insufficiency

Renal
☐ Nephron loss from intrauterine hypoxia

Neurological
☐ Delayed myelination and reduced neuronal connectivity
☐ Reduced brain volume

Endocrinologic
☐ Fetal oxidation of nonglucose substates, including amino acids and lactate, may persist in adult insulin-sensitive tissues
☐ Persistent hormonal aberrations may underly insulin resistance: decreased anabolic hormones (insulin and IGF) and increased catabolic hormones (corticosteroids)
☐ Possibly lower ß-cell mass in FGR
☐ Disturbed cholesterol metabolism due to decreased hepatic growth

31. With focus on the patient's preterm Cesarean section for FGR, what are important _____ maternal aspects of care to address in postpartum counseling? *(1 point per main bullet)*

Max 4

☐ Continue to offer psychosocial support services

☐ Encourage use of reliable contraception; avoidance of a short interpregnancy interval has dual advantages in this clinical context:
  ○ *An interpregnancy interval greater than 18–24 months is preferred for future consideration of vaginal birth after Cesarean section*
  ○ *Short interpregnancy interval is a risk factor for FGR and other adverse obstetric outcomes*

☐ Explain to the patient that prior FGR attributed to placental dysfunction implicates both the future risk of recurrence, as well as risk of other placental complications in future pregnancies, such as placental abruption, preeclampsia, and stillbirth

☐ Encourage maintenance of a healthy lifestyle given the risk of future cardiovascular morbidity, especially after placental-mediated early-onset FGR

☐ Advise early future prenatal care in a high-risk center

TOTAL: **125**

CHAPTER 10

Alloimmunization

Noor Amily, Amira El-Messidi, and Karen Fung-Kee-Fung

A new patient presents for consultation and transfer of care to your high-risk obstetrics unit at a tertiary center. She is a 34-year-old G4P2A1L2 at 14^{+3} weeks' gestation with *anti-c* antibodies detected on routine testing; results have been confirmed at your hospital's laboratory. All other prenatal investigations are unremarkable, including first-trimester sonogram and aneuploidy risk assessment.

LEARNING OBJECTIVES

1. Take a focused prenatal history from a patient with red cell antibodies and initiate timely investigations to assess fetal antigen status
2. Demonstrate a detailed understanding of antenatal maternal-fetal surveillance, mode, and timing of delivery for pregnancies complicated by clinically significant alloantibodies, detailing key differences between non-D and anti-Kell antibodies
3. Recognize aspects involved in preparation, counseling, and performance of intrauterine transfusions for fetal anemia
4. Provide principal elements in preconception counseling for previously alloimmunized pregnancies

SUGGESTED READINGS

1. Brennand J, Cameron A. Fetal anaemia: diagnosis and management. *Best Pract Res Clin Obstet Gynaecol.* 2008;22(1):15–29.
2. Castleman JS, Kilby MD. Red cell alloimmunization: a 2020 update. *Prenat Diagn.* 2020;40(9): 1099–1108.
3. The management of women with red cell antibodies during pregnancy. Green Top Guideline number 65, 2014. Available at www.rcog.org.uk/en/guidelines-research-services/guidelines/ gtg65. Accessed February 22, 2021.
4. Koelewijn JM, Vrijkotte TG, de Haas M, et al. Risk factors for the presence of non-rhesus D red blood cell antibodies in pregnancy. *BJOG.* 2009;116(5):655–664.
5. Moise KJ Jr, Argoti PS. Management and prevention of red cell alloimmunization in pregnancy: a systematic review. *Obstet Gynecol.* 2012;120(5):1132–1139.
6. Scottish National Clinical Guidance: Pregnant women with red cell antibodies, version 2, July 2013. Available at https://nhsnss.org/services/blood-tissues-and-cells/clinical-services/ information-and-manuals-for-clinicians/. Accessed February 22, 2021.

7. Society for Maternal-Fetal Medicine, Mari G, Norton ME, et al. Society for Maternal-Fetal Medicine (SMFM) Clinical Guideline No. 8: the fetus at risk for anemia – diagnosis and management. *Am J Obstet Gynecol.* 2015;212(6):697–710.
8. Webb J, Delaney M. Red blood cell alloimmunization in the pregnant patient. *Transfus Med Rev.* 2018;32(4):213–219.
9. White J, Qureshi H, Massey E, et al. Guideline for blood grouping and red cell antibody testing in pregnancy. *Transfus Med.* 2016;26(4):246–263.
10. Zwiers C, van Kamp IL, Oepkes D. Management of red cell alloimmunization. Chapter 10 in: Kilby MD, Johnson A, Oepkes D, eds., *Fetal Therapy: Scientific Basis and Critical Appraisal of Clinical Benefits*, 2nd ed. Cambridge: Cambridge University Press; 2020.

POINTS

1. With regard to presence of red cell antibody, what aspects of a focused history would you want to know? *(1 point per main bullet, unless specified)*

Max 15

☐ Ascertain the patient's blood type
☐ Presence/absence of previous alloimmunized pregnancies

Current pregnancy:[§]
☐ Most recent antibody titer or quantification *(3 points)*
☐ Recent/remote trauma
☐ Vaginal bleeding

Previous obstetric sources of exposure for alloimmunization:
☐ Details of the prior early pregnancy loss *(e.g., ectopic, fetal demise, spontaneous/therapeutic, and complications)*
☐ Obstetric hemorrhage *(i.e., antepartum or postpartum, of variable causes)* with/without blood transfusions
☐ Spontaneous feto-maternal hemorrhage
☐ External cephalic version
☐ Intrauterine procedures *(e.g., amniocentesis/chorionic villous sampling, transfusions, laser therapy, fetal reduction, manual/surgical removal of the placenta)*
☐ Mode of deliveries and instrumental deliveries

Medical history-related sources of exposure:
☐ Receipt of blood transfusions for any acute/chronic condition including timing, indication, and number of units received
  ○ *Likelihood of alloimmunization increases with volume of allogenic blood exposure; alloimmunization may occur with as little as 0.1 mL of exposure*
  ○ *Transfusion-associated alloimmunization exceeds risk from feto-maternal bleeding*
☐ Previous nonobstetric major surgery *(e.g., orthopedic, abdominal, surgery posttrauma, transplant)*

Neonatal manifestations of alloimmunization:
☐ Jaundice, phototherapy, transfusions

Social history:
- ☐ Occupation *(particularly for risk of blood source contamination)*
- ☐ Prior needlestick injuries *(source of alloimmunization)*
- ☐ Intravenous drug use/tattoos/acupuncture/shared needles *(source of alloimmunization)*

Male partner:
- ☐ Ethnicity *(required for calculating the likelihood of heterozygosity using gene frequency tables)*
- ☐ Establish whether he is the same biologic father for all pregnancies
- ☐ Assess whether his blood type is known or was recently tested

Special note:
§ No evidence that assisted reproductive technology with one's own oocytes increases the risk of red cell alloimmunization *(RCOG[3])*

You learn that the patient is a healthy dental assistant. She had two uncomplicated pregnancies with her first husband, where both sons were born by Cesarean sections six and four years ago, respectively. Since her second marriage 18 months ago, she had a ruptured ectopic pregnancy last year, requiring two units of packed red blood cells intraoperatively. Current pregnancy has been unremarkable. Social history is only significant for work-related needlestick injuries, without transmission of blood-borne pathogens. Although her sons had normal neonatal courses, the patient is aware that her healthy 10-year-old stepson needed postnatal exchange transfusions for unspecified indications.

The patient's blood group is A-negative with an *anti-c* titer at 1:16 (quantified level >7.5 IU/mL[§]) last week. Her husband has not had blood testing. You inform the patient that presence of the alloantibody is not due to her wrongdoing, yet she remains curious as to possible sources of sensitization.

Special notes:
§ In the United Kingdom, levels of anti-c and anti-D antibodies are quantified with an automated analyzer, whereas antibody titers are used for other antibodies; other countries may use titers. Case scenario demonstrates how fetal medicine expertise is indicated at critical antibody titers; referral is also warranted with rising titers, sonographic features of fetal anemia, history of unexplained neonatal features of hemolytic disease, or with anti-Kell antibodies once detected

2.	Ensuring professionalism and maintaining a nonjudgmental approach, identify this patient's risk factors for sensitization to c-antigen. *(1 point each)*	Max 6

- ☐ Red blood cell transfusions
- ☐ Occupational blood-exposure, needlestick injuries
- ☐ Multiparity
- ☐ Prior Cesarean sections
- ☐ At least one prior male child[†]
- ☐ Ectopic pregnancy
- ☐ New partner
- ☐ Stepson's history of neonatal exchange transfusion

Special note:
† Exact mechanism of how a male child is a risk for non-RhD antibodies is unknown – stimulation of immune response to male-specific antigens is possible *(Suggested Reading 4)*

3. Indicate the <u>next best</u> investigation in the diagnostic evaluation of this pregnancy. *(1 point for either approach; international variations exist)*   1

☐ Noninvasive maternal cell-free DNA (cfDNA) for c-antigen[‡]
   ○ Genotyping can be undertaken as of 16 weeks for D, C, c, E, and e antigens; testing can be done as of 20 weeks for K-antigens (Kell) *(RCOG[3])*
      ▪ Ensure laboratory-specific guidance on the earliest reliable gestation for testing is followed
      ▪ Internal laboratory quality assurance may require confirmation of fetal Kell genotype at 28 weeks' gestation (*i.e.*, two samples are sent during gestation)

OR

☐ Paternal phenotyping for the *c*-antigen with estimation of his genotype (i.e., zygosity) based on the gene frequency in the population
   ○ *Followed by cfDNA, where available, for paternal heterozygosity*
   ○ *Individualized consideration for nonpaternity or unknown paternity*

Special note:
‡ *International differences in access exist*

Unfortunately, cfDNA testing for fetal antigen status is not available in your jurisdiction.[‡] As the patient is confident of paternity, genetic testing will be arranged. She understands that if her husband lacks the implied *c-antigen*, her primary care provider may continue routine obstetric care. The patient wonders whether a positive paternal phenotype implies *obligate* fetal *c-antigen* status, and what would management entail with presence of fetal c-antigen.

Special note:
‡ Nonavailability of maternal cfDNA for fetal antigen status is presented for academic interest: *refer to Question 5*

4. Explain the implications of a positive paternal phenotype for *c-antigen* and inform the patient of your recommended fetal diagnostic evaluation, where necessary. *(1 point per main and subbullet)*   3

☐ Paternal serology or DNA testing would be required to determine zygosity
   ○ *Serology determines the **probable** genotype based on population gene frequency*
   ○ Homozygosity implies all fetuses will have the c-antigen, with risk of hemolytic disease (assuming pregnancies with a *c-sensitized* mother)
   ○ Heterozygosity requires fetal genotyping for the *c-antigen* through maternal cfDNA testing or amniocentesis for fetal polymerase chain reaction (PCR)

5. In the event of amniocentesis, indicate aspects to address in <u>counseling and management</u>   Max 3
    of this patient. She understands procedure-related risks. *(1 point per main bullet)*

☐ Anti-D immunoglobulin is indicated for this patient *(Rh-negative status without*
    D-sensitization)
    ○ Ensure the patient consents to receipt of blood products
☐ Inform the patient that invasive testing further increases the risk of alloimmunization
    (e.g., higher anti-c levels or developing new antibodies)
☐ Reassure her that possible minute amounts of non-D antibodies in anti-D
    immunoglobulin do not contribute to alloimmunization

Fetal antigen testing, performed for paternal heterozygosity, confirms a D-positive, c-positive male[‡] fetus. You inform the patient that as *'not all alloantibodies are created equal'*; anti-c antibodies carry a 65% risk of fetal hemolytic disease, warranting close obstetric management.

Special note:
‡ Rh-D-positive male fetuses with clinically significant alloantibodies are more likely to become hydropic than females

6. Explain why certain alloantibodies may not cause clinically significant fetal-neonatal   1
    hemolysis.

☐ Alloantibodies that elicit an <u>IgM</u> response are not transported across the placenta *(e.g.,*
    Lewis, I, P, A and B antigens from the ABO blood group system)

7. Outline the details of your <u>obstetric management</u> for this patient, with focus on   Max 6
    alloimmunization. *(1 point each)*

Maternal:
☐ Serial measurement of anti-c titers/levels every 4 weeks until 28 weeks' gestation, then
    every 2 weeks until delivery *(RCOG[3])*
☐ This patient would require routine antenatal administration of anti-D immunoglobulin in
    the absence of new-onset D-sensitization by 28 weeks' gestation
☐ Early neonatology consultation
☐ Ensure availability of donor blood compatible with the specific antibody *(e.g., anti-c)* is
    available for delivery

Fetal:
☐ Initiate serial sonographic surveillance every one to two weeks for fetal risk of anemia
    using MCA-PSV with anti-c critical antibody titer of 1:16 or quantified level >7.5 IU/mL[‡]
☐ Use MCA-PSV >1.5 MoM *(i.e., <0.65 MoM for fetal hemoglobin)* for gestational age as a
    cutoff for moderate to severe fetal anemia requiring cordocentesis and possible
    intrauterine transfusion
    ○ False-positive rate of MCA-PSV is 12% for predicting moderate to severe anemia with
        100% sensitivity[§]
☐ Consideration for fetal pulmonary corticosteroids

Special notes:

‡   Anti-c level >20 IU/mL correlates with high risk of hemolytic disease of the fetus and newborn *(RCOG³)*

§   Refer to Chapter 59 for sensitivity definition and calculation

Fetal anatomy survey at 19 weeks' gestation revealed normal biometry and morphology, without signs of anemia. Maternal antibody titers were stable until 24^{+0} weeks' gestation when reported titers became 1:64. During sonographic assessment at 24^{+0} weeks' gestation, you use this opportunity to teach your obstetric trainee the technical aspects[†] of the following Doppler acquisition:

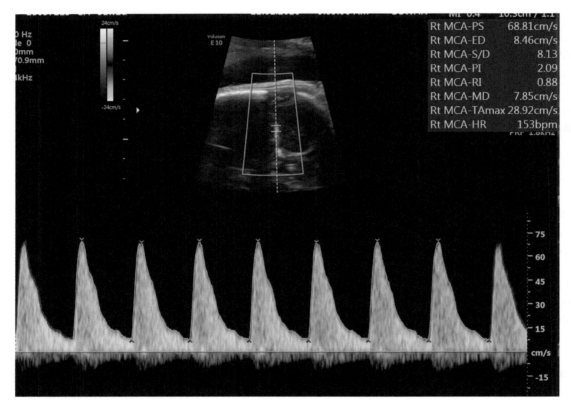

Figure 10.1

Courtesy of Professor K. Fung-Kee-Fung

There is no association between the patient's image and this case scenario. Image used for educational purposes only.

Special note:

† Refer to Chapter 63 for discussion on factors that contribute to false-positive MCA-PSV assessment

8.   Facilitate your trainee's learning by detailing the steps required for adequate MCA image acquisition and assessment. *(1 point per main bullet)*   Max 4

☐   Avoid any unnecessary pressure on the fetal head

☐   Obtain and magnify an axial section of the brain that includes the thalami, cavum septum pellucidum, and greater wing of sphenoid

□ Color flow mapping should be used to identify the circle of Willis and proximal MCA

□ Pulsed-wave Doppler gate is placed within the proximal third of the MCA vessel, just after it bifurcates from the carotid siphon

   ○ *Peripheral placement of the gate leads to false depression of the true MCA-PSV*

□ Maintain an angle of insonation as close as possible to 0°,[‡] and always <30° (preferably by probe positioning and beam steering)

□ Await fetal quiescent states

□ At least 3, and fewer than 10, consecutive waveforms should be recorded

Special note:

[‡] The importance relates to the Doppler shift equation where cosine 0 = 1; angle corrections otherwise introduce error

You share with your obstetric trainee how to utilize this classic curve in the interpretation of this fetus' Doppler assessment portrayed at 24^{+0} weeks' gestation. You highlight that the lower curve represents the median and the upper curve indicates 1.5 MoM.

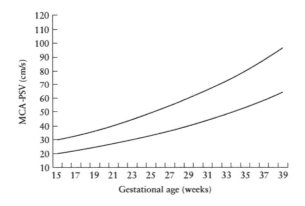

Figure 10.2

With permission: Figure 2, page 324 from Mari G. Middle cerebral artery peak systolic velocity for the diagnosis of fetal anemia: the untold story. *Ultrasound Obstet Gynecol.* 2005;25(4):323–330.

9. Based on your diagnosis, elicit <u>non-Doppler features</u>[†] on imaging that may represent the severe spectrum of this fetus's hemodynamic state. *(1 point each)*

   Max 5

□ Ascites

□ Cardiomegaly

□ Pericardial effusions

□ Pleural effusions

□ Skin edema >5 mm thick

□ Placental thickness ≥4 cm in the second trimester and ≥6 cm in the third trimester

□ Polyhydramnios

Special note:

[†] Refer to Chapter 63 for image representations of each feature indicated above; placental thickness and polyhydramnios may be *associated* findings with hydrops fetalis but do not constitute features in the definition

While surfing the internet, your trainee is surprised to learn that the biological basis for increased MCA-PSV Doppler velocimetry in fetal anemia differs from fetal growth restriction (FGR). He or she is also searching to clarify the interpretation of antibody titers, confused how 1:64 is 'greater' than 1:16.

---

10. Summarize the principal physiological rationale for increased fetal MCA-PSV in anemic states relative to FGR. *(1 point each)*   2

☐ <u>Fetal anemia</u>: Increased flow of low-viscosity blood preserves brain oxygenation
☐ <u>FGR</u>: Increased cardiac output of normal-viscosity blood preserves brain oxygenation

---

11. Facilitate your trainee's understanding of the biological implications of this patient's anti-c antibody titers   2

☐ Antibody is a reciprocal of the greatest dilution of maternal serum where the antibody agglutinates RBCs with the c-antigen
  ○ 1:64 represents seven serial dilutions, a greater maternal antibody concentration, than 1:16 implying five serial dilutions

---

Close follow-up is initiated and with upward trend in MCA-PSV, the patient consents to fetal blood sampling and possible intrauterine transfusion.

Awaiting her husband's presence before continued discussion, you take this opportunity to teach your trainee important considerations in planning for intrauterine transfusion. You highlight that autologous maternal donation will not be feasible as her hemoglobin is <120–125 g/L. As such, donor units will be cross matched with the patient's blood to reduce the risk of further sensitization to non-D alloantibodies.

---

12. List the characteristics of donor packed red blood cells for intrauterine transfusion of this anti-c alloimmunized patient. *(1 point each)*   Max 6

☐ O-negative, or ABO identical with the fetus, as known from amniocyte testing
  ○ *(SMFM[7]): O-positive blood may be needed with anti-c alloimmunization due to the rarity of O-negative, c-negative blood [0.0001%]*
  ○ *(RCOG[3]): Exceptionally, O-positive, c-negative blood is necessary, as with anti-c alloimmunization, where giving RhD-negative blood would be harmful*
☐ *c*-antigen-negative
☐ Hemoglobin-S-negative; K-negative
☐ CMV seronegative
☐ Leukodepleted *(reduces risk of CMV transmission where seronegative donors are unavailable)*
☐ Irradiated *(reduces graft-versus-host reaction)*, and transfused within 24 hours of irradiation
☐ Packed to a hematocrit 70%–85% *(reduces volume of fetal transfusion)*
☐ Washed units
☐ Fresh units, collected within five days *(to enhance level of 2,3-diphosphoglycerate)*
  ○ *Placed in CPD (citrate phosphate dextrose anticoagulant)*

13. Provide your trainee with potential fetal approaches for intrauterine transfusion, illustrating advantages and disadvantages/caveats of various modalities. *(3 points per bullet)*

Max 3

		Advantages	Caveats/disadvantages
☐	Umbilical vein at the placental cord root	# Preferred # Stability for access	# Posterior placentation # Fetal position
☐	Intrahepatic portion of the umbilical vein	# Low risk of fetal bradycardia (artery is distant) # Intraperitoneal bleeding is self-limited, absorbed over 7–10 days, and functions as an intraperitoneal transfusion # Less feto-maternal hemorrhage	# Induces fetal stress hormones (*i.e.,* possibly pain) # Access is dependent on optimal fetal position
☐	Umbilical artery (UA)	—	Fetal bradycardia (vessel wall spasm)
☐	Intraperitoneal	# Early gestational age precluding fetal venous access # Often adjunctive to intravascular transfusion	# Suboptimal blood absorption with ascites or hydrops # Slower uptake, ~10% per day, rendering longer time to optimize fetal hemoglobin
☐	Intracardiac	—	Frequent complications; IUFD

In counseling the couple, you highlight that at this gestational age, fetal pulmonary corticosteroids will be administered 48 hours preprocedure. Neonatology consultation has also been arranged.

You inform them that overall survival generally exceeds 95%, with 5%–12% risk of long-term neurodevelopmental impairment. As they inquire about the general mechanism by which transfusion controls fetal hemolysis, your trainee takes note to ask about technical aspects of intrauterine transfusion after this clinical encounter. The couple understands that 1%–2% of all procedures encounter complications, upon which you elaborate your counseling.

14-A. Relating to the pathophysiology of hemolytic disease, explain the <u>general</u> purpose of intrauterine transfusion.

2

☐ Replace fetal blood volume by adult red blood cells that will not be targeted by maternal alloantibodies; suppress fetal erythropoiesis

14-B. Address the consequences of untreated fetal anemia worthy of discussion in counseling the parents. *(1 point each)*

5

☐ Hydrops
☐ Spontaneous or iatrogenic preterm birth
☐ Perinatal death (IUFD, neonatal death)
☐ Severe neonatal jaundice, kernicterus, deafness, cerebral palsy
☐ Neonatal exchange transfusion

15. Verbalize a comprehensive list of intrauterine transfusion-associated complications, upon which you will structure your approach to couple's counseling. *(1 point each)*

Max 6

☐ Fetal bradycardia**, or tachycardia
☐ Bleeding from a puncture site; cord hematoma
☐ Exsanguination *(related to thrombocytopenia)*
☐ Feto-maternal hemorrhage *(worsening alloimmunization)*
☐ Fetal trauma
☐ Preterm labor/PPROM
☐ Emergency Cesarean delivery *(mostly related to cord complications or exsanguination following needle removal/displacement)*
☐ IUFD
☐ Intrauterine infection

Special note:
**   Most common complications

16. Identify risk factors for intrauterine transfusion-related fetal loss or complications. *(1 point each)*

Max 3

☐ Operator inexperience
☐ Lower gestational age
☐ Hydrops fetalis
☐ Refraining from fetal paralysis
☐ Fetal anomalies
☐ Increased body mass index (BMI)

17. After this patient encounter, inform your trainee of three accepted definitions for fetal anemia. *(1 point per main bullet; severity criteria are provided for academic interest)*

3

☐ Hemoglobin deviation from the mean for gestational age
  ○ *Mild: <20 g/L (<2 g/dL)*
  ○ *Moderate: 20–70 g/L (2–7 g/dL)*
  ○ *Severe: >70 g/L (>7 g/dL) [hydrops generally occurs with actual hemoglobin <50 g/L (>5 g/dL)]*
☐ Hemoglobin values expressed as MoM
  ○ *Mild: 0.84–0.65 MoM*
  ○ *Moderate: 0.64–0.55 MoM*
  ○ *Severe: ≤0.54 MoM*
☐ Hematocrit <30%

18. Further challenging your trainee, you inquire on one formula to calculate infused volume of packed red blood cells, via either the intravascular or intraperitoneal approach. *(5 points for any method)*

5

'Simple method':[†]
☐ EFW (grams) x transfusion coefficient
  ○ *Transfusion coefficient depends on the desired increased increment in hematocrit; refer to designated table*[†]

Mandelbrot Formula:[‡]
☐ Transfused volume (mL) = [Fetoplacental unit volume (mL) × (target – initial hematocrit)]

hematocrit of transfused blood
  ○ *Where fetoplacental unit volume = 1.046 + [EFW (grams) × 0.14]*

Intraperitoneal route:[§]
☐ Transfused volume (mL) = [Gestational age (weeks) – 20] × 10

Special notes:
Refer to Chapter 63 for *general* factors required to calculate intrauterine transfusion volume; **the above-indicated formulas are presented for the advanced learner or reader**
[†] (1) Giannina G, Moise KJ Jr, Dorman K. A simple method to estimate volume for fetal intravascular transfusions. *Fetal Diagn Ther.* 1998;13(2):94–97; (2) Nicolaides KH, Clewell WH, Rodeck CH. Measurement of human fetoplacental blood volume in erythroblastosis fetalis. *Am J Obstet Gynecol.* 1987;157(1):50–53.
[‡] Mandelbrot L, Daffos F, Forestier F, MacAleese J, Descombey D. *Fetal Ther.* 1988;3 (1–2):60–66.
[§] Bowman JM. *Obstet Gynecol.* 1978;52(1):1–16.

The first intrauterine transfusion procedure was unremarkable. Posttransfusion fetal hematocrit is 48%.[§]

You explain that MCA-PSV *may* be used to time the second transfusion, although a predicted decline in fetal hemoglobin may also be considered *(SMFM[7])*. After the second procedure, however, MCA-PSV is less reliable. The couple is interested in the physiological rationale for suboptimal value in fetal Doppler assessment after intrauterine transfusions.

Special note:
§ If the fetus were hydropic, stepwise transfusion would be advised, raising hematocrit initially to ~30% followed by repeat transfusion in ~48 hours

---

19. Detail the physiology of suboptimal value in MCA-PSV assessments post-intrauterine transfusions. *(2 points for main bullet)*   2

☐ Compensatory rise in cerebral blood flow (*i.e.*, MCA-PSV) due to lower fetal hemoglobin concentration and arterial oxygenation with smaller, less viscous adult red blood cells with a lower oxygen carrying capacity than fetal red blood cells
  ○ *Following initial transfusion, MCA-PSV >1.69 MoM is the recommended threshold for diagnosis of fetal anemia needing second transfusion (SMFM[7])*

---

20. Address the couple's inquiry on a physiological rationale for scheduling subsequent fetal transfusions. *(either bullet)*   1

Hemoglobin decline:
☐ Expected decline of fetal hemoglobin is ~0.4 g/dL/d after the first, 0.3 g/dL/d after the second, and 0.2 g/dL/d after the third transfusion

Hematocrit decline:
☐ ~1%/d

Special note:
Main reason for recurrent fetal anemia is fetal growth with increase in total fetoplacental blood volume *(Suggested Reading 10)*

By 35 weeks' gestation, the patient had serial uncomplicated intrauterine transfusions. Fetal growth biometry has been appropriate. Due to her obstetric progress, delivery will be arranged in your tertiary center.

---

21. Discuss aspects of delivery timing and intrapartum care for this patient with known clinically significant antibodies. *(1 point each)*   Max 5

☐ Plan for induction of labor at 37–38 weeks, depending on timing of last transfusion and anticipated decline in hematocrit
☐ Maintain continuous electronic fetal heart monitoring *(RCOG[3])*
☐ Consideration for blood availability in case of need for acute maternal transfusion
☐ Aim for delayed cord clamping, where possible *(appears to be advantageous after intrauterine transfusion for alloimmunization)*

☐ Test cord blood for full/complete blood count (FBC/CBC), serum bilirubin, and direct antiglobulin test, red cell eluate, and ABO and Rh blood group

☐ Maternal sample for Kleihauer-Betke test, taken at least 45 minutes after placental separation to allow distribution of fetal cells in maternal circulation

☐ Ensure presence of neonatology team at delivery, and completion of neonatal consultation

The patient has an uncomplicated induction of labor and vaginal delivery at 36^{+3} weeks' gestation. The newborn is admitted to the NICU for investigations, observation, and possible treatment.

Although you had discussed essential elements of postpartum care in advance of delivery, you visit the patient on postpartum day 1 and review aspects of care.

22. Provide important elements of postpartum counseling and management, in hospital or after discharge, most specific to recent alloimmunization in pregnancy. *(1 point each)*   Max 5

Mental well-being and health maintenance:
☐ Screen for postpartum depression and maintain psychosocial support services *(stressful antenatal events)*
☐ Reassure the patient of no long-term maternal adverse health consequences associated with red cell antibodies *(RCOG[3])*, although future cross-matching may be challenging in the presence of alloantibodies
  ○ *Levels decline over ~12 weeks postpartum*
☐ As the fetus is Rh-D-positive, tested antenatally, maternal administration of postpartum anti-D immunoglobulin should be given in line with established practice

Breastfeeding:
☐ Encourage to decrease dehydration and neonatal jaundice *(RCOG[3])*

Future pregnancy:
☐ Encourage prepregnancy counseling *(RCOG[3])*
☐ Inform the patient that hemolysis may recur earlier with increased severity; likely need of earlier/more frequent transfusions
☐ Address the risk of developing additional alloantibodies
☐ Antibody titers will be unreliable in future pregnancy with the same father; initiation of routine MCA-PSV Doppler at 18 weeks' gestation is recommended

23. Address her inquiry on prophylactic interventions against fetal hemolytic disease in subsequent pregnancies. *(1 point each)*   3

☐ In vitro fertilization with preimplantation genetic diagnosis
☐ Gestational carrier
☐ Donor insemination

Special note:
Consideration for individual cultural implications and jurisdictional policies is advised

You later call her primary care provider to inform him/her of the patient's latter obstetric course. Your colleague is now seeking advice for the care incidentally detected **anti-Kell** antibodies with a titer at 1:4 on routine prenatal screening at 10 weeks' gestation.

---

24. Address how the pathophysiology and obstetric care of anti-Kell antibodies differs from the anti-c alloimmunized pregnancy. Assume a Kell-positive father of the fetus. *(1 point per main bullet)*

Max 3

☐ Referral for MFM expertise is indicated ***upon detection*** of anti-Kell antibodies, irrespective of titers

☐ Risk of severe anemia is due to erythroid suppression with immune destruction of progenitor red cells <u>and/or</u> hemolysis of mature red blood cells

☐ Noninvasive fetal genotyping using cfDNA for Kell antigen can be undertaken from 20 weeks, compared to earlier genotyping at 16 weeks in pregnancies with non-Kell alloimmunization *(RCOG[3])*
   ○ *Risk of false-negative results with earlier testing for Kell antigen using cfDNA*

☐ Critical titer is lower than with other alloantibodies; titers do not correlate well with onset or severity of fetal anemia
   ○ Critical titer is 1:4 or 1:8 *(international variations exist)*

☐ Serial surveillance of antibody titers begins at ~18 weeks' gestation (*i.e.*, similar to non-Kell alloimmunization <u>after</u> an affected pregnancy)
   ○ Surveillance is recommended every 4 weeks until 28 weeks' gestation, then every 2 weeks until delivery *(RCOG[3])*

TOTAL: **100**

CHAPTER 11

Dichorionic Twin Pregnancy

Noor Amily, Amira El-Messidi, and Karen Fung-Kee-Fung

A healthy 35-year-old secundigravida with a history of an uncomplicated Cesarean delivery performed four years ago for fetal malpresentation at term is referred by her primary care provider to your general obstetrics clinic at 11^{+5} weeks' gestation by menstrual age. The physician provided you with a sonographic dating report confirming a viable intrauterine dichorionic diamniotic twin gestation with a crown–rump length (CRL) of twin A and B at 47 mm and 44 mm, respectively. The patient does not have any obstetric complaints and has been taking routine prenatal vitamins for the past four months. Her social and family histories are unremarkable.

LEARNING OBJECTIVES

1. Understand the approach to sonographic dating of a spontaneous twin pregnancy and assessment of chorionicity
2. Provide counseling on noninvasive prenatal screening, diagnostic amniocentesis, and selective termination for a discordant anomaly in a dichorionic pregnancy
3. Present comprehensive antepartum and intrapartum management plans for an uncomplicated dichorionic twin pregnancy, recognizing complex antenatal clinical situations that require maternal-fetal medicine expertise
4. Discuss strategies to optimize the perinatal survival of the remaining dichorionic twin following previable delivery of the co-twin
5. Detect and interpret intertwin fetal growth abnormalities and provide patient counseling on perinatal risks associated with selective fetal growth restriction (sFGR) in dichorionic pregnancies

SUGGESTED READINGS

1. American College of Obstetricians and Gynecologists' Committee on Practice Bulletins – Obstetrics, Society for Maternal-Fetal Medicine. Multifetal gestations: twin, triplet, and higher-order multifetal pregnancies: ACOG Practice Bulletin, No. 231. *Obstet Gynecol.* 2021;137(6): e145–e162.
2. Antonakopoulos N, Pateisky P, Liu B, et al. Selective fetal growth restriction in dichorionic twin pregnancies: diagnosis, natural history, and perinatal outcome. *J Clin Med.* 2020;9(5): 1404.

3. Cheung KW, Seto MTY, Wang W, et al. Effect of delayed interval delivery of remaining fetus (es) in multiple pregnancies on survival: a systematic review and meta-analysis. *Am J Obstet Gynecol.* 2020;222(4):306–319.

4. (a) FIGO Working Group on Good Clinical Practice in Maternal-Fetal Medicine. Good clinical practice advice: management of twin pregnancy. *Int J Gynaecol Obstet.* 2019;144(3):330–337.

   (b) FIGO Working Group on Good Clinical Practice in Maternal-Fetal Medicine. Good clinical practice advice: role of ultrasound in the management of twin pregnancy. *Int J Gynaecol Obstet.* 2019;144(3):338–339.

5. Goodnight W, Newman R. Optimal nutrition for improved twin pregnancy outcome. *Obstet Gynecol.* 2009;114(5):1121–1134.

6. Khalil A, Beune I, Hecher K, et al. Consensus definition and essential reporting parameters of selective fetal growth restriction in twin pregnancy: a delphi procedure. *Ultrasound Obstet Gynecol.* 2019;53(1):47–54. [Correction in *Ultrasound Obstet Gynecol.* 2020 Dec;56(6):967]

7. Khalil A, Rodgers M, Baschat A, et al. ISUOG Practice Guidelines: role of ultrasound in twin pregnancy. *Ultrasound Obstet Gynecol.* 2016;47(2):247–263. [Correction in *Ultrasound Obstet Gynecol.* 2018 Jul;52(1):140]

8. National Institute for Health and Care Excellence (NICE) Guideline No. 137: twin and triplet pregnancy. September 2019.

9. Palomaki GE, Chiu RWK, Pertile MD, et al. International Society for Prenatal Diagnosis Position Statement: Cell free (cf)DNA screening for Down syndrome in multiple pregnancies. *Prenat Diagn.* 2020;41(10):1222–1232.

10. (a) Audibert F, Gagnon A. No. 262 – prenatal screening for and diagnosis of aneuploidy in twin pregnancies. *J Obstet Gynaecol Can.* 2017;39(9):e347–e361.

    (b) Brown R, Gagnon R, Delisle MF. No. 373 – cervical insufficiency and cervical cerclage. *J Obstet Gynaecol Can.* 2019;41(2):233–247.

    (c) Morin L, Lim K. No. 260 – ultrasound in twin pregnancies. *J Obstet Gynaecol Can.* 2017;39(10):e398–e411.

POINTS

1. Given spontaneous conception of twins, outline the approach to pregnancy dating and discuss your calculation of the approximate gestational age. *(1 point each)*   Max 2

☐ Pregnancy dating is preferable when the CRL is 45–84 mm *(i.e., between 11^{+0}- and 13^{+6}-weeks' gestation)*

☐ Among spontaneous pregnancies, estimated gestational age is based on CRL of the larger twin *(i.e., 47 mm for this pregnancy)*

☐ Using the *'rule of thumb'* [*CRL (mm) + 42 = gestational age (days)*],† the patient would be 89 days, or 12^{+4} weeks' gestation

Special note:
Refer to Question 2 in Chapter 9

2. Assuming a spontaneous twin gestation presenting at ≥ 14 weeks' gestation, indicate how gestational age dating would have been selected.

1

☐ At ≥ 14 weeks' gestation, pregnancy dating should be based according to biometry of the fetus with the larger head circumference *(ISUOG[7])*

The patient, a biologist, requests you explain the scientific basis of dichorionic twinning as she wonders whether her twins will be phenotypically identical. Meanwhile, your obstetric trainee inquires about the sonographic basis for determining chorionicity and amnionicity, which he or she is aware should be done by two-dimensional (2-D), not 3-D, imaging. *(NICE [8])*

3. Address the patient' inquiry by detailing the physiology of zygosity in spontaneous dichorionic twins and socio-medical factors known to increase the risk of dichorionic twins. *(1 point per main bullet, unless indicated)*

Max 7

☐ Dichorionic twins may be mono- or dizygotic

Monozygotic, dichorionic twins:
☐ A fertilized ovum (monozygotic) that divides at less than four days postconception results in dichorionic twins that should be phenotypically and genotypically identical *(assuming no postdivision mutation)*
☐ *~18%* of same sex dichorionic twins are monozygotic – 'identical'
☐ The frequency of spontaneous monozygotic twins is consistent worldwide at 1/250 or 4/1000 births

Dizygotic, dichorionic twins:
☐ Fertilization of two separate ova that are genetically dissimilar
☐ Approximately two-thirds of naturally conceived twins are dizygotic
☐ Variables affecting rated of dizygotic twins: *(1 point per subbullet; max 4)*
   o Advanced maternal age
   o Maternal weight (BMI ≥ 30 kg/m^2) and height (≥ 1.65 m)
   o Multiparity
   o Positive maternal family history
   o Ethnicity [African ethnicity (180/10,000 deliveries) relative to the lowest rates seen in Asia (40/10,000 deliveries)]
   o Ovulation-inducing agents **with/without** in vitro fertilization

4. Inform your trainee about sonographic markers used to determine a dichorionic gestation at <10 and >10 weeks' gestation. *(1 point each)*

Max 5

At 6–10 weeks' gestation:
☐ 2 gestational sacs separated by a thick dividing membrane
☐ 2 amniotic sacs,[†] each containing a fetal pole
☐ 2 yolk sacs

Greater than 10 weeks' gestation:
☐ Gender discordance (not routinely used at the 10- to 14-week scan)
☐ 2 distinct placental masses visualized
☐ Intertwin membrane insertion in the placenta appears as a triangular projection of amnion between layers of chorion, giving the appearance of a 'lambda,' 'delta,' or 'twin-peak' sign *(sensitivity >97%, specificity 100% for dichorionicity; this sign disappears by 20 weeks' gestation ~20% of the time)*
☐ Membrane thickness >2 mm

Special note:
† Each amnion is very thin and may be best detected by transvaginal scanning

The patient asks your professional opinion regarding prenatal screening tests for this twin pregnancy. You intend to counsel her in a nondirective manner, respecting her choice to accept or decline available testing options.

5. Without local limitations in availability of tests, counsel the patient on noninvasive screening options for twin gestations, focusing on test characteristics to convey in discussion. *(1 point per bullet and subbullet)*

Max 6

☐ Option A: Maternal serum cell-free DNA (cfDNA)
  ○ The average fetal fraction for each twin is less than that for singletons; this may result in a fetus with a chromosomal abnormality contributing less fetal DNA, thereby masking the aneuploidy result and accounting for test failure
  ○ Test failure rates are 1.6%–13.2% (median 3.6%)
  ○ Differences in fetal fraction between twins (may be at least 1.5-fold in 10% of cases)
  ○ Sensitivity for trisomy 21 appears to be similar to test performance in singletons
☐ Option B: Maternal age and nuchal translucency (NT) values of each twin
  ○ Trisomy 21 detection rate is ~80% at a 5% false-positive rate
☐ Option C: First-trimester combined test using serum β-hCG and PAPP-A and NT values
  ○ Serum protein values are adjusted for twin gestation
  ○ This method decreases the false-positive rate of option B
☐ Option D: Integrated NT plus first- and second-trimester serum screening
  ○ Higher levels of maternal serum biochemistry in twin pregnancies may result in higher rates of invasive prenatal diagnosis
  ○ This would provide a risk estimation *per pregnancy*, rather than *per fetus*

6. Calculate, stepwise, the age-associated risk of at least one trisomy 21 affected fetus in an assumed dizygotic twin pregnancy prior to any aneuploidy screening test. *(1 point per main bullet)*

☐ At age 35 years, the risk of trisomy 21 at term is 1/350 for a singleton[†]
☐ For dizygotic twins, the risk of at least one affected fetus is considered to be twice the risk for a singleton for a given maternal age: $2 \times 1/350$
   ○ *Risk for both affected fetuses would be $1/350 \times 1/350$ at delivery*

Memory trick:
† **35 years 1/350**

2

With informed consent, the patient opts for cfDNA testing. You are pleased to know her body mass index (BMI) is 22 kg/m², as high maternal weight would further contribute to test failure rates.

Although she and her husband are excited about the prospect of having twins, she has read about associated risks with multiple pregnancies, including different norms for antenatal management relative to her last pregnancy.

7. Present a structured outline of risks you may discuss regarding maternal-fetal adverse outcomes with a dichorionic twin pregnancy. *(1 point each)*

[the following list is not exhaustive; learners are encouraged to understand that most medical, obstetrical, or surgical features are more common to multiple pregnancies]

14

Maternal: *(max 10)*

First trimester	Second and/or third trimester	Any trimester or intrapartum/ postpartum
☐ Spontaneous pregnancy loss *(background rate in twins ~6%)*	☐ Spontaneous preterm birth *(in ~60% of twin pregnancies <37 weeks)* or iatrogenic preterm delivery	☐ Iron-deficiency anemia/fatigue
		☐ Carpal tunnel syndrome
☐ 'Vanishing twin'	☐ Preterm prelabor rupture of membranes	☐ Venous thromboembolism
☐ Hyperemesis gravidarum	☐ Gestational diabetes	☐ Operative vaginal delivery
	☐ Acute fatty liver of pregnancy	☐ Cesarean section
	☐ Cholestasis of pregnancy	☐ Peripartum hysterectomy

(cont.)

First trimester	Second and/or third trimester	Any trimester or intrapartum/ postpartum
	☐ Dermatoses of pregnancy	☐ Malpresentation
		☐ Placenta/cord aberrations
	☐ Hypertensive diseases of pregnancy	☐ Postpartum hemorrhage
		☐ Blood transfusion
	☐ Placental abruption	☐ Depression ± anxiety
	☐ Gastroesophageal reflux	☐ Mortality
	☐ Hemorrhoids	

Fetal/neonatal: *(max 4)*

☐ Risk of aneuploidy for either or both fetuses
☐ Structural anomalies

   o *Each dizygotic twin has the same risk as a singleton*
   o *Concordance rate for an anomaly to be present in both fetuses is low*

☐ Fetal growth restriction in either or both fetuses
☐ Cerebral palsy and/or complications of prematurity
☐ IUFD or neonatal death

---

8. Provide a comprehensive discussion of your <u>focused</u> antenatal management, assuming an <u>uncomplicated</u> dichorionic twin gestation. *(1 point per main bullet)*   Max 10

☐ Consideration for planned multidisciplinary antenatal care, depending on individual patient needs (*e.g.*, dieticians, nurses or midwives, sonographers, perinatal health experts, social workers, women's health physiotherapists)

   o *Local variations in practice exist regarding 'specialized antenatal clinics' for multiple pregnancies: maternal-infant health outcomes have not been proven to be better relative to standard antenatal care[†]*

☐ Inform the patient that in the event of maternal-fetal complications, care may be transferred to a tertiary center

Antenatal visits and sonographic surveillance:

☐ Plan monthly clinic visits until 28 weeks, then bimonthly visits until ~36 weeks, followed by weekly until delivery
☐ Screen for hypertensive disorders of pregnancy and signs/symptoms of preterm labor at each antenatal appointment

☐ This patient would be offered additional first-trimester sonography as part of aneuploidy screening (NT measurement) and early detection of major anomalies *(note that only chorionicity and embryonic size was specified in the provided imaging report)*

☐ Routine detailed fetal anatomy scan, biometrics, placental localization, amniotic fluid volume, and cervical length assessment is recommended between 18–22 weeks' gestation
  ○ *NICE[8]*: Although cervical length measurement is <u>supported</u> as predictor of preterm birth in twin pregnancy, <u>no recommendation</u> could be made in the absence of effective intervention(s) for women at risk
  ○ *Mode for cervical length assessment (i.e., transabdominal or transvaginal) may vary by physician or patient factors*
    ▪ *FIGO[4a]* and *SOGC[10c]* advise transvaginal method for cervical length assessment

☐ Inform the patient to anticipate more time for completion of the anomaly scan relative to her previous singleton pregnancy
  ○ *Allow 45 minutes[$] for the anomaly scan in a twin pregnancy*
  ○ *Fetal echocardiography is not routinely indicated for spontaneous dizygous twins*

☐ After the anomaly scan, plan monthly sonographic surveillance for fetal growth biometries, amniotic fluid volumes [using deepest vertical pocket method per amniotic sac], and umbilical artery (UA) Dopplers until planned delivery
  ○ *FIGO[4a]* and *ISUOG[7]* recommend UA Dopplers after routine morphology scan, whereas *SOGC[10c]* does not recommend UA Dopplers in uncomplicated twin pregnancies
  ○ *More frequent sonographic imaging is arranged where required*
  ○ *Allow 35 minutes[$] for growth scans in a twin pregnancy*

☐ Weekly antenatal surveillance may be considered at 36^{+0} weeks' gestation *(ACOG[1])*

Gestational weight gain, physical activity, and nutrition:

☐ With a normal BMI, the National Academy of Medicine *(formerly the Institute of Medicine)* recommends total weight gain is 37 to 54 lbs (16.8 to 24.5 kg)

☐ In the absence of risk factors or pregnancy complications, advise the same exercise recommendations as for singletons**

☐ Dietary expert guidance for patients with twin pregnancies and normal BMI recommends a daily caloric intake of 40–45 kcal/kg/d and additional micronutrients (*e.g.*, iron, calcium, magnesium, zinc, vitamin D) beyond amounts found in typical prenatal vitamins *(Suggested Reading 5)*

Medications:

☐ Advise 1 mg folic acid-containing prenatal vitamins *(Suggested Reading 5)*

☐ *[Consideration for]* Low dose aspirin (LDASA) (~75–160 mg) nightly started preferably at 12 weeks {ideally <16 weeks}
  ○ ISSHP[‡] and SMFM[‡] guidelines: Multiple gestation is a *strong* risk factor for preeclampsia
  ○ NICE[‡] guidelines: Multiple gestation is a *moderate* risk factor, where LDASA would be advised with at least one other moderate risk factor

Specific laboratory tests for multiple pregnancy:

☐ In addition to routine screening at the first visit, repeat CBC (or FBC) for hemoglobin concentration at 20–24 weeks' gestation, as well as the usual 28- and 34-weeks' gestation *(FIGO[4a])*

Special notes:

† Dodd JM, Dowswell T, Crowther CA. Specialised antenatal clinics for women with a multiple pregnancy for improving maternal and infant outcomes. *Cochrane Database Syst Rev.* 2015;(11):CD005300. Published 2015 Nov 6.

§ Recommended by the NHS Fetal Anomaly Screening Program me (FASP) *(NICE[8])*

** Refer to Chapter 1

‡ Refer to Question 11 in Chapter 38; referenced guidelines are indicated in the list of Suggested Readings

SCENARIO A

Routine intrapartum care for dichorionic twins

The patient appreciates your detailed overview of her projected prenatal care for this dichorionic pregnancy. She inquires about delivery plans and the possibility of a trial of VBAC. You take this opportunity to address the patient's concerns as well as teach your trainee strategies for intrapartum care of dichorionic gestations.

9. Indicate your evidence-based advice for delivery planning at term for uncomplicated dichorionic twins, highlighting to your trainee important intrapartum management considerations. *(1 point per main bullet)*

Max 13

Setting and personnel:

☐ Inform the patient that all twin gestations should be cared for in a hospital-based delivery suite when in labor

☐ Ensure obstetric expertise is available for potential twin B's internal podalic version, breech delivery, or need for emergency Cesarean delivery

☐ Consideration for double-set-up delivery (*i.e.,* in the operating room/theater) in case of need for emergency Cesarean section (*e.g.,* umbilical cord prolapse, abnormal fetal heart rate, failed internal/external version)

    ○ *Delivery in a birthing room may also be considered for cephalic/cephalic presentations and where timely maternal transfer to an operating room/theater is feasible in case of an emergency*

☐ Inform anesthesiology personnel upon delivery-admission

☐ Ensure adequate neonatology personnel/equipment for each neonate

Timing of delivery: *(Varying practice recommendations)*

☐ *[ACOG and SMFM][1]*: Anticipate delivery around 38^{+0} to 38^{+6} weeks' gestation

☐ *NICE[8]*: Planning delivery from 37^{+0} to 37^{+6} weeks' gestation does not appear to increase serious neonatal adverse outcomes; continuing pregnancy $>37^{+6}$ weeks increases the risk of fetal death

VBAC:

☐ In the absence of contraindications, her previous Cesarean delivery is not a contraindication to a trial of VBAC with current twin gestation[§]

☐ Reassure the patient that twin-VBAC deliveries have similar success rates and uterine rupture rates as singleton gestations

☐ Discuss the risks and benefits of the use of oxytocin for labor augmentation (*can follow the same protocol used for singleton VBAC pregnancies*)

Labor anesthesia with twins' delivery:

☐ Offer epidural anesthesia with planned vaginal birth *(where no contraindications exist)*

☐ Inform the patient that epidural anesthesia is likely to improve the chance of successful and optimal timing of assisted vaginal birth(s) *(NICE[8])*

☐ Inform the patient that epidural anesthesia is likely to enable a quicker emergency Cesarean delivery if needed *(NICE[8])*

Delivery route and specific equipment:

☐ Explain to the patient that a routine elective Cesarean delivery does not reduce the risks of fetal or neonatal mortalities or serious neonatal morbidities among dichorionic twins >32 weeks where the first twin is cephalic and in the absence of significant intertwin discordance

☐ Vaginal delivery is anticipated where twin A has a cephalic presentation at delivery-admission, and Cesarean delivery is ***preferred*** where the presenting fetus is noncephalic
  ○ *Although not advised, vaginal delivery of a noncephalic presenting twin is practiced in some international jurisdictions; beware of the risk of interlocking fetal chins where twin B is cephalic*

☐ Discuss use of oxytocin for uterine inertia between delivery of first and second twin

☐ Patient should be informed of the ~5% risk of combined delivery (vaginal/Cesarean), based on acute maternal-fetal indications

☐ Ensure availability of an ultrasound machine in the delivery room

☐ Ensure availability of Piper, Neville-Barns (or equivalent) forceps[‡] for delivery of the aftercoming head in the event of a twin B vaginal breech delivery

☐ Plan for 30–60 seconds delayed cord clamping after delivery of each dichorionic twin[**]

☐ Advise adequate intravenous access, blood product availability, and uterotonic agents/ 'postpartum hemorrhage kit' for risks of greater blood loss
  ○ *Patient consent is required, as routine, for blood product administration*
  ○ *Plan for active management of the third stage of labor*

Intrapartum fetal monitoring:

☐ Continuous electronic monitoring for each fetus during labor, ensuring two discernable fetal heart rate patterns are detected
  ○ Simultaneous display of maternal pulse monitoring on the cardtiocography (CTG) tracing or via pulse oximetry is advised
  ○ *NICE[8]*: Dual channel CTG monitors with fetal hearts separated by ≥20 beats/min
  ○ *FIGO[4a]*: Consideration for combined vaginal scalp clip[†] and abdominal tocometry for twin A and B, respectively

Special notes:

§ Refer to Chapter 18

‡ Refer to Questions 14 and 16 in Chapter 20

** Refer to 'Committee Opinion No. 684: Delayed Umbilical Cord Clamping after Birth,' *Obstet Gynecol.* 2017;129(1):1.

† At >34 weeks' gestation and without contraindications

You assure the patient that after delivery, services of the perinatal mental health expert will be available as required, noting that postpartum depression is three times as common among women with multiple pregnancies than singletons.

10. Where twin B is noncephalic in labor, with no major congenital malformations, identify   3
three obstetric features warranting specific consideration for the route for delivery of
diamniotic twins. *(1 point each)*

☐ Gestational age <32–34 weeks
☐ Estimated fetal weight <1500 grams
☐ Discordance ≥20%–25% above twin A *(individualized experts' decisions for % differences)*

SCENARIO B

(This is a continuation of the clinical scenario after Question 8):
Short cervix and previable delivery of a co-twin

The patient appreciates your detailed overview of her projected prenatal care plan.
Noninvasive cfDNA confirmed the twins are discordant in gender with a low risk of trisomy
13, 18, and 21. Pregnancy progresses well with interdisciplinary care. At 20 weeks' gestation,
both fetal morphology surveys and amniotic fluid volumes are normal. A suspected short
cervix on transabdominal scanning is confirmed transvaginally where the cervix is 21 mm; the
patient is asymptomatic, and the cervix is closed on gentle pelvic examination. There is no
clinical suspicion of genitourinary infections.

The patient is concerned, recalling her cervical length being at least 30 mm at this gestation in
her first pregnancy. She would like to consider all interventions possible to prolong her
pregnancy and decrease the risk of spontaneous preterm birth.

11. With focus on her transvaginal cervical length, detail your evidence-based management   Max 4
and clinical controversies for preterm birth prevention in a multiple pregnancy. *(1 point
per main bullet)*

☐ Consideration for consultation with a maternal-fetal medicine expert and/or transfer of
care to a tertiary center *(local variations exist)*
☐ Discuss local practice guidance for progestogen treatment (oral, vaginal, or intramuscular):
    ○ *SOGC*[**]: Recommend vaginal micronized progesterone 400 mg nightly for prevention
      of spontaneous preterm birth given a multiple pregnancy with short transvaginal
      cervical length (≤25 mm) between 16 and 24 weeks' gestation
    ○ *[EPPPIC, SMFM ACOG]:*[§] In multifetal gestations, there is insufficient evidence to
      recommend the use of progestogens regardless of cervical length or prior preterm birth
    ○ *EPPPIC:*[§] Intramuscular 17-alpha hydroxyprogesterone caproate is associated with
      preterm prelabor rupture of membranes in multifetal pregnancies
    ○ *NICE*[8]: No recommendations yet on vaginal progesterone[#] to prevent spontaneous
      preterm birth in twin pregnancies; intramuscular progesterone is not advised
☐ Inform the patient that cerclage is not warranted by current guidelines:
    ○ *SOGC*[10b]: Cerclage placement for short cervix (<25 mm) in twins is not advantageous
      and might increase the risk of preterm birth; limited evidence suggests possible
      advantage to cerclage with cervical length ≤15 mm or rescue procedure with cervical
      dilatation >10 mm[†] at 16–24 weeks[‡]

☐ Current evidence does not support benefit of a cervical pessary for prevention of preterm birth or adverse perinatal outcome, even in the presence of a short cervix

☐ Bed rest or reduced activity is **not** recommended in multifetal pregnancy with a short cervical length (or previous preterm birth) for reduction of spontaneous preterm birth

Special notes:

** Refer to Jain V, McDonald SD, Mundle WR, Farine D. Guideline No. 398: Progesterone for Prevention of Spontaneous Preterm Birth. *J Obstet Gynaecol Can.* 2020;42(6):806–812.

§ EPPPIC Group. Evaluating Progestogens for Preventing Preterm birth International Collaborative (EPPPIC): meta-analysis of individual participant data from randomised controlled trials. *Lancet.* 2021;397(10280):1183–1194.

§ SMFM Statement response. www.smfm.org/publications/383-smfm-statement-response-to-epppic-and-considerations-of-the-use-of-progestogens-for-the-prevention-of-preterm-birth, accessed April 12, 2021.

§ ACOG Practice Advisory. www.acog.org/clinical/clinical-guidance/practice-advisory/articles/2021/03/clinical-guidance-for-the-integration-of-the-findings-of-the-epppic-meta-analysis-evaluating-progestogens-for-preventing-preterm-birth-international-collaborative, accessed April 12, 2021.

\# Evidence for lack of benefit, refer to Norman JE, Mackenzie F, Owen P, et al. Progesterone for the prevention of preterm birth in twin pregnancy (STOPPIT): a randomised, double-blind, placebo-controlled study and meta-analysis. *Lancet.* 2009;373(9680):2034–2040.

† Refer to Roman A, Zork N, Haeri S, et al. Physical examination-indicated cerclage in twin pregnancy: a randomized controlled trial. *Am J Obstet Gynecol.* 2020;223(6):902.e1–902.e11.

‡ Refer to Li C, Shen J, Hua K. Cerclage for women with twin pregnancies: a systematic review and metaanalysis. *Am J Obstet Gynecol.* 2019;220(6):543–557.e1.

After clinical assessment and patient consultation with a maternal-fetal medicine expert, a trial of nightly vaginal progesterone is commenced. Serial clinical and sonographic follow-up is unremarkable until 23^{+6} weeks' gestation when she presents to the tertiary center's obstetric emergency assessment unit with spontaneous onset of uterine contractions, detected on tocometry. There are no other obstetric complaints, and two fetal heart rates are documented. The patient is afebrile and normotensive. The cervix is 4 cm dilated and the amniotic membranes are bulging with twin A, presenting cephalic. Standard investigations and management are commenced. Despite attempted tocolysis,† primarily for completion of corticosteroids, she delivers twin A shortly after the administered bolus of magnesium sulfate (neuroprotection) and intravenous antibiotics. The neonatology team is currently resuscitating the 600-gram newborn, as was dually agreed in counseling.

After delivery of twin A, labor subsides. There is no suspected clinical chorioamnionitis. The patient remains optimistic to maximize outcomes for the remaining twin. She is clinically well, and the heart rate of the remaining twin remains normal. Her treating physician calls you to provide updates after detailed counseling and informed consent.

Special note:

† At this gestational age, a short course of indomethacin is safe; nifedipine is also optional. Beta-agonists would not be recommended due to increased risk of pulmonary edema in multiple pregnancies

12. What nonpharmacologic option could be considered in an attempt to prolong latency time to delivery of the second twin?   1

☐ Delayed interval delivery (DID)

The treating physician informs you that at the present time, there are no maternal-fetal contraindications to DID. With consent, she received prophylactic Rh immunoglobulin for D-negative blood group without respective atypical antibodies. Given the relative rarity of clinical situations and diverse dimensions of decision-making in DID, there are no clinical practice guidelines on counseling and management; clinical care is largely individualized and based on reported cases, reviews, or meta-analyses. You intend to teach your obstetric trainee about DID, as evidence suggests it may significantly prolong[†] pregnancy and improve perinatal survival relative to the first born, especially when a twin delivers prior to mid-gestation.

Special note:
† Reported latency period is highly variable; delays >150 days have been reported

13. Indicate perinatal risks of DID that the treating physician has discussed with the patient.   Max 10
(1 point each, unless specified)

Maternal:
☐ Chorioamnionitis/sepsis *(3)*
☐ Uterine contractions with/without labor
☐ Preterm prelabor rupture of membranes (PPROM) of remaining twin
☐ Placental abruption
☐ Postpartum hemorrhage
☐ Antepartum/postpartum venous thromboembolism[†] *(due to limited physical activity)*
☐ Mortality

Fetal/neonatal:
☐ Abnormal electronic fetal heart tracing
☐ Neonatal morbidity, depending on gestational age at birth and maternal morbidities
   (e.g., chorioamnionitis, placental abruption)
☐ Mortality

Special note:
† Consideration for mechanical and/or pharmacologic thromboprophylaxis

SCENARIO C

(This is a continuation of the clinical scenario after Question 8):
Growth discordance in dichorionic twins

The patient appreciates your detailed overview of her projected prenatal care plan. Noninvasive cfDNA confirmed the twins are <u>discordant</u> in gender with a low risk of trisomy 13, 18, and 21. Pregnancy progresses well with interdisciplinary care. At 20 weeks' gestation, both fetal morphology surveys, amniotic fluid volumes, and transvaginal cervical length are normal. Biometries are concordant and appropriate for gestational age. Complete placenta previa with normal cord insertion is noted for twin A (male), while its co-twin has normal placentation.

You receive her 32 weeks' gestation fetal sonographic report indicating twin A's estimated fetal weight (EFW) is now on the 1232 g (5th percentile), a change from the prior 20th percentile curve maintained to date; twin B's EFW is 1833 g (50th percentile) and growth velocity remains adequate. Twin A's umbilical artery pulsatility index (UA-PI) is >95th percentile while that of its co-twin remains normal; amniotic fluid volumes are normal. The report indicates a 32.8% intertwin growth discordance. Placentation remains unchanged and the patient has no obstetric complaints. To date, multidisciplinary obstetric care has been provided in your level II hospital center.

---

14. What are the two next steps in management of this patient? *(1 point each)*   2

☐ Counsel the patient of the ultrasound findings
☐ Request consultation and/or transfer of care to a hospital center with necessary maternal-fetal medicine and neonatal expertise

---

15. Inform your trainee <u>how</u> the intertwin discordance was obtained.   1

☐ $\frac{\text{EFW(larger twin)} - \text{EFW(smaller twin)}}{\text{EFW(larger twin)}} \times 100$

---

16. Specify the terminology used for the featured growth abnormality in these dichorionic twins.   1

☐ Selective fetal growth restriction (sFGR) of twin A

---

17. With sFGR, list investigations that <u>may</u> be considered in the work-up of this fetus. *(1 point each)*   2

☐ Maternal serum perinatal infections (*e.g.*, cytomegalovirus, toxoplasmosis, rubella)
☐ Consideration for amniocentesis for exclusion of chromosomal abnormalities not detected by routine aneuploidy screening tests

---

You alert your trainee that there is no optimal threshold for defining growth discordance in dichorionic twins that best predicts adverse birth outcomes. The trainee is aware that frequency of maternal-fetal monitoring will be increased relative to routine prenatal care among dichorionic pregnancies.

18. Discuss one definition for intertwin growth discordance. *(1 point each)*   1

☐ Greater than 20%–25% intertwin growth discordance (estimated fetal weight)
  o *Use of either percent discordance may adequately predict the risk of adverse outcomes; practice variations exist*
☐ EFW of either fetus <10th percentile for gestational age
☐ Greater than 20 mm difference in intertwin abdominal circumferences *(SOGC[10c])*

19. In counseling, address her inquiry on perinatal risks associated with sFGR in a dichorionic   Max 4
pregnancy. *(1 point per main bullet)*

Maternal:
☐ Iatrogenic prematurity
☐ Increased risk of Cesarean section due to the growth restriction and larger twin B

Fetal/neonatal:
☐ Risk of fetal demise (IUFD) for the sFGR fetus; the risk of demise in the co-twin is 3%
  o *Note that rates of fetal demise are likely not increased when intertwin discordance is seen without either fetus being growth restricted*
☐ With single fetal demise in a dichorionic pregnancy, the rate of co-twin neurodevelopmental impairment ranges from 2%[†] to 10%[††]
  o *No benefit to prompt delivery after a twin's demise*
☐ Increased neonatal morbidity[§] related to FGR, prematurity,[‡] and multiple gestation

Special notes:
† ISUOG[7]
†† Refer to Mackie FL, Rigby A, Morris RK, Kilby MD. Prognosis of the co-twin following spontaneous single intrauterine fetal death in twin pregnancies: a systematic review and meta-analysis. *BJOG.* 2019;126(5):569–578.
§ Refer to Questions 29 and 31-B in Chapter 9 for neonatal metabolic morbidities and long-term morbidities with FGR, respectively
‡ Refer to Chapter 7 for neonatal morbidities associated with prematurity

20. After the consultation, you take the opportunity to teach your trainee about causes for   Max 2
fetal growth discordances in dizygotic twins where <u>no</u> intrinsic fetal pathology exists.
(1 point each)

☐ Abnormal placental implantation for one twin *(e.g., placenta previa, underlying fibroma or uterine septum at the implantation site)*
☐ Umbilical cord anomalies that are more frequently encountered in multiple gestations *(e.g., vasa previa, marginal or velamentous cord insertions)*
☐ Placental proximity *(i.e., 'crowding')* resulting in suboptimal early placental development of one twin

SCENARIO D

(This is a continuation of the clinical scenario after Question 8):
Discordant anomaly and selective fetocide in dichorionic twins

The patient appreciates your detailed overview of her projected prenatal care for this dichorionic pregnancy. Noninvasive cfDNA confirmed two male fetuses with a low risk of trisomy 13, 18, and 21. Pregnancy progresses well with interdisciplinary care. You referred the patient for detailed second-trimester sonographic fetal morphology at a tertiary center after a fetal anomaly was suspected at your center's imaging unit. Indeed, at 20 weeks' gestation, anomalous findings in twin B include short, curved femurs ('telephone receiver'), short ribs, a small thoracic circumference, platyspondyly, without a cloverleaf skull. Twin A's morphology, both amniotic fluid volumes, and cervical length are normal. Although her care has been transferred to a maternal-fetal medicine expert, you maintain liaison with updated progress of her care.

21. What is the <u>most specific</u> anticipated best next diagnostic step in the care of this patient? 1

☐ Amniocentesis for skeletal dysplasia panel in the affected fetus
  ○ *The fetuses in this scenario may be monozygotic dichorionic twins; twin A may demonstrate phenotypic abnormalities, suggestive of a skeletal dysplasia, in later gestation*
  ○ *Concordance rate for anomalies in monozygotic twins is ~20%*

The patient consents to a senior trainee performing the amniocentesis under supervision of the maternal-fetal medicine expert. Accordingly, the consultant takes this opportunity to review important technical aspects of amniocentesis in a dichorionic pregnancy prior to the patient encounter. The patient is Rh-positive.

22-A. Outline amniocentesis-related risks <u>specific</u> to twin pregnancy. *(1 point each)* 2

☐ The rate of pregnancy loss after amniocentesis in a twin gestation ranges from 1% to 3.1%
☐ Inadvertent septostomy/membrane shearing leading to a monoamniotic cavity

22-B. Detail important aspects related to amniocentesis in dichorionic twins that the consultant is likely to review with the trainee preprocedure. *(1 point each)* 3

☐ Sequential and separate needle techniques for each fetus is preferable, under standard sonographic guidance
☐ The patient should be reassured that the two-needle-entry technique does not increase the procedure-related pregnancy loss rate
☐ Consideration for insertion of 2–3 mL indigo carmine or Evan's blue dye§ (if technically required) after sampling of the first sac

Special note:
§ Methylene blue dye is contraindicated due to risks of neonatal methemoglobinemia, skin staining, and small bowel atresia

Results of the uncomplicated amniocentesis later confirm two normal genetic males, with a discordant mutation for fibroblast growth factor receptor 3 (FGFR3) gene in twin B, consistent with the sonographic anomalies. In addition to the geneticist, a perinatal mental health expert has been involved in her care.

---

23. With regard to twin B's diagnosis and prognosis, outline <u>focused</u> clinical considerations for management of the dichorionic pregnancy. *(1 point per main bullet)*

                        Max 2

☐ Twin B is affected by thanatophoric dysplasia type I, which is the most common *lethal* skeletal dysplasia

☐ As thanatophoric dysplasia type I may be associated with polyhydramnios in 50% of cases, selective fetal termination could be considered for preterm birth prevention, optimizing outcomes for twin A
   ○ *Timing of selective termination is individualized; options include: (a) upon diagnostic confirmation; (b) with onset of polyhydramnios, or (c) in the third trimester where sonographic findings have been stable in pregnancy*

☐ Inform the patient that although a thanatophoric dysplasia is lethal, selective fetal termination may be preferable to the emotional burden of carrying an ultimately nonviable fetus

After comprehensive patient counseling by interdisciplinary team members, she opts for late selective fetal termination in the third trimester or sooner, if polyhydramnios develops; this is permitted by your regional laws and regulations.

With severe polyhydramnios present at 28 weeks' gestation, the procedure has been arranged and will be performed by the maternal-fetal medicine expert.

---

24. What would be the preferred technique for selective termination of this dichorionic pregnancy?

                        1

☐ Ultrasound-guided transabdominal or transvaginal intracardiac or intrafunicular potassium chloride or lidocaine injection until asystole is achieved
   ○ Confirm asystole of the selected twin for at least five minutes postprocedure

Special note:
Contrary to dichorionic twins, umbilical cord occlusion, radiofrequency ablation, or laser ablation of the cord of the affected twin are methods for selective termination of monochorionic twins

---

25. During patient counseling, address the risks and postprocedure follow-up with selective termination of dichorionic twins planned at 28 weeks' gestation.[§] *(1 point each)*

                        Max 5

Risks:[‡]
☐ Low risk of preterm delivery *(especially as the reduced twin not presenting)*
☐ Co-twin neurodevelopmental impairment is ~10% with dichorionic placentation (see Question 19)

- ☐ Inadvertent reduction of the healthy twin *(accurate fetal identification is crucial)*
- ☐ Maternal complications related to invasive procedures *(e.g., PPROM, preterm labor, chorioamnionitis, placental abruption, maternal-fetal hemorrhage, isoimmunization)*
- ☐ Parental stress

Follow-up:
- ☐ Sonographic assessment of the viable twin in approximately one week, followed by serial fetal growth and well-being thereafter *[individualized interval]*

Special notes:
§ Although not relevant to this clinical scenario, the overall pregnancy loss rates after single fetal reduction ranges from 2.4% to 7.9% before 24 weeks' gestation

‡ SOGC[10a]: Monitoring for disseminated intravascular coagulation after selective reduction of dichorionic twins

TOTAL: **105**

CHAPTER 12

Monochorionic Twin Pregnancy

Nimrah Abbasi and Greg Ryan

A 34-year-old primigravida is referred by her primary care provider to your hospital center's high-risk obstetrics unit after sonographic imaging confirmed viable intrauterine spontaneous monochorionic diamniotic (MCDA) twins with crown–rump lengths (CRL) of 47 mm and 44 mm, consistent for 12^{+4} weeks' gestation by CRL of the larger twin. Twin A's and twin B's nuchal translucency (NT) measurements are 1.5 mm and 1.0 mm, respectively, with normal-appearing first-trimester fetal morphologies.

Her medical, surgical, social, and family histories are unremarkable. She has been taking routine prenatal vitamins containing folic acid for the past four months. The patient does not have any obstetric complaints. She is normotensive with a body mass index (BMI) of 26.5 kg/m^2.

Special note: *To avoid overlap of content addressed in* Chapter 11, *this case scenario is presented with a focus on counseling and management of uncomplicated and complicated MCDA twins. An overweight body habitus is intended to highlight different gestational weight gain recommendations for twin pregnancies relative to women with a normal body mass index, as presented in* Chapter 11. *Readers are encouraged to complement subject matter with material in* Chapter 11, *Questions 1, 2, 4, 5, and 7, relevant to all twin gestations.*

LEARNING OBJECTIVES

1. Understand sonographic descriptors of chorionicity and amnionicity that manifest from the basic biology of monochorionic twinning
2. Appreciate the complications of monochorionic twins warranting specialized sonographic expertise and interdisciplinary management
3. Provide detailed antepartum and intrapartum management of uncomplicated MCDA twins
4. Recognize principles of diagnosis and care of selected monochorionic complications, including twin–twin transfusion syndrome (TTTS), twin anemia-polycythemia sequence, selective fetal growth restriction (sFGR), and antenatal counseling and management of a viable twin after spontaneous demise of its co-twin

SUGGESTED READINGS

1. American College of Obstetricians and Gynecologists' Committee on Practice Bulletins – Obstetrics, Society for Maternal-Fetal Medicine. Multifetal gestations: twin, triplet, and

higher-order multifetal pregnancies: ACOG Practice Bulletin, No. 231. *Obstet Gynecol.* 2021;137(6):e145–e162.

2. Bamberg C, Hecher K. Update on twin-to-twin transfusion syndrome. *Best Pract Res Clin Obstet Gynaecol.* 2019; 58:55–65.

3. Bennasar M, Eixarch E, Martinez JM, et al. Selective intrauterine growth restriction in monochorionic diamniotic twin pregnancies. *Semin Fetal Neonatal Med.* 2017;22(6):376–382.

4. FIGO Working Group on Good Clinical Practice in Maternal-Fetal Medicine. Good clinical practice advice: management of twin pregnancy. *Int J Gynaecol Obstet.* 2019;144(3):330–337.

5. Hoskins IA, Combs CA. Society for Maternal-Fetal Medicine Special Statement: updated checklists for management of monochorionic twin pregnancy. *Am J Obstet Gynecol.* 2020;223(5):B16–B20.

6. Khalil A, Rodgers M, Baschat A, et al. ISUOG Practice Guidelines: role of ultrasound in twin pregnancy. *Ultrasound Obstet Gynecol.* 2016;47(2):247–263. [Correction in *Ultrasound Obstet Gynecol.* 2018 Jul;52(1):140]

7. Kilby MD, Bricker L. Management of monochorionic twin pregnancy. *BJOG* 2016;124:e1–e45.

8. Moldenhauer JS, Johnson MP. Diagnosis and management of complicated monochorionic twins. *Clin Obstet Gynecol.* 2015;58(3):632–642.

9. NAFTNet (a) Bahtiyar MO, Emery SP, Dashe JS, et al. The North American Fetal Therapy Network consensus statement: prenatal surveillance of uncomplicated monochorionic gestations. *Obstet Gynecol.* 2015;125(1):118–123.

   NAFTNet (b) Emery SP, Bahtiyar MO, Dashe JS, et al. The North American Fetal Therapy Network consensus statement: prenatal management of uncomplicated monochorionic gestations. *Obstet Gynecol.* 2015;125(5):1236–1243.

10. National Institute for Health and Care Excellence (NICE) Guideline No. 137: Twin and triplet pregnancy. September 2019.

POINTS

1. Inform your obstetric trainee of sonographic markers that may have contributed to confirmation of a MCDA twin gestation. *(1 point per main bullet)*	4

Sonography at 11–14 weeks' gestation:‡
☐ Intertwin membrane insertion in the placenta appears as a T-sign projection of fused amniotic membranes without interspersed chorionic parenchyma
  ○ *'T-sign' has 100% sensitivity and >98% specificity for detecting MCDA gestations*
☐ Thin, <2 mm, two-layered intertwin amniotic membrane
☐ Single placental mass*
☐ Sex concordance§

Special notes:
‡ Twin fetuses should be labeled systematically based on laterality or vertical orientation as well as placental cord insertion sites at the 11–14 weeks' scan to enable accurate longitudinal monitoring of their biometry on serial scans and interpretation of prenatal screening/diagnostic results for each twin. On later scans, any features that may help distinguish the twins should be added, such as *'larger/smaller'* or discordant Doppler waveforms; labeling as 'twin A and twin B' is not advised
* A dichorionic placenta may be a fused single placental mass
§ Although sex discordance is almost invariably consistent with dichorionicity, sex concordance does not exclude dichorionicity.

The patient, a biologist, requests your explanation of the scientific basis for this form of monochorionic twinning, as she wonders whether her twins will be identical and if any features on medical history may have contributed to this placentation. Aware of available noninvasive screening options for aneuploidy,[†] she opts for combined screening using maternal age, first-trimester serum markers, and NT measurements, which will provide a *pregnancy-specific* risk of aneuploidy in monochorionic twins *(RCOG[7]).*

Special note:
† Refer to Question 5 in Chapter 11

2.	Address the patient's inquiries by detailing the physiology of zygosity in MCDA twins, highlighting variables that may affect incidence rates, if any. *(1 point each)*	2

☐ Monochorionic twins are all monozygotic, occurring at a constant rate of ~1/250 pregnancies (*i.e.*, 4/1000)
☐ Chorionicity and amnionicity of monozygotic gestations are determined by the time at which the fertilized ovum divides; for divisions at four to eight days after fertilization, the inner cell mass has formed and cells destined to become the chorion have already differentiated, but those of the amnion have not (MCDA twins)

3.	Although monochorionic twins resulting from a single fertilized egg are monozygotic, explain how MCDA twins may be discordant for genetic and structural abnormalities.	2

☐ Postzygotic (including *de-novo*) mutations may lead to a discordant phenotype or genotype (*e.g., Marfan syndrome in one of a monochorionic twin pair*)

4.	In general terms, describe how the risk of trisomy 21 at term would be determined for such monochorionic twins.	1

☐ The risk of trisomy 21 is calculated *per pregnancy with* monochorionic twins based on the average risk for both fetuses

Although excited about the prospects of having twins, her primary care provider briefed her that monochorionic placentation is associated with specific fetal complications that require close prenatal surveillance. The patient understands that while the relative likelihood of each complication changes with advancing gestation, they can all occur at any gestational age *(NICE[10]).*

You have already elaborated on complications more common to all types of multiple gestations relative to singletons.[§]

Special note:
§ Refer to Question 7 in Chapter 11

5. Which <u>fetal complications</u> of <u>monochorionicity</u> warrant specialized sonographic expertise and clinical management? *(1 point each)*

Max 6

- ☐ Cord entanglement with monoamniotic twins
- ☐ Twin–twin transfusion syndrome (TTTS)
- ☐ Twin anemia-polycythemia sequence
- ☐ Twin reversed arterial perfusion sequence
- ☐ Selective fetal growth restriction (sFGR)
- ☐ Single in utero fetal demise (IUFD)
- ☐ Discordant anomalies
- ☐ Conjoined twins

6. Following her comprehensive first-trimester sonogram, outline your <u>focused</u> antenatal management for this patient, assuming that this is an <u>uncomplicated</u> MCDA twin gestation. *(1 point per main bullet)*

Max 12

- ☐ Inform the patient that once the required sonographic follow-up for monochorionic twins is arranged, antenatal care may be provided by a generalist obstetrician, specialist midwife, or continued with a fetal medicine expert
- ☐ Multidisciplinary care providers would be available based on individual patient needs (*e.g.*, dietician, perinatal health expert, social worker, women's health physiotherapist)
    - ○ *Local variations in practice exist regarding 'specialized antenatal clinics' for multiple pregnancies: maternal-infant health outcomes have not been proven to be better relative to standard antenatal care*[†]

Sonographic surveillance: [*]
- ☐ Serial ultrasound every 2 weeks from 16 weeks' gestation until delivery
    - ○ Assess fetal growth, liquor volume, bladder filling, umbilical artery-pulsatility indices (UA-PI), and middle cerebral artery peak systolic velocities (MCA-PSV)
- ☐ Arrange for detailed fetal anomaly surveys with assessment of placental location/umbilical cord insertions at 18–22 weeks' gestation
    - ○ *Monozygotic twins are two to three times more likely to be affected by fetal structural abnormalities*
- ☐ Fetal echocardiography is recommended at 18–22 weeks' gestation for monochorionic pregnancies (*ACOG*[1])
    - ○ *~5% of monochorionic twins have congenital heart disease in at least one twin, with pregnancies complicated by TTTS at higher risk*
- ☐ Discuss local practice guidance for cervical length assessment
    - ○ *FIGO*[4], *ISUOG*[6]: Cervical length evaluation is recommended at 20 weeks' gestation to identify women at risk of extreme preterm birth
    - ○ Mode for cervical length assessment (*i.e.*, transabdominal or transvaginal) may vary by physician or patient factors
    - ○ *NICE*[10]: Although cervical length measurement is <u>supported</u> as a predictor of preterm birth in twin pregnancy, <u>no recommendation</u> can be made in the absence of effective intervention(s) for women at risk

Maternal clinical care:

□ After the first early-prenatal visit, plan monthly clinical visits until 28 weeks, then bimonthly until delivery

□ Screen for signs/symptoms of hypertensive disorders of pregnancy and preterm labor at each antenatal appointment

□ Inform the patient that monochorionic twin pregnancies have higher rates of pregnancy loss (mainly due to second-trimester loss) than dichorionic twins *(RCOG[7])*

□ Encourage early patient reporting of sudden increases in abdominal girth or breathlessness *(RCOG[7])*

□ *[Consideration for]* Low dose aspirin (~75–160 mg) nightly started preferably at 12 weeks {ideally <16 weeks}

  ○ ISSHP[‡] and SMFM[‡] guidelines: Multiple gestation is a *strong* risk factor for preeclampsia

  ○ NICE[‡] guidelines: Multiple gestation is a *moderate* risk factor, where LDASA would be advised with at least one other moderate risk factor

□ Advise continuation of 1 mg folic acid-containing prenatal vitamins[#]

□ As this patient is overweight, her recommended total weight gain would be 31 to 50 lbs (14.1 to 22.7 kg) with a twin pregnancy, according to the National Academy of Medicine *(formerly the Institute of Medicine)*

□ With dietary expert guidance for an overweight BMI, recommended daily caloric intake with a twin pregnancy would be 30–35 kcal/kg/d, altered as necessary for the ideal weight gain goal and with larger doses of micronutrients (*e.g.*, iron, calcium, magnesium, zinc, vitamin D) than in routine prenatal vitamins[#]

□ In the absence of risk factors or pregnancy complications, advise the same exercise recommendations as for singletons[**]

□ In addition to routine screening at the first visit, repeat CBC (or FBC) for hemoglobin concentration at 20–24 weeks' gestation, as well as the usual 28- and 34 weeks' gestation

Special notes:

* *RCOG[7] and NICE[10]* do not recommend first-trimester screening for TTTS

† Dodd JM, Dowswell T, Crowther CA. Specialised antenatal clinics for women with a multiple pregnancy for improving maternal and infant outcomes. *Cochrane Database Syst Rev.* 2015;(11):CD005300.

‡ Refer to Question 11 in Chapter 38; referenced guidelines are indicated in list of Suggested Readings

Refer to Chapter 11, Suggested Reading 5: Goodnight W, Newman R; Society of Maternal–Fetal Medicine. Optimal nutrition for improved twin pregnancy outcome. *Obstet Gynecol.* 2009;114(5):1121–1134.

** Refer to Chapter 1

SCENARIO A

Routine intrapartum care for MCDA twins

The patient appreciates your detailed overview of her projected prenatal care for this monochorionic pregnancy. She is curious whether delivery involves particularities, as with antepartum care of MCDA twins.

7. Indicate your evidence-based advice for delivery planning of uncomplicated MCDA twins, while highlighting to your trainee important intrapartum management considerations.

Max 13

Timing of delivery:

☐ Optimal timing for delivery of uncomplicated MCDA twins has not been ascertained; practice recommendations vary: *(any subbullet for 1 point; other practice recommendations may be deemed acceptable)*

	Recommended timing for elective delivery
○ ACOG,† [1]	34^{+0} to 37^{+6} weeks' gestation
○ NAFTNet[9b]	36^{+0} to 37^{+6} weeks' gestation
○ NICE[10] and systematic review/meta-analysis[‡]	36^{+0} to 36^{+6} weeks' gestation
○ SMFM[5]	By 37^{+6} weeks' gestation, or earlier if complications, antenatal corticosteroids are advised within seven days of delivery when delivery is anticipated before 34 weeks' gestation
○ RCOG[7] and FIGO[4]	As of 36^{+0} weeks' gestation, with administration of antenatal corticosteroids, unless earlier delivery is indicated

Mode of delivery:[§] *(1 point each, for 3)*

☐ Vaginal delivery is preferred in uncomplicated MCDA twins; Cesarean delivery is reserved for obstetric indications

☐ Patient should be informed of the ~5% risk of combined delivery (vaginal/Cesarean), based on acute maternal-fetal indications

☐ Have Piper, Neville-Barns (or equivalent) forceps[#] available in case they may be necessary for delivery of the aftercoming head if twin B is breech

Protocol for cord clamping: *(1 point)*

☐ *Although limited evidence-based and controversial recommendations,* the first twin of a monochorionic pair may not be an ideal candidate for delayed cord clamping due to the risk of acute feto-fetal transfusion leading to hypovolemia and adverse outcomes for the undelivered twin B

Setting and personnel: *(1 point per main bullet; max 5)*

☐ Inform the patient that all twin gestations should be cared for in a hospital-based delivery suite when in labor

☐ Consideration for double-set-up delivery (*i.e.*, in the operating room/theater) for possible emergency Cesarean section (*e.g.*, umbilical cord prolapse, abnormal fetal heart rate, failed internal/external version)

　　○ *Delivery in a birthing room may also be considered for cephalic/cephalic presentations and where timely maternal transfer to an operating room/theater is feasible in case of an emergency*

☐ Ensure obstetric expertise is available for potential twin B's internal podalic version, breech delivery, or need for emergency Cesarean delivery

☐ Inform anesthesiology personnel upon delivery-admission, and ensure availability of intravenous nitroglycerin

☐ Ensure adequate neonatology personnel/equipment for each twin

☐ Advise adequate intravenous access, blood product availability, and uterotonic agents/ 'postpartum hemorrhage kit' for risks of greater blood loss
  ○ *Patient consent is required, as routine, for blood product administration*
  ○ *Plan for active management of the third stage of labor*

☐ Ultrasound machine availability in the delivery room, even where twin B is cephalic, to confirm twin B's presentation if necessary and to rapidly assess B's fetal heart

Intrapartum fetal monitoring: *(1 point for main bullet)*

☐ Continuous electronic monitoring for each fetus during labor, ensuring two discernable fetal heart rate patterns are detected
  ○ Simultaneous display of maternal pulse monitoring on the cardtiocography (CTG) tracing is advised
  ○ NICE[10]: Dual channel CTG monitors with fetal hearts separated by $\geq$20 beats/min
  ○ FIGO[4]: Consideration for combined vaginal scalp clip[††] and abdominal tocometry for twin A and B, respectively

Labor anesthesia with twins' delivery: *(1 point each; max 2)*

☐ Offer epidural anesthesia with planned vaginal birth *(where no contraindications exist)*

☐ Inform the patient that epidural anesthesia is likely to improve the chance of successful and optimal timing of assisted vaginal birth(s) *(NICE[10])*

☐ Inform the patient that epidural anesthesia is likely to enable a quicker emergency Cesarean delivery if needed *(NICE[10])*
  ○ *Where epidural is declined, pudental block should be available for delivery of the second twin*

Special notes:

† American College of Obstetricians and Gynecologists' Committee on Obstetric Practice, Society for Maternal-Fetal Medicine. Medically Indicated Late-Preterm and Early-Term Deliveries: ACOG Committee Opinion, No. 831. *Obstet Gynecol.* 2021;138(1):e35–e39.

‡ Cheong-See F, Schuit E, Arroyo-Manzano D, et al. Prospective risk of stillbirth and neonatal complications in twin pregnancies: systematic review and meta-analysis. *BMJ.* 2016;354:i4353. Published 2016 Sep 6.

Refer to Questions 14 and 16 in Chapter 20

§ Insufficient evidence for or against delayed cord clamping in monochorionic twins; consideration for risk of intrapartum placental transfusion

†† At >34 weeks' gestation and without contraindications

You assure the patient that after delivery, services of the perinatal mental health expert will be maintained. The obstetric trainee is aware that postpartum depression is three times as common among women with multiple pregnancies than singletons.

SCENARIO B
(This is a continuation of the clinical scenario after Question 6)
Twin–twin transfusion syndrome (TTTS) and Twin Anemia-Polycythemia Sequence
The patient appreciates your detailed overview of her projected prenatal care for this monochorionic pregnancy. Routine maternal prenatal laboratory tests are unremarkable and blood group is O-negative without alloimmunization. Pregnancy progresses well with interdisciplinary care.

At 20 weeks' gestation, both detailed fetal morphology surveys, including echocardiography reports, are normal. External genitalia are consistent with female genders Although twin A is slightly larger than its co-twin, biometric parameters are within normal and discordance is <20%. Amniotic fluid deep vertical pockets (DVPs), bladder fillings, and fetal Doppler indices are normal. Twin B has a velomentous cord insertion[#].

At 22 weeks' gestation, routine fetal sonography reveals *isolated* amniotic fluid volume discordances with DVP-twin A at 11 cm and DVP-twin B at 1.5 cm. All other parameters of comprehensive maternal-fetal assessment are normal.

Special note:
\# Velomentous cord insertions are more common in monochorionic than dichorionic twins

8. Based on your <u>most specific</u> diagnosis, discuss your counseling and management plan.   2
   (1 point each)

Quintero Stage I TTTS:[§]
- ☐ Conservative management with close surveillance (at least weekly ultrasound) is reasonable, as up to 60% of stage 1 disease will deteriorate, requiring intervention[†]
- ☐ Reinforce early patient reporting of increased abdominal girth, breathlessness, or signs/symptoms of preterm labor

Special notes:
§ Refer to Quintero RA, Morales WJ, Allen MH, et al. Staging of twin–twin transfusion syndrome. *J Perinatol.* 1999;19(8 Pt 1):550–555
   In Europe, polyhydramnios is diagnosed when DVP is ≥8 cm at ≤20 weeks' and ≥10 cm after 20 weeks' gestation
† Stirnemann J, Slaghekke F, Khalek N, et al. *Am J Obstet Gynecol.* 2021 May;224(5):528.e1–528.e12

You explain that TTTS occurs in 10%–15% of MCDA twins and thoroughly address its natural history. The patient is keen to salvage both fetuses and agrees to close expectant follow-up with possible intervention, if necessary.

9. Outline essential elements of the natural history and pathophysiology of TTTS, addressing your trainee's inquiry of 'protective' mechanisms against this phenomenon in the majority of monochorionic placentas. *(1 point per main bullet)*

3

□ TTTS tends to occur in the mid-trimester (16–26 weeks) with perinatal mortality rates at 70–100% with mid-trimester severe TTTS without intervention
□ Pathophysiology: Unbalanced arterio-venous placental anastomoses result in unidirectional flow from a donor-to-recipient twin, leading to characteristic volume shifts with volume depletion, oliguria and oligohydramnios in the donor while the recipient has volume overload, polyuria and polyhydramnios
□ Protective mechanisms: arterial-arterial anastomoses that allow for bidirectional flow, balancing the effects of arterio-venous anastomoses

Sonographic findings remain stable the following week. At 24^{+1} weeks' gestation, fetal weight discordance has increased to 25%, with twin B being smaller and with anhydramnios without bladder filling. Twin A's DVP is now at 15 cm with bladder distension. All Doppler indices are normal. Neither fetus is hydropic. Over the past week, the patient has noticed an increase in abdominal girth and uterine discomfort for which she was considering presenting to hospital. Comprehensive clinical assessment, including her oxygen saturation and pelvic examination, are normal.

10. Inform the patient of the <u>most specific</u> diagnosis and discuss your <u>comprehensive</u> management plan. The patient remains keen to salvage both fetuses.[†] *(1 point per main and subbullet)*

Max 7

Diagnosis and possible interventions:[‡]
□ Quintero Stage 2 TTTS
  ○ Fetoscopic laser photocoagulation of placental communicating vessels is the standard of care
  ○ Amnioreduction is an inferior management to laser therapy *(but may be considered in settings where laser therapy or transfer of care is not feasible)*

Essentials of focused comprehensive care:
□ Administer fetal pulmonary corticosteroids after viability
□ Administer maternal anti-D immunoglobulin *(patient is D-negative without alloimmunization)*
□ Neonatology consultation prior to the intended intervention
□ Continue to offer psychosocial support services for the patient and/or support person(s)
□ Arrange for routine gestational glucose screening test at greater than or equal to seven days after administration of the patient's last dose of fetal pulmonary corticosteroids

Special notes:
† Expectant management or selective termination would not be options where the patient chooses to salvage the pregnancy; expectant management in stage II TTTS would invariably result in pregnancy loss or premature labor
‡ Septostomy is of no benefit and should NOT be performed

You highlight to your trainee that Quintero staging **does not** represent a chronological order of deterioration, even though this patient's twins appear to have progressed in sequence. The trainee comprehends that without intervention at this stage II TTTS, stage V may arise without progressing through stages III or IV.

During directive counseling, you inform the patient that among treatment options for TTTS, laser photocoagulation of placental communicating vessels results in improved neurodevelopmental outcomes with higher rates of neurologically intact survival at six years of age, without differences in survival among treatment modalities.[†] She is aware that fetoscopic laser photocoagulation of the placental anastomoses for TTTS has dual fetal survival rates of 65%–75%.

Special note:

† Refer to Roberts D, Neilson JP, Kilby MD, Gates S. Interventions for the treatment of twin–twin transfusion syndrome. *Cochrane Database Syst Rev.* 2014;(1):CD002073. Published January 30, 2014

---

11. Outline short- and long-term complications of fetoscopic laser photocoagulation for TTTS, which you may discuss in the informed consent process. *(1 point per main bullet; max point specified per section)*   10

Maternal: *(max 5)*
- ☐ Spontaneous or iatrogenic preterm birth *(35% of patients deliver at <32 weeks' gestation)*
  - ○ *Consideration for delivery at ~34–35 weeks' gestation*
- ☐ Preterm prelabor rupture of membranes (PPROM)
- ☐ Intrauterine infection
- ☐ Pulmonary edema
- ☐ 'Mirror' syndrome *(rare; only if the recipient is hydropic)*
- ☐ Future risks of alloimmunization

Fetal/childhood: *(max 5)*
- ☐ Recurrence of TTTS (~1%–2%)
- ☐ Postlaser twin-anemia polycythemia sequence (2%–13%; usually one to five weeks after laser)†
- ☐ Fetal demise: single fetus (20%–25%),‡ dual demise (10%–15%)
- ☐ Iatrogenic septostomy creating a monoamniotic pregnancy
- ☐ Chorion/amnion separation and association risks of complications from amniotic bands
- ☐ Antenatal cerebral abnormalities
- ☐ Childhood neurodevelopmental delay (6%–8%; *mainly related to prematurity*)
- ☐ Pulmonary artery stenosis by age 10 years

Special notes:

† Spontaneous twin-anemia polycythemia sequence occurs in ~5% of monochorionic twins, usually diagnosed >26 weeks' gestation

‡ First postoperative week represents the highest risk period for single demise after laser (70%)

12. Inform the patient of planned follow-up and timing of delivery after uncomplicated fetoscopic laser therapy for TTTS. *(1 point per main bullet)*   3

☐ Weekly sonography for the first four weeks after treatment, reducing to alternate weeks following clinical evidence of resolution, continued until delivery
   ○ *Treatment should result in normalization of amniotic fluid by 14 days*
   ○ *When present, normalization of the recipient's cardiac dysfunction is usually expected within one month*
   ○ *At each assessment, amniotic fluid DVP, UA, MCA and ductus venosus (DV) Doppler waveforms will be documented for each fetus*
   ○ *Fetal growth biometries will be performed every two weeks*
☐ Detailed sonographic assessment of the brain, heart, and limbs for each fetus at ~28–32 weeks
   ○ *Assessment of the fetal limbs for amputations is warranted due to risks of ischemic thrombotic event or amniotic bands*
   ○ *Detailed neurosonogram*
☐ Treated TTTS with an intact intertwin membrane should be delivered by 36^{+6} weeks' gestation *(range: 34^{+0} to 36^{+6}; RCOG[7])*

Special note:
Optimal route of delivery following laser therapy has not been determined *(ISUOG)*

Uncomplicated laser photocoagulation is performed at 24^{+3} weeks' gestation.

By three weeks postprocedure, twin A's (former recipient) MCA-PSV is above 1.5 multiples of the median (MoM) while twin B's (former donor) MCA-PSV is below 0.8 MoM. Amniotic fluid DVP have improved and both bladders are visualized. You notice twin B has decreased diminished liver parenchymal echogenicity with clearly identified portal venules, providing a 'starry sky' appearance. Marked placental dichotomy is also noted with twin B's corresponding placental section appearing hypoechoic, while placental sections associated with Twin A territory (donor) appear thicker and hyperechoic.[§]

Special note:
§ Placental descriptions associated with twin-anemia polycythemia sequence are intended for academic purposes, alerting learners of additional featured manifestations.

13. Provide definition(s) of the most consistent diagnosis and brief your trainee on the pathophysiology of this condition. *(1 point per main and subbullets)*   4

Antenatal diagnosis:
☐ Twin anemia-polycythemia sequence
   ○ Combination of MCA-PSV ≥1.5 MoM in the anemic twin and ≤0.8–1.0 MoM in the polycythemic twin
   ○ MCA-PSV discordance ≥1 MoM can also be used to diagnose twin-anemia polycythemia sequence[†]

Pathophysiology:
☐ Chronic feto-fetal transfusion from minute (<1 mm) arterio-venous surface anastomoses located close to the placental edges, allowing for slow unidirectional transfusions of blood that leads to large intertwin hemoglobin differences, without amniotic fluid discordance, which may occur spontaneously or after laser therapy for TTTS

Special note:
† Refer to Khalil A, Gordijn S, Ganzevoort W, et al. Consensus diagnostic criteria and monitoring of twin anemia-polycythemia sequence: Delphi procedure. *Ultrasound Obstet Gynecol.* 2020;56(3):388–394.

In discussion with the patient, you inform her that pregnancy outcomes of twin pregnancies with twin-anemia polycythemia sequence are variable; fetal brain imaging in the third trimester and long-term neurological assessments are recommended. You will ensure follow-up with neonatology expert(s).

In the absence of clearly defined treatment recommendations for twin-anemia polycythemia sequence, you inform the patient that management largely depends on the severity of findings, gestational age at diagnosis, technical feasibility of intrauterine therapy, and parental choice.

14. Outline available treatment[†] strategies for twin-anemia polycythemia sequence. *(1 point per main bullet)*   Max 3

☐ Conservative management
☐ Fetoscopic laser ablation of placental vascular anastomoses, if technically feasible
  ○ *Technical challenges relate to absence of polyhydramnios and presence of only miniscule anastomoses as well as location of the placenta and difficulty in technical access and visualization of vascular equator after previous laser therapy*
☐ Serial intrauterine transfusion for the anemic twin ± partial exchange transfusion to dilute blood of the polycythemic twin
☐ Delivery (gestational-age dependent)

Special note:
† Refer to (a) Tollenaar LS, Slaghekke F, Middeldorp JM, et al. Twin Anemia Polycythemia Sequence: Current Views on Pathogenesis, Diagnostic Criteria, Perinatal Management, and Outcome. *Twin Res Hum Genet.* 2016;19(3):222–233, and (b) Tollenaar LSA, Slaghekke F, Lewi L, et al. Treatment and outcome of 370 cases with spontaneous or postlaser twin anemia-polycythemia sequence managed in 17 fetal therapy centers. *Ultrasound Obstet Gynecol.* 2020 Sep;56(3):378–387

SCENARIO C
(This is a continuation of the clinical scenario after Question 6)
Selective fetal growth restriction (sFGR) and single fetal death in MCDA twins
The patient appreciates your detailed overview of her projected prenatal care for this monochorionic pregnancy. Routine maternal prenatal laboratory tests and first-trimester aneuploidy screening were unremarkable.

At 20 weeks' gestation, both detailed fetal morphology surveys, including echocardiography reports, are normal. External genitalia are consistent with female sex. The placenta is fundal and both umbilical cord insertions are normal.

- Twin A's estimated fetal weight (EFW) is 400 g with normal UA-PI, bladder filling, and DVP.
- Twin B's EFW is 250 g (<10th percentile) with UA Doppler showing persistently absent end-diastolic velocity (AEDV), normal DV Dopplers, bladder filling, and DVP. Twin B does not demonstrate markers of perinatal infection.

15. Identify the <u>most specific</u> diagnosis and explain the underlying <u>pathology</u> of this monochorionic complication. *(1 point for main bullet)*   3

Diagnosis:
☐ Selective fetal growth restriction (sFGR) type II
  ○ *Both defining criteria for sFGR are present in this case scenario: twin B's EFW is <10th percentile and intertwin discordance is 37.5%[†] (i.e., >20%)*
  ○ *Classification is based on the featured UA Doppler waveform*
  ○ *Distinguishing sFGR type II and III is important to guide prenatal prognostication and management; sFGR type III would present with intermittent absent/reversed UA end-diastolic flow velocity (A/REDV)*

Pathology:
☐ Unequal placental sharing/placental discordance[§]
☐ Presence of *fewer* of the large (>2 mm) arterial-arterial (AA) anastomoses[‡] than sFGR type 1

Special notes:
[†] Refer to Question 15 in Chapter 11 for calculation of intertwin discordance
[§] Note that the mechanism for sFGR in monochorionic twins differs from abnormal uteroplacental perfusion featured in dichorionic twins
[‡] AA anastomoses are capable of bidirectional flow

16. Discuss important elements to convey in counseling and options for management of sFGR type II. *(1 point per main bullet)*   Max 4

☐ Inform the patient that arterial and venous Doppler parameters deteriorate in 90% of sFGR type II, with a high risk of fetal/neonatal demise (up to 29%) for the growth restricted twin
☐ Discuss the need for long-term neurological follow-up

Management options:

☐ Conservative management with weekly fetal Doppler studies and bimonthly growth biometry *(increase surveillance frequency as needed)*
  ○ Preterm delivery as dictated by fetal growth and well-being, with a high risk of delivery by 32 weeks' gestation
  ○ Administration of fetal pulmonary corticosteroids, where delivery timing is determined in conjunction with neonatology
☐ Vascular occlusion of the sFGR twin
  ○ At a previable gestation, the patient may choose pregnancy termination depending on severity of selective growth restriction *(jurisdictional policies vary)*
☐ Fetoscopic laser ablation of intertwin placental vascular anastomoses *(high mortality rate of the sFGR twin)*

17. With conservative management, inform your trainee of fetal signs that would imply worsening status of the sFGR twin requiring consideration for intervention. *(1 point each)*

3

☐ Abnormal DV waveform (*e.g.*, absent or reversed a-wave)
☐ Progressive changes in the umbilical artery (UA) Doppler *(REDV)*
☐ Oligohydramnios for sFGR twin

Concerned about *in utero* demise of the sFGR twin, the patient requests an overview of subsequent pregnancy management and possible interventions to avoid spontaneous twin demise.

18. In the event of spontaneous single *in utero* demise after the first trimester, outline the risks for the surviving fetus. *(1 point per main bullet)*

Max 6

Antenatal risks:

☐ Spontaneous and iatrogenic preterm birth
☐ Co-twin demise
☐ Abnormal fetal brain MRI
  ○ Antenatal brain imaging should be performed for the viable twin four to six weeks after co-twin's demise; diffusion-weighted MRI may be considered within 72 hours of demise to detect acute hypoxic changes
☐ Fetal anemia
  ○ *MCA-PSV and fetal CTG for sinusoidal waveforms or other signs of fetal anemia*

Postnatal risks:

☐ Prematurity-related complications
☐ Abnormal brain imaging
☐ Neurodevelopmental delay
☐ Neonatal death

Special note:
Maternal monitoring for coagulopathy is not indicated

19. Name two techniques used for selective fetal termination of monochorionic twins.   2
   (1 point each)

☐ Bipolar umbilical cord occlusion
☐ Radiofrequency ablation
☐ Interstitial laser ablation

Special note:
In contrast to dichorionic twins, intravascular fetal potassium chloride or lidocaine are
contraindicated in monochorionic twins due to the shared fetal circulation

TOTAL: **90**

CHAPTER 13

Prenatal Care of Fetal Congenital Anomalies

Amira El-Messidi and Majed S. Faden

A 29-year-old G1P1L0 presents for preconception counseling with her husband, as the couple had a fetal neural tube defect (NTD)-affected pregnancy three years ago. Pregnancy was terminated at 21 weeks' gestation. They have since been using dual contraception with an intrauterine contraceptive device (IUD) and condoms. The primary care provider recommended consultation in your hospital center's high-risk obstetrics unit prior to removal of the patient's IUD, as the couple wish to conceive.

LEARNING OBJECTIVES

1. Take a focused preconception history from a patient with prior fetal NTD
2. Recognize types of NTDs and associations with numerous sequences or syndromes, and anticipate obstetric outcomes with anencephaly
3. Provide preconception counseling and outline the antenatal management of a patient with prior open fetal NTD of multifactorial origin
4. Understand prenatal management options for fetal myelomeningocele and provide appropriate intrapartum management of patients who do not undergo hysterotomy for in utero surgical repair
5. Discuss important aspects of the consent process for mid-trimester amniocentesis and chromosomal microarray analysis (CMA)

SUGGESTED READINGS

1. (a) American College of Medical Genetics and Genomics (ACMG). Monaghan KG, Leach NT, Pekarek D, et al. The use of fetal exome sequencing in prenatal diagnosis: a points to consider document of the American College of Medical Genetics and Genomics (ACMG). *Genet Med.* 2020;22(4):675–680.
   (b) American College of Medical Genetics and Genomics (ACMG). Palomaki GE, Bupp C, Gregg AR, et al. Laboratory screening and diagnosis of open neural tube defects, 2019 revision: a technical standard of the American College of Medical Genetics and Genomics (ACMG). *Genet Med.* 2020;22(3):462–474.
2. Committee on Genetics and the Society for Maternal-Fetal Medicine. Committee Opinion No. 682: Microarrays and next-generation sequencing technology: the use of advanced genetic diagnostic tools in obstetrics and gynecology. *Obstet Gynecol.* 2016;128(6):e262–e268.
3. Committee Opinion No. 720: Maternal-fetal surgery for myelomeningocele. *Obstet Gynecol.* 2017;130(3):e164–e167.

4. Gardiner C, Wellesley D, Kilby MD, et al. Recommendation for the use of chromosome microarray in pregnancy. Royal College of Pathologists, June 2015.

5. Gotha L, Pruthi V, Abbasi N, et al. Fetal spina bifida: What we tell the parents. *Prenat Diagn.* 2020;40(12):1499–1507.

6. (a) National Institute for Health and Care Excellence: Fetoscopic prenatal repair for open neural tube defects in the fetus; Interventional procedures guidance (IPG667). January 2020. Available at www.nice.org.uk/guidance/ipg667. Accessed May 6, 2021.

   (b) National Institute for Health and Care Excellence: Open prenatal repair for open neural tube defects in the fetus; Interventional procedures guidance (IPG668). January 2020. Available at www.nice.org.uk/guidance/ipg668. Accessed May 6, 2021.

7. Practice Bulletin No. 187: Neural Tube Defects. *Obstet Gynecol.* 2017;130(6):e279–e290.

8. Society for Maternal-Fetal Medicine (SMFM). Dugoff L, Norton ME, Kuller JA. The use of chromosomal microarray for prenatal diagnosis. *Am J Obstet Gynecol.* 2016;215(4):B2–B9. [Correction in *Am J Obstet Gynecol.* 2017 Feb;216(2):180]

9. (a) Society of Obstetricians and Gynecologists of Canada (SOGC) Clinical Practice Guideline: Guideline No. 324. Pre-conception folic acid and multivitamin supplementation for the primary and secondary prevention of neural tube defects and other folic acid-sensitive congenital anomalies. *J Obstet Gynaecol Can.* 2015;37 (6):534–552.

   (b) Society of Obstetricians and Gynecologists of Canada (SOGC) Clinical Practice Guideline. Douglas Wilson R, Van Mieghem T, Langlois S, et al. Guideline No. 410: Prevention, screening, diagnosis, and pregnancy management for fetal neural tube defects. *J Obstet Gynaecol Can.* 2021;43(1):124–139.

10. (a) World Health Organization. Guideline. Optimal serum and red blood cell folate concentrations in women of reproductive age for prevention of neural tube defects. Geneva, Switzerland: World Health Organization; 2015. Available at www.who.int/ nutrition/publications/guidelines/optimalserum_rbc_womenrep_tubedefects/en. Accessed May 6, 2021.

   (b) Cordero AM, Crider KS, Rogers LM, et al. Optimal serum and red blood cell folate concentrations in women of reproductive age for prevention of neural tube defects: World Health Organization guidelines. *MMWR Morb Mortal Wkly Rep.* 2015;64(15):421–423.

POINTS

1. With regard to the obstetric history of a fetal neural tube defect (NTD), what aspects of a focused history would you want to know? *(1 point per main bullet; max point indicated for specific sections)*

20

Sonographic details of the fetal NTD:
☐ Determine the type and/or level of the defect
☐ Presence of other congenital malformations
☐ Gestational age at diagnosis
☐ Determine the results of prenatal genetic tests, if performed

Maternal medical/surgical history: *(max 6)*
☐ Personal history of NTD or non-NTD folic acid-sensitive congenital anomalies *(see Question 7)*
☐ Prepregnancy diabetes mellitus (type 1 or 2)
☐ Renal insufficiency requiring dialysis, as folic acid is cleared by dialysis

- Advanced liver disease
- Malabsorptive condition (*e.g., celiac disease, inflammatory bowel disease bypass surgery, vitamin B12 deficiency*)
- History of early gestational febrile illness
- Epilepsy
- Anorexia nervosa
- Obesity at the time of prior pregnancy (BMI ≥ 30 kg/m^2 or 80 kg prepregnancy weight)

History of medications used during the preconception/antenatal period:

- Determine if the patient took an appropriate amount of folic acid containing prenatal vitamins, particularly starting one to three months preconception to 12 weeks' gestation
- Antifolate agents used in treatment of medical conditions
  - *e.g., sodium valproate, carbamazepine, phenytoin, phenobarbital, primidone, sulfasalazine, methotrexate, trimethoprim, some antimalarial drugs*

Social features: *(max 3)*

- Occupation (*i.e., indoor air pollution from coal*) [WHO]
- Dietary practices associated with low folic acid intake of fortified foods (*i.e., low carbohydrate diets or high consumption of organic foods*)
- Alcohol use disorder
- Smoking
- Illicit substance use/abuse
- Early gestational use of hot tubs/saunas (*consumption of recommended routine folic acid ≥ 0.4 mg/d attenuates this risk*)[‡]
- Ethnicity and geographic location
  - *e.g., open NTDs are more common in Eastern Mediterranean countries and Southeast Asia than in Europe and the Americas*[§]
  - *Interregional differences exist within countries (e.g., Shanxi Province in China has high [est] worldwide rates of NTDs; Texas–Mexico border exposure to fungal toxin fumonisin)*

Family history:

- NTDs in first- or second-degree relatives
- Presence of non-NTD folic acid-sensitive congenital anomalies (*see Question 7*)
- Polymorphisms in the genes encoding methylenetetrahydrofolate reductase enzyme (*e.g., methylenetetrahydrofolate reductase 677C->T)*[†]

Male partner:

- Consanguinity
- Personal history of NTD
- Family history of NTD in other first- or second-degree relatives

Special notes:

[‡] Refer to Kerr SM, Parker SE, Mitchell AA, Tinker SC, Werler MM. Periconceptional maternal fever, folic acid intake, and the risk for neural tube defects. *Ann Epidemiol.* 2017;27(12):777–782.e1.

[§] Refer to Zaganjor I, Sekkarie A, Tsang BL, et al. Describing the Prevalence of Neural Tube Defects Worldwide: A Systematic Literature Review. *PLoS One.* 2016;11(4):e0151586. Published 2016 Apr 11.

[†] Routine dose folic acid 0.4 mg would adequately increase red cell and serum folate levels

You learn that the couple's last pregnancy was unplanned. An exencephaly/anencephaly sequence was discovered at the 12 weeks' sonogram and although comprehensive multidisciplinary counseling was provided, pregnancy continuation was initially chosen until mid-gestation when the patient felt psychologically prepared for termination of pregnancy. She had an uncomplicated vaginal delivery; autopsy was consistent with sonographic findings and the unremarkable cytogenetic results at invasive second-trimester diagnostic testing of the female fetus.[§] The couple understand that this is common to NTDs, where specific abnormal chromosomal causes are only found in ~2%–16% of cases. Detailed fetal sonographic morphology and echocardiography performed in a tertiary-care center were normal.

Comprehensive medical history of the patient and her partner is noncontributory. They are nonconsanguineous, without family histories of NTDs. The patient practices a healthy diet and lifestyle; she indicates her body habitus has always been normal. The couple are not from a geographic area where NTD is more frequent.

You plan to discuss particular aspects of birth defects and relevant obstetric features of anencephaly with your trainee after this consultation visit.

Special note:
§ NTDs are generally more common in female than in male fetuses

2. Differentiate between a '*sequence*' and a '*syndrome*' and provide two examples[§] of each type of birth defect with known association with NTDs. *(1 point per main and subbullet)* *[Examples provided are intended as a guide; other conditions may be correct.]*	Max 6

Sequence:
- ☐ Abnormalities developed sequentially as a result of a primary insult without a known cause
  Examples with risk of NTDs:
  - ○ Amniotic band sequence
  - ○ OEIS (omphalocele, exstrophy, imperforate anus, spinal defects)
  - ○ Limb-body wall complex
  - ○ Cloacal exstrophy sequence
  - ○ Oculo-auriculo-vertebral sequence (Goldenhar sequence)
  - ○ Caudal regression sequence

Syndrome:
- ☐ A cluster of anomalies that have the same cause
  Examples with risk of NTDs:
  - ○ Trisomy 13, 18, or triploidy
  - ○ Noonan syndrome
  - ○ Spina bifida occulta syndrome
  - ○ Meckel-Gruber
  - ○ Waardenburg
  - ○ HARDE (hydrocephalus-agyria-retinal dysplasia-encephalocele)

Special note:

§ Readers are encouraged to refer to the series of seven articles by Chen, CP on syndromes, disorders, and maternal risk factors associated with neural tube defects in *Taiwan J Obstet Gynecol.* 2008

3. In addition to exencephaly/anencephaly, inform your trainee of other types of NTDs. (*1 point each*)

Max 4

Cranial:
☐ Encephalocele
☐ Iniencephaly

Spina bifida/spinal dysraphism:
☐ Spina bifida occulta
☐ Meningocele
☐ Myelomeningocele

Complex defects:
☐ Myeloschisis
☐ Holorachischisis
☐ Craniorachischisis

4. Outline the obstetric outcomes associated with anencephaly that the patient was most probably informed of last pregnancy and indicate the underlying etiologies for these outcomes. (*1 point per main and subbullet*)

Max 6

Obstetric outcomes with anencephaly:
☐ Preterm prelabor rupture of membranes (PPROM) and/or preterm labor
  ○ Secondary to polyhydramnios-associated lack of fetal swallowing
☐ Postterm pregnancy
  ○ Secondary to deficient fetal neurohormonal pathways involved in parturition
☐ Antepartum or intrapartum fetal death
  ○ Secondary to major congenital malformations, aneuploidy, or neurological dysfunction
☐ Complex vaginal delivery mechanics in advanced gestational ages
  ○ Secondary to abnormal cranial volume for vertex presentations or lack of a presenting part

The patient is aware that the prevalence of open NTDs varies by environmental factors, genetic predisposition, social and medical interventions, with prevalence rates ranging from 1/300 to 1/1000 pregnancies in populations without folic acid fortification or supplementation. The couple's prior obstetric event was deemed of multifactorial origin, which they understand is the most common 'etiology.' She is keen to know your clinical recommendations for future pregnancies, as she cannot recall most aspects of counseling provided after her last pregnancy.

5. Describe the characteristics of multifactorial inheritance[†] which you intend to later discuss with your trainee. *(1 point each)*

Max 5

☐ The disorder is familial, but a pattern of inheritance is not apparent
☐ The risk to first-degree relatives is the square root of the population risk
☐ The risk is significantly decreased for second-degree relatives
☐ The recurrence risk is increased if more than one family member is affected
☐ The risk is increased if the defect is more severe (*e.g.*, the recurrence risk for bilateral cleft lip is higher than for unilateral cleft lip)
☐ If the defect is more common in one sex than in the other sex, the recurrence risk is higher if the affected individual is of the less commonly affected sex

Special note:
† Refer to ACOG Technology Assessment in Obstetrics and Gynecology No. 14: Modern Genetics in Obstetrics and Gynecology. *Obstet Gynecol.* 2018;132(3):e143–e168.

6. With focus on prior fetal NTD of multifactorial origin, outline important elements of preconception counseling and future antenatal management plan for this patient. *(1 point per main bullet)*

Max 10

Maternal:[§]
☐ Inform the couple that the baseline recurrence risk for nonchromosomal NTD is ~4% with one affected sibling (or parent) for a population where prevalence is 1/1000 and no food fortification or folic acid supplementation
  ○ *Recurrence risk is ~10% with one affected sibling + one parent, or two affected siblings with neither parent affected*
☐ Advise use of daily oral supplementation with **4.0 to 5.0 mg folic acid in a multivitamin containing vitamin B12**[‡] for at least three months preconception and until 12 weeks' gestation
  ○ Prescribe additional folic acid supplement if needed, rather than taking excess multivitamins, mainly to avoid vitamin A toxicity
  ○ *After 12 weeks' gestation, continued daily supplementations with a multivitamin containing 0.4 to 1.0 mg of folic acid is recommended for the remainder of pregnancy and for 4–6 weeks postpartum or as long as breastfeeding continues*
☐ Advise a diet rich in folate (vitamin B9)
  ○ *e.g., breakfast cereals, bread, pastas, rice, broccoli, asparagus, beef liver, leafy vegetables, Brussel sprouts, avocados, beans, lentils, corn, peas, egg yolk, milk, tomato/orange juice, papaya, cantaloupe, bananas, strawberries*
☐ Mention that a high dose folic acid supplementation may reduce isolated, nonsyndromic NTD recurrence by ~70% (*i.e.*, from an ~4% to ~1% recurrence risk)
☐ Highlight that at least 30% of isolated, nonsyndromic NTDs may not be prevented by appropriate folic acid supplementation (*e.g., patients with poorly controlled diabetes, obesity, certain antiepileptic agents*)
☐ Maintain a normal body weight and healthy lifestyle practices
☐ Consider testing for diabetes mellitus (*if not performed*) and optimize glycemic control if necessary

☐ Advise against use of hot tubs/saunas and antifolate drug treatments in the preconception and early pregnancy period

☐ Advise antipyretic use in the event of febrile illness in the first trimester

☐ Prenatal care may ensue with her primary care provider in the event of normal fetal morphology and continued absence of maternal comorbidities

☐ If high-quality, targeted fetal ultrasound is anticipated to be limited, traditional biomarkers prenatal screening incorporating maternal serum alpha-fetoprotein (MSAFP) level, ideally at 16–18 weeks' gestation, should be considered

   ○ *Screening performance is significantly decreased at 14 weeks' gestation (ACMG[1b])*

Fetal:

☐ With focus on prior fetal NTD, arrange a sonogram at 11^{+0}–13^{+6} weeks' gestation to assess the biparietal diameter (BPD) and identify the intracranial translucency

   ○ *Although crown–rump length (CRL) provides accurate estimates of gestational age, the optimal dating method for open-NTD screening is the BPD, which would be about two weeks earlier than true gestational age dating in affected pregnancies (ACMG[1b])*

   ○ *The BPD is not used to determine the appropriate screening interval for MSAFP assessment due to unreliability of results (ACMG[1b])*

☐ Consideration for early targeted fetal morphology ultrasound (*e.g.*, ~16–18 weeks' gestation) for intracranial and spinal anatomy

   ○ *This may allow further time for counseling and decision-making*

Special notes:

§ According to the World Health Organization, red cell folate <906 nmol/L (<400 ng/mL) at the **population** level, increases the prevalence of NTDs yet this threshold cannot predict **individual** risk of an NTD-affected pregnancy

‡ Daily multivitamin containing 2.6 ug vitamin B12 is recommended *(SOGC[9a])*

The patient appreciates your counseling and future antenatal care plan. To optimize her preconception folic acid intake in accordance with your recommendations based on her obstetric history, she plans to discontinue contraception *after* starting 4.0 to 5.0 mg folic acid in a multivitamin containing vitamin B12. Addressing her inquiry, you explain that the mechanism of action of folate in the prevention of NTDs is largely unknown, although folate is important for the regulation of nucleic acid synthesis and function, and in metabolism of amino acids.

Your obstetric trainee read that some non-NTD congenital anomalies are associated with suboptimal folic acid intake. You highlight that folic acid, alone or in combination with vitamins and minerals, does not have a clear effect on non-NTD birth defects,[†] although a higher dose (1.0 mg/d) folic acid supplementation is suggested, based on low-quality data, for women with a history of certain congenital anomalies in themselves, their male partners, a prior offspring, or in a first- or second-degree relative.

Special note:

† Refer to De-Regil LM, Peña-Rosas JP, Fernández-Gaxiola AC, Rayco-Solon P. Effects and safety of periconceptional oral folate supplementation for preventing birth defects. *Cochrane Database Syst Rev.* 2015;(12):CD007950. Published 2015 Dec 14.

7. Acknowledging that efficacy remains to be proven, elaborate on the non-NTD anomalies for which 1.0 mg oral daily folic acid preconception and during the first trimester is recommended. *(1 point each)*

Max 4

☐ Congenital hydrocephalus
☐ Orofacial clefts (lip and/or palate)
☐ Congenital heart defects
☐ Urinary tract anomalies
☐ Limb reduction defects
☐ Pyloric stenosis *(Controversial)*

Upon discontinuation of contraceptive measures, and after commencing the planned prenatal vitamin supplementation and folate-rich diet, spontaneous conception ensues within one menstrual cycle. The primary care provider transfers you the patient with sonographic confirmation of a viable intrauterine singleton at 8^{+5} weeks' gestation. All baseline prenatal laboratory investigations are unremarkable; her blood group is B-negative. The 12^{+2} weeks' ultrasound shows a normal cranial vault and early morphology, although the intracranial translucency[#] is not visualized. The patient opted for traditional aneuploidy testing with integrated prenatal screening (IPS).[†]

At 17^{+3} weeks' gestation, you receive results of her IPS indicating a trisomy 21 risk at 1/1000 with an MSAFP level at 4.5 multiples of the median (MoM) [normal: 0.25–2.5 MoM].[‡] You teach your trainee that there is a direct correlation between higher MSAFP levels and the frequency of fetal malformations. Early fetal morphology ultrasound is arranged for the following day. Meanwhile, you take this opportunity to review adverse obstetric outcomes associated with *unexplained* MSAFP should the obstetric morphology sonogram be normal.[§]

Special notes:
\# Sonographic equivalent of the fourth ventricle
† Refer to Question 2 in Chapter 5
‡ First-trimester MSAFP screening for open NTD is not recommended due to a 10% false-positive rate and only 50% detection rate
§ Refer to Question 17 in Chapter 5

8. Indicate 10 <u>fetal-neonatal structural conditions</u> associated with an increased MSAFP level. *(1 point each)*

Max 8

Neurologic/musculoskeletal:
☐ NTDs
☐ Cystic hygroma
☐ Sacrococcygeal teratoma
☐ Osteogenesis imperfecta

Hepatic and gastrointestinal:

☐ Ventral wall defect (*e.g.*, omphalocele, gastroschisis)
☐ Esophageal or intestinal obstruction

Genitourinary:

☐ Cloacal exstrophy
☐ Renal agenesis
☐ Polycystic kidney disease
☐ Obstructive uropathy
☐ Finnish-type congenital nephrosis

Integumentary:

☐ Congenital skin abnormality
☐ Pilonidal cyst

Special notes:

Increased MSAFP level is also associated with **maternal** hepatoma or other liver disease, although not reflected upon in this question.
Refer to Question 17 in Chapter 6 for adverse obstetric outcomes associated with *unexplained* increased MSAFP

The following day, at 17^{+4} weeks' gestation, sonography shows a female fetus with normal biometry and the following findings:

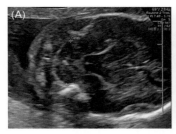 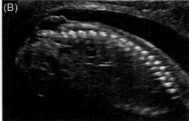

Figure 13.1

With permission: Figure 2 plates A and B from suggested reading #4 – Gotha L, et al. *Prenat Diagn.* 2020;40(12): 1499–1507.

There is no association between the patient's image and this case scenario. Image used for educational purposes only.

Apart from defects on neurosonography, no other malformations are detected.

9. Describe the sonographic findings. *(1 point each)*   3

☐ Obliteration of the cisterna magna
☐ Elongated cerebellum due to herniation in the posterior fossa ('banana sign,' Chiari II malformation)
☐ Cystic or saccular lesion in the lower spine

10. After disclosure of the sonographic finding, which most probably explains the abnormal maternal serum analyte, outline your recommended antenatal care plan at this time. *(1 point each)*

☐ Arrange for fetal echocardiography

☐ Discuss amniocentesis with chromosomal microarray[§] given a major structural malformation

☐ Multidisciplinary consultations for parental counseling on short- and long-term child considerations (*e.g.*, genetics, neonatology; referral to pediatric neurosurgery and urology if pregnancy will be continued)[†]

☐ Individualized consideration for consultation with a perinatal mental health and/or social work expert

☐ Consideration for *adjunctive* fetal MRI in later gestation if more detailed evaluation of the central nervous system is indicated for counseling and antenatal management

Special notes:

§ See Question 12-A

† Transfer of care to a tertiary-care unit with maternal-fetal medicine expertise would be indicated if not already established as implied in this case scenario

11. In obtaining patient consent for amniocentesis under ultrasound guidance, indicate procedure-related complications[§] for this singleton at 17^{+4} weeks' gestation.† *(1 point each)*

☐ Pregnancy loss: *rate is very low at 0.1%–0.3% when performed by experienced operators,*[‡] *yet may be affected by fetal malformation(s), increased MSAFP level, or aneuploidy*

☐ Temporary loss of small volume of amniotic fluid

☐ Overt rupture of amniotic membranes

☐ Vaginal spotting/bleeding

☐ Isoimmunization, particularly if this patient does not receive anti-D immunoglobulin *(recall her blood group is B-negative)*

☐ Amnionitis

☐ Fetal injury or demise *(rare; operator experience is critical)*

Special notes:

§ Although vertical transmission of infection(s) is a complication of invasive diagnostic testing, particularly with suboptimal disease control, prenatal laboratory results for the patient is this case scenario were normal.

† Refer to Question 10 in Chapter 6 for risks associated with early amniocentesis and to Question 22 in Chapter 11 for important features of amniocentesis in dichorionic twins

‡ Practice Bulletin No. 162: Prenatal Diagnostic Testing for Genetic Disorders. *Obstet Gynecol.* 2016;127(5):e108–e122.

12-A. After appropriate pretest counseling, what are two contemporary genetic tests recommended in amniotic fluid analysis for a fetal NTD? *(1 point per main bullet)* — 2

☐ Quantitative fluorescence polymerase chain reaction (QF-PCR) **or** interphase fluorescent in-situ hybridization (FISH)
  ○ *Rapid detection of aneuploidies in chromosomes 13, 18, 21, X and Y*
☐ Chromosomal microarray analysis[†] *(either as a primary test or after normal rapid aneuploidy screening test)*

12-B. Identify two <u>diagnostic tests</u> in amniotic fluid for fetal open NTD, which may be required by some protocols for fetal surgery decision-making. *(1 point each)* — Max 2

☐ Amniotic fluid alpha-fetoprotein[§]
☐ Acetylcholinesterase

Special notes:

† (a) Refer to Question 5 in Chapter 14 for advantages of chromosomal microarray over conventional karyotype; (b) where chromosomal microarray is normal, fetal exome sequencing may be considered after counseling by a provider with expertise in medical genetics

§ While MS-AFP is a *screening* test for fetal NTD, amniotic fluid alpha-fetoprotein is part of a *diagnostic testing protocol.*

Further to the fetal sonographic findings, a genetics counselor/geneticist will meet with the patient; pretest counseling for diagnostic tests will be provided.

13. As a maternal-fetal medicine expert, inform your trainee of the diagnostic value and caveats of prenatal chromosomal microarray analysis (CMA).[†] *(1 point per main bullet; max points specified per section)* — 7

Diagnostic value: *(max 2)*
☐ CMA can identify the large majority of significant abnormalities seen on karyotype
☐ CMA can detect submicroscopic deletions and duplications *[down to a 50- to 100-kilobase level]* that would be missed by routine karyotyping; these finer chromosomal abnormalities, referred to as copy number variants (CNVs) may be pathogenic in ~6% of cases with an *isolated* structural fetal abnormality
  ○ *Microdeletions are smaller than resolution of light microscopy for karyotyping (i.e., >5 megabase pairs); generally, microdeletions are more likely clinically significant than microduplications*
  ○ *Potentially significant CNVs may be detected in ~9% of fetuses with **multiple** anomalies, and in 1%–1.7% of structurally normal fetuses*
☐ CMA identifies nonpaternity or consanguinity not detected by conventional karyotype

Caveats: *(max 5)*

☐ CMA can detect *variants of uncertain significance (VOUS)* for which insufficient or no data exist linking it to a defined clinical phenotype
  ○ *VOUS have an overall prevalence of 1%–2% and pose clinical dilemmas in counseling and greater parental anxiety*
☐ CMA cannot identify balanced translocations (reciprocal and Robertsonian) and inversions give no gain or loss of genomic material, as may be seen with conventional karyotyping
  ○ *If a G-banded karyotype is performed after a negative CMA, the diagnostic yield is 0.78–1.3%*
☐ CMA does not provide information about the chromosomal mechanism of a genetic imbalance, which would be relevant for recurrence risk counseling *(e.g., unable to distinguish between trisomy of an acrocentric chromosome {13, 14, 15, 21, 22} and an unbalanced Robertsonian translocation that might be inherited)*
☐ CMA cannot detect low level mosaicism at <10%–20%
☐ CMA cannot detect point mutations in single gene disorders *(e.g., sickle cell anemia, cystic fibrosis, many skeletal dysplasias)*
☐ Triploidy is only detected by single-nucleotide polymorphism (SNP) array platforms, not comparative genomic hybridization (CGH) arrays
☐ CMA may show a finding unrelated to the ultrasound findings, but which may have future health implications for this offspring and unknowingly affected parent(s)

Special note:

† Refer to Wou K, Levy B, Wapner RJ. Chromosomal Microarrays for the Prenatal Detection of Microdeletions and Microduplications. *Clin Lab Med.* 2016;36(2):261–276.

Interdisciplinary care is initiated; fetal echocardiography is normal, and the patient consented to invasive genetic testing after comprehensive genetic counseling.

At 19^{+1} weeks' gestation, results of genetic tests show fetus 46, XX chromosomal makeup with a normal microarray analysis. Expectedly for breached fetal skin and NTD, alpha-fetoprotein and acetylcholinesterase are detected in the amniotic fluid. The couple was only contemplating repeat termination of pregnancy with a lethal anomaly or in the presence of genetic derangements. They are now keen to maximize their knowledge of management options for the fetal open NTD. Fetal MRI assessment will be arranged.

14. With respect to the open fetal NTD, what are the two main prenatal management options you would discuss in nondirective counseling of this couple who wish to continue pregnancy? *(1 point each)*   2

☐ Expectant prenatal care and planned postnatal surgical repair
☐ Assessment by experts in designated centers with expertise in prenatal fetal surgical repair

15. Until travel plans are arranged to a specialized center in fetal surgical repair, address the patient's queries regarding the benefits of prenatal meningomyelocele repair by hysterotomy[†] relative to postnatal surgery. *(1 point each)*

Max 3

Benefits of hysterotomy for fetal surgical repair relative to postnatal repair:[§‡]
- ☐ Prevention of continued in utero trauma to the exposed central nervous system, leading to improved antenatal sonographic progress
- ☐ Reduced need for ventriculoperitoneal shunting by age one year
- ☐ Reduced neurological conditions (*e.g.*, hindbrain herniation) at age one year
- ☐ Improved lower limb mobility and rates of walking independently
- ☐ Improved long-term quality of life

Special notes:
[†] Research on fetoscopic myelomeningocele repair is ongoing
[§] Controversial effects of fetal spine closure on urinary incontinence
[‡] *Refer to (a)* Adzick NS, Thom EA, Spong CY, et al. A randomized trial of prenatal versus postnatal repair of myelomeningocele. *N Engl J Med.* 2011;364(11):993–1004; *(b)* Tulipan N, Wellons JC 3rd, Thom EA, et al. Prenatal surgery for myelomeningocele and the need for cerebrospinal fluid shunt placement. *J Neurosurg Pediatr.* 2015;16(6):613–620

After comprehensive consultation at an international center with expertise in fetal surgical repair, the couple decided to forego antenatal repair to the postpartum period for nonmedical reasons. The patient is aware of the potential morbidity during the current pregnancy and in subsequent pregnancies. The patient thereby returned for continued multidisciplinary obstetric care in your center, where antepartum liaison with parents of similarly affected children is arranged.

16. With respect of fetal neurosonography and the neuromuscular system, what are the sonographic features associated with open NTDs you need to assess for throughout gestation? *(1 point each)*

Max 5

- ☐ Ventriculomegaly (uni/bilateral), hydrocephalus, or abnormally appearing cerebral ventricles (*e.g.*, pointy appearance of the posterior horns)
- ☐ 'Lemon sign': abnormal skull shape with flattening of the frontal bones
- ☐ Small biparietal diameter (BPD)
- ☐ 'Banana sign,' Chiari II malformation: elongated cerebellum due to herniation in the posterior fossa
- ☐ Obliteration of the cisterna magna
- ☐ Abnormal lower limb movement and/or uni/bilateral talipes equinovarus
- ☐ Scoliosis

By 36 weeks' gestation, monthly fetal sonography has shown normal growth velocity and amniotic fluid volume. Fetal biometry is normal with stable size and appearance of the meningomyelocele. There has not been evidence of macrocephaly or fixed lower limb positioning. Bilateral ventriculomegaly developed at ~26 weeks' gestation and is currently 12–14 mm on each side. Signs of cerebral herniation became evident by cerebellar morphology and small cisterna magna. The fetus has remained in the cephalic presentation. The patient's clinical course has been unremarkable. Multidisciplinary collaboration has been maintained throughout gestation.

17. Outline relevant aspects of intrapartum care and evidence-based mode of delivery, with focus on this fetus with myelomeningocele. *(1 point per main bullet)*   4

☐ Delivery should occur in a tertiary-care center with on-site advanced neonatal care and pediatric neurosurgery services
☐ Plan for vaginal delivery at term (individualized)
  ○ *Cesarean section does not improve neurological outcomes among fetuses with open NTDs (i.e., meningomyelocele)†*
  ○ *Cesarean section is reserved for usual obstetric indications, all patients who have open fetal surgical repair, macrocephaly, or where the NTD is suspected to cause labor dystocia*
☐ Ensure a latex-free delivery and for all team membranes in contact with the newborn
  ○ *Infants with MMC have an ~30% risk of severe, life-threatening latex allergy*
☐ Plan for immediate coverage of the NTD at birth to prevent infectious complications and ongoing trauma

Special note:
† Tolcher MC, Shazly SA, Shamshirsaz AA, et al. Neurological outcomes by mode of delivery for fetuses with open neural tube defects: a systematic review and meta-analysis. *BJOG.* 2019;126(3):322–327.

TOTAL: 100

CHAPTER 14

Intrauterine Fetal Death

Michelle Rougerie and Amira El-Messidi

You are called by your obstetric trainee to assist in the assessment and care of a 33-year-old G2P1 with a singleton pregnancy presenting to the emergency assessment unit at 36^{+3} weeks' gestation with decreased fetal movements. Bedside sonography reveals fetal demise, confirmed by second opinion. Her prenatal chart will be requested from the hospital center affiliated with her obstetric provider.

LEARNING OBJECTIVES

1. Take a focused history, recognizing maternal, fetal, and placental risk factors, for a patient with current late intrauterine fetal death (IUFD)
2. Identify surroundings suitable for counseling and providing in-hospital management for bereaving parents, and understand elements for appropriate interprofessional communication for patients experiencing late fetal loss
3. Detail comprehensive antenatal and postnatal investigations in assessment of late IUFD
4. Counsel on the recurrence of late IUFD and outline the management of a future pregnancy
5. Evaluate patients with perceived decreased fetal movements in the third trimester and provide quality care, recognizing that international practices vary

SUGGESTED READINGS

1. American College of Obstetricians and Gynecologists; Society for Maternal-Fetal Medicine. Management of stillbirth: obstetric care consensus no. 10. *Obstet Gynecol.* 2020;135(3): e110–e132.
2. Flenady V, Oats J, Gardener G, et al. Care around the time of stillbirth and neonatal death guidelines group. Clinical Practice Guideline for Care Around Stillbirth and Neonatal Death. Version 3.4, NHMRC Centre of Research Excellence in Stillbirth. Brisbane, Australia, January 2020.
3. Ladhani NNN, Fockler ME, Stephens L, et al. No. 369 – management of pregnancy subsequent to stillbirth. *J Obstet Gynaecol Can.* 2018;40(12):1669–1683.
4. Leduc L. No. 394 – stillbirth investigation. *J Obstet Gynaecol Can.* 2020;42(1):92–99.
5. Perinatal Society of Australia and New Zealand and Centre of Research Excellence Stillbirth. Clinical practice guideline for the care of women with decreased fetal movements for women with a singleton pregnancy from 28 weeks' gestation. Centre of Research Excellence in Stillbirth. Brisbane, Australia, September 2019.

6. Queensland clinical guidelines: Stillbirth care. Queensland: Queensland government; 2018.
7. Royal College of Obstetricians and Gynaecologists (RCOG). Green-Top Guideline No. 55: Late intrauterine fetal death and stillbirth. London; October 2010, updated February 2017.
8. World Health Organization (WHO). Stillbirths. Available at www.who.int/maternal_child_adolescent/epidemiology/stillbirth/en/. Accessed December 25, 2020.
9. Wojcieszek AM, Shepherd E, Middleton P, et al. Interventions for investigating and identifying the causes of stillbirth. *Cochrane Database Syst Rev.* 2018;4(4):CD012504.

POINTS

1. Knowing that late-onset in utero fetal demise has been confirmed, identify preferred characteristics of the space and surroundings for your interaction with this patient. *(1 point each)*

Max 2

☐ Private and quiet *(ensure privacy, not isolation)*
☐ Suitable for gathering of extended family *(offer patient calls her partner/family's attendance for support)*
☐ Free of items or equipment that could be confronting or upsetting to the patient/family
☐ Separate from other pregnant women and newborns *(communication with the patient is necessary to accommodate variations in personal preferences)*

2. What aspects of a <u>focused</u> history would you want to know?

Max 26

Obstetric signs and symptoms: *(1 point each)*
☐ Duration of time since onset of decreased fetal movements
☐ Current/recent abdominal pain/contractions
☐ Current/recent vaginal bleeding or fluid loss with/without prolapse of the umbilical cord *(including signs of infection, such as fever, abnormal amniotic fluid color or odor)*

Details of current pregnancy: *(1 point each)*
☐ Establish whether artificial reproductive techniques were required
☐ Determine whether gestational age was based on menstrual age or ultrasound dating
☐ Determine gestational age at onset of prenatal care and assess adherence to prenatal care

Medical conditions complicating pregnancy: *(1 point each; max 3)*
☐ Viral illness or sick contacts *(e.g., flu-like symptoms, fever, rash, nausea/vomiting/diarrhea)*
☐ Preeclampsia syndromes
☐ Gestational diabetes
☐ Cholestasis of pregnancy

Associated comorbid maternal medical history: *(1 point per organ system; max 3)*
☐ Sleep-disordered breathing/use of a CPAP *(continuous positive airway pressure)* machine, or presence of other respiratory diseases
☐ Cardiac or renal diseases
☐ Autoimmune disorders or endocrinopathies
  ○ Antiphospholipid antibody syndrome
  ○ Systemic lupus erythematosus

    ○ Pregestational diabetes mellitus
    ○ Thyroid disease (hyper- or hypofunction)
☐ Vascular disorders
    ○ Severe anemia
    ○ Venous thromboembolism
    ○ Chronic hypertension
☐ Celiac disease
☐ Neurologic diseases: *e.g.,* epilepsy
☐ Psychiatric conditions or perceived stress

Substance-use and medications: *(1 point each)*
☐ Cigarette smoking (or second-hand exposure)
☐ Alcohol consumption
☐ Recreational drug use
☐ Medications or use of teratogenic agents

Social history: *(1 point each; max 2)*
☐ Consanguinity and ethnicity *(non-Hispanic black race entail higher risk of stillbirth in developed countries)*
☐ Primipaternity or same partner as prior pregnancy
☐ Recent travel to endemic areas *(e.g., malaria, Zika)*

Associated feto-placental history: *(1 point each; max 3)*
☐ Aneuploidy screening and maternal serum analyte results, if available
☐ Fetal gender (male) and malformation(s) on second-trimester morphology survey
☐ Placental and umbilical cord abnormalities detected at, or subsequent to, the fetal morphology survey *(e.g., placental masses/tumors, velomentous cord insertion, umbilical vein varix)*
☐ Recent spontaneous or provoked abdominal trauma *(screen for domestic abuse)*
☐ Recent obstetrical procedure *(e.g., external cephalic version, amniocentesis)*

Past pregnancy history and presence of adverse outcomes: *(1 point each)*
☐ Determine if patient had prior, *undisclosed*, fetal demise or pregnancy losses
☐ Interval since delivery, mode of delivery, gestational age, and birthweight
☐ Previous pregnancy complications *(e.g., preeclampsia syndromes, placental abruption, or gestational diabetes)*
☐ Previous child with an anomaly, genetic condition, or failure to reach developmental milestones

☐ **Paternal history or maternal family history:** *(1 point)*
    ○ *e.g., stillbirth, medical diseases, hereditary conditions or syndromes, congenital anomalies, aneuploidies, recurrent pregnancy loss, sudden death, sudden infant death syndrome, venous thromboembolism, antiphospholipid syndrome*

Special note:
International variations exist related to gestational age criteria, birthweight threshold, and frequency of causes for stillbirths; generally accepted gestational age cutoff among high-income countries is ≥20 weeks' gestation whereas WHO (World Health Organization) recommends ≥28 weeks' gestation

Expectedly, the patient is distressed with the devastating fetal loss and is initially unable to provide a medical history. Having assured the time and space required for care of this patient, including presence of her partner, you learn she is a healthy Caucasian with unremarkable lifestyle habits. She last felt fetal movements 12 hours ago, without abdominal cramps, vaginal bleeding, or amniotic fluid leakage. The patient has not experienced abdominal trauma or recent obstetric procedures. She does not have symptoms suggestive of preeclampsia syndromes or obstetric cholestasis; routine gestational glucose screening was normal.

This is a spontaneous pregnancy with her nonconsanguineous partner who is the father of her healthy two-year-old daughter. Since first-trimester dating sonography, she has been regularly followed by a colleague. Aneuploidy screening and second-trimester morphology survey of this male fetus were unremarkable; she is not aware of any abnormalities related to the placental unit. Family history is noncontributory.

Her prior antenatal and postnatal course were uncomplicated; she had a spontaneous vaginal delivery at 39 weeks' gestation of a 3000-g newborn in a nearby hospital center under the care of her current obstetric provider.

As you are about to perform a physical examination, the patient asks whether a different protocol of fetal movement counting may have prevented the outcome.

3. Address the patient's query by discussing <u>evidence-based caveats</u> of fetal movement counting.	1

- ☐ Counseling to increase maternal awareness for prompt reporting of decreased fetal movements is unproven to decrease stillbirth[†]
  - ○ *Ensure discussion to dissipate patient's self-blame*

Special note:

[†] (a) Bellussi F, Po' G, Livi A, et al. Fetal Movement Counting and Perinatal Mortality: A Systematic Review and Meta-analysis. *Obstet Gynecol.* 2020;135(2):453–462, and (b) Norman JE, Heazell AEP, Rodriguez A, et al. Awareness of fetal movements and care package to reduce fetal mortality (AFFIRM): a stepped wedge, cluster-randomized trial. *Lancet* 2018;392(10158): 1629–1638

4. Verbalize essentials of the physical examination for this patient with late in utero fetal demise assuming absence of underlying health issues. *(1 point each, unless specified)*	Max 5

- ☐ Vital signs: blood pressure (BP), pulse, temperature, and oxygen saturation
- ☐ Note her body habitus (or, ideally, assess height and weight to calculate BMI)
- ☐ General skin assessment for signs of abuse, trauma, or needle tracks
- ☐ Abdominal examination for fundal height and uterine tenderness *(may consider Leopold maneuvers, although sonographic evaluation will be required)*
- ☐ Vaginal evaluation: *(1 point per subbullet)*
  - ○ Inspection for signs of infection *(e.g., vesicles, ulcerations);* consideration for cervical-vaginal swabs
  - ○ Cervical assessment/Bishop score for delivery planning

Her BP is 147/82 mmHg, pulse is 96 bpm, and she is afebrile with normal oxygenation on room air. Given her distress, you are satisfied by the generally unremarkable body habitus. The uterus is soft, nontender, with fundal height appropriate for gestational age. There is no suggestion of trauma or history of intravenous drug use. The cervix is closed and uneffaced.

Reflecting on your planned investigations, you counsel the couple on possible causes of fetal demise. They are interested to pursue all tests pre- and postdelivery to find an attributable cause for their loss. Results of her routine prenatal tests remain unavailable.

Prior to taking written parental consent for fetal cytogenetic analysis, you inform your trainee that while karyotypic analysis can identify a chromosomal abnormality in 6%–13% of stillbirths, exceeding 20% in fetuses with malformations, international practices vary regarding use of postnatal tissue specimens or performing amniocentesis/chorionic villous sampling upon diagnosis of fetal demise.[†] With up to 50% of cell cultures being unsuccessful for karyotype analysis, many laboratories are using DNA-based methods for chromosomal analysis.

Special note:
† *RCOG*[7] – 'Amniocentesis can also provide cytogenetic results if the mother chooses expectant management, but patient acceptability and safety (infection) of amniocentesis has not been investigated at this time'; *SOGC*[4] – 'An amniocentesis can also be considered for cytogenetic studies when amniotic fluid is present'; *ACOG*[1] – 'One strategy to increase the yield of cell culture is to perform chorionic villous sampling or amniocentesis before the delivery'

5.   Indicate two <u>advantages</u> of chromosomal microarray analysis (CMA) over conventional   Max 2
     karyotyping for prenatal diagnostic testing. *(1 point each)*

Chromosomal microarray analysis *vs.* karyotype:
☐   Higher resolution allows for detection of copy number variants (CNVs) otherwise missed at conventional karyotype
☐   Does not require dividing cells (*i.e.*, uncultured cells), thereby improving detection of causative abnormality for intrauterine fetal demise
☐   Amenable to automation (*i.e.*, reduced failure rate and faster turnaround time)
☐   Greater cost-effective analysis

Special note:
Refer to Question 12 in Chapter 13 for discussion of diagnostic value and caveats with CMA

6. Given your sonographic skills, alert your obstetric trainee's attention to specific aspects of the fetal-placental assessment to note during sonography for planned amniocentesis. *(1 point each)*

☐ Fetal presentation (and possible biometry)
☐ Hydrops fetalis
☐ Collapse of the fetal skull with overlapping bones
☐ Ability to recognize fetal mass *(would be affected by maceration)*
☐ Intrafetal gas (within the heart, blood vessels, or joints)
☐ Amniotic fluid volume
☐ Placental abruption

Special notes:
(1) Consider noting major fetal malformation and placental implantation site, particularly among patients without prior sonographic assessment;
(2) finding nuchal cord(s) may not be the cause of death; this diagnosis should be made with caution, and only after corroborating evidence is sought

Max 4

7. You inform your trainee that although there is no evidence to guide the best investigations for the cause of stillbirth, you outline comprehensive <u>maternal</u> serum/urine evaluation. *(1 point per main bullet or subbullet, where present)*

Serum:
☐ Blood group and antibody screen
☐ Fetal-maternal hemorrhage screen: Kleihauer-Betke test or flow cytometry for fetal cells in maternal circulation (**as soon as possible after stillbirth**, and before delivery)
☐ Antiphospholipid antibodies: [*i.e., acquired thrombophilia*][†] *(RCOG[7]: most tests are not affected by pregnancy – if abnormal, repeat at six weeks)*
   ○ Lupus anticoagulant
   ○ Anticardiolipin antibodies
   ○ ß2-glycoprotein antibodies
☐ TORCH testing: (Controversial utility and varying international recommendations)[§]
   ○ Syphilis
   ○ Parvovirus B19 IgG, IgM serology *(if suspected infection, or fetal hydrops)*
   ○ *Listeria monocytogenes* culture *(if suspected infection)*
   ○ *Zika (if suspected infection)*
☐ CBC
☐ C-reactive protein *(RCOG recommendation)*
☐ Hepatic transaminases and function tests
☐ Creatinine
☐ Coagulation function and fibrinogen for investigation of disseminated intravascular coagulation (DIC) *(RCOG[7]: not a test for cause of late IUFD, although testing is required before regional anesthesia or for case-based indications)*
☐ Hemoglobin electrophoresis *(with fetal hydrops, maternal anemia, or suspected alpha or beta thalassemia)*
☐ HbA1c and/or random glucose
☐ TSH and free T4, free T3 *(if suspected signs or symptoms)*

Max 17

☐ Bile acids *(if suspected obstetric cholestasis)*

☐ Anti-Ro and Anti-La antibodies *(if hydropic fetus or postmortem atrioventricular node calcification or endomyocardial fibroelastosis)*

Urine:

☐ Assessment for proteinuria *(if suspected preeclampsia syndromes)*

☐ Toxicology screen *(with maternal consent, and in cases of placental abruption or suspected drug use)*

☐ Midstream urine culture *(if clinically suspected infection)*

Special notes:

† Inherited thrombophilia is **not** recommended in evaluation of IUFD; consider testing with personal or family history of thromboembolic disease

§ Serology for toxoplasmosis, cytomegalovirus, rubella, and herpes simplex virus are of unproven benefit and not recommended *(ACOG[1])*; serology for toxoplasmosis, cytomegalovirus, and herpes simplex virus may be considered based on clinical suspicion *(SOGC[4])*; serology for toxoplasmosis, herpes simplex virus, parvovirus B19 are recommended routinely *(RCOG[7])*

Sonographic evaluation reveals cephalic presentation without signs of hydrops or nuchal cord(s). Amniotic fluid volume is low-normal range for gestational age and brown-tinged fluid is removed through a transamniotic amniocentesis, without evidence of meconium-stained fluid. The placenta is fundal without sonographic signs of abruption. Reported maternal serum evaluation reveals normal hemoglobin, platelets, coagulation function, renal and hepatic tests; she confirms her blood group is positive for Rh factor.

8. Discuss important psychosocial aspects and interprofessional considerations in the care of this couple. *(1 point per main bullet)*   Max 3

☐ Inform the patient/couple of the nonurgency in starting induction of labor (may prefer to return home for personal/cultural preferences, or to await spontaneous labor)
   ○ *Beware of the ~10% risk of coagulopathy within four weeks of IUFD*
   ○ *Consideration for twice-weekly DIC testing if she chooses expectancy for >48 hours, and inform patient that value of postmortem examination may be reduced*

☐ Arrange for a lead contact trained in bereavement for the patient and health care team *(e.g., counselor, mental health professional, religious support leader)*
   ○ Consider a second member of personnel to avoid compassion fatigue

☐ Arrange for expert morphologic postmortem neonatal examination shortly after delivery *(ideally a geneticist based on institutional availability; neonatologist or perinatal pathologist are additional possibilities)*

☐ Ensure arrangements are made for placement of a discrete bereavement symbol, understood by staff, at the patient's hospital room and in her medical chart

☐ Provide timely communication of the recent IUFD with her primary obstetric provider and ensure cancellation of future obstetric appointments

The patient and her partner meet with a bereavement counselor; plans are made for them to spend time and have memory keepsakes with their infant. Prior to proceeding with induction of labor[†] as the patient wishes, you inform the couple of possible physical abnormalities, including skin peeling and discoloration, at delivery of the infant, and counsel them on postnatal examinations of the infant and placenta. You have informed your trainee that intrapartum antibiotic prophylaxis should not be used routinely, nor is treatment required had she been colonised with group B streptococcus.[‡]

Special notes:
† Refer to Chapter 16
‡ RCOG[7]

---

9. Elaborate on postnatal infant and placental investigations in the setting of antepartum   Max 4
    stillbirth of unidentified etiology. *(1 point per main bullet, unless specified)*

☐ Physical examination of the infant ± clinical photographs with parental consent *(generally performed by individual(s) with expertise in genetics, perinatal pathology, or neonatology)*
☐ Consent the patient for postmortem autopsy
☐ If autopsy is declined, options for infant testing include: *(1 point per subbullet)*
  ○ Imaging studies by X-ray, sonography, or MRI
  ○ Chromosomal analysis through tissue sampling such as blood or skin[†]
☐ Bacterial culture of the fetal surface of the placenta
  ○ Particularly for Group B *Streptococcus, E. coli, L. monocytogenes*
☐ Gross and histopathology examination of the placenta, membranes, and umbilical cord
  ○ *This is the single most useful aspect of the evaluation of stillbirth (Suggested Reading 1)*

Special note:
† With consent for cytogenetic analysis, internal fetal tissue specimens that thrive under low-oxygen tension are preferred, such as costochondral junction, patella, Achilles tendon; fetal skin sampling is not recommended due to risk of contamination during delivery

---

The patient has an uneventful induction of labor and delivery of an appropriately grown male infant weighing 2797 g. There is one loose true knot in the umbilical cord seen at delivery. The placenta appeared intact with normal weight and preliminary gross morphology; laboratory examination is arranged. After parents had the opportunity to hold their infant and perform cultural rituals, prompt examination of the stillborn by a neonatologist is reportedly normal. The patient has consented for chromosomal analysis and autopsy.

After delivery, your trainee is curious whether he or she can document 'cord accident' as the likely cause of death.

10. Explain to your trainee important considerations before a cord accident is attributed to the cause of fetal death. *(1 point each)*

2

Fetal findings:
☐ Evidence of hypoxia and cord occlusion

Histologic findings:
☐ Thrombosis and vascular ectasia in the umbilical cord, chorionic plate, and stem villi

By postpartum day 2, she is ready for discharge; she does not require narcotic analgesics. Available laboratory investigations are only significant for isolated serum anticardiolipin antibodies of the IgA isotype. Her blood group is A+.

11. Discuss aspects of <u>postpartum</u> management *most specific* to consider prior to this patient's hospital discharge. *(1 point each unless specified)*

Max 8

Interprofessional support and follow-up:
☐ Ensure continued access to psychosocial support services
☐ Ensure the primary care/principal obstetric provider receives all clinical documentation, laboratory results, and pathology reports
☐ Consideration for close postpartum follow-up with screening for postpartum depression, anxiety, and posttraumatic stress disorder
☐ Arrange for follow-up appointment for revision of pending investigations

Analysis of current laboratory results: *(3 points)*
☐ Inform the patient that *IgA* isotype for anticardiolipin is of uncertain significance and is not associated with diagnosis of antiphospholipid syndrome

Lactation and contraception:
☐ Considerations for cabergoline or bromocriptine for primary inhibition of milk production
  ○ *Ice packs, support breast binders, or analgesics may still be associated with severe breast pain*
☐ Patient may also wish to lactate and donate breast milk
☐ Discuss contraceptive options

As arranged, the patient presents to clinic when results of investigations are available, which are all normal. You explain that no specific cause is found in almost 50% of stillbirths. She intends to plan another pregnancy soon and requests your advice in prevention of recurrent fetal death.

12. Assuming access and adherence to appropriate obstetric care, identify recommended strategies that may modify the risk of recurrent unexplained stillbirth. [Note: Strategies *may or may not* apply to this patient in particular] *(1 point each)*

☐ Preconceptional attainment of ideal body weight (for both obese and underweight patients)

☐ Preconceptional folic acid supplementation *(by decreasing risk of folic-acid sensitive anomalies)*

☐ Abstinence from alcohol and cessation of illicit substance use *(recreational drugs or nonprescription opioids)*

☐ Smoking cessation *(consider nicotine replacement measures)*

☐ Technical procedures to limit the occurrence of multiple gestations among pregnancies conceived through artificial reproductive technologies

☐ Optimization of chronic medical conditions

Special note:
Reassure the patient that no optimal interpregnancy interval reduces risk of recurrent stillbirth

Max 4

13. Highlight principles of subsequent pregnancy counseling and management in the context of this patient's prior <u>unexplained</u> late stillbirth. *(1 point per main bullet)*

☐ Monitor her mental health and ensure access to required support

☐ Risk of recurrent stillbirth in this context is ~1/1000 births

☐ Mention that risks of other adverse pregnancy outcomes are increased after previous unexplained stillbirth (*e.g.*, preterm delivery, abruption, low birthweight)

☐ After stillbirth at ≥32 weeks' gestation, future antepartum fetal testing is recommended one to two times weekly beginning at 32^{+0} weeks' gestation, or one to two weeks prior to the gestational age of prior stillbirth *(ACOG[1])*

☐ Inform the patient that **no** fetal surveillance intervention or protocol (ultrasound, cardiotocography, kick counting) in a future uncomplicated pregnancy prevents stillbirth

☐ Consideration for gestational diabetes screening early in pregnancy (or preconceptionally) with prior unexplained stillbirth
    ○ *Screening early in gestation may be with HbA1c ± fasting serum glucose*
    ○ *Routine prenatal screening is recommended thereafter if normal in early pregnancy*

☐ Accurate gestational dating with early sonography is advised (minimize risk for FGR)

☐ Inform the patient that term delivery is recommended (37–39 weeks' gestation)
    ○ *Exact timing depends on individual considerations and regional variations*
    ○ *No evidence to support delivery <37 weeks solely for prior IUFD*

☐ LDASA may reduce risks of recurrent perinatal death where previous event may have been attributed to placental insufficiency or preeclampsia

☐ Anticoagulation (*e.g.*, LMWH) is **not** recommended for prevention of stillbirth in the absence of antiphospholipid syndrome

Max 7

TOTAL: **85**

Labor and Delivery

CHAPTER 15

Labor at Term

Amira El-Messidi and Srinivasan Krishnamurthy

During your call duty, a *healthy* 30-year-old primigravida at 40^{+4} weeks' gestation, confirmed by first-trimester sonography, presents to the obstetric emergency assessment unit of your hospital center with possible spontaneous rupture of the chorioamniotic membranes after a two-day history of increased aching in the low back and coccyx. You recall meeting the patient at a routine prenatal visit at 32 weeks' gestation while briefly covering your colleague's practice; you ascertained all aspects of maternal-fetal care had been normal. Electronic health records indicate she has since remained compliant with obstetric care, which has been uncomplicated up to the latest prenatal visit three days ago.

Special note: *For comprehensive presentation of resources, clinical, and academic subject matter addressed in this chapter, the 'Suggested Readings' list exceeds 10.*

LEARNING OBJECTIVES

1. Take a focused history from a patient at term, establish a diagnosis of labor, and confirm suspected rupture of chorioamniotic membranes
2. Discuss evidence-based labor management for a parturient with a singleton pregnancy at term, appreciating diverse means for labor analgesia
3. Provide counseling for, and management of, intrapartum complications, including malpresentation, dystocia, presumed intraamniotic infection, aberrations on electronic maternal-fetal tracing, and obstetric anal sphincter injuries (OASIS)
4. Demonstrate knowledge of important principles of instrumental deliveries
5. Recognize and manage a potentially challenging fetal delivery at Cesarean section

SUGGESTED READINGS

1. ACOG Committee Opinion No. 766: Approaches to limit intervention during labor and birth. *Obstet Gynecol.* 2019;133(2):e164–e173.
2. Alhafez L, Berghella V. Evidence-based labor management: first stage of labor (part 3). *Am J Obstet Gynecol MFM.* 2020;2(4):100185.
3. Alrowaily N, D'Souza R, Dong S, et al. Determining the optimal antibiotic regimen for chorioamnionitis: a systematic review and meta-analysis. *Acta Obstet Gynecol Scand.* 2021;100(5):818–831.

4. American College of Obstetricians and Gynecologists' Committee on Obstetric Practice. Delayed umbilical cord clamping after birth: ACOG Committee Opinion No. 814. *Obstet Gynecol.* 2020;136(6):e100–e106.

5. Ayres-de-Campos D, Arulkumaran S, FIGO Intrapartum Fetal Monitoring Expert Consensus Panel. FIGO consensus guidelines on intrapartum fetal monitoring: physiology of fetal oxygenation and the main goals of intrapartum fetal monitoring. *Int J Gynaecol Obstet.* 2015;131(1):5–8.

6. Ayres-de-Campos D, Spong CY, Chandraharan E, FIGO Intrapartum Fetal Monitoring Expert Consensus Panel. FIGO consensus guidelines on intrapartum fetal monitoring: Cardiotocography. *Int J Gynaecol Obstet.* 2015;131(1):13–24.

7. Bloch C, Dore S, Hobson S. Committee Opinion No. 415: Impacted fetal head, second-stage Cesarean delivery. *J Obstet Gynaecol Can.* 2021;43(3):406–413.

8. Bonapace J, Gagné GP, Chaillet N, et al. No. 355 – physiologic basis of pain in labour and delivery: an evidence-based approach to its management. *J Obstet Gynaecol Can.* 2018;40(2):227–245.

9. Committee on Practice Bulletins-Obstetrics. ACOG Practice Bulletin No. 198: Prevention and management of obstetric lacerations at vaginal delivery. *Obstet Gynecol.* 2018;132(3):e87–e102.

10. Committee Opinion No. 712: Intrapartum management of intraamniotic infection. *Obstet Gynecol.* 2017;130(2):e95–e101.

11. Conde-Agudelo A, Romero R, Jung EJ, et al. Management of clinical chorioamnionitis: an evidence-based approach. *Am J Obstet Gynecol.* 2020;223(6):848–869.

12. Dore S, Ehman W. No. 396 – fetal health surveillance: intrapartum consensus guideline. *J Obstet Gynaecol Can.* 2020;42(3):316–348.e9. [Correction in *J Obstet Gynaecol Can.* 2021 Sep;43(9):1118]

13. Harvey MA, Pierce M, Alter JE, et al. Obstetrical anal sphincter injuries (OASIS): prevention, recognition, and repair. *J Obstet Gynaecol Can.* 2015;37(12):1131–1148. [Correction in *J Obstet Gynaecol Can.* 2016 Apr;38(4):421]

14. Hobson S, Cassell K, Windrim R, et al. No. 381 – assisted vaginal birth. *J Obstet Gynaecol Can.* 2019;41(6):870–882.

15. Ghi T, Eggebø T, Lees C, et al. ISUOG practice guidelines: intrapartum ultrasound. *Ultrasound Obstet Gynecol.* 2018;52(1):128–139.

16. Lee L, Dy J, Azzam H. Management of spontaneous labour at term in healthy women. *J Obstet Gynaecol Can.* 2016;38(9):843–865.

17. Lewis D, Downe S, FIGO Intrapartum Fetal Monitoring Expert Consensus Panel. FIGO consensus guidelines on intrapartum fetal monitoring: Intermittent auscultation. *Int J Gynaecol Obstet.* 2015;131(1):9–12.

18. Money D, Allen VM. No. 298 – The prevention of early-onset neonatal group B streptococcal disease. *J Obstet Gynaecol Can.* 2018;40(8):e665–e674.

19. Murphy DJ, Strachan BK, Bahl R. Assisted vaginal birth. *BJOG* 2020;127:e70–e112.

20. National Institute for Health and Care Excellence. Intrapartum care for healthy women and babies; updated Feb 2017. Available at www.nice.org.uk/guidance/cg190/. Accessed September 13, 2021.

21. Prevention of group B Streptococcal early-onset disease in newborns: ACOG Committee Opinion, No. 797. *Obstet Gynecol.* 2020;135(2):e51–e72. [Correction in *Obstet Gynecol.* 2020 Apr;135(4):978–979]

22. Royal College of Obstetricians and Gynaecologists. The management of third-and-fourth degree perineal tears. Green-Top Guideline No. 29; June 2015. Available at www.rcog.org.uk/globalassets/documents/guidelines/gtg-29.pdf. Accessed September 13, 2021.

23. Tempest N, Navaratnam K, Hapangama D. Management of delivery when malposition of the fetal head complicates the second stage of labour. *Obstetrician and Gynaecologist* 2015;17:273–280.

24. Tsakiridis I, Mamopoulos A, Athanasiadis A, et al. Obstetric anal sphincter injuries at vaginal delivery: a review of recently published national guidelines. *Obstet Gynecol Surv.* 2018;73(12): 695–702.
25. Visser GH, Ayres-de-Campos D, FIGO Intrapartum Fetal Monitoring Expert Consensus Panel. FIGO consensus guidelines on intrapartum fetal monitoring: Adjunctive technologies. *Int J Gynaecol Obstet.* 2015;131(1):25–29.

POINTS

1. What aspects of a focused history would you want to know <u>either</u> from the patient or her electronic obstetrical chart? *(1 point each)*

Max 10

Details related to the clinical presentation:
- ☐ Time interval since possible rupture of chorioamniotic membranes
- ☐ Color of the fluid loss (*i.e.*, clear, bloody, or green-tinged)
- ☐ Presence of vaginal bleeding
- ☐ Presence of uterine contractions or abdominal pains that accompany the back symptoms
- ☐ Normal fetal activity before and after possible rupture of chorioamniotic membranes

General obstetric details:
- ☐ Results of the vaginal-rectal group B *Streptococcus* (GBS) swab performed within five weeks of presentation, or known positive status based on GBS bacteriuria at any time during pregnancy or a positive vaginal-rectal swab resulted during investigations for preterm labor
- ☐ Documented fetal presentation at the most recent antenatal visit
- ☐ Ascertain whether fundal heights until the late third trimester had been appropriate to gestational age, or reported estimate of fetal weight if third-trimester sonography was required

Medical aspects related to intrapartum care:
- ☐ Medications (prescribed and unprescribed)
- ☐ Drug allergies

Social aspects related to intrapartum care:
- ☐ Ascertain whether a labor support person will be present (*i.e.*, husband/partner, family/ friend, doula[‡])

Special notes:
Knowledge of placental localization is implicit to the described normal aspects of maternal-fetal care, the patient's gestational age, and compliance with antenatal care
[‡] 1:1 emotional support by support personnel (*e.g.*, doula) improves outcomes for women in labor

You learn that the patient experienced a vaginal gush of clear fluid approximately one hour prior to presentation, followed by onset of lower abdominal cramps. Meanwhile, her back and coccygeal pains have intensified over the past hour. She has not had any vaginal bleeding. Fetal activity has been normal. The patient only took prenatal vitamins; her obstetric provider informed her of the need for intrapartum antibiotics for GBS bacteria on the vaginal-rectal swab performed at 36 weeks' gestation. She has no drug allergies. You learn from the electronic medical records that fundal heights were normal and the fetus remained in the cephalic presentation by abdominal assessments. Her husband has just returned from their homeland in Asia and will soon be arriving at the hospital.

2. Verbalize essentials of your focused physical examination. *(1 point each, unless specified)*   10

General appearance:
☐ General body habitus; may consider revision of the prepregnancy BMI
☐ Apparent distress from abdominal or back pains

Vital signs:
☐ Blood pressure, pulse rate, temperature, oxygen saturation

Fetal heart rate: *(2 points)*
☐ Intermittent auscultation[§]

Abdominal assessment:
☐ Palpate for the presence, duration, and frequency of uterine contractions
☐ Leopold maneuvers to confirm fetal presentation and determine fetal lie[†]

Gynecologic examination:
☐ Evidence of spontaneous rupture of the chorioamniotic membranes with continued fluid leaking, or speculum examination to visualize fluid leakage from the cervical os or pooling in the posterior vaginal fornix
☐ Perform adjunctive confirmatory test(s), where necessary, to confirm spontaneous rupture of the chorioamniotic membranes *(see Question 4)*
☐ Based on this patient's distress, perform vaginal examination for cervical dilation, effacement, station, position, and consistency[‡] (a digital vaginal examination would also be indicated based on risk factors for umbilical cord prolapse, or presence of palpable contractions; examination could otherwise be deferred, particularly given known GBS-positive status)

Special notes:
§ Routine use of (admission) cardiotocography (CTG) for this low-risk patient is not recommended as it increases Cesarean section rates without improving perinatal outcomes – *refer to* Devane D, Lalor JG, Daly S, et al. Cardiotocography versus intermittent auscultation of fetal heart on admission to labour ward for assessment of fetal wellbeing. *Cochrane Database Syst Rev.* 2017;1(1):CD005122. Published 2017 Jan 26.
† Although ultrasound may assist in fetal assessment, it is not uniformly indicated
‡ Bimanual examination is not always required

The patient appears of normal body habitus, and electronic records indicate her prepregnancy BMI was 21.5 kg/m². Vital signs are unremarkable. She appears in distress, holding her lower abdomen and back during contractions, during which she feels some rectal pressure. Contractions are palpable at five- to six-minute intervals for 30–60 seconds duration. Cephalic presentation is confirmed by abdominal palpation; there is evidence of subumbilical flattening with fetal limbs palpable anteriorly and to the maternal left. Intermittent fetal auscultation is normal. In the absence of visual evidence of spontaneous rupture of amniotic chorioamniotic membranes, you proceed with diagnostic tests, following which vaginal examination reveals the internal cervical os is 2 cm dilated, 50% effaced, with the fetal head 3 cm above the ischial spines. There is no evidence of umbilical cord prolapse. During the examination, you alert your trainee about the importance of remaining vigilant for unanticipated findings on inspection and examination where vaginal delivery would be contraindicated, such as active genital herpes or genital condylomas obstructing the birth canal.

3. Inform your obstetric trainee of the suspected fetal presentation based on your assessment, while eliciting features supporting your impression. *(1 point each, unless specified)*   Max 6

☐ The fetus is suspected to be in the right-occipitoposterior (ROP) position *(4)*

Supporting features:
☐ Subumbilical flattening representing a groove between the fetal head and body
☐ Fetal limbs are palpable anteriorly and to the maternal left
☐ Backache associated with occiput-induced pressure on the sacral nerves
☐ Rectal pressure due to overstimulation of sacral nerves
☐ Fetal head is not applied on the cervix

4. Identify individual noninvasive tests used in clinical practice to <u>support or confirm</u> spontaneous rupture of chorioamniotic membranes, outlining to your obstetric trainee the rationale and caveats of each modality, where known. *(1 point per main and subbullet)*   Max 10

☐ Litmus paper and pH testing
  ○ *Rationale:* The standard pH of vaginal secretions (4.5 to 5.5) increases when contaminated by amniotic fluid (7.0 to 7.5)
  ○ *Caveats:* False-positive results from vaginal infections, blood, semen, alkaline urine or alkaline antiseptics; false-negative results with minimal leakage with chronic chorioamniotic rupture or a 'high fluid leak'
☐ Amniotic fluid crystallization test
  ○ *Rationale:* 'Ferning' appearance on microscopy is due to the sodium chloride and protein content of amniotic fluid
  ○ *Caveats:* False-positive results from semen, cervical mucous, or fingerprints; false-negative results in the presence of blood, meconium, heavy leukorrhea
☐ Placental alpha-microglobulin-1 test (AmniSure™)
  ○ *Rationale:* The placental glycoprotein is abundant in amniotic fluid (2000–25,000 ng/mL), with much lower concentrations in maternal blood (5–25 ng/mL) and negligible amounts in cervicovaginal secretions with intact membranes (0.05–0.2 ng/mL)
  ○ *Caveats:* Nil identified; minimal false-positives and -negatives
☐ Absorbent pad (AmnioSense™)
  ○ *Rationale:* A central strip changes color on contact with fluid pH >5.2; if in contact with urine, the strip revers to its original color when dry due to detached conjugate- based nitrazine molecules by urine ammonium ions
  ○ *Caveats:* Unknown; potential interference with active bacterial vaginosis or trichomonas vaginalis

Special note:
Refer to El-Messidi A, Cameron A. Diagnosis of premature rupture of membranes: inspiration from the past and insights for the future. *J Obstet Gynaecol Can.* 2010;32(6):561–569.

Having confirmed spontaneous rupture of amniotic chorioamniotic membranes by a positive AmniSure™ result, the patient concurs to planned admission for labor pain management and antibiotic treatment for GBS-positive status. You recall the patient mentioning, at the antenatal visit, she chose to birth at your hospital center's labor ward given its known reputation for a supportive environment that fosters the natural hormonal physiology of labor and delivery.

You take this opportunity to teach your trainee that appropriate counseling of this patient would have been necessary in the event of confirmed chorioamniotic membrane rupture in the absence of labor, as evidence for immediate induction of labor appears favorable for maternal-neonatal infectious morbidity.[†]

Special note:
† *Refer to* Middleton P, Shepherd E, Flenady V, McBain RD, Crowther CA. Planned early birth versus expectant management (waiting) for prelabour rupture of membranes at term (37 weeks or more). *Cochrane Database Syst Rev.* 2017;1(1):CD005302. Published 2017 Jan 4.

5. Counsel the patient on techniques, used sequentially or in combination, that *may* help her   Max 8
    cope with labor pain. *(1 point each; max points indicated per section)*

Nonpharmacologic methods of labor pain management: *(max 5)*
☐ Ambulation in labor and assuming vertical/upright positions
☐ Aromatherapy with essential oils (*e.g.,* lavender, jasmine, rose, almond, or mixture)
☐ Acupuncture, acupressure
☐ Accessories for the labor process (*e.g.,* birthing balls, trapeze bars)
☐ Breathing, relaxation and visualization techniques; hypnosis/hypno-birthing
☐ Massage during or between contractions
☐ Music
☐ Warm/cold packs
☐ Water immersion *(offers some analgesic benefit)*
☐ Yoga
☐ Intradermal sterile water injections in the low back, where the patient experiences strong pain
☐ Transcutaneous electrical neurostimulation (TENS) machine

Pharmacologic methods of labor pain management: *(max 3)*
☐ Inhalational anesthetics (nitrous oxide gas)
☐ Injectable opioids[†] or opioid agonist-antagonist agents
☐ Epidural or combined spinal-epidural analgesia
☐ Pudental nerve block

Special note:
† Intrapartum use of opioids with a long half-life (*e.g.,* meperidine) is not recommended due to effects of long-acting active metabolites on neonatal outcomes

6. Noting how this laboring patient innately prefers to ambulate or assume upright positions,   Max 6
   you teach your obstetric trainee its <u>evidence-based benefits</u> in the first or second stages
   of labor where no regional analgesia is used or contraindications to mobility exist.
   (1 point each)

☐ Reduced use of epidural analgesia[†]
☐ Shortened first stage of labor[†]
☐ Decreased likelihood of Cesarean delivery[†]
☐ Reduced number of episiotomies[‡]/diminished perineal trauma[§]
☐ Improved effectiveness of spontaneous contractions[§]
☐ Improved fetal oxygenation[§]
☐ Fewer 'abnormal' fetal heart rate patterns in the second stage[‡] (upright or lateral relative to
   supine positions)
☐ Facilitates fetal descent[#]
☐ Increased likelihood of spontaneous vaginal birth[†]/reduced incidence of operative
   vaginal birth[‡]

Special notes:
[†] *Refer to* Lawrence A, Lewis L, Hofmeyr GJ, Styles C. Maternal positions and mobility
   during first stage labour. *Cochrane Database Syst Rev.* 2013;(10):CD003934. Published
   2013 Oct 9.
[‡] *Refer to* Gupta JK, Sood A, Hofmeyr GJ, Vogel JP. Position in the second stage of labour for
   women without epidural anaesthesia. *Cochrane Database Syst Rev.* 2017;5(5):CD002006.
   Published 2017 May 25.
[§] *SOGC*[8]
[#] *Refer to* Zwelling E. Overcoming the challenges: maternal movement and positioning to
   facilitate labor progress. *MCN Am J Matern Child Nurs.* 2010;35(2):72–80.

7. What is the physiological mechanism by which upright positions in labor facilitates fetal   1
   descent relative to laying supine?

☐ Decreased pressure of the bed that forces the sacrum and coccyx anteriorly promotes
   widening of the pelvic outlet

Special note:
Refer to Zwelling E. Overcoming the challenges: maternal movement and positioning to
facilitate labor progress. *MCN Am J Matern Child Nurs.* 2010;35(2):72–80

Upon admission to the labor ward, continuous one-on-one support is provided by obstetric care
providers in collaboration with her husband. As contraction frequency and intensity are increasing, the patient engages in several nonpharmacologic methods for labor pain management,
preferably delaying or avoiding the need of pharmacologic agents.

8-A.   Review with the patient the importance of intrapartum antibiotics for GBS-positive status.

Max 3

Role of intrapartum GBS prophylaxis: *(2)*

☐ Explain that antibiotic treatment aims to prevent early-onset neonatal GBS disease,[§] with conferred benefit from antibiotic administration **at least two hours** before delivery; lack of intrapartum treatment of women colonized at delivery can result in disease among 1%–2% of neonates[†]

8-B.   Specify the treatment protocol for intrapartum GBS prophylaxis where the patient does not have drug allergies. *(1 point each)*

First-line intrapartum treatment:

☐ Initiate intravenous penicillin G 5 million units as a loading dose, followed by 2.5–3 million units every four hours until delivery

Alternative treatment where penicillin is unavailable:

☐ Intravenous ampicillin 2 g loading dose followed by 1 g every four hours until delivery

Special notes:

§ Defined as vertical transmission-associated neonatal sepsis, pneumonia, or meningitis within seven days of life

† *Refer to* Verani JR, McGee L, Schrag SJ; Division of Bacterial Diseases, National Center for Immunization and Respiratory Diseases, Centers for Disease Control and Prevention (CDC). Prevention of perinatal group B streptococcal disease—revised guidelines from CDC, 2010. *MMWR Recomm Rep.* 2010;59(RR-10):1–36.

9.   In addition to intrapartum GBS prophylaxis, outline your evidence-based plans for admission with regard to maternal-fetal monitoring and nutrition during spontaneous labor of a low-risk singleton gestation, while explaining the rationale to your trainee. *(1 point per main bullet)*

Max 5

Maternal monitoring and nutrition:[§]

☐ Unless clinically indicated, plan four-hourly cervical examinations; there is no benefit from two-hourly assessments on length of labor, use of epidural analgesia, or mode of delivery (*Suggested Reading 2*)

☐ Allow unrestricted intake of fluid or solid food in the first stage of labor as this is associated with shorter duration of labor, no increase in maternal-neonatal adverse outcomes, and the risk of aspiration in low-risk singleton pregnancies is very low, at 1/1,000,000[†]

☐ If fluid restriction is required, plan intravenous dextrose-containing fluid infusion at 250 mL/hr, as this is associated with a shorter duration of labor and lower incidence of Cesarean delivery relative to 125 mL/hr[‡]

☐ Allow for spontaneous urination or perform intermittent bladder catheterization, if required, as continuous drainage can impact ambulation, increase pain and infection without improving labor progress or likelihood of vaginal delivery

☐ Routine monitoring of labor progress by use of any of the available partograms is not recommended in the absence of known improvements in maternal-neonatal features and the inherent difficulty in diagnosing abnormal labor progress[#]

Fetal monitoring:

☐ Intermittent auscultation in the first and second stages of labor, in the absence of indications for electronic fetal monitoring (SOGC[12])

   ○ *Frequency of fetal heart auscultation may vary by institutional protocol*

   ○ *Although of controversial value, intrapartum CTG for low-risk women has become standard of care in many countries (FIGO[6])*

Special notes:

§ Individualized protocols for serial assessment of vital signs

† *Refer to Suggested Reading 2 and Ciardulli A, Saccone G, Anastasio H, Berghella V. Less-restrictive food intake during labor in low-risk singleton pregnancies: A systematic review and meta-analysis. Obstet Gynecol.* 2017;129(3):473–480.

‡ *Refer to (a)* Riegel M, Quist-Nelson J, Saccone G, et al. Dextrose intravenous fluid therapy in labor reduces the length of the first stage of labor. *Eur J Obstet Gynecol Reprod Biol.* 2018;228:284–294, and *(b)* Ehsanipoor RM, Saccone G, Seligman NS, et al. Intravenous fluid rate for reduction of cesarean delivery rate in nulliparous women: a systematic review and meta-analysis. *Acta Obstet Gynecol Scand.* 2017;96(7):804–811.

Refer to Lavender T, Cuthbert A, Smyth RM. Effect of partograph use on outcomes for women in spontaneous labor at term and their babies. *Cochrane Database Syst Rev.* 2018;8 (8):CD005461. Published 2018 Aug 6.

Your obstetric trainee rightly extrapolates from your counseling of the patient that obstetric interventions, including the need to offer oxytocin infusion if labor progress slows, need not be delayed solely to ensure at least four hours of antibiotic administration before delivery, which is the interval known to be highly effective protection against early-onset GBS disease *(Suggested Reading 2 and ACOG[21])*.

Labor progresses well until 5 cm dilatation when spontaneous contractions become less frequent, increasing from every 2–3 minutes to 10-minute intervals. Meanwhile, the patient is feeling increasing low back and rectal pains, no longer alleviated by nonpharmacologic means. She appears frustrated that labor is lengthy, indicating that cervical dilatation has progressed merely 3 cm in eight hours since admission and is requesting a Cesarean delivery. Her vital signs remain normal and intermittent fetal auscultation unremarkable. Pelvic examination reveals persistent ROP position, now at 1 cm above the ischial spines; the cervix has become fully effaced.

10. Refer to the current definitions of dystocia in the first stage of labor with regard to clinical management you would now discuss with the patient. *(1 point per main and subbullet)*   5

☐ Provide reassurance that both maternal and fetal progress are normal to date without features warranting urgent delivery
   ○ Cesarean section is not recommended until labor has arrested in the *active* phase (*i.e.,* ≥6 cm[$]) for at least four hours with adequate uterine contractions or at least six hours with inadequate contractions despite use of oxytocin infusion *(Suggested Reading 2)*

☐ Offer pharmacologic means for analgesia or consultation with the obstetric anesthesiologist

☐ Counsel on commencement of standard intravenous oxytocin infusion (*i.e.,* low-dose or high-dose regimen)

☐ Reassure the patient that intermittent auscultation may continue to be used for fetal monitoring with initiation of patient-controlled epidural (*i.e., low-risk, term pregnancy in spontaneous labor*), unless combined spinal-epidural is planned, where electronic fetal monitoring would be recommended[†] *(SOGC[12])*

Special notes:
§   International variations exist regarding the start of the active phase of labor (*i.e.,* >4–6 cm)
†   Higher risk of abnormal fetal heart tracings warrants closer monitoring

After comprehensive counseling,[†] a low-dose epidural (*i.e.,* implies the dose of local anesthetic) is placed and your hospital center's low-dose[$] intravenous oxytocin protocol commenced at 2 milliunits/min, to be increased by 2 milliunits/min approximately every 30 minutes (not more frequently than every 20 minutes) based on the uterine contraction pattern and fetal tolerance to labor.[$$]

While updating your medical documentation thereafter, you take the opportunity to review aspects of labor physiology with your obstetric trainee.

Special notes:
Refer to Chapter 16, Question 26 (counseling on intravenous oxytocin[†]), Question 25 (elaboration on low- and high-dosing regimens[$]), and the clinical description prior to Question 25 (maximal dose of oxytocin[$$])

11. Discuss the differences between endogenous/natural and exogenous/synthetic oxytocin on labor physiology with your obstetric trainee. *(1 point each)*   Max 2

☐ Contrary to synthetic oxytocin which is not present in significant amounts in the maternal brain, endogenous oxytocin, produced by the hypothalamus and stored for release from the posterior pituitary, has central analgesic properties and promotes a sense of calmness

☐ Synthetic oxytocin is associated with increased labor pains, triggering stronger, longer, and more frequent contractions than physiologic processes

☐ Prolonged exposure to synthetic oxytocin in labor reduces the sensitivity of uterine oxytocin receptors, potentially increasing the risk of postpartum hemorrhage *(SOGC[8])*

12. Review with your obstetric trainee the <u>nonanalgesic benefits</u> of modern low-dose versus high-dose epidurals in labor. *(1 point each)*

Advantages of low-dose versus high-dose epidurals in labor:

Lower risks of:

☐ Interference with ambulation

☐ Hypotension

☐ Urinary retention and need for catheterization

☐ Motor blockade, prolonged second stage, malpresentation, and assisted vaginal birth

When oxytocin is infusing at 12 milliunits/min, you are informed of an abnormal intermittent auscultation, for which electronic fetal monitoring has just been initiated. The nurse reassures you that all vital signs, including urine output, remain normal and there is no vaginal bleeding. Your plan is to revert to intermittent auscultation in ≥20 minutes if the fetal tracing is normal and there are no changes to the patient's overall status *(SOGC[12])*. However, during the first 12 minutes of electronic fetal monitoring, you are called urgently to manage the following CTG tracing with a paper speed at 3 cm/min.

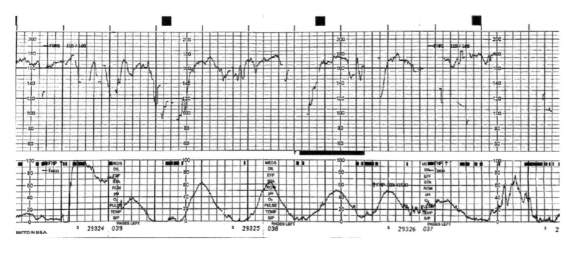

Figure 15.1

With permission: Figure 1 from Hobson SR, Abdelmalek MZ, Farine D. Update on uterine tachysystole. *J Perinat Med.* 2019;47(2):152–160.

There is no association between the patient's cardiotocography and this case scenario. Image only used for educational purposes.

13. Based on your interpretation of CTG tracing, summarize your management with an understanding that interventions are often performed simultaneously, in addition to keeping the patient informed. *(1 point per main bullet; subbullets are provided for academic purposes)*

Max 5

Management of intrauterine resuscitation:
- ☐ Stop the oxytocin infusion
  - ○ *Promotes uterine relaxation to improve fetal oxygenation and uteroplacental perfusion*
- ☐ Maternal repositioning to the left or right side
  - ○ *Alleviates umbilical cord compression and/or improves uteroplacental perfusion*
- ☐ Cervical reassessment
  - ○ *Assess for umbilical cord prolapse*
- ☐ Consideration for acute tocolysis[§] (*e.g.*, intravenous nitroglycerin 50 μg over two to three minutes, repeated every three to five minutes to a maximum of 200 μg; or subcutaneous terbutaline 250 μg; or sublingual[†] nitroglycerin 0.4 mg/spray given once or twice)
- ☐ Consideration for Cesarean section if there is no response to routine corrective measures
- ☐ Explain to the patient recent events and ensure timely documentation

Special notes:
§ Maintain caution for contraindications
† Although frequently used, the sublingual form of nitroglycerin is not effective in the presence of tachysystole *(SOGC[12])*

14. Address your trainee's inquiry as to why you did not administer maternal oxygen supplementation or initiate an intravenous fluid bolus of a non-glucose-containing crystalloid solution. *(1 point each)*

2

- ☐ Supplemental intrapartum oxygen in a normoxemic patient does not improve umbilical artery pH or neonatal outcome, and may lead to free radical formation[†]
- ☐ For a euvolemic, nonhypotensive patient, there is no high-quality evidence that intravenous fluid bolus is beneficial for fetal heart rate abnormalities

Special note:
† (a) Raghuraman N, Temming LA, Doering MM, et al. Maternal oxygen supplementation compared with room air for intrauterine resuscitation: A systematic review and meta-analysis. *JAMA Pediatr.* 2021;175(4):368–376; (b) Fawole B, Hofmeyr GJ. Maternal oxygen administration for fetal distress. *Cochrane Database Syst Rev.* 2012;12(12):CD000136. Published 2012 Dec 12.

The CTG tracing normalizes with intrauterine resuscitation, allowing for reinitiation of oxytocin infusion in 30 minutes based on a half-life of 3–5 minutes (*i.e.,* four half-lives as a washout period).

Your obstetric trainee notifies you that cervical dilatation progressed from 5 to 8 cm over six hours. Oral temperature is 39.2°C [102.6°F][†] and she continues to receive intravenous penicillin G for GBS prophylaxis at four-hourly intervals.

15. Outline your initial clinical examination for the diagnostic evaluation of fever in this   6
    parturient. *(1 point each)*

☐ Obtain comprehensive vital signs
☐ Assess the CTG tracing for fetal tachycardia, excluding accelerations, decelerations, and
   periods of marked variability
☐ Auscultate the lung fields
☐ Palpate for abdominal tenderness in between contractions *(on-going epidural anesthesia
   may mask symptoms)*
☐ Assess for costovertebral angle tenderness
☐ Assess for a change in vaginal fluid loss to purulent or foul-smelling loss

Vaginal fluid is now purulent, foul-smelling, and green-tinged. The abdomen is nontender between contractions and electronic fetal monitoring remains normal. There are no nonobstetric significant findings.

16. Based on the working diagnosis, outline your counseling and management of this patient.   Max 6
    (1 point each)

☐ Inform the patient that an intraamniotic infection (*i.e.,* chorioamnionitis) is suspected
   based on clinical findings
☐ Explain that a Cesarean section is not required to expedite delivery solely for an
   intrauterine infection, as a shorter labor does not improve neonatal outcomes[†] yet
   increases maternal morbidity (*e.g.,* postpartum transfusion, wound infection, or
   endometritis)[‡]
☐ Address the need to modify the intrapartum antibiotic regimen to include broad-spectrum
   antibiotics
☐ Initiate antipyretic treatment with acetaminophen or paracetamol
☐ Maintain continuous electronic fetal monitoring until delivery
☐ Communicate the suspected intraamniotic infection to the neonatology team to provide
   patient counseling and neonatal surveillance for signs of infection
☐ Arrange for postpartum histopathologic examination of the placenta, umbilical cord, and
   chorioamniotic membranes

Special notes:
† Rouse DJ, Landon M, Leveno KJ, et al. The Maternal-Fetal Medicine Units cesarean
  registry: chorioamnionitis at term and its duration-relationship to outcomes. *Am J Obstet
  Gynecol.* 2004;191(1):211–216.
‡ Venkatesh KK, Glover AV, Vladutiu CJ, Stamilio DM. Association of chorioamnionitis
  and its duration with adverse maternal outcomes by mode of delivery: a cohort study.
  BJOG. 2019;126(6):719–727.

17. Address a patient inquiry about potential adverse <u>maternal</u> outcomes associated with clinical chorioamnionitis, with an understanding that neonatal complications will be discussed in specialist consultation. *(1 point each)*

Max 5

<u>Maternal risks of clinical chorioamnionitis:</u>
- ☐ Labor dystocia
- ☐ Uterine rupture
- ☐ Cesarean section
- ☐ Postpartum hemorrhage due to uterine atony
- ☐ Emergency hysterectomy
- ☐ Blood transfusion
- ☐ Endometritis, wound infection, pelvic abscess
- ☐ Septic pelvic thrombophlebitis
- ☐ Admission to the intensive care/treatment unit (ICU/ITU)
- ☐ Rarely, mortality

You elaborate with your trainee on controversies surrounding effects of antipyretic treatment on maternal-fetal and neonatal outcomes. You also acknowledge the wide selection of antibiotic regimens and lack of a most appropriate therapy that optimizes maternal-neonatal outcomes, selecting one of multiple proposed regimens, based on local protocol and drug availability. Reassuringly, the patient has no drug allergies.

While intravenous ampicillin and gentamycin are infusing, your obstetrics trainee indicates that fetal presentation appears unchanged on digital examination, although caput succedaneum now limits palpation of sutures and fontanelles. Your trainee is thereby considering intrapartum ultrasound to verify fetal head station and position, recalling literature demonstrating higher accuracy and reproducibility, in addition to being more acceptable to parturients than digital examination *(ISUOG[15])*.

18. Knowing that <u>intrapartum ultrasound</u> has not (yet) been shown to improve the management of the birthing process, identify circumstances that *may or may not* relate to this patient, where intrapartum ultrasound may serve as an adjunct to clinical examination. *(1 point each)*

Max 2

- ☐ Slow progress in labor or first- or second-stage arrest
- ☐ Ascertainment of fetal head position *(by transabdominal probe)* and station *(by transperineal probe)* before potential instrumental vaginal delivery
- ☐ Visual assessment of fetal head malpresentations *(e.g., deflexed head or asynclitism)*

Three hours later, the patient has reached the second stage with augmentation of labor, an unremarkable fetal tracing, and continued broad-spectrum antibiotic treatment of chorioamnionitis. The epidural is functioning well. Meconium consistency remains thin. Fetal station is now 1 cm below the ischial spines, and the position continues to be right occiput-posterior (ROP) with a known caput succedaneum. There is no asynclitism. Perineal warm compresses[$] and perineal massage[$#] are initiated in the second stage for prevention of obstetric tears.

Currently in the *early* second stage, you consider manual rotation of the fetal head, sharing with your trainee its higher chance of success as a *prophylactic* maneuver rather than for *treatment* of arrest of descent. You suspect the procedure will succeed and briefly explain you awaited full dilation based on higher success rates than when performed earlier in labor,[†] it may occasionally facilitate labor progress.[‡]

Special notes:
§ Recommended by *ACOG*[9], *RCOG*[22]; [#]not advised by *NICE*[20]
† *Refer to* Le Ray C, Serres P, Schmitz T, Cabrol D, Goffinet F. Manual rotation in occiput posterior or transverse positions: risk factors and consequences on the cesarean delivery rate. *Obstet Gynecol.* 2007;110(4):873–879.
‡ *SOGC*[14]

---

19. Address aspects you would review or discuss with the patient prior to attempting a <u>manual</u> <u>rotation</u> of the occiput-posterior position. *(1 point per main bullet unless specified)*

    7

☐ Inquire about the effectiveness of the epidural analgesia
☐ Inform the patient that a successful manual rotation may obviate morbidities of an occiput-posterior delivery: *(1 point per subbullet, with max 2 points per category)*

Maternal:[†]
   ○ Prolonged, or arrest, of labor
   ○ Third- and fourth-degree perineal lacerations
   ○ Postpartum hemorrhage
   ○ Operative delivery (vaginal and Cesarean)

Fetal-neonatal:[‡]
   ○ Acidemia on umbilical cord blood gas analysis
   ○ Birth trauma/brachial plexus injury[§]
   ○ Apgar score <7 at one minute
   ○ Admission to the neonatal intensive care unit (NICU)

☐ Inform the patient that rotation may be unsuccessful, or the head may rotate to its original position
☐ Reassure the patient that complications of manual rotation are slim, yet include skull fracture and maternal tissue trauma

Special notes:
Chorioamnionitis[†] and meconium-stained amniotic fluid[‡] are additional morbidities of occiput-posterior deliveries, already existing in this case scenario
§   Related to malposition rather than shoulder dystocia

20. With successful manual rotation to the occiput-anterior position, counsel this nulliparous patient receiving neuraxial analgesia on timing the active second stage. *(1 point per main and subbullet)*

Max 3

☐ Encourage pushing if the patient feels the urge; otherwise acknowledge conflicting evidence with regard to early (immediate) or delayed pushing in a nulliparous patient receiving epidural analgesia:

Early pushing
   ○ Decreased rates of chorioamnionitis, postpartum hemorrhage, and neonatal acidemia, with similar rates of spontaneous vaginal birth
   ○ Higher rates of OASIS

Delayed pushing
   ○ Decreased total duration of pushing with higher rates of successful vaginal birth
   ○ Possibly lower Apgar scores

With continued one-on-one support, pushing is commenced and you encourage the patient to breath using her preferred and most effective technique, highlighting to your trainee that data regarding superiority of spontaneous versus Valsalva pushing is limited.

Knowing of the high incidence of maternal heart rate artifact,[†] you choose to monitor the maternal pulse simultaneously with the fetal tracing in the active second stage *(FIGO[6] and SOGC[12])*.

After one hour of effective pushing, examination reveals appropriate head descent in the occiput-anterior position and electronic fetal tracing remains unremarkable; treatment of chorioamnionitis continues. After discussion with the patient, you agree to an assisted vaginal delivery for severe maternal exhaustion; you anticipate reasonable chance of success yet prepare, as routine with instrumental deliveries, for potential shoulder dystocia.[‡] The neonatology team will attend delivery and the anesthesiologist has been notified should surgical delivery be required. Currently, the patient is in the lithotomy position with adequate anesthesia and the bladder has just been emptied.

Special notes:
† *Refer to* Paquette S, Moretti F, O'Reilly K, Ferraro ZM, Oppenheimer L. The incidence of maternal artefact during intrapartum fetal heart rate monitoring. *J Obstet Gynaecol Can.* 2014;36 (11):962–968.
‡ Refer to Question 1 in Chapter 19

SCENARIO A
Vacuum-assisted vaginal delivery and episiotomy
Although competent in either type of instrumental vaginal technique for which this patient is eligible, an **outlet** vacuum-assisted procedure is mutually agreed with the patient. You understand that vacuum deliveries are generally less likely to effect vaginal delivery than forceps procedures.

21. Address your trainee's inquiry regarding what you implied by an 'outlet' instrumental delivery for *this*[†] fetus. *(1 point each)*

3

☐ Fetal scalp is visible at the introitus without separating the labia
☐ Fetal skull has reached the pelvic floor
☐ Sagittal suture is in the anterior-posterior position[†]

Special note:
† While maximal rotation of 45° is an additional defining feature of an outlet procedure, it is not pertinent to this case scenario

22. Highlight circumstances that would have prohibited a vacuum-assisted delivery for this gravida at <u>term</u>. *(1 point each)*

Max 6

Maternal contraindications:
☐ Declines to provide verbal consent
☐ Incomplete cervical dilatation
☐ Suspected cephalopelvic disproportion *(maternal or fetal factor)*
☐ Inability to progress to a timely Cesarean delivery *(maternal or fetal factor)*

Fetal contraindications:
☐ Nonvertex presentation (*e.g.,* face or brow)
☐ Unengaged head
☐ Uncertainty of head position
☐ Known or suspected coagulopathy, thrombocytopenia, or brittle skeletal dysplasia
☐ Rotational forces needed to effect delivery

23. What are <u>fetal</u> risks of vacuum-assisted delivery you would disclose in preprocedural counseling? *(1 point each)*

Max 4

☐ Exaggeration of the subcutaneous caput
☐ Scalp lacerations and bruising
☐ Cephalohematoma
☐ Hyperbilirubinemia and neonatal jaundice
☐ Subgaleal hemorrhage (~1/1000 Kiwi™ cup procedures[†])

Special note:
† *Refer to* Baskett TF, Fanning CA, Young DC. A prospective observational study of 1000 vacuum assisted deliveries with the OmniCup device. *J Obstet Gynaecol Can.* 2008;30:573–80

24. With regard to risks of maternal tissue injury that you disclosed in patient consultation, outline technical considerations for its prevention in a vacuum-assisted delivery.[†] *(1 point each)*

4

- ☐ Avoid traumatic insertion, including avoidance of insertion during a contraction
- ☐ Verify for maternal soft tissue entrapment between the fetal scalp and vacuum cup[‡]
- ☐ Maintain a proper angle in traction[‡]
- ☐ Avoid rapid traction and uncontrolled descent[§] and delivery over the perineum[‡]

Special notes:
† Refer to *Advances in Labour and Risk Management (ALARM) Manual* 24th edition, 2017–2018. Published by The Society of Obstetricians and Gynaecologists of Canada (SOGC). ISBN 978–1-897116–53–1
‡ Causative factors for pop-off of the suction cup
§ Provided by countertraction on the suction cup

The patient provides consent and accepts having the obstetric trainee apply your chosen suction cup under supervision. The trainee reassures the patient of prior clinical experience; you also recall providing simulation training where you taught different skills involved based on the type of vacuum device.

Your trainee is verbalizing technical steps during application of the suction cup, having ensured equipment appears normal and is functioning.

25. Explain <u>why</u> the cup must be applied at the flexion point on the fetal scalp. *(1 point each)*

Max 3

Reductions in:
- ☐ Fetal head diameter that must transit the maternal pelvis
- ☐ Required force of traction
- ☐ Likelihood of pop-offs
- ☐ Maternal-fetal trauma

Special note:
Refer to *Advances in Labour and Risk Management (ALARM) Manual* 24th edition, 2017–2018. Published by The Society of Obstetricians and Gynaecologists of Canada (SOGC). ISBN 978–1-897116–53–1

To decrease risks of vacuum-associated fetal injury, vacuum pressure is gradually increased to a maximum of 500–600 mmHg and traction is applied in the direction of the pelvic curve. You corrected one pop-off due to a poor seal. Appropriate fetal descent is noted during the procedure. You aim for delivery in the shortest time possible and within 20 minutes' duration.[‡]

Attentively, you listen to the fetal heart rate and detect a deceleration during a contraction, noting the following on electronic tracing:

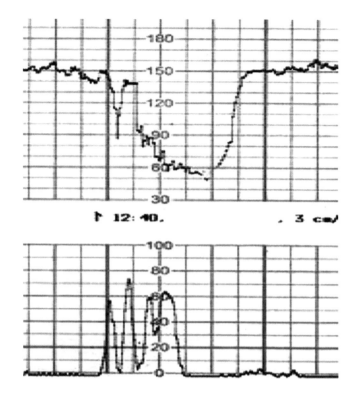

Figure 15.2

With permission. Figure 1 – left panel, from suggested reading #12: Dore S, Ehman W. No. 396-Fetal Health Surveillance: Intrapartum Consensus Guideline [published correction appears in *J Obstet Gynaecol Can.* 2021 Sep;43(9):1118]. *J Obstet Gynaecol Can.* 2020;42(3):316–348.e9.

There is no association between the patient's cardiotocography and this case scenario. Image used for educational purposes only.

Special notes:

Refer to Murphy DJ, Liebling RE, Patel R, et al. Cohort study of operative delivery in the second stage of labour and standard of obstetric care. *BJOG.* 2003;110:610–615.

‡ Refer to *Advances in Labour and Risk Management (ALARM) Manual* 24th edition, 2017–2018. Published by The Society of Obstetricians and Gynaecologists of Canada (SOGC). ISBN 978-1-897116-53-1

26. Interpret this segment of maternal-fetal monitoring, facilitating your labor assistant's live documentation.

2

☐ Complicated variable deceleration based on an abrupt slope of decline in the fetal heart rate, followed by failure of the fetal heart rate to return to baseline by the end of the contraction

27. Refer to fetal physiology and potential impact of this feature on the electronic tracing to validate your intent to hasten delivery. *(1 point each)*   2

Complicated variable deceleration
Physiology:
☐ Umbilical cord compression that leads to a baroreceptor response, and potentially a chemoreceptor component, in a fetus with limited oxygen reserves

Impact:
☐ This feature may be indicative of fetal hypoxia and acidemia

While your trainee is about to perform a digital fetal scalp stimulation during this deceleration, in anticipation of a sympathetic nervous system response, you promptly correct your trainee by indicating that digital scalp stimulation should, in fact, *be avoided* during a deceleration, as it aggravates the vagal response already in effect.

You now notice a thicker meconium consistency. As the fetus is crowning with the next contraction, you advise the patient not to push, indicating to your trainee that this decreases the incidence of OASIS *(SOGC[13])*; simultaneously, your trainee attempts perineal protection *(SOGC[13], RCOG[22])*, yet you notice the beginning of a spontaneous tear in the midline. Keeping the patient informed and ensuring she does not feel '*sharp pain,*' you direct the inadvertent tear in the mediolateral direction.

28. Holding the scissors, explain the technique of mediolateral episiotomy to your obstetric trainee. *(1 point each)*   3

☐ Keep your fingers between the perineum and fetal crown
☐ Direct the episiotomy 60–70° from the midline with the perineum being distended (*i.e.,* at 20–30° off the horizontal) because the angle of the cut performed at crowning decreases after delivery and can lead to OASIS
☐ Make a cut ~2–4 cm in length

Knowing of the important advantage whereby a mediolateral episiotomy decreases the incidence of third- and fourth-degree perineal lacerations, your trainee is curious how it otherwise compares to midline procedures. You indicate your intent to continue clinical teaching of this matter after the patient encounter.

29. Outline the <u>caveats</u> of a mediolateral relative to midline episiotomy that you plan to teach your trainee after this delivery. *(1 point each)*   5

Mediolateral episiotomy is associated with greater risks of:
☐ Blood loss
☐ Difficult surgical repair
☐ Postoperative pain
☐ Faulty healing/suboptimal anatomical results
☐ Dyspareunia and slower resumption of sexual relations at one month postpartum

There is no nuchal cord. The suction cup is removed once the head delivers and the body follows without difficulty. The newborn is pale, tone is poor, and foul odor is evident. Noting the lack of spontaneous breathing immediately after birth, the neonatology team begins ventilation at the bedside, *with the umbilical cord still intact*, to prevent reductions in neonatal cardiac output during the time between cord clamp and initiation of ventilation.[†] Meanwhile, you continue with routine care in the third stage of labor; prophylactic oxytocin has been administered.

Special note:
† *Refer to* Xodo S, Xodo L, Berghella V. Delayed cord clamping and cord gas analysis at birth. *Acta Obstet Gynecol Scand.* 2018;97(1):7–12.

30. Identify the only two currently available methods to <u>objectively quantify</u> possible hypoxia/acidosis just prior to birth. *(1 point each)*   2

☐ Umbilical artery blood lactate concentration *(reference values vary according to the device)*
☐ Umbilical artery blood gas analysis *(pH <7.0 and base deficit ≥12 mmol/L)*

31. During sampling of the umbilical artery and vein as recommended, outline to your trainee findings on blood gas that would support inadvertent sampling of the vein, mixed sampling, or air contamination. *(1 point each)*   2

☐ Difference in pH <0.02 and difference in P_{CO2} <5 mmHg between the two samples suggests blood mixing or sampling the same vessel *(FIGO[5])*
☐ P_{CO2} <22 mmHg indicates contamination from air or the umbilical vein *(FIGO[5])*

The placenta is meconium-stained, foul-smelling but otherwise grossly unremarkable; pathological examination is arranged. After repair of the perineum, you guide a debriefing meeting among delivery care providers and will similarly offer the patient an interdisciplinary meeting. You engage in clinical teaching with your trainee after completing delivery documentation.

Umbilical arterial blood values at delivery revealed: pH 7.0, P_{CO2} 50.3 mmHg, P_{O2} 11 mmHg, HCO_3 17 mEq/L, and base excess of −12 mEq/L.

32. Assist your trainee in interpreting umbilical arterial cord blood values.   1

☐ Metabolic acidosis
  ○ *Normal mean values for umbilical arterial blood: pH 7.27, P_{CO2} 50.3 mmHg, P_{O2} 18.4 mmHg, HCO_3 22 mEq/L, and base excess −2.7 mEq/L*

Special note:
Refer to Question 2 in Chapter 19 for an example of respiratory acidosis on umbilical arterial cord blood analysis

33. Briefly summarize the fetal physiology leading to this type of acidosis.   3

☐ (a) Continued hypoxia leads to lactic acid formation that breaks down to release hydrogen ions
   (b) Hydrogen ions are initially neutralized by substances such as bicarbonate and hemoglobin
   (c) Increasing hydrogen ion formation overwhelms circulating buffers, resulting in cellular enzyme disruption and tissue damage

Knowing that the neonatology team assigned an Apgar score of 3 and 7 at one and five minutes of life, respectively, you decide to elicit *how* this was determined from your obstetric trainee: at one minute of life, pulse was 90 bpm, tone remained poor and without response to stimulation, respirations were slow and irregular; the body color had improved while extremities remained blue. By five minutes of life, pulse was 120 bpm, extremities were well flexed, the newborn was starting to show some response to stimulation, and the body and extremities became pink while respirations remained slow and irregular.

34. Discuss the *general* significance of one- and five-minute Apgar scores and elaborate on this   12
   newborn's calculations.

Significance: *(1 point each)*
☐ One-minute Apgar score is a crucial parameter in deciding the start of newborn resuscitation, but a relatively low association with intrapartum hypoxia/acidosis
☐ Five-minute Apgar score has a stronger association with short- and long-term neurological outcome and neonatal death

Apgar score calculation: *(2 points each)*

Indicator	1-minute	5-minutes
☐ Appearance (skin color)	1 (Pink body and blue extremities)	2 (Pink)
☐ Pulse	1 (Below 100 bpm)	2 (Above 100 bpm)
☐ Grimace (reflex irritability)	0 (Floppy)	1 (Minimal response to stimulation)
☐ Activity (muscle tone)	0 (Absent)	1 (Flexed arms and legs)
☐ Respiration	1 (Slow and irregular)	1 (Slow and irregular)
Total	**3**	**7**

35. Which <u>nonhypoxic factors</u> *may* have potentially contributed to this newborn's Apgar scores? *(1 point each)*

Max 4

☐ Chorioamnionitis
☐ Instrumental delivery-associated birth trauma *(not yet diagnosed)*
☐ Medications administered in labor
☐ Meconium aspiration
☐ Early neonatal interventions, such as vigorous endotracheal intubation
☐ A yet-unidentified congenital anomaly

SCENARIO B
The following is a continuation of the case scenario after the clinical description following Question 20
Forceps-assisted delivery and Obstetric Anal Sphincter Injuries (OASIS)
Although your skillset, scope of practice, and competence allow for either type of instrumental vaginal technique for which this patient is eligible, a **low** forceps-assisted procedure is mutually agreed with the patient.

36. Address your trainee's inquiry regarding what you implied by an 'low' instrumental delivery on the occiput-anterior position.

2

☐ Leading point of the fetal skull is ≥2 cm below the ischial spines (without need for rotation)

37. In addition to performing an instrumental vaginal delivery for decreased maternal expulsive effort, briefly mention to your trainee other clinical contexts whereby assisted delivery may be considered. *(1 point each)*

3

☐ Abnormal fetal heart tracing
☐ Delayed progress in the second stage requiring instrumental rotational to effect delivery
☐ Maternal conditions precluding repetitive expulsive efforts (*e.g.,* New York Heart Association class III or IV, severe respiratory disease, proliferative retinopathy, cerebral arteriovenous malformations, myasthenia gravis, spinal cord injury at risk of autonomic dysreflexia)

The patient understands that rates of shoulder dystocia are lower with forceps compared with vacuum-assisted births, although neonatal risks including facial palsies and lacerations, external eye injury and corneal abrasions, or skull fractures, are more common to vacuum-assisted deliveries. You then address the patient's inquiries on potential adverse outcomes to her well-being while team members maintain contemporaneous documentation.

38. Outline maternal risks of forceps-assisted delivery you may address with the patient during the consent process, <u>or</u> detail in later teaching with your obstetric trainee. *(1 point each)*

Max 5

☐ Bleeding with/without blood transfusions and anemia
☐ Lower genital tract lacerations
☐ Postpartum urinary retention and urinary tract damage
☐ Vulvovaginal hematoma
☐ OASIS and related morbidities (*e.g.,* infection or abscess formations, wound breakdown, anal incontinence, rectovaginal fistula, perineal pain, long-term dyspareunia, and sexual dysfunction)
☐ Increased intrapartum and postpartum pain requiring greater analgesic needs relative to a spontaneous vaginal delivery
☐ Psychological impact on the mother and partner/family; apprehension about future childbearing

The patient subsequently provides consent and accepts having the obstetric trainee apply the blades under supervision. The trainee reassures her that he or she has had prior simulation training and clinical experience.

39. Verbalize how you would verify correct application of the blades prior to applying traction. *(1 point each)*

5

☐ Posterior fontanelle is midway between the sides of the blades
☐ Lambdoid sutures are equidistant from the forceps blades
☐ Lambdoid sutures are one fingerbreadth above the plane of the shanks
☐ With solid blades, no more than a fingertip should be inserted between the blade and the fetal head; with fenestrated blades, the fenestrations should be minimally felt and symmetric to the contrary side
☐ Sagittal suture is perpendicular to the plane of the shanks throughout its length

Having considered the heightened risk of maternal tissue injury associated with a forceps delivery, you maintain a low threshold for a mediolateral episiotomy, yet the maternal perineum inadvertently tears extensively.

Following successful instrumental delivery and active management of the third stage of labor, you inform the patient of the now-confirmed fourth-degree laceration and arrange to perform the surgical repair. You are aware of your trainee's yet limited exposure to validated models and surgical training laboratories known to improve learners' abilities to restore OASIS injuries.[†]

Special note:

† *Refer to (a)* Siddighi S, Kleeman SD, Baggish MS, et al. Effects of an educational workshop on performance of fourth-degree perineal laceration repair. *Obstet Gynecol.* 2007;109(2 Pt 1):289–294, and *(b)* Sparks RA, Beesley AD, Jones AD. 'The sponge perineum:' an innovative method of teaching fourth-degree obstetric perineal laceration repair to family medicine residents. *Fam Med.* 2006;38(8):542–544.

40. Outline surgical principles you would highlight in teaching your trainee with regard to repairing a <u>full-thickness</u> fourth-degree laceration. *(1 point each unless specified)*

Max 12

☐ Consider repairing OASIS in the operating room/theater, ensure adequate anesthesia, lighting, and appropriate instruments

☐ Single dose of intravenous antibiotics may be reasonable **at the time of repair** *(ACOG[9])*

Tissue to repair (3 points per tissue layer)	Suture technique	Suture material
☐ Anorectal mucosal	Continuous or interrupted, with knots tied in the anal lumen[†]	3–0 polyglactin *(RCOG[22])* 3–0 or 4–0 polyglactin or chromic *(ACOG[9])* 3–0 polyglactin or PDS *(SOGC[13])*
☐ Internal anal sphincter	Separate repair[$] with interrupted or mattress sutures[†] without any overlap of the sphincter	3–0 PDS or 2–0 polyglactin *(SOGC[13], RCOG[22])* 3–0 PDS or 3–0 polyglactin *(ACOG[9])*
☐ External anal sphincter and fascial sheath	Overlapping or end to end[†]	3–0 PDS or 2–0 polyglactin *(SOGC[13], RCOG[22])*; use of 3–0 polyglactin is also accepted *(ACOG[9])*

Polyglactin: Vicryl; PDS: polydioxanone

☐ Suture the perineal muscles after repair of the anal sphincter complex, burying surgical knots beneath the muscle to avoid migration through the skin; vaginal mucosa and skin are repaired as per usual technique

☐ Perform a rectal examination after completion of surgical repair to ensure no remaining open defect and sutures do not penetrate the rectal mucosa

Special notes:
[†] Figure-of-eight sutures should be avoided due to risk of tissue ischemia and poor healing
[$] Separate repair improves the likelihood of anal continence

41. Counsel the patient on postprocedural management considerations after an obstetric anal sphincter injury. *(1 point per main bullet)*

Max 8

Pharmacologic care:
- ☐ Prophylactic broad-spectrum antibiotics are recommended **after the repair** to reduce risks of postoperative infection and wound dehiscence *(SOGC[13], RCOG[22])*[†]
  - ○ *Single-dose intravenous second-generation cephalosporin (SOGC[13])*
- ☐ Prescribe oral laxatives and stool-softeners for about 10 days after the repair
  - ○ *Bulking agents are not recommended (SOGC[13], RCOG[22])*
- ☐ Provide analgesia, preferably oral nonsteroidal anti-inflammatory drugs (NSAIDs), acetaminophen/paracetamol and topical perineal anesthetic sprays/creams; caution against risk of constipation if using opioid analgesia
  - ○ *Rectal NSAIDs may theoretically disrupt the repair and impair wound healing; consider avoidance or use cautiously*
- ☐ Consideration for thromboprophylaxis based on medical or obstetric risk factors[‡] *(e.g., obstetric hemorrhage >1000 mL or need for blood product replacement, or prolonged labor >24 hours)*

Nonpharmacologic care:
- ☐ Encourage baths and icepacks to the perineum for analgesia
- ☐ Provide counseling on ways to avoid constipation *(e.g., drink water, eat vegetables and cereals)*
- ☐ Early initiation of pelvic floor physiotherapy to decrease postpartum *urinary* incontinence, while informing the patient that effects on *anal* incontinence is controversial
- ☐ Screen for postpartum depression and offer psychological support
- ☐ Offer a debrief session to review delivery events, discuss short- and long-term implications, and address the patient/family's questions
- ☐ Avoid strenuous activity for at least four to six weeks
- ☐ Reinforce the importance of early and consistent follow-up postpartum (usually 6–12 weeks)[§]
  - ○ *If the patient experiences incontinence or persistent pain at follow-up, arrange early referral to a urogynecologist and/or colorectal surgeon*
- ☐ Provide the patient with an information leaflet, or a suitable alternative, on perineal care after a third- and fourth-degree tear[#]

Special notes:
[†] *ACOG[9] suggests a single dose of antibiotic at the time of repair (see Question 41)*
[‡] Refer to Question 4 in Chapter 52 for risk factors warranting consideration for perinatal thromboprophylaxis
[§] There are no standard guidelines for postpartum follow-up of women with OASIS injuries
[#] An example, provided by the Royal College of Obstetricians and Gynaecologists, 'Care of a third or fourth-degree tear that occurred during childbirth' can be found at www.rcog.org .uk/en/patients/patient-leaflets/?q=tearsandsubject=Pregnancy+and+birthandorderby= title/, accessed September 18, 2021.

On postpartum day 1, the patient appears well and appreciates the comprehensive debrief provided by the team. She is pleased to have obviated neonatal trauma related to an unexpected birthweight of 4040 g. You sense apprehension about future childbearing and plan to address her concerns. Subsequently, you resume clinical teaching provided to your obstetric trainee intrapartum.

---

42. Address a patient inquiry regarding future delivery considerations after an index OASIS injury. *(1 point per main bullet)*

Max 2

Future pregnancy considerations:
- ☐ Provide reassurance that the absolute risk of recurrent OASIS at a subsequent delivery is low, at ~5% [*i.e.,* 3.7%–7.5%] *(ACOG[9], SOGC[13])*
- ☐ Counsel the patient about the possibility of subsequent vaginal delivery, while informing her that a Cesarean section is reasonable after comprehensive discussion, informed consent, or if any of the following is noted after the index OASIS:
  - ○ Anal incontinence
  - ○ Abnormalities are detected on endoanal ultrasound and/or manometry
  - ○ Wound infection or a need for repeat repair
  - ○ Psychological trauma
- ☐ Inform the patient that the role of prophylactic episiotomy at a future delivery is not known; routine clinical indications would prevail

---

43. Acknowledging the difficulty in predicting OASIS, which risks factors[†] would you expect your obstetric trainee to identify in *retrospect* for this patient? *(1 point each)*

Max 7

- ☐ Forceps delivery
- ☐ Macrosomia >4000 g
- ☐ Mediolateral episiotomy could not be performed
- ☐ Second stage duration more than two hours[‡]
- ☐ Nulliparity
- ☐ Asian ethnicity
- ☐ Oxytocin augmentation of labor
- ☐ Epidural analgesia
- ☐ Occiput posterior position in labor, requiring manual rotation
- ☐ Gestational age at delivery *(Controversial)*

Special notes:
- † Other risk factors, ***not*** specific to this case scenario, include shoulder dystocia, induction of labor
- ‡ McLeod NL, Gilmour DT, Joseph KS, Farrell SA, Luther ER. Trends in major risk factors for anal sphincter lacerations: a 10-year study. *J Obstet Gynaecol Can.* 2003;25(7):586–593.

SCENARIO C
The following is a continuation of the case scenario after the clinical description following Question 20
Second-stage Cesarean delivery with impacted fetal head
Despite appropriate application of the vacuum suction cup, there is no fetal descent with traction, leading you to abandon the procedure.

44. Justify your next most appropriate means for delivery. *(1 point per main and subbullet)*   Max 2

☐ Cesarean section is warranted
  ○ *Rationale A:* Sequential use of instruments to achieve delivery is associated with increased neonatal complications (*e.g.,* neonatal intensive care admission, intracranial/retinal hemorrhage, feeding difficulties, and need for mechanical ventilatory support)
  ○ *Rationale B:* This unsuccessful vacuum attempt is *not* due to suboptimal application or technical issues, where forceps (or vice-versa) could have been contemplated

With patient consent, timely Cesarean section is arranged. In response to a query from the anesthesiologist, you explain that routine preoperative prophylactic antibiotics are not required as broad-spectrum antibiotics, commenced for intrapartum chorioamnionitis, were given less than one hour ago. You communicate with your team the potential for a challenging delivery.

45. Outline preincisional preparations you would consider to facilitate fetal delivery at Cesarean section after unsuccessful instrumental delivery. *(1 point each)*   Max 5

☐ Ensure appropriate assistance at surgery and among operating suite health care providers
☐ Ensure neonatal resuscitation personnel are present at delivery
☐ Consider the availability of blood products
☐ Inform the anesthesiologist of the possible need for uterine relaxation during fetal delivery
☐ Inform the anesthesiologist of the potential for longer operating time
☐ Have standing stools available[†]
☐ Consider the modified lithotomy (Whitmore)[‡] position and/or Trendelenburg position

Special notes:
† Facilitates the delivering surgeon's ability to flex and/or direct the fetal head cranially toward the patient instead of directly outward, which risks lateral uterine extensions
‡ Allows a health care provider to dislodge the fetal head at vaginal examination

Proceeding with Cesarean section in the standard fashion, you take the opportunity to alert your obstetric trainee providing surgical assistance, of possible intraoperative maternal complications that merit surgical caution when performing a Cesarean section in the second stage.

46. Indicate <u>maternal</u> surgical complications at Cesarean section focused on greater fetal head impaction after unsuccessful instrumental delivery. *(1 point each)*   3

- ☐ Hemorrhage
- ☐ Inferior or lateral extensions of the uterine incision
- ☐ Injury to the bladder and/or ureters

47. Prior to the uterine incision, review your planned maneuvers with intrapartum care providers to enable delivery in the event of head impaction, with an understanding that the chosen technique(s) depend on fetal positioning and your preference as the surgeon. *(1 point each; max points indicated)*   5

Surgical aspects prior to delivery: *(3)*
- ☐ Ensure adequate surgical space at different tissue layers
- ☐ Make the uterine incision higher in the lower uterine segment
- ☐ Keep the uterus relaxed (*e.g.,* intravenous nitroglycerin 50–200 ug)

Delivery maneuvers: *(max 2)*
- ☐ Option 1: Attempt to elevate the fetal shoulders, if it is encountered after the uterine incision is made
- ☐ Option 2: 'Push technique,' where an experienced heath care provider attempts to dislodge the head by exerting gentle upward pressure on vaginal examination during uterine relaxation; as the delivering surgeon, you simultaneously exert upward traction on the fetal shoulders
- ☐ Option 3: 'Pull technique,'[†] entailing a reverse breech extraction (legs are more accessible in the occiput-posterior position); with occiput-anterior position, consider delivery of the fetal arm first, followed by lateral fetal rotation to access the legs
- ☐ Option 4: Shoulders-first technique (*i.e.,* Patwardhan[‡] technique), where initial delivery is of the anterior shoulder, then posterior shoulder, buttocks, legs, and lastly the head
- ☐ Option 5 *(limited access and data)*: Fetal head elevating device

Special notes:
[†] Consider appropriate expansion of the hysterotomy scar (*i.e.,* inverted T or J)
[‡] *Refer to* Jeve YB, Navti OB, Konje JC. Comparison of techniques used to deliver a deeply impacted fetal head at full dilation: a systematic review and meta-analysis. *BJOG.* 2016;123(3):337–345.

After surgery, you guide a debriefing meeting among delivery care providers and will similarly offer the patient an interdisciplinary meeting.

48. Identify a long-term complication particular to Cesarean section in the second stage of labor that you would address in counseling, among other morbidities of surgical delivery.   1

- ☐ Future risk of cervical insufficiency, preterm prelabor rupture of membranes (PPROM), and/or preterm birth

TOTAL: 220

CHAPTER 16

Induction of Labor at Term

Genevieve Eastabrook and Amira El-Messidi

You are covering the obstetric practice of a colleague who just left on a two-month leave. A 28-year-old primigravida with a spontaneous singleton at 35^{+1} weeks' gestation presents for a routine prenatal visit. Pregnancy dating was confirmed by first-trimester sonography. Your trainee informs you the patient is normotensive, fundal height is appropriate for gestation, and she does not have clinical complaints. Fetal activity has been normal. The patient wishes to discuss labor management with you at this visit.

LEARNING OBJECTIVES

1. Elicit contraindications to vaginal delivery on focused prelabor history in the third trimester with a singleton in the cephalic presentation
2. Recognize prelabor interventions proven to benefit maternal outcomes and increase the likelihood of natural labor
3. Provide comprehensive, evidence-based counseling on methods for cervical ripening and induction of labor, understanding particularities related to different modalities
4. Appreciate international practice variations in recommendations for pharmacologic and nonpharmacologic methods for cervical ripening and induction of labor
5. Recognize and manage intrapartum complications of cervical ripening and induction procedures

SUGGESTED READINGS

1. (a) ACOG Practice Bulletin No. 107: Induction of labor. *Obstet Gynecol.* 2009;114(2 Pt 1): 386–397.
   (b) ACOG Practice Bulletin No. 146: Management of late-term and postterm pregnancies. *Obstet Gynecol.* 2014;124(2 Pt 1):390–396.
2. (a) Berghella V, Di Mascio D. Evidence-based labor management: before labor (Part 1). *Am J Obstet Gynecol MFM.* 2020;2(1):100080.
   (b) Berghella V, Bellussi F, Schoen CN. Evidence-based labor management: induction of labor (Part 2). *Am J Obstet Gynecol MFM.* 2020;2(3):100136.
3. (a) Alfirevic Z, Gyte GM, Nogueira Pileggi V, et al. Home versus inpatient induction of labour for improving birth outcomes. *Cochrane Database Syst Rev.* 2020;8(8):CD007372.
   (b) Boie S, Glavind J, Velu AV, et al. Discontinuation of intravenous oxytocin in the active phase of induced labour. *Cochrane Database Syst Rev.* 2018;8(8):CD012274.

    (c)   Finucane EM, Murphy DJ, Biesty LM, et al. Membrane sweeping for induction of labour. *Cochrane Database Syst Rev.* 2020;2(2):CD000451.

    (d)   Kerr RS, Kumar N, Williams MJ, et al. Low-dose oral misoprostol for induction of labour. *Cochrane Database Syst Rev.* 2021;6(6):CD014484.

    (e)   Middleton P, Shepherd E, Morris J, et al. Induction of labour at or beyond 37 weeks' gestation. *Cochrane Database Syst Rev.* 2020;7(7):CD004945.

    (f)   Smith CA, Armour M, Dahlen HG. Acupuncture or acupressure for induction of labour. *Cochrane Database Syst Rev.* 2017;10(10):CD002962.

4.   Grobman WA, Caughey AB. Elective induction of labor at 39 weeks compared with expectant management: a meta-analysis of cohort studies. *Am J Obstet Gynecol.* 2019;221(4):304–310.

5.   Grobman WA, Rice MM, Reddy UM, et al. Labor induction versus expectant management in low-risk nulliparous women. *N Engl J Med* 2018; 379:513–523.

6.   (a)   National Institute for Health and Care Excellence (NICE). Inducing labour. Draft guideline May 2021, update of CG70, 2008.

    (b)   National Institute for Health and Care Excellence (NICE). Insertion of a double balloon catheter for induction of labour in pregnant women without previous caesarean section (IPG528). July 2015.

7.   Leduc D, Biringer A, Lee L, et al. Clinical Practice Obstetrics Committee; Special Contributors. Induction of labour. *J Obstet Gynaecol Can.* 2013;35(9):840–857.

8.   SMFM statement on elective induction of labor in low-risk nulliparous women at term: the ARRIVE trial. July 2019. Available at www.smfm.org/publications/258-smfm-statement-elective-induction-of-labor-in-low-risk-nulliparous-women-at-term-the-arrive-trial. Accessed June 5, 2021.

9.   WHO recommendations: induction of labour at or beyond term. Geneva: World Health Organization; 2018.

	POINTS
1. Specify features you would review in this patient's chart that would preclude a potential vaginal delivery. *(1 point each)*	10

Maternal:
- ☐ Medical conditions including, but not limited to, HIV with high viral load, active perianal inflammatory bowel disease, Marfan syndrome with aortic dissection/dilatation
- ☐ History of a primary or nonprimary first episode of genital herpes in the third trimester
- ☐ Presence of uterine myomas in the lower segment or cervix likely to obstruct labor
- ☐ Known invasive cervical cancer
- ☐ History of transmural uterine surgery or major reconstruction *(e.g., cornual resection)*

Fetoplacental:
- ☐ Transverse or oblique fetal lie, or footling breech presentation[†]
- ☐ Fetal anomaly that may obstruct labor or increase fetal morbidity at vaginal delivery
- ☐ Placenta previa
- ☐ Placenta accreta spectrum
- ☐ Vasa previa

Special note:
- † Frank or complete beech presentations are not absolute contraindications for vaginal delivery; *provider preference and jurisdictional variations in practice exist*

You learn the patient is healthy and has not had antenatal complications to date. Routine maternal investigations were unremarkable; her blood group is B-positive without alloantibodies. Prenatal aneuploidy screening revealed extremely low maternal serum unconjugated estriol levels on serum biochemistry for which genetic counseling was performed. As fetal risk of aneuploidy was inconclusive, noninvasive cell-free DNA (cfDNA) testing revealed low risks of the common aneuploidies. The patient identified male relatives with a 'scaly skin' disorder and her husband is known to be affected by steroid sulfatase deficiency. She deferred prenatal diagnostic testing (chromosomal microarray) to the postnatal period as fetal diagnosis would not influence the couple's gestational plans. Fetal morphology survey was normal with male external genitalia and fundal placentation. Her obstetric chart indicates fundal heights have been appropriate and fetal presentation cephalic.

You take interest in reviewing the genetic consultation note prior to meeting the patient.

2.   Highlight aspects related to <u>fetal genetic and obstetric risks</u> with abnormally low maternal unconjugated estriol levels and paternal steroid sulfatase deficiency.   6

Genetic risks: *(1 point each)*
☐ Abnormally low maternal serum estriol level, especially in the context of affected male family members, increases likelihood of placental sulfatase deficiency (*i.e.*, offspring with X-linked ichthyosis)
☐ Assuming this mother is a carrier of steroid sulfatase deficiency, 50% of her offspring will bear the X chromosome with the mutation, with 50% of sons affected and 50% of future daughters being carriers
☐ The affected father is <u>not</u> the source of disease transmission to the male fetus, although all his future daughters will be carriers

Obstetric risks: *(3 points)*
☐ Placental sulfatase deficiency is associated with delayed onset of labor (*range of >20 hours to one-week longer pregnancy duration*)

The patient indicates she anticipates a normal vaginal delivery. Her twin sister, who had a similarly uncomplicated pregnancy, recently opted for 'prophylactic'[†] induction of labor at 39 weeks' gestation after discussion with her obstetric provider. The patient requests your professional advice on interventions before and in preparation for labor.

Special note:
† Consideration for terminology change from 'elective' to 'prophylactic' induction among low-risk women at ≥39 weeks with appropriately dated pregnancies; refer to Voutsos L. Prophylactic induction. *Am J Obstet Gynecol.* 2020;222(3):290.

3. Provide <u>evidence-based</u> recommendations from <u>high-quality</u> data for prelabor interventions, including their rationale, to discuss with the patient with a healthy singleton in the cephalic presentation. *(1 point per main bullet and subbullet)*

6

☐ Perineal massage with oil for 5–10 minutes daily starting at 34 weeks' gestation until labor *(Suggested Reading 2a)*
  ○ *Rationale: Associated with reduced incidence of perineal trauma at delivery requiring suturing in women without previous vaginal birth*

☐ Voluntary contractions of pelvic floor muscles for at least 8 weeks' duration prior to anticipated delivery (*i.e.*, starting at 30–32 weeks' gestation) performed as ≥1 daily sets on at least several days of the week *(Suggested Reading 2a)*
  ○ *Rationale: Associated with reduced risk of postpartum urinary incontinence*

☐ Membrane sweeping/stripping starting at 37–38 weeks' gestation *(Suggested Reading 2a)* performed weekly, or from 39^{+0} weeks' gestation with <u>consideration</u> for additional membrane sweeping if labor does not start spontaneously *(NICE guideline[6a])*
  ○ *Rationale: Associated with significant increases in phospholipase A2 activity and prostaglandin F2α levels, leading to greater likelihood of <u>natural</u>[†] labor*

Special note:
[†] Note preferred description of labor onset occurring *naturally*, as opposed to *spontaneously*, after membrane sweeping *(NICE guideline[6a])*

Your obstetric trainee elaborates that although transvaginal ultrasound cervical length at 37–38 weeks' gestation has good accuracy for prediction of spontaneous labor at term,[†] evidence of its cost-effectiveness remains insufficient to recommend this intervention. You highlight that available risk calculators for Cesarean delivery after induction of labor are of limited benefit to an individual patient, thereby not universally practiced at this time.

As she would like time to consider induction of labor at 39 weeks' gestation, she wishes to know its potential advantages, understanding that risks would depend on specific circumstances and proposed induction methods in due course.

Special note:
[†] Saccone G, Simonetti B, Berghella V. Transvaginal ultrasound cervical length for prediction of spontaneous labour at term: a systematic review and meta-analysis. *BJOG.* 2016;123(1):16–22.

4. Despite limited long-term outcome data for children born after induction of labor at 39 weeks, counsel the patient on recognized potential advantages based on results of randomized trials and observational studies. *(1 point each)*

Max 4

Reduced risks of:
☐ Cesarean delivery, whether or not the cervix is favorable
☐ Hypertensive disorders of pregnancy
☐ Meconium-stained amniotic fluid
☐ Maternal peripartum infection
☐ Neonatal respiratory morbidity
☐ Neonatal intensive care unit admission
☐ Perinatal mortality

Special note:
Refer to *Suggested Readings 4 and 5.*

The group B streptococcus (GBS) vaginal-rectal swab taken at 36^{+1} weeks' gestation is positive. Pregnancy remains unremarkable and the patient is adherent to your evidence-based prelabor recommendations.

At 39^{+1} weeks' gestation, the patient requests membrane sweeping with continued expectancy for spontaneous labor unless labor induction becomes clinically indicated. You reassure her of the safety of this practice as she remains a low-risk gravida with a cephalic presentation and normal fetal heart rate. You take the opportunity to alert your obstetric trainee of practical and resource limitations in universal induction of labor for low-risk women with singleton pregnancies who have reached 39 weeks' gestation with accurate pregnancy dating, although patient preferences warrant consideration after appropriate counseling.

5. Provide your recommendations with regard to <u>membrane sweeping</u> in view of her GBS-positive status, explaining the technique and its inherent risks, if relevant. No contraindications to vaginal delivery are apparent. *(1 point each; max points specified where relevant)*

5

GBS-positive status (or unknown):
☐ No evidence of increased risk of maternal or neonatal infection

Technique:
☐ Where the cervix permits, a finger is inserted past the internal os where three circumferential passes of the finger are then made to attempt separation of the membranes from the lower segment
☐ Where the cervix is closed, its surface is massaged with the middle finger and forefinger for 15–30 seconds, or the vaginal fornices are massaged

Risks: *(max 2)*
☐ Discomfort/pain
☐ Bleeding
☐ Irregular uterine contractions within the ensuing 24 hours
☐ Prelabor rupture of membranes *(Controversial)*

6. Inform your trainee of the <u>proposed physiology</u> for membrane sweeping.   1

☐ Increased production of local prostaglandins

Having obtained consent for membrane sweeping, you are only able to massage the cervix, as the internal os is not sufficiently dilated to permit a sweep. The patient tolerated the procedure well and there are not immediate procedure-related complications.

She inquires about possible benefits of *natural or home remedies* to promote labor induction including coitus, hot baths, homeopathy, acupuncture, unilateral nipple stimulation, castor oil, and evening primrose oil.

7. Indicate your evidence-based advice for any three means she inquired upon for labor   1
induction, if differences in recommendations exist.

☐ Evidence does not support any of the stated methods for labor induction

Pregnancy remains uncomplicated until 41^{+0} weeks' gestation when you offer induction of labor in accordance with standard obstetric recommendations *(NICE[6a], SOGC[7b])* to which the patient concurs. She reports normal fetal activity and does not have obstetric complaints. You explain that cervical assessment, as part of the physical examination, will assist in determining the readiness of the cervix and inform the initial choice of method for induction.

8. State the essentials of the focused physical examination to plan the method and   Max 8
anticipated general success rate for her labor induction. *(1 point per main bullet
unless specified)*

☐ Review the prepregnancy BMI and height[§]
☐ Vital signs (*e.g.*, blood pressure, pulse, temperature)
☐ Confirmation of fetal presentation[†]
☐ Doptone for fetal heart rate assessment[†]
☐ Cervical factors[‡] *(1 point per subbullet, for 5 points)*
   ○ Dilation
   ○ Effacement
   ○ Station
   ○ Position
   ○ Consistency

Special notes:
§ As an individual entity, maternal height features in the likelihood of successful labor induction; readers are also encouraged to refer to Question 5 in Chapter 18
† Although ultrasound may assist in fetal assessment, it is not uniformly indicated
‡ Factors to be noted on cervical examination are indicated in sequence of most to least important for predicting successful induction of labor

Vital signs are unremarkable and fetal presentation remains cephalic by abdominal maneuvers with a normal heart rate. On pelvic examination, the cervix is 1 cm dilated, 50% effaced (2 cm long), presenting part is 2 cm above the ischial spines, cervical position is posterior and of medium consistency.

Her prepregnancy BMI was 20.5 kg/m^2 based on a weight of 66.4 kg.

---

9. Identify the patient's <u>modified</u> <u>Bishop</u> score and counsel her on its general implications. *(1 point per main bullet)*   3

☐ The patient's modified Bishop score is 4/10
   ○ *(i.e., One point for each finding on examination, except posterior cervical position which scores 0 points)*
☐ Inform the patient that cervical ripening methods are required prior to labor induction
   ○ *Although there is no universally accepted threshold for favorability of the cervical score, a score of ≥6/10 is deemed favorable*
☐ Explain that an unfavorable cervix does not imply that delaying labor induction would improve the chance of vaginal delivery, as evidence shows improved rates of Cesarean delivery irrespective of cervical status

---

10. Elicit features of this patient's demographic and obstetric history that would <u>increase and decrease</u> the likelihood of labor induction or vaginal birth if spontaneous labor were to occur. *(1 point each)*   Max 8

Positive predictive factors:
☐ Age <35 years
☐ BMI <30 kg/m^2
☐ Greater maternal height *(i.e., based on calculation; her height is 5 feet, 9 inches [1.80 m])*
☐ Absence of diabetes mellitus
☐ Estimated fetal weight is appropriate for gestational age *(i.e., based on clinical fundal height assessments)*
☐ Absence of comorbidities associated with placental insufficiency, such as preeclampsia or fetal growth restriction

Negative predictive factors:
☐ Bishop score <6/10
☐ Nulliparity
☐ Intact amniotic membranes *(i.e., implied given she had no obstetric complaints)*

Prior to discussing options for cervical ripening with the patient, you first highlight to your obstetric trainee that international variations exist regarding the use of pharmacologic methods on an outpatient basis among low-risk gravidas at term with an uncomplicated singleton fetus in the cephalic presentation. Furthermore, there is variance on preferred/first-line versus second-line pharmacologic agents of choice or use of combined pharmacologic and nonpharmacologic modalities.

Earlier in gestation, the patient was informed that midwife-led care is recommended for low-risk women, as evidence shows numerous medical advantages including higher maternal satisfaction rates. She had decided on a hospital-based delivery given the proximity of your hospital center to her residence.

---

11. Outline pharmacologic and nonpharmacologic methods that may be offered for cervical ripening at this time, assuming no contraindications arise. *(1 point each)*

Max 3

Nonpharmacologic methods:
☐ Transcervical balloon catheter insertion

Pharmacologic methods:
☐ Vaginal[†] prostaglandin E2 (dinoprostone) preparations *[gel, tablet, or controlled-release delivery system]*
☐ Prostaglandin E1 (misoprostol) *[oral or vaginal]*[‡]

Combined nonpharmacologic and pharmacologic methods:
☐ Transcervical balloon catheter with a prostaglandin or oxytocin[§]

Special notes:
† Although intracervical dinoprostone is available in Canada, vaginal preparations are preferable as they result in more timely vaginal delivery *(SOGC[7a])*; intracervical dinoprostone is not commercially available in the United States *(ACOG[1])* and use is not supported in the United Kingdom *(NICE[6a])*
‡ Vaginal misoprostol for cervical ripening is practiced in Canada and United States; use in the United Kingdom is not recommended
§ Available evidence does not support intravenous oxytocin alone as an effective method for cervical ripening given lack of smooth muscle in the cervix

---

SCENARIO A
Outpatient induction of labor with transcervical balloon catheter insertion
After offering the patient available options for cervical ripening at term, she opts for nonpharmacologic means. You inform your obstetric trainee that while osmotic cervical dilators can be used in the second trimester, available evidence does not support their use for later induction of labor.

You proceed to discuss outpatient transcervical balloon catheter placement,[§] taking the opportunity to inform your trainee of clinical practice standards while providing patient counseling required for informed consent.

Special note:

§ Note that GBS-positive status, as in this patient, is not a contraindication to use of mechanical cervical ripening.

12. Explain the proposed mechanism(s) of action for transcervical balloon catheter insertion.
(1 point each)

2

The role of pressure applied to the internal cervical os is twofold:
☐ To stretch the lower uterine segment
☐ To increase release of local prostaglandins

13. Discuss the benefits of transcervical balloon catheter for induction of labor and its advantages compared with prostaglandins. [features *may or may not* relate to this patient].
(1 point each)

Max 8

General benefits:
☐ Simplicity of use/application
☐ Potential for reversibility
☐ No specific storage or temperature requirements
☐ No increased rates of maternal infection (*i.e.*, chorioamnionitis, endometritis) in women with intact membranes
☐ No increased rates of neonatal infection
☐ Low cost

Advantages when compared with prostaglandins:
☐ Low risk of tachysystole with or without fetal heart rate changes[†]
☐ Safer for women with previous low transverse Cesarean section in whom use of prostaglandins at term is contraindicated
☐ Lower rates of meconium-stained amniotic fluid *(more common with misoprostol use)*
☐ No interval delay is required between removal of the transcervical catheter and initiation of a secondary method including prostaglandins, amniotomy, or oxytocin
☐ No difference in Cesarean section rates
☐ No difference in overall vaginal births within 24 hours

Special note:
[†] Based on contemporary terminology, *'hyperstimulation'* and *'hypercontractility'* should be abandoned; refer to Macones GA, Hankins GDV, Spong CY, Hauth J, Moore T. The 2008 National Institute of Child Health and Human Development Workshop Report on Electronic Fetal Monitoring. *Obstet Gynecol.* 2008;11:661–6

14. Indicate risks of transcervical balloon catheter you may discuss in counseling.
(1 point each)

Max 3

☐ Discomfort during and after insertion
☐ Bleeding *(especially with low-lying placentation; use in this setting is discouraged)*
☐ Unsuccessful cervical ripening
☐ Increased need for oxytocin in labor
☐ Displacement of the presenting part
☐ Cervical laceration or ischemia, if prolonged use

You teach your trainee that evidence supports single-balloon over double-balloon catheter as the latter is associated with greater pain without reductions in time to delivery or rates of Cesarean section. While variations exist in volume of insufflation from 30 to 80 mL,[§] and in duration of use from 12[†] to 24[‡] hours unless balloon expulsion or spontaneous rupture of amniotic membranes occur, current evidence does not support catheter use for extra-amniotic injection of dinoprostone, prostaglandin F2α, or fluid. The patient's vital signs remain normal; the procedure will be performed under standard sterile techniques.

Special notes:

[§] Larger balloon volumes (60–80 mL) only modestly reduce induction-to-delivery interval time compared with 30 mL balloons volumes, supporting both choices: Refer to Schoen CN, Saccone G, Backley S, et al. Increased single-balloon Foley catheter volume for induction of labor and time to delivery: a systematic review and meta-analysis. *Acta Obstet Gynecol Scand.* 2018;97(9):1051–1060.

[†] *Suggested Reading 2b*

[‡] SOGC[7a]

---

15. Outline pre- and postprocedure observations and care prior to patient discharge with a transcervical balloon catheter, assuming uncomplicated placement. *(1 point per main and subbullet, max points specified per section)*

8

Preprocedure assessment: *(max 2)*

☐ Confirmation of fetal health by a surveillance mechanism; international jurisdictional variations exist (e.g., Doptone only or 30-minute electronic fetal monitoring pre- and posttranscervical catheter insertion[§])

☐ Abdominal assessment of the stability and level of the fetal head in the lower part of the uterus at or near the pelvic brim *(NICE[6a])*

☐ Reevaluate the Bishop score *(individualized need based on clinical history and time interval from initial assessment)*

☐ Consideration for adding membrane sweeping at the beginning of cervical ripening and induction of labor *(Suggested Readings 2b, 7a)*

Postprocedure care: *(6)*

☐ Encourage the patient to seek medical care in the mutually agreed timeframe or if any one of:
   ○ Rupture of amniotic membranes
   ○ Bleeding
   ○ Painful uterine contractions
   ○ Catheter expulsion
   ○ Any other concerns, such as reduced fetal movements

Special note:

[§] *Refer to* Dore S, Ehman W. No. 396-Fetal Health Surveillance: Intrapartum Consensus Guideline [published correction appears in *J Obstet Gynaecol Can.* 2021 Sep;43(9):1118]. *J Obstet Gynaecol Can.* 2020;42(3):316–348.e9.

SCENARIO B

The following is a continuation of the case scenario after Question 11
Induction of labor with dinoprostone

Special note: International practice recommendations vary regarding outpatient use of
dinoprostone

After offering the patient available options for cervical ripening at term, she opts for vaginal
dinoprostone as an inpatient, with the understanding that there is little evidence to
demonstrate superiority of one preparation over another. You proceed to inform your trainee
of relevant pharmacologic aspects related to preparations of dinoprostone while providing
patient counseling for informed consent.

16. Explain the proposed <u>mechanism(s) of action</u> of prostaglandins for cervical ripening.   Max 2
    (1 point each)

□ Dissolution of the collagen structural network
□ Change in cervical glycosaminoglycans
□ Increased inflammatory activity (*e.g.*, cytokine production and white blood cell
  infiltration)

17. Indicate <u>adverse effects</u>[†] of dinoprostone you may discuss in counseling. *(1 point per main*   Max 5
    bullet, unless specified)

□ Tachysystole with or without fetal heart rate changes *(4 points)*
  ○ *More commonly with misoprostol than dinoprostone*
  ○ *More commonly with vaginal than oral misoprostol*
□ Fever, chills[§]
□ Gastrointestinal symptoms, such as vomiting and diarrhea[§]
□ Idiopathic cardiovascular events (rare)

Special notes:
† There is no evidence that use of vaginal prostaglandins (dinoprostone preparations or
  vaginal misoprostol) increases risks of infection in women with ruptured amniotic
  membranes
§ Prophylactic antiemetics, antipyretics, and antidiarrheal agents are usually needed as such
  side effects are common

18. Outline pre- and postprocedure observations and care with vaginal dinoprostone for   6
cervical ripening. *(1 point per main bullet, max points specified per section)*

Preprocedure care and assessment: *(max 3)*
☐ Confirmation of normal fetal heart rate pattern and absence of uterine contractions by
CTG
☐ Abdominal assessment of the stability and level of the fetal head in the lower part of the
uterus at or near the pelvic brim
☐ Encourage maternal voiding prior to starting dinoprostone use as recumbency is required
for at least 30 minutes
☐ Reevaluate the Bishop score *(individualized need based on clinical history and time interval
from initial assessment)*
☐ Consideration for adding membrane sweeping at the beginning of cervical ripening and
induction of labor *(Suggested Readings 2b, 7a)*

Monitoring postinitiation of vaginal dinoprostone: *(max 3)*
☐ Maintain continuous electronic fetal monitoring by CTG for 60 minutes to 120 minutes
after administration of vaginal prostaglandin[§]
☐ Proceed to intermittent auscultation if the CTG tracing is normal and maternal clinical
circumstances are unchanged
☐ Offer analgesia or consultation with an obstetric anesthesiologist, as needed
☐ Periodic reassessment of the Bishop score 6 hours after insertion of gel or 12 hours after
insertion of the controlled-release system, or sooner if clinically indicated

Special note:
§ *Refer to* Dore S, Ehman W. No. 396-Fetal Health Surveillance: Intrapartum Consensus
Guideline [published correction appears in *J Obstet Gynaecol Can.* 2021 Sep;43(9):1118].
J Obstet Gynaecol Can. 2020;42(3):316–348.e9.

You highlight to your trainee the importance of specific time intervals required between use of
dinoprostone preparations and initiation of oxytocin, where clinically indicated.

19. Explain the biological basis for securing a specified time interval between use of   1
dinoprostone gel or the controlled-release insert and initiation of oxytocin.

☐ Prostaglandins increase uterine sensitivity to oxytocin

20. Indicate the time interval after which oxytocin may be initiated after use of dinoprostone gel or the controlled-release insert, if differences in recommendations exist. *(1 point each)*

2

Initiation of oxytocin after dinoprostone:
☐ At least six hours after the final dose of gel
☐ At least 30 minutes after removal of the controlled-release insert

After a 24-hour trial of cervical ripening with dinoprostone has elapsed, cervical assessment remains unchanged without uterine activity and continued normal fetal heart tracing. The patient is clinically well, although frustrated at the time involved. You counsel her to consider subsequent modalities, yet she is requesting Cesarean section for unsuccessful induction of labor.

21. Indicate the evidence-based recommendations by which you would counsel her regarding performing a Cesarean section for unsuccessful induction of labor at this time. *(1 point each)*

2

☐ Duration of time devoted to cervical ripening does not factor in diagnosis of unsuccessful/failed induction of labor
☐ Cesarean section is not *yet* indicated for unsuccessful/failed induction of labor before ~15 hours of oxytocin infusion with amniotomy if feasible, and ideally after 18–24 hours of oxytocin infusion

SCENARIO C
The following is a continuation of the case scenario after Question 11
Induction of labor with misoprostol

Special notes:

(a) Hospitalization is advised when misoprostol is used for third-trimester induction of labor;
(b) international practices vary with regard to supporting vaginal administration

After offering the patient available options for cervical ripening at term, she voices a preference for an oral preparation. She will consider membrane sweeping you offered at the start of labor induction given some evidence supports this intervention; however, she declined combined misoprostol and transcervical catheter insertion, despite your counseling that combination therapy hastens the time to delivery within 24 hours without an apparent effect on rates of Cesarean delivery or adverse effects.

You ascertain your obstetric trainee understands pharmacologic aspects of misoprostol, including its mechanisms of action, adverse effects, and contraindications, having recently discussed prostaglandin use for third-trimester cervical ripening and induction of labor.

22. State one acceptable dosing protocol for cervical ripening and induction of labor with oral misoprostol, knowing that there is no clear consensus on the optimum protocol and that treatment may continue in the absence of painful contractions. *(2 points each)*

Max 2

Oral misoprostol:[†]
- ☐ 25 µg, followed by 25 µg every two to four hours
- ☐ 25 µg, followed by 50 µg, repeated every four to six hours
- ☐ 50 µg, repeated every four hours

Special note:
† Prompt swallowing of the tablet is advised to avoid sublingual absorption until safety data is available.

You remind your trainee that although tachysystole with or without fetal heart rate changes can occur with any dose or route of administration, the occurrence appears to be dose-dependent and less common with oral than vaginal routes.

One hour after the third dose of oral misoprostol 25 µg, the uterine contraction frequency increases to a seven-per-10-minute period over a half-hour, during which fetal CTG tracing has remained normal. The patient received epidural analgesia upon request. Your obstetric trainee now notifies you of new-onset diminished baseline variability and two variable decelerations. The patient is afebrile, oxygen saturation by pulse oximetry is 97%, and amniotic membranes remain intact.

23. Based on the clinical diagnosis, detail your comprehensive management with an understanding that interventions are often performed simultaneously, in addition to keeping the patient informed. *(1 point each)*

Max 5

Tachysystole with fetal heart rate changes:
- ☐ Maternal repositioning to the left or right side
- ☐ Cervical reassessment, unless recently performed
- ☐ Consideration for acute tocolysis[§] *(e.g.,* intravenous nitroglycerin 50 µg over two to three minutes, repeated every three to five minutes to a maximum of 200 µg; or subcutaneous terbutaline 250 µg; or sublingual[†] nitroglycerin 0.4 mg/spray given once or twice)
- ☐ With normalization of fetal heart tracing, maintain continuous CTG monitoring for at least 60 minutes
- ☐ Consideration for Cesarean section if there is no response to routine corrective measures
- ☐ Explain to the patient recent events and ensure timely documentation

Special notes:
(a) Administration of oxygen is only warranted if decreased maternal saturation (*e.g.,* <95%)
(b) Attempted removal of remnants of a misoprostol tablet or dinoprostone insert would be warranted with vaginal routes of administration
§ Maintain caution for contraindications
† Although frequently used, the sublingual is not effective in the presence of tachysystole; *refer to* Dore S, Ehman W. No. 396-Fetal Health Surveillance: Intrapartum Consensus Guideline [published correction appears in *J Obstet Gynaecol Can.* 2021 Sep;43(9):1118]. *J Obstet Gynaecol Can.* 2020;42(3):316–348.e9.

With maternal repositioning to the left lateral side and two doses of 50 µg intravenous nitrogly-cerin at a five-minute interval, the frequency of uterine contractions decreases with resolution of fetal variable decelerations.

Over the next hour, uterine contractions occur at seven- to eight-minute intervals and fetal heart rate tracing remains normal. Spontaneous rupture of amniotic membranes with clear fluid loss occurs at two hours after the administration of misoprostol. You ensure absence of umbilical cord prolapse on examination and find the cervix is now 2 cm dilated, 80% effaced, central and soft, with a presenting part at ischial spines.

24. Indicate important elements to discuss with the patient with regard to labor management. *(1 point each)*   3

☐ Initiate antibiotic prophylaxis for GBS-positive status
☐ Ensure oxytocin is <u>not</u> initiated over the next two hours despite the sporadic contraction pattern *(ie., to allow for a minimum of four hours after the final misoprostol dose)*
☐ Encourage use of oxytocin infusion thereafter over expectancy, if labor progression is not evident

Over the next two hours, maternal-fetal status remains reassuring. Cervical reassessment is unchanged as uterine contraction frequency has diminished. Intravenous antibiotics for GBS prophylaxis have been commenced from the time of spontaneous amniotomy. You proceed to counsel the patient on initiation of oxytocin infusion.

You teach your trainee that oxytocin infusion protocols vary among and within countries, as the regimen that optimizes maternal and perinatal outcomes has not been identified. Regardless of the chosen regimen, practice recommendations agree that oxytocin should be administered by infu-sion pump to ensure accurate minute-to-minute control. You highlight that there is no evidence-based optimal maximal dose of oxytocin, which is gauged to achieve a contraction pattern of 200–250 Montevideo units and maintain normal fetal status on CTG, although most regimens use an upper-limit of 40 mU/min for augmentation of labor in the third trimester with viable fetus(es).

25. Elaborate on the dosing protocols most commonly implicated by 'low dose' and 'high dose' regimens. *(1 point each)*   3

		Low dose	High dose
☐	Starting dose (mU/min)	0.5–2	4–6
☐	Dosage interval (min)	15–40	15–40
☐	Incremental increase (mU/min)	1–2	4–6

26. Elaborate on common risks of oxytocin to mention in patient counseling, in addition to rare/serious adverse effects to teach your trainee. *(1 point each)*

Max 4

☐ Abnormal fetal heart rate tracing

☐ Tachysystole (more commonly with high-dose regimens)

☐ Hypotension and reflex tachycardia (*rare* unless intravenous bolus dose is given)

☐ Hyponatremia[†] and related complications (*e.g., grand-mal seizures, abdominal pain, nausea/vomiting, coma, or even death*) [*rare* with doses below 40 mU/min]

☐ Uterine dehiscence or rupture (*rare* among women with unscarred uteri unless risk factors are present, including multiparity or connective tissue disorders)

☐ Maternal arrhythmias or anaphylaxis (*rare*)

Special note:

† Amino-acid homology with arginine-vasopressin, both of which are synthesized in the hypothalamus, transported and stored in the posterior pituitary for later release

With the patient's consent, your center's oxytocin infusion protocol is started. Fetal heart rate tracing remains normal, and the cervix dilates to 6 cm in an appropriate interval. You alert your trainee that evidence-based management of oxytocin infusion in the active phase of labor among singletons at term with a cephalic presentation continues to emerge, with the purpose of identifying whether discontinuation of infusion reduces maternal-fetal adverse effects and improves birth outcomes relative to continued infusion until delivery.

27. Discuss <u>evidence-based</u> perspectives for management of this patient's oxytocin infusion in the active phase of labor where contractions are adequate. *(1 point each)*

Max 4

Discontinuation of oxytocin relative to continued infusion until delivery:

Pros:

☐ Reduced uterine tachysystole

☐ Reduced rates of Cesarean section

☐ Reduced fetal heart rate tracing abnormalities

Cons:

☐ Longer active phase

☐ Longer second stage of labor

☐ Need to restart oxytocin infusion due to protracted or arrested labor

TOTAL: 115

CHAPTER 17

Cesarean Delivery on Maternal Request

Alexa Eberle and Amira El-Messidi

A healthy 25-year-old primigravida with a spontaneous singleton pregnancy at 32^{+3} weeks' gestation presents for a routine prenatal visit accompanied by her husband. Her primary care provider just left on a three-month sabbatical. Pregnancy dating was confirmed by first-trimester sonography. All maternal-fetal aspects of routine prenatal care have been unremarkable, and the patient has not experienced any pregnancy complications. There is no history of mental health disorders, and the patient practices a healthy lifestyle.

The patient is normotensive with a normal body habitus, ascertained fetal viability, and appropriate fundal height for gestational age, and fetal presentation is cephalic. Her medical chart indicates her obstetric provider attempted to address her request for elective Cesarean delivery, but she wishes her husband to be present for the discussion.

LEARNING OBJECTIVES

1. Explore potential reasons for maternal request for elective Cesarean delivery in the absence of medical or obstetrical indications, recognizing the medical evolution of factors that have contributed to the perceived safety of surgical delivery
2. Provide individualized counseling for a Cesarean delivery on maternal request, respecting patient autonomy while remaining consistent with ethical principles of medical practice
3. Understand that many short-term risks of Cesarean delivery for maternal request are based on nonrandomized trials, raising challenges when engaging in evidence-based directive counseling
4. Recognize that numerous tools are available for assessment of fear of childbirth
5. Appreciate the biopsychosocial impacts, and dimensions for management, of tocophobia

SUGGESTED READINGS

1. ACOG Committee Opinion No. 761: Cesarean delivery on maternal request. *Obstet Gynecol.* 2019;133(1):e73–e77.
2. Alsayegh E, Bos H, Campbell K, et al. No. 361 – Caesarean delivery on maternal request. *J Obstet Gynaecol Can.* 2018;40(7):967–971.
3. (a) D'Souza R, Arulkumaran S. To 'C' or not to 'C'? Caesarean delivery upon maternal request: a review of facts, figures and guidelines. *J Perinat Med.* 2013;41(1):5–15.

   (b) D'Souza R. Caesarean section on maternal request for non-medical reasons: putting the UK National Institute of Health and Clinical Excellence guidelines in perspective. *Best Pract Res Clin Obstet Gynaecol.* 2013;27(2):165–177. [documents (a) and (b) are similar]

4. FIGO Ethics and Professionalism Guideline: decision making about vaginal and caesarean delivery. June 26, 2020. Available at www.figo.org/decision-making-about-vaginal-and-caesarean-delivery. Accessed April 18, 2021.

5. National Institutes of Health state-of-the-science conference statement: Cesarean delivery on maternal request March 27–29, 2006. *Obstet Gynecol.* 2006;107(6):1386–1397.

6. National Institute for Health and Care Excellence (NICE guideline No. 192). Caesarean birth. March 31, 2021. Available at www.nice.org.uk/guidance/ng192. Accessed April 3, 2021.

7. O'Donovan C, O'Donovan J. Why do women request an elective cesarean delivery for non-medical reasons? A systematic review of the qualitative literature. *Birth.* 2018;45(2):109–119.

8. Opiyo N, Kingdon C, Oladapo OT, et al. Non-clinical interventions to reduce unnecessary caesarean sections: WHO recommendations. *Bull World Health Organ.* 2020;98(1):66–68.

9. Richens Y, Smith DM, Lavender DT. Fear of birth in clinical practice: A structured review of current measurement tools. *Sex Reprod Healthc.* 2018;16:98–112. [Correction in *Sex Reprod Healthc.* 2019 Oct;21:108]

10. Royal Australian and New Zealand College of Obstetricians and Gynaecologists (RANZCOG). Cesarean delivery on maternal request (C-Obs 39); July 2017. Available at https://ranzcog.edu.au/statements-guidelines. Accessed April 18, 2021.

POINTS

1. Present a <u>comprehensive</u> outline of aspects to explore with the patient to determine her motivation for an elective Cesarean section. (1 *point per main bullet*)	Max 12

☐ Determine whether her desired mode of delivery was intended *prior* to pregnancy or *after* a medical/social gestational event

Patient-perceived risks with labor and vaginal delivery:

☐ Perineal or abdominal pain

☐ Spontaneous perineal/vaginal lacerations or episiotomy

☐ Symptoms of pelvic organ prolapse, urinary, and/or anal incontinence
  - *The risk of stress urinary incontinence (SUI) does not differ between Cesarean and vaginal delivery at two years postpartum; risks of SUI increase in future pregnancies irrespective of the mode of delivery*
  - *Planned Cesarean delivery protects against anal incontinence compared with forceps-vaginal births and midline episiotomy*

☐ Sexual dysfunction
  - *Any differences in sexual function based on mode of delivery dissipates by six months postpartum*

☐ Need for an emergency intrapartum Cesarean delivery after prolonged labor

☐ Fetal/neonatal morbidity associated with spontaneous vaginal or assisted instrumental delivery (despite low absolute risks)
  - *e.g., brachial plexus injury,[†] cerebral palsy, hypoxic ischemic encephalopathy*

  ○ *Cerebral palsy affects ~1/1000 term births, of which only 10% are believed to be of intrapartum origin; thereby, prelabor Cesarean delivery would only potentially avoid 0.1/ 1000 cerebral palsy events*

  ○ *~10,000 Cesareans would be required to prevent one cerebral palsy event*

☐ Risk of intrauterine fetal death (IUFD) with postterm pregnancy

☐ Risk of peripartum maternal or fetal mortality

Psychosocial contributors to choosing Cesarean delivery:

☐ No intended desire for future childbearing

☐ History of infertility

☐ Convenience of a planned delivery date

☐ Desire to ensure her obstetrical provider's presence at delivery (*i.e.*, fear of 'abandonment')

☐ History of physical or sexual abuse-related aversion to pelvic examinations

☐ Observed or hearing of negative vaginal birth experiences or adverse neonatal outcome

☐ General fear and/or anxiety from vaginal birth (*i.e.*, tocophobia)

☐ Desire to avoid memory of childbirth

☐ Desire for autonomy and control in mode of delivery

☐ Cultural norms and beliefs, media-persons' influence, partner/family's influence

☐ Encounters with health care providers who encouraged Cesarean delivery

Special note:

† Refer to Chapter 19

Although she and her husband desire a large family, you learn that ever since she witnessed a shoulder dystocia at her sister's delivery two years ago, and despite a normal neonatal outcome, the patient has been intending to have a Cesarean delivery in due course. This has been further strengthened by her readings of social media communications regarding difficult experiences with vaginal birth. The patient explains that with *'things that can go wrong at natural birth,'* she prefers to *'prioritize'* her child's wellness given the safety of Cesarean section, where a general anaesthetic would also prevent recollection of the delivery experience. While her husband opts to *'let nature takes its course,'* he appreciates her fears of labor and choice for Cesarean delivery as it is *'her body.'* In confidence, the patient reports no history childhood or adulthood abuse.

2. Identify factors that have contributed to reduced Cesarean-associated morbidity and mortality, positively influencing patients' perceived safety of surgical delivery. *(1 point each)* Max 5

☐ Correction of preoperative maternal anemia

☐ Availability of intraoperative/postoperative blood products

☐ Prophylactic antibiotics

☐ Safer surgical techniques

☐ Safer anesthetic techniques/practices

☐ Careful perioperative planning in cases of placenta previa or accreta

☐ Postoperative thromboprophylaxis or protocols thereof

3. You highlight that Cesarean delivery constitutes major abdominal surgery, with many of the maternal-neonatal outcome variables associated with planned surgical delivery being based on suboptimal quality evidence (nonrandomized studies). Present a structured framework for <u>short-term risks (less than one year)</u> of Cesarean delivery. *(1 point per main bullet)*

Max 10

Maternal:[†]

☐ Longer delivery hospitalization and recovery relative to uncomplicated spontaneous vaginal or instrumental delivery
  ○ *Later ability to drive and resume everyday activities*
☐ Postoperative pain and use of narcotics
☐ Injury to internal organs *(e.g., bladder, ureter, bowel, uterus, cervix)*
☐ Peripartum hysterectomy for postpartum hemorrhage
☐ Postoperative bladder paralysis/ileus
☐ Relaparotomy
☐ Infective morbidity *(e.g., endomyometritis, wound complications, superficial/pelvic hematoma, seroma, abscess, wound disruption, urinary tract infection, puerperal sepsis)*
☐ Amniotic fluid embolism (AFE)
☐ Cardiac arrest *(possibly <u>unrelated</u> to AFE)*
☐ Anaesthetic complications
☐ Postoperative admission to intensive treatment units
☐ Reduced rates of initiation and maintenance of exclusive breastfeeding at six months
☐ Cost of Cesarean delivery (private and state-funded health care systems)
☐ Venous thromboembolism (VTE)
  ○ *NICE[6](Appendix A, Box 1): Thromboembolic disease is likely to be similar for Cesarean or vaginal birth*
☐ *Controversial* risk of mortality (very low absolute risk in developed countries)
  ○ *Preexisting morbidity is likely an important marker for Cesarean-associated maternal mortality*
  ○ *In countries with high surgical delivery rates, Cesarean-associated maternal mortality is <u>not</u> more common than at vaginal delivery*
☐ *Controversial* risk of postpartum depression
  ○ *Reportedly increased rates post-Cesarean delivery may be affected by breastfeeding and maternal-infant bonding relationship*
  ○ *Psychosocial outcomes do not appear to differ between mode of delivery, and may be better with planned Cesarean delivery*

Infant:[‡]

☐ Respiratory morbidities *(e.g., transient tachypnea of the newborn, persistent pulmonary hypertension of the newborn, respiratory distress syndrome, or combined respiratory problems)*
☐ Iatrogenic or inadvertent prematurity
  ○ *Related to inaccurate dating and arranged delivery at suboptimal gestational age*
☐ NICU admission and longer hospital stay than with uncomplicated vaginal birth, incurring health care costs
☐ Superficial skin laceration (1%–2% of Cesarean births)
  ○ *Most common fetal injury at Cesarean delivery*

○ *Related to skin incision-to-delivery interval <3 min, T or J uterine incisions, nonvertex presentations, and ruptured membranes prior to surgical delivery*
  □ Delayed skin-to-skin and parental bonding

Special notes:
† Risks of early postpartum hemorrhage, obstetric shock, and need for blood transfusion are *lower* with *planned* Cesarean than *combined* planned vaginal and intrapartum Cesarean delivery
‡ Neonatal mortality appears the same based on the risk difference between Cesarean and vaginal births *(NICE[6], Table 2);* however, complicated vaginal delivery carries greater risk of neonatal mortality than with planned Cesarean delivery

---

4. Address the patient's misconceptions by discussing the advantages of neuraxial relative to general anesthesia in the event of Cesarean delivery. *(1 point each)*   Max 10

Maternal

Cardiorespiratory risk-reductions:
□ Aspiration
□ Hypertensive response to intubation in the at-risk patient *(e.g., preeclampsia)*
□ Cardiac arrest

Surgical risk-reductions:
□ Intraoperative uterine atony and hemorrhage
□ Surgical site infection

Neurological and psychogenic benefits:
□ Reduced risk of awareness under general anesthesia
□ Reduced chronic postdelivery pain
□ Allows for immediate postdelivery skin-to-skin bonding and breastfeeding *(this has newborn benefit)*
□ Allows for parental participation in birth

Infant risk-reductions
□ Respiratory depression at delivery
□ Apgar score <7 at five minutes of life
□ NICU admission

The patient appreciates your evidence-based counseling and professional approach. Despite her continued fear of labor and vaginal delivery, she is surprised to learn of the complications associated with Cesarean delivery, including risks of general anesthesia. You take this opportunity to provide patient-education articles including a leaflet† for patients choosing to have a Cesarean delivery, realizing that no specific format for patient educational interventions (pamphlets, videos, role play education) is recommended as more effective *(Suggested Reading 8).*

In your socially funded health care system, you remind your trainee of the duty to wisely allocate limited health care resources where there are clear net benefits, while continuing to treat an individual patient fairly and as medically indicated.

†   The following example from the Royal College of Obstetricians and Gynaecologists (RCOG) is available at www.rcog.org.uk/en/patients/patient-leaflets/choosing-to-have-a-caesarean-section/, accessed April 18, 2021.

5. Which ethical principle are you alluding to with your trainee?	2

☐ Justice

6. Indicate <u>long-term risks (more than one year)</u> of Cesarean delivery you may address in counseling. *(1 point per main bullet)*	Max 11

Maternal:
☐ Cesarean scar pregnancy/ectopic pregnancy
☐ Spontaneous early pregnancy loss
☐ Uterine scar dehiscence and/or rupture with/without labor in subsequent pregnancy
☐ Abdominal adhesions and Asherman syndrome
☐ Incisional hernias
☐ Localized numbness at the lateral aspects of transverse skin incisions
☐ Future peripartum hysterectomy
☐ Preterm birth
☐ Subfertility and conception delays
  ○ *Contributing factors may include adhesions, abnormal placentation, psychological factors contributing to the reluctance for future pregnancy, or voluntary delays to optimize uterine wound healing*

Fetal/child:
☐ Unexplained term stillbirth in the second pregnancy at ≥34 weeks' gestation
  ○ *Absolute risk remains low at ~4/1000 women (refer to RCOG patient leaflet indicated above)*
  ○ *Contributing factors to stillbirth may include abnormalities in placentation, uterine blood flow, or placental abruption*
☐ Reduced fetal growth
☐ Childhood morbidities (*e.g.*, asthma, obesity, rhino-conjunctivitis, systemic connective tissue disorders, juvenile arthritis, immune deficiencies)

Placental: *(with associated complications)*
☐ Placenta previa
  ○ *Parity also independently increases the risk for placenta previa, compounded by prior Cesarean delivery*
☐ Placenta accreta spectrum‡
  ○ *Given the couple's desire for a large family, consider the >60% risk of placenta previa accreta after three Cesarean deliveries and possible need for peripartum hysterectomy*
☐ Placental abruption

Special note:
‡   Refer to Question 6 in Chapter 23

At the following week's prenatal visit, she informs you that although the provided resources were valuable and she is cognizant of various risks associated with Cesarean delivery by maternal request, the thought of vaginal childbirth has been anxiety-provoking and affected her sleep over the week. The patient understands that Cesarean delivery based on maternal request would not be performed prior to 39 weeks' gestation.

Knowing of >10 tools specifically designed to assess fear of childbirth *(Suggested Reading 9)*, you decide to administer the two-item 'Fear of Birth Scale' (FOBS), where she scores 60/100. With an estimated 14%[‡] of women experiencing the distinct psychological entity of 'tocophobia,' you teach your trainee that a FOBS cutoff score of 54/100 has a sensitivity and specificity of 89% and 79%, respectively, in identifying women who score >85/165 on the most widely used 33-item Wijma Delivery Expectancy/Experience Questionnaire (W-DEQ) to assess fear of childbirth.[§†]

Prior to discussing prenatal management options with the patient, you take note to later teach your trainee the effects of tocophobia on pregnancy.

Special notes:

‡ O'Connell MA, Leahy-Warren P, Khashan AS, Kenny LC, O'Neill SM. Worldwide prevalence of tocophobia in pregnant women: systematic review and meta-analysis. *Acta Obstet Gynecol Scand.* 2017;96(8):907–920.

§ Haines HM, Pallant JF, Fenwick J, et al. Identifying women who are afraid of giving birth: A comparison of the fear of birth scale with the WDEQ-A in a large Australian cohort. *Sex Reprod Healthc.* 2015;6(4):204–210.

† Wijma K, Wijma B, Zar M. Psychometric aspects of the W-DEQ; a new questionnaire for the measurement of fear of childbirth. *J Psychosom Obstet Gynaecol.* 1998;19(2):84–97.

---

7. Illustrate an understanding of the <u>impact of tocophobia</u> on pregnancy. *(1 point each)* — Max 3

   - ☐ Avoidance of preparation for childbirth, including attendance at prenatal classes
   - ☐ Impact on antenatal and postnatal maternal-infant bonding
   - ☐ Declining appropriate medical interventions related to the process of labor and delivery *(e.g., fetal cardiotocography (CTG) monitor)*
   - ☐ Increased maternal-infant morbidity associated with potential elective Cesarean delivery
   - ☐ Risk of pregnancy termination, even if desires a family *(gestational age and jurisdictional policy influences apply)*

---

8. Propose <u>management</u> options for tocophobia known to enhance patients' capacity for making an autonomous choice, possibly choosing a vaginal birth. *(1 point each)* — Max 5

Biological dimensions:

   - ☐ Offer repeat discussion on the risk-benefit ratio of her request for elective Cesarean section
   - ☐ Refer for antenatal consultation with an obstetric anesthesiologist to discuss analgesic options
   - ☐ Consideration for homebirth with appropriate midwifery care *(requires careful patient selection)*

Psychosocial dimensions:
☐ Emphasize your/provider's support and continuity of medical care
☐ Refer for psychotherapy, cognitive behavioral therapy, or other mental health resources
☐ Consideration for prenatal yoga classes
☐ Consideration for additional emotional support during labor *(e.g., doula or patient-selected individual)* and extended postpartum clinical visits

9. What is the best practice management if, as a professional, you are unwilling to accede to the patient's request for primary elective Cesarean delivery? 2

☐ Referral for a second opinion by an obstetrician

TOTAL: 60

CHAPTER 18

Vaginal Birth after Cesarean Section

Amira El-Messidi and Alan D. Cameron

You are seeing a 29-year-old G2P1 with a singleton pregnancy at 34^{+6} weeks' gestation for a routine prenatal visit. Pregnancy dating was confirmed by first-trimester sonography. She reports normal fetal activity and has no clinical complaints. Your colleague following her obstetric care is now on a two-month leave. Although mode of delivery was addressed early in prenatal care, your colleague left you a note to discuss a trial of vaginal birth after Cesarean delivery (VBAC) with the patient.

LEARNING OBJECTIVES

1. Take a focused history to provide appropriate counseling for a VBAC, identifying factors that affect the likelihood of successful VBAC
2. Recognize situations prohibiting consideration for a VBAC
3. Discuss means for induction of labor in VBAC and provide appropriate intrapartum care, including timely multidisciplinary management in acute obstetric emergency
4. Appreciate the clinical markers of uterine rupture in labor, with an understanding that none are accurate predictors of potentially catastrophic maternal-fetal consequences
5. Counsel on risks of recurrent uterine rupture, and provide recommendations on mode and timing of delivery for future pregnancy

SUGGESTED READINGS

1. American College of Obstetricians and Gynecologists' Committee on Practice Bulletins – Obstetrics. ACOG Practice Bulletin No. 205: Vaginal birth after Cesarean delivery. *Obstet Gynecol.* 2019;133(2):e110–e127.
2. Di Spiezio Sardo A, Saccone G, McCurdy R, et al. Risk of Cesarean scar defect following single- vs double-layer uterine closure: systematic review and meta-analysis of randomized controlled trials. *Ultrasound Obstet Gynecol.* 2017;50(5):578–583.
3. Dodd JM, Crowther CA, Grivell RM, et al. Elective repeat caesarean section versus induction of labour for women with a previous caesarean birth. *Cochrane Database Syst Rev.* 2017;7(7): CD004906.
4. Dy J, DeMeester S, Lipworth H, et al. No. 382 – trial of labour after Caesarean. *J Obstet Gynaecol Can.* 2019;41(7):992–1011. [Corrections in *J Obstet Gynaecol Can.* 2019 Sep;41(9):1395; *J Obstet Gynaecol Can.* 2020 Nov;42(11):1452]

5. Fox NS. Pregnancy outcomes in patients with prior uterine rupture or dehiscence: a 5-year update. *Obstet Gynecol.* 2020;135(1):211–212.

6. Landon MB, Grobman WA; Eunice Kennedy Shriver National Institute of Child Health and Human Development Maternal–Fetal Medicine Units Network. What we have learned about trial of labor after Cesarean delivery from the Maternal-Fetal Medicine Units Cesarean Registry. *Semin Perinatol.* 2016;40(5):281–286.

7. Royal College of Obstetricians and Gynaecologists (RCOG). Birth after previous Caesarean birth. Green-Top Guideline No. 45. London: RCOG; October 2015.

8. Swift BE, Shah PS, Farine D. Sonographic lower uterine segment thickness after prior cesarean section to predict uterine rupture: a systematic review and meta-analysis. *Acta Obstet Gynecol Scand.* 2019;98(7):830–841.

9. Tanos V, Toney ZA. Uterine scar rupture – prediction, prevention, diagnosis, and management. *Best Pract Res Clin Obstet Gynaecol.* 2019; 59:115–131.

10. Tsakiridis I, Mamopoulos A, Athanasiadis A, et al. Vaginal birth after previous Cesarean birth: a comparison of 3 national guidelines. *Obstet Gynecol Surv.* 2018;73(9):537–543.

POINTS

1. What aspects of a focused history would you want to know in order to counsel the patient on a VBAC? *(1 point each)*

Max 15

Details related to prior Cesarean section:
☐ Obtain operative report, *if possible*
☐ Type of previous uterine scar, *if known to the patient and report is unavailable*
☐ Indication for the Cesarean section; if performed for arrest of dilation, inquire about cervical dilation prior to delivery
☐ Interdelivery interval
☐ Gestational age at delivery
☐ Inquire if uterine rupture had occurred
☐ Intraoperative or postpartum complications
☐ Newborn's birthweight

Social, medical, and surgical history:
☐ Race/ethnicity
☐ Height and weight, to calculate the body mass index (BMI)
☐ Maternal medical condition precluding vaginal delivery *(e.g., active perianal inflammatory bowel disease, Marfan syndrome with aortic dissection/dilatation, HIV with high viral load)*
☐ Prior transmural uterine surgery or major reconstruction *(e.g., cornual resection, perforated uterine wall)* and/or abdominal surgery unrelated to prior Cesarean delivery
☐ Presence of uterine myomas in the lower segment or cervix likely to obstruct labor
☐ Current anticoagulation

Current pregnancy:
☐ Absence of a major congenital anomaly that may obstruct labor or increase fetal morbidity at vaginal delivery *(e.g., exomphalos with liver herniation, large fetal teratoma)*
☐ Placental localization
☐ Obstetric complications that may decrease likelihood of successful VBAC *(e.g., preeclampsia)*

You learn that the patient is a healthy Caucasian with an unremarkable pregnancy to date. The fetal morphology survey was normal with fundal placentation. Her obstetric chart indicates appropriate fundal heights on clinical assessments.

Three years ago, prior to immigration, she had a Cesarean delivery for unexplained prolonged fetal bradycardia at 6 cm dilation after presenting in spontaneous labor at term. The operative notes are not available. The patient reports an uneventful surgery and postoperative recovery; her newborn's birthweight was 3550 g. Apart from Cesarean delivery, she has not had other abdominal-pelvic surgeries. She is interested in a vaginal delivery.

Her obstetric chart indicates a BMI of 25 kg/m^2; she is normotensive. Viability is ascertained and fetal presentation is cephalic by abdominal palpation. You note a low transverse *skin* scar. Your obstetric trainee inquires about the patient's candidacy for VBAC despite an inaccessible operative report.

2. Address your trainee's concerns regarding mode of delivery in the context of an unknown uterine scar, and specify reassuring features based on the patient's clinical history.   4

☐ The majority of unknown uterine scars are low transverse and offering VBAC is safe and acceptable after appropriate clinical evaluation *(1 point)*
☐ Reassuringly, based on her history, a low transverse incision is most likely in the context of: *(1 point per subbullet)*
   ○ Term gestation *(Delivery at extreme premature gestational ages increases the likelihood of a prior classical Cesarean delivery)*
   ○ Cephalic presentation
   ○ Intrapartum Cesarean delivery

Special note:
Single- versus double-layer uterine closure is generally not considered in offering a VBAC

3. Identify situations prohibiting VBAC despite a cephalic presentation. *(1 point per main bullet)*   Max 11

Maternal:
☐ Short interdelivery interval
   ○ *RCOG:* <12 months
   ○ *ACOG, SOGC:* ≤18 months
☐ Patient declines VBAC after appropriate counseling, or she requests an elective repeat Cesarean section
☐ Presence of a maternal condition precluding safe vaginal delivery
☐ Prior uterine rupture
☐ Pregestational transmural or major uterine reconstructive surgery

- ☐ Transmural incisions for open fetal surgery
- ☐ Known/suspected prior classical, inverted T/J, or transfundal incisions at Cesarean delivery
- ☐ Patient was informed by surgeon at Cesarean delivery that she is not a candidate for VBAC
- ☐ Prior low vertical uterine incision that extends into the contractile region of the uterus
  - ○ *Low vertical uterine scar that does not extend into the contractile uterus is a relative contraindication to VBAC*
- ☐ Lower uterine segment thickness <2.0–2.3 mm *(relative contraindication)*

Feto-placental:
- ☐ Major fetal malformation where risk of obstructed labor or fetal morbidity would be increased at vaginal delivery
- ☐ Suspected fetal compromise by sonography or CTG with low likelihood of fetal tolerance to labor
- ☐ Placenta previa, percreta, or vasa previa

Special notes:
(ACOG, RCOG, SOGC) Two prior low transverse Cesarean deliveries is not a contraindication to VBAC; individualized discussion and risk assessment of uterine rupture, transfusions, and hysterectomy is warranted

4. Discuss the success rate at VBAC and address the use of predictive models for personalized risk assessment. *(1 point each)*   2

- ☐ The overall chance of successful VBAC is 60%–80%
- ☐ Calculators that predict the probability of successful VBAC based on clinical risk factors and demographics may be considered, recognizing inherent limitations

5. Identify the patient's demographic and prior obstetric factors that increase her likelihood of successful VBAC. *(1 point per main bullet)*   5

- ☐ Young maternal age
  - ○ *ACOG, SOGC:* age ≤30 years
  - ○ *RCOG:* age <40 years
- ☐ BMI <30 kg/m² and/or greater maternal height
- ☐ Caucasian
- ☐ Interpregnancy interval is less than approximately six years
- ☐ Previous Cesarean was performed for a fetal indication as opposed to labor dystocia

Special note:
At least one previous vaginal birth, particularly after Cesarean delivery, would also have factored into her success at VBAC; previous vaginal delivery independently reduces the risk of uterine rupture

6. Elicit *current* obstetric or intrapartum considerations that would increase her likelihood of successful VBAC. *(1 point each)*

Max 5

☐ Spontaneous labor
☐ Cephalic presentation
☐ Bishop score is >6 at hospital delivery admission
☐ Fetal head engagement and/or low station
☐ Oxytocin is not required for labor augmentation
☐ Gestational age at delivery is <40 weeks
☐ Nonmacrosomic infant (estimated fetal weight <4000 g)

She understands the need to deliver in a hospital center with facilities available in case of emergency. The patient seems most motivated at the prospects of shorter recovery after vaginal delivery.

7. In addition to a shorter recovery period, inform the patient of other advantages of <u>successful</u> relative to failed VBAC requiring emergency Cesarean delivery. *(1 point per main bullet, unless specified)*

Max 8

Maternal benefits:
☐ Greater likelihood of *repeat* successful VBAC
☐ Decreased risks of: *(1 point per subbullet)*
   ○ Uterine rupture
   ○ Hemorrhage/blood transfusion
   ○ Thromboembolism
   ○ Postpartum wound infections and endometritis
   ○ Abdominal adhesions and Asherman syndrome
   ○ Maternal consequences related to multiple Cesarean deliveries (*e.g.,* abnormal placentation, hysterectomy, bladder/bowel injury)
   ○ Mortality

Neonatal benefits:
☐ Decreased transient respiratory morbidity (*i.e.,* transient tachypnea of the newborn, respiratory distress syndrome)

Special note:
Refer to Chapter 17 for risks and benefits of Cesarean delivery

Although she is keen to attempt a VBAC, the patient is worried about uterine rupture. Incidentally, your hospital center is participating in a research protocol examining the sonographic lower uterine segment thickness at 35–38 weeks' gestation after one prior Cesarean section in prediction of uterine rupture in labor. The patient understands that until further prospective studies are available, the value, technique, and absolute cutoff value of lower uterine segment thickness are currently unknown. You also indicate that results of her ultrasound will be used with caution in the shared decision-making for VBAC. She provides informed consent for participation in the study.

8. Given a single prior delivery and assuming a low transverse uterine scar, approximate the patient's risk of uterine rupture in spontaneous labor.

1

☐ 0.2%– 0.5%

Special notes:
(a) Uterine rupture risk approximates 1% with oxytocin augmentation;
(b) Classical or inverted-T incisions have an unacceptably high risk of rupture in labor at 4%–9%

9. Counsel the patient on adverse outcomes of uterine rupture in the current pregnancy. *(1 point each)*

Max 8

Maternal:
☐ Hysterectomy
☐ Blood product transfusions
☐ Injury to the bladder or other organs
☐ Mortality

Fetal/neonatal:
☐ Hypoxic ischemic encephalopathy of the newborn/hypoxic brain injury
☐ Admission to the neonatal intensive care unit (NICU)
☐ Five-minute Apgar score ≤ 5
☐ Umbilical artery blood pH ≤ 7.0
☐ Mortality

10. Identify two <u>nonobstetric</u>[†] causes of uterine rupture on an unscarred uterus. *(1 point each)*

2

☐ Maternal abdominal trauma
☐ Connective tissue disorders *(e.g., Ehlers-Danlos syndrome)*

Special note:
† Multiparity is the most common *obstetric* cause of intrapartum rupture of an unscarred uterus

As part of the study protocol, fetal biometry is reported on the 30th percentile at 36^{+6} weeks' gestation with normal amniotic fluid volume. Transvaginal examination of the lower uterine segment, with a full maternal bladder, reveals the following:

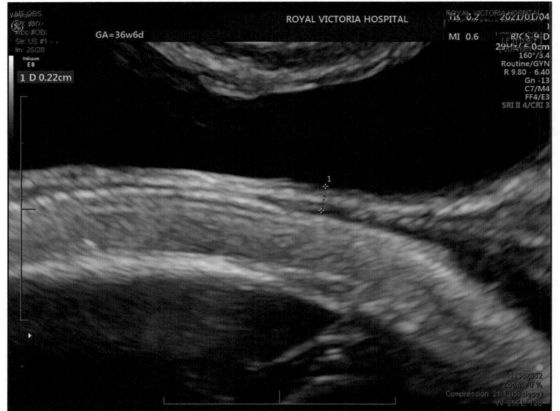

Figure 18.1

With permission: There is no association between the case scenario and this patient's image. Antepartum imaging of the hysterotomy scar remains investigational. Image is used for educational purposes only.

11. Outline the sonographic findings demonstrated in this image. *(1 point each)*   2

☐ Cephalic presentation
☐ Full thickness of the lower uterine segment is 2.2 mm

The routine vaginal-rectal group B *Streptococcus* (GBS) swab is obtained during a prenatal visit, based on practice in your jurisdiction. She remains keen to attempt a VBAC and understands the 1/1000 risk of antepartum stillbirth beyond 39^{+0} weeks' gestation (recommended timing of elective repeat Cesarean section) while awaiting spontaneous labor. She has no obstetric complaints.

12. Particular to patients with prior Cesarean section(s), discuss clinical considerations <u>worthy</u>   1
of mentioning during prenatal visits.

☐ Present early to hospital in the event of incisional pain or painful contractions

Special note:
Homebirths are not recommended for VBAC; hospital facilities should be capable of
performing emergency Cesarean delivery

Prenatal visits are unremarkable until 41^{+1} weeks' gestation. Fetal well-being[§] is ascertained, and
amniotic fluid volume is normal. The patient consents to a membrane sweep[‡] as fetal presentation
is cephalic. Her Bishop score is 4. By institutional protocol, you initiate discussion and plans for
labor induction.

Special note:
§ NST or BPP, jurisdictional variations exist
‡ *Refer to* Chapter 16

13. Counsel the patient on options for, and risks of, labor induction with a planned VBAC in
    the third trimester. *(1 point each; max points indicated where necessary)*   4

Options for induction of labor:[†] *(max 2)*
☐ Amniotomy, *if feasible*
☐ Foley catheter/balloon cervical dilation
☐ Oxytocin IV infusion[‡]

Risks:
☐ Lower rates of successful VBAC particularly with an unfavorable cervix
☐ Risk of uterine rupture

Special notes:
† Prostaglandins should not be used for induction of labor in VBAC in the third trimester
  due to increased risk of uterine rupture; misoprostol may be considered for induction of
  labor in a VBAC up to 26 weeks' gestation, with individualized discussion; *refer to* Morris
  JL, Winikoff B, Dabash R, et al. FIGO's updated recommendations for misoprostol used
  alone in gynecology and obstetrics. *Int J Gynaecol Obstet.* 2017;138(3):363–366.
‡ RCOG does not comment on use of oxytocin specifically for *induction* of labor in VBAC

During your call duty that evening, the patient presents to the hospital with rupture of membranes;
amniotic fluid is clear. Her GBS swab was negative. Fetal CTG is normal and contractions occur
every 10–15 minutes. While preparing for admission, you take this opportunity to teach your
obstetric trainee about clinical monitoring of uterine rupture.

14. Outline essentials of intrapartum management of the patient's trial of VBAC. *(1 point each)*   9

□ Supportive one-to-one nursing or midwifery care in established labor

□ Continuous electronic fetal monitoring and tocometry at the onset of regular uterine contractions

□ Obtain IV access, CBC, and blood group in established labor

□ Consider arranging for availability of blood products, and obtain patient consent in case of emergency

□ Early notification of the anesthesiologist and consideration for early placement of an epidural catheter

□ Reassure the patient that epidural analgesia does not mask signs/symptoms of uterine rupture

□ Regular assessments of cervicometric progress in labor; considerations for use of a labor curve *(e.g., Friedman curve or other validated partogram)*

□ Where oxytocin infusion is indicated, routine institutional labor dosing protocol may be used

□ Continued monitoring for signs/symptoms of uterine rupture *(intrauterine pressure catheters do not assist in detection of rupture)*

15. Discuss the signs and symptoms of uterine rupture with your trainee. *(1 point each)*   Max 10

Signs:
□ Sudden onset of fetal heart rate abnormalities[†] *(e.g., bradycardia, deep or prolonged variable decelerations, sinusoidal waveform)*
□ Loss of fetal station
□ Inability to detect fetal heart rate at the established transducer site
□ Frequent need of anesthetic redosing after effective neuraxial analgesia
□ Abdominal palpation of fetal body parts
□ Altered abdominal contour (due to free-floating fetal body parts)
□ Acute scar tenderness
□ Vaginal bleeding
□ Hematuria
□ Maternal hemodynamic instability
□ Changes in amplitude[§] and frequency of contractions, or decreased uterine tone

Symptoms:
□ Suprapubic pain *(i.e., at the location of the prior hysterotomy)*
□ Sudden onset of abdominal pain, especially if persisting between contractions

Special notes:
† No pathognomonic sign; bradycardia is most common
§ Gradual decline in amplitude of contractions may appear as a 'staircase sign'

Labor ensues spontaneously, and regional analgesia is provided at 3 cm dilation upon maternal request. The patient consents to oxytocin augmentation which becomes clinically indicated at 7 cm dilation. Shortly thereafter, you note a change in fetal variability to ≤ 5 bpm with new-onset repetitive variable decelerations.

16. Recognizing that interventions are performed simultaneously, describe the steps of your clinical management. *(1 point per main bullet)*

Max 7

☐ Discontinue the oxytocin infusion
☐ Assess for signs/symptoms of uterine rupture *(see Question 15)*
☐ Assess the patient's blood pressure, pulse, oxygenation on room air *(i.e., vital signs)*
☐ Maternal repositioning onto the left lateral decubitus (or the right side)
　○ *Aids in relieving cord compression and/or improving uteroplacental perfusion*
☐ Perform a vaginal examination for cervicometric assessment
☐ Consideration for IV bolus of a non-glucose-containing crystalloid solution *(e.g.,* Ringer's lactate or normal saline) with suspected maternal hypovolemia
　○ No evidence to support or refute the benefit of maternal IV fluid boluses on fetal heart rate abnormalities *alone*
　○ Exercise caution in clinical situations sensitive to volume overload
☐ *Controversial* value of oxygen administration by face mask in nonhypoxemic patients
☐ Keep the patient informed and ensure timely documentation

Shortly after your intrauterine resuscitative maneuvers, the patient complains of sudden suprapubic pain; concurrent fetal bradycardia at 80 bpm is noted. She remains alert. Since your most recent examination, the fetal station changed from +1 cm to −1 cm relative to the ischial spines.

17. Indicate your steps in preparation for expedited delivery. *(1 point each)*

6

☐ Call for help *(e.g., anesthesiologist, an experienced surgical assistant, neonatologist, allied health members)*
☐ Inform the patient and/or family member that uterine rupture is probable
☐ Ensure consent for Cesarean delivery with possible hysterectomy has been documented
☐ Call for blood product availability in the operating room and/or mobilize the local massive transfusion protocol
☐ Document fetal viability regularly until the start of surgery
☐ Plan the abdominal incision; midline skin incision may facilitate abdominal exploration and fundal repair *(provider's preference; individualized assessment)*

Timely Cesarean section is performed, and your clinical suspicion is confirmed: all uterine layers have been disrupted in the lower uterine segment and the fetus is promptly delivered from the abdominal cavity. Uterine conservation[†] is achieved and hemoperitoneum is controlled; the uterine rupture has not resulted in bladder injury or damage to other organs. The patient received two U PRBCs, IV crystalloids, and broad-spectrum antibiotics. Postoperative debriefing is performed, and documentation is kept up to date. At birth, umbilical arterial pH was 7.10; the newborn remains stable in the NICU.

Special note:

† Optimal uterine closure (*i.e.,* single- or double-layer) after rupture is unknown

18. In relation to the patient's obstetric events, outline important considerations to address prior to discharge and/or at the postpartum visit. *(1 point per main bullet)*   Max 5

☐ Screen for postpartum depression and offer psychosocial support
☐ Offer reliable contraception

Future pregnancy with prior uterine rupture:
☐ Risk of recurrent uterine rupture appears greatest with fundal or longitudinal rupture (~32%), relative to rupture localized to the lower segment (~6%)
☐ Inform the patient that rates of adverse outcomes are reassuring, provided elective prelabor Cesarean delivery is planned
☐ Aim for Cesarean delivery at 36^{+0} to 37^{+0} weeks after prior uterine rupture
  ○ *Corticosteroids and/or confirmation of fetal lung maturity may be considered accordingly*
  ○ *Prior uterine rupture is an absolute contraindication for VBAC*

Antecedent receipt of blood transfusion:
☐ Observe for the development of atypical antibodies

TOTAL: 105

CHAPTER 19

Shoulder Dystocia

Amira El-Messidi and Robert Gagnon

You are covering an obstetrics clinic for your colleague who left for vacation. A 30-year-old G2P1 at 37^{+2} weeks' gestation by first-trimester sonogram presents for a prenatal visit. Screening tests revealed a male fetus with a low risk of aneuploidy and a normal second-trimester morphology sonogram. Maternal investigations were unremarkable in the first trimester. Your colleague's note from a second-trimester prenatal visit details the counseling provided with regard to prior shoulder dystocia; a recent note indicates the intent to review management during this visit.

LEARNING OBJECTIVES

1. Recognize predisposing factors for shoulder dystocia, appreciating their inability to accurately predict or prevent this obstetric emergency
2. Appreciate the difficulty in establishing consensus definitions for shoulder dystocia
3. Understand the multidimensional aspects of prenatal counseling of a patient with prior shoulder dystocia
4. Provide a structured outline of, and recognize, perinatal complications associated with shoulder dystocia
5. Outline system strategies of known benefit in managing shoulder dystocia, elaborate on intrapartum measures and maneuvers to release shoulder impaction, and detail elements required in postpartum documentation

SUGGESTED READINGS

1. Chauhan SP, Gherman R, Hendrix NW, et al. Shoulder dystocia: comparison of the ACOG practice bulletin with another national guideline. *Am J Perinatol.* 2010;27(2):129–136.
2. Gilstrop M, Hoffman MK. An update on the acute management of shoulder dystocia. *Clin Obstet Gynecol.* 2016;59(4):813–819.
3. Gurewitsch Allen ED. Recurrent shoulder dystocia: risk factors and counseling. *Clin Obstet Gynecol.* 2016;59(4):803–812.
4. Moni S, Lee C, Goffman D. Shoulder dystocia: quality, safety, and risk management considerations. *Clin Obstet Gynecol.* 2016;59(4):841–852.
5. Practice Bulletin No 178: shoulder dystocia. *Obstet Gynecol.* 2017;129(5):e123–e133.

6. Royal College of Obstetricians and Gynaecologists. Shoulder dystocia. Green-Top Guideline No. 42, 2012. 2nd ed. Available at www.rcog.org.uk/en/guidelines-research-services/guidelines/gtg42/. Accessed March 5, 2021.

7. Macrosomia: ACOG Practice Bulletin, No. 216. *Obstet Gynecol.* 2020;135(1):e18–e35.

8. Menticoglou S. Shoulder dystocia: incidence, mechanisms, and management strategies. *Int J Women's Health.* 2018;10:723–732.

9. Ouzounian JG. Shoulder dystocia: incidence and risk factors. *Clin Obstet Gynecol.* 2016;59(4):791–794.

10. Sentilhes L, Sénat MV, Boulogne AI, et al. Shoulder dystocia: guidelines for clinical practice from the French College of Gynecologists and Obstetricians (CNGOF). *Eur J Obstet Gynecol Reprod Biol.* 2016;203:156–161.

POINTS

1. Detail aspects of a focused history with regard to shoulder dystocia that you would obtain from her prenatal chart. *(1 point per main bullet)*

Max 10

Maternal factors in current and prior pregnancy:
☐ Pregestational or gestational diabetes *(RCOG and ACOG)*
☐ Prepregnancy obesity *(RCOG and ACOG)*
☐ Excessive gestational weight gain

Current fetal factors:
☐ Large for gestational age/macrosomia *(RCOG and ACOG)*
  ○ *Most significant risk factor, although the large majority of infants ≥4500 grams do not develop shoulder dystocia*

Past obstetric history:
☐ Gestational age at delivery, particularly >41 weeks *(ACOG)*
☐ Induction versus spontaneous labor *(RCOG and ACOG)*
☐ Oxytocin augmentation *(RCOG)*
☐ Use of epidural analgesia *(ACOG)*
☐ Prolonged first or second stage of labor *(RCOG)*; precipitous[§] labor*(ACOG)*
☐ Operative vaginal delivery *(RCOG and ACOG)*
  ○ *Similar risk for vacuum and forceps[†]*
☐ Procedures used to relieve the shoulder dystocia
☐ Head-to-body interval in minutes
☐ Birthweight *(particularly for large for gestational age (LGA) fetus/macrosomic infant)*
☐ Apgar scores and umbilical cord blood gases
☐ Maternal or neonatal short- or long-term morbidities associated with shoulder dystocia

Special notes:
§ Rapid descent results in insufficient time for fetal bisacromial diameter to rotate to an oblique position
† *Refer to* Dall'Asta A, Ghi T, Pedrazzi G, Frusca T. Does vacuum delivery carry a higher risk of shoulder dystocia? Review and meta-analysis of the literature. *Eur J Obstet Gynecol Reprod Biol.* 2016;204:62–68.

You learn from your colleague's comprehensive records that, similar to her prior pregnancy, the patient is healthy with a normal prepregnancy BMI, gestational weight gain, and negative second-trimester glucose screening test. The prenatal course has been unremarkable and fundal heights have been appropriate.

Two years ago, she had an uncomplicated pregnancy, spontaneous labor, and vaginal delivery at 39^{+1} weeks' gestation in your hospital center. A vacuum-assisted delivery was needed after a 3.5-hour second stage of labor to support maternal fatigue during expulsive efforts. Several maneuvers were performed during the 1.5-minute interval to release the fetal shoulders and deliver her son[§] weighing 3670 grams.[†] Basic steps of resuscitation improved neonatal tone, color, and oxygenation by eight minutes of life. Umbilical arterial blood values at delivery revealed: pH 7.19, P_{CO2} 60.2 mmHg, P_{O2} 18.4 mmHg, HCO_3 23 mEq/L, and base excess of -4 mEq/L. Although there were no maternal-neonatal morbidities from the difficult delivery, your obstetric trainee inquires about potential complications that may have been incurred, realizing that ~50% of shoulder dystocias occur in patients with low clinical suspicion and normal birthweights, hampering prediction to merely 10%–16% in the general population. Being largely a subjective diagnosis, your trainee is curious whether criteria exist for diagnosis of shoulder dystocia.

While the patient is having her prearranged obstetric sonogram for growth biometry, you take this opportunity to address your trainee's queries. You highlight to your trainee that third-trimester ultrasound scans have a 10%–13% margin of error for actual birthweight.

Special notes:
§ Male gender is a risk factor for shoulder dystocia, likely attributed to higher birthweight
† Birthweight <4000 grams is selected to highlight to the learner that ~50% of shoulder dystocias occur in nonmacrosomic infants; the majority of macrosomic infants do not experience shoulder dystocia

2. Assist your trainee in interpreting the provided umbilical arterial blood values from the patient's last delivery.

        1

☐ Respiratory acidosis
  ○ *Normal mean values for umbilical arterial blood: pH 7.27, P_{CO2} 50.3 mmHg, P_{O2} 18.4 mmHg, HCO_3 22 mEq/L, and base excess -2.7 mEq/L*

Special note:
Refer to Question 32 in Chapter 15 for an example of metabolic acidosis on umbilical arterial cord blood analysis

3. Discuss three of the various definitions used in the literature to establish a shoulder dystocia diagnosis.[†] *(1 point per main bullet)*   3

☐ Failure to deliver the fetal shoulders using solely gentle downward traction *(RCOG and ACOG)*

☐ Need for maneuvers in addition to gentle downward traction to affect delivery *(RCOG and ACOG)*

☐ Head-to-body interval greater than or equal to one minute[‡]
   ○ *Objective measure, although may not be the most sensitive to detect significant clinical sequelae*

☐ Tight shoulders

☐ Any difficulty in shoulder extraction after fetal head delivery

☐ Clinical judgement

☐ Inability of the mother to push the shoulders out with her own efforts with the next contraction after delivery of the head, without any traction on the head *(Suggested Reading 8)*

Special notes:

† Readers are encouraged to refer to *Suggested Reading 4* and Gherman RB, et al. *Am J Obstet Gynecol.* 2006;195(3):657–672

‡ Spong CY, Beall M, Rodrigues D, Ross MG. An objective definition of shoulder dystocia: prolonged head-to-body delivery intervals and/or the use of ancillary obstetric maneuvers. *Obstet Gynecol.* 1995;86(3):433–436.

4. Provide a structured approach to teach your trainee the obstetric risks of shoulder dystocia. *(1 point per main bullet unless specified)*   Max 10

Maternal:

☐ Postpartum hemorrhage (PPH) (11%)[†]

☐ Third- and fourth-degree perineal lacerations (3.8%)[†]

☐ Vaginal lacerations

☐ Cervical tears

☐ Bladder rupture

☐ Uterine rupture *(primarily with fundal pressure)*

☐ Symphyseal separation

☐ Sacroiliac joint dislocation

☐ Lateral femoral cutaneous neuropathy

Fetal:

☐ Brachial plexopathies[‡] *(RCOG: 2.3%–16%; ACOG 4%–16%)* **(1 point per subbullet; max 3)**
   ○ Erb's palsy (C5-C6 deficiency)
   ○ Klumpke's palsy (C8-T1 deficiency)
   ○ Horner syndrome
   ○ Phrenic nerve palsy/diaphragmatic paralysis

☐ Fractures of the clavicle or humerus (1.7%–9.5% and 0.1%–4.2%, respectively)

☐ Pneumothoraces

☐ Hypoxic ischemic encephalopathy (0.3%)

☐ Death (<1%)

Special notes:

† The two most common maternal complications

‡ Brachial plexus injuries may occur at Cesarean section (4%) or at vaginal delivery in the absence of shoulder dystocia due to labor forces

During your discussion, your obstetric trainee recalls a patient presenting last week for a routine postpartum visit with her newborn who endured injury after a shoulder dystocia at birth. The patient provided consent for obtaining the following images for publication in a medical journal.

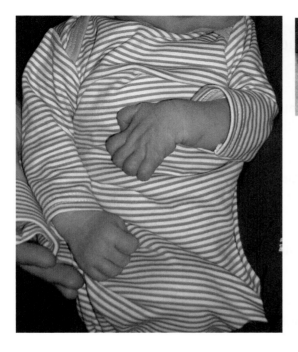
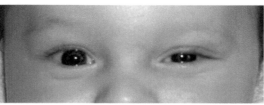

Figure 19.1 and 19.2

With permission: images are from Buchanan EP, et al. *J Hand Surg Am.* 2013;38(8):1567–1570.

There is no association between the patient images and this case scenario. Images are used for educational purposes only

Readers are encouraged to refer to: Coroneos CJ, Voineskos SH, Christakis MK, et al. Obstetrical brachial plexus injury (OBPI): Canada's national clinical practice guideline. *BMJ Open.* 2017;7(1): e014141. Published 2017 Jan 27.

5. Identify the infant's manifestations of birth-associated trauma. *(1 point each)*   2

☐ Figure 19.1 Klumpke's palsy – left claw hand

☐ Figure 19.2 manifestations of Horner syndrome *(miosis and ptosis)*

What is the third component of the Horner syndrome triad that cannot be appreciated by the infant's photograph?   1

☐ Anhidrosis

6. Explain to your trainee the delivery mechanisms causing Klumpke's palsy relative to Erb's brachial plexopathy. *(1 point per main bullet)*

2

Klumpke's palsy (lower lesions, C8-T1 deficiency):
☐ Due to abduction and backward rotation of the shoulder at the time of delivery

Erb's palsy (upper lesions, C5-C6 deficiency):
☐ Due to lateral flexion of the head away from the affected shoulder, with depression of the ipsilateral shoulder
  ○ *'Waiter's tip' palsy appears as an adducted, internally rotated at the shoulder, extended at the elbow, and pronated at the forearm*
  ○ *Grasp reflex is maintained, contrary to Klumpke's palsy*

Special note:
Approximately 90% of brachial plexopathies heal by one year and 10% have permanent disability

Your patient returns to the clinic after her obstetric ultrasound; currently at 37^{+2} weeks' gestation, the estimated fetal weight (EFW) is 3308 grams consistent for the 88th percentile with a normal head circumference-to-abdominal circumference ratio, normal femur length-abdominal circumference ratio, and normal amniotic fluid volume. The patient remains normotensive with appropriate weight gain since last visit; she has no obstetric complaints. Along with your trainee, you proceed to discuss her delivery management in view of prior shoulder dystocia.

Special note:
This case scenario highlights how normal head circumference-to-abdominal circumference and femur length-abdominal circumference ratios do not exclude the risk of shoulder dystocia

7. Discuss important aspects of counseling of this nondiabetic patient regarding her prior delivery complicated by shoulder dystocia. *(1 point per main bullet)*

Max 4

☐ Mention that recurrence risk ranges from 1% to 25% *(RCOG)*, noting that the majority of patients do not experience a recurrence
  ○ *Prior shoulder dystocia is the single greatest risk factor for recurrence*
  ○ *Risk prediction models are currently not recommended*
☐ Inform the patient of the aim to avoid recurrent operative vaginal delivery
☐ Individualized discussion regarding elective Cesarean section: for this nondiabetic patient, elective Cesarean section may be considered when the EFW is >5000 grams *(ACOG)*
  ○ *Consider Cesarean section for an EFW ≥4500 grams in pregnancies complicated by preexisting or gestational diabetes regardless of treatment (RCOG and ACOG)*
☐ Reassure the patient that individualized interventions can minimize intrapartum complications and improve delivery outcomes with a history of shoulder dystocia
☐ Inform the patient that induction of labor (IOL) may have merit given her history of prior shoulder dystocia

8. Recalling that induction of labor (IOL) is not recommended as a means of decreasing the   2
    rate of shoulder dystocia for suspected macrosomia, provide rationale why IOL may have
    merit for the gravida with <u>prior</u> shoulder dystocia. *(1 point each)*

☐ Avoidance of pregnancy beyond the estimated due date *(a modifiable risk factor for
  shoulder dystocia)*
☐ Recurrence risk of shoulder dystocia correlates with similar/greater birthweight at
  subsequent delivery compared with the index shoulder dystocia

9-A. The patient is keen for vaginal delivery. She understands that non-water-based delivery   2
      in a hospital setting is required. Address her inquiry regarding existing <u>predelivery</u>
      strategies proven beneficial in the event of a shoulder dystocia emergency. *(1 point per
      main bullet)*

☐ Multidisciplinary skills-drills improves the function of birth attendants in obstetric
  emergencies
☐ Simulation training using mannequins improves the proportion of delivery completion in
  shoulder dystocia
  ○ *Training models with force-monitoring may reduce traction-injuries*

9-B. Provide your trainee with <u>intrapartum</u> strategies in preparation for possible shoulder   Max 4
      dystocia. *(1 point per main bullet)*

☐ Plan for assistance from multidisciplinary team members at delivery
  ○ *e.g., obstetric, nursing, midwifery, anesthetic and neonatal staff*
  ○ *Clearly state the problem to the team: 'this is a shoulder dystocia' (RCOG)*
☐ **Consider** having a step stool in the event suprapubic pressure is required
☐ Position the patient in the lithotomy‡ position with her buttocks flush at the end of the bed
  for delivery
☐ Keep the bladder empty to maximize vaginal space for the fetus
☐ Ensure availability of uterotonics and blood products in the event of PPH

Special note:
‡ Prophylactic McRoberts' positioning before fetal head delivery is not recommended for
   prevention of shoulder dystocia *(RCOG)*

After a detailed discussion, the patient opts to await spontaneous labor. During your call duty, she presents to the obstetric emergency assessment unit at 39^{+3} weeks' gestation with regular uterine contractions and 6 cm cervical dilatation with clear amniotic fluid from spontaneous amniorhexis. The fetus is in a right occiput-transverse position at 1 cm above the ischial spine with a normal cardiotocography (CTG) tracing.

Oxytocin augmentation is required to achieve full cervical dilatation by six hours of admission. She receives epidural analgesia at 8 cm cervical dilatation, upon her request. The second stage is precipitous, with the station at 2 cm below the ischial spines within 10 minutes of full dilation; the fetus is now in the right occiput-anterior position. At this time, she expresses an urge to push. Fetal CTG remains normal throughout labor.

With the assembly of team members, you prepare for potential recurrent shoulder dystocia. Crowning is achieved within 15 minutes of the second stage. The patient, aware of potential delivery maneuvers and complications, remains motivated.

10. Although not diagnostic, identify and explain the <u>classic sign</u> at the time of delivery that may be *suggestive of* impending shoulder dystocia.

2

☐ 'Turtle-neck sign': due to retraction of the fetal head toward the perineum after expulsion due to reverse traction from the impacted shoulders at the pelvic inlet

11. Detail your first- and second-line maneuvers in management of a shoulder dystocia, knowing that no maneuver is considered superior to another and maneuvers need not be performed in any particular sequence. *(1 point each)*

Max 6

First-line maneuvers: (based on ease of use and noninvasiveness)
☐ *McRoberts position* involves hyperflexing the maternal thighs *(avoid pulling on the fetal head)*
☐ *Mazzanti maneuver (suprapubic pressure)* involves an assistant applying pressure from the side of the fetal back in a downward and lateral direction *(RCOG: there is no clear difference in efficacy between continuous pressure and rocking motion)*

Second-line and other maneuvers:
☐ Consider episiotomy, if it will facilitate internal maneuvers
☐ *Jacquemier maneuver (delivery of the posterior arm)* involves grasping the fetal forearm or wrist and sweeping it across the anterior fetal chest to effect delivery
☐ *Rubin's maneuver* involves the application of pressure to the posterior aspect of the most accessible fetal shoulder toward the fetal chest
☐ *Woods corkscrew maneuver* involves the application of pressure to the anterior aspect of the posterior fetal shoulder to rotate it toward the fetal back
☐ *Menticoglou maneuver* involves downward-and-outward traction of the posterior fetal axilla along the sacral curve using the operator's middle fingers of both hands to guide delivery of the posterior shoulder and arm
  ○ *Described in 1609 by royal midwife Louise Bourgeois (Suggested Reading 8)*
☐ *Couder maneuver* involves attempted delivery of the anterior arm by using provider's fingers as a splint on the anterior surface of the upper humerus to push the humerus backward toward the fetal back; this may flex the elbow and allow grasping of the hand under the symphysis
☐ *Intended fracture of the humerus or clavicle*
☐ *Gaskin maneuver* involves rotating the patient to the all-fours position (hands and knees) to effect delivery by applying downward or upward pressure to effect delivery of the posterior shoulder (against the sacrum) or anterior shoulder (against the symphysis), respectively
☐ *PAST (posterior axilla sling traction)* involves threading of a soft catheter around the posterior shoulder to affect delivery of the posterior shoulder

12. Indicate measures that you would specifically <u>avoid</u> in managing a shoulder dystocia. *(1 point per main bullet)*

Max 4

Avoid:

☐ Fundal pressure *(associated with high neonatal complication rate and uterine rupture)*
☐ Maternal pushing during the shoulder dystocia *(exacerbates shoulder impaction)*
☐ Strong downward traction on the fetal head *(increases brachial plexopathy)*
☐ Inverse rotation of the fetal head *(increases shoulder impaction and brachial plexopathy)*
☐ Immediate clamping of the umbilical cord despite a limp, depressed newborn after shoulder dystocia *(Suggested Reading 8)*
  ○ Instead, advise allowing time for placental autotransfusion to compensate for fetal hypovolemia after blood flow interruption due to compression of the fetal chest or umbilical vein; the problem is not due to lack of oxygen
  ○ Start resuscitation at the mother's bedside

As predicted, a shoulder dystocia ensues. Despite appropriate help, a right mediolateral episiotomy, and several failed maneuvers, you indicate that an intended clavicular fracture is necessary to affect delivery. A two-minute head-to-body delivery interval was recorded for the 3770-gram newborn[†] who required brief resuscitation. During your repair of the episiotomy, the neonatologist attends to the patient's bedside to counsel her on management of her son's clavicular fracture.[‡] There are no suspected brachial plexopathies.

Special notes:
[†] Birthweight is higher among infants of women with prior shoulder dystocia who experience a recurrence
[‡] The rate of injury after recurrent shoulder dystocia is higher than in primary shoulder dystocia

13. Indicate what the neonatologist has mentioned to the patient regarding management and prognosis of obstetric clavicular fractures. *(1 point each)*

3

☐ Neonatal chest radiography will be performed to ensure absence of pneumothorax
☐ Expectant management involves analgesia and immobility
☐ Healing is expected by ~10 days

While completing delivery documentation, your obstetric trainee surprises you that he or she was a physicist prior to pursuing a medical career and is now inquiring how specific maneuvers release shoulder impaction. He or she is also curious what may have been your 'last resort' measures to resolve the shoulder dystocia.

14. Explain to your trainee the physiological mechanisms by which first-line maneuvers, rotational second-line maneuvers, delivery of the posterior fetal arm, and episiotomy aid in management of shoulder dystocia. *(1 point each)*   6

□ McRoberts maneuver straightens the lumbosacral angle, rotates the symphysis pubis cephalad, and increases the *relative* anterior-posterior diameter of the pelvis

□ Suprapubic pressure decreases the fetal bisacromial diameter by adducting the anterior shoulder and bringing the shoulder into the wider oblique pelvic diameter

□ Rubin's maneuver leads to adduction of the fetal shoulder to allow its rotation and delivery from behind the pubic bone where it is impacted

□ Woods corkscrew maneuver attempts to affect a 180 degrees rotation of the fetal shoulder to allow fetal descent during rotation

□ Delivery of the posterior arm reduces the 13-cm bisacromial diameter to 11-cm axillo-acromial diameter

□ An episiotomy creates space to facilitate the operator's maneuvers; it does not release impacted shoulders

15. Address your trainee's inquiry by identifying three measures associated with maternal-fetal morbidity that may release fetal shoulder impaction at delivery. *(1 point each)*   Max 3

□ Intentional cleidotomy *(RCOG and ACOG)*

□ Zavanelli maneuver *(RCOG and ACOG)*

□ Symphysiotomy *(RCOG)*

□ Abdominal rescue through a low transverse hysterotomy through which fetal shoulders are manually rotated to an oblique diameter for subsequent vaginal delivery *(ACOG)*

16. Focusing on the incident shoulder dystocia, provide a structured framework of aspects you would document in your unit-based checklist, starting from the patient's hospitalization for labor. *(1 point each)*   Max 20

Labor and delivery details:

□ Time of onset of active labor, if known

□ Time of onset/duration of second stage

□ Fetal well-being in labor

□ Medication/anesthesia given

□ Specify team members present and note the time they were called for assistance

□ Mode of fetal head delivery and if instrumental, indicate type of instrument, station, indication, duration

□ Time of delivery of the head

□ Time of delivery of the body *(calculate head-to-body interval)*

□ Time when shoulder dystocia diagnosis was made

□ How the diagnosis was made

□ Fetal position during delivery, specifying which shoulder was anterior

   ○ *Brachial plexopathy to the posterior shoulder is unlikely to be provider-related*

☐ Maneuvers performed, their sequence, duration, and result

☐ Specify pertinent negatives (*e.g., no forceful traction on the vertex was used, fundal pressure was avoided*)

☐ Identify whether the umbilical cord was clamped/cut at the perineum prior to or after release of the impacted shoulder

Maternal delivery-related data:

☐ Preparatory strategies (*e.g., step stool, maternal positioning, bladder emptying, patient counseling*)

☐ Laceration or type/time of episiotomy

☐ Estimated blood loss (EBL); occurrence of PPH or other morbidity

☐ Address whether parental debriefing was performed

Neonatal-related data:

☐ Time neonatal care team called/attended

☐ Names of neonatal care provider(s)

☐ Birthweight

☐ Apgar scores

☐ Umbilical cord acid-based measurements

☐ Neonatal assessment *(1 point per subbullet)*

  ○ Sign of arm weakness

  ○ Sign of potential bony fracture

  ○ NICU admission

TOTAL: **85**

CHAPTER 20

Fetal Malpresentation and Breech Delivery

Andrew Zakhari and Amira El-Messidi

You are covering an obstetrics clinic for your colleague who left for vacation. A 26-year-old G2P1 with a singleton pregnancy at 36^{+4} weeks' gestation by first-trimester sonogram presents for a prenatal visit. First- and second-trimester fetal aneuploidy screening tests were low risk. Her primary care provider had arranged for serial obstetric sonograms in the second and third trimesters for decreased fundal height. Imaging today shows a new finding of breech presentation. The patient does not have any obstetric complaints. Your nurse mentions the patient requests an external cephalic version.

LEARNING OBJECTIVES

1. Develop a structured understanding of risk factors for breech presentations in the late third trimester
2. Elicit features on prenatal history to determine eligibility for external cephalic version and describe factors that increase success rates
3. Detail aspects of informed consent for external cephalic version or vaginal breech birth
4. Outline essentials of labor management for safe delivery of vaginal breech birth in the appropriately selected patient
5. Elaborate on techniques for vaginal breech birth, including management of related complications

SUGGESTED READINGS

1. ACOG Committee Opinion No. 745: Mode of term singleton breech delivery. *Obstet Gynecol.* 2018;132(2):e60–e63.
2. Carbillon L, Benbara A, Tigaizin A, et al. Revisiting the management of term breech presentation: a proposal for overcoming some of the controversies. *BMC Pregnancy Childbirth.* 2020;20(1):263.
3. External cephalic version: ACOG Practice Bulletin, No. 221. *Obstet Gynecol.* 2020;135(5): e203–e212.
4. Homafar M, Gerard J, Turrentine M. Vaginal delivery after external cephalic version in patients with a previous Cesarean delivery: a systematic review and meta-analysis. *Obstet Gynecol.* 2020;136(5):965–971.

5. Impey LWM, Murphy DJ, Griffiths M, et al. External cephalic version and reducing the incidence of term breech presentation. Green-Top Guideline No. 20a. *BJOG* 2017; 124(07): e178–e192.

6. Impey LWM, Murphy DJ, Griffiths M, et al. Management of breech presentation: Green-Top Guideline No. 20b. *BJOG* 2017;124(07):e151–177.

7. Kotaska A, Menticoglou S. No. 384 – management of breech presentation at term. *J Obstet Gynaecol Can.* 2019;41(8):1193–1205.

8. Magro-Malosso ER, Saccone G, Di Tommaso M, et al. Neuraxial analgesia to increase the success rate of external cephalic version: a systematic review and meta-analysis of randomized controlled trials. *Am J Obstet Gynecol.* 2016;215(3):276–286. [Correction in *Am J Obstet Gynecol.* 2017 Mar;216(3):315]

9. Royal Australian and New Zealand College of Obstetricians and Gynaecologists. Management of breech presentation at term. Available at https://ranzcog.edu.au/. Accessed March 6, 2021.

10. Tsakiridis I, Mamopoulos A, Athanasiadis A, et al. Management of breech presentation: a comparison of four national evidence-based guidelines. *Am J Perinatol.* 2020;37(11): 1102–1109.

POINTS

1. Which <u>specific</u> aspects in the prenatal chart would you want to review in order to counsel the patient on potential external cephalic version? *(1 point per main bullet)*

Max 12

Maternal medical and prenatal features:
☐ Body mass index (BMI) *(obesity may affect the success rate of external cephalic version$^\$$)*
☐ Rh status and alloimmunization†
☐ Assess for any medical or obstetrical situation where a Cesarean section is indicated† *(e.g., placenta/vasa previa, prior uterine rupture, Classical/T-incision Cesarean section, HIV-positive status with high viral load)*
☐ Antepartum hemorrhage within one week of the potential date of external cephalic version† *(i.e., as of 37^{+0} weeks' gestation)*
☐ Known major uterine anomaly† *(e.g., unicornuate, septate uterus, fibroids causing uterine distortion or obstructing cervical canal)*
☐ Fetal anomaly likely to interfere with, or increase risk of, external cephalic version†
☐ Known placental abruption†
☐ Presence of hypertension or hypertensive syndromes of pregnancy†
☐ Determine whether the patient takes thromboprophylaxis

Details of the most recent obstetric sonogram:
☐ Type of breech presentation (frank, complete or incomplete/footling)
☐ Fetal lie (*i.e.*, longitudinal, oblique, transverse) and spine orientation
☐ Estimated fetal weight (EFW)
☐ Presence of umbilical cord presentation
☐ Amniotic fluid volume (ensure absence of oligohydramnios)
☐ Placental localization

Obstetric history:‡
☐ Previous breech presentation and external cephalic version in her last pregnancy
   ○ *Knowledge of patient's history may have implications on counseling*

Special notes:

§   Chaudhary S, Contag S, Yao R. The impact of maternal body mass index on external cephalic version success. *J Matern Fetal Neonatal Med.* 2019;32(13):2159–2165.

†   There is no general consensus on the eligibility for, or contraindications to, external cephalic version; other clinical contraindications {not pertinent to this case scenario} include multiple pregnancy, rupture of amniotic membranes; external cephalic version is contraindicated in the presence of an abnormal cardiotocography (CTG)

‡   One low transverse Cesarean section is not by itself an absolute contraindication for external cephalic version

You learn from your colleague's comprehensive records that the patient is healthy with a normal BMI; she last weighed 64 kg at her prenatal visit. Her only medications include prenatal vitamins and routine receipt of Rh immunoglobulin at 28 weeks' gestation for her blood type; she does not have alloimmune antibodies. Second-trimester morphology ultrasound showed a normal female fetus; glucose screening test was also normal. Her prenatal course has been unremarkable, and she has been anticipating a repeat uncomplicated term vaginal delivery as with her son two years ago.

Obstetric ultrasound today reveals complete breech presentation; fetal lie is oblique with a flexed head in the maternal left upper quadrant and presenting parts in the right lower quadrant. Estimated fetal weight is on the 45th percentile, amniotic fluid index is 12 cm, and the placenta is posterior, well distant from the internal cervical os without overlying umbilical cord. You are relieved to read that the clinically suspected decreased fundal height is unrelated to fetal growth or fluid volume.

2. Identify three <u>known</u> risk factors for breech presentation in this patient. *(1 point each)*   3

☐ Preterm or late-preterm gestation
☐ Multiparity
☐ Female fetus

3. Prepare a list of <u>other risk factors</u> for breech presentation you intend to teach your trainee   Max 10
after this consultation visit. *(1 point each)*

Maternal: *(max 5)*
☐ Past pregnancy with breech presentation *(recurrence approximates 10% after the first pregnancy and 25% after two consecutive pregnancies with breech presentations)*
☐ Maternal or paternal history of term breech delivery themselves *(possible genetic component)*
☐ Uterine malformations *(e.g.,* septate, uni/bicornuate, or fibroids)
☐ Multiple pregnancy
☐ Contracted pelvis
☐ Connective tissue disorders, such as Ehlers-Danlos syndrome
☐ Use of anticonvulsant drugs

Feto-placental: *(max 5)*
☐ Placental location *(e.g.,* previa or cornual)
☐ Oligohydramnios/polyhydramnios
☐ Fetal growth restriction (FGR)

- ☐ Short umbilical cord
- ☐ Fetal neuromuscular impairment
- ☐ Anomaly causing fetal body distortion (*e.g.*, anencephaly, hydrocephalus, large encephalocele or facial/neck mass, sacrococcygeal teratoma)

As a young woman who is planning a large family, she is motivated to have a vaginal delivery to avoid risks of Cesarean section and implications on future childbearing.§ You inform her that although appropriate expertise for vaginal breech birth is available in your center, an external cephalic version in the appropriately selected patient effectively decreases rates of noncephalic presentations in labor and rates of Cesarean section. Reassuringly, your personal success rate at external cephalic version in the past 100 procedures is consistent with general statistics. She heard of non-external cephalic version methods to achieve fetal version and asks for your evidence-based practice.

Special note:
§ Refer to Chapter 17

4. Provide your evidence-based opinion on non-external cephalic version methods to achieve cephalic version. *(1 point each)*	Max 1

- ☐ Postural methods alone have not been proven to promote successful spontaneous version *(RCOG)*
- ☐ Guided by a trained practitioner, moxibustion at 33–35 weeks' gestation may promote fetal activity to achieve a cephalic presentation *(RCOG)*
  - ○ *Moxibustion is a traditional Chinese medicine therapy*

5. Elicit factors associated with <u>increased</u> likelihood of success at external cephalic version for this patient. *(1 point each)*	Max 8

Clinical factors:
- ☐ Operator experience
- ☐ Complete breech presentation
- ☐ Patient remains <38 weeks' gestation
- ☐ Unengaged presenting part/nonimpacted breech
- ☐ Multiparity
- ☐ Nonobese maternal habitus; weight <65 kg

Ultrasound factors:
- ☐ Nonlongitudinal fetal lie
- ☐ Anterior fetal spine
- ☐ Normal amniotic fluid volume (>10 cm)
- ☐ Posterior placenta location

Special note:
(a) *Refer to* Kok M, Cnossen J, Gravendeel L, et al. Clinical factors to predict the outcome of external cephalic version: a metaanalysis. *Am J Obstet Gynecol.* 2008;199(6): 630.e1–e5, and
(b) Kok M, Cnossen J, Gravendeel L, Van Der Post JA, Mol BW. Ultrasound factors to predict the outcome of external cephalic version: a meta-analysis. *Ultrasound Obstet Gynecol.* 2009;33(1):76–84

6. Detail important <u>procedural aspects</u> of external cephalic version during the patient consent process. *(1 point per main bullet; max points specified where required)*

Timing:
- ☐ Recommended gestational age for external cephalic version is from 37^{+0} weeks *(ACOG and RCOG)*
  - ○ *RCOG: For nulliparous patients, external cephalic version may be offered as of 36^{+0} weeks*
  - ○ External cephalic version at 34–36 weeks' gestation decreases rates of noncephalic presentations by 19% compared with external cephalic version beginning at 37 weeks, at the expense of increased late-preterm births[$]
  - ○ No upper-gestation limit for external cephalic version procedure in the absence of contraindications

External cephalic version success rate and subsequent management: *(max 3)*
- ☐ Indicate that success rates for external cephalic version is ~50%–60% *(RCOG: 50%; ACOG: ~58%)*
  - ○ Overall, multiparas have higher success rates than nulliparas (60% *vs* 40%, respectively)
  - ○ An external cephalic version attempt should not be based on decision-models predicting success
- ☐ Mention that a fetus may revert to breech by the time of labor (3%)
- ☐ Explain that there is no evidence to support routine immediate induction of labor to minimize reversion
- ☐ Mention that despite successful version, the risk of Cesarean section and instrumental delivery are increased relative to a spontaneous cephalic presentation

Management options when external cephalic version is unsuccessful:
- ☐ Arrange for an elective Cesarean section at ≥39 weeks' gestation if persistent breech presentation
- ☐ Attempt retrial of an external cephalic version
- ☐ Await labor and rare finding of spontaneous version after unsuccessful external cephalic version (3%–7%)

Technical aspects: *(max 5)*
- ☐ Procedure is performed in a hospital facility where surgical delivery is available
- ☐ After ensuring this patient has not been sensitized to D-antigen, obtain consent to administer Rh immunoglobulin within 72 hours for Rh-negative status, regardless of procedure success
  - ○ *ACOG: Rh immunoglobulin is not required if the fetus Rh-negative status is known, D-alloimmunization exists, or delivery is planned within 72 hours when assessment can be performed postpartum*
  - ○ *British Committee for Standards in Haematology*: Routine screening for fetomaternal hemorrhage is recommended to determine women who require additional anti-D immunoglobulin*
- ☐ Consideration for neuraxial analgesia to increase success at external cephalic version; inform the patient she may experience pain
  - ○ *RCOG: Regional or neuraxial analgesia is not routinely recommended, although may be considered for a repeat external cephalic version attempt or where women cannot tolerate the procedure*

- ○ *ACOG: Neuraxial analgesia, in combination with tocolysis, can be considered a reasonable intervention to increase external cephalic version success*
- ○ *No statement presented by SOGC or RANZCOG*
- ☐ Tocolysis may improve procedural-success rates:
  - ▪ *Salbutamol 250 ug in 25 mL of normal saline (10 ug/mL) as slow IV dose* **or**
  - ▪ *Terbutaline 250 ug subcutaneously*
  - ▪ *Insufficient evidence for nifedipine relative to betamimetics*
  - ○ *RCOG and ACOG recommend betamimetics, unless contraindicated*
  - ○ *No statement presented by SOGC or RANZCOG*
- ☐ Fetal well-being and contraction pattern should be assessed pre- and postprocedure (*e.g.,* nonstress test (NST)/electronic fetal monitoring)
  - ○ *ACOG: Either a biophysical profile (BPP) or NST may be used*
- ☐ Intermittent use of real-time sonographic guidance
- ☐ Inform the patient of limited evidence to guide practice of external cephalic version: ≤ 4 attempts for a total maximum duration of 10 minutes has been advised (*RCOG; Collins S et al. BJOG 2007; 114:636–8*)

Risks of external cephalic version:
- ☐ Reassure the patient of very low complication rates with appropriate precautions

Fetal complications:[†]
- ☐ Transient heart rate changes [~5%] (*e.g., bradycardia, decelerations*)
- ☐ IUFD [0.2%]

Maternal complications: *(max 5)*
- ☐ Preterm labor
- ☐ Preterm rupture of membranes (PROM), and possible umbilical cord prolapse
- ☐ Feto-maternal hemorrhage; isoimmunization
- ☐ Vaginal bleeding
- ☐ Placental abruption
- ☐ Uterine rupture[‡]
- ☐ Amniotic fluid embolism
- ☐ Emergency Cesarean section [~0.5% within first 24 hours] (*mostly due to vaginal bleeding or abnormal CTG*)

Special notes:
- § Hutton EK, et al. External cephalic version for breech presentation before term. *Cochrane Database Syst Rev.* 2015;(7):CD000084
- * Qureshi H, et al. *Transfus Med* 2014;24:8–20
- † Rates are provided for academic interest; pooled maternal-fetal complications are ~6%
- ‡ No increased rates among women with one previous low transverse Cesarean section

---

7. Address the patient's query regarding why timing of external cephalic version at 37^{+0} weeks' gestation is preferred. *(1 point each)*

3

- ☐ Preterm delivery would be avoided if emergency Cesarean delivery is required
- ☐ Spontaneous version would have likely occurred by this time
- ☐ Spontaneous reversion to breech presentation is less likely after this gestational age

8. Provide four rationales to teach your trainee why successful external cephalic version remains associated with risk of operative delivery (*i.e.*, Cesarean section or instrumental vaginal) compared with spontaneous cephalic presentations. *(1 point each)*

4

Fetal factors:
☐ Increased risk of unengaged, unmolded cephalic presentation in labor and/or asynclitism
☐ Decreased fetal tolerance to labor due to inherent biological differences between breech- and cephalic-presenting fetuses (*e.g.*, lower birthweight, fetoplacental ratio, and fetal heart rate patterns)

Maternal factors:
☐ Increased labor dystocia due to maternal factors (*e.g.*, pelvic configuration, uterine anomalies)
☐ Increased uterine compliance-associated abnormal uterine contractility

Special note:
Refer to de Hundt M, et al. *Obstet Gynecol.* 2014;123(6):1327–1334.

The patient consents to an attempt at external cephalic version at 37 weeks' gestation. She is curious about the possibility of a vaginal breech birth in case of failed external cephalic version or reversion to breech presentation. You recall that the PREMODA[†] study demonstrated that a cautious approach to planned vaginal breech birth in modern, well-supported obstetric units can be safe for many women; a protocol exists in your hospital center where you are among colleagues with expertise in vaginal breech birth. The patient understands that an emergency Cesarean section is required in about 40% of planned vaginal breech births.

Special note:
† *Refer to* Goffinet F, Carayol M, Foidart JM, et al. Is planned vaginal delivery for breech presentation at term still an option? Results of an observational prospective survey in France and Belgium. *Am J Obstet Gynecol.* 2006;194(4):1002–1011.

9. Discuss fetal/neonatal morbidities and mortality associated with vaginal breech birth and compare mortality rates with Cesarean section. *(1 point each)*

11

Morbidities with vaginal breech delivery:
☐ Risk of cerebral palsy is ~1.5/1000 breech births, *regardless* of planned mode of birth
☐ No increased risk of long-term morbidities or adverse neurological outcomes from vaginal breech delivery compared to Cesarean section
☐ Umbilical cord prolapse (*<1% for frank breech; ~10% for footling breech*)
☐ Lower Apgar scores compared to planned Cesarean section
☐ Dysplasia of the fetal hip
☐ Iatrogenic fetal abdominal trauma
☐ Brachial plexus injury (~1/1000 vaginal breech births)
☐ Fracture of the skull, clavicle, humerus, and/or femur
☐ Entrapment of the aftercoming head

Perinatal mortality: *(2 points)*
☐ Risk is ~2.0/1000 deliveries with vaginal breech birth and ~0.5/1000 deliveries with Cesarean section after 39^{+0} weeks

The patient appreciates your evidence-based information. Although she was contemplating a home breech birth, she now understands that perinatal mortality would be ~10-fold higher than with well-supported planned vaginal breech delivery in hospital.

After the patient's consultation visit, you use this opportunity to teach your trainee on specific aspects related to vaginal breech birth. He or she is aware that international practice variations exist surrounding the role of pelvimetry in determining patient suitability for vaginal breech birth, with some jurisdictions advocating clinical assessment *(SOGC)*, whereas others are either unclear on the role of pelvimetry *(RCOG)* or have not stated recommendations *(ACOG and RANZCOG)*. You teach your trainee that magnetic resonance imaging (MRI) is diversely used in Europe, particularly for nulliparous women, with recent studies showing it may be useful for the preselection and counseling of women with breech presentations.[§]

Special note:

§ *Refer to* Klemt AS, et al. MRI-based pelvimetric measurements as predictors for a successful vaginal breech delivery in the Frankfurt Breech at term cohort (FRABAT). *Eur J Obstet Gynecol Reprod Biol.* 2019; 232:10–17

10. Identify responses you would expect from your trainee regarding your query on <u>fetal contraindications</u> to planned vaginal breech birth. *(1 point each)*	Max 5

☐ Umbilical cord presentation
☐ Footling breech presentation
☐ FGR *(avoid vaginal birth with estimated fetal weight <2800 g or <10th percentile)*
☐ High estimated fetal weight >3800–4000 g
☐ Fetal anomaly likely to cause dystocia or increase fetal morbidity/mortality
☐ Hyperextended fetal neck on ultrasound
☐ Evidence of antenatal fetal compromise

11. Provide three reasons why vaginal delivery of complete or frank breech presentations may be considered, whereas Cesarean delivery is advocated for incomplete/footling breech presentations. *(1 point each)*	3

☐ Passing of large presenting parts (*i.e.*, fetal thighs and trunk) through the birth canal in complete or frank presentations generally implies that aftercoming shoulders and head are likely able to pass through
☐ With incomplete breech, one/both feet can slip through an incompletely dilated cervix, followed by entrapment of the aftercoming shoulders or head
☐ Risk of umbilical cord prolapse with passing of one/both feet and knees through the cervix

12. Your trainee asks you to explain why Cesarean section is preferrable for delivery of growth restricted fetuses in the breech presentation. *(1 point each)*	2

☐ Risk of entrapment of the larger after coming head
☐ Increased likelihood of metabolic acidemia due to cord compression and fetal bradycardia

The following day after successful external cephalic version was performed at 37^{+1} weeks' gestation, the patient returns to the obstetric emergency assessment unit in active labor. The patient is 7 cm dilated, amniotic membranes remain intact, and there is no bleeding. Bedside sonography confirms the fetus has reverted to a frank breech presentation. Cardiotocographic monitoring is normal. The patient declines your offer of an urgent Cesarean section; she remains motivated to attempt a vaginal breech birth, as she had indicated during your extensive prenatal counseling. You inform your obstetric trainee that women presenting in advanced labor do not appear to have an increased perinatal risk.

13. <u>Detail</u> essential elements of your labor management protocol for this patient's planned vaginal breech birth. *(1 point per main bullet)*   10

- ☐ Maintain continuous electronic fetal monitoring in labor
  - ○ *Decreased variability and late decelerations are more prevalent than with vertex deliveries*[†]
  - ○ *If required, a fetal cardiotocographic electrode may be placed into the fetal buttocks*
- ☐ Avoid artificial rupture of membranes without clear indication while continuing to monitor for risk of cord prolapse; immediate vaginal examination is required after spontaneous rupture of amniotic membranes
- ☐ Neuraxial analgesia may be offered, provided maternal expulsive effort is not impaired
  - ○ *Pudental nerve block is also an option*
- ☐ With patient consent, oxytocin augmentation may be considered where contraction frequency is <4 in 10 minutes *(according to local protocol)*
- ☐ Allow up to two hours for labor progress with adequate uterine contractions, after which Cesarean section should be considered if labor progress is inadequate
- ☐ Arrange for an experienced clinician to establish the timing of full dilatation given its subjectivity as the cervix remains palpable during descent of the fetal trunk; diagnosis of full dilatation is related to the descent of the breech
- ☐ Allow 90 minutes for the passive second stage to maximize breech descent into the pelvis
  - ○ *RCOG: if the breech is not visible within two hours of passive second stage, Cesarean section should be recommended*
- ☐ Aim to achieve delivery, or ensure delivery is imminent, after 60 minutes of active second stage
- ☐ Birth in an operating room/theater is not routinely recommended *(RCOG)*
- ☐ Ensure multidisciplinary personnel are present for delivery *(i.e., anesthesia, neonatology, nursing/midwifery)*

Special note:

† *Refer to* Toivonen E et al. Cardiotocography in breech versus vertex delivery: an examiner-blinded, cross-sectional nested case-control study. *BMC Pregnancy Childbirth.* 2016;16 (1):319. Published 2016 Oct 21.

14. Elaborate on technical aspects related to vaginal breech delivery which you would teach your trainee either theoretically or using the hands-on breech training model in your unit. *(1 point each)*

Max 10

☐ Ensure an experienced operator is present at the delivery; presence of an assistant is recommended at vaginal breech birth *(particularly when procedures are necessary)*

☐ Avoid fetal traction; effective maternal and uterine power is essential to safe delivery

☐ Await spontaneous descent to the umbilicus prior to performing breech delivery maneuvers, unless there is poor tone, color, or delay more than five minutes from buttocks to the head or more than three minutes from the umbilicus to the head *(RCOG)*

☐ Consider placing a **warm** towel on the breech at delivery *(may help avoid fetal gasping with yet undelivered head)*

☐ Maintain the fetal trunk <45° above the horizontal plane of the birth canal *(neck extension risks cervical spine injury or death)*

☐ Gently guide the breech to remain in, or achieve, a sacrum-anterior position

☐ Exercise care by avoiding trauma to fetal abdominal soft tissues; support the fetus by grasping the pelvic girdle

☐ Perform principal eponymous maneuvers to assist in delivery of the limbs: legs (Pinard) and delivery of nuchal arms (Løveset), as required

☐ Verify umbilical cord pulsation after delivery of the legs

☐ Delivery of the fetal head may occur by three means: (a) spontaneously, with assistance of suprapubic pressure; (b) Mauriceau-Smellie-Veit maneuver; (c) with assistance of Piper forceps

☐ Selective rather than routine episiotomy is recommended

15. Regarding avoidance of fetal traction, you teach your trainee, 'do not pull on a breech': explain the physiological reason for this recommendation.

2

☐ Excessive manipulation can lead to the Moro reflex (extension of the yet undelivered fetal arms and neck)

Labor management ensues according to your intrapartum care plan. The patient progresses well and is brought to the operating room in the active second stage in accordance with your institutional protocol. Attending to your request for Piper forceps, your nursing assistant presents you with the following instruments, as she is uncertain which you prefer.

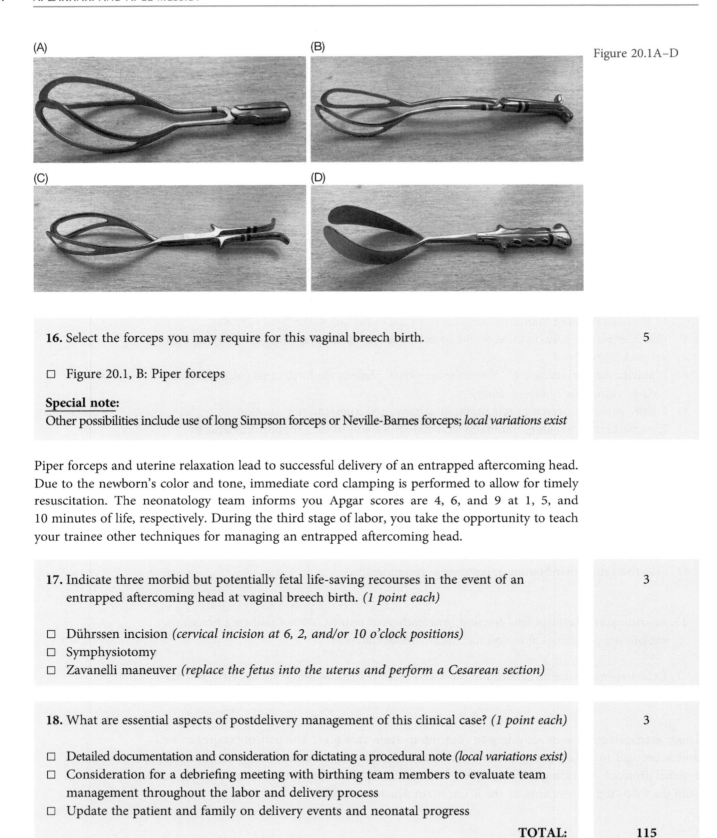

(A)   (B)   Figure 20.1A–D

(C)   (D)

16. Select the forceps you may require for this vaginal breech birth.   5

☐ Figure 20.1, B: Piper forceps

Special note:
Other possibilities include use of long Simpson forceps or Neville-Barnes forceps; *local variations exist*

Piper forceps and uterine relaxation lead to successful delivery of an entrapped aftercoming head. Due to the newborn's color and tone, immediate cord clamping is performed to allow for timely resuscitation. The neonatology team informs you Apgar scores are 4, 6, and 9 at 1, 5, and 10 minutes of life, respectively. During the third stage of labor, you take the opportunity to teach your trainee other techniques for managing an entrapped aftercoming head.

17. Indicate three morbid but potentially fetal life-saving recourses in the event of an   3
entrapped aftercoming head at vaginal breech birth. *(1 point each)*

☐ Dührssen incision *(cervical incision at 6, 2, and/or 10 o'clock positions)*
☐ Symphysiotomy
☐ Zavanelli maneuver *(replace the fetus into the uterus and perform a Cesarean section)*

18. What are essential aspects of postdelivery management of this clinical case? *(1 point each)*   3

☐ Detailed documentation and consideration for dictating a procedural note *(local variations exist)*
☐ Consideration for a debriefing meeting with birthing team members to evaluate team management throughout the labor and delivery process
☐ Update the patient and family on delivery events and neonatal progress

TOTAL: 115

CHAPTER 21

Amniotic Fluid Embolism and Disseminated Intravascular Coagulation

Roupen Hatzakorzian and Amira El-Messidi

During an obstetrics call duty in your tertiary center, you are called urgently to assist in a Cesarean section of a 42-year-old with sudden intraoperative maternal collapse. Your surgical colleague followed her prenatal care.

LEARNING OBJECTIVES

1. Elicit significant risk factors and clinical characteristics in evaluation of intrapartum maternal collapse, recognizing principal pregnancy- and non-pregnancy-related causes
2. Maintain a high index of suspicion for amniotic fluid embolism (AFE) and understand the principles involved in achieving hemodynamic stability
3. Anticipate consumptive coagulopathy, and appreciate the importance of a multidisciplinary team in obstetric emergencies
4. Detail the therapeutic treatments involved in management of AFE and disseminated intravascular coagulopathy (DIC)
5. Appreciate the importance of detailed documentation, generally performed after the acute event; contemporaneous note-keeping should be provided by a designated scriber
6. Recognize that debriefing with the patient and/or family is a component of holistic maternity care, and among staff involved

SUGGESTED READINGS

1. Chu J, Johnston TA, Geoghegan J. Royal College of Obstetricians and Gynaecologists. Maternal collapse in pregnancy and the puerperium: Green-Top Guideline No. 56. *BJOG*. 2020;127(5):e14–e52.
2. Clark SL, Romero R, Dildy GA, et al. Proposed diagnostic criteria for the case definition of amniotic fluid embolism in research studies. *Am J Obstet Gynecol*. 2016 Oct;215(4):408–412.
3. Lipman S, Cohen S, Einav S, et al. The Society for Obstetric Anesthesia and Perinatology consensus statement on the management of cardiac arrest in pregnancy. *Anesth Analg*. 2014 May;118(5):1003–1016.
4. Pacheco LD, Clark SL, Klassen M, et al. Amniotic fluid embolism: principles of early clinical management. *Am J Obstet Gynecol*. 2020 Jan;222(1):48–52.
5. Pacheco LD, Saade GR, Costantine MM, et al. An update on the use of massive transfusion protocols in obstetrics. *Am J Obstet Gynecol*. 2016 Mar;214(3):340–344. [Erratum in *Am J Obstet Gynecol*. 2017 Jan;216(1):76]

6. Royal College of Obstetricians and Gynaecologists (RCOG) Green-Top Guideline No. 47: Blood transfusion in obstetrics, May 2015. Available at www.rcog.org.uk/en/guidelines-research-services/guidelines/gtg47/. Accessed November 22, 2020.

7. Shamshirsaz AA, Clark SL. Amniotic fluid embolism. *Obstet Gynecol Clin N Am.* 2016; 43:779–790.

8. Society for Maternal-Fetal Medicine (SMFM) Clinical Guideline No. 9, with the assistance of Pacheco LD, Saade G, Hankins GD, et al. Amniotic fluid embolism: diagnosis and management. *Am J Obstet Gynecol.* 2016 Aug;215(2):B16–24.

9. Sultan P, Seligman K, Carvalho B. Amniotic fluid embolism: update and review. *Curr Opin Anesthesiol.* 2016; 29:288–296.

10. Wada H, Matsumoto T, Yamashita Y. Diagnosis and treatment of disseminated intravascular coagulation (DIC) according to four DIC guidelines. *J Intensive Care* 2014; 2(15):1–8.

POINTS

1. Which aspects of a focused history would you inquire about, or general observations you would make, upon entering the surgical suite?

12

Observations: *(1 point each; max 6 points)*
☐ Establish whether the fetus has been delivered
☐ Establish if the placenta has been delivered and whether manual removal was performed
☐ Presence of maternal hemorrhage and/or uterine atony
☐ Premonitory symptoms, if conscious (*e.g.*, agitation, restlessness, anxiety, dyspnea)
☐ Mode of anesthesia (general vs regional)
☐ Clinical staff attending for help
☐ BMI
☐ Ethnicity (African)

Maternal characteristics: *(from team members in operating theater) (1 point each; max 3)*
☐ Indication and grade of urgency for Cesarean section
☐ Known placenta previa
☐ Gravidity, parity, gestational age, and number of prior Cesarean deliveries, if any
☐ Preexisting hypertensive disorder of pregnancy or coagulopathy
☐ Allergies

Details of cardiovascular collapse: *(1 point each; max 3)*
☐ Oxygen saturation and supplementation
☐ Hypotension, arrhythmia, or cardiac arrest
☐ Ensure early mobilization of blood products
☐ Resuscitative treatments thus far
☐ Seizure onset, if any

Quickly, you learn the patient is a healthy G6P5 with a spontaneous dichorionic pregnancy who was admitted in early labor at 38^{+1} weeks' gestation. Her prenatal course was unremarkable. Given prior precipitous deliveries, she initially declined regional anesthesia. With recurrent late decelerations on electronic fetal monitoring of the presenting twin, an amniotomy was performed at 4 cm dilatation, revealing thick meconium-stained amniotic fluid. Despite intrauterine resuscitation, fetal heart tracing of this twin remained abnormal, and spontaneous uterine hyperstimulation ensued. The patient verbally consented for an emergency Cesarean section. The patient was not bleeding and did not have intrapartum fever.

You note the patient's obese habitus and her African heritage. The patient is agitated, claiming a sense of doom. A spinal anesthetic was administered, and the surgical procedure recently commenced; the hysterotomy has not yet been performed and you see the patient is not hemorrhaging.

Scrubbed in to assist your colleague and assistant obstetric trainee, the anesthesiologist alerts you of the patient's rapidly deteriorating status:

- Blood pressure (BP) is 60/30 mmHg, unresponsive to a total of 0.6 mg IV phenylephrine,
- Sinus tachycardia at 130 bpm,
- Respiratory rate at 40 breaths/min,
- Oxygen saturation is 82% on 100% mask-FiO2

Both the anesthesia and nursing teams have called for experts' immediate assistance.

With ongoing active resuscitation, you are considering causes of respiratory arrest in this otherwise healthy parturient. In liaison with the anesthetic team, simultaneous investigations and treatments are underway, aiming to achieve hemodynamic stability.

2. Discuss your diagnostic differential for cardiorespiratory collapse in a parturient.

11

Obstetrical causes: *(1 point each; max 5)*
- ☐ AFE
- ☐ Peripartum cardiomyopathy
- ☐ Placental abruption
- ☐ Eclampsia
- ☐ Hemorrhagic shock
- ☐ Uterine rupture
- ☐ Uterine atony

Nonobstetrical causes: *(1 point each; max 4)*
- ☐ Pulmonary embolism
- ☐ Air embolism
- ☐ Septic shock
- ☐ Anaphylaxis
- ☐ Aortic dissection
- ☐ Myocardial infarction

Anesthetic causes: *(1 point each; max 2)*
- ☐ High spinal blockade
- ☐ Aspiration
- ☐ Anesthetic toxicity

3. A 12-lead ECG has been initiated. Indicate which <u>investigations</u> are most relevant in the evaluation and management of this patient.

10

Serum:[‡] *(1 point each; max 7)*
☐ CBC *(hemoglobin and platelet count)*
☐ Coagulation profile *(aPTT, PT, INR, fibrinogen)*
☐ Electrolytes: including calcium, magnesium, and phosphate
☐ Creatinine
☐ Liver enzymes and function tests
☐ Cardiac troponins
☐ Lactate
☐ Mast cell tryptase *(may be useful in confirming if maternal collapse is due to anaphylaxis)*
☐ Brain natriuretic peptide (BNP)

Imaging/other tests: *(1 point each for 3 points)*
☐ Transesophageal or transthoracic echocardiography *(TEE or TTE, respectively)*
☐ Arterial blood gas *(pH, PO$_2$, PCO$_2$, base excess)*
☐ Bedside chest X-ray

Special note:
‡ Blood type and antibody screen should be ordered, if not available at admission by standard institutional protocol

As the intraoperative team awaits test results, the patient has refractory hypotension and continued hypoxemia. Her level of consciousness is fluctuating. In addition to extra anesthesiologists and nurses, other medical experts[†] have promptly arrived, as routine according to your institutional protocol for obstetric emergencies. Apart from tachycardia and ST-segment and T-wave changes consistent for right ventricular strain, there is no suggestion of ischemia or infarction.

Special note:
† Other experts may include intensivists, hematologists, maternal-fetal medicine experts

4. Which blood products do you anticipate might be requested on site? *(1 point each)*

4

☐ Packed red blood cells
☐ Fresh frozen plasma – to correct the INR and PTT
☐ Platelets *(aim >50 × 10^9/L)*
☐ Cryoprecipitate *(aim fibrinogen >150–200 mg/dL)*

Special note:
Packed red blood cells, fresh frozen plasma, platelets given in a 1:1:1 ratio (hemostatic resuscitation) before laboratory results; theoretically, this minimizes dilutional coagulopathy and third spacing

The surgical suite contains many team members. You hear the anesthetic team request blood products be made available as soon as possible, while you proceed with surgery.

5. Describe the best mode of communication in acute situations involving numerous professionals.

2

☐ Closed-loop communication *(directing specific tasks to particular individuals)*

While the request for specific blood products is made by the anesthetic team, your obstetric trainee whispers that another clotting factor may be necessary in the event of hemorrhage.

6-A. What is the most likely clotting factor your trainee is considering?

1

☐ Recombinant activated factor VII (rFVIIa)

6-B. Aside from high cost, respond to your trainee as to why rFVIIa is not a cornerstone of resuscitation. *(1 point each)*

2

☐ Serious arterial and venous thromboses, makes this a last resort to treating hemorrhage
☐ Increased mortality when used in AFE *(Leighton BL et al. Anesthesiology 2011;115:1201–8)*

7. Outline the comprehensive principles involved in the initial management of the patient at this time. *(1 point each)*

Max 8

Fetal health:
☐ Expedite delivery
☐ Ensure presence of the neonatology team, *if not already present* (especially given multiple gestation)

Circulatory compromise:
☐ Ensure adequate peripheral and central venous access
☐ Early activation of institutional 'Massive Transfusion Protocol,' where available
☐ Judicious IV crystalloids; avoid boluses *(worsens right ventricular failure)*
☐ For refractory hypotension, direct-acting vasopressors and inotropes are adjuncts to optimize perfusion pressure[†]
☐ Prepare to initiate cardiopulmonary resuscitation in the event of cardiac arrest and/or severe hypotension

Respiratory compromise:
☐ Correct hypoxemia to maintain oxygenation close to 100% *(anesthesia team to consider intubation and ventilation)*
☐ Sputum or blood aspirates during intubation can be examined for fetal elements to support a diagnosis of AFE

Special note:
† Vasopressors include phenylephrine; inotropes include epinephrine, norepinephrine, vasopressin, dobutamine, and milrinone; vasopressin is generally reserved to the period after delivery

Assisting your colleague, you proceed to deliver the male fetuses expeditiously, both of whom are requiring resuscitation. The placentas deliver spontaneously, and manual uterine exploration is performed, to ensure absence of remaining tissues of conception. You ask for prompt administration of IV oxytocic agents.

Meanwhile, the anesthesiologist indicates that her BP by cuff remains 50/30 mmHg without a detectable pulse and her heart rate is 140 bpm. Intubation and ventilation are in progress; central and arterial lines are placed. Norepinephrine and epinephrine infusions are initiated. As the patient is already in left-lateral tilt for Cesarean delivery, cardiopulmonary resuscitation is initiated, and an intensivist will perform a TEE.

---

8. Identify two advantages of expediting delivery in the resuscitative process. *(1 point each)*   2

☐ Aid to improve perinatal neurologically intact survival
☐ Facilitate maternal resuscitative efforts by improving right heart venous return

---

9. Which anatomical or physiological findings on TEE or TTE could be compatible with an AFE? *(1 point each)*   Max 3

☐ Severe right ventricular dilatation and hypokinetic function (acute cor pulmonale)
☐ Elevated pulmonary artery pressure
☐ Underfilling of the left ventricle with left septal shift
☐ Severe tricuspid regurgitation

Special note:
Right ventricular failure characterizes early phase; left ventricular failure characterises second phase of AFE

After five minutes of cardiopulmonary resuscitation, a pulse is detected and BP is 85/50 mmHg. The patient remains on high doses of inotropic support and on 70% FiO_2. Laboratory investigations reveal the following findings:

		Reference ranges
Arterial blood gas		
pH	7.25	7.40–7.47
PaO_2 (mmHg)	70	90–104
$PaCO_2$ (mmHg)	40	27–34
Bicarbonate (mEq/L)	17	18–22
Lactate (mmol/L)	6.0	0.0–2.0
CBC and coagulation tests		
Hemoglobin (g/L)	75	110–140
Platelets ($\times 10^9$/L)	45	150–400
INR	1.7	0.9–1.0
aPTT (seconds)	55	26.3–39.4
Fibrinogen (mg/dL)	90	200–400

After return of spontaneous circulation, the intensivist performs a TEE: there is right ventricular dilatation with moderate dysfunction, reduced left ventricular function with an ejection fraction (LVEF) of 40% (normal >60%) and underfilling of the left ventricle.

10-A. What are your most likely diagnoses? *(1 point each)*   3

☐ AFE
☐ Coagulation dysfunction/DIC
☐ Metabolic acidosis

10-B. Using the Modified International Society on Thrombosis and Hemostasis (ISTH)   4
      scoring system* for overt DIC in pregnancy, justify your diagnosis of DIC by calculating
      her score. *(1 point each)*

☐ Patient's score is 5 (*i.e.,* ≥3 is compatible with overt DIC)

	score
☐ Platelets <50,000/mL	2
☐ Prothrombin time or INR >50% increased	2
☐ Fibrinogen <200 mg/dL	1

(Suggested Reading 1)

Special note:
Coagulopathy must be detected *before* hemorrhage can itself account for DIC

11-A. Although no clinical or demographic risk factor can predict AFE to justify a change   Max 7
      in obstetric practice, identify possible contributing factors for AFE in *this* patient.
      (1 point each)

☐ Advanced maternal age
☐ Multiple gestation
☐ Grand-multiparity (≥5 *live births or stillbirths*)
☐ Obesity
☐ Cesarean delivery
☐ Ethnic origin
☐ Fetal distress
☐ Male fetal genders

Special note:
Patient's uterine hyperstimulation or tachysystole is not believed to be a risk factor for AFE due to the decrease or arrest in maternal-placental exchange when uterine pressure exceeds maternal venous pressure (*Clark SL et al. Am J Obstet Gynecol 1995; 172:1158–67*)

11-B. Indicate five other possible risk markers for AFE, not particular to this patient.
  (1 point each)

5

- ☐ Hypertensive disorders of pregnancy
- ☐ Abnormal placentation: previa, accreta, or abruptio
- ☐ Abdominal trauma
- ☐ Uterine rupture
- ☐ Cervical lacerations
- ☐ Precipitous labor
- ☐ Instrumental delivery
- ☐ Polyhydramnios
- ☐ Induction of labor *(inconsistent evidence)*

Given the complex pathophysiology of AFE, whereby coagulopathy is a prominent feature in ~85% of patients, your trainee plans to research the proposed inciting factors for DIC among patients with AFE.

12. Provide two evidence-based rationales for the relationship between AFE and coagulopathy.

2

Procoagulant theory:
- ☐ Tissue factor in amniotic fluid binds Factor VII to activate the extrinsic pathway

Anticoagulant theory:
- ☐ Plasminogen activator inhibitor-1 in amniotic fluid causes fibrinolysis

The uterus is now atonic despite multiple uterotonic agents. Bleeding continues throughout the endometrial surface. Although tissues are friable at the hysterotomy site, you manage to perform one-layer incisional closure, although no further surgical maneuvers are possible due to the progressing coagulopathy. The anesthesiologist now notes spontaneous bleeding from venipuncture sites. Although minimal urine output, no hematuria is noted.

Together, your team decides to pack the abdomen, leave sponges in-situ until closure the following day. Broad-spectrum IV antibiotics have been initiated.

13. Apart from uterotonic agents, what is your most conservative temporary approach to provide uterine tamponade?

1

- ☐ Intraoperative Bakri® Balloon placement‡
  - ○ *Inflated with 300–600 mL of fluid*

Special note:
‡ Other devices possible for mechanical compression; patient instability does not favor consideration of transfer for uterine artery embolization or surgical procedures including vessel ligation, B-Lynch or other brace sutures

On pressure support, her BP becomes 110/50 mmHg and heart rate is 100 bpm. The patient received the following blood replacement therapy:

- 6 U packed red blood cells
- 6 U fresh frozen plasma
- 10 U platelets
- 10 U cryoprecipitate

Intubated, she is transferred to the ICU (ITU).

14. After the patient is stabilized for transfer to a monitored setting, what are essential aspects of postacute care? *(1 point per main bullet)*

4

☐ Arrange for a debriefing meeting with the entire multidisciplinary care team
☐ Update family on medical events and offer psychosocial counseling:
  ○ High maternal mortality rate *(overall mortality 20%–60%)*
  ○ Increased neurological morbidity due to cerebral anoxia *(up to 85% of survivors)*
☐ Communicate with the neonatology team for updates on newborns' status
  ○ Neonatal outcome is generally poor: mortality rates may be 25%, with only 50% neurologically intact survival *(among singletons)*
☐ Detailed documentation

Her husband asks whether the primary goal of transferring the patient is due to her intubated status.

15. Outline the immediate measures or goals required in the intensively monitored setting. *(1 point per main bullet)*

Max 5

☐ Maintain oxygenation at pulse oximetry value of 94%–98%
  ○ Avoid 100% oxygen administration after survival of a cardiac arrest *(may worsen ischemia-reperfusion injury)*
☐ Maintain perfusion with a mean arterial pressure of 65 mmHg
☐ Continue correction of the coagulopathy
☐ Maintain mild therapeutic hypothermia at 32°–36°C for 12–24 hours to improve neurologic outcome and decrease maternal mortality
  ○ *Temperature is preferably kept closer to 36°C due to concomitant risk of hemorrhage*
☐ Maintain serum glucose at 8–10 mmol/L (140–180 mg/dL)
☐ Continue to eliminate competing etiologies *(i.e., AFE is a diagnosis of exclusion)*

As the patient is being transferred to a closely monitored setting, your obstetric trainee realizes that this may be the only career encounter of AFE, given its low prevalence at 1–10/100,000 deliveries. He or she thereby wants to maximize the learning experience from this clinical scenario.

16. Although uniform international consensus for the diagnosis of AFE is lacking, discuss the most widely standardized criteria for *research* reporting. *(1 point each)*

SMFM and AFE Foundation, 2016 *(Suggested Reading 2)*[§]

All criteria must be met:[‡]

☐ Acute hypotension (with systolic BP <90 mmHg) <u>OR</u> cardiac arrest
☐ Acute respiratory compromise (*i.e.,* hypoxia <90% saturation, cyanosis, or dyspnea)
☐ Overt DIC
☐ Clinical manifestations occur in labor or Cesarean section, appearing within 30 minutes of placental delivery
   ○ *Rarely occurs at pregnancy termination or amniocentesis*
☐ No fever (≥ 38.0 °C) in labor

Special notes:

§ RCOG Green-Top Guideline No. 56 recommendation for future research is to investigate the best diagnostic and management strategies for AFE

‡ (1) Fetal squames in maternal pulmonary circulation are not diagnostic – may exist without clinical features of AFE *(Lee W, et al. Am J Obstet Gynecol 1986; 155:999–1001)*; (2) laboratory and pathology findings are nonessential elements for diagnosis

17. What are novel, and possibly controversial, approaches in establishing hemodynamic stability in suspected AFE? *(1 point per main bullet)*

☐ Extracorporeal membrane oxygenation (ECMO):
   ○ *Useful in cases without return of spontaneous circulation after cardiac arrest*
   ○ *Associated with bleeding in patients with AFE due to the need for anticoagulation*
☐ Inhaled nitric oxide or inhaled/IV nitroglycerin
   ○ *Decreases pulmonary afterload; allows for direct pulmonary vasodilation*
☐ Ventricular assist device

The patient's body temperature is cooled, and she is closely monitored for end-organ damage. Moderate cardiogenic pulmonary edema appears on chest X-ray, with appropriate furosemide-induced diuresis. Over the next 24 hours, she is gradually weaned from cardio-respiratory support, requiring low-dose norepinephrine to maintain systolic BP >100 mmHg. She is alert and responds appropriately to command. Repeat TTE shows near-normal left ventricular function with mild right-sided dysfunction. Serum laboratory investigations reveal:

- Lactate 2.0 mmol/L
- Hemoglobin 95 g/L
- Platelets 90 × 10^9/L
- INR 1.3
- aPTT 45 seconds

Bleeding has subsided and the patient returns for surgical removal of the packing and abdominal closure.

The patient is extubated 48 hours after this catastrophic life event and has not sustained any organ deficits. After an eight-day hospital stay, she is discharged with resolution of her cardiovascular function.

18. With focus on her <u>delivery events</u>, what are important elements to discuss at this patient's postpartum visit? *(1 point per main bullet, unless specified)*	Max 3

☐ Inform her that risk of recurrence is unknown, though appears low
   ○ Successful pregnancies are reported
☐ Transfusion-related risk of developing alloantibodies causing fetal/neonatal hemolytic disease *(2 points)*
☐ Continue to offer psychosocial support, *as necessary*

                                                      TOTAL: **95**

CHAPTER 22

Postpartum Hemorrhage

Amira El-Messidi and Glenn D. Posner

During an obstetrics call duty in your tertiary center, you are called urgently to assist in the management of vaginal bleeding in a 42-year-old G7P5A2 after recent vaginal delivery of dichorionic twins at term. Although your colleague was anticipating delivery in the operating room/theater, deliveries occurred in the labor suite. Due to a concurrent emergency, the obstetrician has just stepped out of the patient's room, leaving the junior trainee to continue assisting you in the care of this patient.

Special note: _For comprehensive presentation of resources, clinical, and academic subject matter, the 'Suggested Readings' list for this chapter exceeds 10._

LEARNING OBJECTIVES

1. Elicit significant clinical features in evaluation of early (primary) postpartum hemorrhage, recognizing principal etiologies and related management considerations
2. Demonstrate a detailed understanding of pharmaceutical agents, nonsurgical mechanical methods, and surgical approaches for atonic postpartum hemorrhage
3. Understand early and late complications of postpartum hemorrhage
4. Appreciate the importance of interprofessional collaboration and early initiation of protocols in acute obstetric emergencies

SUGGESTED READINGS

1. (a) ACOG: Committee on Practice Bulletins-Obstetrics. Practice Bulletin No. 183: Postpartum hemorrhage. _Obstet Gynecol._ 2017;130(4):e168–e186.
   (b) ACOG: Quantitative blood loss in obstetric hemorrhage: ACOG Committee Opinion No. 794. _Obstet Gynecol._ 2019;134(6):e150–e156.
2. Bienstock JL, Eke AC, Hueppchen NA. Postpartum hemorrhage. _N Engl J Med._ 2021;384(17): 1635–1645.
3. (a) Begley CM, Gyte GM, Devane D, et al. Active versus expectant management for women in the third stage of labour. _Cochrane Database Syst Rev._ 2019;2(2):CD007412.
   (b) Diaz V, Abalos E, Carroli G. Methods for blood loss estimation after vaginal birth. _Cochrane Database Syst Rev._ 2018;9(9):CD010980.
   (c) Gallos ID, Papadopoulou A, Man R, et al. Uterotonic agents for preventing postpartum haemorrhage: a network meta-analysis. _Cochrane Database Syst Rev._ 2018;12(12):CD011689.

(d) Hofmeyr GJ, Mshweshwe NT, Gülmezoglu AM. Controlled cord traction for the third stage of labour. *Cochrane Database Syst Rev.* 2015;1(1):CD008020.

(e) Parry Smith WR, Papadopoulou A, Thomas E, et al. Uterotonic agents for first-line treatment of postpartum haemorrhage: a network meta-analysis. *Cochrane Database Syst Rev.* 2020;11(11):CD012754.

(f) Kumar N, Jahanfar S, Haas DM, et al. Umbilical vein injection for management of retained placenta. *Cochrane Database Syst Rev.* 2021;3(3):CD001337.

(g) Soltani H, Hutchon DR, Poulose TA. Timing of prophylactic uterotonics for the third stage of labour after vaginal birth. *Cochrane Database Syst Rev.* 2010;(8):CD006173.

(h) Shakur H, Beaumont D, Pavord S, et al. Antifibrinolytic drugs for treating primary postpartum haemorrhage. *Cochrane Database Syst Rev.* 2018;2(2):CD012964.

4. (a) FIGO Guidelines. Safe Motherhood and Newborn Health Committee; International Federation of Gynecology and Obstetrics. Non-pneumatic anti-shock garment to stabilize women with hypovolemic shock secondary to obstetric hemorrhage. *Int J Gynaecol Obstet.* 2015;128(3):194–195.

(b) FIGO: Morris JL, Winikoff B, Dabash R, et al. FIGO's updated recommendations for misoprostol used alone in gynecology and obstetrics. *Int J Gynaecol Obstet.* 2017;138(3):363–366.

5. Gerdessen L, Meybohm P, Choorapoikayil S, et al. Comparison of common perioperative blood loss estimation techniques: a systematic review and meta-analysis. *J Clin Monit Comput.* 2021;35(2):245–258.

6. Leduc D, Senikas V, Lalonde AB. No. 235 – active management of the third stage of labour: prevention and treatment of postpartum hemorrhage. *J Obstet Gynaecol Can.* 2018;40(12): e841–e855.

7. Matsubara S, Yano H, Ohkuchi A, et al. Uterine compression sutures for postpartum hemorrhage: an overview. *Acta Obstet Gynecol Scand.* 2013;92(4):378–385.

8. Mavrides E, Allard S, Chandraharan E, et al. Prevention and management of postpartum haemorrhage. Green-Top Guideline No. 52. *BJOG* 2016;124:e106–e149.

9. Muñoz M, Stensballe J, Ducloy-Bouthors AS, et al. Patient blood management in obstetrics: prevention and treatment of postpartum haemorrhage. A NATA consensus statement. *Blood Transfus.* 2019;17(2):112–136.

10. Pacheco LD, Saade GR, Hankins GDV. Medical management of postpartum hemorrhage: An update. *Semin Perinatol.* 2019;43(1):22–26.

11. Sentilhes L, Goffinet F, Vayssière C, et al. Comparison of postpartum haemorrhage guidelines: discrepancies underline our lack of knowledge. *BJOG.* 2017;124(5):718–722.

12. Queensland Clinical Guidelines. Postpartum haemorrhage. Guideline No. MN18.1-V9-R23 Queensland Health. 2020. Available at www.health.qld.gov.au/qcg. Accessed June 17, 2021.

13. Weeks AD, Fawcus S. Management of the third stage of labour: (for the Optimal Intrapartum Care series edited by Mercedes Bonet, Femi Oladapo and Metin Gülmezoglu). *Best Pract Res Clin Obstet Gynaecol.* 2020;67:65–79.

14. Wendel MP, Shnaekel KL, Magann EF. Uterine inversion: a review of a life-threatening obstetrical emergency. *Obstet Gynecol Surv.* 2018;73(7):411–417.

15. (a) WHO Recommendations: Tang J, Kapp N, Dragoman M, et al. WHO recommendations for misoprostol use for obstetric and gynecologic indications. *Int J Gynaecol Obstet.* 2013;121(2):186–189.

(b) *WHO Recommendation on Tranexamic Acid for the Treatment of Postpartum Haemorrhage.* Geneva: World Health Organization; 2017.

(c) *WHO Recommendation on Uterine Balloon Tamponade for the Treatment of Postpartum Haemorrhage.* Geneva: World Health Organization; 2021.

(d) *WHO Recommendations: Uterotonics for the Prevention of Postpartum Haemorrhage.* Geneva: World Health Organization; 2018.

POINTS

1. What aspects of a focused history would you inquire about, or general observations would you make, upon entering the delivery suite? *(1 point per main or subbullet; max points specified per section)*

Max 25

Observations: *(max 8)*
☐ Expeditious visual estimation of blood loss on amniotic fluid-soaked sponges, drapes and presence of ongoing bleeding
☐ Determine whether the placenta(s) delivered, including antenatal sonographic location
☐ Presence of premonitory symptoms (*e.g.*, agitation, restlessness, anxiety, dyspnea)
☐ Note whether oxygen via face mask has been initiated[$]
☐ Assess whether the head of the bed is lowered
☐ Presence of two intravenous access sites *(large bore)*
☐ Presence of an indwelling bladder catheter *(assists uterine contraction and monitoring of output)*
☐ Presence of warming devices (*e.g.*, blankets, warm intravenous crystalloid, room temperature)
☐ Body mass index (BMI)
☐ Other clinical staff attending for help (*e.g.*, nursing, midwifery, anesthetic, obstetric)

Clinical measures and/or maneuvers for bleeding control [*assuming placental delivery*]: *(max 7)*
☐ Blood pressure, pulse rate, and pulse oximetry
☐ Assess the type, dose, and frequency of uterotonic agent(s) used
☐ Assess level of pain control and determine mode of labor analgesia, if any
☐ Inquire about last known hemoglobin concentration[#]
☐ Determine whether bimanual uterine massage has been attempted
☐ Inquire about uterine revision/internal examination to ensure evacuation of clots and/or placental fragments
☐ Inquire if careful inspection for lacerations of the cervix, vagina, and perineum has been performed
☐ Other maneuvers (*e.g.*, intrauterine balloon tamponade)

Details related to labor and delivery: *(max 4)*
☐ Determine whether this is a vaginal birth after previous Cesarean (VBAC)
☐ Labor mode (*i.e.*, induction/spontaneous) and rate (*i.e.*, prolonged active phase[†] or precipitous)
☐ Intrapartum use of oxytocin for labor augmentation or therapeutic use of magnesium sulfate
☐ Use of instrumental vaginal delivery with/without an episiotomy or spontaneous laceration
☐ Known chorioamnionitis

Maternal characteristics: *(max 6)*
- ☐ Prior postpartum hemorrhage and its successful treatments
- ☐ Prior uterine surgeries including dilatations and evacuations *(i.e., at prior deliveries or in relation to prior early pregnancy losses)*
- ☐ Gestational complications or antecedent medical features: *(1 point per subbullet)*
  - ○ Hypertensive disorder of pregnancy
  - ○ Bleeding diathesis or known hypercoagulopathy/gestational thromboembolic event
  - ○ Asthma *(preferred avoidance of 15-methyl-prostaglandin $F_{2\alpha}$ [carboprost])*[‡]
  - ○ HIV status in relation to use of protease inhibitors *(use of ergometrine would be contraindicated)*
- ☐ Recent administration of anticoagulants
- ☐ Allergies

Special notes:
- § Oxygen 10–15 L/min via face mask is recommended regardless of maternal oxygen saturation *(RCOG[8] and Queensland Clinical Guideline[12])*
- # Parturient's hemoglobin should be determined at delivery admission, unless recently available without risk factors for postpartum hemorrhage *(NATA[9])*
- † Defined as >12-hour duration – Nyfløt LT, Stray-Pedersen B, Forsén L, Vangen S. Duration of labor and the risk of severe postpartum hemorrhage: A case-control study. *PLoS One* 2017;12(4):e0175306.
- ‡ Refer to Question 13 in Chapter 35

You observe an excessive amount of blood on the delivery drapes and the floor, where at least 15 bloody sponges lay aligned in sequence. The patient is healthy, body habitus appears normal, and she remains conversant despite complaining of abdominopelvic pain. The well-functioning epidural was inserted just over an hour ago upon admission with spontaneous rupture of amniotic membranes of the presenting twin with idiopathic polyhydramnios. All prior deliveries were spontaneous and uncomplicated. You notice a used vacuum cup on the delivery tray and learn that instrumental delivery was prompted by bradycardia of the second twin. As the patient lays in the dorsal lithotomy position with an intravenous line per arm and an oxygen face mask, continuous pulse oximetry readings show >95% saturation and most recent blood pressure is 90/50 mmHg with a pulse rate at 115 bpm; an indwelling bladder catheter was just inserted, draining a large volume of clear-colored urine.

Actively pulling both short-appearing umbilical cords while simultaneously massaging the uterine fundus, where the placentas are known to be implanted, the novice trainee's arm providing traction appears to tremble. You prompt release of undue cord traction accompanied by *suprapubic* pressure as you prepare to assist in care. The trainee had recently initiated prophylactic oxytocin alone[†] as a component of active management of the third stage of labor.[§] You intend to later teach your trainee that while controlled cord traction can be routinely offered in the third stage of labor (with necessary skill), evidence shows limited benefits in prevention of severe postpartum hemorrhage with use of uterotonic(s); omission of controlled cord traction risks needing manual placental removal *(Cochrane review[3d])*.

Having obtained her verbal consent for examination, bimanual examination reveals a nonpalpable uterine fundus with a soft, congested bleeding mass found in the vagina, beyond the cervical ring yet above the perineum.

Special notes:

† Dual agent uterotonic prophylaxis, or individual use of carbetocin, could be considered in this case scenario *(Cochrane review[3c])* although no uniform recommendations have been made.

§ Timing of oxytocin prophylaxis for active management of the third stage has not been found to be associated with a difference in risk of postpartum hemorrhage (*i.e.*, with delivery of the anterior shoulder, after delayed umbilical cord clamping, or with placental delivery) *(ACOG[1a], Cochrane review[3g])*

2. What is your <u>most specific</u> diagnosis?   2

    ☐ Second-degree uterine inversion

3. Recognizing that high-quality evidence for management of puerperal uterine inversion is   Max 10
    unavailable, provide a comprehensive treatment plan, explaining potential technical
    maneuvers extrapolated from case reports or case series. *(1 point per main bullet; max
    points specified per section)*

Supportive aspects:[†] *(max 5)*
☐ Initiate mobilization of additional staff to assist in resuscitation, including obstetrics, anesthesiology, nursing, and midwifery personnel
☐ Prepare for possible transport to the operating room/theater if conservative uterine replacement is unsuccessful
☐ Communicate the situation to the patient and attendants in the room
☐ Withhold use of any uterotonic agent
☐ Prompt treatment with aggressive crystalloid resuscitation and initiate blood transfusion protocols
☐ Request urgent blood tests including CBC/FBC, creatinine, ionized calcium, liver transaminases and function tests, and coagulation panel (*i.e.*, prothrombin time, activated partial thromboplastin time, fibrinogen level)
☐ Close monitoring of vital signs, including blood pressure, pulse, oxygen saturation, and temperature

Conservative approaches for uterine replacement: *(max 3)*
☐ Preferred avoidance of placental delivery until correction of uterine inversion
  ○ *Manual removal of the placenta prior to correction of uterine inversion may be associated with excessive hemorrhage and maternal shock*
  ○ *If initial placental removal is attempted, the patient would ideally be in the operating room, remain hemodynamically stable and have appropriate anesthesia*

☐ Tocolytic agent (*e.g.*, intravenous nitroglycerin, inhalational anesthetics, intravenous or subcutaneous terbutaline, intravenous magnesium sulfate[‡]) may be considered, although not uniformly required

☐ Cup the inverted uterine fundus in your palm and push it cephalad above the level of the umbilicus *(Johnson maneuver)*
  ○ Simultaneous use of ringed forceps on the cervical ring has been described, serving as countertraction[§]

☐ Use normal saline hung to gravity to exert hydrostatic pressure with a vaginal catheter in-situ to distend vaginal walls and force the fundus upward *(O'Sullivan maneuver)*
  ○ *Uterus gradually returns to its correct position in 10–15 minutes*

Corrective approaches at laparotomy after failed conservative uterine replacement: [#] *(max 2)*

☐ Apply Allis or Babcock clamps sequentially below the previous clamps along the round ligaments, exerting gentle upward traction until the fundus is replaced *(Huntington method)*

☐ Perform a horizontal hysterotomy along the posterior (to avoid the bladder) lower uterine wall through the cervical ring to facilitate the Huntington method *(Haultain method)*
  ○ *Uterine incision is subsequently repaired as routine*

☐ Place the Silastic vacuum cup on the fundus from above, and apply negative pressure to restore the uterus in place *(Antonelli method)*

Special notes:

[†] Flattening of the patient's bed, placing two large-bore intravenous access lines, bladder catheterization, and obtaining adequate pain control are additional fundamental aspects of treatment, which have already been ensured in this case scenario

[‡] Although magnesium sulfate is not considered a tocolytic agent in managing preterm labor, its brief tocolytic effect may be valuable in treatment of uterine inversion

[§] Henderson H, Alles RW. Puerperal inversion of the uterus. *Am J Obstet Gynecol.* 1948;56:133–142.

[#] Vaginal-surgical correction (*e.g.*, Spinelli) is no longer advised

While simultaneous supportive interventions are underway, your attempted immediate uterine replacement is unsuccessful. As the patient remains alert with adequate analgesic control and no change in vital signs, two successive doses of intravenous nitroglycerin 50 μg are administered, promoting uterine relaxation and manual successful correction of the inversion in the delivery room.

You take a mental note to later discuss your preferred selection of nitroglycerin with your trainee, based on its ultra-short half-life in a patient with hemodynamic changes (*i.e.*, hypotension and tachycardia). You also intend to highlight that albeit a rare puerperal complication without precipitating factors in as many as 50% of cases, prompt recognition and management are of utmost importance as morbidity and mortality are seen in ~41% of cases *(Suggested Reading 14)*.

4. Outline your management upon conservative correction of uterine inversion.
(1 point each)

Max 3

☐ Continue grasping the fundus via your palm internally for approximately three to five minutes

☐ Await spontaneous separation of the placenta, as routine, reserving manual removal for standard obstetric indications (*e.g., third stage of labor >30 minutes or active bleeding*)

☐ Upon placental delivery, start a uterotonic agent in prevention or treatment of atony; mechanical intrauterine balloon tamponade may also be considered to preserve the position of the fundus

☐ Consider prophylactic intravenous antibiotics, according to local protocols for intrauterine procedures (*NATA[9]*)

Special note:
If laparotomy was required, the external surface of the uterine fundus would be grasped for several minutes

5. Identify general risk factors for uterine inversion and highlight features that may have synchronously contributed to this patient's event [indicated by *]. *(1 point each)*

Max 10

Maternal:
☐ Primiparity (in relation to increased incidence of fundal placentation in this population)
☐ Uterine structural anomalies
☐ Uterine fibroids
☐ Connective tissue disorder (associated with congenital weakness of the uterine wall and/or cervix)
☐ Preeclampsia (with severe features)

Fetoplacental:
☐ Short umbilical cord *
☐ Fundal placentation *
☐ Morbidly adherent placenta
☐ Macrosomia *(controversial)*

Labor:
☐ Precipitous labor *
☐ Prolonged labor
☐ Uterine atony

Iatrogenic:
☐ Excessive cord traction and inappropriate fundal massage * (*Credé maneuver*)
☐ Use of uterotonic agents prior to placental removal

Spontaneous placental separation[†] follows correction of uterine inversion. You remove remaining placental fragments and clots while continuing to perform bimanual uterine massage and initiate uterotonics. The patient does not have contraindications to any uterotonic agent.

Warmed intravenous Ringer's lactate is infusing; the patient's blood pressure and pulse are stable at 101/55 mmHg and 120 bpm, respectively. Blood products have yet to arrive. The patient continues to tolerate examination well.

Special note:

† Use of intraumbilical vein injection of misoprostol or oxytocin in saline as an alternative intervention before manual placental removal is controversial (*accepted practice by SOGC[6] and Cochrane review[3f]; not recommended by Queensland Clinical Guideline[12]*)

6. Regarding pharmacotherapy for treatment of postpartum hemorrhage, outline one first-line and two second-line agents, detailing route(s) of administration, dose(s), and at least one adverse effect to convey to the patient.

12

	Dose and Route of Administration	Adverse Effects
First-line therapy: *(4 points)*		
☐ Oxytocin[†]	• 10–40 IU/500–1000 mL IV Ringer's lactate crystalloid solution • 5–10 IU IM or IMM up to 4 doses	• Usually none [effects relate to rate and dosage] • vomiting, hyponatremia, SIADH with prolonged dosing • hypotension, tachycardia can result from IV push
Second-line therapies:[‡§] *(4 points for any agent)*		
☐ Methylergonovine/ methylergometrine or ergonovine/ ergometrine	• 0.2 mg IM or IMM every 2–4 hours (maximum 5 doses) • 0.2 mg PO every 6–8 hours for 2–7 days	• severe hypertension, myocardial infarct (particularly when given IV; not recommended) • vomiting • abdominal pain requiring analgesics
☐ Fixed-dose combination of oxytocin and ergometrine	5 IU/500 µg IM one dose	• *See adverse effects above of individual components*
☐ Tranexamic acid[#]	1 g (100 mg/mL) IV over 10-min; may repeat after 30 min if bleeding persists or restarts within 24 hours of completing the first dose [Do not initiate >3 hours after birth {WHO[15b]}]	• new-onset seizures • headache • nausea, diarrhea

(cont.)

	Dose and Route of Administration	Adverse Effects
☐ 15-methyl-prostaglandin F$_{2\alpha}$ (carboprost)	250 µg IM or IMM up to every 15 min (maximum 8 doses); contraindicated IV	• diarrhea • hypertension/headache • bronchospasm • nausea, vomiting, • transient fever/chills
☐ Misoprostol (PGE$_1$)	400–1000 µg S/L, PO, PR, PV repeat doses every 15 min – dose should not exceed 1000 µg *(Suggest alternative route to PV with vaginal bleeding)*	• shivering and transient fever • vomiting, diarrhea
☐ Dinoprostone (PGE$_2$)	20 mg vaginal or rectal suppository; may be repeated at 2-hour intervals	See Question 17 in Chapter 16, *i.e.*, fever, chills, vomiting, diarrhea, idiopathic cardiovascular event (rarely)

Special notes:

IV intravenous, IM intramuscular, IMM intramyometrial, PO per os (orally), PGE$_1$ prostaglandin E$_1$, S/L sublingual, PR per rectum, SIADH syndrome of inappropriate antidiuretic hormone secretion

† Carbetocin would not be indicated in this case scenario based on >1 risk factor for postpartum hemorrhage with vaginal delivery *(SOGC[6])*

‡ Role of recombinant factor VIIa in primary postpartum hemorrhage is controversial; use is reserved for extenuating circumstances or as part of a clinical trial; expert collaboration is advised

§ Desmopressin acetate (DDVAP) may be adjunctive in postpartum hemorrhage for women with type 1 von Willebrand disease or renal dysfunction/uremia; use is not otherwise appropriate in this scenario

Tranexamic acid does not increase risk of thromboembolic events {*Cochrane review[3h]* and Taeuber I, Weibel S, Herrmann E, et al. Association of intravenous tranexamic acid with thromboembolic events and mortality: a systematic review, meta-analysis, and meta-regression. *JAMA Surg.* 2021;156(6):e210884.}; note that the WHO[15b] recommends use of tranexamic acid as a first-line agent with standard treatments in all cases of postpartum hemorrhage, regardless of cause or route of delivery

Uterine tone improves with use of a second-line uterotonic, although vaginal bleeding continues. Intrauterine uterine exploration does not reveal retained products of conception. Subjective blood loss is estimated to be at least 1500 mL. Although quantitative estimation of blood loss does not appear to reduce the need for uterotonic treatment, blood transfusions or use of volume expanders in care of postpartum hemorrhage *(Cochrane review[3b])*, the blood-soaked materials will be weighed for quantification *(ACOG[1b], NATA[9])* where 1 g weight approximates 1 mL of blood. You anticipate that novel calorimetric methods involving electronic artificial intelligence techniques for real-time estimates of blood loss may become mainstay in the clinical setting *(Suggested Reading 5)*.

Interdisciplinary professionals have presented to assist in patient care. The patient remains alert with normal oxygen saturation; blood pressure is 85/60 mmHg, pulse rate is 118 bpm, and temperature is >35°C. Blood products have just arrived; laboratory-based coagulation tests remain pending. You continue to communicate with the patient during resuscitation.

7. Identify two purposes of continued verbal engagement with the patient during resuscitative maneuvers at this time. *(1 point each)*	2

- ☐ Assess her level of consciousness
- ☐ Provide appropriate communication of ongoing medical care

8-A. With continued vaginal bleeding despite increased uterine tone, discuss your subsequent steps in the care of this patient, prior to attempting your next therapeutic treatment. *(1 point per main bullet)*	Max 4

- ☐ Emergency activation of the 'massive obstetric hemorrhage' protocol, including medical and allied health professionals
- ☐ Commence blood product replacement based on maternal clinical status; awaiting results of laboratory tests is not advised
- ☐ Observe for systemic signs of bleeding (*e.g.*, hematuria, intravenous cannulation, subconjunctival, oronasal mucosa)
- ☐ Examine the cervix, vagina, and perineum for lacerations or genital tract hematoma[§] initiate repair
  - ○ *Cervical assessment is fundamental in instrumental deliveries*
- ☐ Initiate/reinforce mechanisms to minimize risk of hypothermia (*i.e.*, removing wet linen, warming the room temperature, applying warm blankets and intravenous fluids)
- ☐ Consider drawing a blood sample to check for clot formation which is expected within five to eight minutes

Special notes:
Refer to Chapter 21
§ Vigilance is warranted given this precipitous and instrumental vaginal delivery

8-B. Address the potential benefits of a point-of-care blood clotting analyzer {*e.g.*, TEG® [thromboelastography] or ROTEM® [rotational thromboelastometry]} if locally accessible. *(1 point each)*	Max 4

- ☐ Decreased time for availability of laboratory-based results of coagulation function
- ☐ Distinguish between causes of bleeding (*i.e.*, coagulopathy *vs.* surgical origin)
- ☐ Facilitate guidance of blood product replacement based on the specific type of coagulopathic defect
- ☐ Reduced need for blood product replacement
- ☐ Reduced morbidity from postpartum hemorrhage

The patient had provided consent for receipt of blood products during the course of pregnancy when she received routine anti-D immunoglobulin for Rh-negative status. As care providers in the delivery room are preparing to administer blood products, your briefly mention to your obstetric trainee that in the absence of high-quality data to guide the ratio for transfusion blood products in postpartum hemorrhage, accepted protocols have been based on trauma literature.

There continues to be no clinical suspicion of disseminated intravascular coagulation. While repairing delivery-associated lacerations, you take the opportunity to review principal aspects of postpartum hemorrhage and blood product replacement with your trainee.

9. Review the traditional definition of <u>primary</u> postpartum hemorrhage and alert your trainee of one contemporary diagnostic criterion, noting differences exist among international organizations.   3

(i) Traditional definition: *(1 point)*
☐ Blood loss > (or ≥) 500 mL after a vaginal delivery or > (or ≥) 1000 mL after a Cesarean delivery within 24 hours of delivery
(ii) Contemporary definitions: *(2 points for any societal definition; other responses may be accepted, based on local jurisdiction)*

ACOG[#1a]
☐ Cumulative blood loss of ≥1000 mL irrespective of the route of delivery within 24 hours of delivery

OR
☐ Blood loss associated with signs or symptoms of hypovolemia irrespective of the route of delivery within 24 hours of delivery
  o *Signs or symptoms of postpartum hemorrhage-associated hypovolemia may only become evident when blood loss is >1500 mL in late pregnancy (i.e., >25% of total blood volume)*

SOGC[6]
☐ Any blood loss that jeopardizes hemodynamic stability; the amount of blood loss depends on preexisting conditions (*e.g.*, iron-deficiency anemia, thalassemia, preeclampsia)

RCOG[8]
☐ Minor (500–1000 mL) and major (>1000 mL) postpartum hemorrhage

NATA[9]
☐ Blood loss >500 mL (severe blood loss >1000 mL, life-threatening blood loss >2500 mL or hypovolemic shock) within 24 hours of delivery, irrespective of the route of delivery
OR
☐ Blood loss associated with signs or symptoms of hypovolemia irrespective of the route of delivery within 24 hours of delivery (*i.e., similar to ACOG above*)

WHO[15]
☐ Blood loss ≥500 mL (severe blood loss ≥1000 mL) within 24 hours of birth

10. Present a structured outline of *this* patient's risk factors for postpartum hemorrhage. *(1 point each)*

Max 7

Tone (atony):
☐ Precipitous labor and delivery
☐ Uterine overdistension based on multiple gestation and polyhydramnios
☐ Bladder distension prior to catheterization
☐ Advanced maternal age of 42 years
☐ Multiparity (>4)

Trauma:
☐ Uterine inversion
☐ Lacerations related to instrumental vaginal delivery and/or spontaneous tears of the cervix, vagina, or perineum

Tissue:
☐ Retained placental fragments and clots

Special note:
Regarding the fourth 'T,' thrombin, in etiology of postpartum hemorrhage, there is no known coagulopathy at this time

11. Packed red blood cells are being infused. Illustrate three accepted protocols for blood product replacement in relation to units of red cells, knowing there is limited available data on best treatment for hemostatic impairment in postpartum hemorrhage. *(1 point each)*

Max 3

Packed red cells: fresh-frozen plasma: platelets in ratios of:
☐ 1:1:1 *(designated to mimic replacement of whole blood)*

OR
☐ 6:4:1

OR
☐ 4:4:1

OR
☐ If eight units of packed red blood cells and fresh frozen plasma are being transfused and tests of hemostasis remain unavailable, consider transfusion for fibrinogen supplementation (*e.g.*, two pools of cryoprecipitate) and one pool of platelets[†]

Special note:
† Collins P, Abdul-Kadir R, Thachil J; Subcommittees on Women's Health Issues in Thrombosis and Haemostasis and on Disseminated Intravascular Coagulation. Management of coagulopathy associated with postpartum hemorrhage: guidance from the SSC of the ISTH. *J Thromb Haemost.* 2016;14(1):205–210; the International Society of Thrombosis and Haemostasis (ISTH) recommends against 1:1:1 ratio

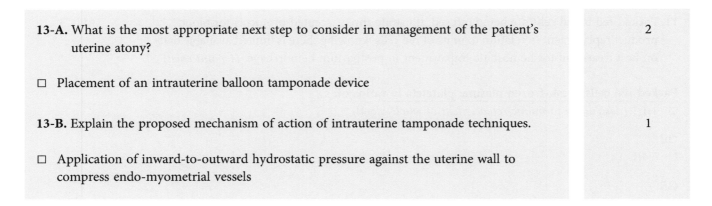

12. While slight variations exist, summarize the main targeted hematologic goals for therapeutic treatment of postpartum hemorrhage. *(1 point each; slight variations in response may be deemed acceptable)*   4

☐ Clauss fibrinogen >2 g/L[†]
☐ Hemoglobin concentration >80 g/L (8 g/dL)
☐ Platelet count >50 × 10⁹/L (50,000/μL)
☐ Activated partial thromboplastin time (aPTT) and prothrombin time (PT) <1.5 times normal

Special notes:
Refer to *Suggested Reading 2*, with reference to Hunt BJ, Allard S, Keeling D, et al. A practical guideline for the haematological management of major haemorrhage. *Br J Haematol.* 2015;170(6):788–803.

† Fibrinogen is first to fall to critical levels during hemorrhage and resuscitation with red cells, crystalloids, and colloids

Despite continued administration of uterotonics, vaginal bleeding restarts with decreased uterine tone. The patient remains hemodynamically stable, packed red blood cells and crystalloids continue to infuse, and her pain is well controlled. Laboratory results are consistent with significant blood loss requiring replacement therapy; coagulation parameters remain normal.

13-A. What is the most appropriate next step to consider in management of the patient's uterine atony?   2

☐ Placement of an intrauterine balloon tamponade device

13-B. Explain the proposed mechanism of action of intrauterine tamponade techniques.   1

☐ Application of inward-to-outward hydrostatic pressure against the uterine wall to compress endo-myometrial vessels

Recognizing multiple commercially available devices for uterine tamponade, you guide your obstetric trainee with technical aspects of insertion of the chosen agent, while simultaneously communicating with the patient during the procedure. You highlight evidence suggests safety and success (~85%) of uterine balloon tamponade systems in management of postpartum hemorrhage.

Special note:
Uterine packing is not routinely recommended due to numerous disadvantages; use may be considered in low resource settings

14. With regard to uterine balloon tamponade, what are important postplacement management considerations? *(1 point each)*

Max 5

☐ At frequent intervals, check uterine fundal height and blood loss through the drainage portal

☐ Serial monitoring of urine output and vital signs (*i.e.*, pulse rate, blood pressure, oxygen saturation, temperature)

☐ Consider point of care testing by TEG® (thromboelastography) or ROTEM® (Rotational thromboelastometry) for adequate coagulation assessment

☐ Consider continued oxytocin infusion to maintain uterine tone

☐ Consider prophylactic intravenous antibiotics, according to local protocols for intrauterine procedures[†]

☐ Plan elective removal of the intrauterine balloon insufflation device, either slowly or all at once, within 24 hours of insertion

Special note:

[†] Although no high-quality evidence on efficacy of antibiotic prophylaxis in this setting exists, readers may refer to Wong MS, Dellapiana G, Greene N, Gregory KD. Antibiotics during intrauterine balloon tamponade is associated with a reduction in endometritis. *Am J Perinatol.* 2019;36(12):1211–1215.

After placement of the uterine tamponade device, you are reassured by being in a center where advanced supportive care is available, should it be required. You inform your trainee that you would have otherwise considered patient transfer if bleeding ensues.

15. If you were providing care in a lower resource setting, identify a recommended invaluable technique that temporarily maintains blood pressure and reduces uterine blood flow while awaiting definitive treatment.

2

☐ Nonpneumatic antishock garment

Special note:

Benefits include potential for avoidance of unnecessary hysterectomy for intractable uterine atony, decreased need for or number of blood transfusions, continued access to assess the perineum and uterine status, and safety when worn for up to 48 hours *(FIGO[4a])*

The patient appears to respond well to the uterine tamponade device with simultaneous oxytocin infusion. You are called two hours postinsertion for increased blood draining through the portal. The patient's clinical and laboratory hemodynamic parameters remain stable; fundal height is appropriate.

16. What is the next most appropriate treatment consideration?   1

☐ Uterine artery embolization (UAE)

Special note:
This case scenario is set in a tertiary-care setting to maximize clinical and academic instruction (refer to the patient stem). Where UAE is not available, the next most appropriate treatment would be laparotomy (*i.e.,* proceed to the clinical scenario prior to Question 18); international variations exist with regard to involvement of the obstetrics team in patient counseling for UAE

17. Address the advantages and caveats/risks of uterine artery embolization you would discuss in patient counseling. *(1 point each)*   Max 6

Advantages:
☐ Fertility-preserving, with reported pregnancy rates of ~43%–48%
☐ High rate of effectiveness (median success rate ~90%)
☐ Risk of significant harm is low (<5%)
   ○ *reported events from small case series include uterine necrosis, deep vein thrombosis, and peripheral neuropathy*
☐ Subsequent pregnancy complications do not appear increased relative to the general population (*e.g.,* preterm birth and fetal growth restriction)

Caveats/risks:
☐ Hemodynamic stability to allow for angiographic intervention of approximately one hour duration in a radiology suite *(hybrid suite is optimal, if available)*
☐ Future pregnancy risk of placenta accreta spectrum
☐ Uterine necrosis, deep vein thrombosis, and peripheral neuropathy

Uterine atony is unresponsive to a tamponade device, uterine artery embolization, and standard intravenous resuscitation. The uterus remains boggy, and bleeding persists. The uterine balloon device has been deflated.[†] Laboratory parameters do not demonstrate a consumptive coagulopathy. The patient remains alert and oriented, although the treating team is uniformly concerned about impending hemorrhagic shock. The anesthesiologist has already inserted arterial and central venous catheters. The patient has been transported to the surgical suite as you plan for laparotomy with the assistance of another surgical expert. Estimated blood loss is now at least 2500 mL.

Although of grand-multiparity, the patient indicates she has not completed childbearing and would prefer attempted conservative surgical approaches prior to hysterectomy. She does, however, consent to hysterectomy as a definitive life-saving measure.

Special note:
† Intrauterine balloon catheter deflation allows for its use after fertility-preserving surgical intervention; 'uterine sandwich' technique involves combined uterine compression suture and balloon catheter.

18. Provide rationale for your choice of surgical incision in management of postpartum hemorrhage after vaginal delivery. *(1 point each)*

2

Midline vertical laparotomy:
☐ Optimizes exposure of the abdomen and pelvis
☐ Minimizes dissection of tissue planes that may bleed if coagulopathy develops

19. Elaborate on fertility-preserving surgical options for control of postpartum hemorrhage. *(1 point each)*

Max 3

☐ Bilateral uterine artery ligation *(O'Leary sutures)*
☐ Uterine compression/brace sutures *(e.g., B-Lynch, Cho, Hayman, Pereira, Esike)*
☐ Bilateral utero-ovarian artery ligation
☐ Internal iliac artery ligation (ipsilateral or bilateral)
   ○ *Surgical skill required for retroperitoneal dissection*
   ○ *Suboptimal success rates of ~50%–60%*

Special notes:
(a) Judicious application of aortic compression may be considered as a temporizing measure in the event of imminent threat of exsanguination
(b) Intraoperative cell savage should be considered for emergency use in postpartum hemorrhage *(RCOG[10])*; although intraoperative cell savage is safe and efficacious, use is limited by availability as the large majority of events are unpredictable *(ACOG[1a])*

After bilateral uterine artery ligations, the decision is made to proceed with a uterine compression suture. Knowing of numerous existing techniques, where none has been deemed superior to another, a plan is made to perform the Cho suture.

20. Regarding surgical technique, explain why a Cho suture may be preferable to the B-Lynch suture as a uterine compression mechanism for this patient.

2

☐ Unlike the B-Lynch suture, the Cho suture obviates the need for hysterotomy as this patient delivered vaginally

21. Indicate important elements to convey in counseling after <u>successful</u> uterine compression suture. *(1 point per main bullet)*

2

☐ Successful future pregnancy rate ranges from 11% to 75%
   ○ *individual variations exist in rates of conception and pregnancy outcome by surgical method and operator technique*
☐ Reported complications[†] include intrauterine synechiae, pyometra, uterine necrosis, bowel herniation through persistent loops of suture after uterine involution

Special note:
† Maternal mortality does not appear to be an associated complication of uterine compression sutures

Uterine atony has responded well to compression suture. Postoperatively, the patient is admitted to an intensive care setting for close hemodynamic monitoring. Debriefing will be arranged with the patient, her family, as well as among interdisciplinary professionals. Meticulous documentation has been maintained.

---

22. Outline complications of primary postpartum hemorrhage for which the patient would be monitored, prophylaxis provided or clinically managed accordingly. *(1 point per main bullet; section-points specified)*   Max 10

Early complications: *(max 7)*
- ☐ Anemia requiring blood transfusion, parenteral iron therapy or oral supplementation
- ☐ Complications of blood product transfusions (*e.g.*, alloimmunization, transfusion-related acute lung injury [TRALI], transfusion-associated circulatory overload [TACO]/pulmonary edema, acute respiratory distress syndrome, hyperkalemia/hypocalcemia, infectious morbidity, mortality)
- ☐ Disseminated intravascular coagulopathy
- ☐ Myocardial ischemia
- ☐ Acute renal failure
- ☐ Hepatic failure
- ☐ Venous thromboembolism
  - ○ *Consideration for early instigation of **mechanical** thromboprophylaxis with postpartum hemorrhage*
  - ○ *Consideration for **pharmacologic** thromboprophylaxis when clinically safe and as soon as feasible after postpartum hemorrhage, in the absence of contraindications; continue therapy for at least 10 days or until other risk factors resolved (i.e., resolution of the postpartum hemorrhage inflammatory syndrome)*[†]
- ☐ Abdominal compartment syndrome
- ☐ Sepsis
- ☐ Limitations in maternal-newborn bonding, skin-to-skin care, or breastfeeding
- ☐ Maternal mortality

Late complications: *(3)*
- ☐ Sheehan syndrome (pituitary necrosis and panhypopituitarism)
- ☐ Postpartum depression associated with anemia and delivery morbidity/posttraumatic stress disorder
- ☐ Asherman syndrome/infertility/subfertility

Special note:
[†] Refer to Collins P, Abdul-Kadir R, Thachil J; Subcommittees on Women's Health Issues in Thrombosis and Haemostasis and on Disseminated Intravascular Coagulation. Management of coagulopathy associated with postpartum hemorrhage: guidance from the SSC of the ISTH. *J Thromb Haemost.* 2016;14(1):205–210

TOTAL: **125**

Placental Complications

CHAPTER 23

Placenta Accreta Spectrum

Cleve Ziegler and Amira El-Messidi

A 37-year-old G6P3A2 at 20^{+3} weeks' gestation is referred from a community hospital center for consultation at your tertiary center's high-risk obstetrics unit for '*anterior placenta previa with abnormal features*' reported on ultrasound evaluation of the morphologically normal female fetus. First-trimester sonography performed in the same center, integrated with maternal serum biomarkers, revealed a low risk of fetal aneuploidy.

Your obstetric trainee informs you that the patient is normotensive with a prepregnancy body mass index (BMI) of 22 kg/m^2; fetal viability has been ascertained. The obstetric chart, including reports of current maternal-fetal investigations, has been requested from her primary care provider.

Special note: *While readers are encouraged to recognize that anterior placenta previa in the second trimester is a principal risk marker for placenta accreta spectrum disorders, comprehensive clinical acumen remains fundamental to risk assessment, as absent sonographic clues do not preclude diagnosis.*

LEARNING OBJECTIVES

1. Demonstrate the ability to take a focused history, and understand elements of comprehensive sonographic assessment, for risk of placenta accreta spectrum disorders
2. Explain pathophysiological concepts for placenta accreta spectrum disorders, including the biological rationale with regard to projected fetal growth potential
3. Illustrate an understanding of maternal-fetal risks with placenta accreta spectrum disorders by developing an appropriate antenatal and surgical care plan
4. Provide patient counseling on possible uterine-preserving techniques and associated short- and long-term risks of conservative management
5. Appreciate the importance of initiating multidisciplinary collaboration in a centralized hospital center for patients with known or strongly suspected placenta accreta spectrum disorders

SUGGESTED READINGS

1. American College of Obstetricians and Gynecologists; Society for Maternal-Fetal Medicine. Obstetric Care Consensus No. 7: Placenta accreta spectrum. *Obstet Gynecol.* 2018;132(6): e259–e275.

2. Cali G, Forlani F, Lees C, et al. Prenatal ultrasound staging system for placenta accreta spectrum disorders. *Ultrasound Obstet Gynecol.* 2019;53(6):752–760.

3. Collins SL, Alemdar B, van Beekhuizen HJ, et al. Evidence-based guidelines for the management of abnormally invasive placenta: recommendations from the International Society for Abnormally Invasive Placenta. *Am J Obstet Gynecol.* 2019;220(6):511–526.

4. Expert Panel on Women's Imaging, Poder L, Weinstein S, et al. ACR Appropriateness Criteria® placenta accreta spectrum disorder. *J Am Coll Radiol.* 2020;17(5S):S207–S214.

5. (a) FIGO Expert Consensus Panel: Jauniaux E, Ayres-de-Campos D, Langhoff-Roos J, et al. FIGO classification for the clinical diagnosis of placenta accreta spectrum disorders. *Int J Gynaecol Obstet.* 2019;146(1):20–24.

    (b) FIGO Consensus Guidelines: Jauniaux E, Ayres-de-Campos D, FIGO Placenta Accreta Diagnosis and Management Expert Consensus Panel. FIGO consensus guidelines on placenta accreta spectrum disorders: Introduction. *Int J Gynaecol Obstet.* 2018;140(3): 261–264.

    (c) FIGO Consensus Guidelines: Jauniaux E, Chantraine F, Silver RM, et al. FIGO consensus guidelines on placenta accreta spectrum disorders: epidemiology. *Int J Gynaecol Obstet.* 2018;140(3):265–273.

    (d) FIGO Consensus Guidelines: Jauniaux E, Bhide A, Kennedy A, et al. FIGO consensus guidelines on placenta accreta spectrum disorders: prenatal diagnosis and screening. *Int J Gynaecol Obstet.* 2018;140(3):274–280.

    (e) FIGO Consensus Guidelines: Sentilhes L, Kayem G, Chandraharan E, et al. FIGO consensus guidelines on placenta accreta spectrum disorders: conservative management. *Int J Gynaecol Obstet.* 2018;140(3):291–298.

    (f) FIGO Consensus Guidelines: Allen L, Jauniaux E, Hobson S, et al. FIGO consensus guidelines on placenta accreta spectrum disorders: nonconservative surgical management. *Int J Gynaecol Obstet.* 2018;140(3):281–290.

6. Hobson SR, Kingdom JC, Murji A, et al. No. 383 – screening, diagnosis, and management of placenta accreta spectrum disorders. *J Obstet Gynaecol Can.* 2019;41(7):1035–1049.

7. Jauniaux E, Alfirevic Z, Bhide AG, et al. Placenta praevia and placenta accreta: diagnosis and management: Green-Top Guideline No. 27a. *BJOG.* 2019;126(1):e1–e48.

8. Jauniaux E, Hussein AM, Fox KA, et al. New evidence-based diagnostic and management strategies for placenta accreta spectrum disorders. *Best Pract Res Clin Obstet Gynaecol.* 2019;61:75–88.

9. Jauniaux E, Kingdom JC, Silver RM. A comparison of recent guidelines in the diagnosis and management of placenta accreta spectrum disorders. *Best Pract Res Clin Obstet Gynaecol.* 2021;72:102–116.

10. Silver RM, Branch DW. Placenta accreta spectrum. *N Engl J Med.* 2018;378(16):1529–1536.

11. Shainker SA, Coleman B, Timor-Tritsch IE, et al. Special report of the Society for Maternal-Fetal Medicine Placenta Accreta Spectrum Ultrasound Marker Task Force: consensus on definition of markers and approach to the ultrasound examination in pregnancies at risk for placenta accreta spectrum. *Am J Obstet Gynecol.* 2021;224(1):B2–B14. [Correction in *Am J Obstet Gynecol.* 2021 Jul;225(1):91]

1. With regard to *'anterior placental previa with abnormal features,'* what aspects of a focused history would you want to know? *(1 point per main bullet; max points specified per section)*

Characteristics of current pregnancy: [#] *(6)*
☐ Determine whether conception occurred by in vitro fertilization
☐ Inquire whether first-trimester sonogram suspected implantation over a Cesarean scar or low implantation of the gestational sac
☐ Current anticoagulation
☐ Assess whether the patient is known for iron-deficiency anemia and specify treatment(s), if any
☐ Current/prior episodes of vaginal bleeding and/or lower abdominal cramping
☐ Current/prior episodes of gross hematuria[†]

Details related to prior obstetric history: *(max 8)*
☐ Mode of deliveries, including the number of Cesarean sections, if any
☐ Type of previous uterine scar(s), if any
☐ Obtain operative reports of Cesarean section(s) and/or intra-abdominal surgeries, if any
   ○ Where operative reports are inaccessible, determine whether surgeon commented to the patient on the extent of intra-abdominal adhesions
☐ Gestational ages at deliveries and indications thereof
☐ Inquire whether placenta accreta was diagnosed antenatally or incidentally discovered intrapartum at any of the prior deliveries
☐ Manual removal of the placenta at any delivery
☐ Postpartum hemorrhage and its successful treatments
☐ Any episode(s) of postpartum endometritis
☐ Need for uterine surgical evacuation in any of the two reported pregnancy losses

General medical/surgical features: *(max 4)*
☐ Blood type and antibody screen, if known to the patient
☐ Receipt of blood transfusions for obstetric or nonobstetric indications
☐ Bleeding diathesis or hypercoagulopathy
☐ Prior use of intrauterine device mechanisms[‡]
☐ Mullerian anomaly (*e.g.*, bicornuate uterus)[‡]
☐ Submucous fibroids,[‡] myomectomy, or fibroid embolization
☐ Adenomyosis[‡]
☐ Hysteroscopy for any indication
☐ Known myotonic dystrophy[‡]
☐ Receipt of prior chemotherapy or exposure to pelvic radiation[‡]
☐ Allergies

Social features: *(2)*
☐ Distance of residence from the tertiary center, access to transportation, and family supports
☐ Smoking *(a risk factor for placenta previa)*

> **Special notes:**
> \# Multiple gestation is a risk factor for placenta accreta spectrum disorders, yet not relevant to this case scenario
> † Clinical symptoms of bladder invasion by the placenta are rare
> ‡ Reported associated 'nonsurgical scar' risks for placenta accreta spectrum disorders

You learn that conception occurred via in vitro fertilization, as with the couple's three children, due to male-factor infertility. She had three uncomplicated elective low-transverse Cesarean sections at term, after a previous abdominal full-thickness myomectomy. Subsequent to her last delivery, the patient required brief hospitalization for postpartum endometritis; she recalls her physician mentioning the placenta was somewhat adherent, yet manual delivery was feasible without intraoperative complications. Since the last delivery four years ago, two spontaneous conceptions resulted in one requiring a suction curettage for early pregnancy failure and a tubal ectopic pregnancy treated by methotrexate.

Her fertility expert had provided preconception counseling on the risk of invasive placentation. First-trimester sonography sought to ensure absence of Cesarean scar pregnancy. Pregnancy has been clinically uncomplicated to date. Apart from routine prenatal vitamins, the patient takes oral iron supplementation for known iron-deficiency anemia. Although qualifying for preeclampsia prophylaxis based on maternal age criteria by your local guidance,† aspirin-induced bronchospasm precluded its use. Medical history is otherwise unremarkable and the patient practices healthy social habits. You are pleased to know she lives in close proximity to your hospital center.

As you prepare to perform a detailed sonographic evaluation at this consultation visit, you take the opportunity to discuss with your obstetric trainee the patient's clinical features that raise suspicion for, and may contribute to, the pathophysiology of placenta accreta spectrum disorders. You highlight that while current evidence is limited with regard to the predictive value of maternal first- and second-trimester biomarkers in screening for placenta accreta spectrum, some studies have demonstrated patterns of abnormalities and international literature continues to evolve.

Special note:
† Refer to Question 10 in Chapter 38

---

2. Elicit the patient's risk factors for placenta accreta spectrum disorders or related morbidity. *(1 point each)*

Max 8

Obstetric features:

Characteristics relevant to prior pregnancies:
□ Cesarean deliveries, particularly increasing number of surgical deliveries
□ Manual placental removal with a history suggestive of adherent placentation
□ Postpartum endometritis
□ Suction curettage

Characteristics relevant to current pregnancy:
□ Anterior placenta previa
□ Advanced maternal age ≥35 years†

☐ In vitro fertilization
☐ Multiparity
☐ Iron-deficiency anemia
☐ Female fetus

Nonobstetric features:
☐ Uterine fibroids and abdominal myomectomy

Special note:
† Effect of advanced maternal age may be due to multiparity, risk of placenta previa, or greater odds of having had uterine surgery

---

3. Regarding maternal serum biomarkers used in screening for Down syndrome, discuss the derangements which *may be* associated with placenta accreta spectrum disorders. *(1 point each)*

Max 3

☐ Increased levels of first-trimester pregnancy-associated plasma protein A (PAPP-A)
☐ Decreased levels of first-trimester beta-human chorionic gonadotropin (ß-hCG)
☐ Increased levels of second-trimester ß-hCG
☐ Increased levels of second-trimester maternal serum alpha-fetoprotein (MSAFP)

Special note:
The amount of maternal serum cell-free DNA (cfDNA) is unchanged in women with placenta accreta spectrum disorders *(FIGO[5d], based on* Samuel A, Bonanno C, Oliphant A, Batey A, Wright JD. Fraction of cell-free fetal DNA in the maternal serum as a predictor of abnormal placental invasion-a pilot study. *Prenat Diagn.* 2013;33(11):1050–1053.)

---

4. Address your trainee's inquiry on pathophysiological concepts for placenta accreta spectrum disorders. *(1 point each)*

Max 2

Maternal origins:
☐ Prior uterine surgery disrupts endometrial reepithelialization, resulting in a defective zona spongiosa layer of the decidualized endometrium, and prompting myometrial infiltration by extravillous trophoblast
☐ Abnormal vascularization and tissue oxygenation of the uterine scar defect may be a precursor or contributor to focal myometrial degeneration and abnormal endometrial reepithelialization

Placental origins:
☐ Primary defective trophoblast biology leads to myometrial invasion *(evidence does not support this theory, contrary to pathophysiological origins of molar pregnancy and placental insufficiency)*

Special note:
Readers are encouraged to refer to Jauniaux E, Collins S, Burton GJ. Placenta accreta spectrum: pathophysiology and evidence-based anatomy for prenatal ultrasound imaging. *Am J Obstet Gynecol.* 2018;218(1):75–87.

Although the patient has numerous risk markers for placenta accreta spectrum disorders, you alert your trainee that the condition may remain undiagnosed antenatally in ~50%[†]–70%[‡] of cases. While multimodal ultrasound is the mainstay for screening and diagnosis, with a sensitivity and specificity of 90.7% and 96.9%, respectively,[§] several factors contribute to its high diagnostic accuracy in placenta accreta spectrum disorders.

Special notes:

[†] (a) Bailit JL, Grobman WA, Rice MM, et al. Morbidly adherent placenta treatments and outcomes. *Obstet Gynecol.* 2015;125(3):683–689; (b) Fitzpatrick KE, Sellers S, Spark P, et al. The management and outcomes of placenta accreta, increta, and percreta in the UK: a population-based descriptive study. *BJOG.* 2014;121(1):62–71.

[‡] Thurn L, Lindqvist PG, Jakobsson M, et al. Abnormally invasive placenta-prevalence, risk factors and antenatal suspicion: results from a large population-based pregnancy cohort study in the Nordic countries. *BJOG.* 2016;123(8):1348–1355.

[§] D'Antonio F, Iacovella C, Bhide A. Prenatal identification of invasive placentation using ultrasound: systematic review and meta-analysis. *Ultrasound Obstet Gynecol.* 2013;42(5): 509–517.

---

5. Identify factors that impact the effectiveness of ultrasound in screening and diagnosis of placenta accreta spectrum disorders. *(1 point per main bullet)*   Max 5

☐ Awareness of clinical risk factors
  ○ *Without an appropriate clinical context, ultrasound sensitivity is ~53%*[†]
☐ Operator's technical skills, including probe pressure
☐ Interpretation of what constitutes the sonographic marker being assessed
☐ Ultrasound equipment
☐ Machine settings *(i.e., gain and velocity scale)*
☐ Transducer type and probe frequency *(i.e., higher frequency [5–9 MHz] and linear probe are preferable)*
☐ Independent use of gray-scale imaging or in combination with Doppler imaging
☐ Scanning route *(i.e., abdominal, vaginal, perineal)*
☐ Body mass index (BMI)
☐ Adequate bladder filling
☐ Gestational age
☐ Depth of placental invasion and lateral extension of villous tissue

Special note:

[†] Bowman ZS, Eller AG, Kennedy AM, et al. Accuracy of ultrasound for the prediction of placenta accreta. *Am J Obstet Gynecol.* 2014;211(2):177.e1–7

6. Provide your trainee with an evidence-based percent estimate for the patient's risk of placenta accreta spectrum disorder based on her obstetric history and known placenta previa, relative to nonprevia placentation.

2

☐ For her fourth Cesarean section in the presence of placenta previa, the estimated rate of placenta accreta spectrum is 61%, relative to 0.8% in the absence of placenta previa

Special note:
Silver RM, Landon MB, Rouse DJ, et al. Maternal morbidity associated with multiple repeat cesarean deliveries. *Obstet Gynecol.* 2006;107(6):1226–1232.

With a full bladder, transabdominal sonography is remarkable for features suggestive of placenta accreta spectrum disorders, which you explain to the patient. You highlight, however, that there is no known set combination or single sign that accurately differentiates between adherent and invasive placental conditions. You teach your trainee that transvaginal scanning is recommended in conjunction with the transabdominal modality for this patient to improve evaluation of the uteroplacental architecture in the anterior lower uterine segment *(ACR[4])*; cervical length is 33 mm after bladder emptying. Fetal biometry, morphology, and amniotic fluid volume are unremarkable.

The patient understands that although she may opt for mid-pregnancy termination at this previable period based on your local guidance, the procedure in the setting of suspected placenta accreta spectrum also carries risk and there is no data to support the magnitude of risk reduction, if any *(ACOG[1])*.

(A)

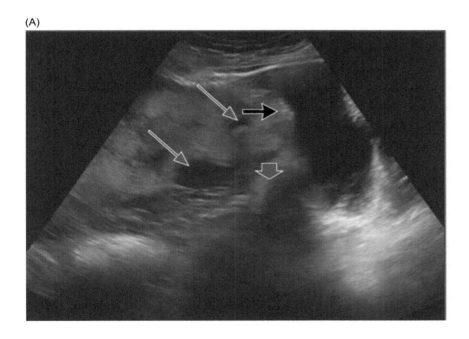

Figure 23.1
With permission: Figures 23.1 and 23.2 are from *Silver RM, Branch DW. Placenta accreta spectrum. N Engl J Med. 2018;378(16):1529–1536.*

There is no association between this case scenario and this patient's image. Image used for educational purposes only.

(B)

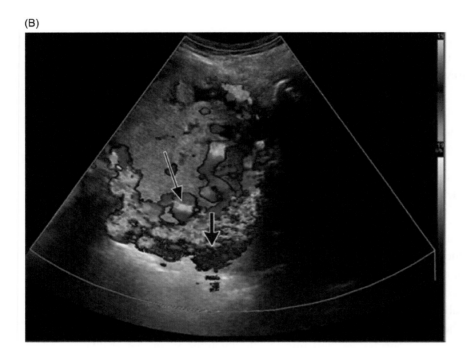

Figure 23.2
There is no association between this case scenario and this patient's image. Image used for educational purposes only.

7. Explain to your trainee the sonographic findings depicted by your designated arrows in Figures 23.1 and 23.2, including other pertinent findings not otherwise labeled in these figures. *(1 point per main bullet)*

Max 6

Figure 23.1 – grayscale imaging:
☐ Placenta previa *(blue arrow)*
☐ Abnormal placental lacunae *(green arrows)*
  ○ *The risk of placenta accreta spectrum increases with the number of lacunae*
  ○ *Presence of multiple, large, and irregularly shaped lacunae raises clinical suspicion*
☐ Interruption of the uterine serosa-bladder interface *(black)*
  ○ *i.e., the normally visualized hyperechoic line between the uterine serosa and bladder lumen is lost or interrupted*
☐ Loss or irregularity of the normal hypoechoic retroplacental myometrial zone (*i.e.,* 'clear zone')[†]
☐ Thinning of the myometrium overlying the placenta to <1 mm or undetectable

Figure 23.2 – color Doppler imaging:
☐ Turbulent vascular flow within lacunae *(thin arrow)*
☐ Subplacental hypervascularity *(thick arrow)*
  ○ *The striking color Doppler signal indicates multidirectional flow and aliasing, likely representing dense vascularity*
☐ Bridging vessels[‡] from the placenta, traveling perpendicular through the myometrium to the serosal interface

Special notes:
† Excessive probe pressure results in artifactual loss of the clear zone
‡ May also be assessed by three-dimensional ultrasound ± power Doppler

8. Assuming no additional ultrasound features of placenta accreta spectrum disorders are visualized at this time, what are other signs to indicate as pertinent negatives in your report? *(1 point per main bullet)*

Max 3

Grayscale imaging:
☐ Placental bulge[‡] *(i.e., the 'snowman sign'[§] at laparotomy)*
   ○ *Ballooning of the uterine wall-containing placenta into an adjacent organ, usually bladder, with an <u>intact-appearing uterine serosa</u>*
☐ Focal exophytic mass[‡]
   ○ *Placenta invasion <u>beyond the uterine serosa</u> into an adjacent organ, most commonly the bladder; this is only featured in placenta percreta*

2-dimensional color Doppler imaging:
☐ Uterovesical hypervascularity[‡] *(see description for subplacental hypervascularity, Question 7)*
☐ Placental lacunae feeder vessels
   ○ *High-velocity flow vessels arising from radial or arcuate arteries in the myometrium feeding lacunae*

3-dimensional ultrasound ± power Doppler:
☐ Intraplacental hypervascularity

Special notes:
§ Matsuo K, Conturie CL, Lee RH. Snowman sign: a possible predictor of catastrophic abnormal placentation. *Eur J Obstet Gynecol Reprod Biol.* 2014;181:341–342.
‡ Signs may also be assessed by three-dimensional ultrasound ± power Doppler

Having recently learned that the diagnostic value of magnetic resonance imaging (MRI) is similar to ultrasound for detection of placenta accreta spectrum, when performed with appropriate expertise *(RCOG[7])*, your trainee contemplates whether MRI may provide supplementary information for comprehensive assessment and planning of this patient's management.

9. Address the role of MRI in diagnosis and/or evaluation of placenta accreta spectrum disorders. *(1 point each)*

Max 2

Roles of MRI:
☐ Staging of disease, namely depth and lateral extension of myometrial invasion; added value also includes assessment of parametrial extension
☐ Determining presence of an accreta spectrum disorder with posterior or fundal implantation
☐ Assessment of lateral aspects of the former hysterotomy site(s) in relation to myometrial involvement by the placenta
☐ Obesity limits ultrasound assessment *(ACR[4])*

You counsel the patient that based on the high probability of clinically significant placenta accreta spectrum disorder with likely diffuse involvement, you will collaborate with her primary care provider to designate comprehensive care to your hospital center with regional excellence in management of these conditions.

The patient is aware of the potentially life-threatening nature of placenta accreta spectrum especially in the context of placenta previa; she understands that multidisciplinary collaboration is fundamental, guided by your center's protocol checklists to promote uniform care.

10. Highlight the evidence-based advantages of regional organization of care for placenta accreta spectrum disorders. *(1 point each)*   3

Benefits of centralized care include decreased rates of:
- ☐ Large volume blood transfusion
- ☐ Reoperation within seven days
- ☐ Intensive care admission

11. With centralized care at your regional hospital, detail essential aspects of the patient's antenatal management with focus on suspected placenta accreta spectrum disorder. *(1 point per main bullet)*   Max 25

Maternal management

Antenatal counseling and aspects of clinical care:
- ☐ Discuss her desires for future fertility versus planning Cesarean-hysterectomy, as determined by antenatal imaging (ultrasound/MRI), symptoms of regionally invasive disease (*e.g.,* hematuria) and intraoperative findings
- ☐ Counsel the patient that in the event of placenta percreta, uterine-preserving surgery is associated with high risks of peri/postpartum complications and secondary hysterectomy
- ☐ Inform the patient to present to hospital immediately if *any* vaginal bleeding, contractions, or abdominal aches/pains arise
- ☐ Discuss that avoidance of intercourse in the setting of placenta previa is often advised, although efficacy is unproven
- ☐ Advise avoidance of aerobic exercise after 26 weeks with placenta previa[‡]
- ☐ Provide the patient with a medical letter indicating high-risk features, in case of emergency
- ☐ Obtain surgical consent in advance of the planned procedure, should an emergent situation arise
- ☐ Obtain consent for receipt of blood product transfusion, should an emergent situation arise
- ☐ Optimize the preoperative hemoglobin concentration

☐ Inform the patient that should she remain asymptomatic[§] from placenta accreta spectrum, evidence is insufficient to recommend *optimal* timing of delivery that balances maternal-fetal risks; recommendations include:

○ ACOG[1]	34^{+0} to 35^{+6} weeks
○ SOGC[6]	34 to 36 weeks
○ RCOG[7]	35^{+0} to 36^{+6} weeks
○ SMFM[#]	34 to 37 weeks
○ *International Society for Abnormally Invasive Placentation (IS-AIP)*[3]	Individualized timing: plan delivery around 34^{+0} weeks if increased risk of emergent delivery, otherwise expectancy until after 36^{+0} weeks is reasonable

○ *Amniocentesis confirmation of fetal lung maturity is not required*

Laboratory-related care:

☐ Confirm results of prenatal blood-borne viral screening (*i.e.*, hepatitis B and C, HIV)
☐ Confirm blood type and antibody screen, with anti-D immunoglobulin prophylaxis as needed; consideration for serial antibody screen where antenatal transfusions are needed
☐ Complete/full blood count (CBC/FBC)
☐ Serum ferritin level

Potential multidisciplinary consultations: *(assuming your expertise in maternal-fetal medicine and obstetric expertise in sonographic imaging)*

☐ Surgical gynecology/gynecologic oncology
☐ General surgery
☐ Vascular surgery
☐ Urology
☐ Anesthesiology
☐ Intensive care medicine
☐ Hematology and transfusion medicine (blood product considerations and/or cell savage)
☐ Interventional radiology
☐ Neonatology
☐ Affiliated health care professionals, including specialized nurses and/or midwives

Psychosocial well-being:

☐ Offer social work support with anticipated frequent visits for antenatal care or elective/emergency hospitalizations *(individualized care based on patient needs)*
☐ Screen for depression and/or anxiety disorders; offer consultation with a mental health expert

Fetoplacental management:

☐ Serial sonographic follow-up to detect interval change and possible progression of invasion to guide patient management on timing and type of delivery
  ○ *Optimal timing of interval sonography has not been established (ACR[4])*

☐ Consideration for MRI, preferably after 24 weeks' gestation, may contribute to *staging*, rather than diagnosis, of this patient's disease
  ○ *Earlier imaging can be considered where termination of pregnancy is planned or for evaluation of suspected severe disease (ACR[4])*

☐ Serial fetal sonographic imaging for growth biometry and amniotic fluid assessment is guided by this patient's mode of conception with in vitro fertilization
  ○ *There is no clinical evidence of an association between placenta previa with/without grades of placenta accreta spectrum disorders and impaired fetal growth[†]*

☐ Arrange for elective maternal administration of a single course of fetal pulmonary corticosteroids between 34^{+0}- and 35^{+6}-weeks' gestation (or up to 36^{+6} weeks**); corticosteroids for fetal pulmonary maturity are most effective within seven days of delivery

Special notes:

‡ ACOG Committee Opinion No. 650: Physical activity and exercise during pregnancy and the postpartum period. *Obstet Gynecol.* 2015;126(6):e135–e142.

§ There is no evidence for routine elective antenatal hospitalization for placenta accreta spectrum with or without placenta previa provided patients remain asymptomatic and have received counseling; consider resources to allow rapid hospital return where needed

Society for Maternal-Fetal Medicine (SMFM) Consult Series #44: Management of bleeding in the late preterm period. *Am J Obstet Gynecol.* 2018;218(1):B2–B8.

† Jauniaux E, Dimitrova I, Kenyon N, et al. Impact of placenta previa with placenta accreta spectrum disorder on fetal growth. *Ultrasound Obstet Gynecol.* 2019;54(5):643–649.

** Committee on Obstetric Practice. Committee Opinion No. 713: Antenatal corticosteroid therapy for fetal maturation. *Obstet Gynecol.* 2017;130(2):e102-e109.

Your obstetric trainee appreciates participating in your counseling of the patient; he or she would have otherwise presumed that serial sonographic monitoring for risk of fetal growth restriction would be required with placenta previa accreta disorders based on a premise that uteroplacental insufficiency and suboptimal spiral artery remodeling may be accentuated in this patient.

12. Present a rationale to explain why fetal growth is not impaired in placenta accreta spectrum disorders.

☐ Incomplete spiral artery remodeling in adherent and invasive placentation is limited to the affected area, rather than affecting the entire placental function; this may relate to areas with absent decidua, disrupting maternal immune activation for spiral artery remodeling

The patient consents to receipt of blood products where clinically indicated. She requests discussion of uterine conservation procedures and associated postoperative care, as she is uncertain about completion of childbearing.

13. Provide a brief discussion of options for conservative management of an adherent placenta that you *may consider,*[$] depending on intraoperative findings and with appropriate intra/postoperative interprofessional support. *(1 point per main bullet and for appropriate explanation of each technique)*

6

☐ Expectant management or 'leaving the placenta in-situ' approach
  ○ *Spontaneous resolution and expulsion of the placenta is expected at a mean of 6 months (range from 4 to 12 months)*
  ○ *Delayed curettage or hysteroscopic resection of retained tissue may be considered to shorten recovery time*
☐ One-step conservative surgery approach – partial myometrial resection of the area with invasive accreta
  ○ *Consider local resection if there is no parametrial or cervical involvement and if the region of abnormality is <50% of the anterior uterine surface (IS-AIP³)*
  ○ *Vascular disconnection of feeder vessels and separation of affected uterine from vesicle tissues is performed prior to upper segment hysterotomy for fetal delivery and surgical reconstruction*
☐ Triple-P procedure
  ○ *Similar to the one-step conservative approach where affected myometrial tissue is excised and reconstructed, yet incision of placental vascular sinuses is avoided; preoperative balloons are placed in the anterior divisions of the internal iliac arteries to achieve intraoperative pelvic devascularization*

Special note:
[$] Extirpative technique would not be considered and is not advised; forceful removal of an adherent placenta risks massive hemorrhage and is associated with maternal morbidities

14. Outline risks associated with conservative management in adherent placenta to discuss in patient counseling. *(1 point each)*   Max 10

Systemic or infectious morbidity	Hematologic morbidity	Urologic/gynecologic morbidity	Other
☐ Fever ☐ Sepsis/ shock ☐ Peritonitis	☐ Consumptive coagulopathy ☐ Complications of blood transfusions[§] ☐ Venous thromboembolism	☐ Delayed hemorrhage ☐ Uterine necrosis ☐ Vesico-uterine fistula ☐ Urethral strictures ☐ Prolonged retention of placental fragments and associated uterine polyps ☐ Postpartum uterine rupture ☐ Need for emergent hysterectomy ☐ Long-term development of intrauterine synechiae ± amenorrhea ☐ Recurrence of placenta accreta spectrum disorders (*i.e.*, up to 29%) ☐ Other future pregnancy complications including uterine rupture, postpartum hemorrhage, peripartum hysterectomy	☐ Acute renal failure *(via prerenal, renal insult, or postrenal obstructive mechanism)* ☐ Maternal mortality

Special note:

§   Refer to Question 22 in Chapter 22 for discussion of blood product complications

15. Address the patient's inquiry regarding <u>postoperative management considerations</u> with uterine conservation. Psychosocial support services will be maintained. *(1 point each)*   7

☐ Inform the patient that compliance with care and reliability with follow-up is paramount given a 6% risk of severe maternal morbidity *(IS-AIP[3])*

☐ Ensure the patient remains in close proximity to the hospital center and reports any fever, bleeding, or abdominopelvic pain

☐ Plan regular follow-up (*e.g.*, weekly visits for approximately two months followed by monthly visits until resorption)

☐ Arrange for serial CBC/FBC, vaginal cultures, and ultrasound monitoring[†]

☐ Prophylactic antibiotics (*e.g.*, amoxicillin and clavulanic acid may be considered for this patient without related drug-allergy[§])

☐ Provide mechanical and daily pharmacologic thromboprophylaxis with low molecular weight heparin (LMWH) *(individualized duration)*

☐ Advise the patient that while breastfeeding is encouraged, she may experience difficulty as estrogen is produced by yet functional placental tissue *(SOGC[6])*

Special notes:
† Evidence is insufficient to recommend serial MRI or serum ß-hCG to monitor placental resorption; prophylactic uterine artery embolization is not a recommended aspect of conservative management
§ Clindamycin may be used in case of penicillin allergy *(FIGO[5e])*

The patient recalls that methotrexate was used for devascularization and trophoblastic resorption of her ectopic pregnancy. Despite unpleasant side effects, known inability to breastfeed on treatment, and its toxicities, she inquires about the role of methotrexate in conservative management of placenta accreta spectrum disorders.

16. Refer to drug pharmacokinetics to illustrate why methotrexate is not indicated in expectant management of placenta accreta spectrum disorders.   2

☐ With specific blockade of the S-phase (synthesis) of the cell cycle, methotrexate inhibits proliferation of actively dividing trophoblastic cells, which is limited in third-trimester placental cells and ceases after delivery of the fetus

Special note:
Refer to Question 2 in Chapter 42 for discussion on gestational risks and recommendations with methotrexate treatment

At 25 weeks' gestation, the patient undergoes an MRI of the abdomen and pelvis without gadolinium contrast.[†] You teach your obstetric trainee that timing the MRI after 24 weeks' gestation improves accuracy, sensitivity, and positive predictive values of diagnosis *(ACR Appropriateness Criteria[® 4])*.

Consistent with sonography, MRI demonstrates placenta previa with numerous findings suggestive of invasive placentation including bladder wall involvement; there is no evidence of cervical or parametrial involvement. The patient has remained clinically well and is compliant with the care plan.

After comprehensive considerations of risks related to uterine conservation, she opts for elective peripartum hysterectomy for which consent is obtained. The patient is informed about *delayed-interval hysterectomy* as a means to minimize blood loss and tissue damage in the event that extensive placenta invasion (percreta) precludes immediate hysterectomy. Counseling of interim risks, including the potential for complications at second surgery in a stable patient, are considered.

An interdisciplinary meeting is arranged to coordinate elective surgical planning, as well as develop a contingency plan in case of an obstetric emergency. Delivery is intended for 35^{+2} weeks' gestation with surgical suite and maternal-fetal equipment being reserved in advance. The anesthesiologist will counsel and consent the patient on the safety of regional anesthesia (SOGC[6], RCOG[7]) with possible conversion to general anesthetic.

Special note:
† Refer to Chapter 42 for discussion of obstetric considerations of MRI and intravenous gadolinium contrast in pregnancy

---

17. Explain the advantages of total hysterectomy for definitive management of placenta accreta spectrum disorders. *(1 point each)*   3

Advantages of total hysterectomy:
- ☐ Cervical stump bleeding or infection if contains placenta disease
- ☐ Continued risk of future malignancy in the cervical stump, necessitating routine cervical cytology
- ☐ No increased rates of iatrogenic urinary tract injury relative to a supracervical procedure

---

18. Maintaining interprofessional collaboration, discuss technical and therapeutic considerations once inside the delivery suite. Surgical debriefing has been completed, blood products and cell saver equipment available, intraoperative point-of-care testing available, vascular access sites initiated, and epidural anesthetic placed. *(1 point per main bullet)*   Max 12

Preoperative aspects:
- ☐ Use either the modified lithotomy position or place the legs straight, but parted
  - ○ *There are no publications to address maternal position for surgery for placental accreta spectrum*
  - ○ *Beware of risks of compartment syndrome and obstetric neuropraxia with prolonged use of stirrups*
- ☐ Pneumatic compression stockings
- ☐ Use ultrasound mapping to locate the upper anterior placental edge and guide the upper margin of the skin incision for uterine exposure (IS-AIP[3], FIGO[5f])
- ☐ Selective consideration for ureteric stents to reduce urinary tract injury when bladder invasion is suspected by antenatal imaging (ACOG[1], IS-AIP[3], FIGO[5f], SOGC[6], RCOG[7])
  - ○ *Routine preoperative cystoscopy is not recommended as the appearance of the bladder should not change imaging-based management (IS-AIP[3])*
- ☐ Insert a three-way bladder catheter; the access channel allows for partial intermittent insertion of methylene blue dye to facilitate surgical dissection of the vesicouterine plane

- ☐ Routine surgical antibiotic prophylaxis *(i.e., based on BMI and allergy status)* at skin incision or within one hour before the skin incision[†]
- ☐ Ensure availability of the same antibiotic given potential need for additional intraoperative dose as blood loss is anticipated to be ≥1500 mL[†]
- ☐ Prophylactic intravenous tranexamic acid 1 g (100 mg/mL) IV over 10 min[††] is recommended by some authorities as an adjunctive therapy in placenta accreta spectrum based on its benefit in established postpartum hemorrhage and lack of increased maternal-fetal adverse events; timing of administration includes:
  - ○ At the start of surgery *(SOGC[6])*
    OR
    At delivery after cord clamping *(ACOG[1], FIGO[5f])*
  - ○ *Prophylactic tranexamic acid remains unstudied in the context of placenta accreta spectrum*

Surgical aspects:[§]

- ☐ Use of either a vertical midline abdominal incision or wide transverse incisions *(e.g., Maylard of Cherney incision)* is accepted for cases of antenatally diagnosed placenta accreta spectrum
  - ○ *No evidence of benefit for routine vertical midline incision (IS-AIP[3]) and comparative data of skin incisions is lacking (ACOG[1])*
- ☐ Consideration for intraoperative sterile ultrasound, if required, to optimize uterine incision away from the placental site
- ☐ Uterine incision is more commonly a fundal transverse hysterotomy; use of a high upper-segment transverse uterine incision above the upper margin of the placenta may also be selected *(FIGO[5f])*
- ☐ Plan for routine delayed umbilical cord clamping, if appropriate
- ☐ Ensuring the placenta would not **spontaneously** deliver, leave the placenta and secured segment of the umbilical cord in-situ[#]
- ☐ Close the uterus expeditiously in one layer to limit blood loss
- ☐ *Controversial* use of uterotonic agents after delivery *{see Question 19}*
- ☐ *Controversial* effectiveness of surgical pelvic devascularization [*e.g., (i)* surgical ligation of the anterior division of the internal iliac arteries, *(ii)* temporary arterial balloon occlusion[‡]] *{see Questions 20 and 21, respectively}*

Special notes:

† Committee on Practice Bulletins-Obstetrics. ACOG Practice Bulletin No. 199: Use of prophylactic antibiotics in labor and delivery [published correction appears in *Obstet Gynecol.* 2019 Oct;134(4):883–884]. *Obstet Gynecol.* 2018;132(3):e103–e119.

†† Refer to Question 6 in Chapter 22

§ For complications related to disseminated intravascular coagulation (DIC) or postpartum hemorrhage, refer to Question 10-B in Chapter 21 for revision of the Modified International Society on Thrombosis and Hemostasis (ISTH) scoring system for overt DIC in pregnancy and to Questions 11 and 12 in Chapter 22 for discussion of concepts related to blood product replacement in postpartum hemorrhage

Where conservative management is planned, the umbilical cord segment is cut short, close to the placental insertion site

‡ Options include more selective occlusion of the anterior division of the internal iliac artery, less selective occlusion in the common iliac artery, or occlusion of the infrarenal abdominal aorta

After partaking in the interdisciplinary meeting for surgical delivery planning, your trainee performs an internet search for literature on controversial aspects of care in placenta accreta spectrum.

You share with your trainee that elective intra-arterial balloon placement may have also been considered perioperatively, with some evidence suggesting decreased surgical blood loss and need for transfusion, although routine consideration remains controversial.

---

19. Review with your trainee arguments for and against routine use of prophylactic uterotonics at Cesarean hysterectomy for placenta accreta spectrum disorders. *(1 point per main bullet)*

3

Against use of prophylactic uterotonics:[†]
- ☐ Uterotonics promote partial placental separation in regions of normal implantation; this may contribute to increased blood loss at the beginning of the hysterectomy
  - ○ *Routine administration is indicated if the placenta separates fully or partially, or if hemorrhage ensues*

Favored use of prophylactic uterotonics:[§]
- ☐ After delivery, uterine decompression may spontaneously promote partial separation of a placenta previa
- ☐ Component of active management of the third stage in prevention of postpartum hemorrhage

Special notes:
† Refer to (a) IS-AIP[3]; (b) Matsubara S. Measures for peripartum hysterectomy for placenta previa accreta: avoiding uterotonic agents and 'double distal edge pickup' mass ligation. *Arch Gynecol Obstet.* 2012;285(6):1765–1767; and (c) Matsubara S, Kuwata T, Usui R, et al. Important surgical measures and techniques at cesarean hysterectomy for placenta previa accreta. *Acta Obstet Gynecol Scand.* 2013;92(4):372–377.
§ Ngene N, Titus J, Onyia C, Moodley J. Should uterotonic agents be avoided during cesarean hysterectomy for placenta previa accreta?. *Acta Obstet Gynecol Scand.* 2013;92 (11):1338.

---

20. In addition to the advanced surgical skill involving retroperitoneal dissection for internal iliac artery ligation, address its potential complications or caveats that contribute to its controversial practice. *(1 point each)*

Max 3

- ☐ Ureteral injury
- ☐ Internal iliac vein laceration
- ☐ Buttocks and thigh claudication if inadvertent ligature of its posterior branch
- ☐ Precludes possibility of postoperative selective pelvic angiography and embolization

21. Identify <u>maternal-fetal morbidity</u> that has been associated with prophylactic <u>internal iliac artery balloon catheters</u> for prenatal diagnosis of placenta accreta spectrum disorders. *(1 point per main bullet; section-specific points as specified)*

Max 4

Maternal:[§] *(max 3)*

☐ Femoral artery puncture site hematoma, dissection, or pseudo-aneurysm formation *(all rare events, though most frequent complications)*

☐ Internal iliac arterial thrombus, rupture, or perforation

☐ Lower extremity embolism

☐ Distal ischemia reperfusion injury

☐ Sciatic nerve ischemic nerve injury

☐ Increased surgical bleeding from dense collateral vascular circulation

Fetal:[§]

☐ (Low dose) radiation exposure from fluoroscopy

   o *Pulsed fluoroscopy and last-image-hold decrease fetal risk*

   o *e.g., average dose of 4.4 mGy (0.44 rad) has been reported[†]; note that background risk of child leukemia of ~1/3000 may increase by a factor of 1.5–2 if the fetus is exposed to 10–20 mGy[‡]*

Special notes:

§ Petrov DA, Karlberg B, Singh K, Hartman M, Mittal PK. Perioperative internal iliac artery balloon occlusion, in the setting of placenta accreta and its variants: The role of the interventional radiologist. *Curr Probl Diagn Radiol.* 2018;47(6):445–451.

† Teixidor Viñas M, Chandraharan E, Moneta MV, Belli AM. The role of interventional radiology in reducing haemorrhage and hysterectomy following caesarean section for morbidly adherent placenta. *Clin Radiol.* 2014;69(8):e345–e351

‡ Committee Opinion No. 723: Guidelines for diagnostic imaging during pregnancy and lactation [published correction appears in *Obstet Gynecol.* 2018 Sep;132(3):786]. *Obstet Gynecol.* 2017;130(4):e210–e216.

Arrangements for operative delivery proceed according to the interdisciplinary plan; a vertical midline abdominal incision is performed, and the fetus is delivered through a fundal transverse hysterotomy. The umbilical cord is secured after one-minute delayed cord clamping, following which peripartum hysterectomy is successful without surgical complications. An additional intraoperative antibiotic dose was given; total estimated blood loss was 2500 mL and warmed blood product replacement was started intraoperatively. The patient is aware of the need for postpartum pharmacologic thromboprophylaxis, bladder care aspects as arranged by the urologist, and continued access to psychosocial support services. She will be carefully monitored and counseled for short- and long-term complications related to the potential for hypoperfusion, surgical- and transfusion-related complications.[†] Parental and interdisciplinary debriefing have been arranged and meticulous documentation ensured.

Special note:
† Refer to Question 22 in Chapter 22

TOTAL: 130

Neurological Disorders in Pregnancy

CHAPTER 24

Epilepsy in Pregnancy

Raluca Pana and Amira El-Messidi

A 30-year-old nulligravida with epilepsy is referred by her primary care provider to your hospital center's high-risk obstetrics unit for preconception counseling.

LEARNING OBJECTIVES

1. Take a focused history and provide preconception counseling of a patient with epilepsy, identifying features of seizure control and antiepileptic drugs (AEDs) associated with optimal perinatal outcome
2. Understand pregnancy-associated triggers for breakthrough seizures among women with epilepsy, and be able to provide appropriate investigations based on clinical descriptors
3. Appreciate differential etiologies for unexplained seizures in pregnancy, and initiate necessary treatment for suspected status epilepticus
4. Demonstrate the ability to plan antepartum and intrapartum care of a patient with epilepsy, maintaining continued interdisciplinary collaboration
5. Formulate home-safety measures and highlight important aspects for contraception among postpartum mothers with epilepsy

SUGGESTED READINGS

1. Campbell E, Kennedy F, Russell A, et al. Malformation risks of antiepileptic drug monotherapies in pregnancy: updated results from the UK and Ireland Epilepsy and Pregnancy Registers. *J Neurol Neurosurg Psychiatry*. 2014;85(9):1029–1034.
2. Committee on Practice Bulletins-Obstetrics. Practice Bulletin No. 187: Neural tube defects. *Obstet Gynecol*. 2017;130(6):e279–e290.
3. Douglas Wilson R, Van Mieghem T, Langlois S, et al. Guideline No. 410: Prevention, screening, diagnosis, and pregnancy management for fetal neural tube defects. *J Obstet Gynaecol Can*. 2021;43(1):124–139.e8.
4. Harden CL, Hopp J, Ting TY, et al. Practice parameter update: management issues for women with epilepsy – focus on pregnancy (an evidence-based review): obstetrical complications and change in seizure frequency: report of the Quality Standards Subcommittee and Therapeutics and Technology Assessment Subcommittee of the American Academy of Neurology and American Epilepsy Society. *Neurology*. 2009;73(2):126–132. Reaffirmed 2013.

5. Harden CL, Pennell PB, Koppel BS, et al. Practice parameter update: management issues for women with epilepsy – focus on pregnancy (an evidence-based review): vitamin K, folic acid, blood levels, and breastfeeding: report of the Quality Standards Subcommittee and Therapeutics and Technology Assessment Subcommittee of the American Academy of Neurology and American Epilepsy Society. *Neurology.* 2009;73(2):142–149.

6. Patel SI, Pennell PB. Management of epilepsy during pregnancy: an update. *Ther Adv Neurol Disord.* 2016;9(2):118–129. Reaffirmed 2013.

7. Rajiv KR, Radhakrishnan A. Status epilepticus in pregnancy – can we frame a uniform treatment protocol? *Epilepsy Behav.* 2019;101(Pt B):106376.

8. Royal College of Obstetricians and Gynaecologists. Epilepsy in pregnancy. Green-Top Guideline No. 68. London: RCOG; 2016.

9. Tomson T, Battino D, Bromley R, et al. Management of epilepsy in pregnancy: a report from the International League Against Epilepsy (ILAE) Task Force on Women and Pregnancy. *Epileptic Disord.* 2019;21(6):497–517.

10. Viale L, Allotey J, Cheong-See F, et al. Epilepsy in pregnancy and reproductive outcomes: a systematic review and meta-analysis. *Lancet.* 2015;386(10006):1845–1852.

POINTS

1. With regard to epilepsy, what aspects of a focused history would you want to know?   21
(1 point each, with section-specific max points)

General aspects of seizure disorder: *(max 5)*
☐ Duration of time since diagnosis
☐ Classification of seizure type(s)/epilepsy syndrome(s)
☐ Change in disease activity over time
☐ Results of most recent electroencephalogram or brain imaging
☐ Need for hospitalizations/prior status epilepticus
☐ Name and contact of treating neurologist

Medical/surgical risk factors for, or morbidities of, epilepsy: *(max 4)*
☐ Perinatal asphyxia, personal neurodevelopment
☐ Febrile seizures
☐ Central nervous system infections, intracranial mass lesions
☐ Traumatic brain injury
☐ Neurosurgery or placement of vagal nerve stimulator
☐ Psychiatric conditions; current mood
☐ Antiphospholipid syndrome

Manifestations of seizure episodes: *(max 2)*
☐ Time since last seizure, average frequency and duration of episodes
☐ Presence/absence of auras
☐ Description and duration of the post-ictal phase
☐ Known triggers/exacerbating factors *(e.g., fatigue, sleep deprivation, stress, photosensitivity)*

Current/prior medications, clinical response and side effects: *(max 4)*
☐ **Enzyme-inducing AEDs:** *e.g.,* phenytoin, primidone, phenobarbital, carbamazepine, oxcarbazepine, eslicarbazepine

☐ **Non-enzyme-inducing AEDs:** *e.g.,* sodium valproate, topiramate, lamotrigine, levetiracetam, gabapentin, pregabalin, tiagabine, vigabatrin, clonazepam/clobazam

☐ Assess for initiation of folic acid-containing prenatal vitamins[‡]

☐ Use of agents for comorbid conditions *(e.g., psychiatric diseases)*

☐ Contraceptive method, *if any*

Social aspects and routine health maintenance: *(max 4)*

☐ Occupation *(i.e., particularly for risk of fatigue, sleep deprivation)*

☐ Living arrangements and support persons

☐ Driving permission

☐ Smoking, alcohol consumption, and use of illicit substances

☐ Balanced nutritional diet

☐ Vaccination status *(e.g., influenza, hepatitis B, tetanus)*

Male partner/family history: *(2)*

☐ Epilepsy *(aides to assess fetal inheritance risk)*

☐ Family history of febrile seizures

☐ Partner's history of a neural tube defect

Special note:

‡ Inconsistent evidence regarding best periconceptional dose of folic acid supplementation; recommendations vary from 0.4 mg to 4–5 mg daily for women with epilepsy:

- ACOG, SOGC, American Academy of Neurology/American Epilepsy Society, and the International League Against Epilepsy support routine 0.4 mg supplementation *(Suggested Readings 2, 3, 4, and 9 respectively)*
- RCOG *(Suggested Reading 8)* advises folic acid 5 mg/d preconception until at least the end of the first trimester

Ten years ago, the patient was diagnosed with idiopathic temporal lobe epilepsy causing focal to bilateral tonic-clonic seizures. Neuroimaging and disease activity were stable on long-term twice-daily dosing of valproic acid, topiramate, and lamotrigine, respectively. Her treating neurologist had advised reliable contraception, for which she chose the levonorgestrel-releasing intrauterine system (LNG-IUS). Average seizure frequency was twice weekly; the patient was never a candidate for weaning or discontinuation of AEDs.

In anticipation of becoming pregnant, her neurologist modified treatment nine months ago, currently maintained on twice-daily lamotrigine 100 mg and levetiracetam 1000 mg respectively[†]; seizure activity increased with attempted lowering of these dosages. Her neurologist recently initiated folate-containing vitamins. Given quiescent disease activity since the new medication regimen, she anticipates approval for discontinuation of her contraceptive device. The patient maintains a healthy diet and life habits. Common to ~70% of patients, there is no family history of epilepsy. Her husband is healthy, without prior neural tube defect, and is supportive of the patient.

Special note:

† Fetal risks with polypharmacy likely depend on *actual* AED agents, *dose, and timing* of exposure rather than *number* of medications; lamotrigine and levetiracetam confer lowest risks of fetal malformations

2. With the aim of teaching your obstetric trainee, discuss the neurologist's rationale for pregestational replacement of valproic acid and topiramate by <u>detailing obstetric risks</u> of exposure.

8

Valproic acid:[†]
- ☐ In utero teratogenicity (up to 10%), including: *(1 point per subbullet; max 3)*
  - ○ Neural tube defects
  - ○ Craniofacial defects *(e.g., craniosynostosis, orofacial clefts, microcephaly)*
  - ○ Congenital heart malformations *(e.g., atrial septal defects)*
  - ○ Genitourinary defects *(e.g., hypospadias)*
  - ○ Limb defects *(e.g., polydactyly, clubfeet)*
- ☐ Nonteratogenic effects of in utero exposure (~40%), including: *(1 point per subbullet; max 2)*
  - ○ Neonatal coagulopathy due to hypofibrinogenemia
  - ○ Lower IQ scores *(more marked with polytherapy)*
  - ○ Impaired psychomotor development
  - ○ Increased educational needs
  - ○ Autism spectrum disorders
  - ○ Attention-deficit hyperactivity disorder

Topiramate: *(1 point each; max 3)*
- ☐ Orofacial clefts (~1%)
- ☐ FGR or small for gestational age newborns (~20%)
- ☐ Microcephaly (less than third percentile)
- ☐ IUFD (related to maternal metabolic acidosis)

Special note:
- † March 2018: Co-ordination Group for Mutual Recognition and Decentralised Procedures – Human (CMDh) endorsed the contraindication for valproate exposure in pregnancy or among women of child-bearing potential; Pregnancy Prevention Program is advised. Refer to www.ema.europa.eu/en/news/new-measures-avoid-valproate-exposure-pregnancy-endorsed, accessed January 1, 2021.

3. Identify three <u>disease-related</u> features that justify your professional recommendation related to this patient's anticipation of pregnancy. *(1 point each)*

Max 3

Current reassuring features:
- ☐ Patient has been seizure-free for 9 months *(ideally 9- to 12-month interval)*
- ☐ Patient's AEDs include new-generation agents with reassuring fetal safety profiles (*i.e.,* lamotrigine and levetiracetam)
- ☐ Patient is taking the lowest-effective dose
- ☐ Controversial benefit of periconceptional folic acid supplementation on IQ scores of children *with in utero exposure to AEDs*

The patient appreciates your evidence-based opinion for removal of her LNG-IUS. She believes that adherence to prepregnancy folic acid supplementation will mitigate risks of major congenital malformations associated with AEDs, including possible effects of epilepsy on pregnancy.

4. International variations exist regarding high-dose periconceptional folic acid supplementation for epileptic women. Troubleshoot her misconceptions by highlighting two mechanisms for AED-associated teratogenicity, unrelated to folate deficiency. *(1 point each)*   2

☐ Cytotoxic damage to DNA from oxidation of drugs forming free radical intermediates
☐ Genetic deficiency in epoxide hydrolase leading to accumulation of toxic metabolites

5. You inform the patient that excluding congenital abnormalities, several maternal-fetal complications remain of *controversial association* with epilepsy. What remains uncertain is whether they are a consequence of the epilepsy itself or an effect of the AEDs. Among your discussion on overall prospects for her pregnancy, the patient also wishes to know of possible maternal-fetal complications. *(1 point per main bullet, with section-specific max points)*   10

Reassuring maternal/fetal aspects: *(2)*
☐ Over 90% of women with epilepsy have an uncomplicated pregnancy
   ○ *Short episodes of hypoxia generally do not adversely affect the fetus*
   ○ *Fetal bradycardia may occur during/after generalized tonic-clonic seizures without long-term cerebral damage*
☐ Rates of early pregnancy loss are generally not greater than unaffected women

Maternal risks: *(max 5)*
☐ Depression (antepartum or postpartum); anxiety conditions
☐ Preterm labor *(greatest among smokers with epilepsy)*
☐ Antepartum and postpartum hemorrhage
☐ Placental abruption
☐ Preeclampsia/eclampsia; other hypertensive syndromes of pregnancy
☐ Cesarean delivery *(generally reserved for recurrent generalized seizures in late pregnancy or labor)*
☐ Trauma from seizure-related activity
☐ Sudden unexpected death in epilepsy (SUDEP) or event-related mortality[§]

Fetal risks: *(max 3)*
☐ FGR or suboptimal growth velocity
☐ Prematurity[†] *(iatrogenic or spontaneous preterm labor)*
☐ Injury from maternal abdominal trauma related to seizure activity
☐ Inheritance of seizure disorder *(4%–5% given only the patient is affected; risk increases to ~20% if both parents are affected)*
☐ IUFD

Special notes:
† AEDs may independently increase risks of preterm birth
§ Absolute increase in risk of maternal mortality is <0.1%

The patient is content knowing of the overall reassuring outlook for her planned pregnancy, albeit with inherent risks related to epilepsy and possibly AEDs, lamotrigine and levetiracetam. She recalls her neurologist's discussion of the impact of pregnancy on her disease control, although requests your input. The patient appreciates that her gestational care will be arranged in a multidisciplinary fashion.

6-A. Address the patient's inquiry on general periconceptional effects on seizure activity.   3
   (1 point each)

☐ Reassure the patient that ***antepartum*** seizure activity is unchanged in ~50%–60% of women, and may increase in ~15% of women
☐ Inform the patient that the ***intrapartum*** risk of seizure is ~1%–2%[‡]
☐ Inform the patient that the risk of seizures in the first 24 hours ***postpartum*** is ~1%–2%[‡]

Special note:
[‡] Advise against leaving a patient unattended during this time

6-B. Identify two main risk factors that may account for antepartum seizures in *this* patient.   2
   (1 point each)

☐ Focal epilepsy (*i.e., temporal lobe epilepsy*)
☐ Delays in adjustment of AED dosages (*e.g.,* serum levels of lamotrigine decrease as early as five weeks' gestation)
   ○ *Neurologist's collaboration is advised*

7. In anticipation of pregnancy, present a model for your <u>antepartum</u> management of the   14
   patient's epilepsy, while on levetiracetam and lamotrigine AED therapy.

Maternal: *(1 point per first nine main bullets)*
☐ Counseling on prevention, and provide early treatment, of nausea/vomiting
☐ Ensure the patient redoses AEDs if emesis occurs shortly after AED intake
☐ Serial screening for depression and anxiety
☐ Anticipate more frequent obstetric appointments
☐ Serial clinical monitoring for hypertensive syndromes of pregnancy
   ○ *Neither epilepsy nor AEDs are recognized major/moderate risk factors for preeclampsia to warrant prophylactic LDASA*[†]
☐ At-least routine dose folic acid supplementation
☐ Anticipate AED dose increases, in collaboration with her neurologist
☐ Considerations for serum monitoring of AED levels vary by agent and individual practices; collaboration with a neurologist is advised:
   ○ *American Academy of Neurology/American Epilepsy Society*[5]: Therapeutic antenatal monitoring of AED helps prevent seizure deterioration
   ○ *RCOG*[8]: Routine serum AED monitoring is generally not recommended, although individual circumstances may vary
   ○ *ILAE*[9]: For this patient on lamotrigine and levetiracetam, monthly serum drug-monitoring is indicated; marked declines in serum concentrations start in the early first trimester[§]

- ☐ Consideration for antenatal consultation with anesthesiologist (or early upon hospitalization)
- ☐ No benefit for routine oral vitamin K to prevent hemorrhagic disease of the newborn *(i.e., this patient is not taking enzyme-inducing AEDs)*
  - ○ *RCOG:* Evidence is insufficient for supplementation even among women taking enzyme-inducing AEDs
- ☐ No benefit for routine oral vitamin K to prevent postpartum hemorrhage

Fetal: *(1 point each)*
- ☐ First-trimester sonography for early detection of structural anomalies *(epilepsy/AEDs do not increase risks of aneuploidy)*
- ☐ Second-trimester detailed morphology scan
- ☐ Fetal echocardiography *(jurisdictional variations exist)*
- ☐ Serial growth scans *(given patient exposure to AEDs)*
  - ○ *No role for routine antepartum fetal surveillance with cardiotocography (CTG)*
- ☐ Consideration for neonatology consultation, where clinical concerns exist

Special notes:
† *Refer to Chapter 38*
§ Practice settings may lack resources for AED blood levels

After removal of her LNG-IUS, she conceives spontaneously within six months. During this time, she experienced three tonic-clonic seizures related to community-acquired pneumonia. She continues to be compliant with her comprehensive epilepsy care plan. There have not been changes to her focal epilepsy syndrome.

As a high-risk obstetrician, you follow her antenatal care with the established preconceptional plan. Pregnancy is unremarkable until 16^{+2} weeks' gestation when she complains of a typical breakthrough focal seizure, commonly manifesting with an aura. Witnessed by her husband who placed her in the recovery position to prevent aspiration and ensure her safety, the tonic-clonic component lasted 30 seconds and was followed by a postictal phase. She is currently well, and examination is unremarkable. She has no obstetric complaints and fetal viability is ascertained. First-trimester serum AED levels were therapeutic; she was planning to repeat blood testing in several days.

8. Although often multifactorial, illustrate an understanding of the causes for breakthrough seizures during pregnancy. *(1 point each)*	Max 5

- ☐ Reduced plasma concentration of AEDs
- ☐ Sleep deprivation
- ☐ Nausea/vomiting, common to early pregnancy
- ☐ Poor adherence to AEDs due to concerns over teratogenesis
- ☐ Psychosocial stress
- ☐ Intrapartum hyperventilation/pain
- ☐ *'Other'* causes: intercurrent illness, infections, metabolic disturbances, alcohol consumption/illicit substance use

9. In collaboration with her neurologist, <u>detail</u> your agreed-upon investigations in evaluation of the patient's seizure event. *(1 point each)*

Serum:
☐ CBC
☐ Creatinine
☐ Calcium
☐ Sodium
☐ Glucose
☐ Levetiracetam and lamotrigine levels
☐ Hepatic transaminases and function tests

Urine:
☐ Urinalysis ± urine culture

Neuro-testing:
☐ Electroencephalogram *(poses no fetal risk)*

Special note:
Brain imaging is not indicated as the seizure was described in its typical form

Investigations reveal a serum lamotrigine at 6 µmol/L (1.5 µg/mL), relative to a prepregnancy of 10 µmol/L (2.5 µg/mL). Levetiracetam is therapeutic, and all other investigations are unremarkable. The neurologist explained that given her lamotrigine concentration decreased to **65% or less**[§] of her target prepregnancy concentration, this is the most attributable cause for the recent breakthrough seizure. He or she thereby increased lamotrigine to 175 mg and 200 mg in the morning and evening, respectively.

Special note:
§ Refer to (a) *Suggested Reading 5*, (b) Reisinger TL, et al. *Epilepsy Behav.* 2013; 29(1): 13–8, (c) Voinescu PE, et al. *Neurology* 2018; 91(13): e1228–36.

10. Refresh your obstetric trainee's knowledge of the <u>physiologic</u> bases for reductions in gestational plasma concentrations of AEDs. *(1 point each)*

☐ Increased renal blood flow and glomerular filtration rate
☐ Increased hepatic metabolism (*e.g.*, glucuronidation, cytochrome P450 enzymes)
☐ Decreased gastrointestinal absorption

Pregnancy progresses well and fetal growth remains on the 11th–20th percentile with reassuring markers of fetal well-being. At 32 weeks' gestation, the patient presents to the obstetric emergency assessment unit by ambulance, after her husband found her unconscious on the floor at home. Paramedics indicate she had three generalized tonic-clonic seizures en route. At presentation, the patient remains unconscious, already positioned on her left lateral decubitus. Rectal temperature is 39°C (102°F), blood pressure is 110/70 mmHg, pulse is 100 bpm, and oxygen saturation is 94% on room air. There are no signs of trauma, needle tracks, vaginal bleeding, or overt evidence of ruptured amniotic membranes. On continuous CTG tracing, fetal heart baseline is 110 bpm, variability is minimal without decelerations or a sinusoidal waveform. Uterine quiescence is noted. The neurology team on duty presents urgently to assist in her care.

---

11. As simultaneous comprehensive investigations are underway, you contemplate numerous causes being tested. List six possible etiologies for the patient's clinical presentation. *(1 point each)*

   Max 6

☐ Status epilepticus
☐ Eclampsia
☐ Infection related to the central nervous system or other systemic etiology
☐ Posterior reversible leukoencephalopathy syndrome
☐ Thrombotic thrombocytopenic purpura (TTP)
☐ Antiphospholipid syndrome
☐ Stroke *(ischemic or hemorrhagic)*
☐ Cerebral venous sinus thrombosis
☐ Reversible cerebral vasoconstriction syndrome
☐ Acute intermittent porphyria
☐ Metabolic derangements *(e.g., alcohol/drug withdrawal, hypoglycemia, hypocalcemia, hyponatremia)*
☐ Space-occupying lesion

Special note:
The above list serves as a guide; other etiologies may be appropriate

---

Capillary blood glucose is normal; urinalysis reveals leukocyte esterase and nitrites with minimal proteinuria. Results of other investigations are pending.

---

12. Outline two <u>therapeutic</u> regimens that would be considered part of this patient's initial <u>maternal</u> stabilization. *[1 point per main and subbullet; accept one regimen from (A) and one regimen from (B)]*

   2

Status epilepticus:
☐ **(A)** First-line benzodiazepine is lorazepam 4 mg IV over 2 minutes, repeated once after 10–20 minutes if ongoing confusion or seizures
   ○ If unavailable, use diazepam 10–20 mg IV at 2 mg/min *or* 10–20 mg rectal gel; midazolam 10 mg IM is optional
☐ **(B)** If benzodiazepine fails, AED of choice is levetiracetam IV 60 mg/kg loading dose (max 4500 mg/dose)
   ○ If unavailable, use phenytoin IV 20 mg/kg (max 1500 mg/dose)

Special note:
Standard magnesium sulfate protocols (refer to Chapter 38) for eclampsia would be indicated until definitive diagnosis, where seizures cannot be clearly attributed to epilepsy

---

The patient regained consciousness after two doses of lorazepam, with concurrent normalization of the fetal tracing within five minutes. A loading dose of levetiracetam was given. Serum AED levels were therapeutic and oral treatments have been resumed. A routine course of prophylactic betamethasone[‡] was given for fetal pulmonary maturity. Evaluation of potential precipitants was only significant for an *E. coli* urinary tract infection, for which IV ceftriaxone was administered until defervescence. The patient will complete an oral antibiotic regimen and one-week follow-up is arranged.

While timing of delivery is controversial after status epilepticus in pregnancy, an interdisciplinary plan is made for close monitoring of maternal-fetal well-being, aiming for spontaneous labor at term. The patient understands that iatrogenic prematurity may otherwise be indicated.

At 35 weeks' gestation, you review her intrapartum care plan and address postpartum home-safety strategies previously discussed in pregnancy.

Special note:
‡ Doubling the dose of prophylactic antenatal corticosteroids is not recommended, even with enzyme-inducing AEDs *(RCOG[8])*

13. Recognizing that delivery will take place in a consultant-led unit, provide essentials of <u>intrapartum</u> management with regard to her epilepsy. (*1 point per main bullet*)	Max 8

☐ Advise *early* presentation to hospital in labor
☐ Early notification of the anesthesiologist, ensuring adequate analgesia and hydration to minimise risks for seizures *(e.g., hyperventilation, sleep deprivation, fatigue, pain, stress)*
   ○ *Meperidine (pethidine) may decrease seizure threshold; caution is advised*
   ○ *Morphine analgesia is preferable*
☐ Continued liaison with the neurology team/expert involved in her care
☐ Continue AED treatment during labor, or provide parenteral alternatives where required
☐ Arrange for continuous observation with one-to-one care *(RCOG)*
☐ Consider keeping bed rails raised in event of seizure
☐ Ensure written guidelines have been prepared in the event of intrapartum seizures
☐ Continuous electronic fetal monitoring
☐ Anticipate risk of postpartum hemorrhage; ensure uterotonics are available at delivery
   ○ *Individualized plans for presence of blood products on delivery unit*
☐ Consideration for delayed pushing in the second stage of labor *(fatigue-induced seizures)*
☐ Maintain a low threshold for assisted second stage *(fatigue-induced seizures)*

Special notes:
(a) Water birth would not be recommended for <u>this</u> patient; individualized assessment is advised for women not requiring AEDs and seizure-free for a significant period *(RCOG[8])*.
(b) All neonates should receive intramuscular vitamin K 1 mg

14. Formulate a list of <u>home-safety</u> measures for <u>the postpartum period</u> of mothers with epilepsy and their newborns. (*1 point each*)	Max 7

☐ Avoid sleep deprivation *(e.g., pump milk in advance for family members to care for newborn)*
☐ Presence of a support person at all times at home should be considered

☐ Use the floor or middle of a bed while feeding/changing the newborn

☐ Use shallow water to bathe the newborn with supervision available

☐ Discourage co-sleeping in same bed

☐ Avoid walking/performing activities while carrying the newborn; use of a stroller is advised

☐ Organize newborn care items on different levels of the home

☐ Discourage mother from taking baths behind a closed, locked door or without an adult in the home

☐ *Other general precautions:* keep rooms free of clutter or individual carpets; use a microwave or crockpot instead of a stove; no driving

The patient presents at 36^{+5} weeks' gestation in early spontaneous labor. In accordance with the prearranged intrapartum care plan, the patient has an uneventful labor and vaginal delivery of a healthy male weighing 2500 g at birth.

You visit her on postpartum day 1; she plans to ask her neurologist about gradual conversion to a carbamazepine-including regimen, which her friend is taking.

15. In relation to seizure disorder, delineate important elements for the <u>postpartum</u> care of your patient. *(1 point per main bullet)*

Max 7

Mental health and support:

☐ Screen for postpartum depression and offer psychosocial support contacts in the event of symptoms
  ○ *The risk of postpartum depression and anxiety is increased among women with epilepsy*

AED treatments:

☐ Collaborate with a neurologist to ensure tapering of AEDs to prepregnancy levels (plus 50 mg to the baseline lamotrigine dose)
  ○ Empiric tapering of levetiracetam/lamotrigine over 10–14 days postpartum

Breastfeeding:

☐ Generally, encouraged for maternal-infant benefits

☐ Consider feeding **before** taking AEDs to decrease infant adverse symptoms (*e.g., sedation, poor suckling, hypotonia, vomiting, apnea*)

☐ Inform her that breastfeeding while on AEDs can improve child neurodevelopmental and cognitive outcomes

Contraception:[‡]

☐ In standard doses, depot medroxyprogesterone acetate (DMPA) decreases seizure frequency

☐ While taking **non-enzyme-inducing AEDs**, there are no restrictions on contraceptive methods

☐ Higher dose lamotrigine is required with estrogen-containing contraceptives; consider minimizing the hormone-free interval as lamotrigine side effects may manifest
  ○ *(lamotrigine is the only AED whose metabolism is affected by estrogen)*

☐ If patient converts to an **enzyme-inducing AED** regimen, promote use of copper-IUD,[†] LNG-IUS, or DMPA injections

○ *UK-MEC:* Combined oral contraceptives, progesterone-only pills or implants, transdermal patches, or vaginal ring are not advised due to decreased efficacy with concurrent enzyme-inducing AEDs

○ *US-MEC:* Progesterone implants are an option to be considered for women on enzyme-inducing AEDs (category 2)

○ Promote dual contraception (*e.g.,* condoms) where hormonal contraceptives are used with enzyme-inducing AEDs

○ Consider *(unconfirmed efficacy)* higher dose estrogen compounds, longer half-life progesterone agents, and decreasing hormone-free intervals when hormone contraceptives are used with enzyme-inducing AEDs

Follow-up:

☐ Arrange postpartum clinic appointment *(individualized timing)*, and ensure planned follow-up with her neurologist

☐ Promote future preconception counseling to optimize timing of conception with regard to seizure control and treatments

Special notes:

‡ Refer to (a) Gynecologic management of adolescents and young women with seizure disorders: ACOG Committee Opinion Summary, No. 806. *Obstet Gynecol.* 2020;135(5): 1242–1243; (b) UK Medical Eligibility Criteria (MEC) for contraceptive use 2016, revised Sept 2019; (c) US-MEC 2016, amended 2020

† Preferred emergency contraceptive agent if patient reverts to enzyme-inducing AED regimens

TOTAL: **110**

CHAPTER 25

Headache and Stroke in Pregnancy

Isabelle Malhamé, Amira El-Messidi, and Catherine Legault

During your on-call duty, a 34-year-old primigravida at 23 weeks' gestation with no systemic condition presents to the obstetric emergency assessment unit with a one-day history of a headache.

Your colleague follows her prenatal care, and pregnancy has been unremarkable. Routine prenatal laboratory investigations, aneuploidy screening, and fetal morphology sonogram were normal.

LEARNING OBJECTIVES

1. Take a focused history of headache in pregnancy, eliciting characteristics that warrant prompt evaluation
2. Recognize clinical features with, triggers for, and management of a common primary headache syndrome in pregnancy
3. Appreciate causes of secondary headaches with 'red flag' signs in pregnancy requiring timely interdisciplinary collaboration for evaluation, investigations, and acute management of a stroke in the antepartum period
4. Understand the elements of focused obstetric counseling and management throughout the perinatal period after a sustained acute antepartum ischemic stroke
5. Highlight important features to communicate in preconception counseling of a patient with a prior cryptogenic ischemic stroke during the antenatal period

SUGGESTED READINGS

1. (a) Burch R. Headache in pregnancy and the puerperium. *Neurol Clin*. 2019;37(1):31–51.
   (b) Burch R. Epidemiology and treatment of menstrual migraine and migraine during pregnancy and lactation: a narrative review. *Headache*. 2020;60(1):200–216.
2. Camargo EC, Feske SK, Singhal AB. Stroke in pregnancy: an update. *Neurol Clin*. 2019;37(1):131–148.
3. Grear KE, Bushnell CD. Stroke and pregnancy: clinical presentation, evaluation, treatment, and epidemiology. *Clin Obstet Gynecol*. 2013;56(2):350–359.
4. Ladhani NNN, Swartz RH, Foley N, et al. Canadian stroke best practice consensus statement: acute stroke management during pregnancy. *Int J Stroke*. 2018;13(7):743–758.
5. Miller EC, Leffert L. Stroke in pregnancy: a focused update. *Anesth Analg*. 2020;130(4): 1085–1096.

6. O'Neal MA. Headaches complicating pregnancy and the postpartum period. *Pract Neurol.* 2017;17(3):191–202.

7. Roth J, Deck G. Neurovascular disorders in pregnancy: A review. *Obstet Med.* 2019;12(4): 164–167.

8. Scottish Intercollegiate Guidelines Network (SIGN). Pharmacological management of migraine. Edinburgh: SIGN publication no. 155. February 2018.

9. Swartz RH, Ladhani NNN, Foley N, et al. Canadian stroke best practice consensus statement: secondary stroke prevention during pregnancy. *Int J Stroke.* 2018;13(4):406–419.

10. van Alebeek ME, de Heus R, Tuladhar AM, et al. Pregnancy and ischemic stroke: a practical guide to management. *Curr Opin Neurol.* 2018;31(1):44–51.

POINTS

1. With regard to her headache, what aspects of a focused history would you want to know? *(1 point per main bullet)*	Max 20

☐ Establish whether this is a new headache or whether the patient has a known history of headaches

Characteristics warranting prompt evaluation ('Red flags'):
☐ New onset of a severe/thunderclap headache *(e.g., 'worst headache of my life')*
  o *Thunderclap headaches are sudden in onset with acute maximal intensity*
☐ Headache awoke her from sleep/worse in the morning
☐ Focal neurological symptoms, such as visual changes, motor/sensory loss, dysarthria, or abnormal gait
☐ Nonfocal neurological symptoms, such as altered mental status/cognition
☐ Seizure activity
☐ Headache after head trauma
☐ Fever or signs of infection

Associated signs and symptoms:
☐ Postural and/or exertional features *(e.g., Valsalva, coughing)*
☐ Nausea and/or vomiting
☐ Pulsatile tinnitus or phonophobia
☐ Epigastric or right upper quadrant pain

Characteristics of the headache:
☐ Description of the quality of the headache *(e.g., throbbing, pulsatile, sharp/dull, constant)*
☐ Location/pattern of spread, if any
☐ Chronology
☐ Severity grading and progression

Social history:
☐ Occupation *(i.e., particularly for risks of fatigue, sleep deprivation, and toxic exposure)*
☐ Cigarette smoking
☐ Alcohol consumption
☐ Illicit substance use *(e.g., cocaine, marijuana, amphetamines)*

Medications and allergies:
- ☐ Nonprescription drug use (current/prior and side effects encountered)
- ☐ Narcotic use (current/prior and side effects encountered)
- ☐ Anticoagulant use, or nonmedicinals with anticoagulant activity
- ☐ Allergies

Family history:
- ☐ Headache
- ☐ Thrombophilia or venous thromboembolism (VTE)

You learn that the patient's headache was of spontaneous onset this morning, gradually increasing in intensity throughout the day. Despite resting in a quiet, dark room, she has been seeing lights and zigzag lines that she knows are not real. Last night, she experienced insomnia after a stressful three-hour work-related meeting on an electronic platform. Her headache is described as a severe, right-temporal throbbing pain accompanied by phonophobia and nausea. She has not been able to tolerate oral intake all day. There are no other systemic features. The patient has not taken any medications, in fear of pregnancy-associated risks. Her medications only constitute prenatal vitamins; she practices healthy life-habits and recently discontinued her small cup of morning coffee. The patient feels her symptoms simulate her long-standing catamenial headaches she experienced since her teenage years and was initially pleased with pregnancy-associated symptom resolution.

On physical examination, she is afebrile, normotensive, and has a BMI of 22 kg/m^2. Upon her request, lights have been dimmed throughout the clinical assessment. Fetal viability is ascertained. There are no abnormal obstetric features on assessment. In collaboration with an obstetric internist/neurologist, the patient's neurological examination is normal. Bedside random capillary glucose is normal.

2. Based on your discussion with the obstetric internist/neurologist, identify the triggers and clinical features that are consistent with the most probable diagnosis for this patient. *(1 point each)*   10

Triggers:
- ☐ Stress
- ☐ Insomnia
- ☐ Visual stimuli
- ☐ Recent discontinuation of caffeine
- ☐ Pregnancy-associated hormonal changes

Clinical features consistent with a migraine:
- ☐ Unilateral, severe throbbing headache of gradual onset
- ☐ Light sensitivity/photophobia
- ☐ 'Fortification spectra' (*i.e., the appearance of light phenomena before the eye/zigzag lines*)
- ☐ Nausea and vomiting[†]
- ☐ History of catamenial headaches with similar symptoms to the current presentation

Special note:
† Dehydration may also trigger a headache, although this is likely a result of, rather than a cause for, this patient's presentation.

3. Outline your clinical management and first- or second-line treatment options to abate her   9
acute migraine episode in pregnancy. *(1 point each)*

Nonpharmaceutical: *(max 4)*
- ☐ Oral hydration
- ☐ Provide a calm environment
- ☐ Avoid known triggers
- ☐ Ice or heat
- ☐ Biofeedback techniques *(helpful as traditional acute therapy and as prophylaxis)*

Pharmaceutical: *(max 5)*
- ☐ Parenteral hydration
- ☐ Acetaminophen (paracetamol) 1 g
- ☐ Prochlorperazine[§]
- ☐ Metoclopramide[§§]
- ☐ Combined [acetaminophen (paracetamol) and metoclopramide] or [acetaminophen (paracetamol) and prochlorperazine]
- ☐ Triptans [5-HT1 agonists] *(e.g., sumatriptan, naratriptan, rizatriptan)*
- ☐ Intravenous magnesium sulfate *(limit duration to less than five days to avoid fetal bone malformations)*
- ☐ Ondansetron[§§§]
- ☐ A nonsteroidal anti-inflammatory agent *(e.g., ibuprofen, naproxen, diclofenac)* may be considered in the second trimester for a maximum of 48–72 hours duration
- ☐ Prednisone for limited duration
- ☐ Occipital nerve blocks (may be helpful in both rescue and prophylaxis)
- ☐ Butalbital (a barbiturate) in combination with acetaminophen (paracetamol) and low-dose caffeine (40–50 mg)
  - ○ *Barbiturate availability varies by jurisdiction; agents are unavailable in the UK*

Special note:
Refer to Questions 6[§] and 7[(§§,§§§)] in Chapter 4 for drug regimens

In discussion with the obstetric internist/neurologist, your obstetric trainee inquires about theoretical risks of uteroplacental vasoconstriction and increased uterine contractions with triptan use.

4. Elaborate on the safety profile of triptan agents for treatment of acute migraine in   3
pregnancy.

Triptans in pregnancy:
- ☐ No increased risk of pregnancy loss, congenital anomalies, or prematurity

5. Alert your obstetric trainee of pharmaceutical agents to <u>always or preferentially avoid</u> for treatment of acute migraine in pregnancy and justify your evidence-based opinion.
(2 points per main bullet, and 1 point per subbullet)

☐ Ergotamine agents
  ○ Uteroplacental vasoconstriction
  ○ Uterine contractions
☐ High-dose aspirin[‡]
  ○ Fetal-neonatal bleeding
  ○ Closure of the patent ductus arteriosus in the third trimester
☐ Opiates and codeine
  ○ Analgesic-rebound headache
  ○ Worsens nausea/vomiting in pregnancy
  ○ Worsens constipation in pregnancy
  ○ Neonatal opiate withdrawal syndrome with chronic use

Special note:
[‡] Aspirin, in doses for treatment of acute migraine (~900 mg), is not an analgesic of choice during pregnancy *(Suggested Reading 9)*

Max 12

Within several hours, the patient responds well to an analgesic and antiemetic in combination with nonpharmaceutical measures. She is concerned about the risk of migraine recurrence and inquires about preventative therapies in pregnancy. Meanwhile, you find your obstetric trainee surfing the internet for the effects of migraine on pregnancy. You indicate that although women with migraines should be monitored for associated pregnancy complications, there are no studies to support any specific intervention.

6. Address the effects of migraine on pregnancy.

Max 4

Maternal risks: *(1 point each; max 3)*
☐ Hypertensive syndromes of pregnancy *(irrespective of migraine treatment or prophylaxis)*
☐ Stroke
☐ Preterm delivery
☐ Early pregnancy loss

Fetal risks: *(1 point for either)*
☐ Low birthweight *(without FGR)*
☐ No increased risk of congenital anomalies

7. Discuss important aspects of your counseling on the general course of migraine during the obstetric period. *(1 point each)*   Max 5

Antepartum:
☐ Migraines generally improve over the course of pregnancy in ~60%–70% of women
☐ The patient's history of menstrual migraines and absence of auras confer positive features for symptomatic improvement in pregnancy
☐ Encourage nonpharmacological interventions and avoidance of triggers
☐ Consideration for expert consultation for biofeedback and cognitive behavioral therapy training

Postpartum:
☐ Indicate that migraine recurrences can occur postpartum *(lack of sleep, stress, falling estrogen levels, endothelial changes)*
☐ Address the protective effects of breastfeeding on postpartum migraine recurrence *(possibly due to greater stability of serum estrogen levels)*

8. In collaboration with the obstetric internist/neurologist, address the indications for pharmacological migraine prophylaxis in pregnancy. *(1 point each)*   Max 3

☐ Frequent use of acute migraine treatment (*e.g.*, more than twice weekly)
☐ Regular onset of disabling headaches (*e.g.*, more than twice monthly)
☐ Migraines with neurological sequelae
☐ Suboptimal response to symptomatic treatment

The patient appreciates your detailed counseling of nonmedicinal remedies for prevention of migraines and is optimistic about expected improvement during the antenatal period. In addition to the multiple maternal-infant benefits of breastfeeding, she is further motivated by your migraine-based discussion. Prior to discharge, you ensure a follow-up is arranged in your clinic, as her primary care provider will soon be away for vacation.

Unfortunately, migraines without auras or neurological sequelae continued to occur two to three times weekly over the following three weeks.

9. In collaboration with the obstetric internist/neurologist, outline four agents that can be used as migraine prophylaxis in pregnancy and alert your trainee of four agents to avoid. The patient remains otherwise healthy and has no allergies. Her obstetric progress is unremarkable.   8

Safe prophylactic agents: *(1 point each; max 4)*
☐ Beta-blockers *(preferably propanolol; avoid atenolol due to the greater risk of low birthweight)*
☐ Tricyclic antidepressants (*e.g., preferably amitriptyline; nortriptyline is optional as well*)
☐ Low-dose aspirin 75 mg daily
☐ Vitamin B2 (riboflavin) in physiologic doses
☐ Oral magnesium

- ☐ Calcium channel blockers *(e.g., verapamil)*
- ☐ Lamotrigine
- ☐ Occipital nerve block
- ☐ Coenzyme 10, cyclobenzaprine, and memantine are likely safe *(limited data)*

Advise against: *(1 point each; max 4)*
- ☐ Valproic acid[†]
- ☐ Topiramate[†]
- ☐ Angiotensin-converting enzyme inhibitors (ACEi)[‡] or angiotensin receptor blocking agents
- ☐ Feverfew
- ☐ Onabotulinum toxin A *(not currently recommended due to limited information; no known risks of fetal malformations)*

Special notes:
[†] Refer to Question 2 in Chapter 24 for obstetric risks of valproic acid and topiramate
[‡] Refer to Question 5 in Chapter 47 for prenatal management of, and fetal risks with, ACEi agents

At 26 weeks' gestation, the patient was started on nortriptyline 25 mg nightly. Prophylactic treatment and continued behavioral modifications have led to remission of migraines by 28 weeks' gestation.

At 33 weeks' gestation, the patient presents to the obstetric emergency assessment unit with a three-day history of headache and blurry vision in her left eye. This episode started with unilateral left bright sparkling lights of 20 minutes duration and a simultaneous severe right-sided occipital headache, which is of a different character from her standard migraine headaches. Although the visual changes are also new to her, the patient assumed this was a migraine with aura. She decided to seek care after unsuccessful attempts to resolve this event. She has not experienced other neurological or systemic symptoms. The fetus continues to move well, and she has no obstetric complaints. The fetal cardiotocography (CTG) tracing is normal at presentation.

Upon your request, the obstetric internist/neurologist promptly attends to her care. On examination, the patient is afebrile and her blood pressure (BP) is 145/95 mmHg. Comprehensive neurological, including fundoscopic, examination reveals left homonymous hemianopia *(vertical visual loss on the left side of both eyes)*.

10. After informing the patient of the clinical findings and concerns, identify the next most appropriate steps in management. You reassure her that your institution has the necessary specialization in place for rapid access to diagnostic tests and interventions.[†] *(1 point each)*   Max 2

- ☐ 'Code stroke' or urgent neurological evaluation
- ☐ Patient transfer to an emergency department or unit capable of close neurological monitoring of vital signs
- ☐ Participate in the interdisciplinary discussion to arrange safe neuroimaging in pregnancy, while counseling the patient on the potential imaging modalities

Special note:
[†] Timely transfer to a medical center with both stroke and obstetric specialization would otherwise be warranted

While the stroke team is attending to the patient, you reflect on possible causes of her clinical features.

11. Formulate a differential diagnosis for causes of secondary headaches in the third trimester that may explain the patient's presentation and clinical findings. *(1 point each)*

Max 5

☐ Ischemic or hemorrhagic stroke
☐ Hypertensive syndromes of pregnancy
☐ Subarachnoid hemorrhage
☐ Cerebral venous sinus thrombosis
☐ Posterior reversible leukoencephalopathy syndrome
☐ Reversible cerebral vasoconstriction syndrome
☐ Idiopathic (benign) intracranial hypertension
☐ Carotid artery dissection
☐ Pituitary apoplexy

12. Based on the three potential neuroimaging modalities being considered for this obstetric patient, indicate important considerations for patient counseling and management. *(1 point per main and principal subbullet)*

Max 6

☐ CT-head **without** contrast:
  ○ Estimated fetal radiation exposure is very low, at 0.001–0.01 mGy,[†] which is far below the 50 mGy threshold for fetal radiation complications
  ○ Routine abdominal shielding should be avoided in imaging modalities where ionizing radiation does not directly expose the fetus because (1) most of the fetal dose results from internal (rather than external) scatter, and (2) automatic control can cause increased dose exposure if the shield is inadvertently in the field of view during the scan.[§]
  ○ Abdominal shielding may be considered on a case-by-case basis if it offers patient reassurance after appropriate counseling.[§§]

☐ CT-head **with** contrast (CT angiography):
  ○ There is no evidence for harm from iodinated contrast media
    ▪ *Theoretical concerns about potential adversity of free iodide on the fetal thyroid gland have not been found in human studies*
  ○ Despite a higher dose of radiation than CT-head without contrast, fetal radiation exposure remains below the threshold for pregnancy complications

☐ MRI:[‡]
  ○ Noncontrast MR angiography (time-of-flight imaging modalities) can often provide sufficient vascular information for emergency stroke decision-making in pregnancy, and is preferable to contrast scanning

Special notes:
[†]   Refer to table 3 in <Committee Opinion No. 723: Guidelines for diagnostic imaging during pregnancy and lactation [published correction appears in *Obstet Gynecol.* 2018 Sep;132(3):786]. *Obstet Gynecol.* 2017;130(4):e210–e216.>
[§]   Tirada N, Dreizin D, Khati NJ, et al. Imaging pregnant and lactating patients. *Radiographics* 2015;35:1751–65
[§§]   *Refer to* (a) American Association of Physicists in Medicine. AAPM position statement on the use of patient gonadal and fetal shielding, 2019, and (b) British

Institute of Radiology, Institute of Physics and Engineering in Medicine, Public Health England, Royal College of Radiologists, Society and College of Radiographers, the Society for Radiological Protection. Guidance on using shielding on patients for diagnostic radiology applications. 2020.

‡ *Refer to* Question 10 in Chapter 42 for discussion on use of MRI in pregnancy; fetal risks of gadolinium contrast agent are also addressed

In follow-up of the MRI results, you learn she has a subacute right posterior cerebral artery infarct involving the right occipital lobe.

13. In collaboration with the neurology team, enumerate <u>investigations</u> for evaluation of the acute ischemic stroke in pregnancy. *(1 point each)*

6

Laboratory tests: *(max 4)*
☐ CBC/FBC
☐ Liver aminotransferases and function tests
☐ Cardiometabolic profile, including HbA1c and lipid profile
☐ Antiphospholipid antibody screening *(refer to Chapter 49)*
☐ Inherited thrombophilia screening *(refer to Chapter 52)*

Imaging modalities: *(max 2)*
☐ Transthoracic echocardiogram *(may consider a bubble study for assessment of a patent foramen ovale or atrial defect; transesophageal echocardiogram may otherwise be performed)*
☐ Carotid imaging
☐ Leg compression ultrasound with Doppler interrogation *(selected cases)*
☐ Transesophageal echocardiogram *(selected cases)*
☐ CT-angiography of the chest for possible arteriovenous malformations *(selected cases)*

14. Until results of investigations become available, provide management of the patient's ischemic stroke in the third trimester, as planned in affiliation with her treating neurology team. There are no signs or symptoms of preterm labor. *(1 point each)*

Max 8

☐ Hospitalization in a unit with expertise in neurology

Maternal:
☐ Maintain maternal blood pressure within safe target values in pregnancy[†]
☐ Antiplatelet therapy is recommended, as for nonpregnant patients
☐ Neurology interdisciplinary management: physical and occupational therapy, sleep language pathology, psychology, social work consultations for stroke rehabilitation; ophthalmology assessment for formal visual field testing and possibility for future driving capacity
☐ Obstetric-anesthesiology consultation
☐ Screening for depression and consideration for liaison with a perinatal mental health expert *(high incidence of depression among pregnant/postpartum women with a stroke)*
☐ Consideration for compression stockings if ambulation is limited

Fetal:
- ☐ Arrange for CTG monitoring at least once daily
- ☐ Sonographic growth biometry and Doppler interrogation given the likelihood of underlying maternal vascular disease and/or other comorbidities
- ☐ Neonatology consultation

Special note:
- † Refer to Question 2 in Chapter 38

You highlight to your obstetric trainee that prophylactic low molecular weight heparin (LMWH) is not advised in the first two weeks after an ischemic stroke. They are curious about the safety of medical or mechanical interventions for antenatal acute stroke management.

---

15. Discuss the safety of, and important clinical considerations for, systemic thrombolysis and endovascular thrombectomy in pregnancy. *(1 point per main bullet)*

    Max 3

Intravenous alteplase:
- ☐ Although treatment in pregnancy is not contraindicated, decision-making can be complex in the antenatal period and requires interdisciplinary consultation
  - ○ No known risk of fetal intracranial or systemic bleeding (alteplase is a large molecule that does not cross placenta)
  - ○ Unknown risk of placental abruption; continue close monitoring for prompt recognition
- ☐ Treatment would have been considered with patient presentation within 4.5 hours of symptoms (*i.e.*, hyperacute stroke)

Endovascular thrombectomy:
- ☐ Angiography with thrombectomy is not contraindicated in pregnancy
- ☐ Treatment is considered for proximal large vessel occlusions within 24 hours of an acute stroke where salvable tissue is noted on imaging

---

Comprehensive investigations are unremarkable. As with ~30% of all ischemic strokes, the patient's stroke is deemed cryptogenic *(no identifiable cause)*.

During the latter third trimester, the patient responds well to intensive rehabilitation with demonstrable improvements in functional recovery. A residual small left visual field defect remains. There has not been hemorrhagic transformation of the ischemic stroke. Fetal growth and well-being have remained normal.

---

16. Address the mode of delivery and important intrapartum management considerations for this patient. All antenatal interdisciplinary consultations have been performed. Delivery is planned at your facility equipped to treat patients with stroke. *(1 point per main bullet)*

    5

- ☐ Aim for vaginal delivery at term, with Cesarean section performed for obstetric indications
  - ○ *Surgical delivery increases the risk of peripartum and postpartum stroke recurrence*

- ☐ Plan induction of labor after withholding the antiplatelet agent, if necessary, for five to seven days to maximize the opportunity for neuraxial blockade and minimize the risk of maternal bleeding
- ☐ Neuraxial blockade (epidural) is optimal *(avoid sedation and general anesthesia, if possible)*
- ☐ Maintain continuous electronic fetal monitoring in labor *(Suggested Reading 4)*
- ☐ Consider delayed pushing in the second stage of labor and maintain a low threshold for instrumental vaginal delivery *(to minimize increased maternal intracranial pressure and hypertension)*

Induction of labor ensues at term after having withheld antiplatelet therapy for one week. The patient receives epidural analgesia and intrapartum care proceeds as per the arranged plan. A healthy vigorous neonate is delivered with vacuum assistance after maximal passive descent.

17. In relation to having sustained an acute stroke in pregnancy, delineate important elements for the patient's postpartum care. *(1 point per main bullet)*

Max 10

Mental health and support:
- ☐ Screen for postpartum depression and continue to offer psychosocial support
  - ○ *The risk of postpartum depression and anxiety is increased with pregnancy-associated stroke*

Stroke precautions and secondary prevention:
- ☐ Avoid sedating analgesics
- ☐ Reinitiate antiplatelet therapy postpartum and for at least 12 weeks
- ☐ Educate the patient/family about signs of stroke recurrence, emphasizing the need to immediately contact emergency health services in the event of difficulty breathing, sudden and severe headaches, sudden change in consciousness, speech, strength, vision, balance, or sensation
- ☐ Maintain BP control, as established antepartum
- ☐ Continue her migraine prophylaxis with nortriptyline and/or occipital nerve blocks
- ☐ Promote a healthy lifestyle that incorporates a balanced diet, weight control, physical activity tailored to the patient's abilities, and avoidance of smoking and alcohol

Breastfeeding:
- ☐ Encourage breastfeeding; consultation with lactation support experts can be helpful to facilitate breastfeeding, particularly where the patient has residual physical or cognitive deficits

Contraception:‡
- ☐ Estrogen-containing contraceptives remain contraindicated
- ☐ Progesterone-only oral agents, either progesterone or copper intrauterine devices, or barrier methods are safe

Follow-up:
- ☐ Arrange appointments with her stroke-neurologist, affiliated care team, and postpartum obstetric care provider prior to her delivery discharge
- ☐ Promote future preconception counseling

Special note:

‡   Depot medroxyprogesterone acetate contraception is category 3 among patients with history of stroke; refer to (a) UK Medical Eligibility Criteria (MEC) for Contraceptive Use 2016, revised Sept 2019, and (b) US-MEC 2016, amended 2020

Two years later, the patient is referred to you for preconception counseling and potential discontinuation of her levonorgestrel intrauterine system. She has now fully recovered and has been driving again for the past year, as approved by her neuro-ophthalmologist.

18. With regard to a previous antenatal cryptogenic ischemic stroke, highlight issues you would address with the patient and communicate with the referring physician(s) in your preconception consultation note. *(1 point each)*	Max 6

☐ *Antenatal* recurrence risk of an ischemic stroke is very low
☐ *Postpartum* period poses the greatest risk for recurrent stroke
☐ Low-dose aspirin is advisable during the antepartum and postpartum periods for secondary stroke prevention after a cryptogenic stroke
☐ Thromboprophylaxis is not required for secondary stroke prevention unless other indications exist, such as multiple strokes or antiphospholipid antibody syndrome
☐ Target BP in pregnancy to <140 mmHg systolic and <90 mmHg diastolic given previous stroke *(Suggested Reading 9)*
☐ Optimize migraine prophylaxis and management
☐ Close multidisciplinary follow-up is advised for management of medical (*e.g.,* hypertension, diabetes) and lifestyle risk factors that may increase recurrence stroke risk during future pregnancy or during the postpartum period

                                           TOTAL: **125**

CHAPTER 26

Multiple Sclerosis in Pregnancy

Alexa Eberle, Meena Khandelwal, and Amira El-Messidi

A 34-year-old G2P1 with long-standing multiple sclerosis (MS) is referred by her neurologist for prenatal care of a spontaneous pregnancy at 10 weeks' gestation by dating sonography. She takes prenatal vitamins and has no obstetric complaints.

LEARNING OBJECTIVES

1. Take a focused prenatal history for a patient with MS and be able to plan and manage antepartum, intrapartum, and postpartum considerations, recognizing the importance of interdisciplinary care
2. Identify selected disease-modifying drug therapies currently approved for antepartum maintenance treatment among patients with MS, where required
3. Counsel on the bidirectional relationship between pregnancy and MS
4. Recognize clinical features of pregnancy that can suggest pseudo-relapse manifestations of MS
5. Understand essentials of treatment and management of MS flares during pregnancy, and identify factors that increase the risk for postpartum exacerbations

SUGGESTED READINGS

1. Bove R, Alwan S, Friedman JM, et al. Management of multiple sclerosis during pregnancy and the reproductive years: a systematic review. *Obstet Gynecol.* 2014;124(6):1157–1168.
2. Coyle PK, Oh J, Magyari M, et al. Management strategies for female patients of reproductive potential with multiple sclerosis: an evidence-based review. *Mult Scler Relat Disord.* 2019; 32:54–63.
3. Dobson R, Dassan P, Roberts M, et al. UK consensus on pregnancy in multiple sclerosis: 'Association of British Neurologists' guidelines. *Pract Neurol.* 2019;19(2):106–114.
4. Fang X, Patel C, Gudesblatt M. Multiple sclerosis: clinical updates in women's health care primary and preventive care review. *Obstet Gynecol.* 2020;135(3):757–758.
5. Kalinowska A, Kułakowska A, Adamczyk-Sowa M, et al. Recommendations for neurological, obstetrical and gynaecological care in women with multiple sclerosis: a statement by a working group convened by the Section of Multiple Sclerosis and Neuroimmunology of the Polish Neurological Society. *Neurol Neurochir Pol.* 2020;54(2):125–137.
6. Liguori NF, Alonso R, Pinheiro AA, et al. Consensus recommendations for family planning and pregnancy in multiple sclerosis in Argentina. *Mult Scler Relat Disord.* 2020; 43:102147.

7. Pozzilli C, Pugliatti M, ParadigMS Group. An overview of pregnancy-related issues in patients with multiple sclerosis. *Eur J Neurol.* 2015;22 Suppl 2:34–39.

8. Thöne J, Thiel S, Gold R, et al. Treatment of multiple sclerosis during pregnancy – safety considerations. *Expert Opin Drug Saf.* 2017;16(5):523–534.

9. Toscano M, Thornburg LL. Neurological diseases in pregnancy. *Curr Opin Obstet Gynecol.* 2019;31(2):97–109.

10. Varytė G, Zakarevičienė J, Ramašauskaitė D, et al. Pregnancy and multiple sclerosis: an update on the disease modifying treatment strategy and a review of pregnancy's impact on disease activity. *Medicina (Kaunas).* 2020;56(2):49. Published 2020 Jan 21.

POINTS

1. With respect to MS, what aspects of a focused history would you want to know?   Max 18
(1 point per main bullet; max points specified where required)

General disease-related details: *(max 5)*
☐ Duration of time since diagnosis *(i.e., specify 'long-standing')*
☐ Primary presenting clinical and imaging features
☐ Classification of her MS pattern or subtype
☐ Frequency and her typical manifestations of relapses
☐ Time since last relapse
☐ Rate of disease progression, *if any*
☐ Presence of residual disability *(e.g., according to the Expanded Disability Status Scale [EDSS], or other scale of functional assessment)*

Medications and routine health maintenance:
☐ Current/prior disease-modifying drug (DMD) therapies, clinical response and side effects
☐ Vitamin D supplementation
☐ Vaccination status

MS-related manifestations or functional morbidities: *(findings related to four bullets; 4 points)*
☐ *Cerebral and mental function: (e.g., fatigue, mood and cognitive changes, seizures)*
☐ *Pyramidal: (e.g., paresis, Lhermitte sign[†])*
☐ *Cerebellar: (e.g., gait impairment, limb ataxia, tremor, vertigo)*
☐ *Brainstem: (e.g., speech, swallowing, or respiratory dysfunction)*
☐ *Visual: (e.g., scotoma, diplopia, visual loss, pain, nystagmus)*
☐ *Sensory: (e.g., presence and location of decreased vibration, touch, or position sense, tingling)*
☐ *Bladder and bowel: (e.g., detrusor hyper/hypoactivity, dyssynergia, constipation, fecal incontinence)*
☐ *Other disease-attributed neurologic phenomena: (e.g., insomnia, restless-leg syndrome, sexual dysfunction, spasticity, hyperreflexia, pain phenomena, Uhthoff phenomenon[‡])*

Past pregnancy features related to MS:[§]
☐ Antenatal/postnatal disease flares and treatment received
☐ Need for operative delivery, either assisted vaginal delivery or Cesarean section, for disease-related features

Social history: *(max 3)*

☐ Ethnicity and upbringing in a geographic location associated with increased risk of MS
  ○ *Prevalence of MS increases at farther distances from the equator; exceptions exist*
☐ Dietary and nutritional intake
☐ Smoking, alcohol consumption, and use of illicit substances
  ○ *Smoking is associated with increased progression of relapsing-remitting to secondary progressive disease*
☐ Social support *(particularly related to physical limitations or during disease exacerbations)* and current/recent stressors

Male partner/family history:

☐ MS *(presence of MS in **both** parents is associated with >20% offspring risk of MS later in life; presence of MS in one parent is associated with ~2% offspring risk of MS)* **

Special notes:

† Refers to electric shock-like sensation that runs down the back and/or limbs with neck flexion
‡ Heat intolerance, aggravating neurologic symptoms
§ Overall, women with MS do not seek assisted reproductive technology more than unaffected women
** General population risk of MS is 0.13%

Four years ago, the patient experienced an episode of painful monocular visual loss with spontaneous recovery within a few weeks. Associating it to the stress of having recently moved from Canada, her native homeland, she did not seek medical care. Over the following year, she had two bouts of scotomas, fatigue, constipation, and burning pains in her feet; comprehensive investigations revealed demyelinating lesions on neuroimaging compatible with relapsing-remitting MS. Within eight months of conception, she had a flare lasting one week, treated with intermittent therapy. She preferred to defer long-term disease-modifying drugs (DMDs) while planning pregnancy. Her husband maintains physical and emotional support during disease exacerbations.

Her perinatal course was complicated by an MS-flare and postpartum endometritis. Initiation of interferon beta/glatiramer acetate (IFN-B/GA) was later required at 2 months after vaginal delivery; treatment maintained her relapse-free for the past 10 months. Excited, albeit concerned, with current pregnancy on her DMD therapy, the patient met her neurologist and after thorough counseling, antenatal treatment with IFN-B/GA will be maintained. Vaccinations are up to date, she practices healthy habits, and family history is noncontributory.

The patient requests your reassurance regarding antenatal continuation of her designated DMD therapy. She mentions that ever since her MS flared postpartum, she *feels* that gestation impacted the course of her disease. Your obstetric trainee assures her that up to 25% of women experience relapse during the first three months postpartum, while you take note to elaborate on potential explanations for this phenomenon.

2. Suggest three contributors or predictors for postpartum MS exacerbations. *(1 point each)*   3

- ☐ Infection *(i.e., endometritis)*
- ☐ Relapse within the year preceding pregnancy
- ☐ Relapse during pregnancy
- ☐ Rapid postpartum decline in estradiol levels
- ☐ Loss of antenatal immunotolerance *[i.e., postpartum return in the T-helper (Th) cell profile to the predominantly Th1 (pro-inflammatory cytokines) rather than Th2 (anti-inflammatory cytokines) dominant state during pregnancy]*
- ☐ Exhaustion/psychosocial stress

3. Recognizing the need for contraception with many DMD agents with varying washout   3
periods, indicate the safety and rationale her neurologist likely discussed regarding
continuation of IFN-B/GA during pregnancy. *(1 point each)*

Interferon beta/glatiramer acetate (IFN-B/GA):
- ☐ No association with miscarriage
- ☐ Nonteratogenic in humans
- ☐ Possibly decreased efficacy in reducing postpartum relapse rate when restarted after antenatal discontinuation

Special note:
In September 2019, the Committee for Medicinal Products for Human Use (CHMP)
recommended approval of interferon beta treatments during pregnancy and breastfeeding for
relapsing MS

4. Discuss the impact of pregnancy on the course of MS. *(1 point each)*   Max 2

- ☐ No change in overall risk of relapse during a pregnancy year (*i.e.*, nine months' gestation and three months postpartum)
- ☐ No worsening of disease progression due to pregnancy
- ☐ No long-term disability due to pregnancy

The patient appreciates your reassurance and evidence-based counseling. She vaguely recalls possible detrimental effects to pregnancy due to MS, preferring to review such risks with you. Although she knows that relapse rates of MS generally decrease during pregnancy, the patient indicates she was often concerned with common pregnancy-related symptoms that overlap with manifestations of MS.

5. Discuss pregnancy complications associated with MS, reassuring the patient where appropriate. *(1 point each; max points specified per section)*   3

Maternal: *(max 2)*
☐ Urinary tract infections
☐ Venous thrombosis, where associated with limited mobility
☐ Possibly increased risk of anemia during pregnancy
☐ Possible association with operative vaginal delivery or Cesarean section *(due to neuromuscular/perineal weakness or spasticity)*
☐ Possible association with induction of labor

Fetal/neonatal: *(max 1)*
☐ No adverse outcomes including early pregnancy loss, ectopic pregnancy, congenital malformations, preterm birth (PTB), or IUFD
☐ Controversial/possible association with low birthweight *(individualized decision-making regarding sonographic fetal growth assessments)*

6. While encouraging the patient to report any signs or symptoms concerning her during pregnancy, review features common to pregnancy which may overlap with manifestations of MS-flares. *(1 point each)*   Max 4

☐ Fatigue
☐ Abnormal gait, imbalance, or spasticity
☐ Respiratory difficulty
☐ Restless leg syndrome
☐ Paresthesia in the extremities or other parts of the body
☐ Nerve entrapment syndromes *(e.g., carpal tunnel syndrome, sciatica)*, and Bell's palsy
☐ Mood disturbance *(e.g., depression or anxiety)*
☐ Urinary symptoms *(e.g., frequency, urgency, incontinence)*
☐ Constipation

7. Highlight to your obstetric trainee two infections, routinely tested among prenatal baseline investigations, where clinically advanced disease can mimic features of MS. *(1 point each)*   2

☐ HIV
☐ Syphilis *(neurosyphilis)*

After addressing her concerns, and with an intent to teach your accompanying obstetric trainee, you decide to *summarize* the antenatal care plan for this patient. Disease-modifying drug therapy with IFN-B/GA will be continued.

8. Outline essential elements of <u>maternal antenatal</u> management particular to patients with MS. *(1 point per main bullet)*   Max 5

☐ Maintain multidisciplinary collaboration[†] *(e.g., neurology, obstetrics/maternal-fetal medicine, anesthesiology, physiotherapy, nutrition, social work, mental health expert, and neonatology)*

☐ Support individual patient needs to decrease psychosocial stressors, perform serial screening for depression/anxiety

☐ Encourage maintenance of physical activity and safe exercises

☐ Counsel on healthy sleep habits

☐ Encourage, or maintain, abstinence from smoking

☐ Provide supplementary vitamin D 1000–2000 units orally daily

☐ Serial screening for urinary tract infections and maintain a low threshold for treatment of asymptomatic or symptomatic infection

☐ Advise nonpharmacologic strategies to manage MS symptoms throughout pregnancy *(Suggested Reading 4)*

  ○ Preferred avoidance of pharmacologic treatment of symptoms associated with MS

Special note:

[†] Having MS does not automatically imply a 'high-risk' pregnancy; antenatal care can usually be led by a midwife *(UK consensus, Suggested Reading 3)*; international variations may exist

Pregnancy progresses well until 26 weeks' gestation when the patient reports a one-week[†] history of left lower extremity weakness with decreased sensation in her legs, affecting ambulation. You notify her neurologist who attends to the patient with you; examination is notable for leg weakness and decreased touch and position sense. The patient is afebrile without suggestion of infectious causes to explain her physical findings. She has no obstetric complaints and fetal viability is ascertained. Last week, her glucose screening test was normal. Although she has been adherent to her DMD regimen, she reports increased recent stress related to an ill family member. She is willing to comply with the recommended management to ameliorate her symptoms.

Special note:

[†]According to the McDonald criteria for MS relapse, minimum required duration of symptoms with objective findings is 24 hours, in the absence of fever, infection, or other explanations

9. With focus on her clinical manifestations and physical findings, detail the counseling and management you agreed upon with her neurologist. *(1 point per main bullet)*

Max 7

☐ Inform the patient that the goal of treatment is to speed the recovery time from the MS-flare, without any effect on long-term function or disease stability

☐ Consideration for hospitalization *(particularly if known diabetes for care of glycemic control)*

☐ Maintain heightened awareness for signs or symptoms of depression, and provide psychosocial support services *(particularly given her known social stressors)*

☐ *First-line treatment:* Intravenous methylprednisolone 1 g daily for three to five days
  ○ Dose-tapering is not necessary
  ○ Preferred avoidance of *oral* glucocorticoids,[†] due to the recurrence risk of optic neuritis
  ○ Dexamethasone is contraindicated *(maternal-fetal transfer decreases treatment efficacy)*

☐ *Second-line treatment:* Corticosteroid-refractory symptoms may be managed with intravenous immunoglobulin (IVIG) or plasmapheresis (plasma exchange)

☐ Consideration for neuroimaging with an MRI of the brain/spinal cord (without gadolinium contrast)[§]; neuroimaging is unnecessary where clinical suspicion of disease flare is high, or with mild symptoms
  ○ Individualized considerations and local availability of MRI is advised

☐ Neuro-physiotherapist consultation *(e.g., optimize mobility and care for labor and delivery, assess need for cane or ambulatory supports)*

☐ Consideration for compression stockings ± thromboprophylaxis if prolonged, restricted mobility

☐ With decreased lower body sensation, educate the patient on symptoms suggestive of labor *(e.g., gastrointestinal upset, increased spasticity, flushing, back pain)*[‡]

Special notes:
§ For discussion on use of MRI in pregnancy, including risks of gadolinium contrast, refer to Chapter 42
† For fetal and maternal effects of maternal corticosteroids refer to Chapter 45 and Chapter 46, respectively
‡ For signs or symptoms of labor among patients with spinal cord involvement, refer to Chapter 28

Magnetic resonance imaging did not show new lesions relative to prior imaging. The patient responded well to five-day treatment with intravenous methylprednisolone and will be resuming her treatment with IFN-B/GA. She complains of residual paresthesia and mild leg weakness, although neurological examination is reassuringly normal. The remainder of pregnancy is unremarkable.

In collaboration with her neurologist, you discuss mode and management of delivery during the 36 weeks' antenatal visit. She presents in spontaneous labor at 39^{+5} weeks' gestation. The fetal cardiotocography is normal. Her routine vaginal-rectal group B streptococcal swab was negative.

10. Outline essentials of <u>delivery management</u> with respect to MS. *(1 point each)*   Max 3

☐ Offer epidural in labor, assuring the patient that neuraxial anesthesia does not increase the risk of MS relapse
☐ Benzodiazepines (diazepam) may be used for intrapartum bladder spasticity
☐ Consideration for delayed pushing in the second stage of labor, if decreased maternal expulsive effort
☐ Consideration for maintaining a low threshold for assisted vaginal delivery, where indicated for poor maternal expulsive effort

Special note:
Umbilical cord blood collection and banking specifically for future MS-related treatments or stem-cell therapies remains investigational; individualized discussion is advised

Expectedly for a multiparous woman, accelerated progress of labor ensues at 6 cm dilation. A vacuum-assisted delivery is required for perineal weakness and a healthy neonate is delivered weighing 3150 g. The placenta delivers spontaneously and there are no immediate postpartum complications.

11. Address important <u>postpartum</u> considerations for the care of this patient with MS. *(1 point per main bullet, unless specified)*   10

Mental health care:
☐ Screen for postpartum depression and continue to offer psychosocial support services
  ○ *The risk of postpartum depression is increased among parents with MS*

MS-related medications:
☐ Continuation, or resumption of pregestational regimen, of IFN-B/GA treatment to decrease risks of relapse
☐ Continuation of supplementary vitamin D *(UK consensus, Suggested Reading 3)*
  ○ *Recommended infant administration of vitamin D in line with standard advice*

Breastfeeding:
☐ Encourage breastfeeding for standard maternal-infant benefits
  ○ *Controversial benefit of exclusive breastfeeding on postpartum MS relapse rate*
☐ Advise pumping and storage of breast milk supply *(3 points)*

Contraception:
☐ No restrictions on contraceptive method for patients with MS *without* immobilization
  ○ Currently, there are no known negative interactions between combined oral contraceptives and DMD
  ○ Possible, *yet controversial*, association between low-dose combined oral contraceptives and slowed disease progression, relapse rates, or MRI activity in relapsing-remitting MS
  ○ Individualized assessment of drug–drug interactions with hormonal agents is advised for treatment of specific MS-related manifestations
  ○ Long-acting reversible contraception is advised with DMD therapies contraindicated in pregnancy

Follow-up:
- ☐ Arrange routine postpartum clinical appointment, and encourage follow-up with her MS team
- ☐ Advise future preconception counseling, and discourage self-initiated discontinuation of medical therapy in the event of unplanned pregnancy

12. Provide three justifications for your advice to store her breast milk, as particular to patients with MS. *(1 point each)*   **3**

- ☐ Severe fatigue
- ☐ Relapse-associated disability to breastfeed
- ☐ Need for medical therapy incompatible with breastfeeding

The patient selects the levonorgesterol-releasing intrauterine system as she is not contemplating pregnancy within five years. Expecting to be of advanced maternal age, she asks about particularities related to her disease should reproductive treatments be necessary.

13. Counsel the patient on the effects of disease on fertility and address her concerns related to artificial reproductive technologies specific to MS. *(1 point each)*   **Max 2**

- ☐ Reassure her that neither MS nor DMD therapies affect fertility
- ☐ Increased risk of flares with GnRH *(gonadotropin-releasing hormone)* agonists rather than antagonists; preferred avoidance with relapsing-remitting MS is advised
- ☐ Increased MS relapse rates with failed cycles of assisted reproductive technologies

You later receive a telephone call from a colleague in a remote center seeking advice regarding potential discontinuation of the disease-modifying drug, **natalizumab,** for a 30-year-old with rapidly evolving severe MS with a viable, unplanned eight-week pregnancy. The physician is awaiting the neurologist's assistance.

14. Indicate your evidence-based advice regarding antenatal recommendations particular to MS treatment with <u>natalizumab</u> infusions. *(1 point per main and subbullet)*   **Max 5**

- ☐ Reassure the physician of no human evidence for related teratogenicity
- ☐ Advise <u>against current discontinuation</u> of therapy due to:
  - ○ High risk of relapse/rebound
  - ○ Gestational benefits in decreased MS relapse rates may not occur with severe disease requiring natalizumab
- ☐ Maternal monitoring for brain-MRI is required for progressive multifocal leukoencephalopathy
- ☐ Plan to hold treatment at ~34 weeks' gestation, and restart it soon after birth *(keep interval at 8–12 weeks maximum between last dose and resumption postpartum to minimize rebound disease)*
- ☐ Ensure neonatology consultation with antenatal treatment *(infant risk of anemia and thrombocytopenia)*

TOTAL: **70**

CHAPTER 27

Myasthenia Gravis in Pregnancy

Andrea S. Parks and Amira El-Messidi

Your next patient is a new referral for consultation and transfer of care. The transfer note indicates she is a 28-year-old G1P0 with known myasthenia gravis (MG) who is at 12 weeks' gestation by sonographic dating.

LEARNING OBJECTIVES

1. Take a focused history and verbalize essentials of a focused physical examination for a prenatal patient with MG
2. Discuss potential pregnancy-related changes to MG symptoms and its course
3. Provide counseling on prenatal risks associated with MG
4. Manage acute neuromuscular deterioration in a pregnant patient with MG
5. Formulate a plan for delivery for a patient with MG
6. Be familiar with medications commonly used to treat MG, including their side effects and/or contraindications pertinent to prenatal and postpartum care

SUGGESTED READINGS

1. Ciafaloni E. Myasthenia gravis and congenital myasthenic syndromes. *Continuum (Minneap Minn).* 2019;25(6):1767–1784.
2. Hamel J, Ciafaloni E. An update: Myasthenia gravis and pregnancy. *Neurol Clin.* 2018; 36:355–365.
3. Massey JM, De Jesus-Acosta C. Pregnancy and myasthenia gravis. *Continuum (Minneap Minn).* 2014;20(1):115–127.
4. Norwood F, Dhanjal M, Hill M, et al. Myasthenia in pregnancy: best practice guidelines from a UK multispecialty working group. *J Neurol Neurosurg Psychiatry.* 2014; 85: 538–543.
5. Sanders DB, Wolfe GI, Benatar M, et al. International consensus guidance for management of myasthenia gravis: executive summary. *Neurology.* 2016; 87:419–425.
6. Varner M. Myasthenia gravis and pregnancy. *Clin Obstet Gynecol.* 2013;56(2): 372–381.
7. Waters J. Management of myasthenia gravis in pregnancy. *Neurol Clin.* 2019; 37: 113–120.

POINTS

1. With regard to MG, what aspects of a focused history would you want to know?
    (1 point each, unless specified)

    Max 10

Disease-related details:
- [ ] Time elapsed since onset of symptoms *(85% progress to generalized weakness within three years of onset)*
- [ ] Antibody status: anti-acetylcholine receptor antibody, anti-muscle specific kinase antibodies, others, or seronegative
- [ ] Past surgical history of thymectomy
- [ ] Current and prior medications, dosages, and any side effects encountered

Current symptoms: *(2 points each)*

Associated with myasthenia gravis:
- [ ] Ocular: diplopia, ptosis
- [ ] Facial weakness
- [ ] Oral: dysarthria, dysphagia, choking, or nasal regurgitation
- [ ] Respiratory: shortness of breath
- [ ] Proximal muscle weakness that worsens with repetitive activity

Associated with pregnancy:
- [ ] Nausea/ vomiting, cramping, vaginal bleeding

Family history:
- [ ] MG or other autoimmune condition

Social features and routine health maintenance:
- [ ] Occupation, smoking, drug use, alcohol consumption
- [ ] Vaccination status *(live virus vaccines are generally avoided particularly in the setting of immunosuppressive therapy)*
- [ ] Allergies

You learn that she was diagnosed with myasthenia gravis six months ago when she presented with diplopia and mild proximal weakness. Serum anti-acetylcholine receptor antibody antibodies are positive. The patient has been symptom-free since starting pyridostigmine 30 mg PO four times daily, and she has not experienced side effects. CT chest showed no thymoma and she has not had a thymectomy. Her pregnancy is unremarkable to date, with no nausea or vomiting.

2-A. What are two pertinent pregnancy management considerations at this time? *(1 point each)*

2

- [ ] Notify her treating neurologist of the current pregnancy
- [ ] Encourage regular rest periods and stable environment

2-B. Name two tests you would recommend with regard to MG? *(1 point each)*

2

- [ ] Obtain thyroid function tests, if not recently done
- [ ] Obtain baseline respiratory functional tests (*i.e.,* forced vital capacity [FVC] testing)

3. Which symptoms or signs on history and physical examination *may* be associated with side effects of pyridostigmine? *(1 point each)*

Max 2

☐ Increased salivation
☐ Abdominal cramping/diarrhea
☐ Muscle cramps or twitching (fasciculations)
☐ Bradycardia

4. Highlight aspects you would discuss in counseling the patient with regard to the effect of pregnancy on MG. *(1 point each)*

Max 4

☐ The long-term outcome of MG is not affected by pregnancy
☐ ~40% of women experience worsening of symptoms, mostly in the first trimester or postpartum, while 20% remain unchanged, and 20% improve
☐ Improvement, or even remission, may occur in the second trimester *(likely due to α-fetoprotein-induced immunosuppression)*
☐ Nausea or vomiting should be reported early in onset due to decreased drug absorption
☐ Physiologic changes of early pregnancy *(increased blood volume and renal function, decreased gastrointestinal absorption)* may require increased medication dosages
☐ Respiratory function may be compromised due to diaphragmatic restriction from the enlarging uterus

The patient responded well to oral treatment of pregnancy-induced vomiting, and the dose of pyridostigmine was increased to 60 mg PO four times daily. Baseline tests for thyroid and respiratory function were normal. You receive the report of her routine 20-week fetal anatomy survey.

5. Which two aspects of the obstetric ultrasound are of particular importance in relation to maternal MG? *(1 point each)*

2

☐ Evidence of arthrogryposis *(rare, but may occur with transplacental antibody transfer against the fetal acetylcholine receptors)*
☐ Presence of polyhydramnios

At 25 weeks' gestation, the patient presents to hospital with generalized fatigue, diplopia, and progressive difficulty climbing stairs over the past week. She choked twice on her dinner last night and had difficulty chewing her food. The patient has no obstetric complaints and fetal viability has been ascertained.

6. Outline your focused physical exam with regard to the status of her MG. (*1 point each, unless specified*) Max 4

☐ Vital signs (must specify respiratory rate and temperature; *note that changes in oxygen saturation are late-findings*) – **2 points**
☐ Assess for dysarthria or shortness of breath with prolonged speech
☐ Assess extraocular eye movements and ptosis
☐ Assess lip seal, facial/jaw/tongue weakness
☐ Assess proximal strength, including neck flexion and extension

The patient's vital signs, including respiratory rate and oral temperature, are normal. She is able to speak full sentences without abnormal articulation or hyponasality but is unable to whistle and she sneers when asked to smile. She has vertical diplopia with sustained upgaze. It was easy to provide resistance when she was asked to squeeze her eyes shut, with more pronounced weakness on the right side. It was also easy to provide resistance on her strength assessment including neck flexion.

7. What are your next steps in the management of the patient? (*1 point each*) Max 3

☐ Immediate consultation with her neurologist (or neurology team)
☐ Notify respiratory therapist to perform MIPs and MEPs (*maximal inspiratory pressures and maximal expiratory pressures, respectively*)
☐ Keep the patient fasting (nil per os) until swallowing assessment performed
☐ Ensure absence of reversible triggers for myasthenic crisis, such as infections, electrolyte imbalance, or medications used in pregnancy that may exacerbate MG (*e.g.*, magnesium-containing laxatives/antacids, calcium channel blockers, β-blockers, macrolides, penicillins, nitrofurantoin)

As her neurologist is on the way, the respiratory therapist's test results show maximal inspiratory pressure -50 cmH$_2$O and maximal expiratory pressure 60 cmH$_2$O. (*maximal inspiratory pressure <-30 cmH$_2$O and maximal expiratory pressure <40 cmH$_2$O are usually used to determine if intubation is necessary, however testing requires proper mouth closure which may be compromised*)

8. What is the immediate best next step in management of this patient? 1

☐ ICU (ITU) consultation and admission

Neurology and ICU (ITU) teams assess the patient and diagnose a myasthenic crisis.

9. Identify 2 treatments for acute exacerbations of MG that have the most reassuring safety profiles in pregnancy. *(1 point each)*   2

☐ IVIG *(treatment of choice)*

☐ Prednisone *(risk of hypertension, gestational diabetes; transient worsening of MG may occur with initiation of therapy)*

☐ Plasmapheresis *(may be considered, but is not preferred due to theoretical obstetrical risks)*

Special note:

Do not accept **IV** acetylcholinesterase inhibitors as these should be avoided in pregnancy due to risk of uterine contractions

The patient is admitted to ICU and receives IVIG 2 g/kg divided over five days. Her neurologist also starts prednisone 30 mg daily. Her symptoms begin to improve on day 3 of treatment. By day 7, she has been moved to the ward and her symptoms have largely resolved.

The neurology team inquires about the use of high-dose pyridostigmine in pregnancy.

10. What is an important potential side effect of very high doses of pyridostigmine in pregnancy?   2

☐ Preterm labor

You are later called urgently because the patient inadvertently took extra pyridostigmine and is now sweating heavily, has muscle twitches, and she complains of increased proximal limb weakness. The nurse tells you her oxygen saturation remains 95% on room air and her heart rate is 55 beats per minute. The patient denies any abdominal pain and the fetus is moving well.

11. What is your working diagnosis for her current symptoms?   1

☐ Cholinergic crisis

She receives appropriate treatment for the cholinergic crisis. Prior to discharge, she is concerned that MG may impose risk of preterm delivery. A friend told her she would need a Cesarean section to avoid respiratory muscle weakness in labor.

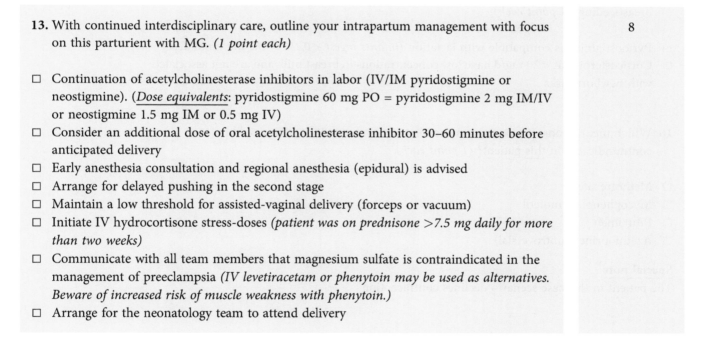

12. How would you address her concerns and troubleshoot misconceptions? *(1 point each)*   Max 3

☐ MG itself does not increase risk for pregnancy complications (*No evidence for increased risk of preterm birth, early spontaneous pregnancy loss, low birthweight, fetal growth restriction, preeclampsia, or eclampsia*)

☐ Polyhydramnios, if present, may increase risks of preterm labor and/or preterm prelabor rupture of membranes (*serial fetal ultrasound scans are advised to ensure normal limb movements and amniotic fluid volume*)

☐ MG is not an indication for Cesarean section, which is reserved for obstetrical indications

The patient progresses well in pregnancy on pyridostigmine and oral prednisone 30 mg daily. Fetal sonography remains normal. At 39 weeks' gestation, she presents with a new-onset occipital headache, epigastric pain, and a generalized feeling of unwellness. Her blood pressure is 190/105 mmHg and she has proteinuria. Cardiotocography is normal. Laboratory tests reveal elevated transaminases, normal platelet counts, and normal renal function.

After counseling the patient, she is admitted for induction of labor.

13. With continued interdisciplinary care, outline your intrapartum management with focus on this parturient with MG. *(1 point each)*   8

☐ Continuation of acetylcholinesterase inhibitors in labor (IV/IM pyridostigmine or neostigmine). (*Dose equivalents*: pyridostigmine 60 mg PO = pyridostigmine 2 mg IM/IV or neostigmine 1.5 mg IM or 0.5 mg IV)

☐ Consider an additional dose of oral acetylcholinesterase inhibitor 30–60 minutes before anticipated delivery

☐ Early anesthesia consultation and regional anesthesia (epidural) is advised

☐ Arrange for delayed pushing in the second stage

☐ Maintain a low threshold for assisted-vaginal delivery (forceps or vacuum)

☐ Initiate IV hydrocortisone stress-doses (*patient was on prednisone >7.5 mg daily for more than two weeks*)

☐ Communicate with all team members that magnesium sulfate is contraindicated in the management of preeclampsia (*IV levetiracetam or phenytoin may be used as alternatives. Beware of increased risk of muscle weakness with phenytoin.*)

☐ Arrange for the neonatology team to attend delivery

During labor, her blood pressure responded well to IV hydralazine and she received IV levetiracetam as prophylaxis for eclampsia. She has an uneventful vacuum-assisted delivery. Shortly after delivery, the baby boy is having difficulty suckling. The nurse notes he has poor generalized tonus and ptosis, with increased use of his respiratory muscles. The neonatology team is currently assessing the newborn.

14-A. What is the most probable diagnosis?   1

☐ Transient neonatal myasthenia

14-B. What is the medical management you anticipate this neonate may require for transient   Max 2
myasthenia? *(1 point each)*

☐ Neostigmine or pyridostigmine may be used if mild symptoms or prior to feeding
☐ Plasmapheresis or IVIG should be considered if respiratory involvement
☐ Ventilatory support and nasogastric feeding, *if needed*

After a two-week neonatal admission, the baby is well and ready for discharge. The patient is exclusively breastfeeding. She declines contraception. Her neurologist has decreased the pyridostigmine to her baseline prepregnancy dose and she continues to take concurrent prednisone 20 mg daily.

15. Discuss the drug-safety profiles of acetylcholinesterase inhibitors and steroids in   2
breastfeeding. *(1 point each)*

☐ Pyridostigmine is compatible with lactation *(infants ingest <0.1% of the maternal dose)*
☐ Corticosteroids at <20 mg/d have low concentrations in breast milk and are not associated
with newborn risks

16. Which medications, *if any*, used in the long-term treatment of MG, would be   Max 2
contraindicated in <u>this</u> patient? *(1 point each)*

☐ Methotrexate
☐ Mycophenolate mofetil
☐ Rituximab
☐ Azathioprine (controversial)

Special note:
The patient in this case scenario declines contraception

17. What two specific aspects related to the obstetric care of a patient with MG would you   2
address during this patient's postpartum visit? *(1 point each)*

☐ Suggest consideration for elective interval thymectomy, as this may decrease the likelihood
of recurrent neonatal myasthenia *(baseline recurrence risk approximates 75%)*
☐ Encourage preconceptual counseling to optimize treatment prior to future pregnancies

TOTAL: 55

CHAPTER 28

Pregnancy with Spinal Cord Injury

Rasha Abouelmagd and Amira El-Messidi

A 33-year-old primigravida at 16 weeks' gestation is referred by her primary care provider for obstetrical care. She was in a car accident four years ago that resulted in paraplegia due to a T4 spinal cord injury (SCI).

LEARNING OBJECTIVES

1. Understand the unique challenges of pregnancy in a patient with SCI
2. Detect autonomic dysreflexia (ADR), and differentiate it from mimicking pregnancy-related disorders
3. Recognize ADR as a medical emergency, and understand principles of immediate management
4. Appreciate the importance of multidisciplinary collaboration in caring for a pregnant patient with SCI

SUGGESTED READINGS

1. Andretta E, Landi LM, Cianfrocco M, et al. Bladder management during pregnancy in women with spinal-cord injury: an observational, multicenter study. *Int Urogynecol J.* 2019;30:292–300.
2. Berghella, V. *Maternal-Fetal Evidence Based Guidelines.* Boca Raton, FL: CRC Press; 2017.
3. Dawood R, Atlanis E, Ribes-Pastor P, Ashworth F. Pregnancy and spinal cord injury. *Obstetr Gynaecol.* 2014;16:99–107.
4. Krassioukov A, Warburton DER, Teasell R, et al. A systematic review of the management of autonomic dysreflexia following spinal cord injury. *Arch Phys Med Rehabil.* 2009 April;904(4):682–695.
5. Kuczkowski KM. Labor analgesia for the parturient with spinal cord injury: what does an obstetrician need to know? *Arch Gynecol Obstet.* 2006 May;274(2):108–112.
6. McLain AB, Massengill T, Klebine P. Pregnancy and women with spinal cord injury. *Arch Phys Med Rehabil.* 2016;97(3):497–498.
7. Obstetric management of patients with spinal cord injuries. Committee Opinion No. 808. American College of Obstetricians and Gynecologists. *Obstet Gynecol.* 2020 May;135(5): e230–e236.
8. Periera L. Obstetric management of the patient with spinal cord injury. *Obstet Gynecol Surv.* 2003;58:676–687.

9. Petsas A, Drake J. Perioperative management for patients with a chronic spinal cord injury. *BJA Education*. 2015;15(3):123–130.

10. Sharpe EE, Arendt KW, Jacob AK, et al. Anesthetic management of parturients with pre-existing paraplegia or tetraplegia: a case series. *IJOA*. 2014;11:77–84.

POINTS

1. With respect to SCI, what aspects of a focused history would you want to know? *(1 point each)*   Max 15

Details related to SCI:
☐ Prior spinal or bladder surgery
☐ Intermittent bladder catheterization, or need for indwelling catheter
☐ Occurrence and frequency of urinary tract infections, response to treatment and presence of drug allergies
☐ Baseline blood pressure and heart rate *(patients with SCI frequently have low basal blood pressure)*
☐ Presence of constipation and treatment(s)
☐ Presence of decubitus ulcers
☐ History of venous thromboembolism
☐ Symptoms and triggers of ADR, including any serious consequences *(e.g., intracranial hemorrhage, retinal detachment, seizures)*
☐ Names and contacts of her care team *(e.g., physical and occupational therapist, spinal rehabilitation physicians, nurses)*

Features related to pregnancy:
☐ Determine whether gestational age was established by menstrual dating or sonography
☐ Current or recent vaginal bleeding, nausea and/or vomiting, palpable contractions
☐ Inquire about results of routine prenatal investigations, if initiated by the referring medical professional
☐ Current/recent medications, including whether prenatal vitamins have been commenced

Social history:
☐ Living arrangements *(i.e., patients with SCI risk unattended labor)*, and presence of a supportive partner and/or family
☐ Occupation
☐ Smoking, alcohol consumption, illicit drug use

You learn that the patient receives regular home-visits from her multidisciplinary care team. She has been living with her husband for 10 years, who is an instrumental support. The patient self-catheterizes multiple times daily and was treated for two *E. coli* urinary tract infections within the past six weeks. She has never had a thromboembolism. The patient has not had any surgeries.

Pregnancy dating was established by ultrasound four weeks ago and was consistent with menstrual dates. Prenatal vitamins were initiated approximately three months prior to conception; the patient does not smoke, drink alcohol, or use illicit substances. Her only complaint to date has been increasing constipation, which triggers headaches, flushing and muscle spasticity. Routine prenatal investigations will be performed.

The patient understands that prenatal care will occur in a multidisciplinary fashion and delivery will occur in a tertiary center.

2. Indicate the investigations you would consider in relation to SCI in this obstetric patient. *(1 point each)*

4

☐ Full/complete blood count and ferritin[†]
☐ Pulmonary function tests (baseline and serial vital capacity)
☐ Renal function tests *(baseline and serial)*
☐ Urinalysis and/or urine culture

Special note:
† ~12% of women with SCI have anemia

3. Outline the prenatal management of this patient in relation to SCI, recognizing that interdisciplinary care will be maintained. *(1 point each; max points indicated per section where necessary)*

Max 15

Management of SCI-related morbidities:

Hematologic: (max 2)
☐ Correction of anemia, if present
☐ Individualized discussion for thromboprophylaxis *(nonuniversal recommendation)*
☐ Consideration for compression stockings, while maintaining vigilance that tight clothing may also trigger ADR

Pulmonary:
☐ Breathing exercises and incentive spirometry

Urinary: (max 3)
☐ Encourage maintenance of adequate hydration
☐ Increase use of intermittent self-catheterization, possibly with topical anesthetic – *some patients need indwelling catheter*
☐ Consideration for antibiotic suppression for recurrent urinary tract infections and increased need for self-catheterization in pregnancy
☐ Consideration for catheters with hydrophilic coating for prophylaxis against infections associated with frequent intermittent catheterizations

Gastrointestinal:
☐ Recommend stool softeners and a high fiber diet

Musculoskeletal and dermatologic: (max 4)
☐ Resize her wheelchair and increase cushioning to accommodate pregnancy
☐ Encourage frequent position changes

☐ Perform regular exams for decubitus ulcers
☐ Encourage regular exercises for range-of-motion and extremities
☐ Consider supplemental vitamin D

Obstetric features in relation to maternal SCI: *(max 5)*
☐ Encourage regular uterine palpation practices
☐ Encourage early reporting of symptoms such as headache, prickling sensation of the skull, nausea, new-onset anxiety, diaphoresis, increased nasal congestion, or spasticity
☐ Inform the patient of the possibility for elective hospitalizations
☐ Consideration for cervical examinations or ultrasound cervical length assessment in late second or early third trimester
☐ Individualized consideration for frequency of sonographic fetal growth assessments
☐ Arrange for consultation with an obstetric anesthesiologist

4.   Highlight to your obstetric trainee the essential elements or most significant concerns of anesthesiologists in caring for an obstetric patient with SCI. *(1 point each)*   Max 3

☐ Airway difficulties, especially in patients with cervical spine fusion; as such, avoidance of the emergent need for general anesthesia is preferred
☐ Risk of deterioration in respiratory function with growth of a gravid uterus
☐ Ascertain the patient's history of ADR, including triggers, frequency of episodes, and treatment responses
☐ Determine the level of spinal surgery, if any, to consider the feasibility and success of neuraxial blocks

The patient remains compliant with prenatal care and fetal investigations are unremarkable. She responds well to antibiotic suppression for recurrent urinary tract infections. Iron-deficiency anemia demonstrated on routine prenatal investigations improves with parenteral and oral therapy.

At 31^{+3} weeks' gestation, the patient presents to the obstetric emergency assessment unit with a two-hour history of a pounding headache accompanied by vomiting. She palpated uterine contractions in between episodes of vomiting. There are no other obstetric complaints. Your obstetric trainee informs you that the patient appears unwell and had one episode of nonbilious vomiting upon arrival. She is afebrile, respiratory rate is normal, and oxygen saturation is 97%; blood pressure is 168/111 mmHg and pulse rate is 60 bpm. Urine dipstick shows trace proteinuria. Cardiotocography demonstrates uterine contractions, as palpated by the patient, and a normal fetal heart tracing. Your trainee opted to perform the pelvic examination in your presence.

An obstetric sonogram performed one day ago reported a cephalic presentation with normal fetal growth biometry and amniotic fluid volume. Interdisciplinary professionals from neurology, anesthesiology, and neonatology services are being notified in a timely manner while her obstetric admission is being arranged.

5. Review the <u>maternal</u> investigations you would request as you promptly attend to the care of this patient.

    3

☐ Full/complete blood count, AST, ALT, LDH, serum creatinine, coagulation profile, and urine protein-creatinine ratio

6. Indicate what you intend to teach your obstetric trainee, after stabilizing the patient, regarding the two principal differential diagnoses of the patient's clinical presentation. *(1 point per bullet)*

    Max 5

	Autonomic dysreflexia (ADR)	Preeclampsia
Hypertension	☐ Synchronous with contractions ☐ Often associated with reflex bradycardia	Unrelated to contractions
Cutaneous changes	☐ Above the lesion, the skin is warm, flushed and diaphoretic, whereas below the lesion, the skin is cool, and piloerection is present	
Laboratory findings	☐ Normal platelet count ☐ Normal hepatic transaminases ☐ Urine norepinephrine is present	Proteinuria is featured rather than norepinephrine
Management	☐ Improves with removal of the triggering features	Consideration for magnesium sulfate; definitive treatment requires delivery

7. Given serial programming of vital signs, detail aspects of <u>initial</u> clinical assessment, maintaining the patient informed of ongoing care. *(1 point each)*

    6

☐ Assess if hypertension is synchronous with contractions
☐ Elevate the head of the bed to improve hypertension-associated with ADR
☐ Optimize analgesia <u>prior</u> to vaginal examination to block the neurologic stimuli from pelvic organs; if neuraxial analgesia is used, maintain vigilance in pelvic examination based on the potential inefficacy of the blockade
☐ Loosen any tight clothing
☐ Catheterize the bladder
☐ Use a warm speculum and glove for pelvic examination

Episodes of severe hypertension occur regularly at 15-minute intervals, together with uterine contractions. Bladder catheterization drained 500 mL. The anesthesiologist places an epidural and initiates continuous pulse oximetry and electrocardiogram monitoring. Pelvic examination reveals the cervix is 6 cm dilated and chorioamniotic membranes are intact. Cephalic presentation is confirmed. Maternal-fetal findings on cardiotocography are stable since initial presentation. Results of laboratory investigations are in progress.

8. Identify the two most probable working diagnoses. *(1 point each)*   2

☐ Autonomic dysreflexia
☐ Preterm labor

9. List five signs and symptoms, respectively, of ADR that *may or may not* be featured at this time in this parturient. *(1 point each)*   10

Signs	Symptoms
☐ Hypertension	☐ Severe, pounding headache
☐ Hyperthermia	
☐ Piloerection	☐ Nausea and vomiting
☐ Respiratory distress	
☐ Altered level of consciousness	☐ Nasal congestion
☐ Seizures	☐ Blurred vision
☐ Increased spasticity of extremities	☐ Facial flushing
☐ Reactive bradycardia	☐ Diaphoresis
☐ Sinus tachycardia	☐ Increased anxiety
☐ Arrhythmias (*e.g.*, premature ventricular contractions, atrio-ventricular conduction abnormalities)	☐ Muscle fasciculations
☐ Fetal decelerations or bradycardia	

Given persistent severe hypertension, pharmacologic intervention is planned in collaboration with the anesthesiologist.

10. Provide three <u>initial pharmacologic regimens</u> accepted for treatment of hypertension in this gravida, given no contraindications exist for any potential agent. *(3 points each)*   9

☐ Intravenous hydralazine 5–10 mg slowly over two minutes
☐ Intravenous labetalol 20–40 mg slowly
☐ Sublingual nifedipine capsules or tablets 10 mg
☐ Sublingual nitroglycerin 0.3 mg, or infusion 5 mcg/min

Labor progresses rapidly to the second stage; time is permitted for passive head descent, as this preterm gestational age prohibits consideration for instrumental vaginal delivery. You alert your obstetric trainee that avoidance of an episiotomy in a parturient with SCI is paramount, as it may otherwise trigger ADR.

Spontaneous vaginal delivery ensues, and a vigorous newborn is subsequently admitted to the neonatal intensive care unit (NICU), based on gestational age. A spontaneous second-degree laceration is repaired, without signs or symptoms of recurrent ADR.

11. Identify postpartum considerations to discuss, either prior to discharge or at the routine postpartum visit in relation to the medical and obstetric course of this patient. *(1 point each)*	Max 8

General maternal-fetal well-being:
- ☐ Screen for postpartum depression and continue to offer psychosocial support services
- ☐ Ensure the patient has appropriate support in caring for the newborn
- ☐ Encourage breastfeeding, while alerting the patient to monitor for onset of ADR
- ☐ Individualized consideration for thromboprophylaxis
- ☐ Individualized consideration for contraception
- ☐ Encourage future preconception counseling for known SCI and preterm delivery

SCI-related care:
- ☐ Alert the team involved in the postpartum care of this patient that uterine fundal massages or fundal height assessments may trigger ADR
- ☐ Encourage frequent bladder catheterization, as overdistention may trigger ADR
- ☐ Provide analgesia for the healing laceration, or consider delaying removal of the epidural, if relevant
- ☐ Perform regular assessments of the healing perineal wound, based on the risk of delayed wound healing in a patient with SCI

TOTAL:	**80**

Psychiatric Disorders in Pregnancy

CHAPTER 29

Mood Disorders in Pregnancy and Postpartum Depression

Victoria E. Canelos, Amira El-Messidi, and Charlotte S. Hogan

A 21-year-old G1P1 with an uncomplicated pregnancy and vaginal delivery presents to your obstetrical assessment unit one week postpartum with concerns regarding the care of her newborn. She informs the nurse of difficulty with breastfeeding, which triggers a sense of worthlessness. The patient also complains of sleeplessness, even when the baby is asleep, and thereby is constantly exhausted. She shares with the nurse that she is 'worried all the time about everything' and finds herself crying randomly throughout the day for no apparent reason. The patient complains of intense 'mood swings,' which have led to frequent argumentation with her partner.

Your nurse was able to elicit a remote history of depression and cannabis use during her college years. The patient had declined elective perinatal mental health services. Her medical history is otherwise unremarkable.

As you attend to see the patient, your nurse mentions that the patient is tearful, asking what is wrong with her.

LEARNING OBJECTIVES

1. Take a focused history related to a mood disorder in a perinatal patient, recognizing essential components of the psychiatric evaluation
2. Identify critical risk factors that guide your screening, differential diagnosis, and treatment paradigm, dually timing psychiatric consultation and concurrent obstetric care
3. Recognize the obstetric morbidities involved in the care of patients with mood disorders
4. Understand the possible causality between medical conditions and dysregulated mood in the prenatal period
5. Develop an appreciation for drug-safety profiles for the mother, fetus, and newborn

SUGGESTED READINGS

1. ACOG Committee on Practice Bulletins – Obstetrics. ACOG Practice Bulletin: Clinical management guidelines for obstetrician-gynecologists No. 92, April 2008. Use of psychiatric medications during pregnancy and lactation. *Obstet Gynecol.* 2008;111(4):1001–1020. Reaffirmed 2013.

2. American College of Obstetricians and Gynecologists Committee on Obstetric Practice. Screening for perinatal depression. Committee Opinion. No. 757. *Obstet Gynecol*. 2018; 132: e208–e212.

3. Becker MA, Weinberger TE, Chandy A, et al. Mood disorders. Chapter 21 in: Berghella V, ed., *Maternal-Fetal Evidence Based Guidelines*. Boca Raton, FL: CRC Press; 2017.

4. Hogan CS, Freeman MP. Adverse effects in the pharmacologic management of bipolar disorder during pregnancy. *Psychiatr Clin North Am*. 2016 Sep;39(3):465–475.

5. Howard LM, Megnin-Viggars O, Symington I, et al. Antenatal and postnatal mental health: summary of updated NICE guidance. *BMJ*. 2014 Dec 18;v349:g7394.

6. Learman LA. Screening for depression in pregnancy and the postpartum period. *Clin Obstet Gynecol*. 2018;61(3):525–532.

7. Molyneaux E, Howard LM, McGeown HR, et al. Antidepressant treatment for postnatal depression. *Cochrane Database Syst Rev*. 2014;(9):CD002018.

8. Pearlstein T. Depression during pregnancy. *Best Pract Res Clin Obstet Gynaecol*. 2015;29(5):754–764.

9. O'Connor E, Senger CA, Henninger ML, et al. Interventions to prevent perinatal depression: evidence report and systematic review for the US Preventive Services Task Force. *JAMA*. 2019;321(6):588–601.

10. Smith B, Dubovsky SL. Pharmacotherapy of mood disorders and psychosis in pre- and post-natal women. *Expert Opin Pharmacother*. 2017;18(16):1703–1719.

POINTS

1. What aspects of a focused history would you explore with the patient? *(1 point per main bullet, unless specified)*

Max 30

Social network:
☐ Living conditions, support from family members
☐ Screen for domestic violence and abuse *(i.e., elaborate 'argumentation' with her partner)*
☐ Assess for safety of children, or other persons, that may be under the care of the patient *(identify who is caring for the children during the time of the interview and who provides their care when the patient's symptoms flare)* **(3 points)**

Postpartum depression screening tool: *(5 points per main bullet)*
☐ Edinburgh Postnatal Depression Scale (EPDS) questionnaire *(or other validated, standardized tool)*
  ○ *EPDS is a self-administered tool of 10 questions, requiring less than five minutes to complete*
  ○ *Addresses emotional symptoms over the past seven days*
  ○ *Score ranges from 0 to 30 with increasing severity; ≥9 requires evaluation*

Suicidal thoughts and/or homicidal ideations (Current and/or prior): *(6 points)*
☐ Current thoughts of self-harm:
  ○ *Assess if the patient has a plan for committing suicide (when and how)*
  ○ *Identify the reasons stopping her from the suicide act*
☐ Determine what her prior action plans for self-harm have been, if any

Screen for past or present symptoms of an affective illness *(i.e., depression or mania)*:

A: Characteristics of depressive episodes: *(max 7)*

☐ Depressed mood

☐ Changes in sleep pattern (insomnia or excessive sleep)

☐ Feeling of guilt and/or hopelessness and worthlessness

☐ Changes in weight or appetite

☐ Changes in psychomotor function

☐ Decreased energy

☐ Poor concentration

☐ Anhedonia

☐ Suicidal thoughts or self-harm behaviors[†]

B: Characteristics of manic episodes: *(max 4)*

☐ Distinct period of abnormally and persistently elevated, expansive, or irritable mood with persistently elevated energy

☐ Grandiosity

☐ Decreased need for sleep

☐ Talkativeness

☐ Racing thoughts

☐ Involvement in at-risk behaviors *(e.g., spending sprees, sexual indiscretions, business investments, substance use)*

Medications:

☐ Current/ previous therapies *(specifically related to psychiatric illness)*, including reasons for discontinuation

Health maintenance:

☐ Current/ previous alcohol consumption, cigarette smoking, or use of recreational drugs

Past psychiatric history:

☐ Psychosis *(delusions, hallucinations, thought disorder, disorganized behavior)*

☐ Compulsive behaviors and/or obsessive or intrusive thoughts

☐ Anxiety *(uncontrolled worrying, nervousness or feeling 'on the edge')*

☐ Prior hospitalizations for mental illness

Family history:

☐ Severe postpartum mental illness in a first-degree relative

☐ Suicide

☐ Substance use

Special note:

† Current or prior suicidal ideation/self-harm behaviors are key components to ascertain in *isolation* from screening for affective disorders, which are indicated separately as elements of a focused history

The patient reports feeling guilty about not bonding well with her son, which makes her sad. She is frequently and intermittently irritable. Her symptoms started three days postpartum. She denies suicidal and homicidal ideations, and specifically indicates she would like to improve her 'mother-hood' feeling. The patient denies domestic violence. Her EPDS score is 22. You learn that the patient was depressed during her college years, which she attributed to 'extreme stress.' She would often feel irritable and was constantly fatigued despite sleeping longer than average. She became withdrawn from her activities of interest, lacking the desire to associate with friends or engage in hobbies. Resorting to significant amounts of cannabis hoping it would resolve her issues, she became more lethargic and depressed. She sought medical care and was prescribed sertraline 50 mg daily, to which she responded well. In planning for conception, the patient tapered herself off the medication and has not been on treatment in over a year. There is no history of other affective illness, suicidality, and she has never been hospitalized for psychiatric health. Family history is significant for bipolar disorder in a paternal aunt who is currently 57 years of age, and her mother remains in remission from thyroid cancer.

2-A. With respect to the patient's history and current symptoms, what is the most probable diagnosis?   2

☐ Postpartum depression

2-B. Identify four other diagnostic possibilities. *(1 point each)*   4

☐ Postpartum blues *(mild symptoms; resolve within two weeks but warrant close follow-up for risk of postpartum depression)*
☐ Normal postpartum changes
☐ Substance-induced mood disturbance
☐ Postpartum psychosis
☐ Medically related factors

In consultation, the perinatal psychiatry team presents to assess the patient and identify her presentation is compatible with postpartum depression.

While the psychiatry team is counseling the patient, your obstetric trainee is keen to learn more about postpartum depression from this clinical encounter. Your trainee had read that postpartum depression is common, in up to 20% of women, although trainees are uncommonly exposed to similar clinical situations in the postpartum period.

3. Which factors raise this patient's susceptibility for a postpartum mood illness? *(1 point per main bullet, unless specified)*   Max 5

☐ Personal history of depression
☐ Self-initiated, preconception discontinuation of her antidepressant
☐ Family history of bipolar disorder
☐ Symptom onset within four weeks of delivery
☐ Current symptoms: *(1 point per subbullet; max 3 points)*
  ○ Irritability
  ○ Feelings of guilt and worthlessness
  ○ Frequent and intermittent crying
  ○ Excessive anxiety over parenting
  ○ Obsessive thoughts
  ○ Difficulty bonding with the newborn

4. Indicate *other* risk factors, social or medical, that may contribute to the onset of postpartum mental illness. *(1 point each)*   3

☐ History of perinatal depression and/or anxiety
☐ Inadequate social support during the antenatal or postpartum period
☐ Stressful life events during pregnancy and/or proximal to delivery *(associated with risk of postpartum depression, not postpartum psychosis)*

Although the working diagnosis is postpartum depression, you teach your trainee that investigations assessing for medical causes that may account for the clinical presentation should not be overlooked.

5. For *this* patient, which medical investigations would be <u>most</u> indicated to ensure absence of organic pathology contributing to her mental illness? *(1 point each)*   3

☐ Complete blood count
☐ Thyroid function tests including thyroid autoantibodies
☐ Urine toxicology screen *(drug abuse)*

As the patient is being counseled by the psychiatry team, she provides consent for urine toxicology screening and serum tests are drawn as well.

During counseling, the psychiatry team acknowledges that the literature on selective serotonin reuptake inhibitor (SSRI) agents in pregnancy appears nonuniform, which may instill fear and confusion among both patients and medical personnel.

The patient is assured that SSRI agents are first line for depression in the pregnant population, and that discontinued treatment is associated with a relapse rate of up to 70%.

6. Discuss the safety of SSRI agents in the perinatal period. *(2 points per main bullet)*   4

☐ SSRI agents have a reassuring safety profile in pregnancy *(individualized therapy)*:
  ○ Single agent with increasing dose adjustments as necessary is preferable to polypharmacy *(this concept applies to treatment of all psychiatric illnesses during pregnancy)*
  ○ Data on risk of exposure to SSRIs during embryogenesis initially suggested an association between paroxetine and right ventricular outflow defects, however, large meta-analyses show absent association
  ○ No associated risk of early pregnancy loss
  ○ Reassuring maternal side-effects profile
☐ Transient neonatal withdrawal symptoms may occur with late prenatal exposure (e.g., mild respiratory distress, transient tachypnea of the newborn, weak cry, poor tone, leading to NICU admissions)

In communication with the patient, a plan is made to resume the sertraline agent. She voices concern regarding the possibility of continuing lactation with this medication.

---

7. Address the patient's inquiry regarding the safety and possible implications of SSRI agents during lactation. *(1 point per main bullet, unless specified)*   Max 3

☐ All psychotropic medications are excreted in breast milk, at varying concentrations
☐ Reassuring safety data for use of SSRIs while breastfeeding
☐ Factors affecting breast milk exposure to consider in counseling patients include:
   (1 point per subbullet)
   ○ Frequency and timing of feeds
   ○ Dosage of medication
   ○ Rate of maternal drug metabolism

Results of medical tests are normal. Given her good insight, absence of suicidal or homicidal thoughts, assurance that her family is supportive, and her home environment is safe, the psychiatry team deems her safe for close follow-up as an outpatient.

---

8. Outline important aspects of management for this patient. *(1 point each)*   Max 2

☐ Encourage compliance with treatment and follow-up, as arranged by the psychiatry team
☐ Liaison with resources for psychotherapy (including cognitive behavior therapy and interpersonal therapy)
☐ Consideration for social services support and/or assistance with childcare

---

The remainder of her postpartum course is unremarkable, and she responds well to sertraline and personal therapy sessions.

Three years later, the patient has a second healthy pregnancy and delivery. You followed her obstetric care jointly with her psychiatrist. She was well controlled on a stable dose of sertraline throughout pregnancy.

---

9. If, during her second pregnancy, this patient experienced a major depressive episode, indicate maternal and fetal, short-term and long-term effects of this mental illness. *(1 point each)*   Max 10

Maternal:
☐ Less compliance with prenatal care
☐ Use of illicit drugs, alcohol, and tobacco
☐ Risk of postpartum hemorrhage due to sertraline use at time of delivery *(Palmsten K, et al. BMJ 2013; 347: f4877)*
☐ Risk of suicide or self-harm

Fetal:
☐ Early pregnancy loss
☐ Growth restriction
☐ Preterm birth
☐ Suboptimal fetal growth velocity

Neonatal:
☐ Increased rates of NICU admission
☐ Neonatal adaptation syndrome *(mild, self-limiting adverse neurobehavioral effects with in utero third-trimester exposure to SSRIs)*

Child and long-term:
☐ Emotional instability
☐ Impaired cognitive function
☐ Conduct disorders and attention-deficit hyperactivity disorder
☐ Risk of suboptimal vaccinations
☐ Suicidal tendencies, depression, schizophrenia
☐ Suboptimal growth and development *(low- to middle-income countries)*
☐ Overweight/obesity *(high-income countries)*

Thankfully, the mother and fetus did well antenatally; however, two weeks postpartum, the patient is brought to the obstetric emergency unit accompanied by family members who are concerned about her mental health. They indicate she is 'not acting like herself,' constantly irritable and confused. Her sleep rituals are greatly disturbed. She is no longer capable of caring for the newborn independently, and the family occasionally resorts to bottle-feeding when the patient is not capable of feeding the newborn. You learn that the patient was never committed to religious practice, but she now talks about God and demons. On the day of presentation, the family became most concerned when she complained that her children are 'looking at her funny,' wondering if they are her own. Her blood pressure and temperature are normal, with no clinical suspicion of sepsis.

10. Indicate the most probable condition and best next step in management of this patient. *(1 point each)*   2

☐ Postpartum psychosis‡
☐ The patient should be escorted by medical personnel to the E.R department *(A&E)* for urgent care, including hospitalization *(this is a medical emergency that requires immediate care, admission, and intervention)*

Special note:
‡*Postpartum psychosis is not a 'diagnosis'; it does not appear in the international classification system*

The patient is very disorganized and paranoid during your encounter. After you counsel the family, she is accompanied to the urgent psychiatric care unit and is admitted to hospital.

11. What is the rationale for urgent admission for patients with postpartum psychosis? *(1 point each)*   2

☐ Increased risk of suicide *(~1/2000 patients with postpartum psychosis)*
☐ Increased risk of infanticide *(~4% of patients with postpartum psychosis)*

12. If, during pregnancy, this patient experienced a flare of mental illness not responsive to medication, with increasing agitation and catatonia, what would be the quickest, nonpharmacological intervention, to abate her symptoms?   1

☐ Electroconvulsive therapy

13. List three risk factors for postpartum psychosis, which *may or may not* be identified in this patient. *(1 point each)*   Max 3

☐ History of postpartum depression
☐ History of bipolar disorder, schizophrenia, or schizoaffective disorder
☐ Family history of postpartum psychosis
☐ Family history of bipolar disorder
☐ Primiparity
☐ Discontinuation of psychiatric medications during pregnancy

Special note:
There is *no* association between a stressful life event and postpartum psychosis

During her admission, the psychiatrist updates you that although the working diagnosis is postpartum psychosis, the patient may indeed have an underlying affective illness, which commonly is bipolar disorder. The psychiatrist tells you they will continue to provide close long-term care for risk of an emerging affective illness.

Later, the junior psychiatry trainee telephones you to ask whether you have any reservations to lithium therapy during her postpartum period. The SSRI agent needed to be discontinued.

14. Outline your advice regarding the postpartum use of lithium.   1

☐ Optimal treatment of her mental illness is the principal goal: Breastfeeding is discouraged with lithium treatment due to high levels of drug excretion

15. In addition to mood stabilizers, which other agents are part of the mainstay of treatment for postpartum psychosis?   1

☐ Second-generation (atypical) antipsychotics *(e.g., olanzapine, quetiapine)*

Special note:
Preferred avoidance of risperidone in treatment of postpartum psychosis due to its hormonal influences which affect the ability to discontinue lactation

You receive a telephone call from a colleague seeking advice for his preconception patient with well-controlled bipolar illness for over two years with maintenance lithium therapy.

16. Discuss the maternal-fetal risks of gestational lithium treatment, including particular antenatal management that you would share with your colleague. *(1 point each; max points indicated per section)* — Max 9

Lithium exposure during organogenesis: *(max 2)*
- ☐ Teratogenic agent, most characterized by Epstein's cardiac anomaly *(small absolute risk estimates at 1/1500 among exposed neonates, although significantly increased relative risk from general population at 1/20,000)*
- ☐ Fetal echocardiography is advised if continued antenatal treatment

Fetal and/or neonatal risks of second- and third-trimester lithium exposure: *(max 4)*
- ☐ Polyhydramnios
- ☐ Fetal and neonatal cardiac abnormalities
- ☐ Hypoglycemia
- ☐ Hyperbilirubinemia and jaundice
- ☐ Nephrogenic diabetes insipidus
- ☐ Reversible thyroid dysfunction and neonatal goiter
- ☐ Floppy baby syndrome
- ☐ Neonatal lithium toxicity *(lethargy, flaccidity, and poor suckling reflex which may last >7 days)*

Maternal risks and management: *(max 3)*
- ☐ Monitor lithium serum levels during pregnancy *(recommended monitoring is approximately monthly until 36 weeks and weekly thereafter)*
- ☐ Periodic assessment of thyroid and renal function
- ☐ Assess serum lithium levels intrapartum and postpartum
- ☐ Consideration for decreasing drug dose intrapartum
- ☐ Consideration for intrapartum IV hydration

17. What are the principal elements to outline in conversation with your colleague regarding the decision to continue lithium treatment during pregnancy? *(1 point each)* — Max 2

- ☐ Discontinuation of lithium due to fetal risks should be balanced against the maternal risks of disease exacerbation *(psychiatrist's advice is crucial)*
- ☐ Mild and infrequent episodes of illness: Women could be gradually tapered prior to conception
- ☐ More severe episodes of illness but only moderate risk of short-term relapse: Women should be tapered prior to conception and treatment reinstituted after organogenesis
- ☐ Frequent and severe episodes of illness: Continuation of gestational lithium therapy with patient's informed decision

Incidentally, although your colleague awaits a call back from the patient's psychiatrist, he or she asks if the patient can continue taking her olanzapine (Zyprexa®, Zyprexa Zydis®) during pregnancy.

18. Discuss the safety of atypical antipsychotics during pregnancy and lactation. *(1 point each)*	Max 2
☐ Generally reassuring risks regarding absence of teratogenicity *(overall limited data)* ☐ Maternal risks of weight gain, gestational diabetes, and hypertension *(primarily associated with olanzapine and clozapine)* ☐ Generally low levels in breast milk, with the exception of clozapine *(lactation is not recommended; theoretical risk of neonatal agranulocytosis)*	
19. Identify the *antiepileptic agent* with the safest fetal toxicity profile and which is efficacious in preventing bipolar depression during pregnancy.	1

☐ Lamotrigine, at the lowest most effective dose
  ○ Generally reassuring reproductive safety, with possible association with congenital malformations with doses >200 mg daily
  ○ Not recommended with breastfeeding *(breast milk concentration up to 50% of maternal serum levels)*	

TOTAL:	**90**

CHAPTER 30

Schizophrenia in Pregnancy

Amira El-Messidi and Nicolas Beaulieu

A 30-year-old primigravida with schizophrenia is referred by her primary care provider to your high-risk obstetrics unit at a tertiary center. Her mental illness is controlled by clozapine, and she takes routine prenatal vitamins. The patient is at 12^{+2} weeks' gestation by dating sonography; first-trimester fetal anatomy was normal with a low risk of aneuploidy. Results of routine prenatal investigations are unremarkable. The patient does not have any obstetric complaints.

You briefly recall seeing this patient for preconception counseling 10 months ago. Along with your obstetric trainee, you start seeing the patient until your consultation report is made available.

Special note: *Although pregnant women with schizophrenia have increased rates of concomitant alcohol consumption, illicit substance use, and medical morbidities, the case scenario is presented as such for academic purposes and to avoid overlap of content addressed in other chapters. Smoking cessation interventions are addressed in* Chapter 76 *and are presented in this scenario to highlight their physiological contribution to psychiatric complications with particular antipsychotic treatment for schizophrenia.*

LEARNING OBJECTIVES

1. Elicit salient points on history from a prenatal patient with schizophrenia, recognizing associated maternal-fetal benefits and morbidities with respective antipsychotic agent(s)
2. Appreciate the importance of multidisciplinary collaboration in preconception, antenatal, and postnatal management of schizophrenia to optimize perinatal outcomes
3. Recognize essential aspects to deem capacity for consent to treatment
4. Understand that physiological factors may complicate psychosocial stressors, contributing to acute psychosis
5. Initiate management of the obstetric patient with acute psychosis

SUGGESTED READINGS

1. ACOG Committee on Practice Bulletins – Obstetrics. ACOG Practice Bulletin: Clinical management guidelines for obstetrician-gynecologists No. 92. Use of psychiatric medications during pregnancy and lactation. *Obstet Gynecol.* 2008;111(4):1001–1020.
2. Appelbaum PS. Clinical practice: assessment of patients' competence to consent to treatment. *N Engl J Med.* 2007;357(18):1834–1840.

3. Birnbaum R, Weinberger DR. Pharmacological implications of emerging schizophrenia genetics: can the bridge from 'genomics' to 'therapeutics' be defined and traversed? *J Clin Psychopharmacol*. 2020;40(4):323–329.
4. Breadon C, Kulkarni J. An update on medication management of women with schizophrenia in pregnancy. *Expert Opin Pharmacother*. 2019;20(11):1365–1376.
5. Chisolm MS, Payne JL. Management of psychotropic drugs during pregnancy. *BMJ*. 2016;532: h5918.
6. Hasan A, Falkai P, Wobrock T, et al. World Federation of Societies of Biological Psychiatry (WFSBP) Guidelines for biological treatment of schizophrenia. Part 3: Update 2015 Management of special circumstances: Depression, suicidality, substance use disorders and pregnancy and lactation. *World J Biol Psychiatry*. 2015;16(3):142–170.
7. Jones I, Chandra PS, Dazzan P, et al. Bipolar disorder, affective psychosis, and schizophrenia in pregnancy and the post-partum period. *The Lancet*. 2014 Nov 15;384(9956):1789–1799.
8. Poo SX, Agius M. Atypical antipsychotics for schizophrenia and/or bipolar disorder in pregnancy: current recommendations and updates in the NICE guidelines. *Psychiatr Danub*. 2015;27(Suppl 1):S255–S260.
9. Rasic D, Hajek T, Alda M, et al. Risk of mental illness in offspring of parents with schizophrenia, bipolar disorder, and major depressive disorder: a meta-analysis of family high-risk studies. *Schizophr Bull*. 2014;40(1):28–38.
10. Robinson GE. Treatment of schizophrenia in pregnancy and postpartum. *J Popul Ther Clin Pharmacol*. 2012;19(3):e380–e386.

POINTS

1. With respect to schizophrenia and her atypical antipsychotic agent, what aspects of a focused history would you want to know or specific assessments would you make during your communication with the patient?

Max 35

(1 point per main bullet, unless otherwise specified; max points are indicated per section)

History related to schizophrenia: *(max 6)*
☐ Age at onset
☐ Frequency of psychotic episodes, and time interval since the most recent episode
☐ Severity of psychotic episodes
  ○ *Severity may be related to aggression, suicidality, or intense disorganization during the episodes*
☐ Determine social or medical triggers for psychotic episodes
☐ Most common clinical manifestations during psychotic episodes
☐ Name and contact of her treating psychiatrist and mental health team
☐ Suicidality *(3 points)*

Pregnancy: *(2)*
☐ Assess her attitudes toward pregnancy
☐ Determine if patient had prior, *undisclosed*, spontaneous, or therapeutic pregnancy losses

Current/recent *positive symptoms* of schizophrenia: *(4)*
☐ Delusions
☐ Hallucinations *(auditory hallucinations are typical of schizophrenic disorders, while visual hallucinations are more common with other medical etiologies, such as delirium)*
☐ Assess for disorganized appearance/behavior
☐ Assess for disorganized/disjointed speech patterns or thought processes

Assess for presence of *negative symptoms* of schizophrenia: *(2)*
- ☐ Diminished expression (*e.g.*, flat affect, poverty of speech, latency in response)
- ☐ Avolition-apathy (*e.g.*, poor hygiene, little interest to socially engage)

Assess for presence of comorbid *psychiatric* illness with schizophrenia: *(3)*
- ☐ Depression
- ☐ Anxiety disorders
- ☐ Assess for suicidality and heteroaggression

Medical history:

Metabolic comorbidities with schizophrenia: (4)
- ☐ Type 2 diabetes mellitus
- ☐ Chronic hypertension
- ☐ Hyperlipidemia
- ☐ Obesity

Medical conditions that may contribute to psychosis: (1)
- ☐ Examples include autoimmune diseases, stroke, HIV, and syphilis infection

Social factors: *(3)*
Stressors are associated with increased relapse of psychosis
- ☐ Involvement of partner, and assess for domestic violence/abuse/neglect
- ☐ Current housing situation
- ☐ Socioeconomic status/occupation

Health maintenance: *(max 4)*
- ☐ Engagement in physical exercise *versus* sedentary lifestyle (*clozapine and schizophrenia itself increase risks of obesity*)
- ☐ Assess her nutritional status and amount of caffeine intake
- ☐ Current/recent cigarette smoking (*common to ~90% of patients with schizophrenia*)
- ☐ Current/recent alcohol consumption or use of recreational drugs (*polysubstance use is highly comorbid with schizophrenia*)
- ☐ Vaccination status (*e.g., influenza, hepatitis A and B, tetanus*)

Medications: *(4)*
- ☐ Determine which antipsychotics have been tried in the past and treatment-response
  - ○ *the patient likely has treatment-resistant schizophrenia given current clozapine treatment*
- ☐ Assess adherence to clozapine, and current side effects
- ☐ Ensure close monitoring of absolute neutrophil count
  - ○ *Clozapine-associated risk of agranulocytosis, at <500/microliter*
  - ○ *Absolute neutrophil count is generally monitored every one to four weeks, depending on treatment duration and prior neutrophil count*
- ☐ Concomitant antipsychotic polypharmacy, opioids, benzodiazepines, or anxiolytics
- ☐ Prior attempts at physician-guided discontinuation or change of antipsychotic therapy

Family/partner history: *(2)*
- ☐ Presence of schizophrenia or other severe mental illness in her family, including postpartum psychosis or depression
- ☐ Presence of psychiatric illness in her male partner

The patient was diagnosed with schizophrenia eight years ago, and after failed trials with different first- and second-generation antipsychotics, she has been in remission for three years on clozapine monotherapy at 450 mg daily. Her psychiatrist's attempts to lower the maintenance dose was not successful. With stabilization of her illness, she has maintained an administrative assistant position at a small company and quit smoking two years ago after a four pack-year history. The patient does not consume alcohol or use recreational drugs. You note she is well groomed and engages appropriately in conversation. The patient does not have any positive symptoms of schizophrenia and is not suicidal. Maintaining close follow-up with her psychiatrist, she reports normal serial blood tests and has not been diagnosed with depression or anxiety disorders. Her mother experienced postpartum psychosis after delivering the patient, and her father died aged 47 years from sudden cardiac arrest.

The patient acknowledges that your motivating approach during prepregnancy consultation prompted her to engage with exercise and nutritional professionals, which helped her lose almost 50 lbs (23 kg) prior to conception leading to menstrual cycle regularity. She also completed your recommended investigations; she does not have chronic medical conditions often associated with schizophrenia or clozapine treatment. She maintains a healthy 18-month marital relationship; her husband does not have psychiatric illness.

Physical examination is unremarkable and fetal viability is ascertained. Your preconception consultation note has just been made available: you note a decrease in BMI to 26.0 kg/m^2, and improvement in blood pressure to 126/78 mmHg from 141/90 mmHg.

---

2. As you review your consultation note, inform your obstetric trainee of the preconception investigations you had suggested given this patient's schizophrenic illness and clozapine treatment. (*1 point per main bullet*)   9

Serum:
- ☐ Complete/full blood count
- ☐ Fasting plasma glucose or glycosylated hemoglobin (HbA1c)
- ☐ Fasting lipid profile
- ☐ Liver function tests
- ☐ Prolactin level
- ☐ Thyroid stimulating hormone (TSH)
- ☐ Luteinizing hormone and follicle stimulating hormone
- ☐ Free testosterone, and dehydroepiandrosterone sulfate

Imaging:
- ☐ Electrocardiogram (ECG) ± echocardiogram
- ☐ Pelvic ultrasound
  - ○ *for detection of sonographic features of polycystic ovarian syndrome given prepregnancy obesity and menstrual irregularity*

---

3. Apart from the patient's initial obese habitus and hypertension, your trainee is curious whether other factors prompted your recommendation for cardiac monitoring. (*1 point each*)   3

- ☐ Antipsychotic-associated QTc prolongation
- ☐ Risk of clozapine-induced cardiomyopathy/myocarditis
- ☐ First-degree relative with sudden early cardiac death

4. Identify <u>maternal</u> side effects of clozapine (or other atypical antipsychotics) most relevant to obstetric morbidity. *(1 point per main bullet)* — Max 4

☐ Excessive weight gain
☐ Hypertension
☐ Gestational diabetes mellitus (GDM)
☐ Cardiomyopathy
☐ Pulmonary thromboembolism
☐ Constipation
   ○ *Compounded with constipation in pregnancy, severe manifestations may lead to adynamic ileus*

Recalling maternal risks with gestational use of clozapine, the patient expresses concern over its continuation in pregnancy. Being in remission for three years, she wishes to consider antenatal weaning, discontinuation, or change in her regimen to minimize pregnancy complications. Although you note this was discussed at preconception consultation, in collaboration with her psychiatrist, you realize the need to readdress counseling.

5. Troubleshoot the patient's concerns by addressing the effect of decreasing or discontinuing clozapine during the antenatal period. *(1 point each)* — 2

☐ Inform her that ≥50% of patients relapse with discontinuation of antipsychotics, which incurs greater risks to maternal-fetal well-being
☐ Indicate that untreated psychosis during the antenatal period would also increase her risk of postpartum psychosis, especially given her family history

6. To further encourage the obstetric patient to continue her antipsychotic agent, you elaborate on basic pharmacokinetic principles in pregnancy. *(1 point per main bullet)* — Max 3

☐ She is on monotherapy
☐ She takes the lowest effective dose to achieve symptom reduction and fewest side effects
   ○ *Recommend against the use of <u>depot</u> antipsychotics due to inflexible dosing and for purpose of limiting prolonged exposure of the fetus to drugs with potential toxicity*
☐ Inform the patient that drug changes during pregnancy incur fetal exposure to more agents and increase relapse rates until control is achieved
☐ With advancing pregnancy, hepatic CYP1A2 enzymes that metabolize clozapine (and olanzapine) are downregulated, resulting in possible need to <u>decrease</u> doses *(Suggested Reading 5)*

The patient comprehends the importance of adherence to drug therapy. Prior to refreshing her memory on fetal risks related to her mental illness and drug therapy, the patient asks about the antenatal management plan.

7. Maintaining collaboration with her mental health team, outline <u>maternal</u> aspects of management *with focus* on schizophrenic illness and her clozapine treatment. *(1 point per main bullet)*

Max 7

Biological:
☐ Encourage the patient to maintain liaison with her nutritionist during pregnancy; advise referral if needed
☐ Close monitoring of gestational weight gain
☐ Early screening for GDM; and consideration for repeat screening in latter pregnancy if early results are normal
☐ Close monitoring for hypertensive syndromes of pregnancy
☐ Serial blood tests (usually every one to four weeks at this stage) for clozapine-associated risk of agranulocytosis (~0.8%)
  ○ *With initiation of clozapine, CBC is recommended weekly for the first six months, then every two weeks for the following six months, then every one to four weeks thereafter*
☐ Titrate clozapine dosage based on clinical response
  ○ *When therapeutic drug monitoring is performed, a clozapine plasma level of 250–350 ng/mL serves as a guide*

Psycho-social:
☐ Engage family and parent education groups to avoid patient isolation, poor self-care, or substance use; consideration for arranging home visits
☐ Consideration for other evidence-based nonpharmacological treatments for schizophrenia, such as cognitive behavioral therapy
☐ At least monthly assessment for signs and symptoms of relapse

8. Address the patient's inquiry regarding fetal genetic risks of schizophrenia and the possibility of in utero testing for risk prediction. *(1 point each)*

2

☐ In general, the risk of schizophrenia in offspring of one affected parent is 10% *(relative to 1% with unaffected parents)*
☐ Inform the patient that despite known genetic contribution, identification of etiological genes to predict onset of schizophrenia have not been identified, unless there is a known genetic mutation, such as 22q11.2, which is strongly associated with schizophrenia

You remind the patient and your obstetric trainee that although increased rates of perinatal complications occur in women with schizophrenia, it is often unclear whether outcomes are due to the illness itself or confounded by concomitant use of medications or medical conditions.

9. Indicate the <u>fetal</u> risks with clozapine and review your antenatal plan for fetal monitoring. *(1 point each)*

   4

☐ Reassure the patient of <u>no confirmed</u> pattern of teratogenicity[‡] attributed to clozapine despite known placental drug transfer

☐ Atypical (second-generation) antipsychotics are associated with large for gestational age fetuses, compared to first-generation agents more commonly associated with fetuses that are smaller for gestational age or have low birthweight

☐ After the second-trimester fetal morphology scan, arrange for serial fetal growth assessments in the second and third trimesters *(individualized frequency)*

☐ Arrange for antenatal neonatology consultation

Special note:
‡ First-trimester exposure to *risperidone* has been associated with a small increased risk in overall malformations, and nonsignificant risk of cardiac malformations

Pregnancy progresses well until 22^{+1} weeks' gestation when the patient presents, accompanied by her husband, to the obstetric emergency assessment unit. Since unexpectedly losing her job three weeks ago, she has been very worried about their finances, despite her husband's reassurance of their socioeconomic stability. Three weeks ago, the day prior to losing her job, fetal morphology survey was normal.

Over the past few weeks, he ascertains witnessing her take clozapine daily. You note therapeutic serum levels last performed one month ago. The patient's husband found cigarette butts and smelled smoke in the house over the past few weeks. He has not found evidence of alcohol or illicit substance use. He reports the patient's behavior has been bizarre with increasing paranoia over the past two days. Being convinced she is secretly monitored by their television, she switched off all household electronics. At presentation now, she appears guarded, muttering to herself and avoiding eye contact. Her vital signs[†] are normal and fetal viability is ascertained, and no obstetric complications are suspected. You notify her psychiatrist and agree on necessary investigations until he or she attends shortly to assist you in the care of the patient. While her nurse is drawing blood tests, the patient accuses her of trying to implant a tracking device.

Special note:
† Vital signs consist of blood pressure, pulse, respiratory rate, temperature and oxygen saturation

10. Based on your discussion with her psychiatrist, indicate your agreed-upon investigations in the work-up of the patient's presentation. *(1 point each, unless specified)*

   10

☐ Clozapine serum levels *(3 points)*
☐ CBC/FBC
☐ TSH
☐ Random glucose level
☐ Serum electrolytes
☐ Alcohol blood level
☐ Urinalysis/urine culture
☐ Urine drug screen

11. Until results of investigations are available, explain to her husband the <u>biophysiological</u> basis for your working diagnosis.

 ☐ Compounds in cigarette tar (*e.g.*, polycyclic hydrocarbons) induce CYP1A2 hepatic enzymes to increase clozapine metabolism, inducing acute psychosis from subtherapeutic drug levels

5

The patient is now insisting on terminating her pregnancy, following the 'grand power's' instruction. She threatens to self-induce pregnancy loss if her request is denied. Results of laboratory investigations remain unavailable. The psychiatrist is yet to attend to the patient as he or she is momentarily occupied with another acute psychiatric emergency.

12. Assuming that pregnancy terminations are permitted and medically feasible in your jurisdiction, <u>justify</u> your agreement or disagreement with the patient's wish. *(1 point each)*

 ☐ Her reason for pregnancy termination is irrational and based on a psychotic delusion; a surrogate decision maker *(her husband in this instance)* is delegated to make medical decisions on her behalf until resolution of her psychotic episode
 ☐ She lacks capacity to consent given her inability to communicate a clear, consistent, and rational choice in keeping with her values
 ☐ She lacks capacity to consent given her inability to demonstrate a reasonable understanding of risks, benefits, and alternative treatments

Max 2

13. With focus on acute psychosis, outline your initial approach to management and stabilization of this obstetric patient. She has no drug allergies. *(1 point per main bullet)*

 ☐ Do not allow the patient to leave against medical advice *(she presents a danger to herself and the fetus, and made a credible threat for self-harm based on delusional ideations)*
 ☐ Clear the room of sharp objects
 ☐ Maintain continued surveillance until she is transferred to a psychiatric unit
 ☐ Treatment options include (a) administration of haloperidol (first choice agent) 2–10 mg IV/IM ideally once, with possible repeat dosing in approximately six hours, **OR** (b) consideration for offering the patient oral antipsychotic medication, provided she is not acutely agitated, presenting a danger to herself or fetus, or refusing oral medication
  ○ Pharmacologic management is less risky to the patient and fetus relative to physical restraints; where restraints are required, use them for the shortest possible time
 ☐ ECG monitoring for risk of long QTc with IV haloperidol

Max 4

Special note:
Where acute psychosis occurs at more advanced gestational ages, electronic monitoring for fetal heart rate and uterine tocometry is indicated if tolerated by the patient, or once stabilized

In collaboration with the psychiatrist, the patient's clozapine serum levels are found to be subtherapeutic, most likely secondary to interactions with cigarette smoking. All other investigations are unremarkable. After one week of admission at the inpatient psychiatric unit, maintaining the same dose of clozapine, her symptoms resolve, and the patient is safely discharged home. Fetal viability has been regularly confirmed during admission and sonographic imaging was normal prior to discharge.

---

14. During your patient visit prior to discharge, identify elements of your counseling to   Max 3
minimize her risk of further psychotic episodes. *(1 point each)*

☐ Provide counseling regarding risks of smoking with concomitant clozapine treatment
☐ Educate the patient on stress reduction techniques (*e.g.,* prenatal yoga, mindfulness, meditation)
☐ Encourage and reassure the patient about use of nicotine replacement therapy (transdermal patch, gum, nasal spray, lozenges) which does not induce CYP1A2 enzymes given absence of cigarette tar
☐ Continue to offer psychosocial support services

Special note:
Refer to Question 12-B in Chapter 76 for discussion on smoking cessation interventions for the obstetric patient

---

With continued support from her husband, family, and health professionals, remaining prenatal care is unremarkable. The patient remains compliant with care and adherent to socio-medical management plan. With multidisciplinary affiliation, her clozapine levels are kept in the therapeutic range and her absolute neutrophil counts remain normal. During the prenatal visit at 35 weeks' gestation, she requests you review neonatal risks after in utero clozapine exposure.

---

15. Discuss <u>neonatal/child</u> effects of in utero clozapine exposure, or risks with third-trimester   Max 3
exposure to antipsychotics. *(1 point each)*

☐ Agranulocytosis
☐ Floppy baby syndrome
☐ Seizures
☐ Hypoglycemia *(may be confounded by maternal metabolic effects of clozapine)*
☐ Extrapyramidal *(e.g., agitation, tremor, hypertonia)* and/or withdrawal symptoms may occur after third-trimester exposure to antipsychotics
☐ Clozapine and other atypical antipsychotics may cause neurodevelopmental delay for the first 6 months of life, resolving by 12 months

---

At 38^{+4} weeks' gestation, the patient has an uncomplicated spontaneous vaginal delivery[§] of a healthy neonate in your tertiary center. The newborn is being closely monitored for complications from in utero exposure to antipsychotics and maternal hospitalization has been electively extended to accommodate mother–infant bonding.

Special note:
§ Although rates of Cesarean section are increased among women taking antipsychotics, Cesarean section is reserved for obstetric indications

16. Regarding the patient's schizophrenic illness and postnatal continuation of clozapine, as arranged by her psychiatrist, what are important postpartum considerations in the care of this patient? *(1 point per main bullet)*

Breastfeeding:
- ☐ Not recommended with use of clozapine given risks of severe neutropenia (agranulocytosis), sedation, and cardiovascular effects (long QTc)
  - ○ *Breastfeeding while on other antipsychotics depends on specific drug-excretion in breast milk; individualized assessment is advised*
  - ○ *For women for whom breastfeeding is permitted, measuring serum levels in the neonate is not recommended*
  - ○ *Typical (first-generation) antipsychotics are excreted in breast milk at <3% of maternal levels; the majority of typical antipsychotics are not associated with adverse events*

Mental health monitoring:
- ☐ Screen for postpartum depression, anxiety, and psychosis and continue to offer psychosocial support services
- ☐ Close postdischarge follow-up for risk of relapse *(e.g., at two weeks postpartum)*; the presence of significant stressors warrant very close follow-up to avoid gaps in care

Contraception:
- ☐ Reassure the patient that contraceptive counseling serves to empower her to achieve the desired interpregnancy interval, and is not a judgement of her suitability for parenting
- ☐ Although no hormonal contraceptive mechanism is *contraindicated* with schizophrenic illness or antipsychotic treatment, consideration should be given to offering long-acting reversible contraception
  - ○ *Emerging evidence suggests combined hormonal contraceptives can have major effects on mental health, specifically depression, even in women without prior history; individualized assessment is advised*
  - ○ *There are promising studies suggesting that estrogen could be useful as an adjunct for treatment refractory schizophrenia*
- ☐ Encourage use of condoms for dual contraception to decrease risks of sexually transmitted infections

Infant care:
- ☐ At discharge, educate the patient and family on signs and symptoms of withdrawal or extrapyramidal symptoms
  - ○ *Symptoms may appear up to several weeks after delivery*
- ☐ Consider local child welfare services to ensure safe care at home

Maternal outpatient follow-up:
- ☐ Ensure arrangements are made for the obstetric visit

TOTAL: **105**

9

SECTION 6

Cardiopulmonary Conditions in Pregnancy

CHAPTER 31

Valvular Heart Disease in Pregnancy

Anita Banerjee, Hannah Douglas, and Amira El-Messidi

A 32-year-old nulligravida with a history of mitral valve replacement is referred by her cardiologist to your high-risk obstetrics clinic for preconception consultation.

LEARNING OBJECTIVES

1. Take a focused history, and identify risk-stratifying features for preconception counseling of a patient with a prosthetic heart valve
2. Appreciate the importance of shared decision-making for maintenance of antenatal therapeutic anticoagulation with a metallic heart valve given the lack of an equally safe strategy for both mother and fetus
3. Demonstrate the ability to manage, with multidisciplinary collaboration, the antepartum and intrapartum periods based on different anticoagulation regimens
4. Recognize differences in antenatal care of a patient on high-dose and low-dose vitamin K antagonist therapy for a metallic heart valve, in contrast to a bioprosthetic valve
5. Understand essentials of pregnancy management for selected complications of prosthetic heart valves or related treatments

SUGGESTED READINGS

1. Aggarwal SR, Economy KE, Valente AM. State of the art management of mechanical heart valves during pregnancy. *Curr Treat Options Cardiovasc Med.* 2018;20(12):102.
2. Bhagra CJ, D'Souza R, Silversides CK. Valvular heart disease and pregnancy part II: management of prosthetic valves. *Heart.* 2017;103(3):244–252.
3. Daughety MM, Zilberman-Rudenko J, Shatzel JJ, et al. Management of anticoagulation in pregnant women with mechanical heart valves. *Obstet Gynecol Surv.* 2020;75(3):190–198.
4. D'Souza R, Ostro J, Shah PS, et al. Anticoagulation for pregnant women with mechanical heart valves: a systematic review and meta-analysis. *Eur Heart J.* 2017;38(19):1509–1516.
5. Güner A, Kalçık M, Gürsoy MO, et al. Comparison of different anticoagulation regimens regarding maternal and fetal outcomes in pregnant patients with mechanical prosthetic heart valves (from the Multicenter ANATOLIA-PREG Registry). *Am J Cardiol.* 2020;127:113–119.
6. Mehta LS, Warnes CA, Bradley E, et al. Cardiovascular considerations in caring for pregnant patients: a scientific statement from the American Heart Association. *Circulation.*

2020;141(23):e884–e903. [Corrections in *Circulation*. 2020 Jun 9;141(23):e904; *Circulation*. 2021 Mar 23;143(12):e792–e793]

7. Otto CM, Nishimura RA, et al. 2020 ACC/AHA guideline for the management of patients with valvular heart disease: a report of the American College of Cardiology/American Heart Association Joint Committee on Clinical Practice Guidelines. *J Thorac Cardiovasc Surg.* 2021;162(2):e183–e353.

8. Regitz-Zagrosek V, Roos-Hesselink JW, Bauersachs J, et al. 2018 ESC Guidelines for the management of cardiovascular diseases during pregnancy. *Eur Heart J.* 2018;39(34): 3165–3241.

9. Steinberg ZL, Dominguez-Islas CP, Otto CM, et al. Maternal and fetal outcomes of anticoagulation in pregnant women with mechanical heart valves. *J Am Coll Cardiol.* 2017;69(22):2681–2691.

POINTS

1. What aspects of a focused history would you want to know? *(1 point each; max points indicated per section)*   20

Details related to the prosthetic heart valve: *(6)*
- ☐ Ascertain the type of valve, biosynthetic or mechanical; for a mechanical valve, identify the model (*i.e.*, first-generation, or newer generation)
  - ○ *this provides crucial information regarding thrombogenicity of the valve*
- ☐ Date of cardiac valve replacement and need for reoperation
- ☐ Congenital or acquired indication for valve replacement
- ☐ History of valve thrombosis, thromboembolism, or atrial fibrillation
- ☐ Latest left ventricular ejection fraction (LVEF) and comprehensive functional assessment of all cardiac valves on [transthoracic] echocardiography
- ☐ Latest results on 12-lead ECG and/or exercise tolerance test

Medications: *(3)*
- ☐ Anticoagulant regimen, adherence to therapy, side effects and complications *(if any)*
- ☐ Contraceptive method
- ☐ Allergies *(particularly in relation to later need of endocarditis prophylaxis)*

Current cardiopulmonary symptoms and signs: *(max 5)*
- ☐ Establish her New York Heart Association Classification (NYHA)
- ☐ Chest pain or palpitations at rest or with exertion
- ☐ Dyspnea at rest or with exertion
- ☐ Cyanosis
- ☐ Orthopnea
- ☐ Paroxysmal nocturnal dyspnea
- ☐ Leg edema

Medical and social morbidities with heart disease:[†] *(max 5)*
- ☐ Hypertension (or other concurrent cardiovascular condition)
- ☐ Hyperlipidemia

- ☐ Obstructive sleep apnea (OSA)
- ☐ Cigarette smoking, illicit drug use, chronic alcohol abuse
- ☐ Antiphospholipid antibody syndrome/thrombophilia(s)
- ☐ Current level of physical activity

Family history: *(max 1)*
- ☐ Premature sudden cardiac death
- ☐ Congenital heart disease

Special note:
† As a comorbidity, obesity is an aspect of the physical examination

2. Attentive to your conversation with the patient, your obstetric trainee requests your elaboration on <u>etiologies for acquired valvular disease</u> which may have accounted for cardiac surgery. *(1 point each)*

Max 2

- ☐ Rheumatic fever
- ☐ Chest irradiation
- ☐ Systemic illness-induced valvulitis

SCENARIO A
Metallic heart valve, requiring high-dose warfarin >5 mg/d
You learn that seven years ago, a *first-generation* metallic prosthesis replaced her native severe mitral valve stenosis which had progressed during the decade after experiencing rheumatic fever as a child. Cardiac surgery, performed in your high-risk hospital center, was uncomplicated and she did not experience any medical or surgical complications. The patient takes warfarin 8 mg daily which maintains the INR in the therapeutic range. A recent echocardiogram, as requested by her cardiologist, showed a LVEF of 61% without valvular dysfunction. She has no cardiopulmonary symptoms and NYHA is class I. The patient uses levonorgesterol intrauterine system (LNG-IUS) for contraception ever since starting warfarin treatment, understanding its teratogenic associations. She has no drug allergies or medical comorbidities; she practices healthy life habits, including swimming twice weekly. Family history is noncontributory.

3. What is her modified World Health Organization (mWHO) risk classification upon which counseling and future prenatal care would be based?

2

- ☐ mWHO risk class III *(i.e., mechanical valve replacement)*

4. Inform the patient of potential <u>cardiac complications</u> in pregnancy with a mechanical valve. *(1 point each)*

☐ Valve thrombosis (~5%)
☐ Thromboembolism
☐ Arrhythmia
☐ Prosthetic valve dysfunction *(e.g., valve obstruction and/or regurgitation)*
☐ Prosthetic valve endocarditis
☐ Left ventricular dysfunction, heart failure, cardiogenic shock
☐ Other acute cardiac pathologies, such as coronary dissection
☐ Maternal mortality (risk varies between 1% and 15%; *Suggested Reading 2*)

Max 3

As the patient is aware that warfarin is associated with embryo-fetal malformations and complications, you take note to later review with your obstetric trainee characteristics of teratogens, focusing on in utero effects of warfarin exposure.

5. Present the criteria and principle(s) to consider in classifying an agent as a teratogen. *(1 point each)*

Max 6

Essential criteria:
☐ Careful delineation of clinical cases, particularly if there is a specific defect or syndrome; this is preferably done by a geneticist or dysmorphologist
☐ Proof that exposure occurred at a critical time of organogenesis
☐ Consistent findings by at least two epidemiological studies of adequate power, after exclusion of bias, adjustment for confounding variables, demonstrating a relative risk of ≥ 3.0 (some recommend ≥ 6.0), with prospective ascertainment if possible
OR
☐ For a rare environmental exposure associated with a rare defect, at least three cases have been reported; this is easiest if the defect is severe

Ancillary criteria:
☐ The association is biologically plausible for a causal, and not only temporal, relationship
☐ Teratogenicity in experimental animals is important but not essential
☐ The agent acts in an unaltered form in an experimental model

Principle to consider:
☐ Agent crosses placenta sufficiently to directly influence embryonic or fetal development or alter maternal or placental metabolism

Special note:
Refer to (i) Shepard TH. Annual commentary on human teratogens. *Teratology*. 2002a; 66:275.
(ii) Shepard TH. Letters: 'proof' of human teratogenicity. *Teratology*. 1994; 50:97.

6. Present a structured approach of embryo-fetal pathologies of in utero warfarin exposure to later teach your trainee. *(1 point each)*

Max 7

Embryotoxic effects *(i.e., exposure at six to nine weeks' gestation)*:
- ☐ Chondrodysplasia punctata (stippled epiphyses)
- ☐ Nasal hypoplasia with a depressed nasal bridge; upper airway obstruction
- ☐ Limb hypoplasia
- ☐ Congenital heart defects
- ☐ Choanal atresia

Fetotoxic effects:
- ☐ Intracranial hemorrhage
- ☐ Microcephaly
- ☐ Agenesis of the corpus callosum
- ☐ Cerebellar atrophy and vermian agenesis
- ☐ Optic atrophy
- ☐ Microphthalmia

7. Apart from its teratogenicity, address a patient inquiry regarding <u>adverse obstetric outcomes</u> that have been associated with warfarin. *(1 point each)*

Max 7

Maternal:
- ☐ Retroplacental bleeding/subchorionic hemorrhage
- ☐ Preterm labor and birth (spontaneous and iatrogenic)
- ☐ Antepartum and postpartum hemorrhage
- ☐ Cesarean section *(in cases where labor begins, or urgent delivery required, when the patient is on warfarin or within two weeks of its discontinuation; fetal INR is likely still increased)*
- ☐ Wound hematoma, intra-abdominal bleeding
- ☐ Maternal mortality (1.1%–1.8%; *Suggested Reading 2*)

Embryo-fetal:
- ☐ Early pregnancy loss >30% with warfarin >5 mg/d *(2020 ACC/AHA Guideline[7])*
- ☐ Fetal growth restriction (FGR)
- ☐ Stillbirth and neonatal death

You further counsel her that given a metallic heart valve, she has an approximate 60% chance for uncomplicated pregnancy with a live birth.[§]

With the decision-making dilemma between the lifelong need of anticoagulation with a metallic heart valve and obstetric risks of warfarin, the patient inquires about potential treatments that could obviate detrimental effects of vitamin K antagonists.

Special note:
§ In the ROPAC registry, event-free pregnancy with a live birth was found in 58% of women with metallic heart valve; this is in contrast to counseling related to bioprosthetic valves discussed in

Question 18 [van Hagen IM, Roos-Hesselink JW, Ruys TP, et al. Pregnancy in women with a mechanical heart valve: Data of the European Society of Cardiology Registry of Pregnancy and Cardiac Disease (ROPAC). *Circulation*. 2015;132(2):132–142.]

8. Counsel the patient on preconception and antenatal particularities of care regarding the need of at least 8 mg daily warfarin for an in-situ mechanical heart valve.

13

Warfarin – preconception: *(5 points)*
☐ Treatment must continue until pregnancy is achieved, regardless of the dose, because the risk of warfarin embryopathy is low in the first five weeks of pregnancy

Antenatal particularities: *(1 point per main bullet; max 8)*

***i.* Maternal**
☐ Current evidence indicates that continuation of warfarin throughout pregnancy is most effective for prevention of valve thrombosis, with risk estimates at 0%–4%; the trade-off is that maternal safety is jeopardized for that of embryo-fetal well-being
☐ Incidence of hemorrhagic complications in the mother is lower with vitamin K antagonist therapy throughout pregnancy than with unfractionated or low molecular weight heparin (UFH, LMWH, respectively)
☐ With known dose-dependent warfarin embryotoxicity,[§] consider withholding warfarin and using adjusted-dose IV UFH (maintaining aPTT $\geq 2\times$ control) or adjusted-dose LMWH twice daily between 6 and 12 weeks' gestation; the patient must understand that this poses a greater threat to her health
   ○ Risk of valve thrombosis on LMWH in the first trimester (5.8%–7.4%) is similar to the risk where LMWH is used throughout pregnancy (4.4%–8.7%) *(ESC Guidelines[8])*
   ○ Risk of valve thrombosis on UFH in the first trimester or throughout pregnancy varies from 9% to 33% *(ESC Guidelines[8])*
☐ Should the patient wish to prevent first-trimester warfarin embryotoxicity, advise her that warfarin therapy *should be considered* from 12 to 36 weeks in view of her high-risk cardiac features *(i.e., first-generation metallic valve in the mitral position)*
☐ Mention the suboptimal option of continuing twice-daily LMWH from early pregnancy until 36 weeks' gestation to minimize embryo-fetal effects of warfarin, at the expense of maternal valve thrombosis; *the patient must understand that valve thrombosis may occur despite therapeutic anti-Xa levels*
☐ At ~36 weeks' gestation, warfarin must be changed in anticipation of delivery; options include

   ○ UFH to keep the aPTT $\geq 2\times$ control, then weekly monitoring

OR
   ○ LMWH twice daily to target anti-Xa levels four- to six-hour postdose 1.0–1.2 IU/mL[†]; monitoring of predose anti-Xa level ≥ 0.6 IU/mL may be considered
☐ Counsel the patient that brief antenatal hospitalization is recommended *[local practices may vary]* during changes to the anticoagulant regimen *(ESC Guidelines[8])*
☐ Explain the need for INR monitoring every one to two weeks
☐ Explain the need for weekly anti-Xa or aPTT monitoring while on LMWH or UFH, respectively

ii. Fetal

☐ Rates of warfarin embryopathy are time- and dose-dependent in relation to exposure; however, a dose-dependent relationship for early pregnancy loss or fetopathy is controversial:[§§]

    ○ Risk of embryopathy with first-trimester exposure is 0.6%–10%, while risks with second- and third-trimester exposure are 0.7%–2% *(ESC Guidelines[8])*

☐ Serial fetal sonographic surveillance for complications of embryopathy and/or fetopathy would be warranted

Special notes:

§ High-dose vitamin K antagonists include warfarin >5 mg/d, phenprocoumon >3 mg/d, or acenocoumarol >2 mg/d

† This postdose anti-Xa target is specific for mitral or right-sided valves; target levels would be 0.8–1.2 IU/mL for metallic aortic valves

§§ In the ROPAC registry, rates of miscarriage or fetal loss among women taking high-dose or low-dose vitamin K antagonists were similar [van Hagen IM, Roos-Hesselink JW, Ruys TP, et al. Pregnancy in women with a mechanical heart valve: Data of the European Society of Cardiology Registry of Pregnancy and Cardiac Disease (ROPAC). *Circulation.* 2015;132(2):132–142.]

You reinforce the importance of strict adherence to an agreed-upon treatment, frequent monitoring for dose-adjustments, and maintenance of therapeutic anticoagulation in pregnancy, highlighting that, based on evidence-based recommendations, you would otherwise counsel against pregnancy *(2020 ACC/AHA Guideline[7]).*

As she contemplates risk-benefit profiles of antenatal therapeutic regimens based on her values and preferences, she addresses your suggested alternatives to pregnancy; neither adoption nor surrogacy are options to the couple. She is curious whether low-dose aspirin can help prevent valve thrombosis when taken concurrently with heparin in the first trimester to protect against embryotoxicity.

9. Discuss recommendations for routine[§] supplementary low-dose aspirin in prevention of valve thrombosis with antenatal therapeutic vitamin K antagonists or heparins.
(1 point each)   2

Controversy exists:

☐ Although limited data is available on safety and efficacy of low-dose aspirin plus anticoagulation in preventing metallic valve thrombosis, routine addition of low-dose aspirin is not recommended based on lack of proven advantages

    ○ *(Refer to 2020 ACC/AHA Guideline[7] and ESC Guidelines[8])*

☐ Supplementary low-dose aspirin may be associated with significantly more maternal hemorrhagic complications, including fatal events

Special notes:

§ Excluding other medical or obstetric risk factors

Some clinicians choose to use low-dose aspirin with heparins or vitamin K antagonist anticoagulation in women with mechanical heart valve(s)

10. Assuming an uncomplicated pregnancy with in-hospital change from warfarin to therapeutic LMWH at 36 weeks' gestation, detail the crucial aspects of <u>delivery management</u> of a mother with a metallic heart valve that need to be addressed in counseling <u>or</u> included in the consultation note to the referring physician. *(1 point each)*

Max 5

☐ Delivery will be arranged in a setting with simultaneous maternal-fetal cardiac monitoring
☐ Inform the patient and the referring physician that from a cardiac perspective, vaginal delivery is preferred for most women
☐ At 36 hours before planned delivery, IV UFH will be initiated to maintain aPTT $\geq$2x control[†]
☐ When IV UFH is stopped four to six hours before delivery to minimize time off anticoagulation for a patient at high risk of valve thrombosis, epidural would be contraindicated until the aPTT returns to normal; antenatal consultation with an obstetric anesthesiologist is warranted
☐ Anticoagulation is restarted four to six hours postpartum in the absence of bleeding
☐ Passive descent of the fetal head is favored over early pushing in the second stage *(i.e., minimize Valsalva maneuver)*
☐ Although neither vaginal nor Cesarean delivery are indications for routine prophylaxis against infective endocarditis, antibiotics administration 30–60 minutes prior to delivery is *reasonable* for a patient with a prosthetic heart valve given heightened risk of adverse outcomes from endocarditis *(e.g., mortality can reach 40%)*

Special note:
[†] With reference to clinical description after Question 28 in Chapter 52, protamine sulfate offers complete reversal of anticoagulation with UFH relative to LMWH; treatment is required for maternal bleeding complications

Spontaneous conception of an intrauterine viable singleton occurs by four months after your consultation visit during which you removed the LNG-IUS, in collaboration with her cardiologist and initiated daily folic acid supplementation. In accordance with the mWHO risk classification, cardiology review, including maternal echocardiography, is planned at least monthly. The patient recalls details of the preconception consultation in which you outlined significantly increased risks of maternal mortality or severe morbidity.

11. In addition to allied health professionals, indicate <u>medical</u> experts *likely* to constitute the 'pregnancy heart team' based on the patient's mechanical valve-associated mWHO class III. *(1 point each)*

Max 5

☐ Obstetrician/maternal-fetal medicine expert
☐ Adult cardiologist
☐ Cardiac imaging or interventional cardiologist
☐ Cardiac surgeon
☐ Obstetric (± cardiac) anesthesiologist
☐ Neonatologist
☐ Mental health expert *(case-based)*
☐ Family medicine expert or specialist midwife *(international variations exist)*

Special note:
American College of Obstetricians and Gynecologists' Presidential Task Force on Pregnancy and Heart Disease and Committee on Practice Bulletins—Obstetrics. ACOG Practice Bulletin No. 212: Pregnancy and heart disease. *Obstet Gynecol.* 2019;133(5):e320–e356.

With multidisciplinary collaboration, the patient deferred risks of warfarin embryopathy and was admitted to hospital upon confirmation of a viable intrauterine pregnancy at six weeks' gestation for conversion to LMWH until anti-Xa levels were therapeutic. There were no contraindications or situations warranting caution with selection of LMWH.[†] Based on its side-effect profile,[‡] the patient had also provided informed consent for use of LMWH over UFH.[§] Close outpatient clinical and echocardiographic follow-up was maintained until readmission at 12 weeks' gestation as her regimen was reverted to warfarin. First-trimester screening for fetal aneuploidy was unremarkable.

At 16 weeks' gestation, the patient presents to the obstetric emergency assessment unit with an isolated new-onset dyspnea. Her NYHA is class III. She has no obstetric complaints and fetal viability is ascertained. Her vital signs and physical examination were unremarkable; INR was on target. The cardiologist promptly assists you in evaluation, which confirms an obstructive metallic valve thrombosis on echocardiography. As maternal hemodynamic stability is maintained, the patient will be counseled by the 'heart valve team' for receipt of a low-dose slow infusion of tissue-type plasminogen activator (tPA), followed by IV UFH. You learn that the designated protocol is based on limited observational studies and will constitute tPA 25 mg over 6 hours, without a bolus dose; treatment may be repeated every 24 hours, based upon echocardiographic findings, to a maximum of 150 mg.[#]

Special notes:
Refer to Questions 16[†] and 26-B[§] and last section of Question 27[‡] in Chapter 52
Özkan M, Çakal B, Karakoyun S, et al. Thrombolytic therapy for the treatment of prosthetic heart valve thrombosis in pregnancy with low-dose, slow infusion of tissue-type plasminogen activator. *Circulation.* 2013;128(5):532–540.

12. Elicit this patient's risk factors for metallic valve thrombosis. *(1 point each)*   4

☐ Pregnancy *(hypercoagulable state)*
☐ Mitral valve position
☐ First-generation mechanical prosthetic valve
☐ Use of LMWH in the first trimester

Special note:
Risk factors not specific to this patient would be prior valve thromboembolic complication, tricuspid mechanical valve, atrial fibrillation/flutter (persistent or paroxysmal), small valve size, and multiple mechanical heart valves

13. Counsel the patient on obstetric aspects of tPA therapy and summarize its obstetric advantages over surgery. *(1 point each)*

Max 2

☐ Provide reassurance that the compound does not cross placenta due to a high molecular weight
☐ Address the risk of embolization (10%), subplacental bleeding, and placental abruption
☐ Mention that medical treatment is preferred to cardiac surgery in pregnancy, where fetal mortality rate is 30%–40% and maternal mortality rate is reported to be up to 9%
  ○ *(Refer to 2020 ACC/AHA Guideline[7] and ESC Guidelines[8])*

She responds well to one dose of fibrinolysis. You learn from the cardiologist that although two of three criteria define successful treatment of an obstructive thrombus, the patient's dyspnea resolved, the thrombus' length[†] decreased by ≥50%, and Doppler interrogation of the previously increased transvalvular gradient has also resolved.

The patient is later transitioned back to warfarin with an increased INR goal now at 3.5 to 4.5 for mitral prosthesis, and maternal-fetal care is unremarkable thereafter for the remainder of pregnancy. Induction of labor, arranged for 38 weeks' gestation, proceeds well and the patient has an unremarkable vaginal delivery. Maternal hemodynamic status is being closely monitored in the cardiac care unit during the early postpartum period.[‡] Bridging of therapy to resume therapeutic warfarin anticoagulation will be established with multidisciplinary collaboration.

Special notes:
† Decreased thrombus *area* by ≥50% is also an accepted feature of resolution
‡ Refer to Question 16 in Chapter 32 for discussion of early postpartum changes in gestational physiology

14. Identify postpartum considerations to discuss, either prior to discharge or at the routine postpartum visit in relation to a mechanical heart valve. *(1 point each)*

Max 7

General maternal-fetal well-being:
☐ Screen for postpartum depression and continue to offer psychosocial support services
☐ Counsel the patient that return to nonpregnant cardiovascular dynamics may take weeks to months, necessitating long-term care with the cardiac team and primary care provider
☐ Encourage a healthy lifestyle to mitigate long-term cardiovascular risk factors
☐ Reassure the patient that breastfeeding is safe with vitamin K antagonists, LMWH, and UFH

Contraceptive recommendations:
☐ Suggest consideration for permanent methods of contraception
☐ No restrictions on use of barrier methods although they are the least effective agents and should not be relied upon in women in whom unintended pregnancy carries significant maternal-fetal risks
☐ Review with the patient that estrogen-containing contraceptives are contraindicated due the antenatal thrombotic event (*in the absence of prior thrombosis, estrogen-containing*

contraceptives would also not be recommended in a patient with a metallic heart valve due to risks of arterio-venous thrombosis)

☐ Safe modalities include LNG-IUS, progestin implants, DMPA, and progestin-oral contraceptives; recognizing the high failure rate of progestin-only pills, these agents may not provide optimal contraception for this patient

☐ Although safe, copper IUD is suboptimal for this patient on indefinite anticoagulation due to increased vaginal bleeding and anemia

SCENARIO B

Mechanical valve on low-dose warfarin (i.e., ≤5 mg/d)

You learn that seven years ago, a *second-generation* metallic valve replaced her native severe mitral valve stenosis which progressed during the decade after experiencing rheumatic fever as a child. Cardiac surgery, performed in your high-risk hospital center, was uncomplicated and she has not had medical or surgical complications. The patient takes warfarin 3 mg daily which maintains the INR in the therapeutic range. A recent echocardiogram, as requested by her cardiologist, showed a LVEF of 61% without any valvular dysfunction. She has no cardiopulmonary symptoms and NYHA is class I. The patient has been relying on levonorgesterol intrauterine system (LNG-IUS) for contraception ever since starting warfarin treatment. She has no drug allergies or medical comorbidities; she practices healthy life habits, including swimming twice weekly. Family history is noncontributory.

15. Highlight the <u>differences</u> in preconception counseling and evidence-based antenatal management of this patient relative to the former in 'scenario A.' *(1 point each)*

3

☐ Inform the patient that warfarin ≤5 mg/d is associated with lower risks of embryopathy (<3%)

☐ Contrary to the patient on high-dose warfarin, where discontinuation between 6 and 12 weeks' gestation *should be considered*, continuation of warfarin where needs are ≤5 mg/d[†] for therapeutic anticoagulation *should be considered (ESC Guidelines[8])*

☐ From 12 to 36 weeks' gestation, a vitamin K antagonist *is recommended* for this patient on low-dose warfarin therapy *(ESC Guidelines[8])*

Special note:

† Low-dose vitamin K antagonists include warfarin ≤5 mg/d, phenprocoumon ≤3 mg/d, or acenocoumarol ≤2 mg/d

Spontaneous conception of an intrauterine viable singleton occurs by four months after your consultation visit during which you removed the LNG-IUS, in collaboration with her cardiologist, and initiated daily folic acid supplementation.

Pregnancy progresses well on low-dose warfarin maintained in the therapeutic range, without maternal-fetal complications. The patient presents to the obstetric emergency assessment unit in advanced active labor at 31^{+0} weeks' gestation; amniotic membranes are intact and there is no vaginal bleeding. Fetal cardiotocography is normal. A bolus dose of magnesium sulfate is administered for fetal neuroprotection; however, labor progress limits benefit from fetal pulmonary corticosteroids. Timely multidisciplinary experts are notified to assist in maternal-fetal care, as warfarin was therapeutic two days ago.

16. Outline urgent pharmacologic treatment and obstetric management for this parturient on therapeutic warfarin. *(1 point per main bullet)*

5

Pharmacologic treatment:
☐ Vitamin K 1–2 mg orally or intravenously
☐ Four-factor prothrombin complex concentrate to target an INR at 2.0; three-factor prothrombin complex concentrate is feasible if the former is unavailable
 ○ *The time required for administration of fresh frozen plasma makes it an unattractive option and insufficient in this emergent situation*

Obstetric management:
☐ Consider having a senior surgical assistant given the potential for bleeding
☐ Proceed with Cesarean delivery after reversal of anticoagulation, recognizing the risk of intracranial bleeding as fetal INR is incompletely reversed
 ○ *Fetal INR is higher than maternal INR due to immaturity of fetal liver metabolism*
☐ Ensure availability of blood products

SCENARIO C
Bioprosthetic valve
You learn that seven years ago, a bioprosthetic valve replaced her native severe mitral valve stenosis which progressed during the decade after experiencing rheumatic fever as a child. Cardiac surgery, performed in your high-risk hospital center, was uncomplicated; she has not developed complications such as valve thrombosis or arrhythmia warranting anticoagulation. A recent echocardiogram, as requested by her cardiologist, showed a LVEF of 61% without valvular dysfunction. She has no cardiopulmonary symptoms and NYHA is class I. The patient has no drug allergies or medical comorbidities; she practices healthy life habits, including swimming twice weekly. Family history is noncontributory.

17. What is her mWHO risk classification upon which prenatal care and counseling is based?

2

☐ mWHO risk class II *(i.e., bioprosthetic valve)*

18. Highlight <u>differences</u> in preconception counseling and evidence-based antenatal management of this patient relative to one with a metallic heart valve. *(1 point each)*

Max 5

☐ Counsel the patient of the small increased risk of maternal mortality or moderate increase in morbidity, consistent with mWHO class II
☐ Based on an mWHO class II risk classification, cardiology follow-up is recommended at least every trimester *(more frequent visits as individually required)*
☐ With a bioprosthetic valve, event-free pregnancy with a live birth can approximate 80%[§]

☐ Low-dose aspirin is *routinely* recommended during the antenatal period with a known bioprosthetic valve

☐ Anticoagulation is generally not required for bioprosthetic valves; exceptions include concurrent atrial fibrillation or prior bioprosthetic valve thrombosis

☐ *Controversial* effect of pregnancy on the risk of bioprosthetic valve loss; valve degeneration may be attributable to the natural course of the bioprosthesis

Special note:

§ In the ROPAC registry, event-free pregnancy with a live birth was found in 79% of women with bioprosthetic valve [van Hagen IM, Roos-Hesselink JW, Ruys TP, et al. Pregnancy in women with a mechanical heart valve: Data of the European Society of Cardiology Registry of Pregnancy and Cardiac Disease (ROPAC). *Circulation.* 2015;132(2):132–142.]

TOTAL: **100**

CHAPTER 32

Ischemic Heart Disease and Acute Coronary Syndrome in Pregnancy

Hannah Douglas, Amira El-Messidi, and Anita Banerjee

A 38-year-old G7P7 is referred by her primary care provider to your high-risk obstetrics clinic for preconception consultation after having angiography and percutaneous coronary intervention (PCI) in your tertiary center for a non-ST elevation myocardial infarction (NSTEMI) 18 months ago. All her children, the youngest aged four years, were delivered vaginally at term prior to emigrating from Africa.

LEARNING OBJECTIVES

1. Obtain a focused history and identify risk-stratifying tests necessary for preconception counseling of a patient with known ischemic heart disease
2. Appreciate the importance of multidisciplinary collaboration in discussing maternal-fetal outcomes among women with ischemic heart disease or pregnancy-associated acute coronary syndrome
3. Appreciate the availability of invasive and conservative management deemed safe during pregnancy
4. Detail fundamental aspects of intrapartum care for a parturient with recent or prior ischemic heart disease
5. Understand antenatal and postpartum maternal cardiac hemodynamics in relation to the clinical care plan

SUGGESTED READINGS

1. Baris L, Hakeem A, Moe T, et al. Acute coronary syndrome and ischemic heart disease in pregnancy: data from the EURObservational Research Programme – European Society of Cardiology Registry of Pregnancy and Cardiac Disease. *J Am Heart Assoc.* 2020;9(15):e015490.
2. Campbell KH, Tweet MS. Coronary disease in pregnancy: myocardial infarction and spontaneous coronary artery dissection. *Clin Obstet Gynecol.* 2020;63(4):852–867.
3. Cauldwell M, Baris L, Roos-Hesselink JW, et al. Ischaemic heart disease and pregnancy. *Heart.* 2019;105(3):189–195.
4. Chavez P, Wolfe D, Bortnick AE. Management of ischemic heart disease in pregnancy. *Curr Atheroscler Rep.* 2021;23(9):52.
5. Lameijer H, Burchill LJ, Baris L, et al. Pregnancy in women with pre-existent ischaemic heart disease: a systematic review with individualised patient data. *Heart.* 2019;105(11):873–880.
6. Nallapati C, Park K. Ischemic heart disease in pregnancy. *Cardiol Clin.* 2021;39(1):91–108.

7. National Institute for Health and Care Excellence (NICE): Intrapartum care for women with existing medical conditions or obstetric complications and their babies. Evidence reviews for women at high risk of adverse outcomes for themselves and/or their baby because of existing maternal medical conditions, September 2018. Available at www.nice.org.uk/guidance/ng121/documents/evidence-review-14. Accessed July 18, 2021.

8. Park K, Bairey Merz CN, Bello NA, et al. Management of women with acquired cardiovascular disease from pre-conception through pregnancy and postpartum: JACC Focus Seminar 3/5. *J Am Coll Cardiol.* 2021;77(14):1799–1812.

9. Regitz-Zagrosek V, Roos-Hesselink JW, Bauersachs J, et al. 2018 ESC Guidelines for the management of cardiovascular diseases during pregnancy. *Eur Heart J.* 2018;39(34):3165–3241.

10. Tweet MS, Lewey J, Smilowitz NR, et al. Pregnancy-associated myocardial infarction: prevalence, causes, and interventional management. *Circ Cardiovasc Interv.* 2020. https://doi.org/10.1161/CIRCINTERVENTIONS.120.008687

POINTS

1. With respect to her background history of ischemic heart disease, what aspects of a focused history would you want to know? *(1 point each)* — Max 25

Details of the revascularization procedure:
☐ Document the date of intervention
☐ Determine the affected vessel(s)
☐ Ascertain which stent type was used (*i.e.*, drug-eluting or bare metal)
☐ Results of latest cardiac function tests

Current cardiopulmonary symptoms:
☐ Establish the New York Heart Association Classification (NYHA) functional status
☐ Dyspnea at rest or with exertion
☐ Orthopnea
☐ Paroxysmal nocturnal dyspnea
☐ Chest pain or palpitations
☐ Leg edema

Ischemic heart disease-related comorbidities[†] and their current/prior medical treatments:
☐ Antecedent cardiac conditions such as arrhythmia or heart failure prior to the ischemic event
☐ Diabetes mellitus
☐ Hypertension
☐ Hyperlipidemia
☐ Anemia
☐ Antiphospholipid antibody syndrome/thrombophilia(s)
☐ Depression (*post-myocaridal infarction period is an independent risk factor for major depression found in ~18% of patients)*[‡]

Current/prior social features and routine health maintenance:
☐ Cigarette smoking
☐ Alcohol consumption
☐ Substance use, particularly cocaine and/or amphetamines
☐ Current level of physical activity and exercise ability

Obstetric complications associated with future heart disease:
☐ Preeclampsia and other hypertensive conditions of pregnancy
☐ Gestational diabetes mellitus
☐ Obstetric hemorrhage with/without transfusion
☐ Peripartum cardiomyopathy
☐ Postpartum infectious morbidity

Family history:
☐ Cardiac disease or comorbidities (*i.e., diabetes mellitus, hypertension, hyperlipidemia, thromboembolic disease*)
☐ Sudden cardiac death

Special notes:
† As a comorbidity, obesity is an aspect of the physical examination
‡ Refer to Ziegelstein RC. Depression in patients recovering from a myocardial infarction. *JAMA.* 2001;286(13):1621–1627.

You learn that the patient had new-generation drug-eluting stents inserted in the culprit left anterior descending artery, for which she takes dual antiplatelet therapy with aspirin and ticagrelor. The patient remains adherent to treatment, which also includes ramipril, a titrated dose of bisoprolol, atorvastatin for dyslipidemia, and oral supplementation for iron-deficiency anemia. Spironolactone was discontinued nine months after the ischemic cardiac event, as her ejection fraction improved from 38% to 55%, with complementary 12-week cardiac rehabilitation. The patient is free from cardiopulmonary symptoms, although she still leads a sedentary lifestyle and has not managed to lose weight (BMI 32 kg/m²). She quit cigarette smoking after the cardiac event; she does not consume alcohol or use illicit substances. Over the past year, the insulin regimen was adjusted to normalize glycemic control, as shown on recent investigations; she remains free of noncardiac macro/microvascular morbidities associated with type 2 diabetes mellitus.

Her medical history is otherwise only remarkable for pregnancy-associated cardiac comorbidities, namely postpartum hemorrhage requiring blood transfusions at her last three deliveries, gestational diabetes mellitus that persisted after the third pregnancy, postpartum sepsis secondary to endometritis. She did not experience early or late transfusion-related complications. Family history is noncontributory.

With the prospects of pregnancy, her cardiologist recently discontinued the angiotensin-converting enzyme inhibitor (ACE*i*)† and angiotensin receptor blocking agents; ticagrelor has been replaced by clopidogrel 75 mg daily. As the ejection fraction normalized, the patient was reassured that spironolactone is not required. The physician also reassured her regarding the safety and importance of continuing her designated ß-blocker throughout pregnancy as it is not associated with similar fetal morbidity as atenolol.‡

Special notes:
† Refer to Question 5 in Chapter 47 for discussion on obstetric aspects of counseling and management of ACE*i* in pregnancy
‡ Refer to Question 5 in Chapter 48 for discussion on obstetric aspects of atenolol

2. From an obstetric perspective, explain to the patient the importance of having discontinued the aldosterone antagonist prior to conception.   1

☐ Spironolactone is contraindicated in pregnancy due to the risk of feminizing a male fetus

3. Address why clopidogrel was substituted for ticagrelor in anticipation of conception and inform the patient why heparin/low molecular weight heparin (LMWH) cannot replace antiplatelet agents. *(1 point each)*   3

Ticagrelor:
☐ No[†] (or limited[‡]) pregnancy safety data limits its use at this time

Clopidogrel:
☐ Available data has not shown an association with early pregnancy loss, teratogenicity, or adverse fetal outcomes

Heparin/LMWH:
☐ Ineffective in prevention of stent thrombosis

Special notes:
[†] 2018 ESC Guidelines[9]
[‡] Refer to Verbruggen M, Mannaerts D, Muys J, Jacquemyn Y. Use of ticagrelor in human pregnancy, the first experience. *BMJ Case Rep*. 2015;2015:bcr2015212217. Published 2015 Nov 25.

The patient intends to remain adherent to therapy and compliant with multidisciplinary care in future pregnancy; she understands that resumption of smoking may predict the occurrence of new ischemic events during pregnancy *(Suggested Reading 1)* and has improved her dietary regime after recent expert consultation.

You inform her that in the absence of high-quality data regarding the duration of postponing pregnancy after an acute myocardial infarction, policy makers generally advise 12 months, contingent upon comorbidities and cardiac status *(2018 ESC guidelines[9])*.

4. In addition to diabetic control, indicate the recommended investigations related to preconception assessment of the patient's cardiovascular status. *(1 point each)*   Max 4

☐ Full/complete blood count (FBC/CBC)
☐ Brain natriuretic peptide (BNP), N-terminal pro-BNP (NT-pro-BNP)
☐ 12-lead electrocardiogram (ECG)
☐ Echocardiogram
☐ Exercise stress testing (preferable) or dobutamine stress testing[†]

Special note:
[†] Both are also safe during pregnancy provided no obstetric complications prohibit exercise

5. Excluding effects of therapeutic treatments and in collaboration with her cardiologist,   5
    counsel the patient on pregnancy outcomes associated with prior ischemic heart disease.
    (1 point each)

Maternal: *(max 3)*
☐ Recurrent acute coronary syndrome,[†] most of which is in the third trimester or
  postpartum (regardless of prior coronary revascularization)
☐ Progressive left ventricular dysfunction/heart failure/pulmonary edema or
  cardiogenic shock
☐ Ventricular arrhythmias
☐ Hypertensive diseases of pregnancy
☐ Increased risk of Cesarean delivery
☐ Mortality [reported incidences between 0% and 23% *(2018 ESC guidelines[9])*]

Fetal: *(max 2)*
☐ Exposure to radiation associated with maternal angiography (albeit low doses), if needed
☐ Iatrogenic prematurity
☐ IUFD/neonatal mortality *(dependent upon timing of a pregnancy-associated acute
  myocardial infarction and gestational age)*

Special note:
† By definition, acute coronary syndrome includes ST elevation myocardial infarction
  (STEMI), non-ST elevation myocardial infarction (NSTEMI), and unstable angina

---

6. Outline to your trainee principal physiological mechanisms that may contribute to the   Max 2
    heightened risk for acute coronary syndromes during pregnancy and postpartum. *(1 point
    per category/bullet)*

☐ Prothrombotic state of pregnancy[†]
☐ Hemodynamic changes *(i.e., increased cardiac output, stroke volume, heart rate, and
  decreased systemic vascular resistance)*
☐ Neurohormonal changes *(i.e., increased estrogen, progesterone and relaxin levels alter
  arterial architecture)*

Special note:
† Refer to Question 5 in Chapter 52

---

7. Identify this patient's nonmodifiable risk factors for future pregnancy-associated acute   6
    coronary syndrome. *(1 point each)*

☐ Maternal age >35 years
☐ Multiparity
☐ Ethnicity (non-Hispanic black race)
☐ Prior ischemic heart disease
☐ Prior obstetric hemorrhage requiring transfusion
☐ Prior postpartum infection

With adequate glycemic control, normal baseline cardiovascular investigations, and clinical examination, spontaneous conception of an intrauterine viable singleton occurs by four months after your consultation visit. Multidisciplinary collaboration is initiated, and the patient has been provided with emergency contacts to the maternal assessment unit. She remains adherent to the following regimen:

- Low-dose aspirin 81 mg daily
- Clopidogrel 75 mg daily
- Bisoprolol titrated to keep heart rate at 50–60 bpm
- Insulin titrated to glycemic control
- Oral iron and folate-containing prenatal vitamins

8. Indicate potential cardiovascular 'red flag' warning signs warranting early medical care to communicate with the patient at the initial prenatal visit. *(1 point each)*   Max 4

☐ Exertional chest pain
☐ Chest pain at rest *(descriptors include dull, heavy, tight, sharp, stabbing, squeezing, gripping)*
☐ Need for rescue sublingual nitrate
☐ New or worsening dyspnea
☐ New or worsening palpitations
☐ Acute bilateral lower extremity edema

Maternal-fetal aspects of prenatal care remain unremarkable until 35^{+4} weeks' gestation when the patient presents to the obstetrics emergency assessment unit with progressively increasing retrosternal chest pain at rest over the past three hours, accompanied by new-onset dyspepsia and nausea. She has no respiratory symptoms above mild baseline gestational dyspnea. There are no obstetric complaints; fetal heart tracing on cardiotocography is normal at presentation. As you are on obstetrics call duty at the tertiary center, you recall that the patient had resumed smoking cigarettes mid-gestation upon the sudden cardiac death of her healthy 43-year-old brother.

You initiate a physical examination and preliminary investigations while awaiting the cardiologist's assistance in the care of this patient.

9. Verbalize essentials of the focused <u>cardiovascular</u> examination based on her presenting complaints. *(1 point each)*

Max 12

General appearance:
☐ Beware of patient's preferred positioning *(e.g., leaning forward, tugging at location of pain)*
☐ Diaphoresis
☐ Cyanosis

Vital signs:
☐ Blood pressure in both arms
☐ Pulse rate and rhythm
☐ Oxygen saturation
☐ Respiratory rate
☐ Temperature

Cardiopulmonary assessment:
☐ Cardiac heart sounds and presence of a murmur
☐ Assess for jugular venous distension
☐ Bilateral air entry on auscultation of both lung fields
☐ Peripheral pulses
☐ Differential swelling of the lower extremities or pitting edema

The patient is conversant yet appears diaphoretic, grasping her mid-chest and leaning slightly forward in apparent pain. During the conversation, you note absence of central or peripheral cyanosis. Vital signs include blood pressure of 148/92 mmHg, and oxygen saturation of 93% on room air, for which oxygen supplementation by nasal prongs is initiated. Acknowledging your limited expertise in cardiac auscultation, you await the cardiologist and ECG's confirmation of your possible findings on examination. There is no appreciable distal edema. Abdominal-fundal assessment is unremarkable.

SCENARIO A

ST-elevation myocardial infarction (STEMI)

With assistance of the cardiologist (or obstetric anesthesiologist), you learn that immediate ECG shows a new left bundle branch block with markedly increased cardiac troponins. The cardiologist indicates that in addition to antihypertensive treatment to maintain blood pressure <130/80–85 mmHg, opiate analgesia, anti-emetic therapy, and oxygen supplementation, timely reperfusion therapy to the occluded artery is required.

You take note to later alert your obstetric trainee that troponins (troponin-T and troponin-I) are preferable to creatine kinase MB fraction as cardiac biomarkers in pregnancy.

10. Among medical reperfusion with thrombolysis versus coronary angiography with percutaneous coronary intervention (PCI), explain the rationale for the preferred treatment in pregnancy. *(1 point each)*

Max 2

PCI is preferred in pregnancy over thrombolysis:
☐ Risk of maternal-fetal hemorrhage with thrombolysis, particularly in peripartum
☐ Thrombolysis may worsen coronary artery dissection, which accounts for a significant portion of acute coronary syndrome in pregnancy
☐ Thrombolysis could be obviated by normal coronary arteries on angiography

11. Counsel the patient on fetal risks with PCI and outline important obstetric considerations to discuss with the cardiologist with regard to the procedure at this gestational age. *(1 point per main bullet)*

4

Fetal risks with PCI:
☐ Estimated fetal radiation exposure can be as low as <1 mGy with radiation dose reduction strategies, which is far below the 50 mGy (5 rad) threshold associated with fetal radiation complications

Procedure-related obstetric considerations: *(max 3)*
☐ Coordinate a standby obstetric team for possible emergency resuscitative Cesarean delivery in the event of maternal decompensation
   ○ *Individualized considerations for fetal pulmonary corticosteroids*
☐ Maintain continuous electronic fetal heart monitoring during the procedure
☐ Use a preferential radial approach arterial access to minimize risks of bleeding with femoral puncture proximal to a gravid uterus
☐ Position the patient in the left lateral decubitus position/left uterine displacement
☐ Reduce fluoroscopic frame rate to minimize fetal radiation exposure
☐ Avoid steep angulated views to minimize fetal radiation exposure
☐ Keep the intensifier as close as possible to the patient to minimize fetal radiation exposure
☐ Avoid routine abdominal shielding in imaging modalities where ionizing radiation does not directly expose the fetus because (1) most of the fetal dose results from internal (rather than external) scatter, and (2) automatic control can cause increased dose exposure if the shield is inadvertently in the field of view during the scan. Abdominal shielding may be considered on a case by case basis if it offers patient reassurance after appropriate counseling. (Refer to the Special Notes section of Question 3 in Chapter 73)

Percutaneous coronary angiography is uncomplicated, and a bare-metal stent is implanted with the purpose of reducing the duration of anticoagulation in view of upcoming delivery. Fetal well-being was maintained.

Left ventricular function is preserved, without ongoing cardiac ischemic events.

SCENARIO B

This is a continuation of the case scenario after the clinical description associated with Question 9

Unstable Angina

You confirm absence of pathologic findings on ECG, beyond pregnancy-associated physiological changes. Troponin levels are normal. Remaining comprehensive investigations are not suggestive of a complementary diagnosis and the cardiologist confirms the patient presented with symptoms consistent with cardiac ischemia.

---

12. Review the normal changes potentially seen on resting ECG in pregnancy. *(1 point each)*   Max 4

- ☐ Sinus tachycardia
- ☐ Supraventricular and ventricular ectopic beats
- ☐ 15° left axis deviation
- ☐ T-wave inversion in leads II and aVF
- ☐ Small nonpathological Q-wave
- ☐ Transient nonspecific ST-depression at Cesarean section under regional anesthesia

---

13. Based on the most consistent cardiac diagnosis, outline principal <u>medical</u> management for this pregnant patient. *(1 point each)*   7

Unstable angina:
- ☐ Admission to a unit with cardiac monitoring in the tertiary center
- ☐ Maintain maternal oxygenation ≥95% to improve both maternal cardiac and uteroplacental oxygenation
- ☐ Initiate a short course of therapeutic LMWH
- ☐ Provide nitrate antianginal agent *(reassuring the patient of its safety in pregnancy)*
- ☐ Administer opiate analgesic *(e.g., morphine)*
- ☐ Continuation of low-dose aspirin
- ☐ Continuation of clopidogrel 75 mg daily

SCENARIO C

This is a continuation of the clinical scenario after either scenario A or B

14. With multidisciplinary collaboration, discuss particularities related to the patient's delivery after recent myocardial infarction. *(1 point each)*

Max 10

- ☐ Optimize control of maternal anemia prior to delivery, as this may otherwise exacerbate underlying ischemia
- ☐ Aim to defer delivery for at least two weeks, if possible, to allow for myocardial healing and reduce risks of delivery complications associated with an acute myocardial infarction
- ☐ Withhold clopidogrel five to seven days prior to planned delivery and/or therapeutic heparin for 24 hours prior to induction of labor
- ☐ Plan mode of delivery based on obstetric indications *(i.e., aim for vaginal delivery)*
- ☐ Arrange for delivery in a setting with simultaneous continuous maternal-fetal cardiac monitoring and postpartum maternal observation for 24–48 hours prior to transfer to an obstetric unit
- ☐ Provide supplemental oxygenation to minimize cardiac workload during labor and delivery
- ☐ Early initiation of epidural analgesia to minimize pain-induced tachycardia, provided the patient has appropriately discontinued the P2Y12 inhibitor *(i.e., her clopidogrel)*
  - ○ *Avoid single-bolus epidural due to risk of profound hypotension*
- ☐ Maintain a left lateral decubitus position to improve cardiac output
- ☐ Consideration for an arterial line for invasive blood pressure monitoring
- ☐ Maintain tight blood pressure control and continue the ß-blocker agent to prevent maternal tachycardia
- ☐ Close monitoring of fluid balance *(due to risk of pulmonary edema)*
- ☐ Allow passive descent of the fetal head in the second stage
- ☐ Consideration for instrumental delivery to minimize maternal pushing
- ☐ Plan active management of the third stage of labor to minimize blood loss, preferably by a slow oxytocin infusion rather than a bolus dose *(risk of hypotension and ventricular arrhythmia)*; misoprostol can be used as a second-line agent in the absence of acute thrombosis
- ☐ In the event of postpartum hemorrhage, avoid carboprost *(risk of secondary hypertension)* and ergonovine *(risk of coronary arterial spasm)*

15. Highlight to your obstetric trainee the cardiovascular conditions warranting consideration for Cesarean delivery. *(1 point each)*

Max 3

- ☐ Significant pulmonary hypertension
- ☐ Fixed obstructive left-sided valvular lesions *(e.g., severe aortic stenosis)*
- ☐ Clinically significant aortopathies *(e.g., Marfan syndrome or other collagen vascular disorders)*
- ☐ Acute heart failure

Consequent to known type 2 diabetes mellitus as well as anticoagulant treatments for cardiac care, induction of labor is arranged at 38–39 weeks' gestation. Being grand-multiparous, labor and vaginal delivery are precipitous with diligent care provided to avoid postpartum hemorrhage. Maternal hemodynamic status is being closely monitored in the cardiac care unit during the early postpartum period.

16. With reference to gestational physiology, discuss the importance of maintaining diligent maternal hemodynamic monitoring in the early postpartum period for this patient with heart disease. *(1 point each)*

Max 3

☐ Cardiac output increases up to ~50%–80% in the early postpartum period
☐ Significant physiological intravascular-extravascular fluid redistribution
☐ Increased venous return to the heart occurs after decompression of the gravid uterus
☐ Blood loss at delivery can exacerbate cardiac ischemia

Special note:
Maternal echocardiography may be required prior to delivery discharge

17. Identify important postpartum considerations to discuss, either prior to discharge or at the routine postpartum visit in relation to ischemic heart disease. *(1 point each)*

5

General maternal-fetal well-being: *(max 3)*
☐ Screen for postpartum depression and continue to offer psychosocial support services
☐ Ensure arrangements are made for maternal outpatient follow-up with the necessary medical experts
☐ Encourage a healthy lifestyle to mitigate long-term cardiovascular risk factors
☐ Discuss that breastfeeding is contraindicated while taking antiplatelet agents other than low-dose aspirin due to lack of data *(2018 ESC Guidelines[9])*

Contraceptive recommendations: *(max 2)*
☐ No restrictions on use of barrier methods although they are the least effective agents, particularly as unintended pregnancy may pose increased health risks
☐ Review with the patient that estrogen-containing contraceptives are contraindicated due to increased risk of thrombosis *(UK and US-MEC, category 4)[†]*
☐ Use of copper intrauterine device for this patient with current and prior ischemic heart disease appears safest among options for hormonal and intrauterine contraception *(UK and US-MEC, category 1)[†]*
☐ Long-term use of progesterone contraceptive agents (*i.e.*, levonorgesterol intrauterine system, DMPA, progestin implants, and progestin-oral contraceptives) may be associated with theoretical or proven risk among women with current/prior ischemic heart disease *(UK and US-MEC, category 3)[†]*

Special note:
[†] UK and US Medical Eligibility Criteria (MEC) for Contraceptive Use, 2016; UK-MEC amended September 2019, US-MEC updated 2020

TOTAL: 100

CHAPTER 33

Pulmonary Hypertension in Pregnancy

Marwa Salman, Amira El-Messidi, and Anita Banerjee

A 28-year-old primigravida at 27 weeks' gestation is referred by her primary care provider to your tertiary center's high-risk obstetrics unit with a four-week history of worsening exertional dyspnea, marked fatigue with limited daily activities, and a recent syncopal episode, witnessed by her husband. She describes palpitations immediately prior to this brief event. She is asymptomatic at rest and has not experienced chest pain. Her medical history appears non-contributory, and although she practices healthy social habits, she has long-standing exercise intolerance in the non pregnant state with breathlessness after running a few meters.

Prepregnancy body mass index (BMI) was 22 kg/m²; routine first- and second-trimester maternal laboratory investigations, fetal aneuploidy screening, and morphology survey of the female fetus were unremarkable. The patient does not have obstetric complaints.

LEARNING OBJECTIVES

1. Elicit clinical features on medical history most focused to determining the cause of pulmonary hypertension, while recognizing the importance of genetic counseling for heritable pulmonary arterial hypertension
2. Appreciate the importance of multidisciplinary collaboration for diagnostic evaluation and treatment of pulmonary hypertension first presenting in pregnancy
3. Understand the effects of pregnancy on pulmonary hypertension, including pathophysiological bases for increased maternal mortality
4. Discuss the impact of pulmonary hypertension on maternal-fetal outcomes, and arrange antenatal, intrapartum, and postpartum management, focusing on obstetric aspects of care

SUGGESTED READINGS

1. American College of Obstetricians and Gynecologists' Presidential Task Force on Pregnancy and Heart Disease and Committee on Practice Bulletins—Obstetrics. ACOG Practice Bulletin No. 212: Pregnancy and heart disease. *Obstet Gynecol.* 2019;133(5):e320–e356.
2. Anjum H, Surani S. Pulmonary hypertension in pregnancy: a review. *Medicina (Kaunas).* 2021;57(3):259.

3. Aryal SR, Moussa H, Sinkey R, et al. Management of reproductive health in patients with pulmonary hypertension. *Am J Obstet Gynecol MFM.* 2020;2(2):100087.

4. Ballard W 3rd, Dixon B, McEvoy CA, et al. Pulmonary arterial hypertension in pregnancy. *Cardiol Clin.* 2021;39(1):109–118.

5. Galiè N, Humbert M, Vachiery JL, et al. 2015 ESC/ERS guidelines for the diagnosis and treatment of pulmonary hypertension. *Rev Esp Cardiol (Engl Ed).* 2016;69(2):177.

6. Kiely DG, Condliffe R, Wilson VJ, et al. Pregnancy and pulmonary hypertension: a practical approach to management. *Obstet Med.* 2013;6(4):144–154.

7. Low TT, Guron N, Ducas R, et al. Pulmonary arterial hypertension in pregnancy-a systematic review of outcomes in the modern era. *Pulm Circ.* 2021;11(2):20458940211013671.

8. Martin SR, Edwards A. Pulmonary hypertension and pregnancy. *Obstet Gynecol.* 2019;134(5):974–987. [Correction in *Obstet Gynecol.* 2020 Apr;135(4):978]

9. Običan SG, Cleary KL. Pulmonary arterial hypertension in pregnancy. *Semin Perinatol.* 2014;38(5):289–294.

10. Regitz-Zagrosek V, Roos-Hesselink JW, Bauersachs J, et al. 2018 ESC Guidelines for the management of cardiovascular diseases during pregnancy. *Eur Heart J.* 2018;39(34): 3165–3241.

POINTS

1. State the essentials of your focused physical examination based on her presenting complaints. *(1 point each)*   15

General appearance:
☐ Apparent distress, including inability to provide complete sentences *(i.e., work of breathing)*
☐ Cyanosis

Vital signs:
☐ Blood pressure
☐ Respiratory rate
☐ Pulse rate and rhythm
☐ Oxygen saturation
☐ Temperature

Cardiopulmonary assessment:
☐ Assess for jugular venous distension
☐ Cardiac heart sounds and presence of a murmur
☐ Bilateral air entry on auscultation of both lung fields
☐ Parasternal heave

Abdominal assessment:
☐ Evaluation of fetal heart rate and rhythm
☐ Fundal height measurement
☐ Right upper quadrant tenderness *(hepatic congestion)* or hepatomegaly *(may be masked by gravid uterus)*

Extremities assessment:
☐ Pitting edema

The patient converses well at rest. She is normotensive and afebrile with a regular pulse rate at 105 beats/min, respiratory rate at 20 breaths/min, and oxygen saturation at 97% on room air. You suspect a loud pulmonary component of the second heart sound, a right ventricular heave, and find obvious jugular venous distension at 8 cm above the sternal angle *(normal <4 cm)*. Bi-basal crepitations are evident on lung fields. Fetal viability is ascertained and fundal height is appropriate; there are no other significant findings on abdominal examination. Bilateral pitting edema in the distal extremities compounds gestational fluid retention.

You notify an obstetric physician (internist) who will promptly attend to assist in the care of this patient.

2. With interdisciplinary collaboration, outline initial maternal non laboratory investigations in the diagnostic evaluation of this patient. *(1 point each)*   3

☐ Transthoracic echocardiography (TTE)
☐ Electrocardiogram (ECG)
☐ Computed tomographic pulmonary angiogram

You learn that the ECG shows evidence of right axis deviation with a strain pattern and right ventricular hypertrophy. With appropriate counseling and maternal consent, a computed tomographic pulmonary angiogram is performed,[†] revealing prominent pulmonary vasculature without evidence of pulmonary emboli.

While the patient is having a TTE, you explain to your obstetric trainee that clinical symptomatology and findings on examination raise suspicion for pulmonary hypertension, where TTE is the screening modality of choice, being non-invasive, readily available, and free of radiation exposure. Significant findings on TTE reveal a left ventricular ejection fraction of 61%, right ventricular dilatation, pulmonary artery systolic pressure at 89 mmHg *(normal ≤40 mmHg)*, and increased peak tricuspid regurgitant jet velocity; there is no evidence of right ventricular failure or left-sided heart disease.

Pregnancy will be managed according to the most probable diagnosis, with definitive gold-standard right heart catheterization planned for approximately four months postpartum.

Special note:
† Refer to Question 25 in Chapter 52 for maternal-fetal aspects to address in counseling for computed tomographic pulmonary angiogram

3. What is her pulmonary hypertension functional class according to the World Health Organization (WHO) classification?   2

☐ Class III[†]

Special note:
† No symptoms at rest, but less than ordinary activity causes undue dyspnea or fatigue, chest pain or near syncope *(Suggested Reading 3)*

4. Elicit features on medical history most focused to determining the etiology of pulmonary hypertension. *(1 point each)*   Max 8

Screening for etiology of pulmonary hypertension:
- ☐ HIV status
- ☐ Use of drugs or exposure to toxins *(e.g., appetite suppressants, chronic cocaine, or amphetamines)*
- ☐ Known chronic hemolytic anemia
- ☐ Connective tissue diseases *(e.g., systemic lupus erythematosus or scleroderma)*
- ☐ Liver disease/history of portal hypertension
- ☐ Congenital heart disease *(e.g., left-to-right shunt-associated conditions including ventricular septal defect, atrial septal defect, or patent ductus arteriosus)*
- ☐ Chronic lung disease (obstructive or restrictive)
- ☐ History of sleep disordered breathing *(i.e., hypoxia)*
- ☐ Prior pulmonary emboli
- ☐ Assess current/prior geographic habitat *(i.e., hypoxia associated with high altitudes)*
- ☐ Exposure to contaminated water, depending on geographic location *(i.e., schistosomiasis)*[†]
- ☐ Family history of pulmonary hypertension

Special note:
[†] Although schistosomiasis appears to be the most common cause of pulmonary arterial hypertension worldwide, most cases are either idiopathic or heritable in regions of the world without endemic schistosomiasis.

While her personal medical history is noncontributory, the patient now recalls two family members with pulmonary hypertension, for which evaluation by a genetic expert is planned.

You teach your obstetric trainee that pregnancy poses hemodynamic challenges in a patient with pulmonary hypertension, raising maternal-fetal risks of adverse outcomes.

5. Pending consultation, address the patient's inquiry regarding genetic predisposition and inheritance of heritable pulmonary arterial hypertension. *(1 point each)*   Max 2

- ☐ Pulmonary arterial hypertension can have autosomal dominant inheritance with variable penetrance
- ☐ Testing for gene mutation(s) may be considered, especially *BMPR2*,[†] being most common and with greater penetrance in women
- ☐ Detection of a genetic mutation may have future implications for the expected female fetus

Special note:
[†] Other mutations associated with heritable pulmonary arterial hypertension include *CAV1*, *KCNK3*, and *EIF2AK4*

6. In collaboration with experts involved in her medical care, counsel the patient on how pregnancy may affect pulmonary hypertension. *(1 point per main bullet)*   5

- ☐ High risk of maternal mortality (20%–56%), with the greatest risk periods being the puerperium and early postpartum
- ☐ Right ventricular failure
- ☐ Eisenmenger syndrome[†]
- ☐ Cardiac arrhythmias
- ☐ Iron-deficiency anemia
  - ○ *Common in ~50% of patients with pulmonary arterial hypertension, although no guidelines exist for threshold warranting treatment among obstetric patients with pulmonary hypertension*

Special notes:
(a) † Thrombocytopenia may be seen with Eisenmenger syndrome.
(b) There is no definitive data to indicate the impact of pregnancy on the natural history and long-term prognosis of disease

7. Identify the three most common causes of maternal mortality associated with pulmonary hypertension. *(1 point each)*   3

- ☐ Pulmonary hypertensive crisis
- ☐ Pulmonary thrombosis
- ☐ Refractory right heart failure

The medical team explains to the patient that where pulmonary hypertension is diagnosed at a previable gestational age, termination of pregnancy would be advocated regardless of disease status due to the high risk of maternal mortality and difficulties in identifying *'lower-risk'* pregnancies. However, with diagnosis now at 27 weeks' gestation, maternal prognosis would not be improved by imminent delivery, unless clinically indicated.

The patient understands that detailed contraceptive counseling will be provided in later gestation and/or postpartum.

8. Explain to your obstetric trainee the physiological changes related to pregnancy that interplay in the heightened risk of maternal mortality with pulmonary hypertension. *(1 point each)*

Max 6

Antepartum:
- ☐ Cardiac output usually peaks at ~28 weeks' gestation (in relation to increased heart rate and stroke volume); patients with pulmonary hypertension have reduced ability to accommodate this increase given high right ventricular afterload
- ☐ Physiologic increase in stroke volume is compromised by high right ventricular afterload
- ☐ Increased blood volume up to 50%, peaking at ~32 weeks' gestation
- ☐ Physiologic pulmonary vasodilation and decreased pulmonary vascular resistance is compromised with pulmonary hypertension

Intrapartum and/or postpartum:
- ☐ Physiologic rapid rise in cardiac output intrapartum and immediately postpartum risks rapid decompensation of the right heart
- ☐ Decreased venous return associated with Valsalva maneuver compromises right heart filling which is needed to overcome high pulmonary resistance
- ☐ Physiologic rapid increases in pulmonary vasoconstriction that occur postpartum further contributes to high risk of mortality during this period
- ☐ Major fluid shifts postpartum including autotransfusion and decompression of the arterial-venous vasculature increase right atrial pressure, and may adversely affect right ventricular function

All stages of pregnancy:
- ☐ Risk of venous thromboembolic phenomena *(i.e. pulmonary emboli)*

9. Excluding effects of pharmaceuticals, counsel the patient on the potential impact of pulmonary hypertension on her pregnancy. *(1 point each)*

Max 7

Maternal:
- ☐ Low threshold for hospitalization
- ☐ Increased frequency of clinical visits and serial investigations
- ☐ Risk of venous thromboembolic phenomena *(pulmonary emboli)*
- ☐ Preterm delivery *(iatrogenic or spontaneous)*
- ☐ Greater risk of Caesarean section or assisted vaginal delivery
- ☐ Possible psychosocial stressors associated with disease and/or complications

Fetal-neonatal:
- ☐ Fetal growth restriction or low neonatal birthweight *(i.e., <2500 g)*
- ☐ Intrauterine fetal death (IUFD)
- ☐ Neonatal mortality
- ☐ Offspring risk of inheritance of the heritable form of pulmonary arterial hypertension, *if present*

In collaboration with medical experts, the patient is informed that in the absence of a standardized approach by clinical practice guidelines for obstetric care with pulmonary hypertension, prenatal management is largely individualized, based on case series and reviews. She understands the importance of continued multidisciplinary care at your center where access to advanced cardio-pulmonary support measures is available.

10. Outline <u>supportive and conventional therapies</u> that may be advocated in this obstetric patient with pulmonary hypertension. *(1 point per main bullet; max points indicated per section)*

8

Supportive: *(max 4)*
- ☐ Completion of immunizations *(e.g., tetanus, influenza, pneumococcus)*
- ☐ Provide supplemental oxygen if saturation is <91%[§] or pO_2 is <60 mmHg *(Suggested Reading 8)*
- ☐ Encourage rest periods and avoidance of excessive physical activity which cause symptoms
- ☐ Avoid vasovagal triggers in pregnancy *(i.e., right ventricular function is preload dependent to overcome increased pulmonary vascular resistance)*
- ☐ Avoid air-travel
- ☐ Control salt and fluid intake
- ☐ Supervised exercise guidance
- ☐ Psychosocial support services

Conventional:[‡] *(4)*
- ☐ Correction of iron-deficiency anemia
- ☐ Consideration for antepartum and postpartum anticoagulation[†]
  - ○ *Anticoagulation has a role to play in some, though not all, forms of pulmonary hypertension; consideration is warranted for heritable, idiopathic, and appetite-suppressant pulmonary arterial hypertension, as well as chronic thromboembolic disease (Suggested Reading 5)*
- ☐ Calcium channel blockers for vasodilation of the pulmonary vasculature
  - ○ *e.g., long-acting nifedipine, diltiazem, or amlodipine*
  - ○ *Avoid verapamil due to potential negative inotropic effect*
- ☐ Diuretic treatment for volume overload or right heart failure
  - ○ *Loop diuretics are preferred to thiazides due to risk of neonatal hemorrhagic complications and hyponatremia among neonates exposed to thiazides*

Special notes:
§ Target level of ideal oxygen saturation among pregnant women with pulmonary hypertension is uncertain, with supplementation advised to maintain a target of at least 90% based on expert opinion
† Anticoagulation may not be advocated with onset of Eisenmenger syndrome due to associated risk of thrombocytopenia
‡ Initiation of low-dose aspirin prophylaxis for preeclampsia would be considered in earlier gestation

11. With reference to disease pathogenesis, outline the two accepted drug classifications for targeted therapy in pregnancy with pulmonary arterial hypertension. *(1 point per main bullet)*

☐ Prostaglandin I_2 (PGI_2) via inhibition of smooth muscle proliferation and enhanced vasodilation
  ○ *e.g., epoprostenol, iloprost*
☐ Phosphodiesterase-5-inhibitors via enhanced vasodilatory effect of nitric oxide
  ○ *e.g., sildenafil*

Special note:
Endothelin receptor antagonists (*e.g., bosentan*) and soluble guanylate cyclase stimulators (*e.g., riociguat*), are contraindicated for use in pregnancy

2

Given a new gestational diagnosis of pulmonary hypertension with functional class III, the treating team opts to commence targeted treatment with nebulized iloprost and oral sildenafil, in addition to conventional and supportive therapies arranged.

As the patient is in the late second trimester, multidisciplinary antenatal visits are planned every one to two weeks until delivery.

12. Further to continued antenatal assessment of clinical history and physical examinations, indicate serial <u>investigations</u> focused on prenatal care and follow-up of pulmonary hypertension. *(1 point each)*

Max 8

Maternal:

Serum tests:
☐ CBC/FBC
☐ Iron studies
☐ Brain natriuretic peptide (BNP)
☐ Troponin levels
☐ Creatinine
☐ Hepatic transaminases and function tests

Imaging/other tests:
☐ Electrocardiogram (ECG)
☐ Pulmonary function tests
☐ Transthoracic echocardiogram (TTE)
☐ Exercise testing with incremental shuttle walking test or six-minute walk test
☐ Consideration for outpatient monitoring of blood pressure and pulse oximetry

Fetal:
☐ At least monthly sonographic surveillance for growth biometry; individualized additional surveillance by nonstress tests and/or third-trimester biophysical profile

As optimal timing and mode of delivery with pulmonary hypertension remains uncertain and largely individualized, an interdisciplinary meeting is arranged to plan accordingly. You mention that expert recommendations suggest that vaginal delivery appears to be equally safe with appropriate obstetric and anesthetic expertise, without specific recommendations on optimal timing of delivery with or without right ventricular failure *(Suggested Reading 10)*.

Elective hospitalisation is planned 24–48 hours prior to delivery to allow for detailed assessment of maternal-fetal status and preparation of noninvasive and invasive measures for continuous blood pressure and hemodynamic monitoring. The team similarly concurs that prophylactic antibiotics for cardiac prophylaxis is not warranted, with routine antibiotic prophylaxis for group B streptococcus (GBS) positivity, as clinically indicated. Consideration for maternal administration of fetal pulmonary corticosteroids will similarly follow standard indications.

13. Provide an accepted gestational window for delivery with known pulmonary hypertension.	1

- ☐ Recommendations range from 32 to 37 weeks' gestation
  - ○ *Delivery in the later window (i.e., 34–37 weeks) is accepted for stable patients, without further elevations in pulmonary pressures*

14. Outline significant factors that would be taken into consideration during decision-making for mode of delivery. *(1 point each)*	Max 5

- ☐ Obstetric history and likelihood of vaginal delivery
- ☐ WHO functional class
- ☐ Classification of pulmonary hypertension
- ☐ Hemodynamic indices
- ☐ Response to drug therapies
- ☐ Fetal growth and well-being
- ☐ Timely availability of extended multiprofessional team members and necessary equipment at delivery in case of urgent intrapartum Cesarean section

15. Provide essential elements of the <u>obstetric</u> care focused on management of maternal disease with anticipated <u>vaginal delivery</u>. *(1 point per main bullet)*	Max 7

- ☐ Withhold low molecular weight heparin (LMWH) prophylaxis, as required prior to cervical ripening and induction of labor
- ☐ Labor in the left lateral decubitus position to avoid decreased venous return from aortocaval compression
- ☐ Close monitoring of maternal fluid balance
- ☐ Continuous maternal pulse oximetry and blood pressure monitoring
- ☐ Continuous electronic fetal monitoring
- ☐ Early initiation of regional anesthesia, preferably with slow-dose epidural or combined spinal-epidural
  - ○ *Avoid single-bolus epidural due to risk of profound hypotension*

☐ Delay pushing in the second stage of labor
☐ Consideration for instrumental vaginal delivery *(where no contraindications exist)*
☐ Avoid postpartum bolus of oxytocin due to an associated increase in pulmonary vascular resistance and tachycardia
☐ Avoid use of methylergometrine (methylergonovine) due to an associated increase in vasoconstriction and hypertension

16. Discuss the arguments in favor of <u>elective Caesarean delivery</u> with pulmonary hypertension. *(1 point each)*   Max 5

☐ Elective preparation of advanced surgical and medical teams, including preparation for extracorporeal membrane oxygenation (ECMO), if required
☐ With patient consent, tubal sterilization may be performed simultaneously as future pregnancy is not recommended
☐ Decreased risks of autotransfusion associated with uterine contractions and Valsalva maneuver
☐ Surgical planning to minimize operative blood loss
☐ Potential for use of bimanual compression and suture compression of the uterus, as appropriate, to minimize use of vasoactive agents
☐ Avoidance of increased risks of maternal morbidity and possible mortality with intrapartum emergent Caesarean delivery, particularly if general anesthesia is necessary

An elective Caesarean delivery is performed at 36 weeks' gestation with combined spinal-epidural analgesia. Despite comprehensive counseling, the patient declined tubal sterilization. Meticulous hemostasis is ensured, nonpharmaceutical maneuvers employed to promote uterine tone after delivery, and judicious use of oxytocin infusion assured. Consistent with antenatal sonographic assessments, the female newborn is on the 10th percentile of weight for gestational age.

Extended maternal admission in the intensive care setting is planned for *at least* 72 hours (range: three to seven days) to allow for close monitoring when fluid shifts and hormonal changes pose highest risk for heart failure and maternal mortality. Subsequently, continued hospitalization is planned for several days.

17. Discuss <u>postpartum</u> considerations most specific to a patient with pulmonary hypertension. *(1 point per main bullet)*   Max 8

Care for pulmonary hypertension and related morbidities:
☐ With expert collaboration and continued close surveillance, encourage maternal continuation of pharmaceutical treatment for pulmonary hypertension
☐ Continue prophylactic thromboprophylaxis for six to eight weeks postpartum, particularly given Caesarean delivery
☐ Continue dietary sodium restriction and controlled fluid intake

Contraception:

☐ Category 1 (no restrictions) for progestin-only oral contraception, implants, and depot medroxyprogesterone acetate (DMPA) injections[†]
   ○ *Beware of decreased patient adherence to oral progestin agents*
   ○ *Avoid use of bosentan (endothelin receptor antagonist) with oral progesterone and implants due to decreased serum progestin concentrations*

☐ Although both the levonorgesterol intrauterine system and copper intrauterine device are safe contraceptive methods among women with pulmonary hypertension (US-MEC category 1),[†] insertion process may be associated with a vasovagal reaction (UK-MEC category 2)[†]
   ○ *Consideration for insertion of intrauterine contraceptives in a hospital setting (Suggested Reading 6)*

☐ Use of combined hormonal contraception is contraindicated[†]

☐ Use of barrier methods as solitary contraceptives is not advised for patients with pulmonary hypertension

Breastfeeding:

☐ Controversial, and dependent on maternal cardiac status and chosen treatment agents; *2018 ESC Guidelines*[10]
   ○ *Informed, case-based decision-making is required*

Psychosocial wellness:

☐ Screen for postpartum depression and continue to offer psychosocial support services

Special note:

† Indicated recommendations are based on UK and US Medical Eligibility Criteria (MEC) for Contraceptive Use, 2016; UK-MEC amended September 2019, US-MEC updated 2020

TOTAL: **95**

CHAPTER 34

Peripartum Cardiomyopathy

Isabelle Malhamé and Amira El-Messidi

During your call duty, a 38-year-old G5P4 with a spontaneous dichorionic pregnancy presents to the obstetric emergency assessment unit of your tertiary center at 37^{+5} weeks' gestation with dyspnea and noticeable bilateral leg edema. She has no obstetric complaints. Your colleague follows her prenatal care. Routine prenatal laboratory investigations, aneuploidy screening, fetal morphology surveys, and serial sonograms have all been unremarkable. She had four uncomplicated pregnancies and term vaginal deliveries in your hospital center.

LEARNING OBJECTIVES

1. Take a focused history, and verbalize essentials of a physical examination for a prenatal patient with cardiopulmonary symptoms
2. Initiate investigations for heart failure in pregnancy, and establish a diagnosis of peripartum cardiomyopathy (PPCM)
3. Demonstrate the ability to plan and manage the antepartum, intrapartum, and postpartum care of a patient with PPCM, recognizing the importance of a multidisciplinary team
4. Provide counseling on contraceptive options and future pregnancy risks in postpartum women with PPCM

SUGGESTED READINGS

1. Bauersachs J, Arrigo M, Hilfiker-Kleiner D, et al. Current management of patients with severe acute peripartum cardiomyopathy: practical guidance from the Heart Failure Association of the European Society of Cardiology Study Group on peripartum cardiomyopathy. *Eur J Heart Fail.* 2016 Sep;18(9):1096–105.
2. Bauersachs J, König T, van der Meer P, et al. Pathophysiology, diagnosis and management of peripartum cardiomyopathy: a position statement from the Heart Failure Association of the European Society of Cardiology Study Group on peripartum cardiomyopathy. *Eur J Heart Fail.* 2019 Jul;21(7):827–843.
3. Bozkurt B, Colvin M, Cook J, et al. Current diagnostic and treatment strategies for specific dilated cardiomyopathies: a scientific statement from the American Heart Association. *Circulation.* 2016 Dec 6;134(23): e579–e646.
4. Cunningham FG, Byrne JJ, Nelson DB. Peripartum cardiomyopathy. *Obstet Gynecol.* 2019 Jan;133(1):167–179.

5. Davis MB, Arany Z, McNamara DM, et al. Peripartum cardiomyopathy: JACC state-of-the-art review. *J Am Coll Cardiol.* 2020 Jan 21;75(2):207–221.
6. Haghikia A, Schwab J, Vogel-Claussen J, et al. Bromocriptine treatment in patients with peripartum cardiomyopathy and right ventricular dysfunction. *Clin Res Cardiol.* 2019 Mar;108(3):290–297.
7. Honigberg MC, Givertz MM. Peripartum cardiomyopathy. *BMJ.* 2019 Jan 30; 364:k5287.
8. Koczo A, Marino A, Jeyabalan A, et al. Breastfeeding, cellular immune activation, and myocardial recovery in peripartum cardiomyopathy. *JACC Basic Transl Sci.* 2019 Jun 24;4(3):291–300.
9. Regitz-Zagrosek V, Roos-Hesselink JW, Bauersachs J, et al. 2018 ESC Guidelines for the management of cardiovascular diseases during pregnancy. *Eur Heart J.* 2018; 39(34):3165–3241.
10. Schaufelberger M. Cardiomyopathy and pregnancy. *Heart.* 2019 Oct;105(20):1543–1551.

POINTS

1. What aspects of a focused history would you want to know? *(1 point each)*   Max 15

Cardiorespiratory symptoms or manifestations:
- ☐ Duration of dyspnea and leg edema
- ☐ Establish whether dyspnea occurs at rest or with exertion
- ☐ Orthopnea
- ☐ Paroxysmal nocturnal dyspnea
- ☐ Chest pain, palpitations, cough
- ☐ Prior episodes of similar presentation/investigations
- ☐ Symptoms suggestive of preeclampsia

Associated conditions or manifestations:
- ☐ Fever or signs of infection *(ensure absence of sepsis)*
- ☐ Pain, erythema, or differential swelling of extremities
- ☐ Thyroid dysfunction
- ☐ Upper gastrointestinal symptoms or known gastroesophageal reflux disease

Past medical/family history:
- ☐ Known history of asthma *(even if deemed inactive disease)*
- ☐ Prior personal or family history of cardiac disease
- ☐ Prior personal or family history of thromboembolic disease

Pregnancy-particularities:
- ☐ Antecedent preterm labor requiring tocolysis
- ☐ Iron-deficiency anemia and antenatal treatment

Social history and allergies:
- ☐ Alcohol consumption
- ☐ Cigarette smoking
- ☐ Recreational drugs
- ☐ Ethnicity
- ☐ Allergies

This is the first incident where the patient describes increasing breathlessness on exertion over the past few hours, aggravated by laying down. Simultaneously, she noticed progressive swelling of both legs. There are no other pertinent positive features related to her presentation. Her social history and family history are also noncontributory.

Unique to her current pregnancy, she developed late gestational hypertension two weeks ago, well controlled on oral nifedipine 30 mg once daily. She takes long-term oral iron supplementation during pregnancy.

As you discuss her presenting features, you note that the cardiotocography (CTG) is normal for both fetuses and there are no detectable contractions on tocometry.

2. With focus on the patient's presenting features, outline your physical examination. *(1 point each)*	Max 12

General appearance:
- ☐ Distress, including ability to provide complete sentences
- ☐ Beware of patient's preferred positioning (*i.e., supine, sitting, leaning forward*)
- ☐ Cyanosis
- ☐ Current or most recent BMI

Vital signs:
- ☐ Blood pressure
- ☐ Respiratory rate
- ☐ Pulse
- ☐ Oxygen saturation
- ☐ Temperature

Cardiopulmonary assessment:
- ☐ Elevated jugular venous pressure (*right-heart congestion*)
- ☐ Pulmonary rales (*left-heart congestion*)
- ☐ Heart murmurs
- ☐ S3 hear sound (*may be normal in pregnancy*)
- ☐ Lower extremity assessment for differential swelling, warmth, erythema, or pitting edema

Despite her inability to complete full sentences, she is capable of providing your requested information while seated. During conversation, you are attentive, noting absence of central or peripheral cyanosis. The patient has an obese habitus. She is afebrile, respiratory rate is at 22 breaths/min, blood pressure is 141/87 mmHg with a pulse at 125 bpm. Her oxygen saturation on room air is 91%, requiring 4 L of nasal supplementation to maintain saturation >95% for optimal fetoplacental oxygenation. Jugular pressure is elevated, and lung auscultation is notable for bibasilar crackles, without wheezing. Nearly equal pitting edema of the feet and ankles is noted, without erythema or tenderness.

You seek consultation by the obstetric physician (internist); in conversation, you discuss the patient's presentation and clinical findings. You also mention that the CTG is normal for both fetuses and she does not have obstetric issues. On bedside sonography, the fetuses are in the cephalic presentation; growth biometries, Doppler velocimetry, and amniotic fluid volumes are normal.

You will initiate the agreed-upon investigations until your colleague's arrival.

3. Keeping in mind the diagnostic differential you considered in conversation with the obstetric physician, indicate which investigations are <u>most</u> relevant in the evaluation of a patient with new-onset dyspnea and lower extremity edema. *(1 point each, unless specified)*	Max 20

Serum:
☐ Investigations for preeclampsia: CBC, ALT, AST, bilirubin, LDH, serum creatinine *(4 points)*
☐ Brain-natriuretic peptide (BNP), N-terminal-proBNP (NT-proBNP) *(4 points)*
☐ Electrolytes: sodium, calcium, potassium
☐ Thyroid function tests (TSH, free T_4 and T_3)
☐ Cardiac troponins *(may be considered if myocardial infarction suspected)*
☐ C-reactive protein *(may be considered if myocarditis suspected)*
☐ D-dimers *(may be considered if pulmonary embolism suspected)*

Urine:
☐ Urine protein/creatinine ratio (UPCR)
☐ Toxicology screen *(case-based; patient consent required)*

Imaging/other tests:
☐ Maternal echocardiography[‡] *(4 points)*
☐ Arterial blood gases
☐ 12-lead ECG
☐ Chest X-ray
☐ Doppler interrogation of the lower extremities *(if venous thromboembolism is suspected)*

Special note:
‡ *Echocardiography is the gold standard for diagnosis of PPCM*

After assessment by the obstetric internist, you engage in jointly reviewing results of her investigations alongside the allied consultant. The patient's ECG shows sinus tachycardia with non-specific ST-segment changes on V3–4–5 leads. With available testing in your laboratory, serum BNP[†] is reportedly markedly elevated.

The cardiologist attends to perform an echocardiogram on your obstetric unit.

Special note:
† Cutoff for acute heart failure: BNP >100 pg/mL, NT-proBNP >300 pg/mL

4-A. Which feature on maternal echocardiography is most reproducible and widely used to establish a diagnosis of PPCM?   3

☐ Left ventricular ejection fraction (LVEF) <45%

4-B. Your trainee is curious as to other physiologic or anatomic features on echocardiography that *may* occur with PPCM. Address this inquiry. *(1 point each)*   Max 4

☐ Left atrial, or biatrial, enlargement
☐ Atrioventricular valvular regurgitation (mitral and/or tricuspid)
☐ Pulmonary hypertension
☐ Ventricular dilatation (left and/or right)
☐ Hypokinetic right ventricle
☐ Pericardial effusion

Her echocardiogram shows left ventricular end-diastolic diameter (LVEDD)† at 5.2 cm with an ejection fraction of 33%. There is no arrhythmia, right ventricular involvement, or cardiac thrombus.

Chest X-ray discloses the following:

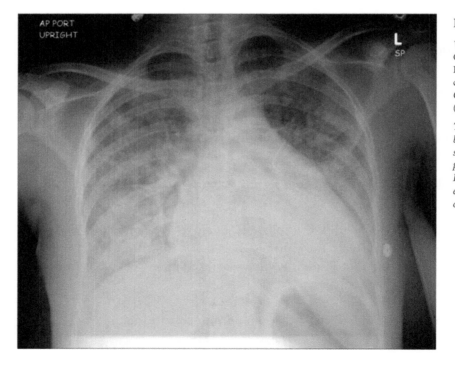

Figure 34.1

With permission: From Cunningham FG, et al. Peripartum cardiomyopathy. *Obstet Gynecol.* 2019;133 (1):167–179.

There is no association between this case scenario and this patient's chest X-ray. Image used for educational purposes only

Special note:
† Marked dilatation is defined by a LVEDD ≥6.0 cm

5. What are two notable findings on her chest X-ray? *(1 point each)*

□ Enlarged cardiac silhouette (cardiomegaly)
□ Pulmonary edema/pleural effusions

2

In the absence of an underlying cause for heart failure and otherwise unremarkable diagnostic work-up, you counsel the patient with the obstetric internist that the working diagnosis is PPCM. You inform her she requires transfer to your hospital's critical care setting where cardiac monitoring is available.

Meanwhile, she is started on furosemide 20 mg intravenously, with appropriate response. Serum electrolyte levels are within normal. Continuous fetal CTG monitoring is normal. Her oxygen supplementation is titrated down to 1 L and saturation is 96%. Oral metoprolol 12.5 mg twice daily has been initiated.

You inform your obstetric trainee that although pulmonary edema is also featured in preeclampsia, the pathobiological distinction from that in PPCM is important.

6. Elicit the underlying pathophysiological mechanisms of pulmonary edema associated with preeclampsia and/or PPCM. *(1 point each)*

□ Impaired systolic function *(PPCM)*
□ Increased afterload *(preeclampsia)*
□ Decreased oncotic pressure *(preeclampsia)*
□ Impaired diastolic function *(preeclampsia and PPCM)*

4

While the patient is in transfer to a monitored setting, you use this prime educational opportunity to discuss PPCM with your obstetric trainee.

7. Explain the diagnostic components of PPCM.[†] *(1 point per main bullet)*

□ Heart failure due to left ventricular systolic dysfunction, most often with a LVEF <45%
□ Heart failure in the last month of pregnancy (or toward the end of pregnancy) or within five months following delivery
  ○ *Majority are diagnosed within one month postpartum*
  ○ *May also occur following spontaneous pregnancy loss or termination*
□ Idiopathic; a diagnosis of exclusion
  ○ *Absence of a specific confirmatory test for PPCM*

3

Special note:
† This represents the broadened definition since the year 2010 by Heart Failure Association of the European Society of Cardiology Working Group (*Eur J Heart Fail* 2010; 12:767–8)

8-A. Which factors raise *this* patient's susceptibility for PPCM? *(1 point each)*   Max 6

- ☐ Gestational age at presentation
- ☐ Maternal age >30 years
- ☐ Multiple gestation
- ☐ Multiparity *(While multiparity is a risk factor for PPCM, most patients who develop PPCM do so during the first or second pregnancy)*
- ☐ Hypertensive disorder of pregnancy
- ☐ Obesity
- ☐ Iron-deficiency anemia

8-B. Indicate six <u>other</u> possible risk markers for the development of PPCM, not particular to this patient. *(1 point each)*   Max 6

- ☐ Geographic hotspots *(incidence may be up to 1/100 in Africa and 1/300 in Haiti, although global impact was shown)*
- ☐ Autoimmune conditions
- ☐ Recreational substance-use *(e.g., maternal cocaine use)*
- ☐ Prolonged tocolysis with an oral beta-adrenergic agonist *(more than four weeks' duration)*
- ☐ Asthma
- ☐ Thyrotoxicosis
- ☐ Chronic kidney disease
- ☐ Diabetes mellitus

Recognizing that multiple factors contribute to PPCM, your trainee researched the possible etiologies of disease. He or she has read about the postulated linkage to hemodynamic stresses of pregnancy and wishes to elaborate on this theory with you.

9. Illustrate an understanding of the hemodynamic alterations in pregnancy which may oppose the theoretical link to PPCM.   1

- ☐ Stroke volume and cardiac output peak in the second trimester (~16 weeks), then plateau
  - ○ *As such, hemodynamic stresses account for symptomatic heart failure in the context of preexisting disease*

After interprofessional discussions among the pregnancy heart team,[†] you attend to counsel the patient on current management plans. Relative to her initial presentation, you note that her breathing is less labored, to which she concurs.

Special note:
[†] *'Pregnancy heart team' was introduced by the ESC 2018 guidelines*[9]

10. At this time, in addition to oxygen, a loop diuretic, and a beta-blocker, outline elements to consider in counseling and management of this patient with PPCM.

8

Obstetric management: *(1 point each; max 5)*

☐ Induction of labor *(Cesarean delivery is reserved for obstetric indications)*
☐ Labor in the lateral decubitus position *(to limit aortocaval compression)*
☐ Continuous CTG monitoring
☐ Consideration for early regional anesthesia
   ○ *Beware of opioid-induced respiratory depression*
   ○ *Limit fluid administration*
☐ Consideration for passive descent of the fetal head in the second stage of labor
☐ Consideration for elective assisted vaginal delivery *(to decrease negative effects of Valsalva)*
☐ Select mode of administration of a uterotonic agent with care to limit IV fluids in the immediate postpartum period
   ○ *Anticipate risk of postpartum fluid overload and recurrent/worsening of pulmonary edema*

Cardiac management in the absence of cardiopulmonary distress: *(1 point each; max 3)*

☐ Sodium restriction
☐ Maternal hemodynamic monitoring
☐ Close monitoring of fluid balance *(input and urine output)*
☐ May require addition of hydralazine and nitrates *(vasodilator)*

Labor ensues by an amniotomy for the presenting twin. Oxytocin augmentation is needed at 5 cm dilatation, following standard guidelines. You inform the nursing team that dilution of oxytocin is not required. The newborns are vigorous at vaginal delivery.

11. Identify important postpartum management considerations and issues to discuss, either prior to discharge or at the routine postpartum visit in relation to PPCM and treatments the patient received. *(1 point per main bullet)*

Max 12

General maternal-fetal well-being:

☐ Screen for postpartum depression and continue to offer psychosocial support services
☐ Breastfeeding is controversial: Limited recent studies suggest safety *(Suggested Reading 7)*, however, 2018 ESC Guidelines[9] discourage breastfeeding with severe heart failure or NYHA Class III/IV
   ○ *Informed, case-based decision-making is required*
☐ Inform the patient that future pregnancy entails maternal morbidity and possible mortality despite full recovery of PPCM* *(informed decision process is necessary)*
   ○ *Prepregnancy LVEF is the strongest predictor of outcome*

   ○ *ESC 2018 guidelines[9]: future pregnancy is discouraged if LVEF has not recovered to >50%–55%*

   ○ *With full recovery, the risk of relapse is ~20%*

  □ If further pregnancy is desired, advise preconceptional counseling, particularly for cardiac assessment and discussion of cardioprotective medication

Cardiovascular-related care:

□ Consideration for postpartum anticoagulation for six to eight weeks, at least in prophylactic dose *(assuming absence of strong indication for treatment, including cardiac thrombus, atrial fibrillation, or systemic embolism)*

  ○ *ESC 2016[1]: With LVEF ≤35%*

  ○ *AHA 2016[3]: With LVEF <30%*

□ Start Angiotensin-converting enzyme inhibitor (ACE*i*) *(reassuring lactation data for short-acting ACEi such as captopril and enalapril);* may choose angiotensin receptor blocking agent if not breastfeeding or have an intolerance to ACE*i*

□ Continue ß1-selective blocking agent

  ○ *Neonatal observation in the initial 24–48 hours of life (hypotension, bradycardia, hypoglycemia)*

□ Start mineralocorticoid receptor antagonist, given LVEF ≤35%

  ○ *Compatible with breastfeeding*

□ Assess for resolution of gestational hypertension, or disease chronicity

□ Promote healthy lifestyle, including weight loss *(patient's increased BMI)*

□ Continue dietary sodium restriction

□ Promote long-term follow-up with her cardiologist; serial echocardiography for six months postpartum, and at least yearly thereafter

  ○ *Recovery often occurs within three to six months, but may take up to two years after diagnosis*

  ○ *Indefinite therapy for heart failure without recovery of LVEF*

  ○ *Optimal duration of treatment is unknown after full recovery*

Contraceptive recommendations: *(counseling would ideally be prior to delivery-discharge)*

□ Absence of an ideal method, although consistent use of a method should be encouraged

□ With impaired cardiac function due to cardiomyopathy, the advantages of using any progesterone method outweighs the risks; estrogen-containing contraceptives are contraindicated[†]

Special notes:

*   Full recovery implies LVEF ≥50%

†   UK and US Medical Eligibility Criteria (MEC) for Contraceptive Use, 2016; UK-MEC amended September 2019, US-MEC updated 2020

Her partner has been searching the internet for treatment options in PPCM and asks about the current stance on bromocriptine therapy.

12. Address the role of prolactin in the pathogenesis of PPCM and provide current guidance on use of bromocriptine therapy.   4

Theoretical role of prolactin: *(1 point for either bullet)*
- ☐ Oxidative stress stimulates cardiomyocytes to express cathepsin-D enzyme
- ☐ Cathepsin-D fragments prolactin, which are cardiotoxic

Bromocriptine: *(1 point per main bullet)*
- ☐ Controversial expert opinions in treatment of PPCM[‡]
  - ○ For consideration with LVEF <25%, right ventricular involvement, and/or cardiogenic shock
- ☐ *At least prophylactic* anticoagulation is recommended in conjunction with bromocriptine
- ☐ Discuss implications of not breastfeeding with the patient

Special note:
‡ US Food and Drug Administration does not endorse use of bromocriptine in treatment of PPCM and the 2020 JACC State-of-the-Art Review[5] views use of bromocriptine as investigational. Both the ESC 2018 guidelines[9] and 2019 Heart Failure Association of the ESC Study Group[2] on PPCM include weak recommendation for use of bromocriptine in PPCM

TOTAL: **100**

CHAPTER 35

Asthma in Pregnancy

Maria Loren Eberle, Amira El-Messidi, and Andrea Carlson

During your call duty, a 29-year-old primigravida at 19^{+2} weeks' gestation by early ultrasound dating presents to the obstetrics emergency assessment unit of your hospital center with a one-week history of dyspnea. She has not refilled her asthma treatments, as she was busy changing residences. The patient converses well, without signs of distress.

Your colleague follows her obstetric care, and pregnancy has been unremarkable to date. Routine prenatal laboratory investigations and results of aneuploidy screening were unremarkable. There are no current obstetric complaints, and fetal viability has been ascertained.

LEARNING OBJECTIVES

1. Take a focused history from an obstetric patient with antecedent asthma, recognizing risk factors for exacerbation
2. Provide detailed counseling of the effects of poorly controlled asthma on risks of obstetric complications
3. Understand evidence-based pharmacotherapy for management of acute asthma exacerbations, life-threatening disease activity, and maintenance therapy during pregnancy
4. Recognize the importance of multidisciplinary management of an obstetric patient with asthma, and highlight relevant considerations during the intrapartum and postpartum periods

SUGGESTED READINGS

1. British Thoracic Society and Scottish Intercollegiate Guidelines Network (BTN/SIGN 158). British guideline on the management of asthma: a national clinical guideline. July 2019. Available at www.brit-thoracic.org.uk/quality-improvement/guidelines/asthma/. Accessed May 16, 2021.
2. Bonham CA, Patterson KC, Strek ME. Asthma outcomes and management during pregnancy. *Chest.* 2018;153(2):515–527.
3. Chan AL, Juarez MM, Gidwani N, et al. Management of critical asthma syndrome during pregnancy. *Clin Rev Allergy Immunol.* 2015;48(1):45–53.
4. Cusack RP, Gauvreau GM. Pharmacotherapeutic management of asthma in pregnancy and the effect of sex hormones. *Expert Opin Pharmacother.* 2021;22(3):339–349.

5. Global Initiative for Asthma (GINA). 2021 GINA Report, global strategy for asthma management and prevention. Available at https://ginasthma.org/gina-reports/. Accessed May 18, 2021.

6. McLaughlin K, Foureur M, Jensen ME, et al. Review and appraisal of guidelines for the management of asthma during pregnancy. *Women Birth.* 2018;31(6):e349–e357.

7. Middleton PG, Gade EJ, Aguilera C, et al. ERS/TSANZ Task Force Statement on the management of reproduction and pregnancy in women with airways diseases. *Eur Respir J.* 2020;55(2):1901208.

8. Namazy JA, Schatz M. Management of asthma during pregnancy: optimizing outcomes and minimizing risk. *Semin Respir Crit Care Med.* 2018;39(1):29–35.

9. National Heart, Lung, and Blood Institute; National Asthma Education and Prevention Program Asthma and Pregnancy Working Group. NAEPP expert panel report. Managing asthma during pregnancy: recommendations for pharmacologic treatment-2004 update. *J Allergy Clin Immunol.* 2005;115(1):34–46. [Correction in *J Allergy Clin Immunol.* 2005 Mar;115(3):477]

10. Wang H, Li N, Huang H. Asthma in pregnancy: pathophysiology, diagnosis, whole-course management, and medication safety. *Can Respir J.* 2020:9046842.

11. Xu Z, Doust JA, Wilson LF, et al. Asthma severity and impact on perinatal outcomes: an updated systematic review and meta-analysis. *BJOG.* 2021. https://doi.org/10.1111/1471-0528.16968

POINTS

1. With respect to her clinical presentation and antecedent asthma, what aspects of a focused history would you want to know? *(1 point per main bullet unless specified; max points indicated where necessary)*

Max 40

Cardiorespiratory symptoms or manifestations: *(max 9)*
☐ Determine temporality of symptoms over the past week
☐ Loss of consciousness
☐ Auditory wheezing
☐ Chest tightness
☐ Paroxysmal nocturnal dyspnea
☐ Nighttime awakenings
☐ Nocturnal cough
☐ Orthopnea
☐ Chest pain
☐ Palpitations
☐ Symptoms of venous thromboembolism

Assessment of asthma control in pregnancy:[§]
☐ Frequency of symptoms
☐ Frequency of nighttime awakening
☐ Interference with normal activity
☐ Frequency of using short-acting β-agonist for symptom-control
☐ Percent of the personal best peak expiratory flow rate (PEFR) or percent predicted by forced expiratory volume in the first second of expiration (FEV1)
  ○ *Ideal FEV1 or PEFR is >80%*
  ○ *Typically, predicted PEFR in pregnancy is 380–550 L/min*

General details related to asthma:
- ☐ Age and context at diagnosis
- ☐ Duration since, and results of, last pulmonary function tests
- ☐ Need for hospitalizations, ICU (ITU) admissions or intubations secondary to asthma
- ☐ Duration of time since last asthma exacerbation requiring systemic corticosteroid

Medical comorbidities or causes of dyspnea in pregnancy: *(max 6)*
- ☐ Increased weight gain during the first trimester, or prepregnancy overweight/obese habitus
- ☐ Fever or signs of infection
- ☐ Depression/anxiety *(greater likelihood and incidence of uncontrolled asthma in pregnancy)*
- ☐ Iron-deficiency anemia and antenatal treatment
- ☐ Presence of cardiac or other respiratory conditions, past or present *(e.g., obstructive sleep apnea, rhinosinusitis, pneumonias, tuberculosis, interstitial lung disease)*
  - ○ *Features may represent diagnostic differentials or triggers of asthma*
- ☐ Gastroesophageal reflux disease *(bronchial irritation)*
- ☐ Endocrine disease *(e.g., thyrotoxicosis, diabetes-associated hyperventilation)*
- ☐ Renal insufficiency/metabolic acidosis-associated compensatory hyperventilation

Allergies:
- ☐ Drug allergies, or exposure to medicinal triggers of asthma *(e.g.,* aspirin, β-blockers)
- ☐ Nonmedicinal allergies *(e.g.,* environmental or dietary features)

Social factors, asthma triggers, and routine health maintenance:
- ☐ Occupation *(particularly for occupational lung disease)* and number of days missed from work due to asthma
- ☐ Household triggers of asthma: *(1 point per subbullet; max 3)*
  - ○ Location is proximal to pollutant industries
  - ○ Pets/animal dander or stuffed animals
  - ○ Lack of a ventilation system
  - ○ Fireplace, wood-burning stove
  - ○ Strong odors, aerosol sprays, or use of cleaning products
  - ○ Carpets, dust mites, mold, cockroach antigens
  - ○ Lack of allergen-impermeable covers for mattresses/pillows
- ☐ Smoking tobacco or illicit substances
- ☐ Exposure to second-hand smoke
- ☐ Symptom-onset with strenuous physical activity
- ☐ Up-to-date vaccination status *(e.g.,* pertussis, flu, COVID-19)
  - ○ *Patients with asthma do not appear to be at higher risk of acquiring COVID-19; systematic reviews have not shown an increased risk of severe COVID-19 in people with asthma (GINA[5])*

Current/prior medical treatments, clinical responses and side effects: *(max 5)*

Therapies compatible with pregnancy:
- ☐ Short-acting β2-agonists[†]- *e.g.,* albuterol, salbutamol
- ☐ Anticholinergics – *e.g.,* ipratropium bromide[†]
- ☐ Inhaled corticosteroids[‡]– low, medium, or high dose
- ☐ Oral/intravenous corticosteroids[†‡]

☐ Long-acting β2-agonists,[‡] *e.g.,* salmeterol, formoterol

☐ Mast cell stabilizers,[‡] *e.g.,* sodium cromoglicate, nedocromil sodium

☐ Leukotriene antagonists,[‡] *e.g.,* montelukast, zafirlukast

☐ Magnesium sulfate[†] *(potential adjunct in severe exacerbations)*

☐ Heliox[†] [80% helium/20% oxygen] *(potential adjunct in severe exacerbations, although unknown efficacy in pregnancy)*

Therapies not preferred for gestational use:

☐ Methylxanthines,[‡] *e.g.,* theophylline *(see Question 11 for particularity with use)*

☐ Monoclonal antiimmunoglobulin-E antibody, *e.g.,* omalizumab- *(risk of anaphylaxis; do not initiate in pregnancy although limited human data appears reassuring)*

☐ Monoclonal anti-interleukin-5 antibody preparations, *e.g.,* benralizumab, reslizumab, mepolizumab *(little or no human safety data)*

☐ Allergen immunotherapy, *e.g.,* subcutaneous/sublingual venom *(risk of anaphylaxis; do not initiate in pregnancy except in special circumstances such as prior anaphylaxis to Hymenoptera venom)*

☐ 5-lipoxygenase inhibitor, *e.g.,* zileuton *(teratogenic in animals; contraindicated in pregnancy)*

☐ Parenteral β-agonists, *e.g.,* epinephrine *(risk of uteroplacental vasoconstriction due to its alpha-adrenergic effect; reserve use for treatment of anaphylaxis in pregnancy);* subcutaneous terbutaline

Asthma-care provider/team:

☐ Record name(s) and contact information

Special notes:

§ For a multiparous patient, the effect of prior pregnancy on asthma severity or control would be significant in history-taking because 60% have similar course of asthma in first and subsequent pregnancies

† Rescue therapy

‡ Long-term control medication

Diagnosed at the age of 14 years with environmental-induced bronchospasm, she has since had recurrent exacerbations requiring *brief* urgent medical care, mostly secondary to low adherence to therapy. The patient has never been hospitalized and does not have medical comorbidities or drug allergies. She generally requires the albuterol metered dose inhaler (MDI) three to six days/week, with nighttime awakenings three times monthly. With a busy lifestyle as a hairdresser, she admits to forgetting to use long-term maintenance agent, an inhaled corticosteroid. Asthma barely limits normal activity, yet moderate intensity exercise aggravates her symptoms.

Her FEV1 was >80% predicted in early pregnancy at the last visit with her respiratory physician. This was an improvement since an exacerbation one month preconception required a 10-day course of oral corticosteroids. Neither she nor her husband smoke. They spent the past week moving from the countryside to a new residence in the city. The couple has been cleaning and plan to install a ventilation system. Without access to albuterol MDI, she presents for urgent care due to increasing fluctuations in dyspnea over the past week and a new-onset night cough. Clinical manifestations and systemic features are otherwise unremarkable.

Special note:

This patient's description of baseline severity is compatible with mild persistent asthma

2. Verbalize essentials of your focused physical examination based on her medical history and presenting complaints. *(1 point each)*	Max 14

General appearance:
- ☐ Beware of patient's preferred positioning
- ☐ Distress, including ability to provide complete sentences *(i.e., work of breathing)*
- ☐ Use of accessory muscles, nasal flaring *(i.e., work of breathing)*
- ☐ Cyanosis or diaphoresis
- ☐ Any manifestation of an atopic dermatitis

Vital signs:
- ☐ Blood pressure
- ☐ Respiratory rate
- ☐ Pulse
- ☐ Oxygen saturation
- ☐ Temperature

Cardiopulmonary assessment:
- ☐ Bilateral air entry on auscultation of both lung fields
- ☐ Wheezing or rhonchi, especially with prolonged expiration

Oculo-rhino-laryngeal features:
- ☐ Increased nasal discharge, pale nasal mucosa, or presence of nasal polyps
- ☐ Pharyngeal edema
- ☐ Signs suggestive of conjunctivitis *(e.g., red or teary eyes)*

With hunched shoulders, the patient has frequent nasal discharge and flaring, without suprasternal retractions. You find her sentences are becoming shorter from breathlessness, relative to earlier conversation. She is normotensive, afebrile, with a respiratory rate of 20 breaths/min, pulse of 105 beats/min, and oxygen saturation at 97% on room air. The patient is not coughing. You auscultate expiratory wheezing in all lung fields.

You highlight to your obstetric trainee that assessment of FEV1 would require a spirometer. Instead, PEFR, which correlates well with FEV1, is reliably measured with a disposable portable peak flow meter: the patient's PEFR is at 65% of her predicted value. A respirologist/urgent care physician has been notified to assist you in the management of this patient; the expert reminds you that recommended treatment of asthma exacerbations is the same as nonpregnant states, for all gestational ages.

3. With interdisciplinary collaboration, outline an approach to the <u>initial pharmacologic</u> <u>management</u> of this gravida's acute asthma exacerbation. *(1 point per main bullet, unless specified)*

Max 5

Pharmacologic management of moderate acute asthma[†]:

☐ Inhaled short-acting β2-agonist *(any accepted regimen for 3 points; other possibilities may apply)*

　○ Albuterol MDI: two to eight puffs, where each puff provides 90 ug, given every 20 minutes for one hour, then repeated every one to four hours as needed

　OR

　○ Albuterol 0.083% 2.5–5 mg nebulizer, given every 20 minutes for one hour, then repeated every one to four hours as needed

　OR

　○ Albuterol continuous nebulization 10–15 mg/hr

☐ May add nebulized ipratropium bromide (anticholinergic) 0.5 mg every 20 minutes for one hour, then on an as-needed basis

☐ Hydration (oral or parenteral) to maintain euvolemia

☐ Supplemental oxygen as needed, to maintain saturation at 94%–98% *(BTS/SIGN[1])*, and/or arterial oxygen tension (PaO2) ≥70 mmHg

　○ Maintaining oxygen saturation >95% is also appropriate

☐ Initiate systemic[‡] corticosteroids if inadequate response to treatment within the first hour

　○ *Corticosteroids would be initiated without delay if the patient were on chronic oral glucocorticoids or with severe exacerbations (see Question 11)*

Special notes:

Continuous electronic fetal monitoring would be indicated at viable gestational ages (refer to Question 11)

† Based on PEFR >50%–75% predicted, oxygen saturation ≥92%, and no features of acute severe asthma

‡ Refer to Question 3 in Chapter 45 for fetal risks associated with maternal corticosteroids

Over the first hour of treatment, while the patient receives albuterol MDI via a spacer, you address your trainee's inquiry regarding disease severity and review the contributing factors for the patient's asthma exacerbation. You inform your trainee that although standard chest radiographs[†] may be performed in pregnancy, imaging is not commonly needed unless the patient does not respond to standard regimens or if there is suspicion of other etiologies.

Special note:

† Refer to Question 3 in Chapter 73 for counseling on maternal-fetal exposure to ionizing radiation associated with chest radiography

4. Specify the clinical markers which would have classified this exacerbation as 'acute severe asthma.' *(1 point each)*

☐ Peak expiratory flow 33%–50% best or predicted
☐ Respirations $\geq$25/min
☐ Pulse $\geq$110 beats/min
☐ Inability to complete a sentence in one breath

4

5. Identify factors raising *this* patient's susceptibility for an asthma exacerbation. *(1 point each)*

Patient-specific risk factors:
☐ Pregnancy
☐ Gestational age *(greatest risk for exacerbations ranges from 17 to 36 weeks)*
☐ Low adherence to therapy/failure to renew her treatment agents
☐ Suboptimal preconception/baseline disease control
☐ Occupation as a hairdresser *(exposure to chemicals)*
☐ Environmental exposure associated with change of residence to the center of town from the countryside
☐ Exposure to allergens while cleaning residence
☐ Stress
☐ Lack of adequate ventilation system

Max 8

6. With reference to respiratory physiology, elaborate on the <u>pathogenesis</u> of asthma aggravation in pregnancy. *(1 point each)*

☐ Increase in uterine size and abdominal pressure raises the diaphragm, leading to decreased functional residual capacity
☐ Hormonally mediated mucosal vasodilation leads to airway congestion and increased rhinosinusitis
☐ Progesterone-associated stimulation of the respiratory center and sensitivity to carbon dioxide
☐ Pregnancy-associated changes in immunity, favoring a Th2-type humoral response (mandatory for fetal survival), contributes to exacerbation of bronchial asthma during pregnancy

Max 3

After one hour of treatment, the patient's PEFR improved to 77% with normal findings on physical examination. She reports feeling similar to her respiratory baseline; fetal viability is reascertained after resolution of the exacerbation. As the patient will be observed for a sustained response until one hour after the last treatment, you highlight that active management of asthma during pregnancy is generally associated with excellent perinatal outcomes. Reassuringly, you explain that available studies give little cause for concern regarding treatment side effects and that conventional asthma medications are safer than symptoms and exacerbations.

7. Detail specific <u>asthma-related features</u> that represent <u>optimal control</u> in an obstetric   Max 5
    patient. *(1 point each)*

☐ Minimal or no chronic symptoms during the day or night
☐ Minimal or no exacerbations
☐ No activity limitations
☐ Maintenance of (near) normal pulmonary function
☐ Minimal use of short-acting inhaled β2-agonist
☐ Minimal or no adverse effects from medications

8. Recognizing existing controversies, identify adverse perinatal outcomes that have   10
    been associated with maternal asthma, particularly with inadequate control or
    exacerbations. *(1 point each; max points specified per section)*

Maternal: *(max 5)*
☐ Viral respiratory infections (frequency and severity)
☐ Early pregnancy loss
☐ Hyperemesis gravidarum
☐ Preeclampsia, superimposed preeclampsia, or eclampsia
☐ Gestational diabetes mellitus
☐ Spontaneous or iatrogenic preterm delivery
☐ Obstetric hemorrhage (antepartum and postpartum)
☐ Cesarean delivery
☐ Pulmonary embolism
☐ ICU (ITU) admission
☐ Mortality

Fetoplacental/neonatal: *(max 5)*
☐ Fetal growth restriction (FGR) or low birthweight
☐ Breech presentation
☐ Placental abruption
☐ Placenta previa
☐ Preterm prelabor rupture of membranes
☐ Congenital malformations associated with first-trimester exacerbations
☐ NICU admission
☐ Neonatal hypoxia
☐ Fetal or neonatal mortality

Special note:
Rates of asthma in childhood are also increased

9. In liaison with the respirology/urgent care physician, provide comprehensive discharge counseling and plan for subsequent antenatal care. *(1 point per main bullet)*   Max 10

Deterrence and patient education:

☐ Highlight treatment adherence, reassuring patient of drug safety and lack of teratogenicity of prescribed agents

☐ Asthma trigger avoidance *(including smoking cessation, where appropriate)*

☐ Verify inhaler technique – *i.e.,* take a maximal inspiration while standing and note the measurement on the peak flow meter

☐ Renew/provide supply of short-acting inhaled β2-agonist (reliever inhaler) and corticosteroid (prevention inhaler)

☐ Encourage daily peak expiratory flow monitoring, with consideration for maintenance of an 'asthma diary' containing daily assessments of asthma status (PEFR and symptoms), activity limitations, and record use of regular and as-needed medications
  ○ *Consideration for objective assessment of asthma control using validated questionnaires such as ACQ (Asthma Control Questionnaire), ACT (Asthma Control Test), p-ACT (pregnancy-specific ACT), or GINA (Global Initiative for Asthma)*

☐ Arrange follow-up with an asthma liaison nurse or at the chest clinic

☐ Provide the patient with a written asthma action plan[†] for home treatment of asthma and indications for seeking medical care
  ○ *Systematic reviews show that patient education and action plans improve asthma control, thereby reducing emergency medical help and hospitalizations*

Obstetric plan for asthma care:

☐ Communicate with and/or plan follow-up with her primary care provider

☐ Monthly assessment of asthma control is recommended *(GINA[5])*

☐ Consideration for high-dose vitamin-D supplementation[‡] for risk-reduction of asthma/recurrent wheezing in early childhood (up to age three years)
  ○ *Dose range is vitamin D₃ 2400–4000 IU daily, in addition to standard dose in routine prenatal vitamins (i.e., vitamin D 400–600 IU daily)*
  ○ *Greatest benefit appears to be for women who maintain 25(OH)Vitamin D level ≥30 ng/mL*

☐ Encourage exercise to reduce asthma-associated obstetric morbidities *(e.g., FGR, gestational diabetes, excessive weight gain, preeclampsia)*

☐ Discuss fetal sonographic growth surveillance given suboptimal asthma control *(risk of FGR)*

☐ Avoid indomethacin (nonsteroidal anti-inflammatory agent) in case of preterm labor as may precipitate bronchospasm

Special notes:

† An example of patient resource form is available at www.asthma.org.uk/advice/manage-your-asthma/pregnancy/#takeactionsymptoms, accessed May 18, 2021

‡ Wolsk HM, Chawes BL, Litonjua AA, et al. Prenatal vitamin D supplementation reduces risk of asthma/recurrent wheeze in early childhood: A combined analysis of two randomized controlled trials. *PLoS One.* 2017;12(10):e0186657. Published 2017 Oct 27.

The patient adheres to use of inhaled β2-agonist and inhaled corticosteroid treatment for mild persistent asthma. Second-trimester morphology of the known female[§] fetus, and subsequent biometric assessments have been normal. She has not had any obstetric complaints or complications.

At 30 weeks' gestation, the patient presents by ambulance to your tertiary center's E.R (A&E) department after returning from a trip where she forgot to bring her inhalers. While on-duty in the birthing center, you are called to assist in the management of this patient with 'life-threatening asthma.'

Special note:

§ A sexual dimorphic response occurs – maternal asthma tends to worsen with a female fetus: explanations may relate to reduced placental enzyme 11β-hydroxysteroid dehydrogenase type 2 (positively correlated with birthweight) and reduced testosterone levels compared to male fetuses, and to female fetus-induced promotion of maternal inflammatory pathways

10. As you promptly attend to the patient, alert your obstetric trainee to life-threatening features of asthma. *(1 point each)*

6

Clinical signs: *(max 3)*
- ☐ Altered level of consciousness
- ☐ Poor respiratory effort/exhaustion
- ☐ Hypotension
- ☐ Arrhythmia
- ☐ Cyanosis
- ☐ Silent chest

Measurements: *(max 3)*
- ☐ Oxygen saturation <92%
- ☐ PEFR <33% best or predicted
- ☐ Severe hypoxia on arterial blood gas (PaO2 <70 mmHg)
- ☐ 'Normal' or increased arterial tension of carbon dioxide on arterial blood gas (PaCO2>32 mmHg)

You learn from the treating urgent care team that upon admission, oxygen saturation was 91% with a PEFR of 31% predicted, and blood pressure was 100/60 mmHg with an inspiratory decrease in systolic blood pressure by 12 mmHg (pulsus paradoxus). The patient was diaphoretic with peripheral cyanosis. She was sitting, leaning forward due to breathlessness, using her accessory muscles. Her husband described audible wheezing prior to presentation, although none were auscultated upon admission. Results of serum investigations, arterial blood gas, and chest radiography are pending. Doptone revealed a fetal heart rate of 140 beats/min at presentation.

11. In collaboration with the urgent care team, outline principal maternal-fetal management considerations for this gravida with an asthma exacerbation. *(1 point per main bullet, unless specified)*

Max 6

Life-threatening asthma:

☐ Early consultation with critical care services for potential ICU/ITU admission and ventilatory support

☐ Deliver oxygen to maintain saturation 94%–98% (goal of >95% is also acceptable) to prevent maternal-fetal hypoxia

☐ Continuous electronic fetal monitoring is recommended with uncontrolled/severe asthma to aid in recognizing fetal distress
  ○ *Although permissive hypercarbia may be tolerated by the mother in pregnancy, the risk of fetal respiratory acidosis warrants attention*
  ○ *Delivery may become necessary for maternal respiratory support*

☐ Start concomitant treatment with inhaled β2-agonist and ipratropium via nebulizer with oxygen, at 15-minute intervals (continuous β2-agonist nebulizer is also optional)

☐ *Early* initiation of systemic corticosteroids

(1 point for any regimen; other possibilities may be deemed acceptable)
Possibilities include:

  ○ Prednisone or prednisolone 40 to 60 mg orally for 3–10 days, <u>or</u>
  ○ Hydrocortisone 100 mg intravenously every eight hours, <u>or</u>
  ○ Methylprednisolone 40 to 60 mg intravenously every six hours

☐ Replete the volume status and correct electrolyte derangements, as needed

☐ Intravenous magnesium sulfate 2 g over 20 minutes for maternal bronchodilation may be considered if poor response to above treatments; other considerations include theophylline and intravenous/subcutaneous β2-agonists
  ○ *Beware that recommended dosing for fetal neuroprotection differs – i.e., magnesium sulfate **4 g** intravenous loading dose with/without 1 g/hr maintenance[‡]*
  ○ *Theophylline has a narrow therapeutic index (maintain serum levels at 5–12 ug/mL), with potential select drug–drug interactions (e.g., erythromycin) and neonatal tachycardia/irritability*

☐ Consider initiating fetal pulmonary corticosteroids

☐ Consider the left lateral decubitus position to improve venous return

Special note:

[‡] Refer to Magee LA, De Silva DA, Sawchuck D, Synnes A, von Dadelszen P. No. 376-Magnesium sulphate for fetal neuroprotection. *J Obstet Gynaecol Can.* 2019;41(4):505–522.

In the intensive care unit, salmeterol, a long-acting β2-agonist, at one puff twice daily is started as an add-on[§] controller therapy to her baseline treatments. Fetal monitoring was unremarkable, and sonography performed upon transfer to the antepartum unit showed a cephalic presentation with normal growth velocity and amniotic fluid volume. After a five-day hospital stay, the patient is discharged on a tapered course of oral corticosteroids; she will continue use of the inhaled treatments. You highlight to your obstetric trainee that contemporary recommendations place a low priority on stepping down treatment given evidence of adverse outcomes from exacerbations during pregnancy, as well as medication-safety data *(GINA[5])*. Timely follow-up is arranged with her respirologist.

At 39^{+2} weeks' gestation, you advise induction of labor for late gestational hypertension. Fetal presentation is cephalic and sonographic monitoring has been normal. The patient completed the course of oral corticosteroids more than three weeks ago[†] and has been responding well to inhaler therapies. You reassure the patient that although asthma exacerbations during labor and delivery are rare, you will ensure an appropriate management plan prior to delivery admission.

Special notes:
§ Should not be used as monotherapy
† Patients on oral corticosteroids ≥5 mg daily for more than three weeks prior to delivery require intrapartum stress doses; refer to Question 14 in Chapter 45 for dosing at planned vaginal delivery, and Question 16 in Chapter 46 for dosing at Cesarean delivery. (National Institute for Health and Care Excellence (NICE) Guideline 121: Intrapartum care for women with existing medical conditions or obstetric complications and their babies. 2019. Available at www.nice.org.uk/guidance/ng121, accessed May 18, 2021.) BTN/SIGN[1] recommends parenteral corticosteroids for women receiving oral prednisolone >7.5 mg/d for more than two weeks prior to delivery

12. Rationalize the rarity of intrapartum asthma exacerbations. 3

☐ Increase in endogenous corticosteroid production

13. Outline <u>intrapartum</u> considerations for this patient, with focus on asthma exacerbations in pregnancy and gestational hypertension requiring induction of labor. *(1 point per main bullet; max points specified)*

12

General: *(max 7)*

☐ Assess peak expiratory flow upon admission and consider repeat testing every 12 hours in labor

☐ Continued liaison with the respirology team involved in her care

☐ Early ICU (ITU) consultation is advised if warranted by the patient's status

☐ Ensure adequate hydration to avoid risk of bronchospasm

☐ Continue asthma medications during labor and delivery

☐ Continuous maternal pulse oximetry, providing supplemental oxygen as required

☐ Continuous electronic fetal monitoring

☐ Plan for early labor analgesia with the same options as women without asthma: *(NICE guideline[§])*

   ○ Entonox (50% nitrous oxide + 50% oxygen)

   ○ Intravenous and intramuscular opioids *(no evidence for opioid-induced bronchospasm from labor analgesia)*

   ○ Epidural analgesia

   ○ Combined spinal-epidural analgesia

☐ Alert the neonatology team if large doses of short-acting β-agonist are used within 48 hours prior to delivery (especially if preterm); neonatal blood glucose monitoring is warranted for the first 24 hours *(GINA[5])*

Treatment of hypertension *(if needed)*:

☐ Avoid labetalol (β-blocker); calcium channel blocker or hydralazine are preferred agents

Induction of labor:

☐ Prostaglandin E1 (misoprostol) and E2 (dinoprostone) are safe; they do not cause bronchoconstriction

   ○ *Prostaglandin E1 (misoprostol) may also be used in management of postpartum hemorrhage (PPH)*

☐ Delay pushing in the second stage of labor to decrease Valsalva maneuvers

☐ Maintain a low threshold for assisted second stage

In case of PPH:

☐ Recommend active management of the third stage of labor, given asthma-associated risks of hemorrhage

☐ Preferred avoidance of 15-methyl-prostaglandin F2α (carboprost) due to risk of bronchospasm

☐ Although ergometrine may cause bronchospasm particularly in association with general anesthesia, this is not a problem encountered when syntometrine (syntocinon/ergometrine) is used for PPH prophylaxis *(BTS/SIGN[1])*

Special note:

§ National Institute for Health and Care Excellence (NICE) Guideline 121: Intrapartum care for women with existing medical conditions or obstetric complications and their babies. 2019. Available at www.nice.org.uk/guidance/ng121.

14. Provide evidence-based counseling for <u>postpartum</u> care with focus on the obstetric patient with asthma. *(1 point per main bullet)* | Max 4

☐ Encourage breastfeeding, reassuring the patient that asthma treatment agents are safe *(small amount of drug transfer to breast milk is not clinically significant)*
  ○ *Breastfeeding may delay onset of childhood asthma but does not protect offspring*
☐ Exercise caution with use of nonsteroidal anti-inflammatory drugs (NSAIDs) for analgesia due to risk of bronchospasm
☐ Encourage a pet-, smoke-, and allergen-free environment
☐ Ensure follow-up is arranged with her asthma-treating teams
☐ Encourage future preconception counseling to optimize asthma control and perinatal outcomes

TOTAL: | **130**

CHAPTER 36

Tuberculosis in Pregnancy

Amira El-Messidi and Alan D. Cameron

A patient is referred by her primary care provider for consultation and transfer of care to your high-risk obstetric unit at a tertiary center. She is a 32-year-old primigravida at 15^{+3} weeks' gestation with new abnormalities on chest X-ray and a positive sputum smear for acid-fast bacilli, performed as part of investigations for a four-week history of cough and night sweats. You have arranged to see her at the end of your clinic, with appropriate infection precautions. Referral to an infectious disease expert has also been instigated. A copy of the routine maternal prenatal investigations is unavailable at this time. First-trimester sonogram and aneuploidy screen were unremarkable. She has no obstetric complaints.

LEARNING OBJECTIVES

1. Take a focused history from a prenatal patient with active tuberculosis (TB), appreciating challenges that pregnancy may incur in diagnosing active disease
2. Recognize the importance of continued multidisciplinary collaboration in the obstetric care of a patient with active TB or latent TB infection
3. Be familiar with the diagnostic evaluation for active TB and first-line treatments for drug-susceptible disease, and counsel on adverse drug effects that warrant early reporting
4. Provide comprehensive counseling on potential perinatal risks of untreated active TB and the effect of pregnancy on TB disease or latent infection
5. Demonstrate the ability to provide evidence-based advice for breastfeeding mothers taking first-line anti-TB agents, and highlight contraceptive particularities with specific anti-TB agents or disease

SUGGESTED READINGS

1. Canadian Tuberculosis Standards, 7th ed; 2014. Available at www.canada.ca/en/public-health/services/infectious-diseases/canadian-tuberculosis-standards-7th-edition.html. Accessed January 20, 2021.
2. Centers for Disease Control and Prevention (CDC). TB in specific populations: pregnancy. Available at www.cdc.gov/tb/topic/populations/pregnancy/default.htm. Accessed January 17, 2021.
3. El-Messidi A, Czuzoj-Shulman N, Spence AR, et al. Medical and obstetric outcomes among pregnant women with tuberculosis: a population-based study of 7.8 million births. *Am J Obstet Gynecol.* 2016;215(6): 797.e1–797.e6.

4. International Union against Tuberculosis and Lung Disease. Management of tuberculosis – a guide to essential practice. 7th ed., 2019. Available at https://theunion.org/technical-publications/management-of-tuberculosis-a-guide-to-essential-practice. Accessed January 17, 2021.

5. Public Health England. Pregnancy and tuberculosis – information for clinicians. Available at www.gov.uk/government/publications/tuberculosis-and-pregnant-women. Accessed January 17, 2021.

6. Miele K, Bamrah Morris S, Tepper NK. Tuberculosis in pregnancy. *Obstet Gynecol.* 2020;135(6):1444–1453.

7. Sobhy S, Babiker Z, Zamora J, et al. Maternal and perinatal mortality and morbidity associated with tuberculosis during pregnancy and the postpartum period: a systematic review and meta-analysis. *BJOG.* 2017;124(5):727–733.

8. Queensland guidelines for the treatment of tuberculosis in pregnant women and newborn infants, version 3.1. September 2016. Available at www.health.qld.gov.au/clinical-practice/guidelines-procedures/diseases-infection/diseases/tuberculosis/guidance/guidelines. Accessed January 17, 2021.

9. World Health Organization (WHO). Guidelines on TB. Available at www.who.int/tb/publications/9789241547833/en/. Accessed January 17, 2021.

10. Zha BS, Nahid P. Treatment of drug-susceptible tuberculosis. *Clin Chest Med.* 2019;40(4):763–774.

POINTS

1. What aspects of a focused history would you want to know? *(1 point per main bullet, unless specified)*

Max 25

Current/prior respiratory TB symptoms or manifestations: *(max 5)*
- ☐ Characterize the cough *(i.e., productive/nonproductive)* and assess for change
- ☐ Hemoptysis *(late finding; occurs when granulomas erode blood vessels)*
- ☐ Shortness of breath
- ☐ Chest pain *(from tuberculous pleurisy)*
- ☐ History of TB disease and treatment *(reinfection with TB is possible; past treatment and cure does not provide immunity)*
- ☐ BCG (bacillus Calmette–Guerin) vaccination[$] *(part of an Extended Program on child Immunization [EPI] in many countries)*

Cardinal systemic symptoms, [in addition to night sweats]: *(3)*
- ☐ Fever
- ☐ Malaise, fatigue
- ☐ Unintended weight loss *(>10% body weight in past six months)*

Medical comorbidities predisposing to progression of latent to active TB: *(inquiry about HIV status is obligatory; max 6)*
- ☐ Result of routine prenatal HIV screening *(4 points)*
- ☐ Pregestational diabetes mellitus *(increases risk, severity, and suboptimal treatment of TB)*
- ☐ End-stage renal disease on hemodialysis
- ☐ Presence of mental health disorders
  - ○ *Existing disorders increase the risk of TB (Suggested Reading 4)*
  - ○ *Psychiatric side effects are associated with some anti-TB agents*
  - ○ *Depression may affect the patient if she requires treatment for TB*

☐ Current treatment with immunomodulator/immunosuppressive therapy (e.g., corticosteroids, biologic agents)

☐ Recipient of a solid organ transplant

☐ Prior malignancy (particularly of the head, neck, lung, or lymphoma/leukemia)

☐ Chronic malnutrition

☐ Prior jejunoileal bypass surgery or gastrectomy

Social factors, routine health maintenance, medications, and allergies: (max 6)

☐ Place of birth

☐ Migration within the past five years from TB-endemic country, or frequent travel to TB-endemic countries

☐ Current housing/socioeconomic status/partner or family support

☐ Occupation (particularly for occupational lung disease or risk of silicosis)

☐ Prior incarceration

☐ Alcohol consumption, tobacco smoking, or recreational substance use

☐ Vaccination status (e.g., influenza, hepatitis A and B, tetanus, COVID-19)

☐ Medications and allergies

Current/prior nonrespiratory TB symptoms or manifestations: (pelvic and one other organ manifestation for max 3 points)

☐ Peripheral lymphadenitis (e.g., most often an isolated, unilateral, nontender neck mass)

☐ Neurologic manifestations of TB (e.g., tuberculous meningitis, myelitis, abscess)

☐ Ocular TB

☐ TB pericarditis

☐ TB mastitis

☐ Pelvic involvement of TB: (2 points for subbullet)
   ○ Assess for history of infertility or assisted reproductive techniques due to pelvic TB

☐ Urinary tract involvement of TB (e.g., gross hematuria, frequency, dysuria)

☐ Enteric TB (most commonly involving the ileocecal area; variable presentations account for difficult diagnosis)

☐ Bones/joints (e.g., vertebral TB [Pott's disease], tuberculous arthritis, osteomyelitis)

☐ Other (TB may affect any other organ or organ system)

Family/contact history:

☐ Household contact or close contact with TB disease, including their treatment regimen
   ○ Knowledge of treatment regimens helps identify multidrug resistant TB (MDR-TB)[‡]
   ○ Contacts are traced up to three months prior to TB treatment initiation (Suggested Reading 4)

Special notes:

§ Live viral vaccine; contraindicated in pregnancy

‡ Resistance to isoniazid (INH) and rifampin (RIF)

You learn that the patient emigrated three years ago with her husband from their native country of birth where TB is endemic. Five months ago, she returned from her yearly trip to visit family in a rural village where up to 10 individuals cohabit per household. Ever since six weeks' gestation of this spontaneous conception, she recalls severe fatigue, loss of appetite, and occasional respiratory discomfort, which she attributed to pregnancy. She subsequently noticed a dry cough, nonresponsive to conservative treatment, and later developed night sweats. She had a negative tuberculin skin test (TST)[§] 18 months ago when she started working at a long-term care facility. She practices a healthy lifestyle and diet; she only takes routine prenatal vitamins. She hands you original copies of her routine prenatal investigations which you note are normal, specifically attentive to her recently performed HIV test. Despite limited nutritional intake, she was reassured gestational weight gain has been adequate. Medical history is unremarkable for tuberculous comorbidities or nonrespiratory diseases. She lives with her husband whom she says has not had any medical complaints. Just prior to returning from her most recent trip, she recalls her niece's discomfort with a long-term cough.

The patient inquires about how infection is acquired and the potential impact of pregnancy on progression of infection or disease. She has been trying to rationalize the months' delay in confirming active TB since the onset of her symptoms.

Special note:
§ TST is synonymous with Mantoux test or purified protein derivative

2. Elaborate on challenges that pregnancy may incur on confirmation of active TB. *(1 point per main bullet)*

3

☐ Unfounded fears of chest radiography[†]
  ○ *Posterior-anterior and lateral chest X-ray views*
☐ Overlapping clinical manifestations between TB disease and pregnancy (*e.g.*, loss of appetite, fatigue, malaise, shortness of breath)
☐ Masked TB-associated weight loss from gestational increases in abdominal girth and body volume

Special note:
† Refer to Question 3 in Chapter 73 for discussion on common misconceptions regarding fetal risks from chest radiography

3. Detail the pathogenesis of TB infection and extrapolate her medico-social risk factors for active disease. *(1 point per main bullet; points specified per section)*

5

TB pathogenesis: *(1)*
☐ Airborne infectious droplets of one of seven mycobacterium acid-fast bacilli may remain asymptomatic in alveolar macrophages, forming granulomas (latent infection; noncontagious), or progress to active pulmonary or extrapulmonary TB disease most commonly where risk factors exist
  ○ *Within alveolar macrophages, most bacilli are inhibited or destroyed*
  ○ *Release of remaining viable bacilli when macrophages die may travel to any organ by way of lymphatics or bloodstream*

Patient's risk factors for active TB: *(max 4)*
☐ Foreign-born
☐ Emigration within five years from a country with high prevalence of TB
☐ Recent travel to a country where TB is endemic
☐ Staff member of a long-term care facility
☐ *Probable* household contact with infectious pulmonary TB (*i.e.*, her niece)
☐ *Controversial* effect of **pregnancy** itself on risk of progression of latent to active TB
  ○ Recent studies suggest that reduced helper T-cells (Th1) activity may contribute to increased risk of TB by at least twofold relative to nonpregnant states

4. Recognizing the controversial effect of pregnancy, *in general,* on the onset on active TB, discuss other aspects you would mention to her in this regard. *(1 point each)*

Max 2

☐ Pregnancy does not affect treatment response to TB disease
☐ Pregnancy has been associated with increased incidence of extra-pulmonary TB and multiorgan involvement *(active pulmonary disease is usually the most symptomatic and contagious)*
☐ Immune reconstitution inflammatory syndrome accounts for the apparent greater incidence of TB disease manifestations in the immediate postpartum

Despite a noticeable dry cough, the patient converses without distress. She has a normal habitus, is afebrile with a normal respiratory rate and oxygenation. Respiratory examination is completely normal; you inform your trainee that this is common in suspected pulmonary TB, even for relatively advanced cases. Nonrespiratory assessment does not reveal lymphadenopathy or other abnormality. Fetal viability is ascertained.

Although the patient anticipates treatment will be recommended by the infectious disease expert in consultation the following day, she is reticent about therapy. She wishes to understand laboratory tests performed in the diagnostic evaluation of active TB.

5. Where a patient is referred for TB treatment, what are important potential <u>social barriers</u> to overcome to optimize patient-centered care? *(1 point each)*

Max 3

☐ Perceived discrimination
☐ Financial access
☐ Means for transportation *(i.e., direct-observed therapy is advised)*
☐ Unfamiliarity with local health care systems
☐ Language barriers

6. Outline three <u>laboratory</u> tests used in the diagnostic evaluation of active TB. *(1 point per main bullet)*

3

☐ At least three sputum specimens (either spontaneous or induced) tested for acid-fast bacilli on microscopy
　○ Where feasible, sputum samples are collected on the same day, with a minimum of one hour apart
　○ One morning sputum sample is preferred for its quality and higher number of acid-fast bacilli
☐ *M. tuberculosis* sputum culture and phenotypic drug susceptibility testing
　○ Culture is <u>gold standard</u> for detection of active TB disease despite a long turnaround period of six weeks or longer for results
　○ In general, a single positive culture for *M. tuberculosis* is definitive for active disease, although culture is recommended for every sputum sample sent for microscopy (occasional risk of false positive results)
☐ Molecular-based tests – Nucleic acid amplification tests for *M. tuberculosis* complex, commonly using polymerase chain reaction (PCR)
　○ Rifampin resistance can be rapidly detected using molecular tests
　○ Not considered confirmatory diagnosis; definitive sputum culture is advised

The following day, the infectious disease expert calls to inform you that the patient has bacteriologically confirmed TB by rapid molecular testing in addition to her positive smear microscopy, the latter of which makes her infectious. He or she agrees with your physical examination findings, although the chest X-ray shows the classic triad of typical findings in immunocompetent adults: there is volume loss, apical infiltrates of the upper lobes, and cavitary lesions.

The physician counseled the patient on immediate treatment initiation with the empiric four-drug regimen for six months' duration; vitamin supplements specific to anti-TB treatment are advised. A patient-centered approach where directly observed therapy is practiced will be arranged by the TB-treating team to optimize adherence and achieve durable cure. As required by local health regulations, the patient's TB diagnosis will be reported and contact tracing initiated. She has been informed of common side effects and adverse drug reactions.

7. Provide rationale for immediate treatment initiation of pregnant women diagnosed with active TB. *(1 point per main bullet; max points specified per section)*   10

☐ Inform the patient that an early start of anti-TB treatment may decrease risks of adverse maternal-fetal outcomes and lead to cure. *(1 point)*

Maternal risks with untreated active TB: *(max 6)*
- **Existing controversy regarding perinatal outcome**
- **Perinatal outcome depends on type of TB disease**

☐ Disease dissemination and progression to more severe forms that may be more difficult to treat *(treatment initiation is also recommended as of the first trimester)*

☐ Community spread

☐ Early pregnancy loss

☐ Antenatal hospitalization

☐ Preterm labor

☐ Preeclampsia

☐ Anemia

☐ Postpartum hemorrhage

☐ Cesarean delivery

☐ Mortality

Fetal/neonatal risks with untreated active maternal TB: *(max 3)*

☐ FGR, low birthweight, or suboptimal fetal growth velocity

☐ Congenital TB[†]
- *Very rare phenomenon with high mortality rates*
- *Occurs via transplacental bacterial spread or fetal aspiration of infected amniotic fluid*

☐ Neonatal TB
- *~50% chance of infection in the first year of life without maternal treatment of active disease*
- *Occurs via exposure to aerosolized secretions*

☐ IUFD or neonatal mortality

Special note:

† Primary focus of the tuberculous bacilli develops in the fetal liver and periportal lymph nodes, followed by secondary pulmonary infection, unlike adults where >80% of primary infections are of pulmonary origin

8. In addition to an HIV-negative result, outline other required tests prior to treatment initiation and discuss serial monitoring of TB treatment response during pregnancy. *(1 point per main bullet)*   4

☐ Pretreatment HBV and HCV testing *(recommended component of routine prenatal care)*
☐ Pretreatment liver transaminases and function tests
☐ Monthly serum liver transaminases and function tests *(more frequent monitoring with risk factors for hepatotoxicity or abnormal serum tests)*
  ○ Isoniazid (INH) should be discontinued in the asymptomatic patient where ALT is more than five times the upper-normal limit or more than three times upper-normal limit with hepatitis symptoms
☐ At least monthly sputum samples until two consecutive negative cultures

9. In collaboration with the TB expert, discuss the <u>preferred empiric</u> four-drug regimen for TB susceptible disease, indicating the <u>purpose</u> of each phase of therapy. *(1 point per main and each subbullet)*   6

☐ Initial two-month intensive phase:
  ○ Isoniazid (INH), rifampin (RIF), ethambutol (EMB), pyrazinamide (PZA)[†]
  ○ *Purpose* is to eliminate most of the micro-organisms, shortening time of infectivity and to decrease risks of bacterial drug-resistance
☐ Subsequent four-month maintenance phase:
  ○ INH and RIF
  ○ *Purpose* is to ensure permanent cure without disease relapse posttreatment

Special note:
Drug doses are weight-based; although daily administration is optimal, thrice weekly regimens are available for HIV-negative patients
[†] PZA is recommended by the WHO as part of the standard regimen for treatment of active TB in pregnancy, although not routinely used in the United States due to limited safety data; use is gaining acceptance in severe disease, extrapulmonary TB, or HIV coinfection. In the absence of PZA in the treatment regimen, maintenance phase is continued for seven months' duration

10. Elaborate on the TB expert's recommended two vitamin supplements with particular anti-TB agents in treatment of the obstetric patient. *(2 points each)*   4

☐ <u>Vitamin B6 (Pyridoxine)</u> 25–50 mg/d is advised with INH as prophylaxis against peripheral neuropathy due to risk of demyelination
☐ <u>Vitamin K</u> 10 mg/d during the last four weeks of pregnancy with rifampin[‡] to protect against hemorrhagic disease of the newborn

Special note:
[‡] Rifampin is a potent hepatic enzyme inducer

The patient consents to thrice weekly anti-TB directly observed four-agent empiric therapy, which has been initiated at 15^{+4} weeks' gestation, the same day she met the infectious disease expert. She has been informed to isolate for the first two weeks of therapy, following which she would be considered noninfectious. Given absence of obstetric complaints warranting presentation for medical care, she calls your office for advice on maternal-fetal monitoring during treatment.

11. With focus on anti-TB treatment, review important aspects of health maintenance with the patient, including adverse reactions where prompt reporting is advised. *(1 point per main bullet)*

Max 4

☐ Encourage continued abstinence from alcohol consumption and other hepatotoxic agents

Prompt reporting is advised with any of the following:
☐ Severe reactions, such as fever, shock, or purpura
  ○ *very rare; may be caused by RIF or PZA*
☐ Hepatitis manifestations (*e.g.*, jaundice, abdominal/right upper quadrant discomfort, dark urine, bleeding/easy bruising, nausea/vomiting, severe fatigue/weakness)
  ○ *INH, RIF or PZA may cause drug-induced hepatitis, more common in the third trimester*
☐ Visual impairment or changes (*e.g.*, decreased color discrimination, blurring, spots)
  ○ *usually associated with EMB*
☐ Neuropsychiatric manifestations (*e.g.*, mania, depression, memory loss, seizures)
  ○ *possibly associated with INH*

12. Specify your <u>fetal</u> management plan during the antepartum period and at delivery, assuming the patient *remains adherent* and has an *appropriate response* to anti-TB therapy. *(1 point each)*

Max 3

☐ Routine antepartum fetal care: there are no specific indications for more frequent monitoring[§]
☐ Antepartum NICU consultation
☐ Testing of umbilical cord blood for acid-fast bacilli at delivery
☐ Arrange for histopathological examination of the placenta and umbilical cord (*assess for congenital TB*)

Special note:
§ *Rarely*, rifampin has been associated with limb reduction defects and central nervous system abnormalities

With directly observed therapy by a trained community health care worker using in-person visits and digital modalities, the patient remains adherent during the intensive treatment phase. At 23 weeks' gestation, after completing two months of therapy, her morning sputum sample is negative for acid-fast bacilli. She has not experienced adverse effects warranting interruption or alternative treatment. Obstetric course has been unremarkable, and she is keen to continue the next four months of maintenance therapy to optimize the chance for cure. Daily oral vitamin K supplementation will be given in the last month of pregnancy.

13. In collaboration with the infectious disease expert, explain to the patient when and how she would be considered <u>cured</u> from bacteriologically confirmed TB.

1

☐ Microscopy smear-negative (or culture-negative) in the last month of treatment and on at least one previous occasion

Special note:
Molecular techniques cannot be used to diagnose cure because results can remain positive for up to five to six years after TB micro-organisms have been effectively killed

14. Address your obstetric trainee's inquiry regarding situations where anti-TB treatment response would be considered <u>inadequate</u>.[†] *(1 point each)*

Max 2

☐ Nonconversion of sputum smear acid-fast bacilli after two to three months of therapy
☐ Sputum cultures are positive at four months (United States) or five months (Europe/ WHO) after initiation of therapy, or revert to positive after completion of treatment
☐ Clinical deterioration or lack of symptomatic improvement

Special note:
† For the scope of this document, '*inadequate*' treatment response includes slow response, drug-resistance or relapse of infection

At 37 weeks' gestation, spontaneous labor results in an unremarkable vaginal delivery of a vigorous newborn with normal birthweight. The delivering physician sampled the umbilical cord blood and the placenta has been sent to the pathology laboratory as planned. Vitamin K has been administered to the newborn and tests will be performed to assess for TB infection.

One month prior to delivery, the patient's sputum sample remained negative for acid-fast bacilli.

15-A. Discuss your recommendations regarding the separation of this newborn from the patient with active TB disease.

1

☐ No mother–infant separation is required as the patient had more than two weeks of RIF and INH-containing treatment and her sputum smear is negative for acid-fast bacilli

15-B. Identify the rare situations warranting careful risk assessment for possible mother–infant separation. *(1 point each)*

2

☐ Untreated (or suboptimally treated) active *respiratory* TB disease at delivery
☐ Multi-drug-resistant types of TB

16. Counsel this patient on breastfeeding recommendations and provide general contraceptive particularities for patients with TB or on treatment. *(1 point per main bullet)*

Max 5

Breastfeeding while taking first-line anti-TB treatments:

☐ Encourage breastfeeding as the patient has had more than two weeks of treatment, sputum smear is negative for acid-fast bacilli, and she does not have HIV infection

☐ Reassure the patient that no infant toxic effects occur with *first-line* anti-TB treatment regimens *(although infant serum levels are highest for INH, they remain below therapeutic levels)*

☐ Suggest consideration for taking anti-TB agents *immediately after* breastfeeding

☐ *Controversial* practice recommendations on the need for pyridoxine supplementation for breastfed infants who are not **themselves** on INH[†]

   ○ Infant pyridoxine supplementation is uniformly indicated for infants taking INH

General contraceptive issues with active TB or on treatment:

☐ Rifampin increases contraceptive failure of estrogen-containing oral agents

☐ No contraindications to hormonal/intrauterine contraception with **nonpelvic** TB

   ○ With **pelvic-TB**, IUD insertion represents an unacceptable health risk (UK and US-MEC,[§] category 4)

Special notes:

† Pyridoxine supplementation is not required according to the American Academy of Pediatrics Committee on Infectious Disease. Red Book 2018–2021: report on the committee on infectious diseases. 31st ed. Elk Grove Village, IL: American Academy of Pediatrics; 2018

§ UK and US Medical Eligibility Criteria (MEC) for Contraceptive Use, 2016; UK-MEC revised September 2019, US-MEC amended 2020

Three weeks later, an obstetric care provider calls you seeking advice for an early prenatal patient with reportedly latent TB.

Refer to:
Malhamé I et al. Latent Tuberculosis in Pregnancy: A Systematic Review. *PLoS One.* 2016;11(5): e0154825.

17. Indicate important aspects you would discuss prior to providing safe advice for the prenatal management of your colleague's patient. *(1 point each)*

4

☐ Ensure absence of HIV infection

☐ Absence of medico-social risk factors for progression to active disease

☐ Normal chest radiograph

☐ Absence of any respiratory or nonrespiratory signs/symptoms featured in active TB disease

Special note:
Respiratory specimens for smear microscopy and culture would only be required with abnormal chest X-ray or clinical suspicion of TB disease

18. Indicate your recommended pregnancy management if the patient is asymptomatic with an unremarkable medical history and a normal chest X-ray.   1

☐ Deferral of TB treatment until three months postpartum due to increased risk of INH-related hepatotoxicity during pregnancy and early postpartum period

19. Your colleague is keen to know the <u>preferred</u> regimen if antenatal treatment of latent TB infection was warranted.   2

☐ INH 5 mg/kg (max 300 mg) daily for nine months combined with pyridoxine 25–50 mg/d, with appropriate monitoring of liver enzymes
  ○ *Directly observed therapy is advised*

Special notes:
(a) RIF-based regimens for latent TB infection treatment in pregnancy may be used for INH-resistant/RIF-sensitive strains
(b) Currently, there is no data to support use of *rifamycin*-based regimen for treatment of latent TB infection in pregnancy

Your colleague appreciates your evidence-based recommendations and wishes to further benefit from your expertise: he or she wonders about the safety of the tuberculin skin test (TST) during pregnancy and whether test interpretation is affected by pregnancy.

20. Troubleshoot the physician's concerns regarding TST performance during pregnancy.   1

☐ TST is safe in pregnancy without impact on clinical response

21. Alert your colleague of an alternative TB screening test, highlighting its advantages over traditional skin testing. *(1 point per main bullet)*   4

☐ Interferon gamma-release assay (IGRA) is performed on whole blood; it detects the presence of the cytokine 'interferon gamma,' produced in response to stimulation with *M. tuberculosis*-specific antigens *{ESAT-6 and CFP-10}*

Advantages of IGRA over TST:
☐ IGRA results are not influenced by previous BCG vaccination
  ○ *BCG vaccine and TST use M. bovis inactivated antigens; cross reactivity may lead to false-positive results*
☐ Objective blood test results avoid human error in assessing skin reactions
☐ Only one clinical visit is necessary

Special note:
Readers may refer to the online TST/IGRA interpreter (version 3.0) based on an individual's clinical profile, available at www.tstin3d.com/en/calc.html, accessed January 17, 2021.

TOTAL: 95

CHAPTER 37

Cystic Fibrosis in Pregnancy

Jennifer Landry and Amira El-Messidi

A 26-year-old Caucasian primigravida with cystic fibrosis (CF) is referred by her primary care provider for prenatal care of her desired pregnancy. Dating ultrasound has just confirmed a viable singleton intrauterine pregnancy at 8^{+0} weeks' gestation.

LEARNING OBJECTIVES

1. Take a focused prenatal history from a patient with CF, and be able to recognize disease-related factors that may predict poor obstetric outcome
2. Identify disease-associated absolute contraindications to pregnancy
3. Understand the genetics of CF inheritance, and provide preliminary calculations for fetal risk of transmission
4. Discuss the effects of pregnancy on CF-related complications, as well as the effects of CF on obstetric risk
5. Demonstrate the ability to plan and manage the antepartum, intrapartum, and postpartum care of a patient with CF, recognizing the importance of continued multidisciplinary collaboration

SUGGESTED READINGS

1. Edenborough FP, Borgo G, Knoop C, et al. European Cystic Fibrosis Society. Guidelines for the management of pregnancy in women with cystic fibrosis. *J Cyst Fibros.* 2008;7 (Suppl 1): S2–32.
2. Geake J, Tay G, Callaway L, et al. Pregnancy and cystic fibrosis: approach to contemporary management. *Obstet Med.* 2014; 7(4):147–155.
3. Grigoriadis C, Tympa A, Theodoraki K. Cystic fibrosis and pregnancy: counseling, obstetrical management and perinatal outcome. *Invest Clin.* 2015; 56(1):66–72.
4. Heltshe SL, Godfrey EM, Josephy T, et al. Pregnancy among cystic fibrosis women in the era of CFTR modulators. *J Cyst Fibros.* 2017;16(6):687–694.
5. Lau EMT, Moriarty C, Ogle R, et al. Pregnancy and cystic fibrosis. *Paediatr Respir Rev.* 2010; 11:90–94.
6. McArdle J. Pregnancy in cystic fibrosis. *Clin Chest Med.* 2011; 32:111–120.

7. Middleton PG, Gade EJ, Aguilera C, et al. ERS/TSANZ Task Force Statement on the management of reproduction and pregnancy in women with airways diseases. *Eur Respir J.* 2020;55:1901208.

8. Panchaud A, Di Paolo ER, Koutsokera A, et al. Safety of drugs during pregnancy and breastfeeding in cystic fibrosis patients. *Respiration.* 2016;91(4):333–348.

9. Roe AH, Traxler S, Schreiber CA. Contraception in women with cystic fibrosis: a systematic review of the literature. *Contraception.* 2016; 93:3–10.

10. Whitty JE. Cystic fibrosis and pregnancy. *Clin Obstetr Gynecol.* 2010;53(2):369–376.

	POINTS
1. With respect to CF, what aspects of a focused history would you want to know? *(1 point each unless indicated; max points specified where required)*	Max 32

☐ Names and contacts of multidisciplinary CF-treating team

Pulmonary manifestations: *(max 8)*
☐ Recent lung function (mainly forced expiratory volume at one second (FEV1))
☐ Bacterial colonization with *Pseudomonas aeruginosa* or *Burkholderia cepacia* or other multidrug resistant bacteria
☐ Presence/ absence of pulmonary hypertension or cor pulmonale
☐ Asthma *(up to 32% of patients with CF will have asthma)*
☐ Chronic rhinosinusitis *(in almost 100% of patients with CF)*
☐ Nasal polyps
☐ Prior pneumothorax
☐ Hospitalizations/ ICU (ITU) admissions
☐ Prior lung transplant

Extrapulmonary manifestations: *(2 points per system)*
☐ *Endocrine*: diabetes mellitus, osteoporosis, bone disease (arthropathy)
☐ *Gastrointestinal:* pancreatic insufficiency, malabsorption, malnutrition, gastroesophageal reflux disease, constipation, distal ileal obstruction syndrome, liver cirrhosis or portal hypertension
☐ *Nutritional status:* presence of malnutrition
☐ *Renal:* calculi, chronic kidney disease (CKD) *(secondary to diabetes mellitus or aminoglycosides)*
☐ *Psychiatric:* anxiety, depression

Medications and allergies: *(max 10)*
☐ Oral, IV, inhaled antibiotics *(including assessment of possibly teratogenic agents)*
☐ Bronchodilators and inhaled corticosteroids
☐ Inhaled hypertonic saline
☐ Sinus rinses and nasal corticosteroids
☐ Cystic fibrosis transmembrane conductance regulator (CFTR) modulators – *individualized assessment for risk-benefit ratio if continued use in pregnancy*
☐ Mucolytic agents: inhaled dornase alfa *(no safety data in pregnancy, however unlikely to affect the fetus)*

- ☐ Pancreatic enzyme replacements
- ☐ Insulin
- ☐ Fat-soluble vitamin supplements (Vitamin A, D, E, and K) and calcium supplements
- ☐ Prenatal vitamins, antiemetics, antacids
- ☐ Nonprescription, over the counter and herbal treatments to be noted
  - ○ Compliance with medication (**Key component** *of discussion as it impacts prognosis of the patient with CF and pregnancy outcome*)
- ☐ Allergies

Social features and routine health maintenance:
- ☐ Occupation, smoking tobacco, alcohol consumption, recreational drugs, support-systems, habitat (*i.e., proximity to factories/ pollutant industries*)
- ☐ Vaccination status

Family history (as specific to CF):
- ☐ Affected family members
- ☐ Medical diseases

Male partner: (*max 1*)
- ☐ Ethnicity[†]
- ☐ Genetic screening

Special note:
- † Ethnicity and genetic defects of CF do not have prognostic/management value for the affected mother and are not relevant aspects in her focused history but are relevant for the partner in fetal risk assessment of CF

The patient is compliant with her CF-multidisciplinary care in your tertiary-care hospital. She has bronchiectasis and is colonized with *Pseudomonas aeruginosa;* she also suffers from chronic rhinosinusitis. The patient is pancreatic insufficient.

Two months ago, her FEV1 was 2.05 L (68% predicted). To date, she has screened negative for CF-related diabetes, but has trouble maintaining her weight. She has not had prior surgeries.

She currently takes suppressive inhaled tobramycin, inhaled dornase alfa, pancreatic enzymes replacements, nasal saline rinses, and supplemental vitamins and minerals (Vitamin A, D, E, and K as well as calcium supplements) to which she responds well. She performs daily chest physio-therapy. She is not currently taking a CFTR modulator, as she was concerned about starting new medications in the preconceptional period yet is now inquiring about its safety profile and recommendations during the antenatal period.

2. What is one of the most likely CFTR mutations in this patient, and why?   1

- ☐ ΔF508, Caucasian race

3. The patient's menarche occurred at age 16 years and her menstrual cycles are often irregular. Which tissue containing CFTR proteins may be associated with subfertility in this population? *(1 point each)*

    ☐ Hypothalamus *(anovulation)*
    ☐ Endometrium
    ☐ Cervical mucosa
    ☐ Fallopian tubes

Max 3

4. Indicate six CF-related factors that, when present, may predict poor obstetric outcome, and specify which are absolute contraindications to pregnancy *(1 point each, unless specified)*

    ☐ Cor pulmonale (absolute contraindication) **(2 points)**
    ☐ Pulmonary hypertension (absolute contraindication) **(2 points)**
    ☐ Hypoxemia (absolute contraindication) **(2 points)**
    ☐ Hypercarbia or the presence of chronic respiratory failure (absolute contraindication) **(2 points)**
    ☐ Severe malnutrition (BMI <18 kg/m^2, or $>15\%$ from predicted ideal body weight for height)
    ☐ Diabetes mellitus
    ☐ FEV1 $<60\%$ predicted/advanced lung disease
    ☐ Colonization with *B. cepacia*
    ☐ Liver disease *(limited literature to guide this relative contraindication)*

Max 10

5. How would you best address her inquiry about starting a CFTR-modulator? *(1 point each)*

    ☐ Seek the opinion of her treating respirologist
    ☐ Treatment considerations depend on the genotype of her CFTR mutation and whether she fulfills criteria for therapy. Orkambi™ (lumacaftor/ivacaftor) is indicated for patients that are homozygous for the ΔF508 mutation. Symdeko™ (tezacaftor/ivacaftor) and the newly released Trikafta™ (elexacaftor, tezacaftor and ivacaftor) are also indicated for patients who are homozygous for the ΔF508 mutation but these two drugs are also indicated for many other combinations of CFTR mutations, even in the absence of one ΔF508 mutation
    ☐ Currently there is no scientific data to support the use of CFTR-modulators in pregnancy and their safety remains unknown. Treatment with CFTR-modulators is not recommended in pregnancy but are generally continued if they have been initiated preconception in a female patient with severe lung disease because of the significant risk of exacerbation and lung function decline when the drug is discontinued. The risk-benefit ratio of continuing the medication merits comprehensive discussion with the patient and the treating medical team for management planning during the antenatal period.

Max 2

6. She asks you about the safety of continuing her inhaled tobramycin therapy during pregnancy, as she is concerned about recurrent or worsening lung infections if she discontinues her medication. Discuss your counseling and best practice management. *(1 point each)*

Max 2

☐ Recommend continuation of inhaled tobramycin, generally maintained at the same dose
☐ Inform the patient of the *rare* risk of fetal ototoxicity and nephrotoxicity
☐ May switch to nebulised colistin *(experience suggests safety in pregnancy)*

The patient is homozygous for the ΔF508 mutation. Six months ago, she and her Caucasian partner were sent for genetic counseling. Due to anxiety, he did not present for his screening test.

7. Given an untested partner, what is their baseline risk of a CF-affected fetus?   2

☐ 1/50 = (1/2 x 1/25)

8. During your first prenatal visit, her partner continues to decline genotype testing. What is her best option for early prenatal diagnosis of CF?   1

☐ Chorionic villus sampling†

Special note:
† Refer to Questions 10 and 11 in Chapter 64

9. If the patient opts out of prenatal diagnosis, which ultrasound marker might her geneticist be most attentive to?   1

☐ Echogenic bowel *(low specificity)*

In view of their current pregnancy, her partner decides to get screened for CF; the test has a 90% sensitivity. There is no mutation detected among the genetic panel performed. They appear concerned about potential obstetric and disease adversities that may result from the gestational process.

10. Given this information, what is the couple's current risk of a CF-affected fetus?   2

☐ 1/492 = (1/2 x 1/246)

11. Apart from risks of disease inheritance, outline obstetric aspects to discuss with the couple.   3
    (1 point each)

☐ No increased baseline risk of congenital anomalies due to CF itself *(risk factor based)*
☐ Preterm delivery *(delivery at <37 weeks' gestation in 10%–25% of patients)*
☐ Fetal growth restriction (FGR) or low birthweight less than 2500 g

12. Provide comprehensive patient counseling on pregnancy-associated disease morbidities. *(1 point each unless specified)*

☐ Essential aspect of discussion with this patient and her partner is the decreased life expectancy of the mother *(mean survival age: 38 years)* and its impact on the couple and the child **(3 points)**

☐ Pregnancy may not affect long-term survival in patients with CF unless advanced or poorly controlled disease exists

Address the risk of health deterioration in pregnancy:

☐ Increased frequency of lung infections and need for aggressive treatments, hospitalizations, and ventilation support *(mechanical ventilation, non-invasive ventilation)*

☐ Decline of FEV1 *(baseline spirometry function usually resumes postpartum)*

☐ Increased oxygen demands

☐ Increased risk of diabetes mellitus

☐ Increased risk of heart failure

☐ Increased risk of pneumothorax

☐ Increased physical and emotional fatigue

☐ Discuss potential difficulty in regaining pre-pregnancy health status

☐ Maternal mortality *(especially if FEV1 is less than 60% predicted)*

The couple appreciates your detailed counseling, and the patient mentions she opts to remain compliant with care and adherent to treatments.

13. With multidisciplinary collaboration, present your management plan for pregnancy with focus on CF. *(1 point per main bullet unless indicated; max points specified per section)*

Prenatal visits, maternal health maintenance, and focused investigations: *(max 8)*

☐ Antenatal visits at least every four weeks in the first and second trimesters, then every two weeks or weekly thereafter as progress dictates, with low threshold for hospitalizations

☐ Updating immunization records, if required

☐ Baseline maternal echocardiography

☐ Maternal weight at each visit *(although a component of routine prenatal care)* is particularly important for patients with CF

☐ Random glucose measurement at every prenatal visit

☐ Early and serial screening for (gestational) diabetes mellitus
  ○ *(European CF Society):* oral glucose tolerance testing (OGTT) at 20 weeks and repeat at 28 weeks
  ○ *(USA/ Australian guidelines):* OGTT at 12–16 weeks and repeat at 24–28 weeks

☐ Serial laboratory tests: serum albumin, total protein, CBC, liver function tests, transaminases, PT, PTT

☐ Obtain assessment of vascular access and consider securing a long-term access site

☐ Encourage increased fiber and fluid intake and/or medical treatment with laxatives as constipation requires particular attention in pregnancy for a patient with CF *(risk of distal intestinal obstruction syndrome)*

Respiratory-related care: *(max 5)*

☐ Baseline spirometry and oximetry

☐ Assess oxygen saturation at every prenatal visit

- [ ] Sputum culture at every prenatal visit
- [ ] Inhalation therapy and airway clearance therapy – *timing of inhalation therapy to airway clearance therapy is important for women who produce large quantities of sputum*
- [ ] Effective clearing of potential nasal obstruction: safe and effective treatments in pregnancy include nasal spray, nasal lavage, suction, topical nasal steroids
- [ ] Chest physiotherapy (*premeal physiotherapy may minimize reflux*)
- [ ] Pelvic floor physiotherapy

Nutrition: *(max 5)*
- [ ] Increased energy intake by ~120% to 150% above non-CF pregnant patient's increased demands by ~300 kcal/d
- [ ] Oral route preferred, with nasogastric tube or total parenteral nutrition reserved if necessary
- [ ] Prophylactic acid-suppressive therapy (protein pump inhibitors or histamine type-2 receptor antagonists)
  - Decreases aggravation of airway inflammation
  - Decreases vomiting with coughing in patients with CF
- [ ] Serial fasting serum levels of fat-soluble vitamins and supplementation as appropriate (Vitamins A, D, E, K)- *Vitamin A supplementation should be less than 10,000 IU/d*
- [ ] Assessment of serum iron levels at 20 weeks' gestation, with supplementation if needed; optimize iron absorption in patients with CF by increasing vitamin C intake
- [ ] Continuation of pancreatic enzyme replacements is essential

Fetal monitoring: *(2 points)*
- [ ] Serial sonographic growth assessments with consideration for Doppler velocimetry and cervical length assessment

At 36^{+0} weeks' gestation, her FEV_1 has declined by 13% to 1.65L (55% predicted). Oxygen saturation is maintained at 96% without supplementation, but the patient complains of shortness of breath and feels congested. Her oral secretions have become increasingly copious and thick, and she has difficulty with expectoration despite frequent airway clearance therapy.

Fetal growth biometry is on the 8th percentile for gestational age with adequate growth velocity and normal Doppler velocimetry. The cardiotocographic tracings remain normal.

Multidisciplinary experts concur that delivery is indicated in view of declining respiratory status. The patient is reassured with regard to expected fetal outcome in relation to this *late-preterm* gestational age.

14. What is your recommended mode of delivery?   1

- [ ] Aim for vaginal delivery; Cesarean section is reserved for obstetric indications or severe compromise in lung function

Similar methods for induction of labor as patients without CF

15. In affiliation with the respiratory treating team, plan <u>intrapartum management</u> focused on care of a parturient with CF. *(1 point per main and subbullet)*

Max 10

☐ Careful management of IV fluids to avoid fluid overload
☐ Early ICU consultation is advised if warranted by the patient's status
☐ Sputum culture at delivery admission
☐ IV antibiotics to cover common CF pathogens such as *Pseudomonas aeruginosa* started prior to delivery and typically continued for a 14-day course *(ideally selecting an agent compatible with breastfeeding, therefore favoring cephalosporins, penicillins with beta-lactamase inhibitors and/or carbapenems and avoiding IV aminoglycosides and respiratory quinolones such as ciprofloxacin)*
☐ Continuous monitoring of her oxygen saturation
☐ Raise the head of the bed in labor (or if Cesarean is indicated)
☐ Consideration for CPAP *(continuous positive airway pressure)* or BiPAP *(bilevel positive airway pressure)* in between contractions *(facilitates large tidal volumes and reduces respiratory rate to mobilize secretions and improve gas exchange)*
☐ Maintain continuous electronic fetal monitoring
☐ Early, low-dose epidural *(aim to reduce the risk of blockade above T10 dermatome)*
   ○ Caution with opioids *(due to respiratory depression)* and nitrous oxide *(due to barotrauma and gas trapping)*
☐ Inhalation therapy and airway clearance therapy is advised before anesthesia
☐ Delay pushing in the second stage of labor to decrease Valsalva maneuvers
☐ Maintain a low threshold for an assisted second stage *(decreases risk of pneumothoraces)*

The patient undergoes induction of labor and receives early epidural analgesia. She has an assisted vaginal delivery of a vigorous male newborn with a birthweight of 2200g.

16. What are important <u>postpartum considerations</u> to discuss, either prior to discharge and/or at the routine postpartum visit in relation to CF? *(1 point each)*

Max 10

General maternal and/or fetal well-being:
☐ Screen for postpartum depression *(particularly important for mothers with CF)*
☐ Offer psychosocial support services for maternal and newborn care
☐ Delayed removal of regional analgesia to allow for early respiratory physiotherapy
☐ Encourage breastfeeding *(individual assessment for the mother with CF is required, in consideration of her clinical status and personal preferences)*
☐ Calcium and vitamin D supplementation is an essential consideration for mothers with CF who are breastfeeding, even though all patients with CF are instructed to take calcium- and vitamin D-containing multivitamins to decrease their heightened risks of osteoporosis and osteopenia
☐ Encourage increased fluid intake if a patient with CF opts to breastfeed
☐ Complete the 14-day course of IV antibiotic *(see Question 15)*
☐ Promote early physical activity and an exercise program
☐ Provide stabilizing binders for support of pregnancy-induced abdominal hernias or diastasis recti, aggravated by repetitive coughing
☐ Offer future prenatal diagnosis, or preimplantation genetic screening

Contraceptive recommendations:

☐ Careful consideration with depot medroxyprogesterone acetate (DMPA) in a patient with CF due to inherent risks of premature osteoporosis

☐ *Theoretical* concerns of decreased hormonal absorption in a patient with CF-associated pancreatic insufficiency *(non-oral contraceptive methods will avoid hepatic first-pass metabolism)*

☐ For women who are not breastfeeding, avoid estrogen-containing contraceptives in patients with permanent venous access

☐ Significant drug interactions exist with oral contraceptives and first- and second-generation CFTR-modulators, such as Kalydeko® (Ivacaftor) and Orkambi® (Lumacaftor/Ivacaftor), with less drug interactions with Symdeko® (Tezacaftor/Ivacaftor)

TOTAL: **110**

CHAPTER 38

Chronic Hypertension and Preeclampsia/HELLP Complications of Pregnancy

Amira El-Messidi, Isabelle Malhamé, Genevieve Eastabrook, and Stella S. Daskalopoulou

A 35-year-old G2P1 with chronic hypertension is referred by her primary care provider to your tertiary-care center for prenatal care of a singleton intrauterine pregnancy at 8^{+2} weeks' gestation by dating sonography. The patient has no obstetric complaints to date. Her last pregnancy was 10 years ago.

LEARNING OBJECTIVES

1. Take a focused prenatal history of a patient with chronic hypertension, recognizing risk factors for superimposed preeclampsia to address in counseling and management
2. Understand the potential value of maternal serum biomarkers and Doppler velocimetry in predicting preeclampsia
3. Identify antihypertensive agents commonly used in pregnancy and in obstetric hypertensive crises
4. Detail prophylactic management of eclampsia, and incur emergent treatment of magnesium toxicity
5. Provide counseling on future health risks after hypertensive disorders of pregnancy

SUGGESTED READINGS

1. ACOG Committee Opinion No. 767. Emergent therapy for acute-onset, severe hypertension during pregnancy and the postpartum period. *Obstet Gynecol.* 2019;133(2):e174–e180.
2. American College of Obstetricians and Gynecologists' Committee on Practice Bulletins – Obstetrics. ACOG Practice Bulletin No. 209: Obstetric analgesia and anesthesia. *Obstet Gynecol.* 2019;133(3):e208–e225.
3. Brown MA, Magee LA, Kenny LC, et al. The hypertensive disorders of pregnancy: ISSHP classification, diagnosis and management recommendations for international practice. *Pregnancy Hypertens.* 2018;13:291–310.
4. Combs CA, Montgomery DM. Society for Maternal-Fetal Medicine (SMFM) Special Statement: Checklists for preeclampsia risk-factor screening to guide recommendations for prophylactic low-dose aspirin. *Am J Obstet Gynecol.* 2020 Sept;223(3):B7–B11.
5. Gestational hypertension and preeclampsia: ACOG Practice Bulletin No. 222. *Obstet Gynecol.* 2020;135(6):e237–e260.
6. Lauder J, Sciscione A, Biggio J, et al. Society for Maternal-Fetal Medicine Consult Series No. 50: The role of activity restriction in obstetric management: *Am J Obstet Gynecol.* 2020;223(2):B2–B10.

7. Magee LA, Pels A, Helewa M, et al. Diagnosis, evaluation, and management of the hypertensive disorders of pregnancy: executive summary. *J Obstet Gynaecol Can.* 2014;36(5):416–441.

8. National Institute for Health and Care Excellence (NICE). Hypertension in pregnancy: diagnosis and management (NICE guideline NG133). 2019. Available at www.nice.org.uk/guidance/ng133. Accessed September 10, 2020.

9. Poon LC, Shennan A, Hyett JA, et al. The International Federation of Gynecology and Obstetrics (FIGO) initiative on pre-eclampsia: A pragmatic guide for first-trimester screening and prevention. *Int J Gynaecol Obstet.* 2019;145(Suppl 1):1–33. [Correction in *Int J Gynaecol Obstet.* 2019 Sep;146(3):390–391]

10. Rabi DM, McBrien KA, Sapir-Pichhadze R, et al. Hypertension Canada's 2020 comprehensive guidelines for the prevention, diagnosis, risk assessment, and treatment of hypertension in adults and children. *Can J Cardiol.* 2020;36(5):596–624.

11. Sotiriadis A, Hernandez-Andrade E, da Silva Costa F, et al. ISUOG Practice Guidelines: role of ultrasound in screening for and follow-up of pre-eclampsia. *Ultrasound Obstet Gynecol.* 2019;53(1):7–22.

POINTS

1. What aspects of a focused history would you want to know? *(1 point each)*　　　Max 10

Chronic hypertension:
- ☐ Chronology of development of chronic hypertension in relation to prior pregnancy
- ☐ Determine the cause of hypertension *(i.e., essential or secondary hypertension)*
- ☐ Assess for the presence of end-organ complications: *(i.e., cardiovascular, renal, neurologic, metabolic diseases)*
- ☐ *Medications:* elicit current and prior use
- ☐ Name and contact of treating physician

Current pregnancy:
- ☐ Establish whether artificial reproductive techniques were used
- ☐ Determine if primipaternity
- ☐ Prepregnancy weight

Prior pregnancy:
- ☐ Assess for maternal-fetal complications
- ☐ Delivery details: gestational age, mode of delivery, birthweight

Social history:
- ☐ Smoking tobacco, alcohol consumption, substance use aggravating hypertension *(e.g., cocaine, amphetamines)*

Allergies and contraindications to potential therapeutic agents:
- ☐ Asthma *(contraindication to aspirin, labetalol)*
- ☐ Nasal polyps *(contraindication to aspirin)*

Family history:
- ☐ First-degree relative with preeclampsia *(i.e., mother or sister)*
- ☐ Cardiovascular diseases *(e.g., stroke, coronary artery disease, hypertension)*, metabolic syndrome, type 1 or type 2 diabetes mellitus

The patient developed essential hypertension six years ago and has since been taking hydrochlorothiazide 25 mg daily. She has no end-organ dysfunction, ascertained on routine serial investigations nine months ago. She does not smoke cigarettes, drink alcohol, or use recreational drugs. Last year, her sister delivered at 27 weeks' gestation due to preeclampsia.

Current pregnancy was conceived spontaneously with her partner of four years.

On exam, blood pressure (BP) is 145/93 mmHg and BMI is 27.5 kg/m^2.

2. Although no universal agreement exists for target BP range in pregnancy, provide the patient with a safe antenatal target value. *(Any adequate range)*   1

Examples include:
☐ BP $\leq$110–140/85 mmHg *(ISSHP[3])*; 130–155/90–105 mmHg *(SOGC[7])*;135/85 mmHg *(NICE[8])*

3. With interdisciplinary collaboration, outline your suggestions for management of the diuretic agent. *(either practice recommendation)*   1

Thiazide agents: *(controversial; no universal consensus)*
☐ Alternative therapies preferred; increased risk of congenital abnormalities and neonatal complications *(NICE[8])*
☐ Accepted as second-line antihypertensives in pregnancy *(ISSHP[3], Hypertension Canada[10])*

Plans are made to replace the hydrochlorothiazide. You inform her that there is no difference in clinical outcome among preferred first-line agents.

4. Provide one pharmacologic first-line oral agent and indicate its starting and maximum dose. *(Any bullet for 3 points)*   Max 3

	First-line oral drugs	Initial dose	Max dose
☐	Labetalol	100 mg twice daily	2400 mg/d
☐	Long-acting nifedipine	30–60 mg once daily	120 mg/d
☐	Methyldopa	250 mg every 8–12 hours	3000 mg/d

Special note:
Other first-line β-blockers include acebutolol, metoprolol, pindolol, and propanolol

5. Regarding chronic hypertension, indicate laboratory investigations you would perform at the initial prenatal visit. *(1 point each)*

Max 6

Serum:
☐ Full or complete blood count (FBC, CBC)
☐ Liver enzymes (AST, ALT), and lactate dehydrogenase (LDH)
☐ Liver function tests: INR, serum bilirubin, serum albumin
☐ Serum creatinine and electrolytes
☐ Serum uric acid[‡]

Urine:
☐ Urinalysis and microscopy
☐ Urine protein-to-creatinine ratio (UPCR)

Special note:
‡ While serum uric acid is not a diagnostic criterion for preeclampsia, increased gestation-corrected values are associated with worse maternal and fetal outcomes

6. Detail your counseling and management regarding the risk of superimposed preeclampsia. *(1 point per main bullet)*

Max 7

☐ Advise the patient of at least 25% risk of superimposed preeclampsia on chronic hypertension
☐ Recommend home BP monitoring, and encourage early reporting of symptoms or signs suggestive of hypertensive diseases
　○ *Instruct the patient that decreased dosing of antihypertensive agents in the second trimester is consistent with physiological changes in BP*
☐ Advise maintenance of a low salt diet based on chronic hypertension
☐ Anticipate serial laboratory testing, at least at 28 and 34 weeks' gestation
☐ Advise low-dose aspirin (LDASA) 75–162 mg, taken nightly (*exact dosing varies by jurisdiction*), as this is currently the only evidence-based preventative strategy for preeclampsia among high-risk women, providing up to 60% reduction in preterm preeclampsia
　○ Ideally initiated prior to 16 weeks' gestation, although there may be benefit from initiation up to 28 weeks' gestation
　○ Discontinue at delivery or diagnosis of preeclampsia
　○ Not a contraindication to neuraxial analgesia
☐ Consideration for high-dose calcium supplementation (*e.g.,* elemental calcium 1.2–2.5 g/d) for women with low calcium intake, defined as less than four daily servings or less than 600–800 mg/d[†]
☐ Plan first-trimester sonography with consideration for uterine artery Doppler (UtAD) velocimetry *(refer to Question 13)*
☐ Plan second-trimester fetal morphology sonography with subsequent serial monitoring of fetal growth biometry, amniotic fluid volume, fetal Doppler velocimetry (where indicated), and assessment of sonographic signs of placental abruption

☐ Encourage moderate intensity physical activity as a meaningful means to reduce the risk of preeclampsia; advise at least 150 minutes/week, over a minimum of three to four days per week, unless otherwise contraindicated

☐ Encourage compliance with multidisciplinary care and adherence to treatment

Special note:

† Recommended by the ISSHP[3] and SOGC[7]; *refer to* Hofmeyr GJ, Lawrie TA, Atallah ÁN, Torloni MR. Calcium supplementation during pregnancy for preventing hypertensive disorders and related problems. *Cochrane Database Syst Rev.* 2018;10(10):CD001059. Published 2018 Oct 1.

---

7. Explain to your trainee plausible biological mechanisms for the circadian benefit of nightly aspirin intake. *(1 point each)*   Max 2

☐ Reduction of the renin-angiotensin-aldosterone system activity
☐ Reduction in excretion of urinary cortisol, dopamine, and norepinephrine
☐ Enhanced release of nitric oxide (vasodilatory chemical) during the night

---

8. Address your trainee's inquiry regarding the proposed relationship between low calcium intake and hypertensive disorders of pregnancy.   1

☐ Increased secretion of renin and parathyroid hormone due to a low calcium environment results in increased intracellular calcium within vascular smooth muscle, stimulating vasoconstriction

---

After this consultation, you take the opportunity to elaborate on 'clinical risk factor'-based assessment with your trainee, upon which decisions for prophylaxis are based.

---

9. Discuss the relationship, *if any*, between maternal age and gestational age at onset of preeclampsia. *(1 point each)*   Max 1

☐ Maternal age has no effect on <u>early-onset</u> disease requiring delivery prior to 34^{+0} weeks
☐ Maternal age increases the risk of <u>late-onset</u> preeclampsia requiring delivery at $\geq 34^{+0}$ weeks (risk increases by 4% per year greater than 32 years of age)

---

10. Based on the patient's demographics and history, elicit the risk factors for preeclampsia, justifying prophylaxis. *(1 point each)*   4

☐ Chronic hypertension
☐ Primipaternity
☐ Interpregnancy interval >10 years (or short interval <12 months)
☐ Age ≥ 35 or 40 years *(varies by jurisdiction)*

11. Identify <u>other</u> strong or moderate risk factors for preeclampsia that play a role in the clinical decision for administration of prophylactic LDASA. *(1 point each; max points specified per category)*

Max 6

Strong: *(max 3)*
☐ Pregestational diabetes mellitus
☐ Autoimmune disease *(e.g., systemic lupus erythematosus, antiphospholipid antibody syndrome)*
☐ Chronic kidney disease
☐ Previous pregnancy with preeclampsia
☐ Multiple gestations (either a strong or moderate risk factor, depending on jurisdictional practice recommendation[†])
☐ Artificial reproductive technology *(ISSHP[3])*

Moderate: *(max 3)*
☐ Obesity[‡] (BMI $\geq$30–35 kg/m^2) prepregnancy or at the first prenatal visit
☐ Nulliparity
☐ Sociodemographic characteristics, including low socioeconomic status, Afro-Caribbean or South Asian ethnicity
☐ Low maternal birthweight
☐ Cocaine or methamphetamine use *(SOGC[7])*
☐ First-degree family history of preeclampsia *(i.e., mother/sister)*

Special notes:
† Strong risk factor by ISSHP[3], SMFM[4], and ACOG[5]; a moderate risk factor by NICE[8]
‡ Strong risk factor by ISSHP[3]

You inform your trainee that prediction models for preeclampsia remain investigational with limited universal availability. Your tertiary center offers early pregnancy biomarker testing and maternal Doppler assessments, which you have discussed with the patient.

Special notes:
ACOG and SOGC do not currently recommend screening for early-onset preeclampsia using screening algorithms outside of a research setting; ISSHP, FIGO, ISUOG support first-trimester screening for preeclampsia (varying combinations)

12. State the currently known best biochemical marker for preeclampsia prediction.

1

☐ Placental growth factor (PlGF)

Serum laboratory investigations requested at the first prenatal visit are unremarkable, and UPCR is below 30 mg/mmol (265 mg/g).

Attending in the ultrasound unit for the patient's sonogram at 12^{+2} weeks' gestation, the following is noted.

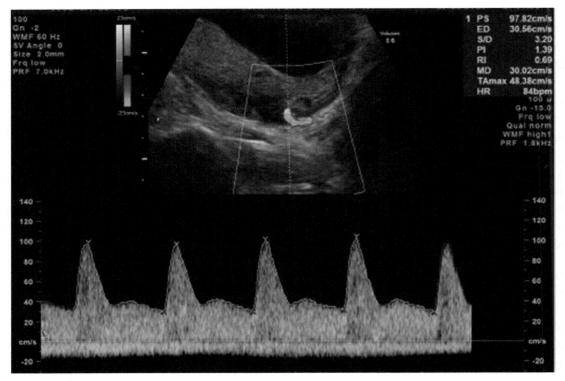

Figure 38.1

With permission: Figure 1 from ISUOG practice guidelines: role of ultrasound in screening for and follow-up of pre-eclampsia. Ultrasound Obstet Gynecol. 2019;53(1):7–22.

There is no association between this case scenario and this patient's image. Image used for educational purposes only.

13-A. Identify the image representation and explain to your obstetric trainee what would constitute an abnormality. *(1 point per main bullet)*   2

☐ Uterine artery Doppler waveform (UtAD)[†]
☐ Increased resistance is implied by a pulsatility index (PI) >95th percentile, with cutoff values being based on technique:
  ○ PI >2.35 *(transabdominal scan at 11^{+0} to 13^{+6} weeks)*[§]
  ○ PI >3.10 *(transvaginal scan up to CRL of 65 mm, declining to PI >2.36 by CRL of 84 mm)*[‡]

Special notes:
† Peak systolic velocity (PSV) >60 cm/s ensures sampling of the uterine rather than arcuate artery
§ UtAD PI >1.44 *(transabdominally at second-trimester scan)*
‡ UtAD PI >1.58 *(transvaginally at second-trimester scan)*

13-B. Explain the preferred use of PI compared to the systolic/diastolic ratio or resistive index parameters. *(1 point each)*   2

☐ PI includes an averaged value of all maximum velocities in the cardiac cycle
☐ PI remains stable despite absent or reversed diastolic flow

Your trainee noticed the diastolic notch and is curious about possible implications.

14. Discuss the caveats of UtAD notching as an index in preeclampsia screening, assuming appropriate scanning technique and waveform representation. *(1 point each)*

Max 1

☐ First-trimester notching is present in ~43% of cases and may be normal; notching is abnormal on second-trimester scans
☐ Subjectivity is involved in determining presence of a notch

15. Refer to physiologic changes to explain the increased resistance in the UtAD among pregnancies at risk of preeclampsia.

1

☐ Incomplete migration of interstitial and endovascular trophoblast into the walls of spiral arterioles, which would normally lead to a low-resistance, low-pressure and high-flow system
  ○ Unique conversion of decidual segments of spiral arterioles, without myometrial changes

Ultrasound shows a nuchal translucency (NT) of 1.3 mm with normal fetal morphology. Serum PlGF is 0.25 multiples of the median (MoM) and pregnancy-associated plasma protein-A (PAPP-A) is <0.41 MoM. Uterine artery Doppler PI is <95th percentile. Aneuploidy screening is negative for trisomy 21.

Given abnormal serum biomarkers, you inform the patient of the increased risk of superimposed preeclampsia and reinforce compliance with the prearranged maternal-fetal care plan.

The patient was hopeful the normal UtAD PI, as a standalone test, would be reassuring regarding pregnancy-related risks.

16. Assuming appropriate skill, list maternal factors that may affect the UtAD PI and limit its value as a standalone test in preeclampsia risk assessment. *(1 point each)*

Max 5

☐ BMI *(inverse relation with UtAD PI)*
☐ Ethnicity *(individuals of African origin have increased PI)*
☐ Uterine contraction during assessment
☐ Maternal heart rate
☐ Gestational age
☐ Maternal age
☐ Type 1 diabetes mellitus
☐ Prior preeclampsia

Routine second-trimester fetal morphology survey reveals biometry on the 15th percentile and normal amniotic fluid volume for gestational age. Home BP is maintained <135/85 mmHg with oral labetalol 200 mg twice daily. She is asymptomatic. Serial laboratory investigations and urine proteinuria remain unremarkable. Fetal growth scans show adequate growth velocity on the 12th–15th percentile, normal amniotic fluid volume, umbilical artery (UA) Doppler; there are no sonographic signs of abruption. Routine screening for gestational diabetes mellitus (GDM) at 25 weeks' gestation is normal.

At 30^{+1} weeks' gestation, the patient presents to the obstetric emergency assessment unit with a three-hour history of new-onset, localized, epigastric pain without accompanying gastroesophageal reflux, nausea, or vomiting. She denies any headache, visual changes, chest pain, or shortness of breath. Blood pressure is 160/105 mmHg, and 15-minute repeat testing is 155/102 mmHg.

Upon admission, nifedipine XL is started and titrated to 60 mg orally twice daily to maintain the BP at 130–140/85 mmHg. The epigastric pain improved with nonnarcotic analgesics.

17. Although not universally endorsed, which biomarker(s) *may* help determine whether presenting features are due to preeclampsia? *(1 point per main bullet)*   2

☐ sFlt-1/PlGF ratio ≥85 at <34 weeks *(preeclampsia likely)*
   ○ *Ratio ≤38 can rule out preeclampsia within the next week*
   ○ *Ratio 38–84 = high likelihood of preeclampsia within four weeks*
☐ PlGF <12 pg/ml *(preeclampsia likely)*
   ○ *12–100 pg/ml = suggestive of preeclampsia*

Special note:
Cutoff levels of ratio are dependent on gestational age

In the obstetric emergency assessment unit, fetal cardiotocography (CTG) is normal and uterine quiescence is ascertained. The patient has no obstetric complaints.

Your trainee informs you of the patient's laboratory results:

		Reference
ALT (IU/L)	62	6–45
AST (IU/L)	89	6–35
Platelets (x 10^9/L)	150	150–429
Creatinine (umol/L)	65	40–70
Normal coagulation function		
UPCR	47 mg/mmol (474 mg/g)	< 30 mg/mmol (265 mg/g)

Affiliated medical consultants involved in her care have been notified.

18. Indicate the most likely <u>pregnancy-related</u> causes of liver enzyme elevation at this stage of pregnancy. *(1 point each)*   Max 2

☐ Preeclampsia with severity features
☐ HELLP syndrome
☐ Intrahepatic cholestasis of pregnancy
☐ Acute fatty liver of pregnancy (AFLP)

19. Inform your trainee of required investigations to assess for the presence of a hemolytic process. *(1 point each)*

Max 3

☐ Serum LDH
☐ Serum haptoglobin
☐ Serum total bilirubin
☐ Blood smear for schistocytes

There is no evidence of hemolysis. The patient is admitted for expectant management of 'chronic hypertension with superimposed early-onset preeclampsia.'

During patient management, your trainee inquires about existing heterogeneity in the definitions of preeclampsia.

20. Outline essential attributes of 'preeclampsia superimposed upon chronic hypertension.' *(4 points for first bullet; 2 points for any **one** subsequent bullet)*

Max 6

☐ Chronic hypertension accompanied by **one or more** signs of maternal organ dysfunction at >20 weeks' gestation
☐ Proteinuria: UPCR ≥30 mg/mmol (265 mg/g) or ≥1–2+ on urine dipstick[‡]
  ○ Note that proteinuria is **not** mandatory for the diagnosis of preeclampsia
  ○ Urine albumin/creatinine ratio ≥8 mg/mmol is an alternative to UPCR *(NICE[8])*
☐ Hematological findings: disseminated intravascular coagulation (DIC), hemolysis, platelets <150 × 10^9/L
☐ Acute kidney injury: serum creatinine ≥90 umol/L (1 mg/dL)
☐ Liver dysfunction (ALT or AST >40 IU/L), with or without right upper quadrant or epigastric pain
☐ Neurological manifestations: blindness, altered mental status, stroke, clonus, severe headache, persistent scotomata
☐ Fetal growth restriction (FGR) **cannot** be used as a diagnostic criterion for superimposed preeclampsia as it may be part of chronic hypertension *(ISSHP[3])*

Special note:
‡ 24-hour urine protein collection (≥300 mg/d) is practically replaced by UPCR to eliminate inherent difficulties in 24-hour urine collections and delays in decision-making; 24-hour urine collection is generally reserved for low-resource settings

21. Although there is no universal consensus for timing of magnesium sulfate prophylaxis, identify two clinical features warranting consideration for use in this patient. *(1 point each)*

2

☐ Epigastric pain
☐ Progressive deterioration in laboratory tests

Special note:
NICE[8] recommends other features including ongoing or recurring severe headaches, scotomata, nausea/vomiting, oliguria, severe hypertension

22. List maternal and fetal-neonatal risks associated with preeclampsia. *(1 point each; max points specified per section)*

Max 13

Maternal (max 10)

Hematologic:
- ☐ DIC
- ☐ Microangiopathic hemolysis

Central nervous system:
- ☐ Eclampsia
- ☐ Posterior reversible encephalopathy syndrome
- ☐ Intracerebral hemorrhage

Ocular:
- ☐ Blindness
- ☐ Retinal detachment

Cardio-respiratory:
- ☐ Acute pulmonary edema/acute respiratory distress syndrome
- ☐ Myocardial infarction
- ☐ Mortality *(mostly due to intracranial hemorrhage)*

Hepatic:
- ☐ HELLP syndrome
- ☐ Hematoma and subcapsular rupture
- ☐ Infarction

Renal:
- ☐ Cortical or tubular necrosis
- ☐ Acute renal failure

Placental:
- ☐ Abruption
- ☐ Infarction

Fetal/neonatal (max 3)
- ☐ Preterm birth (PTB)
- ☐ Fetal growth restriction (FGR)
- ☐ Oligohydramnios
- ☐ Abnormal CTG and need for Cesarean delivery
- ☐ Intrauterine fetal demise (IUFD)

23. In addition to antihypertensive treatment, what are important <u>maternal</u> considerations for antenatal admission? *(1 point per main bullet, unless specified)*   Max 14

☐ Maintain dim lighting and decrease visual stimulation from electronic devices

☐ Blood pressure monitoring approximately every four hours, while awake

☐ Notify physicians if BP is ≥160/110 mmHg (*i.e.,* severe hypertension)

☐ Perform regular assessments for clonus

☐ Encourage reporting of signs or symptoms of severe disease: *(1 point per subbullet; max 4 points)*
  ○ Visual disturbances
  ○ Severe incapacitating headache or unresolved by analgesia
  ○ Nausea and/or vomiting
  ○ Shortness of breath
  ○ Epigastric or right upper quadrant pain
  ○ Subjective deterioration in urine output *(ideally, urine output volume is recorded)*
  ○ Uterine tenderness or vaginal bleeding

☐ <u>Discourage</u> activity restriction during hospital admission, or in the outpatient setting *(ACOG[5], SMFM[6], SOGC[7], NICE[8])*
  ○ *Evidence of physiological and psychological adverse effects of activity restriction*
  ○ *Lack of definitive data for improved perinatal outcome*

☐ Consideration for compression stockings and/or thromboprophylaxis; avoid thromboprophylaxis with worsening thrombocytopenia

☐ Provide a salt restricted diet as the patient has chronic hypertension

☐ Consideration for magnesium sulfate administration for dual benefits of eclampsia prophylaxis and fetal neuroprotection

☐ Discontinuation of low-dose aspirin with diagnosis of preeclampsia

☐ <u>Avoid</u> diuretics based on oliguria *(diuretic treatment is used in the context of pulmonary edema)*

☐ Regular serum laboratory evaluation *(frequency is case dependent)*[‡]

☐ Group B *Streptococcus* (GBS) vaginal-rectal swab, in anticipation of vaginal delivery within five weeks

☐ Offer psychosocial support services

Special note:

[‡] *Controversy* exists regarding serial quantification once significant proteinuria is established. Monitoring of the degree of proteinuria is **not** indicated, as neither the rate of increase nor quantity affect clinical management and delivery decisions; however, neonatal outcomes have been shown to be worse with nephrotic range proteinuria (*e.g.,* >5 g/d; *ISSHP[3]*)

24. Identify important management considerations for <u>fetal</u> health during antenatal admission. *(1 point each, unless specified)*   4

- ☐ At least once daily CTG monitoring
- ☐ Obstetric ultrasound *(frequency is case based)*
- ☐ Administration of fetal pulmonary corticosteroids, based on the increased risk of delivery within seven days[†] *(either bullet for 1 point)*
  - ○ Betamethasone 12 mg intramuscularly, repeated once in 24 hours,

  OR

  - ○ Dexamethasone 6 mg intramuscularly (or intravenously) for four doses at 12-hour intervals
- ☐ Neonatology consultation

Special note:
† Refer to Question 18 in Chapter 9 on international practice guidance recommendations for timing of fetal pulmonary corticosteroids

25. What are the <u>temporary</u> maternal or fetal effects of fetal pulmonary corticosteroids? *(1 point each)*   Max 3

Maternal:
- ☐ Improved platelet count
- ☐ Hyperglycemia, requiring insulin adjustments among treated patients

Fetal:
- ☐ Improved fetal Doppler velocimetry of the umbilical artery and ductus venosus
- ☐ Decreased fetal heart rate variability

During the hospital admission, obstetric ultrasound shows fetal biometry on the 12th percentile with normal amniotic fluid volume and fetal Doppler indices. The GBS swab is negative.

26. Elaborate on sonographic placental findings which may be seen with preeclampsia. *(1 point each)*   Max 3

- ☐ Thickened placenta with diffuse echogenicity, secondary to edema
- ☐ Thinned placenta, possibly due to reduced vascularization
- ☐ Cystic regions, reflecting infarctions or hematomas
- ☐ Signs of placental abruption

At 30[+6] weeks' gestation, the patient complains of generalized malaise and nausea. Her BP is 162/112 mmHg despite adherence to the treatment protocol and compliance with management plan. She has no obstetric complaints and the CTG is unremarkable.

Laboratory results reveal the following:

		Normal				*Normal*
Hemoglobin	101	110–140 g/L		ALT	282	6–45 IU/L
Hematocrit	0.2	0.28–0.39 L/L		AST	519	6–35 IU/L
Leukocytes	15.6	$5–16 \times 10^9$/L		LDH	801	110–210 U/L
Platelets	32	$150–429 \times 10^9$/L		Uric acid	490	150–350 umol/L
Creatinine	95	40–70 umol/L		Bilirubin	20	1.7–18.9 umol/L
Haptoglobin	<0.3	50–220 mg/dL		D-Dimer	675	551–3333 µg/L
Fibrinogen	420	300–690 mg/dL		Smear	1% reticulocytes	
INR	1.0	0.9–1.0				

Multidisciplinary teams are involved in the patient's care.

---

27. Detail your counseling and management plan at this time. *(1 point per main bullet, unless specified)*

Max 12

- ☐ Recommend induction of labor based on the onset of HELLP syndrome
- ☐ Inform the patient that while the route of delivery is based on obstetric indications, individualized decision-making is required if prolonged induction or low likelihood of successful induction is anticipated
- ☐ Maintain continuous CTG monitoring
- ☐ Serial intrapartum serum laboratory monitoring
- ☐ Close monitoring of fluid balance (*i.e.,* input and output)
- ☐ Start acute antihypertensive treatment for BP ≥160/110 mmHg *(see Question 33)*
- ☐ Limit intravenous fluid hydration to 60–80 mL/hr and **avoid** fluid boluses
- ☐ Counsel on administration of magnesium sulfate for eclampsia prophylaxis, while informing her of possible side effects: *(1 point for this main bullet, and any two subbullets)*
  - o Flushing
  - o Diaphoresis
  - o Palpitations
  - o Headaches
  - o Nausea/vomiting
  - o Visual changes
  - o Muscle weakness

☐ Advise platelet transfusion as level is 20–49 × 10⁹/L, and based on mode of delivery:
(1 point for either subbullet)
  ○ *Transfuse if vaginal delivery planned with active bleeding, platelet dysfunction, falling platelet counts, or coagulopathy*
  ○ *Transfuse if Cesarean delivery is required*
☐ Avoid obstetric invasive procedures at vaginal delivery, such as pudental block and episiotomy‡
☐ Arrange for availability of blood products at delivery, in anticipation of the risk of postpartum hemorrhage
☐ Early consultation with an anesthesiologist

Special note:
‡ Assisted vaginal delivery is contraindicated for this patient by virtue of gestational age

28-A. Discuss significant concerns of anesthesiologists involved in the delivery care of patients with preeclampsia. *(1 point each)*   Max 2

☐ Thrombocytopenia precluding neuraxial anesthesia, as in this patient
☐ Difficult or failed intubation if general anesthesia is required at Cesarean delivery, based on pharyngeal edema
☐ Acute hypertensive episode during intubation
☐ Acute hypotension at administration of anesthesia

28-B. Indicate options for labor analgesia based on the presence of severe thrombocytopenia in this patient. *(1 point each)*   Max 2

☐ Nitrous oxide
☐ Patient-controlled analgesia pump
☐ Reconsideration for neuraxial analgesia after increasing the platelet count with transfusion†

Special note:
† Although there is no established safe lowermost threshold for neuraxial anesthesia, ≥70 × 10⁹/L is considered acceptable

Blood pressure responded well to intravenous labetalol and the patient consents to induction of labor and platelet transfusion or need of additional blood products. Fetal CTG is reassuring. Seizure prophylaxis is initiated.

29. Specify your orders regarding administration and clinical monitoring of magnesium sulfate for eclampsia prophylaxis. *(1 point each)*

5

Magnesium sulfate dosing: *(either bullet)*
☐ *Intravenous*: Loading dose 4–6 g over 20–30 minutes, then 1 g/hr maintenance dose

OR

☐ *Intramuscular*: 5 g of 50% solution in each buttock, then 5 g every four hours (consideration for local anesthesia with injections)

Treatment duration:
☐ Continue treatment for 24 hours postpartum, although earlier discontinuation may be appropriate *(individualized decision-making is necessary)*

Routine clinical assessments for signs of hypermagnesemia:
☐ Patellar (deep tendon) reflex is required before starting maintenance dose and every two hours; suppressed or absent reflex suggests magnesium sulfate toxicity
☐ Respiratory rate assessment every 30 minutes, where hypo-respiration is implied by <12/min
☐ Urine output, with abnormal amount being <100 mL in four hours

Special note:
Magnesium sulfate is contraindicated in patients with myasthenia gravis or pulmonary edema; substitution by antiepileptic agents provides inferior prophylaxis or treatment of eclampsia

Having noticed that you do not intend to routinely monitor serum magnesium levels, your trainee inquires about its potential role in adjustment of magnesium sulfate infusion protocol.

30. Elaborate on clinical situations requiring monitoring of serum magnesium levels to ensure therapeutic levels. *(1 point each)*

3

☐ Chronic renal disease or acquired renal insufficiency with serum creatinine >110 umol/L (1.1 mg/dL)
☐ Onset of eclampsia during magnesium sulfate administration
☐ Clinical signs of magnesium toxicity

Intrapartum assessment reveals a respiratory rate at 9 breaths/min, urine output of 20 mL in two hours, and suppressed patellar reflex. Serum creatinine is stable at 97 umol/L. Oxygen saturation is normal on room air. She is alert, responsive, and denies chest pain. Fetal cardiotocography is unremarkable.

31. What are your next best steps in management after patient counseling? *(1 point each)*   2

☐ Hold the magnesium sulfate infusion
☐ Administer intravenous calcium gluconate 10 mL of 10% solution over two to five minutes

Special note:
Intravenous diuretic *may be considered* to enhance magnesium excretion

Labor progresses well and acute platelet transfusions provide a temporary rise to 90×10^9/L. The patient has a spontaneous vaginal delivery of a male neonate weighing 1220 g. Prophylactic uterotonic agents are administered, obviating postpartum hemorrhage.

At four hours postpartum, you are notified that the total urine output is 60 mL since delivery. You teach your obstetric trainee that a urine output averaging 15 mL/hr is normal in the early postpartum period due to the innate synthesis of oxytocin and antidiuretic hormone from adjacent hypothalamic nuclei, followed by their release from storage in the posterior pituitary.

32. In addition to urine output considerations, what are other particularities of <u>maternal</u>   8
management in the early postpartum period? *(1 point each)*

☐ <u>Avoid</u> intravenous fluid boluses
☐ <u>Avoid</u> ergometrine
☐ Avoid nonsteroidal anti-inflammatory agents (NSAIDs) for postpartum analgesia if BP is uncontrolled, or in the presence of acute kidney injury or thrombocytopenia
☐ Monitoring of BP and clinical condition every four hours while awake
☐ Aim to keep BP <140/90 mmHg *(NICE)*
☐ Resumption of oral antihypertensive regimen
☐ Judicious use of simultaneous administration of opioid analgesics and magnesium sulfate based on the risk of cardiorespiratory depression
☐ Serial postpartum laboratory testing is required in HELLP syndrome

On postpartum day 3, you receive an urgent call from your trainee as the patient's BP is 180/115 mmHg, unchanged after repeat testing in 15 minutes, at 182/117 mmHg. She complains of an isolated mild frontal headache. You inform her of the expeditious need to start antihypertensive treatment for severe hypertension.

33. Outline the acute treatment plan for one antihypertensive agent used in obstetric emergencies. *(5 points for one agent)*

5

	Starting dose	Dose adjustments[†]	Maximum dose
☐ Labetalol IV	10–20 mg (continuous infusion of 1-2 mg/minute can be used instead of intermittent therapy or started after 20 mg IV dose; infusion pump and continuous noninvasive monitoring of blood pressure and heart rate would be required)	20–80 mg every 10–30 minutes	300 mg cumulative
☐ Nifedipine PO (short acting)	10–20 mg	May repeat in 20 minutes, then 10–20 mg every 2–6 hours	180 mg daily
☐ Hydralazine IV	5 mg	5–10 mg every 20–40 minutes	20 mg cumulative (constant infusion 0.5–10 mg/hr)

† *Consider switching the antihypertensive agent if BP not at target after three doses*

She responds well to two doses of intravenous hydralazine. You explain that BP may rise three to five days postpartum due to physiologic changes, and close observation is required until a safe BP target is established. You also inform her that titration of her antihypertensive regimen will be needed over the coming weeks.

By postpartum day 8, the patient's BP is well controlled with labetalol 200 mg twice daily and nifedipine XL 60 mg daily. There are no obstetric issues and she continued to breastfeed the newborn, admitted to the NICU.

Outpatient serum laboratory tests normalize over two weeks, with residual proteinuria. She weaned off labetalol, currently requiring only nifedipine XL 60 mg daily for chronic hypertension.

The patient presents for a routine six weeks' postpartum obstetric visit.

34. With respect to her prenatal morbidities, what are important postpartum considerations to discuss, either prior to discharge or at the routine postpartum visit? *(1 point each; max points specified per section)*

Max 10

General maternal-fetal well-being: *(max 5)*
☐ Screen for postpartum depression and continue to offer psychosocial support services
☐ Encourage a healthy lifestyle to promote weight loss and normalization of her body habitus
☐ Elaborate on future risk of cardiovascular and renal morbidity, metabolic syndrome, and mortality; follow-up is advised
☐ Request laboratory testing for antiphospholipid antibodies *(i.e., lupus anticoagulant, anticardiolipin antibodies, ß2-glycoprotein-1 antibodies)* based on a premature birth before 34 weeks' gestation due to preeclampsia with a morphologically normal fetus
☐ Discuss the delayed resolution of proteinuria, with possibility of persistent microalbuminuria
☐ Promote future preconception counseling
☐ Allude to the Barker hypothesis to promote future child health

Breastfeeding: *(max 1)*
☐ Encourage extended breastfeeding to improve BP control and decrease cardiovascular morbidity
☐ Reassure the patient that antihypertensive concentrations in breast milk are mostly very low and deemed safe for the infant; labetalol,[†] methyldopa, long-acting nifedipine, enalapril, or captopril have been shown to be safe with breastfeeding (diuretics are avoided)

Contraceptive recommendations for women with hypertension:[§#] *(max 4)*
☐ No restrictions on use of barrier methods
☐ Use of copper or levonorgesterol intrauterine contraception is safe (Category 1)
☐ Progestin-only oral contraceptives and progestin implants are safe (Category 1)
☐ Unlike other progestins, DMPA is associated with a theoretical risk of unfavorable lipoprotein changes that could contribute to cardiovascular risk among women with hypertension of systolic ≥ 160 mmHg or diastolic ≥ 100 mmHg (UK-MEC, Category 2 and US-MEC Category 3)
☐ Combined hormonal contraceptives should not be used among women with hypertension of systolic 140–159 mmHg or diastolic 90–99 mmHg unless no other method is appropriate or acceptable to the patient (Category 3), and are contraindicated among women with systolic ≥ 160 mmHg or diastolic ≥ 100 mmHg (Category 4)[#]

Special notes:
† There is a theoretical risk of bradycardia in neonates of women taking β-blockers
§ UK and US Medical Eligibility Criteria (MEC) for Contraceptive Use, 2016: *(a)* UK-MEC amended September 2019, *(b)* US-MEC updated 2020; *(c)* ACOG Practice Bulletin No. 206: Use of hormonal contraception in women with coexisting medical conditions [published correction appears in *Obstet Gynecol.* 2019 Jun;133(6):1288]. *Obstet Gynecol.* 2019;133(2):e128–e150.
# Refer to Question 17 in Chapter 32 for contraceptive recommendations among women with ischemic heart disease

TOTAL: 155

SECTION 7

Hepato-Renal and Gastrointestinal Conditions in Pregnancy

CHAPTER 39

Renal Stones, Pyelonephritis, and Urosepsis in Pregnancy

Nader Fahmy and Amira El-Messidi

During your on-call duty, a healthy 24-year-old primigravida at 17 weeks' gestation presents to the obstetric emergency assessment unit with a six-hour history of intermittent right flank pain.

Your colleague follows her prenatal care, and pregnancy has been unremarkable. Routine prenatal laboratory investigations and aneuploidy screening were normal. She takes only prenatal vitamins and has no allergies.

LEARNING OBJECTIVES

1. Take a focused history, and elicit investigations relevant to various complications of renal calculus diseases in the antenatal period
2. Identify sonography as the primary diagnostic test in the prenatal evaluation of nephrolithiasis; magnetic resonance urography may be additive with noninformative ultrasound, and low-dose CT is reserved as a third-line investigation
3. Understand conservative and invasive treatments for obstetric urolithiasis
4. Counsel on maternal and fetal complications related to renal stone disease
5. Recognize maternal sepsis/urosepsis as a medical emergency requiring prompt multidisciplinary resuscitative efforts

SUGGESTED READINGS

1. Assimos D, Krambeck A, Miller NL, et al. Surgical management of stones: American Urological Association/Endourological Society Guideline, PART I. *J Urol*. 2016;196(4): 1153–1160.
2. Bonet M, Nogueira Pileggi V, Rijken MJ, et al. Towards a consensus definition of maternal sepsis: results of a systematic review and expert consultation. *Reprod Health*. 2017;14(1):67. [Correction in *Reprod Health*. 2018 Jan 8;15(1):6]
3. Bowyer L, Robinson HL, Barrett H, et al. SOMANZ guidelines for the investigation and management of sepsis in pregnancy. *Aust N Z J Obstet Gynaecol*. 2017;57(5):540–551.
4. Bridwell RE, Carius BM, Long B, et al. Sepsis in pregnancy: recognition and resuscitation. *West J Emerg Med*. 2019;20(5):822–832.
5. Dion M, Ankawi G, Chew B, et al. CUA guideline on the evaluation and medical management of the kidney stone patient – 2016 update. *Can Urol Assoc J*. 2016;10(11–12):E347–E358.

6. Foeller ME, Gibbs RS. Maternal sepsis: new concepts, new practices. *Curr Opin Obstet Gynecol.* 2019;31(2):90–96.

7. Grette K, Cassity S, Holliday N, et al. Acute pyelonephritis during pregnancy: a systematic review of the aetiology, timing, and reported adverse perinatal risks during pregnancy. *J Obstet Gynaecol.* 2020;40(6):739–748.

8. Masselli G, Derme M, Bernieri MG, et al. Stone disease in pregnancy: imaging-guided therapy. *Insights Imaging.* 2014;5(6):691–696.

9. Society for Maternal-Fetal Medicine (SMFM) Consult Series No. 47: Plante LA, Pacheco LD, Louis JM. Sepsis during pregnancy and the puerperium. *Am J Obstet Gynecol.* 2019;220(4): B2–B10. [Correction in *Am J Obstet Gynecol.* 2020 Oct 6]

10. Türk C, Petřík A, Sarica K, et al. 2020 EAU guidelines on diagnosis and conservative management of urolithiasis. Available at https://uroweb.org/guideline/urolithiasis/. Accessed October 31, 2020.

POINTS

1. What aspects of a focused history would you want to know? *(1 point each; max points per section indicated, where relevant)*   18

Characteristics of the flank pain:
- ☐ Intensity/severity
- ☐ Pattern (*i.e.*, colicky)
- ☐ Radiating to the lower back, abdomen
- ☐ Aggravating/alleviating factors
- ☐ Past similar episodes/investigations

Renal-related manifestations: *(max 7)*
- ☐ Dysuria
- ☐ Urgency
- ☐ Hematuria
- ☐ Stone-passage
- ☐ Sense of incomplete voiding
- ☐ Frequency *(symptom overlap with pregnancy)*
- ☐ Known history of renal calculi
- ☐ History of frequent urinary tract infections

Other systemic manifestations: *(max 2)*
- ☐ Fever, malaise, nausea/vomiting
- ☐ Chronic hypertension *(more common among patients with nephrolithiasis)*
- ☐ Respiratory or lower gastrointestinal symptoms

Pregnancy-related manifestations:
- ☐ Abdominal pain/cramping
- ☐ Vaginal bleeding or fluid loss

Social history:
- ☐ Cigarette smoking, alcohol consumption, or recreational drug use

Family history:
- ☐ Renal calculi

The patient describes a spontaneous first episode of colicky pain radiating to her lower abdomen and groin, now unresponsive to acetaminophen (paracetamol). She has irritative lower urinary tract symptoms including urgency and incomplete voiding; you note that her complaint of frequency overlaps both lower urinary tract symptoms and pregnancy. The patient does not have hematuria and is not known for prior urinary tract infections. She reports new-onset nausea, concurrent with her pain. She recalls a remote episode where three black pebbles were expelled at urination. She does not smoke or drink alcohol while pregnant. Family history is only significant for recurrent paternal renal calculi.

During your patient encounter, she had an episodic bout of pain, holding her right flank, and temporarily incapable of conversing with you. In the brief time you took to arrange for an antiemetic and intramuscular analgesic, her pain had resolved. On examination, the patient has a normal body habitus, is afebrile and normotensive without costovertebral angle tenderness; her pulse is 95 bpm. Obstetrical assessment is unremarkable.

2. Indicate five investigations in the work-up of your most suspected diagnosis. *(1 each)*   Max 5

Serum:
☐ CBC *(i.e., leukocyte count)*
☐ Creatinine
☐ Uric acid
☐ Ionized calcium, sodium, potassium

Urine:
☐ Urinalysis *(i.e., leukocyte count, red blood cells nitrites, bacteria, and casts)*
☐ Culture and sensitivity

Imaging:
☐ Abdominal-renal ultrasound *(i.e., renal calculi and/or hydronephrosis)*

Your obstetric trainee recognizes the patient likely has renal colic but is curious to know sonographic details of interest.

3. Specify the features of interest on sonographic imaging for suspected urolithiasis. *(1 point each)*   4

☐ Hydroureteronephrosis (including the level and degree)
☐ Absence of ureteral jets in bladder
☐ Echogenic foci along the urinary tract
☐ Hypoechoic acoustic shadowing

Ultrasound shows moderate right hydroureteronephrosis, traced to the distal ureter, without definitive visualization of calculi. Both urinary jets are visible in the bladder.

Urinalysis is significant for leukocytes and red blood cells, without bacteria, nitrites or casts; urine pH is 6.

Over a few hours of observation, the pain has not recurred. Although keen for discharge, she inquires about your diagnostic suspicion despite the lack of visible stones on imaging. She is keen to follow your expert advice to prevent recurrence and wonders if she may have caused the flare of renal colic during pregnancy.

4. Rationalize your suspicion of renal colic. *(1 point each)*	Max 6

☐ Patient had prior renal calculi
☐ Consistent clinical presentation of acute flank pain, including referral to the abdomen/groin
☐ Lower urinary tract symptoms are likely related to proximity of calculi to the ureterovesical junction
☐ Afebrile status
☐ Absence of costovertebral angle tenderness
☐ Urinalysis consistent with sterile pyuria without casts
☐ Ultrasound may not detect ~40% of renal stones

5. Discuss the renal physiologic changes in pregnancy that contribute to stone formation. *(1 point per main bullet)*	Max 4

☐ Increased renal <u>filtration</u> of calcium, sodium, uric acid, and oxalate *(increased glomerular filtration rate)*
☐ Increased renal calcium <u>excretion</u> *(placental vitamin D leads to intestinal calcium absorption and parathyroid hormone inhibition)*
☐ Decreased renal tubular calcium <u>resorption</u> *(parathyroid hormone suppression)*
☐ Lesser increases in urinary citrate, magnesium, and glycosaminoglycans *(stone-formation inhibitors)*
☐ Higher urinary pH without increase in urine volume
☐ Hydronephrosis and ureteric dilation *(hormonal and physiologic causes)*
  ○ *Stone migration leads to obstruction and/or pain*
☐ Urinary stasis *(decreased oral hydration and bladder capacity)*
  ○ *Crystal aggregation*

6. Discuss the conservative measures and medical management of this prenatal patient with suspected renal colic. *(1 point each)*	Max 10

Conservative measures for stone prevention:
☐ Encourage daily hydration[†]
☐ Low-salt diet
☐ Moderate intake of animal protein (~200 g/d)
☐ Moderation in dietary calcium intake[§]
☐ Avoid >1 g/d of vitamin C *(prevents hyperoxaluria)*
☐ Consideration for supplementary vitamin D to the standard prenatal vitamins

Management:
☐ Consultation with urology team prior to discharge
☐ Outpatient oral antiemetics and analgesics *(e.g., acetaminophen [paracetemol], lowest effective dose and shortest duration of opioids, if required)*[‡]

□ Lying on her side, with symptomatic side-up *(i.e., her right side-up)*
   o *Relieves ureteric pressure by gravid uterus*
□ Routine sieving of urine, and retain spontaneously passed stones for analysis
□ Encourage early presentation for medical care with onset of fever/chills, nausea/vomiting, or if pain is unresponsive to analgesics

Special notes:
† Efficacy of calcium channel blockers or alpha-blockers as medical expulsive therapies among pregnant women is unknown; Tamsulosin is not advised.
‡ Obstetric considerations require judicious use of NSAIDs
§ Restrict dietary calcium if ureteral stents are placed to minimize encrustation

The patient appreciates your explanations.

Upon her discharge, you find your trainee searching the internet for other causes that may explain the patient's urinalysis.

7. Excluding pregnancy itself and nephrolithiasis, list five etiologies for <u>sterile</u> <u>pyuria</u> among reproductive-aged women.

       5

[the following is a guide; other responses may be acceptable] *(1 point per etiology)*
□ Renal: *e.g., foreign body, polycystic kidneys, papillary necrosis*
□ Infectious: *e.g., STIs, TB, viral, fungal*
□ Autoimmune conditions: *e.g., SLE, diabetes mellitus, Kawasaki disease*
□ Other systemic conditions: *e.g., malignant hypertension, sarcoidosis, malignancy*
□ Drug-induced: *e.g., nitrofurantoin, penicillin-agents, aspirin, protein-pump inhibitors*

Two weeks later, now 19 weeks' gestation, the patient returns to the urgent care unit with recurrent right flank pain unresponsive to hydration and oral analgesia. She is afebrile, abdominal exam is normal and the costovertebral angle is nontender. Obstetric assessment is normal and fetal viability is confirmed.

The patient agrees to intravenous analgesics. Repeat ultrasound shows stable hydroureteronephrosis without calculi. Becoming increasingly frustrated, the patient asks about other diagnostic modalities in view of inconclusive sonographic findings.

8. What is the second-line imaging modality for assessment of possible urolithiasis after noninformative sonography in pregnancy?

       1

□ Magnetic resonance urography, without gadolinium†

Special note:
† Refer to Chapter 42 for effects of gadolinium in pregnancy

While your patient is having the magnetic resonance urography, a physician from an external center calls you in a panic after a pregnancy was discovered inadvertently on abdominal CT that was performed to evaluate renal stone disease. Dating sonography for your colleague's patient confirmed a single, viable fetus with biometry consistent for 14 weeks' gestation. The physician is panicking as he or she trusted the patient's claim for perfect use of oral contraception.

9. Provide your best recommendations regarding fetal exposure to an abdominal CT and indicate other practice management advice for your colleague. *(1 point per main bullet)*	Max 5

☐ Reassure your colleague that pregnancy termination is <u>not</u> recommended solely with exposure to diagnostic radiation

☐ Fetal radiation exposure from abdominal CT is 0.13–3.5 rads (1.3–35 mGy); this is below the threshold limit of 5 rads (50 mGy) for teratogenicity, increasing thereafter with cumulative dose
  ○ *Low-dose CT can be used in the second or third trimester, with high sensitivity and specificity for detecting uretero-renal calculi, if the investigation will impact management decisions (individualized discussion is advised)*

☐ Teratogenicity from diagnostic imaging also depends on gestational age, decreasing after ~15 weeks' gestation *(or prior to eight weeks' gestation)*

☐ No threshold exists for radiation effects of carcinogenesis and mutagenesis; probability increases with doses and may be independent of gestational age

☐ Advise routine pregnancy tests for all reproductive-aged women prior to having radiation-prone imaging tests

☐ Recommend patient disclosure and local revision of protocol

Your patient's magnetic resonance urography demonstrates a 7-mm stone in the right distal ureter. Intravenous analgesics have not alleviated her pain. The urologist saw the patient and discussed the subsequent management plan with you.

10. Based on your discussion with the urologist, indicate the best next step in the management of this patient with obstetric urolithiasis who failed conservative treatment.	1

☐ Urinary diversion procedure *(i.e., percutaneous nephrostomy tube or double-J stent)*

After the urologist counseled the patient on placement of a nephrostomy tube, for which she provided informed consent, you are called to see her. Being stressed and in pain, she cannot recall some information about her upcoming minor procedure, although keenly awaits its therapeutic effects.

11. Rationalize the urologist's choice of percutaneous nephrostomy over ureteral stenting.   Max 5
(1 point each)

☐ Minimally invasive
☐ Provides immediate decompression of the obstruction
☐ Can be performed with acute sepsis
☐ Avoids difficult ureteral manipulation with impacted stones
☐ Decreased risk of forming mineral deposits (*i.e.,* encrustation) relative to stents
☐ Decreased lower urinary tract symptoms relative to stents
☐ Less invasive tube changes *(both require changes at approximate four- to six-week intervals)*
☐ Established access for postpartum percutaneous definitive stone dissolution
☐ Cost-effectiveness

12. List five indications for active interventions of nephrolithiasis, which *may or may not* be   Max 5
applicable to this patient. *(1 point each)*

☐ Nephrolithiasis-induced obstetric complications
☐ Persistent pain
☐ Infection (local or systemic)
☐ Obstructed solitary kidney
☐ Progressive renal obstruction (unilateral or bilateral)
☐ Acute kidney injury or worsening renal function
☐ Bilateral urolithiasis

After assuring normal coagulation function, percutaneous nephrostomy is performed, providing instant relief. She is now able to engage in conversation regarding the fetal implications of renal stone disease.

13. Discuss your counseling of the <u>obstetric</u> risks associated with symptomatic nephrolithiasis.   2
(1 point each)

☐ Preterm labor with/without preterm delivery
☐ Preterm prelabor rupture of membranes (PPROM)

<u>**Special note:**</u>
Perinatal outcomes are not adversely affected *(Rosenberg E et al. World J Urol 2011; 29:743–47)*

At hospital discharge, community medical services have been arranged to care for her urinary bag, outpatient multidisciplinary appointments made, and the patient has been informed when to seek urgent care.

At 23 weeks' gestation, the patient returns for urgent care due to chills and blood in her nephrostomy tube. She is alert but appears unwell; her vital signs are:

- Blood pressure (BP): 80/40 mmHg
- Pulse: 110 bpm

- Respirations: 26/min
- Temperature: 39.2°C (oral)

Her obstetrical course has been unremarkable, and the fetal morphology survey was normal two weeks ago. She has no obstetrical complaints at presentation and the fetal status is normal.

---

14. What is the most probable diagnosis?   1

☐ Maternal sepsis
  ○ *maintain a low threshold for early suspicion and treatment*

While you inform the patient of your clinical suspicion, your obstetric trainee alerts the intensivist and urologist on-call who promptly attend to her care.

---

15. With multidisciplinary collaboration, outline essentials of the <u>initial</u> management of   Max 17
maternal sepsis. *(1 point each unless specified)*

☐ Hospitalization in a monitored setting *(e.g., ICU/ITU)*
☐ Comprehensive investigations including, *but not limited to:* **(1 point per subbullet unless specified; max 10)**
  ○ Bacterial culture from the nephrostomy catheter line **(2 points)**
  ○ Urine culture from the nephrostomy tube
  ○ Urine culture from self-voided sample
  ○ Blood and sputum cultures
  ○ Vaginal cultures
  ○ Arterial blood gases
  ○ CBC/FBC
  ○ Serum creatinine and electrolytes
  ○ Serum lactate level (arterial, venous, or capillary)
  ○ Liver transaminases and function tests
  ○ Coagulation studies
  ○ Repeat abdominal sonography to assess positioning of the nephrostomy tube, and ensure absence of obstruction
☐ Hemodynamic resuscitation; 1–2 L IV crystalloid hydration
☐ Empiric broad-spectrum IV antibiotics as soon as possible (ideally within one hour of presentation)
  ○ *Cover aerobic and anaerobic gram-positive and -negative bacteria*
☐ Administer antipyretics after antibiotics commenced *(i.e., patient is febrile)*
☐ Maintain maternal oxygenation >94% *(for fetal considerations)*
☐ Consideration for vasopressors/inotropic support, if needed
☐ Initiate prophylactic anticoagulation *(e.g., compressions devices/thromboprophylaxis)*
☐ Maintain serum glucose at 8–10 mmol/L (140–180 mg/dL)
☐ Monitor urine output
☐ Avoid delivery of the fetus for the sole indication of sepsis
  ○ *Delivery is based on obstetric indications*
☐ Regular fetal monitoring, guided by gestational age

The patient is admitted to the ICU/ITU; volume resuscitation and meropenem are started. Initial investigations show an elevated serum leukocyte count at 25×10^9/L with normal renal, hepatic, and coagulation function; serum lactate is <2 mmol/L. Blood cultures and voided urine specimen grew penicillin-sensitive *E. coli*. Sonography shows increasing hydronephrosis with extra-renal displacement of the nephrostomy tube, which is corrected under ultrasound guidance.

You present with your obstetric trainee to the ICU/ITU for updates on the patient's status, just in time to attend the treating team's discussion on maternal sepsis.

Despite existing multiple clinical decision tools for recognition and risk prediction of sepsis, none is optimal.

16. As defined by the WHO (2016), what are the elements comprising the evidence-based definition of maternal sepsis? *(1 point each)*

2

Antepartum, intrapartum, postpartum, or postabortion presence of:
- ☐ Organ dysfunction, **plus**
- ☐ Infection (suspected or confirmed)

17. Based on the SIRS[†] *(systemic inflammatory response syndrome)* decision tool, elicit the early warning signs for sepsis in pregnancy, as noted upon her clinical presentation. *(1 point each)*

4

- ☐ Temperature >38°C[$] *(or <36°C)*
- ☐ Pulse >90 bpm
- ☐ Respirations >20 breaths/min *(or $PaCO_2$ <32 mmHg)*
- ☐ Serum leukocyte count >12 × 10^9/L *(or <4 × 10^9/L, or >10% bands)*

Special notes:
† ≥2 features are required
§ Note that fever is neither necessary nor sufficient to confirm sepsis

As an obstetric provider, you inform the group of related scoring systems in the obstetric literature and your Australian-born[§] trainee refers to his or her nation's devised omqSOFA score *(obstetrically modified quick Sequential Organ Failure Assessment)*, with adjusted parameters based on pregnancy-related physiologic changes.

Special note:
§ A UK-born trainee may refer to the 'sepsis 6 care bundle,' available at Red Flag Sepsis!! - Sepsis Trust. https://sepsistrust.org/wp-content/uploads/2018/06/ED-adult-NICE-Final-1107.pdf

18. Using the omqSOFA score, indicate the early warning signs for sepsis in pregnancy, highlighting (*) those fulfilled upon her clinical presentation. *(1 point each)*   3

☐ Respirations ≥25 breaths/min *
☐ Systolic BP ≤90 mmHg *
☐ Altered mentation (not alert)

After treatment for urosepsis, the patient is observed for 48 hours on the ward. You use this opportunity to debrief her hospital course with her and counsel on perinatal morbidities.

19. Identify the <u>perinatal</u> risks associated with sepsis in pregnancy. *(1 point each)*   4

☐ PTL ± PTD
☐ Fetal growth restriction (FGR)
☐ Intrauterine fetal death (IUFD)
☐ Maternal mortality

She is well until 27 weeks' gestation when she presents urgently with recurrent right flank pain, now accompanied by dysuria with turbid urine from her nephrostomy tube and on spontaneous void. Your obstetric trainee informs you that she is febrile at 38.5°C, with normal BP and oxygenation. The patient leaped in pain when your trainee elicited costovertebral angle tenderness. The cardiotocography (CTG) tracing at presentation is normal, and obstetric assessment is unremarkable. Two days ago, fetal growth biometry and amniotic fluid volume were normal.

Her urinalysis is positive for nitrites, bacteria, proteins, and casts; results of other laboratory investigations are pending. The treating urologist will attend to the patient.

20. What is your most probable diagnosis?   1

☐ Acute pyelonephritis

As discussed with the urologist, the patient understands that hospitalization is indicated for prenatal pyelonephritis. Renal sonography$ will be performed, primarily given her complicated renal history. You use this time to address your trainee's curiosity regarding possible radiological findings in pyelonephritis.

Special note:
§ Imaging is *not* routinely indicated to diagnose pyelonephritis

21. With focus on pyelonephritis, discuss the sonographic findings of most interest to you. *(1 point each)*   Max 3

- ☐ Hydronephrosis, relative to prior imaging
- ☐ Debris in the collecting system
- ☐ Changes in renal echogenicity suggesting edema, hemorrhage, or masses
- ☐ Gas bubble formation *(emphysematous pyelonephritis)*
- ☐ Doppler flow: decreased renal cortical vascularity, or absent flow with infarction
- ☐ Renal abscess
- ☐ Perinephric collection

Special note:
Most patients have normal findings on imaging

22. Counsel the patient on the <u>maternal</u> complications of acute pyelonephritis. *(1 point each)*   Max 5

- ☐ Respiratory distress syndrome
- ☐ Sepsis
- ☐ Disseminated intravascular coagulation
- ☐ Anemia
- ☐ Acute kidney injury/renal abscess
- ☐ PTL ± PTD[‡]
- ☐ Chorioamnionitis
- ☐ Mortality

Special note:
‡   Case-based considerations for fetal lung maturity with corticosteroids or neuroprotection

She receives three days of IV ceftriaxone, tailored to the susceptibility profile of urinary *Klebsiella* infection; an oral regimen is continued after clinical improvement.

Exhausted from the complicated course with renal stones, the patient is interested in definitive treatment.

23. In collaboration with her urologist, identify the safest, definitive treatment for obstetric nephrolithiasis.   1

- ☐ Ureteroscopy and stone fragmentation/retrieval[‡]

Special notes:
Shock wave lithotripsy is contraindicated in pregnancy
‡   Suboptimal with multiple calculi or size >1 cm

The urologist counsels the patient who consents to endoscopy upon resolution of the acute infection.

24. Outline important obstetric considerations to review with the endourologist prior to uteroscopy at this gestational age. *(1 point per main bullet, unless specified)*   Max 6

☐ Ideally, utilize ultrasonographic-uteroscopy *(requires equipment and expertise)*
☐ If fluoroscopy will be utilized, beware of fetal safety: *(1 point per subbullet)*
  ○ Radiation source should be <u>beneath</u> the patient
  ○ Lead apron shielding should be kept <u>beneath</u> the patient *(fetal shielding)*
  ○ Minimize radiation dose and duration *(i.e., ALARA principle)*
☐ Pre- and postprocedural monitoring of the fetus and uterine activity on CTG
☐ Ensure back-up obstetric and neonatology expertise is arranged in case of emergency
☐ Single dose of perioperative IV antibiotic with reassuring safety profile in pregnancy
  ○ *Coverage of gram-positive and gram-negative uropathogens*

Uteroscopy is successful and the patient is now asymptomatic and free of renal stones. Follow-up abdominal sonography in four weeks showed physiologic obstetric-hydronephrosis without ureteric stricture formation postuteroscopy.

The remainder of pregnancy is unremarkable, and she has a term, spontaneous vaginal delivery of a healthy newborn.

25. Regarding her history of urolithiasis, what are two long-term recommendations you may suggest prior to delivery-discharge or at the postpartum visit? *(1 point each)*   2

☐ Incorporate measures of stone prevention into her routine lifestyle habits *(Question 6)*
☐ Serum and urinary metabolic investigations for renal calculi formation

TOTAL: 120

CHAPTER 40

Intrahepatic Cholestasis of Pregnancy

Amanda Malik, Meena Khandelwal, and Amira El-Messidi

During your overnight call duty, a 37-year-old G2P1 with a spontaneous pregnancy presents to the obstetrics emergency assessment unit of your tertiary center at 32^{+3} weeks' gestation with pruritis preventing her from sleep. She has no obstetric complaints; cardiotocography initiated upon the patient's presentation shows a normal fetal heart tracing and uterine quiescence.

Your colleague follows her prenatal care; pregnancy has been unremarkable to date. Routine fetal aneuploidy screening and second-trimester morphology survey were unremarkable. Gestational diabetes testing was normal. Three years ago, she had a term vaginal delivery in your hospital center.

LEARNING OBJECTIVES

1. Take a focused history of prenatal pruritis, recognizing clinical signs and symptoms of intrahepatic cholestasis of pregnancy (ICP)
2. Develop a differential diagnosis for gestational causes of abnormal transaminases, and initiate the most relevant investigations for suspected ICP
3. Understand the diagnostic characteristics of obstetric cholestasis, and be able to outline medical treatments and delivery controversies
4. Counsel on ICP-related maternal morbidity and fetal morbidity and mortality in the incident pregnancy
5. Provide safe contraceptive advice for women with prior cholestasis, and appreciate that antecedent ICP is associated with long-term maternal hepatobiliary and cardiovascular disease

SUGGESTED READINGS

1. ACOG Committee Opinion No. 764: Medically indicated late-preterm and early-term deliveries. *Obstet Gynecol.* 2019 Feb;133(2):e151–e155.
2. Bicocca MJ, Sperling JD, Chauhan SP. Intrahepatic cholestasis of pregnancy: Review of six national and regional guidelines. *Eur J Obstet Gynecol Reprod Biol.* 2018 Dec; 231:180–187.
3. Chappell LC, Bell JL, Smith A, et al. Ursodeoxycholic acid versus placebo in women with intrahepatic cholestasis of pregnancy (PITCHES): a randomised controlled trial. *Lancet.* 2019 Sep 7;394(10201):849–860.
4. Geenes V, Chappell LC, Seed PT, et al. Association of severe intrahepatic cholestasis of pregnancy with adverse pregnancy outcomes: a prospective population-based case-control study. *Hepatology.* 2014 Apr;59(4):1482–1491.

5. Ovadia C, Seed PT, Sklavounos A, et al. Association of adverse perinatal outcomes of intrahepatic cholestasis of pregnancy with biochemical markers: results of aggregate and individual patient data meta-analyses. *Lancet.* 2019 Mar 2;393(10174):899–909. [Erratum in *Lancet.* 2019 Mar 16;393(10176):1100]

6. Royal College of Obstetricians and Gynaecologists. Obstetric cholestasis: Green-Top Guideline No. 43. London: Royal College of Obstetricians and Gynaecologists; 2011.

7. Walker KF, Chappell LC, Hague WM, et al. Pharmacological interventions for treating intrahepatic cholestasis of pregnancy. *Cochrane Database Syst Rev.* 2020 Jul 27;7(7):CD000493.

8. Society for Maternal-Fetal Medicine (SMFM). Lee RH, Greenberg M, Metz TD, et al. Society for Maternal-Fetal Medicine Consult Series No. 53: Intrahepatic cholestasis of pregnancy: Replaces Consult No. 13, April 2011. *Am J Obstet Gynecol.* 2021;224(2):B2–B9.

9. Tran TT, Ahn J, Reau NS. American College of Gastroenterology (ACG) clinical guideline: liver disease and pregnancy. *Am J Gastroenterol.* 2016; 111(2):176–194.

10. Williamson C, Geenes V. Intrahepatic cholestasis of pregnancy. *Obstet Gynecol.* 2014 Jul;124(1):120–133.

POINTS

1. With regard to the clinical presentation, what aspects of a focused history would you want to know? *(1 point each)*   Max 17

Characteristics of pruritis:
☐ Onset and duration
☐ Timing and whether symptoms affect sleep
☐ Location and/or progression
☐ Aggravating and alleviating factors

Associated manifestations:
☐ Fever, malaise, nausea/vomiting, systemic pains
☐ Presence and description of a rash
☐ Jaundice
☐ Presence of pale stools or dark urine

Medical and obstetric histories:
☐ Ensure negative prenatal test results for HIV, hepatitis B and C
☐ Gallstones or cholecystectomy[†] *(personal or family history)*
☐ History of obstetric or nonobstetric cholestasis *(personal or family history)*
☐ Dyslipidemia, autoimmune diseases, atopic diseases *(personal or family history)*

Social features:
☐ Change in dietary or hygienic habits
☐ Alcohol or intravenous drug use
☐ Recent travel
☐ Exposure to pets
☐ Geographic origin

Medications and allergies:

☐ Recent use of antibiotics, narcotics, over-the-counter agents, or vaccination

☐ Inquire about history of combined oral contraceptive use

☐ Allergies (drug and nonpharmacologic reactions)

Special note:

† ICP has been reported after cholecystectomy

You learn that the patient developed new-onset nocturnal pruritis one week ago, mostly on her palms and soles. Despite topical remedies, symptoms have been progressively worsening. She has no other associated systemic manifestations. The patient takes prenatal vitamins, does not consume alcohol, and indicates there has not been a change in her dietary or hygiene habits. She does not recall ever experiencing such pruritis, although her sister had ICP in each of her three pregnancies. You verify results of prenatal serologies, which were negative for HIV, hepatitis B and C in the first trimester.

You notice she appears uncomfortable, constantly scratching her palms and rubbing her feet together. She is afebrile, normotensive and pulse rate is normal. The patient does not appear jaundiced and there are no rashes or skin lesions on examination.

2. Indicate the serum investigations that may <u>best</u> support the probable diagnosis.

   (1 point each, unless specified)

   Max 6

☐ Total bile acid concentration† *(3 points)*

☐ Transaminases: ALT and AST§ *(2 points)*

☐ Total bilirubin

☐ Prothrombin time

☐ Gamma-glutamyl transferase (GGT)‡

Special notes:

† Serum bile acid concentration is the most sensitive and specific marker for ICP

§ ALT is more sensitive than AST in the diagnosis of ICP, although elevated transaminases are not necessary for diagnosis

‡ GGT is diagnostic if levels are increased *(RCOG[6])*

The laboratory informs you that results of serum bile acids will be available within a week. Meanwhile, investigations show the following:

		Normal range
ALT	62	6–32 IU/L **
AST	40	11–30 IU/L **
Bilirubin	11	3–14 umol/L **
Prothrombin time	11.5	11–13.5 seconds
GGT	20	3–41 IU/L

** *Pregnancy reference ranges: from Girling, J.C., et al. Br J Obstet Gynecol 1997;104:246–250 and Nelson-Piercy, C. Handbook of obstetric medicine. 5th ed. London (UK): Informa Healthcare; 2015*

3. Identify three <u>pregnancy-specific</u> hepatic conditions that can account for the hepatic enzyme elevations. *(1 point each)*   3

- ☐ Acute fatty liver of pregnancy (AFLP)
- ☐ Preeclampsia with severe features
- ☐ HELLP syndrome
- ☐ Hyperemesis gravidarum

Special note:
As intrahepatic cholestasis may occur in nongestational states, it is not considered a pregnancy-specific condition

In the absence of a definitive cause for her pruritis and based on results of investigations presently available, you counsel the patient that the working diagnosis is ICP. Vividly distressed from pruritis, she agrees to try oral hydroxyzine.

You decide to observe the patient's clinical response to antihistamines prior to hospital discharge. Meanwhile, you use this prime opportunity to discuss ICP with your obstetric trainee.

4. Discuss the diagnostic components of ICP. *(1 point each)*   4

Controversial diagnostic criteria – most expert guidance include the following:
- ☐ Pruritis appearing in the second or third trimester in the absence of a rash
- ☐ Increased total serum bile acids >10 umol/L‡
- ☐ Diagnosis of exclusion of other hepatobiliary conditions presenting with the same clinical and biomarker derangements
- ☐ Resolution of pruritis and biomarkers within four weeks postpartum

Special note:
‡   Reference range for bile acids depends on the assay technique and timing (*i.e.*, random vs fasting). Reference range may be reduced to between 6 and 10 umol/L in fasting women; jurisdictional variations in practice exist

5-A. Elicit the factors that raise *this* patient's susceptibility for ICP. *(1 point each)*   4

- ☐ Third trimester
- ☐ Multiparity
- ☐ Family history of ICP
- ☐ Maternal age >35 years

5-B. Teach your obstetric trainee of other risk factors for ICP, *not* particular to this patient. *(1 point each)*

Max 4

- ☐ Prior gestational or nongestational ICP
- ☐ Multiple gestation
- ☐ In vitro fertilization
- ☐ Chronic hepatitis C virus infection
- ☐ Cholelithiasis
- ☐ Vitamin D deficiency
- ☐ Nonalcoholic liver cirrhosis
- ☐ Nonalcoholic pancreatitis

Over the next two hours, the patient manages to sleep; upon wakening, she reports slight improvement in symptoms. Fetal cardiotocography (CTG) monitoring remains normal. Bedside sonography reveals normal fetal biometry and amniotic fluid volume.

Intending to counsel her on the condition and management plan, the patient expresses concern about the effect of ICP on her obstetric well-being.

6. Address the patient's inquiry regarding pregnancy complications associated with ICP. *(1 point each)*

Max 7

Maternal:
- ☐ Late-preterm delivery (spontaneous or iatrogenic)
- ☐ Postpartum hemorrhage (PPH)
- ☐ Coagulopathy (vitamin K malabsorption)
- ☐ Mild jaundice
- ☐ Preeclampsia, typically two to four weeks after diagnosis of ICP *(women with total bile acid levels ≥ 40 umol/L appear to be at highest risk)*

Fetal/neonatal:
- ☐ Abnormal CTG
- ☐ Meconium-stained amniotic fluid *(associated with bile acid induced bowel motility)*
- ☐ Respiratory distress syndrome
- ☐ Neonatal unit admissions
- ☐ Intrauterine fetal demise (IUFD), primarily after 37 weeks' gestation among singletons[‡]

Special note:
[‡] While stillbirth may be unrelated to biochemical investigations or fetal monitoring, the incidence of stillbirth after 37 weeks' gestation attributable to ICP is estimated at ~1.2%; the risk is ~3.4% when total serum bile acids are ≥100 umol/L

7. With focus on obstetric cholestasis, outline your *initial* management plan for this gravida. (*1 point each*)   8

Maternal:
- ☐ Offer treatment for symptom-control[‡] (*e.g.*, cool compresses, oral or topical antihistaminic agents, emollients, aqueous cream with 2% menthol)
- ☐ Provide precautions on symptoms of preterm labor
- ☐ Encourage early reporting of decreased fetal activity[§]
- ☐ Arrange for follow-up laboratory testing, which may help guide timing of delivery, especially in severe cases[†]; prothrombin time should be assessed in the presence of steatorrhea
- ☐ Arrange follow-up in one week with her obstetric care provider
- ☐ Consideration for neonatology consultation
- ☐ Reassure the patient that although delivery provides definitive treatment, expectant management is advised at this gestational age to promote fetal maturity

Fetal:
- ☐ Mode and frequency of surveillance from diagnosis is based on expert opinion; most experts advise weekly fetal surveillance until delivery[#] (*e.g.*, nonstress test or biophysical profile)

Special notes:
- ‡ In the setting where clinical presentation is characteristic for ICP with normal laboratory results, starting empiric bile acid lowering treatment may mask biochemical evidence of cholestasis
- § No known benefit in decreasing adverse fetal outcome among women with ICP
- † Frequency of testing total bile acid concentration varies; SMFM does not recommend
- # While fetal surveillance testing provides reassurance to patients and care providers, there is no definitive benefit in prevention of sudden fetal demise in the context of ICP

The patient expresses concern about preterm delivery, recalling how her sister required early planned deliveries for all three pregnancies affected by obstetric cholestasis.

8. Illustrate an understanding of management strategies for delivery timing with ICP. (*1 point per main and subbullets*)   Max 5

- ☐ Timing of delivery is controversial; individualized judgement is advised
- ☐ Most expert recommendations advise delivery at 37–38 weeks' gestation, or sooner (with documented pulmonary maturity) for circumstances including:
  - ○ Total serum bile acids ≥40 umol/L
  - ○ Recurring ICP in a current pregnancy after history of stillbirth before 36 weeks due to obstetric cholestasis
  - ○ Severe, unremitting maternal pruritis not relieved by pharmacotherapy
  - ○ Preexisting or acute hepatic disease with clinical or laboratory evidence of worsening hepatic function

The following week the patient presents to your office for prenatal care and follow-up at 33^{+1} weeks' gestation, as her obstetric care provider is now on a holiday for one month. The patient describes pruritis becoming increasingly resistant to oral hydroxyzine, preventing her from sleep despite diphenhydramine 50 mg nightly. She shows you excoriations on her palms and soles. The patient has been attentive to fetal activity which has been normal; she has no obstetric complaints. Fetal CTG performed at this office visit shows a normal tracing with uterine quiescence.

Last week's serum bile acid level is reported at 28 umol/L. You address her concern, informing her that the risk of stillbirth continues to approximate the general population risk until total bile acids are ≥40 umol/L, defining severe disease.

9-A. Describe two proposed pathophysiological <u>associations</u> between conjugated bile salts and fetal death, which you intend to discuss with your obstetric trainee after this clinical visit. *(1 point each)*   2

☐ Sudden fetal arrhythmia from myocardial toxicity induced by transplacental transfer of bile salts from the maternal to the fetal compartment
☐ Vasoconstriction of the placental chorionic vessels caused by high serum bile salts

9-B. Explain the apparent <u>dissociation</u> between the patient's symptom severity and serum bile acid levels.   1

☐ Clinical symptoms of ICP may appear up to three weeks prior to increases in serum bile acid levels

The patient's hepatic biomarkers will be repeated at this prenatal visit. Given clinical symptoms are nonresponsive to topical agents and antihistamines, she agrees to start additional pharmacologic intervention. You highlight that although numerous treatment possibilities exist, none are considered *definitive* resolution of disease.

10-A. Identify the most widely used agent and regimen in management of ICP.   2

☐ Oral ursodeoxycholic acid 10–21 mg/kg/d in two to three divided doses

10-B. List two other nonherbal treatments which *may* improve the symptoms or signs of ICP. *(1 point each)*   2

☐ Rifampin
☐ Cholestyramine (oral)*
☐ S-adenosylmethionine*
☐ Guar gum*
☐ Activated charcoal*
☐ Dexamethasone*

Special note:
* Insufficient evidence for effective treatment in women with ICP *(Cochrane Collaboration[7])*

You opt to initiate oral ursodeoxycholic acid 300 mg twice daily.

11. Inform the patient of the important aspects of counseling prior to initiating ursodeoxycholic acid. *(1 point each)*	4

☐ Provide reassurance of its fetal and neonatal safety
☐ Inform the patient that there is no conclusive evidence on reduction of adverse perinatal outcomes
☐ Indicate that symptomatic relief from pruritis is usually seen within one to two weeks, although some women are nonresponsive; biochemical improvement may take three to four weeks
☐ Reassure her that treatment is generally well tolerated; side effects include mild nausea, dizziness, and headache

The patient is keen to start the treatment, hoping to achieve symptomatic relief. She learned her sister was prescribed vitamin K in each of her pregnancies and wishes to know your professional opinion.

12. Inform the patient of the indications for vitamin K in management of ICP. *(2 points each)*	4

☐ Elevated prothrombin time
☐ Steatorrhea

Special note:
Suggested treatment entails oral vitamin K 5–10 mg daily from diagnosis until delivery; there is no current indication for treatment of this patient

The patient continues weekly investigations and maternal-fetal assessments. Over two weeks, you increased her ursodeoxycholic acid to 500 mg orally thrice daily for control of now widespread pruritis.‡ Vitamin K supplementation has not been required. Fetal sonographic monitoring has been unremarkable and presentation has remained cephalic.

At 36^{+6} weeks' gestation, the patient reports increasing pruritis. Fetal monitoring remains normal. Laboratory personnel calls to inform you that serum results taken four days prior revealed total bile acid level at 113 umol/L and ALT at 150 IU/L. Prothrombin time remains normal.

Special note:
‡ Dose-adjustments would not be advised solely for increasing laboratory tests

13. Outline your counseling and management plan with focus on obstetric cholestasis. *(1 point each)*

Max 5

☐ Recommend induction of labor[†] *(Cesarean delivery is reserved for obstetric indications)*

☐ Advise discontinuation of ursodeoxycholic acid at labor onset

☐ Continuous electronic fetal monitoring is advised in labor due to the higher risk of stillbirth

☐ Case-based considerations for risk of PPH; risk may not be increased among women treated with ursodeoxycholic acid[‡]

☐ Consideration for histopathologic examination of the placenta

☐ Plan for the neonatology team to attend the delivery, primarily if meconium-stained liquor or abnormal fetal tracing develops in labor

Special notes:

† Corticosteroid administration for fetal lung maturity and magnesium sulfate for neuroprotection are not required based on this patient's gestational age; jurisdiction protocols would apply if delivery at earlier gestational age was needed

‡ Furrer R et al. *Obstet Gynecol.* 2016; 128: 1048

The patient is keen to induce labor, recalling this should provide symptom resolution.

Induction of labor proceeds uneventfully and continuous fetal heart monitoring remains normal. The group B *Streptococcus* (GBS) swab was negative one week prior to delivery. Amniotomy reveals meconium-stained amniotic fluid. Spontaneous vaginal delivery ensues with a vigorous neonate at birth. Active management of the third stage of labor was performed as planned to mitigate the risk of PPH.

Breastfeeding is initiated and the patient is discharged from hospital based on routine practice; the newborn is safely discharged from hospital at four days of life, upon recovery from a brief episode of respiratory distress syndrome.

14. Outline postpartum management and counseling of short-term and long-term   Max 7
implications of obstetric cholestasis. *(1 point each)*

Maternal care after ICP:
- ☐ Repeat liver transaminases at two to six weeks postpartum to ensure values normalized and provide specialist referral if test results remain abnormal
- ☐ Consider repeating hepatitis C antibody two to six weeks postpartum to ensure no seroconversion occurred
- ☐ Address future risks of hepatobiliary diseases after ICP *(e.g, cholelithiasis, liver fibrosis, cirrhosis, cholangitis, hepatitis C, or pancreatic diseases)*, where the period of greatest risk appears to be within the first year after an ICP diagnosis
- ☐ Address long-term risks of cardiovascular and immune diseases with prior ICP
- ☐ Inform the patient that the risk of recurrent obstetric cholestasis in future pregnancies may be up to 90%[†]; preconception counseling is advised
- ☐ Consider referral for genetic evaluation based on the patient's family history of obstetric cholestasis and disease severity; genetic variants in bile acid pathway transport proteins have been implicated in ICP

Contraceptive recommendations:
- ☐ There are no restrictions on use of progesterone-only contraceptive agents based on history of obstetric cholestasis or cholestasis related to combined oral contraceptives
- ☐ Combined oral contraceptives remain optional after obstetric cholestasis, where advantages generally outweigh theoretical or proven risks[§]; however, use of combined oral contraceptive agents is not recommended after contraceptive-related cholestasis

Special notes:
† Insufficient evidence to counsel on specific ranges for recurrent risk of ICP
§ UK and US Medical Eligibility Criteria (MEC) for Contraceptive Use, 2016; UK-MEC revised September 2019

<u>**TOTAL:**</u>   **85**

CHAPTER 41

Acute Fatty Liver of Pregnancy

Neel S. Iyer, Meena Khandelwal, and Amira El-Messidi

During your call duty, a *healthy* 40-year-old primigravida with a spontaneous dichorionic pregnancy presents, accompanied by her husband, to the obstetric emergency assessment unit of your hospital center at 33^{+1} weeks' gestation with new-onset abdominal pain and vomiting after a two-day history of nausea and general malaise. She has no obstetric complaints, and fetal viabilities are ascertained upon presentation. Her face appears yellow tinged relative to her last clinical visit one week ago. You recall that routine prenatal laboratory investigations, aneuploidy screening, morphology surveys of the male fetuses, and serial sonograms have all been unremarkable.

Special note: *Although women with acute fatty liver of pregnancy have increased rates of medical and obstetric morbidities, including but not limited to disseminated intravascular coagulation, pancreatitis, concomitant hypertensive disorders of pregnancy, and postpartum hemorrhage, the case scenario avoids overlap of content addressed in other chapters. Readers are encouraged to complement subject matter where clinically required.*

LEARNING OBJECTIVES

1. Take a focused history, and verbalize essentials of a physical examination focused to a typical prenatal presentation of acute fatty liver of pregnancy (AFLP)
2. Recognize laboratory derangements in AFLP, including distinguishing features from HELLP syndrome and preeclampsia
3. Appreciate potential maternal-fetal adverse outcomes with AFLP, highlighting the importance of timely multidisciplinary care
4. Outline critical obstetric and medical aspects of management for a parturient with AFLP
5. Understand clinically relevant features of disease pathogenesis for current maternal-infant care and future prenatal counseling

SUGGESTED READINGS

1. Chang L, Wang M, Liu H, et al. Pregnancy outcomes of patients with acute fatty liver of pregnancy: a case control study. *BMC Pregnancy Childbirth.* 2020;20(1):282.
2. Donck M, Vercruysse Y, Alexis A, et al. Acute fatty liver of pregnancy – a short review. *Aust N Z J Obstet Gynaecol.* 2021;61(2):183–187.
3. Guarino M, Cossiga V, Morisco F. The interpretation of liver function tests in pregnancy. *Best Pract Res Clin Gastroenterol.* 2020;44–45:101667.

4. Liu J, Ghaziani TT, Wolf JL. Acute fatty liver disease of pregnancy: updates in pathogenesis, diagnosis, and management. *Am J Gastroenterol.* 2017;112(6):838–846.

5. Nelson DB, Byrne JJ, Cunningham FG. Acute fatty liver of pregnancy. *Clin Obstet Gynecol.* 2020;63(1):152–164.

6. Nelson DB, Byrne JJ, Cunningham FG. Acute fatty liver of pregnancy. *Obstet Gynecol.* 2021;137(3):535–546.

7. Nelson DB, Yost NP, Cunningham FG. Acute fatty liver of pregnancy: clinical outcomes and expected duration of recovery. *Am J Obstet Gynecol.* 2013;209(5):456.e1–456.e4567.

8. Naoum EE, Leffert LR, Chitilian HV, et al. Acute fatty liver of pregnancy: pathophysiology, anesthetic implications, and obstetrical management. *Anesthesiology.* 2019;130(3):446–461.

9. Rath W, Tsikouras P, Stelzl P. HELLP syndrome or acute fatty liver of pregnancy: a differential diagnostic challenge: common features and differences. *Geburtshilfe Frauenheilkd.* 2020;80(5):499–507.

10. Tran TT, Ahn J, Reau NS. acg clinical guideline: liver disease and pregnancy. *Am J Gastroenterol.* 2016;111(2):176–196. [Correction in *Am J Gastroenterol.* 2016 Nov;111(11):1668]

POINTS

1. What aspects of a focused history would you want to know? *(1 point per main bullet; max points specified per section)*   Max 15

Features related to gastrointestinal symptoms: *(5)*
☐ Characteristics of the abdominal pain
  ○ *i.e., pattern, relation to meals, radiation, aggravating/alleviating factors*
☐ Details of vomitus
  ○ *i.e., bilious, hematemesis, amount and frequency*
☐ Lower gastrointestinal changes
☐ History of cholelithiasis *(i.e., or other hepatobiliary conditions where clinically relevant; this patient is noted to be 'healthy')*
☐ Prior episodes of similar symptoms or presentations

Associated manifestations: *(max 6)*
☐ Fever or chills
☐ Headache or visual changes
☐ Cardiorespiratory symptoms *(e.g., worsening dyspnea, chest pain)*
☐ Pruritis, particularly nocturnal and of the palms/soles
☐ New-onset bruising or nonvaginal bleeding
☐ Polydipsia/polyuria
☐ Pale/concentrated urine, dysuria, hematuria
☐ Confusion, lethargy, obtundedness *(e.g., noted by husband)*

Medications: *(2)*
☐ Excessive use of paracetamol/acetaminophen or another offending agent
☐ Allergies (pharmacologic/nonpharmacologic)

Social features: *(max 2)*
☐ Chronic alcohol abuse
☐ Illicit drug use
☐ Recent travel

You learn that the abdominal pain, limited to the epigastrium and right upper quadrant, has been increasing in intensity since spontaneous onset earlier today; abdominal pain and nonbilious vomitus are unrelated to meals. Her husband remarked that strangely, she appeared unaware of the directions to hospital. Comprehensive medical and social histories are otherwise unremarkable; she only takes routine prenatal vitamins and oral iron supplements. In conversation with the patient, she asks for a large cup of water and voided her bladder twice within 15 minutes of presentation. Uterine quiescence is ascertained on cardiotocography (CTG) and fetal heart tracings show variability is ≤5 bpm in amplitude without decelerations.

2. Verbalize essentials of your <u>focused</u> physical examination. *(1 point each)*   Max 12

Vital signs:
☐ Blood pressure
☐ Pulse
☐ Temperature
☐ Oxygen saturation
☐ Respiratory rate

General appearance and mental status:
☐ Lucidity in conversation; if required, ask the patient to draw a clock face or a five-pointed star[†]
☐ Body habitus

Skin assessment:
☐ Jaundice or scleral icterus
☐ New-onset petechiae/bruising or needle track marks

Cardiorespiratory examination:
☐ Air entry on both lung fields *(i.e., pleural effusion)*

Abdominal examination[‡]:
☐ Assess for focal tenderness at the sites associated with pain
☐ Elicit Murphy's sign
☐ Assess for ascites

Neurologic examination:
☐ Liver flap (asterixis)
☐ Deep tendon reflexes

Special notes:
† Clinical assessment for encephalopathy; refer to Nelson-Piercy, C. *Handbook of Obstetric Medicine*; 5th ed. London (UK): Informa Healthcare; 2015 [page. 219]
‡ Based on this case scenario, there is no indication for pelvic examination at this time

With a known small body habitus, the patient appears excessively lethargic and has brief twitches of both arms where you notice multiple new petechiae. She is normotensive, afebrile, and oxygen saturation is normal. In addition to noticeable jaundice, examination is significant for scleral icterus and tenderness in the upper abdomen, with a negative Murphy's sign. Remaining findings on comprehensive physical examination are unremarkable.

3. Highlight to your obstetric trainee the <u>clinical</u> signs and symptoms compatible   4
    with <u>diagnostic</u> criteria of your most probable pregnancy-associated complication.
    (1 point each)

Swansea Criteria – Clinical:
☐ Vomiting
☐ Abdominal pain
☐ Polyuria/polydipsia (*i.e., 'she asks for a large cup of water and voided her bladder twice within 15 minutes of presentation'*)
☐ Encephalopathy (*i.e., '...strangely, she appeared unaware of the directions to hospital' and '... brief twitches of both arms...'*)

4. Elicit this patient's <u>risk factors</u>[†] that would be consistent with the most likely diagnosis.   6
    (1 point each)

☐ Nulliparity
☐ Multiple gestation
☐ Male fetus(es) *[M:F ratio is 3:1 for risk of AFLP]*
☐ Third-trimester onset of symptoms
☐ Low body mass index (BMI)[‡]
☐ Advanced maternal age

Special notes:
[†] (a) Although prior AFLP or known fetal fatty acid oxidation disorders are risk factors for disease, such aspects will only be relevant in future counseling of this primigravida
[†] (b) Concurrent hepatic disorders (e.g. intrahepatic cholestasis) or diabetes mellitus, are weaker risk factors
[‡] Obesity is also a risk factor for AFLP *(Suggested Reading 6)*

5. In comprehensive work-up related to the differential diagnoses being considered, outline maternal <u>laboratory derangements and imaging features</u> that would be consistent with <u>diagnostic</u> criteria of the most probable diagnosis. *(1 point each)*

10

Swansea Criteria:

Biochemical	Radiological	Histological
Hepatic[†]	☐ Bright liver echo or ascites on abdominal ultrasound	☐ Microvesicular steatosis with periportal sparring
☐ Elevated bilirubin		
☐ Elevated transaminases[‡]		
☐ Elevated ammonia		
Renal		
☐ Elevated urate		
☐ Elevated serum creatinine		
Endocrine		
☐ Hypoglycemia		
Hematological		
☐ Leucocytosis		
☐ Coagulopathy or prolonged prothrombin time		

Special notes:

† Serum cholesterol, which is normally significantly increased by the third trimester, is abnormally low in AFLP, though this is not a diagnostic feature in the Swansea criteria

‡ ALT is more specific than AST AFLP

You inform your trainee that in the absence of a universal standardized diagnostic approach, characteristic clinical features and results of investigations may establish the diagnosis when a total of ≥6 criteria are present. You highlight how imaging modalities are nonspecific and nondiagnostic in isolation. Although liver biopsy is diagnostic, it is rarely required, being invasive and associated with maternal morbidity, particularly in the presence of coagulopathy.

Results of *serum biochemistry* show the following:

Bilirubin	1.6 mg/dL (27.4 μmol/L)
ALT	400 IU/L
AST	200 IU/L
Ammonia	40 μmol/L
Urate	350 μmol/L
Creatinine	1.5 mg/dL (132.6 μmol/L)
Glucose	56 mg/dL (3.1 mmol/L)
Leucocyte count	12.3 × 10⁹/L
Prothrombin time	11 seconds

Hemoglobin and platelet concentrations are within normal on full/complete blood count (FBC/CBC); lactate dehydrogenase (LDH) is mildly increased. Proteinuria is within physiological limits for pregnancy.

6. In the absence of other causes, what is the most responsible diagnosis?   1

   ☐ Acute fatty liver of pregnancy (AFLP)

7. Among the resulted investigations, identify the three laboratory findings that remain   3
   within normal based on diagnostic thresholds associated with this potentially fatal
   pregnancy complication. *(1 point each)*

   ☐ Ammonia remains below 27.5 mg/dL (47 μmol/L)
   ☐ Creatinine remains below 1.7 mg/dL (150 μmol/L)
   ☐ Prothrombin time remains below 14 seconds

   Special note:
   Laboratory parameters consistent with diagnostic thresholds for AFLP include bilirubin
   >0.8 mg/dL (14 μmol/L), transaminases >42 IU/L, urate >5.7 mg/dL (340 μmol/L), glucose
   <72 mg/dL (4 mmol/L), and leukocyte concentration >11 × 10⁹/L

8. Which <u>pregnancy-related disorders</u> may be initially confused with AFLP?   4
   (1 point each)

   ☐ Hyperemesis gravidarum
   ☐ HELLP syndrome or preeclampsia
   ☐ Intrahepatic cholestasis of pregnancy
   ☐ Thrombotic microangiopathy

Recalling the significant overlap between AFLP and HELLP syndrome or preeclampsia, with coexisting disease in 20% and 20%–40% of patients respectively, your trainee inquires about features that may facilitate their challenging distinction. While delivery is the mainstay of management, there may be substantial differences in clinical course, associated sequalae, intrapartum and postpartum management of AFLP and these hypertensive conditions of pregnancy. You take note to address your trainee's queries after timely counseling and management of the patient.

---

9. Outline <u>distinctive features</u> of AFLP that *may aid* in distinguishing it from HELLP syndrome <u>or</u> preeclampsia. *(1 point each)*   Max 11

- ☐ Jaundice
- ☐ Polyuria
- ☐ Polydipsia
- ☐ Ascites
- ☐ (Profound) hypoglycemia
- ☐ Hypocholesterolemia
- ☐ Elevated ammonia levels
- ☐ Leucocytosis
- ☐ Increased *direct* bilirubin levels (as opposed to increased *indirect* bilirubin with HELLP-associated hemolysis)
- ☐ Coagulopathy in the absence of thrombocytopenia
- ☐ Initial absence of hemolysis
- ☐ Encephalopathy with rapid progression to liver failure
- ☐ Progressive course to acute liver failure irrespective of gestational age, without potential for episodic exacerbations/transient remissions
- ☐ Sonographic description of a 'bright liver' or ascites in AFLP, relative to subcapsular hematoma or liver rupture more typical of preeclampsia or HELLP syndrome
- ☐ Histological finding of microvesicular steatosis with periportal sparing and minimal hepatocyte necrosis on liver biopsy in AFLP, relative to periportal hemorrhagic necrosis characteristic of preeclampsia
- ☐ Normal sFlT-1/PlGF level

---

10. Explain the pathophysiological basis for the patient's polydipsia and polyuria.   2

- ☐ Hepatic dysfunction in AFLP leads to decreased metabolism of placental vasopressinase, resulting in increased circulating concentrations of enzyme to metabolize antidiuretic hormone, lowering serum levels of antidiuretic hormone

---

In counseling the patient and her husband, you mention that AFLP is neither predictable nor preventable; you highlight the seriousness of the disorder where multispecialty teams are simultaneously being activated. Nurses and midwives are already collaborating to optimize care of the mother and fetuses.

The patient has no known drug allergies.

11. As a senior obstetrician, identify other <u>interprofessional teams</u> that would be notified for <u>acute</u> care of the patient. *(1 point each)*   5

- ☐ Anesthesiology
- ☐ Neonatology
- ☐ Critical care physicians
- ☐ Hepatology
- ☐ Transfusion medicine/hematology

12. With reference to health care teams, summarize potential complications of AFLP.   10
(1 point each; max points specified per section)

Maternal antenatal or postnatal complications: *(max 7)*
- ☐ Metabolic acidosis
- ☐ Gastrointestinal hemorrhage
- ☐ Postpartum hemorrhage
- ☐ Disseminated intravascular coagulation (DIC)[†]
- ☐ Pulmonary edema/acute respiratory distress syndrome
- ☐ Acute pancreatitis
- ☐ Acute kidney injury
- ☐ Encephalopathy
- ☐ Liver failure requiring transplantation *(rare)*
- ☐ Mortality *(<5% with early diagnosis, prompt delivery and maternal stabilization)*

Fetal/neonatal: *(max 3)*
- ☐ Abnormal CTG monitoring
- ☐ Prematurity and related complications
- ☐ Intrauterine fetal demise (IUFD)
- ☐ Infant demise from nonketotic hypoglycemia among those with long-chain-3-hydroxyacyl CoA dehydrogenase (LCHAD) deficiency

Special note:
[†] 80% of women with AFLP had a diagnostic scoring system; refer to Nelson DB, Yost NP, Cunningham FG. Hemostatic dysfunction with acute fatty liver of pregnancy. *Obstet Gynecol.* 2014;124:40–6.

13. Maintaining multidisciplinary collaboration, detail important aspects of the <u>obstetric and medical management plan</u> for this primiparous patient with AFLP at 33^{+1} weeks' gestation who remains normotensive. *(1 point per main bullet; max points specified per section)*   Max 16

Timing and mode of delivery: *(max 3)*
- ☐ Expedite delivery after maternal hemodynamic stabilization
- ☐ Cesarean section may be preferable where induction of labor will likely to be prolonged or unsuccessful; route of delivery is otherwise based on obstetric indications
- ☐ Consideration for a midline abdominal incision in the setting of coagulopathy (or high risk thereof), as this may offer dual benefits: *(Suggested Reading 6)*
  - ○ *(a)* decreased risk of subfascial hematoma that occurs with a Pfannenstiel incision
  - ○ *(b)* allows for exploration of the upper abdomen, where necessary

☐ Maintain a low threshold for use of a surgical drain if significant surgical oozing or ascites is found at operative delivery

Principles of medical and anesthetic management:[†] *(max 9)*
☐ Continuous monitoring of maternal mental status *(risk of rapidly progressive encephalopathy)*
☐ Obtain two large-bore intravenous catheters *(anticipate PPH or DIC)*
☐ Strict attention is required for fluid balance; bladder catheterization is required
☐ Arrange for potential need of blood product replacement
☐ Low threshold for use of general anesthesia based on platelet concentration, coagulopathy, mental status, or where mandated by abnormal fetal CTG status
☐ Administer an antiemetic treatment with continued vomiting
☐ Administer antacids/H2-receptor antagonists to protect the gastrointestinal tract from stress-induced hemorrhage
☐ Normalize serum glucose levels prior to delivery with 10% or 50% dextrose infusions; serial serum testing is required
☐ Start broad-spectrum antibiotics due to susceptibility to infection; base the choice of pharmacologic agent on renal function *(given no drug allergies)*
☐ Consideration for lactulose or neomycin to treat increased serum ammonia levels
☐ Consideration for intranasal/subcutaneous desmopressin to treat the diabetes insipidus, particularly with hypernatremia, increased serum osmolality, or excessive urine output

Fetal care: *(4)*
☐ Maintain continuous electronic fetal monitoring until delivery
☐ Maternal administration of magnesium sulfate for fetal neuroprotection[‡]
  ○ *ACOG and WHO: <32 weeks*
  ○ *RCOG: upper gestational age limit not specified*
  ○ *SOGC: up to 33[+6] weeks*
☐ Maternal administration of fetal pulmonary corticosteroids,[§] based on gestational age considerations
  ○ *Cesarean section [or induction of labor] should not be delayed*
☐ Ensure presence of neonatology team at delivery for both short- and long-term care of the newborns whose mother has AFLP

Special notes:
† Based on acetaminophen/paracetamol-related hepatotoxicity, N-acetylcysteine may be considered to improve tissue oxygenation and hemodynamics, although evidence of benefit in AFLP is lacking
‡ Magnesium sulfate would also be considered for eclampsia prophylaxis at any gestational age where a diagnosis of preeclampsia is also being considered
§ Refer to Question 18 in Chapter 9

Based on the agreed-upon multidisciplinary care plan, maternal hemodynamic status is stabilized prior to Cesarean delivery, where another senior obstetrician presents to assist you in her care. After delivery of the liveborn twin boys, in the presence of the neonatology team, intrapartum coagulopathy ensues. The patient responds well to blood product replacement, obviating the need for hysterectomy. Postpartum, she is transferred to the intensive care/treatment unit (ICU/ITU) for close monitoring of potential complications.

You debrief with her husband shortly after the neonatologist, who has just discussed planned infants' investigations, particular to maternal AFLP.

14. Elaborate on the significance of the intended neonatal investigations, most specific to maternal AFLP. *(1 point per main bullet)*   2

- ☐ Neonatal screening for LCHAD deficiency is particularly important as it is the culprit in ~20% of AFLP
- ☐ Homozygous LCHAD deficiency causes a mitochondrial fatty acid oxidation defect in offspring that can result in a Reye-like syndrome and death from nonketotic hypoglycemia
  - ○ *Homozygous G1528C mutation, causing a glutamate-to-glutamine amino acid change, is the most common genotype-cause for AFLP*

15. Rationalize why only a subset of AFLP is linked to LCHAD deficiency by identifying other enzyme deficiencies of fetoplacental mitochondrial oxidation that have been associated with AFLP. *(1 point each)*   Max 3

- ☐ Carnitine palmitoyltransferse-1(CPT-1) deficiency
- ☐ Short-chain acyl-CoA dehydrogenase (SCAD) deficiency
- ☐ Medium-chain acyl-CoA dehydrogenase (MCAD) deficiency
- ☐ Very long-chain acyl-CoA dehydrogenase (VLCHAD) deficiency
- ☐ Mitochondrial trifunctional protein deficiency

16. Based on pathophysiology, explain to the patient's husband how a *fetal* enzymatic deficiency of mitochondrial oxidation would lead to a *maternal* life-threatening disorder.   4

- ☐ Defective ß-oxidation of mitochondrial fetal fatty acids results in accumulated intermediate products that enter the maternal circulation; heterozygous mothers for the enzymatic defect cannot complete fatty acid oxidation, leading to hepatocyte toxicity, multiple morbidities, and risk of maternal mortality *(fetal free fatty acids increase in the third trimester to support fetoplacental growth)*

Considering your communication with her husband, your obstetric trainee later contemplates the rationale for the approximate 18% **perinatal mortality**[†] in AFLP, presuming that transplacental transfer of toxic unoxidized fetal fatty acid intermediates would serve as a fetal 'protective mechanism.'

Special note:
† *Suggested Reading 5*

17. Excluding prematurity, present a disease-specific etiology for fetal mortality in AFLP. 2

☐ Maternal acidosis and hypoxia affect uteroplacental blood flow and fetal oxygenation

As the patient recovers over the week postpartum, you intend to provide debriefing with her and routine postpartum counseling.

18. With focus on AFLP and related gestational morbidities experienced by the patient, what are important postpartum considerations to discuss either prior to discharge and/or at the routine outpatient clinical visit? *(1 point per main bullet)* Max 10

General maternal-fetal well-being:
☐ Encourage breastfeeding/pumping
☐ Alert the patient on future pregnancy risk of alloantibodies associated with her receipt of intrapartum blood transfusions
☐ Screen for postpartum depression and continue to offer psychosocial support
☐ Offer social work support based on recent gestational complications, prematurity, and multiple pregnancy *(individualized)*

Aspects related to AFLP:
☐ Inform her that in *most* cases, AFLP resolves completely within 7–10 days postpartum
☐ Maternal LCHAD testing would be indicated with positive neonatal homozygous enzymatic defects
☐ Although the exact risk of future recurrence is unknown, AFLP may recur despite negative maternal testing for enzymatic defects of fatty acid oxidation
☐ Recurrence risk may be up to 25% with positive result for a maternal molecular defect of fatty acid oxidation[†] (autosomal recessive inheritance)
☐ Ensure arrangements are made for maternal outpatient follow-up with necessary medical experts
☐ Encourage future preconception counseling and prenatal care with a maternal-fetal medicine expert

Contraceptive recommendations:
☐ There are no contraceptive contraindications associated with *complete* resolution of organ dysfunction after AFLP
  ○ Combined hormonal contraception is not recommended with decompensated liver disease requiring transplantation

Special note:
† *Refer to* Thann NN, Neuberger J. Liver abnormalities in pregnancy. *Best Pract Res Clinic Gastroenterol.* 2013;27:565–75

TOTAL: 120

CHAPTER 42

Crohn's Disease in Pregnancy

Waseem Ahmed, Amira El-Messidi, and Robert Battat

A 26-year-old G2P1 with Crohn's disease (CD) is referred by her primary care provider to your high-risk obstetrics unit for transfer of care at 10 weeks' gestation by dating sonography. Routine prenatal investigations are unremarkable. She has no obstetric complaints.

Special note: *To avoid overlap, the reader is encouraged to complement subject matter with content presented in Chapter 43.*

LEARNING OBJECTIVES

1. Take a focused prenatal history from a patient with CD, and verbalize essentials of the physical examination for suspected antenatal disease flare
2. Appreciate the importance of multidisciplinary collaboration in caring for the obstetric patient with CD, particularly during hospitalization management of disease flare, and understand relevant CD-related and obstetric considerations in delivery decision-making
3. Identify potential paternal, fetal, and neonatal effects, or reassuring safety profile, of various therapeutics used in inflammatory bowel disease
4. Provide evidence-based counseling recommendations for use of various radiologic studies or endoscopic evaluation of active CD in the obstetric setting
5. Highlight the benefits of preconception counseling of patients with inflammatory bowel disease, and appreciate possible particularities with oral or injectable progesterone-only contraception

SUGGESTED READINGS

1. ASGE Standard of Practice Committee, Shergill AK, Ben-Menachem T, et al. Guidelines for endoscopy in pregnant and lactating women. *Gastrointest Endosc.* 2012;76(1):18–24. [Correction in *Gastrointest Endosc.* 2013 May;77(5):833]
2. Foulon A, Dupas JL, Sabbagh C, et al. Defining the most appropriate delivery mode in women with inflammatory bowel disease: a systematic review. *Inflamm Bowel Dis.* 2017;23(5): 712–720.
3. Mahadevan U, McConnell RA, Chambers CD. Drug safety and risk of adverse outcomes for pregnant patients with inflammatory bowel disease. *Gastroenterology.* 2017 Feb;152(2): 451–462.

4. Mahadevan U, Robinson C, Bernasko N, et al. Inflammatory bowel disease in pregnancy clinical care pathway: a report from the American Gastroenterological Association IBD Parenthood Project Working Group. *Am J Obstet Gynecol.* 2019;220(4):308–323.

5. Mahadevan U, McConnell RA, Chambers CD. Drug safety and risk of adverse outcomes for pregnant patients with inflammatory bowel disease. *Gastroenterology.* 2017 Feb;152(2): 451–462.

6. Mahadevan U, Wolf DC, Dubinsky M, et al. Placental transfer of anti-tumor necrosis factor agents in pregnant patients with inflammatory bowel disease. *Clin Gastroenterol Hepatol.* 2013 Mar;11(3):286–92; quiz e24.

7. Nielsen OH, Gubatan JM, Juhl CB, et al. Biologics for inflammatory bowel disease and their safety in pregnancy: a systematic review and meta-analysis. *Clin Gastroenterol Hepatol.* 2020; S1542–3565(20):31281–31287.

8. Nguyen GC, Seow CH, Maxwell C, et al. The Toronto consensus statements for the management of inflammatory bowel disease in pregnancy. *Gastroenterology.* 2016;150(3): 734–757.

9. Restellini S, Biedermann L, Hruz P, et al. Update on the management of inflammatory bowel disease during pregnancy and breastfeeding. *Digestion.* 2020;101(Suppl 1):27–42.

10. van der Woude CJ, Ardizzone S, Bengtson MB, et al. The second European evidence-based consensus on reproduction and pregnancy in inflammatory bowel disease. *J Crohns Colitis.* 2015;9(2):107–124.

POINTS

1. If anemia is the only abnormal laboratory finding in this patient with Crohn's disease, what aspects of a focused history would you want to know?[†] *(1 point per main bullet, unless specified)*

35

General disease-related details:
☐ Chronology between age at CD diagnosis and last pregnancy
☐ Time-interval since last CD flare
☐ Presence of active disease at conception
☐ Anatomical location of disease
☐ Name and contact of treating gastroenterologist

Current gastrointestinal symptoms:
☐ Quantification of daytime and nocturnal bowel movements
☐ Presence of rectal bleeding
☐ Stool consistency
☐ Incontinence
☐ Abdominal pain *(overlap with pregnancy)*
☐ Nausea/vomiting, weight loss *(overlap with pregnancy)*

History of CD-related complications:
☐ Perianal manifestations *(unique to CD):* **(1 point per subbullet; max 2)**
   ○ *Anorectal fistulizing or abscess process*
   ○ *Anal fissures or stenosis*
   ○ *Rectovaginal fistula*

☐ Intestinal manifestations: *(1 point per subbullet; max 2)*
  ○ *Small bowel obstruction (medical or surgical treatment)*
  ○ *Strictures*
  ○ *Ileal resection status*
☐ Current/prior colonic dysplasia, and findings on most recent colonoscopy
☐ Specify the type of anemia
☐ Disease-related hospitalizations
☐ Personal history of venous thromboembolism

Surgery:
☐ Number of disease-related abdominoperineal surgeries, *if any*
☐ Appendectomy

Past pregnancy features related to CD:
☐ Antenatal/postnatal course and treatment
☐ Mode of delivery
☐ Postpartum disease-related complications

Current/prior medical treatments, clinical response and side effects:
☐ **Therapies not compatible with pregnancy:** methotrexate, tofacitinib
☐ **Therapies compatible with pregnancy:** biologics, thiopurines, corticosteroids, aminosalicylates
☐ Opioid dependence

Social history:
☐ Ethnicity
☐ Cigarette smoking, alcohol, recreational drugs (especially cannabis)

Routine health maintenance:
☐ Vaccination status *(postpartum live viral vaccines, if required, would be avoided with immunosuppressant treatment)*
☐ Recent Papanicolaou smear

Family history: *(max 3 points)*
☐ Inflammatory bowel disease
☐ Earliest age at diagnosis among affected family members
☐ Autoimmune disease
☐ Colorectal cancer
☐ Venous thromboembolism

Male partner history:
☐ Known inflammatory bowel disease *(2 points)*

You learn the patient was diagnosed at age 15 years when she presented with weight loss and perianal pain. Examination under anesthesia revealed a perianal abscess requiring incision and drainage, and a fistula for which a seton was placed to promote healing. Colonoscopy was notable for discontinuous ulcerations involving the terminal ileum, with normal intervening mucosa; histological assessment confirmed CD. Several years ago, the patient had one resection for small bowel obstruction and after several suboptimal treatment responses to methotrexate for attempted disease-control, she was subsequently well-controlled on azathioprine.[†]

Your colleague, who followed her prenatal care two years ago, is now on sabbatical. The patient indicates that azathioprine monotherapy was optimized preconceptionally and continued throughout pregnancy. A perianal fistula developed midgestation for which she had an elective Cesarean delivery at term. The current pregnancy was conceived while the patient was taking a progesterone-only oral contraceptive agent.

Five months prior to her current pregnancy, moderately active disease was found on colonoscopy and magnetic resonance enterography showed a chronic perianal fistula without an abscess. The patient's symptoms responded well to a course of oral prednisone. Her perianal fistulae persisted, and she currently remains on azathioprine monotherapy. She takes replacement therapies for various anemias and daily prenatal vitamins. She currently has two to three nonbloody bowel movements daily; her body mass index is stable at 20 kg/m^2 and she practices healthy lifestyle habits. Several family members are affected with CD, with the earliest age of onset being 17 years, consistent with their ethnicity. Her partner also has Crohn's disease.

At eight weeks' gestation, she saw her gastroenterologist; her fecal calprotectin was elevated at 350 ug/g.[‡]

Special notes:
[†] Testing to ensure normal TPMT (*thiopurine methyltransferase*) enzyme activity is required prior to the initiation of thiopurines
[‡] Optimal cutoff of fecal calprotectin to predict disease activity in pregnancy is unknown: may range from >50 to >250 ug/g

2. Regarding immunomodulators used to stabilize CD in this patient, discuss their associated fetal/neonatal risks, including pregnancy recommendations.   6

Methotrexate: *(1 point each for 3 points)*
☐ Antifolate, teratogenic, contraindicated in pregnancy/breastfeeding
☐ Abortifacient
☐ Ideally discontinued at least three months preconception *(inadvertent use in pregnancy requires referral to a high-risk obstetrics expert for individualized discussion; termination may be considered)*

Azathioprine: *(1 point each; max 3)*
☐ No increased risk of congenital anomalies
☐ Possible risk of preterm delivery *(inconsistent finding)*
☐ No increased risk of infections within the first year of life
☐ No proven concerns of neonatal anemia
  ○ Antenatal pediatric consultation is advised

Special note:
Continuation of azathioprine is permissible; however, initiation during pregnancy carries risks of medication side effects (leukopenia, hepatitis, pancreatitis) which may incur risk to the pregnancy

Prior to counseling the patient and planning antenatal management, your trainee searched for the results of investigations performed earlier in pregnancy to assess the status of her anemia.

3. Identify four etiologies that may explain anemia in this patient with CD. *(1 point each, unless specified)*

    ☐ Iron deficiency *(2 points)*
    ☐ Anemia of chronic disease
    ☐ Vitamin B12 deficiency
    ☐ Drug-induced anemia

5

Laboratory investigations performed recently by her gastroenterologist confirmed iron, folate, and B12 deficiency for which treatment adjustments were made. Although excited about the pregnancy, she is concerned if her children will inherit inflammatory bowel disease and how her disease can affect pregnancy outcome.

4. Which factors specific to *this* patient may influence her offspring's future risk of inflammatory bowel disease? *(1 point each)*

    ☐ Having two affected parents raises the risk of inflammatory bowel disease in their offspring
    ☐ Multiple affected family members with CD
    ☐ Young age at diagnosis of inflammatory bowel disease among family members
    ☐ Ethnicity

4

5. Elicit four <u>disease-related</u> factors that may predict pregnancy outcome, identifying factors specific to *this* patient. *(1 point each, unless specified)*

    ☐ Active disease at conception or during gestation *(2 points)*
    ☐ Prior disease-related surgery
    ☐ Location of disease
    ☐ Presence of perianal fistulae

5

The patient is content with planned multidisciplinary collaboration, similar to her prior pregnancy. She can still detail the fetal risks[†] and management given maternal CD. Albeit early in gestation, she is keen to explore the possibility of a vaginal birth after Cesarean (VBAC) as her online literature search reassured her that the interdelivery interval and prior low transverse uterine scar are in her favor.

Special note:
† *Refer to* Question 6 in Chapter 43

6. Discuss both disease and obstetric considerations in guiding the mode of delivery for patients with CD.

10

CD-related delivery considerations: *(1 point per main bullet and subbullet; max 4)*
    ☐ Cesarean delivery is recommended in the presence of <u>active</u> perianal disease around the time of delivery
    ☐ Mention that the risk of a fourth-degree perineal laceration is increased 10-fold with active perianal disease

□ Inform the patient that with <u>inactive</u> perianal fistulizing disease *(i.e., all fistulas closed on physical exam, magnetic resonance pelvic imaging and/or exam under anesthesia)*, vaginal delivery may be possible, depending on multifactor assessment for risk of perianal tears *(shared decision-making)*:
  ○ Chronicity of perianal lesions
  ○ Other types of fistulizing lesions *(e.g., Cesarean delivery is advised for prior rectovaginal fistula)*
  ○ Characteristics of fistulous tract *(i.e., simple, complex, location)*

Obstetric considerations in deciding the preferred mode of delivery:

Maternal: *(1 point each; max 4)*
□ Primiparity
□ Need for induction of labor
□ Short ano-pubic distance
□ Prior perineal tears or episiotomy
□ Consistency of the perineal body
□ Systemic conditions affecting connective tissues

Fetal: *(1 point each; max 2)*
□ Suspected macrosomia (>4000 g)
□ Complex cephalic presentations *(i.e., face, compound, brow)*
□ Breech delivery of a second twin

As a high-risk obstetrician, you follow her antenatal care in collaboration with her gastroenterologist and nutritionist. The patient remains on maintenance azathioprine and pregnancy is unremarkable until 26^{+4} weeks' gestation when she presents to the obstetric emergency assessment unit with a two-day history of bloody diarrhea, intermittent abdominal pain, and recurrent drainage from her perianal fistula. Last week, her glucose test was normal. She reports fetal activity and has no obstetric complaints. Routine cardiotocography (CTG) monitoring initiated upon her arrival shows an appropriate fetal tracing for gestational age without uterine contractions. You notify a gastroenterologist who presents to assess the patient with you.

7. In conjunction with the gastroenterologist, outline your focused physical exam regarding her presenting complaints. *(1 point each)*   5

□ General appearance and vital signs *(i.e., blood pressure [BP], pulse, temperature)*
□ Current weight in comparison with that at latest prenatal visit
□ Assess for bowel sounds
□ Abdominal tenderness/distension *(may be confounded by pregnancy)*
□ Perianal inspection and digital rectal examination

On exam, the patient appears pale and in distress from abdominal pain. Her BP is 98/60 mmHg, pulse is 105 bpm, and she has a low-grade fever at 37.8°C. She has lost 1.5 lb since the last prenatal visit two weeks ago.

Laboratory investigations are notable for the following:

		Normal
Hemoglobin (g/L)	100	97–148*
Mean copuscular volume (fL)	78	85.8–99.4*
C-reactive protein (mg/L)	25	0.4–20.3*
Erythrocyte sedimentation rate (mm/hr)	40	<30*
Serum albumin (g/dL)	2.2	2.6–4.5*
Fecal calprotectin (ug/g)	2000	<100§

* Pregnancy reference ranges for second trimester, available at www.perinatology.com/Reference/Reference%20Ranges/Reference%20for%20Serum.htm, accessed October 29, 2020
§ Optimal cutoff to predict disease activity in pregnancy is unknown; may range from >50 to >250 ug/g

You perform an obstetric sonogram: fetal biometry is on the 13th percentile and growth velocity is appropriate since the 20-week morphology scan. Fetal markers of well-being are normal. Her cervical length is normal.

After discussion with the gastroenterologist, you concurrently attend to counsel the patient. In conversation, the patient consents to MRI and flexible sigmoidoscopy to assess her disease activity. She alerts the team that she always requires sedation at endoscopic evaluation. The patient undergoes an uncomplicated flexible sigmoidoscopy revealing of deep, serpiginous ulcers extending from the rectum to the sigmoid colon.

8. After counseling her based on clinical findings and laboratory assessment thus far, detail your medical plan and orders for this patient. *(1 point per main bullet)*   10

☐ Hospitalization for CD flare
☐ Perform stool cultures, *C. difficile* toxin assay, and CMV immunohistochemistry on colonic biopsy
☐ Flexible sigmoidoscopy can be performed without sedation or preparation throughout pregnancy
☐ Consider measuring thiopurine drug levels *(6-thioguanine and 6-methylmercaptopurine)* with active disease
☐ Perform daily laboratory investigations: CBC/FBC, C-reactive protein, erythrocyte sedimentation rate, and electrolytes
☐ Start IV solumedrol 20 mg three times daily *(or, lowest effective dose and for the shortest duration)* for active disease found on endoscopic evaluation
☐ Provide analgesia: paracetamol (acetaminophen) as needed
  ○ Discourage use of opioids and NSAIDs‡
☐ Thromboprophylaxis *(e.g., LMWH)* is indicated among patients admitted for flares of inflammatory bowel disease *(and after Cesarean delivery)*
☐ Consideration for antibiotics if perianal disease is suspected in this patient:
  ○ *Amoxicillin/metronidazole is preferred over ciprofloxacin†*

☐ Nutritionist consultation *(indicated for hospitalizations related to inflammatory bowel disease activity)*
☐ Neonatology consultation

Special notes:

† Data is reassuring, showing no increased risk of major birth defects, or adverse fetal and maternal outcomes following ciprofloxacin use during pregnancy

‡ NSAIDs are discouraged in patients with inflammatory bowel disease, irrespective of routine obstetric guidance

Your obstetric trainee recalls having an antenatal patient with an inflammatory bowel disease-related flare where the gastroenterologist preferred initiation of a tumor necrosis factor inhibitor (anti-TNF) agent to induce remission relative to a course of corticosteroids. Your trainee is confused about the considerations involved in this decision-making process.

9. Elicit <u>two reasons</u> that may have guided the gastroenterologist's choice of corticosteroids to induce disease remission in this patient. *(1 point each)*　　　2

☐ Known steroid-responsive patient based on treatment of prior flares
☐ Cost and feasibility of obtaining medication, depending on local resources

On admission day 2, at 26^{+6} weeks, the patient's partner requests to see you. Despite knowing that magnetic resonance enterography is first-line in evaluation of the draining fistula, he is worried about heat exposure or other potential fetal risks.

10. Clarify her partner's understanding of obstetric considerations and general safety recommendations for the use of magnetic resonance imaging (MRI) in evaluating inflammatory bowel disease. *(1 point each)*　　　Max 3

MRI:

☐ No evidence of human fetal teratogenicity, nonthermal effects of tissue heating, or acoustic damage
☐ Nonionizing radiation
☐ No special considerations for any trimester
☐ Reassure patient/partner that gadolinium contrast is generally avoided in pregnancy, limited only to situations where benefit outweighs risks *(fetal risks of gadolinium may include nephrogenic systemic fibrosis, rheumatological, inflammatory, or infiltrative skin conditions, as well as stillbirth and neonatal death)*

Special note:
For lactating women, breastfeeding should <u>not</u> be interrupted after gadolinium administration

While your patient is in the imaging department, a physician from an external center calls you in a panic after a pregnancy was discovered inadvertently on an abdominal X-ray film for possible small bowel obstruction. Your colleague is anxious and wants to know if pregnancy termination is advised.

11. Provide your best recommendations regarding fetal exposure to abdominal X-ray and indicate other practice management advice for your colleague, *if any.* *(1 point each)*   4

- ☐ Reassure your colleague that pregnancy termination is <u>not</u> recommended solely with exposure to diagnostic radiation
- ☐ Fetal radiation exposure from one abdominal X-ray film is 0.01–0.3 rads (0.1–3.0 mGy), below the threshold limit of 5 rads (50 mGy) for fetal effects
- ☐ Risk of carcinogenesis with diagnostic radiation is also very small *(does not influence pregnancy management decisions)*
- ☐ Advise your colleague that patient disclosure is required, as well as system evaluation to ensure β-hCG testing among reproductive-aged women

At 27^{+0} weeks' gestation, the magnetic resonance enterography confirms a perianal fistula without abscess collection, and inflammation in the rectum and sigmoid colon, consistent with the flexible sigmoidoscopy performed during hospitalization. Biopsy stains confirm active CD, without CMV-colitis.

12. With focus on her current gestational period, delineate the general principles you would have discussed with the endoscopist prior to flexible sigmoidoscopy. *(1 point each)*   5

- ☐ Ensure the procedure is performed in a hospital setting with neonatology and obstetric back-up in case of emergency *(case-based obstetric considerations for fetal lung maturity with corticosteroids, or neuroprotection)*
- ☐ Lowest, effective sedative dose *(co-manage with obstetric anesthetist)*
- ☐ Minimize procedure time
- ☐ Pre- and postprocedural monitoring of the fetus and uterine activity on CTG
- ☐ Positioning the patient with a left lateral tilt

With minimal clinical improvement on three days of IV corticosteroids, her gastroenterologist recommends certolizumab[†] to induce remission.

Special note:
† Although infliximab is the most commonly used anti-TNF biologic therapy, certolizumab is chosen for academic purposes; refer to Chapter 43 where infliximab was administered.

13. Suggest why the gastroenterologist may have preferred certolizumab in pregnancy, relative to other anti-TNF biologics. *(1 point each)*   2

Certolizumab:
- ☐ Minimal placental transfer makes it unique among other anti-TNF agents
  - ○ *Certolizumab undergoes passive diffusion, relative to active transport of other agents*
- ☐ No *theoretical* need to adjust live-vaccine schedules among infants with in utero exposure, although may be preferable to delay live vaccines until six months of age

The patient responds to biologic induction therapy and at 28^{+1} weeks' gestation, is discharged on combined azathioprine and certolizumab. She now has four to five semiformed bowel movements per day without abdominal pain, diarrhea, or blood per rectum; fecal calprotectin decreased to 30 ug/g and C-reactive protein is normal. She has ongoing serous drainage from the fistula. The remainder of pregnancy proceeds uneventfully. At her routine 36-weeks prenatal visit, the patient asks about delivery plans.

14. Outline your counseling of delivery recommendations for this patient with CD. *(1 point each)*   4

☐ Elective Cesarean delivery is required due to active perianal disease
☐ Timing delivery as per obstetric indications *(i.e., ~39 weeks)*
☐ Consideration for back-up colorectal surgeon during Cesarean delivery
☐ Thromboprophylaxis *(e.g., LMWH)* is required during hospitalization and after Cesarean delivery

At 38^{+6} weeks' gestation, the patient has an uneventful repeat Cesarean delivery, despite prolonged surgical time due to dense adhesions. Luckily, you did not require the colorectal surgeon's operative assistance.

You visit the patient on postoperative day 1 and find her breastfeeding. Her gastroenterologist informed her that little evidence supports the notion of deferring breastfeeding for four hours after drug ingestion. As you are about to discuss contraceptive options, she requests progesterone-only injectables.

15. Rationalize why some guidance policies allow use of DMPA contraception without   2
restriction, while other experts may have concerns. *(2 points for main bullet)*

☐ Extraintestinal manifestations of osteopenia/osteoporosis among patients with inflammatory bowel disease may be aggravated by DMPA
  ○ *UK-MEC§ allows unrestricted use of DMPA among women with inflammatory bowel disease, while US-MEC§ suggests that advantages generally outweigh theoretical or proven risks*

Special note:
§   UK and US Medical Eligibility Criteria (MEC) for Contraceptive Use, 2016; UK-MEC was revised September 2019

During the six-weeks' postpartum visit, you mention that future preconception counseling is recommended, particularly in relation to inflammatory bowel disease. The patient, however, feels well experienced, having had two pregnancies.

16. With focus on inflammatory bowel disease, what are the known benefits of preconception counseling that you may discuss to address her misconceptions? *(1 point each)*   Max 3

☐ Disease activity is inconsistent among pregnancies *(i.e., avoid false reassurance)*
☐ Improved perinatal adverse outcomes when pregnancy is planned after a minimum of six months of remission and optimized nutrition
☐ Improved adherence to maintenance treatment with reassuring pregnancy safety profile decreases relapse
    ○ *Start higher-dose folic acid (2 g/d) among patients on sulfasalazine maintenance*
    ○ *Preconception period is an opportunity to discontinue teratogenic therapy*
☐ Preconception counseling allows for objective evaluation of disease activity *(i.e., endoscopy or stool calprotectin)* to help decrease risks of antenatal flares

TOTAL: 105

CHAPTER 43

Ulcerative Colitis in Pregnancy

Talat Bessissow, Amira El-Messidi, and Cynthia H. Seow

A 30-year-old nulligravida with ulcerative colitis (UC) is referred by her primary care provider to your hospital center's high-risk obstetrics unit for preconceptional counseling.

Special note: *To avoid overlap, the reader is encouraged to complement subject matter with material covered in Chapter 42.*

LEARNING OBJECTIVES

1. Take a focused history, and provide effective preconception counseling for a patient with UC, identifying factors associated with adverse perinatal outcome
2. Demonstrate the ability to collaborate with gastroenterologists in caring for the obstetric patient with UC
3. Elicit investigations to evaluate disease activity, and understand the work-up in assessing disease flares
4. Recognize that active disease has greater detriment to maternal-fetal outcome relative to treatments with reassuring safety profiles, highlighting adherence to therapeutics throughout the obstetric course
5. Plan a safe mode for delivery

SUGGESTED READINGS

1. Bressler B, Marshall JK, Bernstein CN, et al. Clinical practice guidelines for the medical management of nonhospitalized ulcerative colitis: the Toronto consensus. *Gastroenterology*. 2015;148(5):1035–1058.
2. De Lima A, Zelinkova Z, Mulders AG, et al. Preconception care reduces relapse of inflammatory bowel disease during pregnancy. *Clin Gastroenterol Hepatol*. 2016; 14:1285–1292.
3. Magro F, Gionchetti P, Eliakim R, et al. Third European Evidence-based Consensus on Diagnosis and Management of Ulcerative Colitis. Part 1: Definitions, diagnosis, extra-intestinal manifestations, pregnancy, cancer surveillance, surgery, and ileo-anal pouch disorders. *J Crohns Colitis*. 2017;11(6):649–670.
4. Mahadevan U, Robinson C, Bernasko N, et al. Inflammatory bowel disease in pregnancy clinical care pathway: a report from the American Gastroenterological Association IBD Parenthood Project Working Group. *Am J Obstet Gynecol*. 2019;220(4):308–323.

5. Nielsen OH, Gubatan JM, Juhl CB, et al. Biologics for inflammatory bowel disease and their safety in pregnancy: a systematic review and meta-analysis. *Clin Gastroenterol Hepatol.* 2020; S1542–3565(20):31281–31287.

6. Nguyen GC, Seow CH, Maxwell C, et al. The Toronto Consensus Statements for the management of inflammatory bowel disease in pregnancy. *Gastroenterology.* 2016;150(3):734–757.

7. Picardo S, Seow CH. A pharmacological approach to managing inflammatory bowel disease during conception, pregnancy and breastfeeding: biologic and oral small molecule therapy. *Drugs.* 2019;79(10):1053–1063.

8. Singh S, Picardo S, Seow CH. Management of inflammatory bowel diseases in special populations: obese, old, or obstetric. *Clin Gastroenterol Hepatol.* 2020;18(6):1367–1380.

9. Tandon P, Leung K, Yusuf A, et al. Noninvasive methods for assessing inflammatory bowel disease activity in pregnancy: a systematic review. *J Clin Gastroenterol.* 2019; 53(8):574–581.

10. van der Woude CJ, Ardizzone S, Bengtson MB, et al. The second European evidence-based consensus on reproduction and pregnancy in inflammatory bowel disease. *J Crohns Colitis.* 2015;9(2):107–124.

POINTS

1.   With regard to UC, which aspects of a focused history would you want to know? *(1 point per main bullet; max points specified per section)*   Max 30

General disease-related details: *(4)*
- ☐ Age at diagnosis
- ☐ Duration since last UC flare
- ☐ Anatomical extent of disease (Montreal classification)
   - ○ *Proctitis in ~30% of patients (E1)*
   - ○ *Left-sided colitis (involvement distal to splenic flexure) in ~40% of patients (E2)*
   - ○ *Pancolitis (involvement beyond splenic flexure) in ~30% of patients (E3)*
- ☐ Name and contact of treating gastroenterologist

Gastrointestinal manifestations: *(max 4)*
- ☐ Abdominal pain
- ☐ Tenesmus
- ☐ Urgency
- ☐ Quantification of daytime and nocturnal bowel movements
- ☐ Quantification of episodes with hematochezia
- ☐ Stool consistency
- ☐ Incontinence
- ☐ Weight loss

History of UC-related complications: *(max 3)*
- ☐ Gastrointestinal hemorrhage
- ☐ Colonic dysplasia/colon cancer
- ☐ Toxic megacolon
- ☐ Disease-related hospitalizations

Surgical history: *(max 1)*
- ☐ Appendectomy
- ☐ UC-related surgery (colectomy)

Extraintestinal manifestations: *(max 4)*
☐ *Oral:* aphthous ulcers
☐ *Hematologic:* anemia, venous thromboembolism
☐ *Musculoskeletal: e.g.* ankylosing spondylitis (gene *HLA-B27*), sacroiliitis, osteoporosis/osteopenia, peripheral or axial arthritis
☐ *Dermatologic: e.g.* erythema nodosum, pyoderma gangrenosum, aphthous stomatitis, anal skin tags
☐ *Ocular: e.g.* uveitis, episcleritis, iritis
☐ *Cardio-pulmonary: e.g.* inflammatory processes, bronchiectasis, reactive amyloidosis
☐ *Pancreatico-hepatobiliary: e.g.* pancreatitis, cholelithiasis, primary sclerosing cholangitis, primary biliary cirrhosis, nonalcoholic steatohepatitis
☐ *Genitourinary: e.g.* nephrolithiasis, ureteral obstruction

Current/prior medical treatments, clinical response and side effects: *(4)*
☐ **Therapies <u>not</u> compatible with pregnancy:** methotrexate, tofacitinib, ozanimod
☐ **Therapies compatible with pregnancy:** biologics, thiopurines, corticosteroids, mesalamine, cyclosporine
☐ Opioid dependence
☐ Current contraceptive method

Social history and routine health maintenance: *(5)*
☐ Ethnicity‡
☐ Smoking, alcohol consumption, illicit drug use (especially cannabis)
☐ Recent travel *(contact with enteric infections)*
☐ Vaccination status *(live viral vaccines are avoided with immunosuppressant treatment)*
☐ Most recent cervical smear, prior human papilloma virus vaccination, prior condyloma *(especially important with immunomodulator therapy)*

Family history: *(max 4)*
☐ Inflammatory bowel disease‡
☐ Earliest age at diagnosis among affected family members‡
☐ Auto-immune disease‡
☐ Colorectal cancer
☐ Unprovoked venous thromboembolism

Male partner: *(1)*
☐ Inquire about the presence of inflammatory bowel disease‡

Special note:
‡ Factors affecting offspring's genetic risk of inflammatory bowel disease

You learn that the patient was diagnosed at age 23 years when she presented with >10 daily bouts of crampy abdominal pain associated with diarrhea and mucus-containing hematochezia. Her symptoms were accompanied by red eyes, and nodules on her legs; the patient recalls losing 18 pounds in a two-week period of her presentation and diagnosis. Her disease has been limited to below the splenic flexure on serial colonoscopies.

She is followed by a gastroenterologist in your hospital center, and after several years of poor disease control related to poor adherence to therapy, she achieves clinical disease remission with combined oral sulfasalazine and tofacitinib. Her gastroenterologist had advised reliable contraception, and she chose the copper-IUD. Five months ago, the tofacitinib was discontinued for pregnancy planning. She started high-dose folate supplementation.

The disease is now quiescent on sulfasalazine alone with two nonbloody bowel movements per day. Her weight is stable, and BMI is 22 kg/m². She does not smoke, and other lifestyle habits are unremarkable. The patient has not experienced complications of UC. Her extraintestinal symptoms remained quiescent for several years. There is no personal or family history of venous thromboembolism and her partner does not have inflammatory bowel disease.

Special note:

Although mesalamine is more commonly used clinically, sulfasalazine remains an option and is used for educational purposes related to this scenario

2.   In liaison with her gastroenterologist, indicate the recommended investigations to evaluate preconception disease activity and nutritional status. *(1 point each, unless specified)*

12

Serum:
☐ CBC/FBC
☐ C-reactive protein
☐ Red cell folate
☐ Vitamin B12
☐ Iron studies/serum ferritin
☐ 25-hydroxy vitamin D

Stool: *(5 points)*
☐ Fecal calprotectin
  ○ *Released by neutrophils; identifies inflammation*
  ○ *May correlate with disease activity and treatment response in all trimesters (emerging literature)*
  ○ *May predict flares within three months*

Imaging:
☐ Endoscopy (sigmoidoscopy or colonoscopy)

As you were outlining these investigations before agreeing on the intent to conceive, the patient shares results of recently completed tests. Reassuringly, she is in biochemical and endoscopic remission; however, you note the following:

		Normal
Hemoglobin (g/L)	105	110–140
Serum ferritin (ng/mL)	9	>15
Red cell folate (pg/mL)	5	2–20
Total serum cobalamin (ng/L)	240	>200

She expresses concern that the multiple inflammatory processes impacted her fertility. Although counseled by her gastroenterologist, she remains worried about fetal risks related to her amino-salicylate or former 'small molecule' agent.

---

3. Discuss the <u>fetal/neonatal</u> risks associated with sulfasalazine and tofacitinib. (*1 point each*)   5

Sulfasalazine:[†]
☐ No increased risk of congenital anomalies, despite interference with folate absorption
☐ No increased risks of adverse perinatal outcome
☐ Diarrhea in breastfed infants *(resolves with drug discontinuation)*
☐ Hemolysis in infants with glucose-6-phosphate dehydrogenase (G6PD) deficiency

Tofacitinib:[§]
☐ Teratogenic in animals; not recommended in pregnancy or breastfeeding *(limited human data)*

Special notes:
† DBP *(dibutyl phthalate)*-containing formulations are discouraged; may cause precocious puberty; animal studies show fetal skeletal and male urogenital anomalies
§ Discontinued more than four to six weeks preconception

---

4. Outline the effects of UC on *this* patient's fertility.[†] *(2 points each)*   4

☐ Patient's fertility rate should be equal to the general population, especially given disease remission and absence of prior surgery
☐ Reassure the patient that medical therapies for inflammatory bowel disease do not affect fertility

Special note:
† Crohn's disease generally has greater impact on fertility than ulcerative colitis, although this may be confounded by the more frequent need for operative management

---

Attentive to the discussion, your obstetric trainee addresses her curiosity regarding how active inflammatory bowel disease impacts fertility.

---

5. Identify factors that may affect fertility among women with active inflammatory bowel disease. *(1 point each)*   Max 4

☐ Tubal inflammation and scarring due to the disease process or surgeries, particularly ileo-anal pouch procedures
☐ Ovulatory dysfunction due to nutritional deficiency
☐ Decreased libido
☐ Depression
☐ Voluntary infertility is generally more common among women with inflammatory bowel disease, often due to misconceptions about disease and treatments

6. Discuss important elements of your preconception counseling and <u>antenatal</u> management of UC.

<u>Maternal:</u> *(1 point per main and subbullet; max 14)*
- ☐ Reassure patient there is no contraindication to conception given good prognosticators:
  - ○ Cessation of tofacitinib
  - ○ At least three months of sustained remission on alternate therapy for inflammatory bowel disease
  - ○ More than three months of steroid-free remission
  - ○ Stable nutritional status
- ☐ Pregnancy may influence UC disease course, with antepartum/postpartum flares
- ☐ Risks of flare in pregnancy are greater with active disease at conception
- ☐ Multidisciplinary care, frequent clinic visits/investigations, and possibly hospitalizations
- ☐ Advise 2 mg/d folic acid supplementation given sulfasalazine therapy *(Suggested Readings 4, 6, 10)*
- ☐ Discourage antenatal use of antidiarrheals
- ☐ Optimize iron replacement, usually by means of intravenous iron supplementation among patients with inflammatory bowel disease
- ☐ Offer early nutritionist consultation and discuss the disease-related significance of monitoring gestational weight gain
- ☐ Recommend vaccination for influenza, pneumococcal, COVID-19, hepatitis B virus *(if indicated)*, including routine antenatal pertussis vaccine
- ☐ Discuss venous thromboprophylaxis if the patient needs hospitalization or Cesarean delivery
- ☐ Mode of delivery depends on obstetric indications and patient preferences; interdisciplinary decision-making is advised

<u>Fetal/neonatal:</u> *(1 point per main and subbullet; max 6)*
- ☐ Risks of adverse outcomes is increased with active disease:
  - ○ Early pregnancy loss
  - ○ Preterm prelabor rupture of membranes (PPROM), preterm birth (PTB)
  - ○ Low birthweight or small for gestational age newborn
  - ○ Intrauterine fetal death (IUFD)
- ☐ Consideration for serial fetal growth biometry in the second and third trimesters, especially with active colitis or inadequate maternal weight gain
- ☐ Early neonatology consultation

<u>Genetic risks:</u> *(1 point each for 2 points)*
- ☐ Excluding family history and ethnicity, the offspring's risk of UC is 1.6% given one affected parent
- ☐ No genetic tests reliably predict risk of inflammatory bowel disease

The patient appreciates your counseling and will comply with multidisciplinary management. Albeit adequate control, she recognizes the inherent risk of flares in pregnancy and is eager to know when, and if, surgery may be considered.

7. Albeit rare with well-controlled disease, address the patient's inquiry regarding the indications for UC-related surgery during pregnancy. *(1 point each)*   4

☐ Severe hemorrhage
☐ Acute refractory colitis
☐ Toxic megacolon/perforation
☐ Strongly suspected/known cancer

Special note:
Bowel obstruction and abscess are additional surgical indications, although more commonly related to Crohn's disease

In addition to folic acid, she starts iron and prenatal vitamins. After removing the intrauterine contraceptive device (IUD), spontaneous conception occurs within four months. She was in remission at conception, well controlled on sulfasalazine.

As a high-risk obstetrician, you follow her antenatal care with the established preconceptional plan. Pregnancy is unremarkable until 13^{+2} weeks' gestation when she experiences spontaneous onset of 8–10 bowel movements daily, including two nightly episodes; most of the time, she finds blood in her stool. The patient complains of abdominal cramps related to defecation, with significant tenesmus; she is not febrile. Obstetric assessment is normal. In collaboration with her gastroenterologist, you inform her of required investigations.

8. Based on your discussion with her gastroenterologist, indicate the recommended tests to evaluate her clinical presentation. *(1 point each)*   8

Laboratory investigations: *([†]limited value in antenatal management of inflammatory bowel disease-related flares)*
☐ CBC/FBC[†]
☐ C-reactive protein[†]
☐ Serum albumin[†]
☐ Fecal calprotectin
☐ Stool cultures
☐ *C. difficile* toxin assay
☐ CMV histology/immunohistochemistry *(finding multiple intranuclear inclusions is significant)*

Endoscopy: *(performed when results will dictate management)*
☐ Flexible sigmoidoscopy *(preferred over colonoscopy)*

Stool cultures and *C. difficile* toxin assay are negative. Laboratory tests show:

		Normal
Hemoglobin (g/L)	107	110–140
Fecal calprotectin (ug/g)	1800	<100[§]
C-reactive protein (mg/L)	12	<10

§ Optimal cutoff to predict disease activity in pregnancy is unknown; may range from >50 to >250 ug/g

The patient underwent a flexible sigmoidoscopy demonstrating complete loss of vascular pattern, erosions with mucosal friability consistent with moderately active colitis (Mayo score 2).

Considering a colonoscopy provides complete assessment relative to sigmoidoscopy, your trainee is uncertain why the latter was chosen.

---

9. Rationalize why flexible sigmoidoscopy is preferred over colonoscopy in pregnancy. *(1 point each)*   Max 3

☐ Provides sufficient information about disease activity as the disease starts in the rectum
☐ Performed in any trimester
☐ No sedation required
☐ No oral bowel preparation needed

Having been informed by the gastroenterologist of her UC flare, he or she plans outpatient therapy; the patient will add a rectal aminosalicylate to her oral sulfasalazine and start oral prednisone 40 mg daily.[†]

At 18^{+5} weeks, the patient indicates symptom improvement with now two to three bowel movements per day of formed to semiformed stools without blood. Repeat investigations show fetal calprotectin is 180 ug/g and C-reactive protein is normal. In affiliation with her gastroenterologist, algorithmic weaning off prednisone is planned.

By 20^{+2} weeks, the patient reports inability to tolerate decreasing corticosteroids below prednisone 20 mg. Symptoms worsen and given a corticosteroid-resistant flare, her gastroenterologist recommends anti-TNF therapy with infliximab to induce symptomatic remission. Routine fetal morphology scan is normal; biometry is on the 19th percentile and the cervix is long and closed.

Special note:
† Patient does not require thromboprophylaxis given outpatient treatment of disease flare without history of thromboembolism *(Suggested Reading 6)*

---

10. Name the three classes of biologic agents used in inflammatory bowel disease. *(1 point each)*   3

☐ Anti-TNF-α agents
☐ Anti-interleukin 12 to 23
☐ Anti-integrins

11. Discuss the medical and obstetric benefits of anti-TNF biologics in pregnancy. *(1 point each)*

Max 6

Inflammatory bowel disease-related reductions:
☐ Antenatal flares
☐ Postnatal flares
☐ Disease activity
☐ Hospitalizations
☐ Surgery

Obstetric advantages:
☐ No increased risk of congenital anomalies
☐ No increased risks of adverse perinatal outcomes including early pregnancy loss, PTB, IUFD, low birthweight compared to the general population
☐ Safely continued use across all trimesters *(Suggested Readings 6, 10)*
☐ No short-term or long-term risks of infections with in utero exposure

By 30 weeks' gestation, the UC flare has resolved, and fecal calprotectin normalized. She remains on therapeutic levels of infliximab. The patient has now successfully weaned off prednisone. Serial fetal growth velocity has been appropriate with normal amniotic fluid volume. She remains hopeful for a term, vaginal delivery.

12. In planning for vaginal delivery and in conjunction with her gastroenterologist, outline pertinent intrapartum and postpartum disease-related considerations.

8

Vaginal delivery: *(1 point per main and subbullet; max 5)*
☐ No corticosteroid-stress doses in labor are required for this patient given she discontinued treatment more than three weeks before delivery[†]
☐ Encourage adequate labor and postpartum analgesia, preferably limiting postpartum nonsteroidal anti-inflammatory agents (NSAIDs) which may provoke disease flare
☐ Avoid episiotomy or lacerations, *if possible*
☐ Judicious use of assisted instrumental vaginal delivery *(obstetrical indications)*
☐ Consideration for prophylactic stool-softeners, particularly given the risk of opioid-induced constipation

Particularities for UC-drug therapy: *(1 point each for 3 points)*
☐ Given disease flare requiring antepartum initiation of infliximab, advise continuation of therapy throughout pregnancy until delivery to maintain disease remission (this is fundamental to the care of obstetric patients)
☐ In the absence of postpartum infectious complications, plan resumption of infliximab 24 hours after vaginal delivery, or 48 hours if a Cesarean section was required
☐ Reassure the patient regarding breastfeeding and pharmacologic therapy

Special note:
[†] NICE 2019 Guidelines for Intrapartum Complex Care, National Guideline Alliance (UK). Intrapartum care for women with existing medical conditions or obstetric complications and their babies. London: National Institute for Health and Care Excellence (UK); 2019 Mar. PMID. 31194308.

Spontaneous labor and vaginal delivery with epidural analgesia occur at 38^{+4} weeks. An unavoidable second-degree laceration is repaired without complications. Early ambulation is encouraged, and the patient receives a dose of infliximab on postpartum day 1.

You visit the patient before hospital discharge and find her comfortably breastfeeding.

13. In relation to inflammatory bowel disease, what are important postpartum considerations   Max 6
to discuss, either prior to discharge or at the routine postpartum visit? *(1 point each)*

General maternal-fetal well-being:
☐ Screen for postpartum depression and continue to offer psychosocial support services
☐ Current recommendations advise avoidance of live-viral vaccines for the first six months of life with in utero exposure to biologics**, except with certolizumab[†]
☐ Reassure the patient that all routine non-live-viral vaccines may by administered to infants with antenatal exposure to biologic agents

Disease-related care:
☐ Maintain adequate hydration
☐ Encourage early reporting of disease flare
☐ Encourage a well-balanced diet, weight maintenance, and consider continued nutritional counseling
☐ Arrange follow-up with gastroenterology for approximately three months postpartum

Contraceptive recommendations: (*hormonal and intrauterine options*)
☐ No restrictions exist on progesterone-only or intrauterine contraception[‡§]
☐ Controversial recommendations regarding combined oral contraception: although advantages generally outweigh theoretical or proven risks (*UK-MEC*[§]), continued use of estrogen-containing oral contraceptives may incur increased risk of thrombosis (*US-MEC*[‡])

Special notes:
[†] Certolizumab is not actively transported across the placenta like other biologics
[**] Studies show promising results, challenging this recommendation: *refer to* (a) Beaulieu DB, et al. *Clin Gastroenterol Hepatol.* 2018;16:99–105 and (b) Bendaoud S et al. *J Crohn's Colitis.* 2018; 12(Suppl 1): S527
[§] UK Medical Eligibility Criteria (MEC) for Contraceptive Use, 2016, revised September 2019
[‡] US-MEC 2016

TOTAL: **115**

CHAPTER 44

Biliary Diseases in Pregnancy

Bruno De Souza Ribeiro, Amira El-Messidi, and Maged Peter Ghali

A 34-year-old G3P2 at 20 weeks' gestation presents to the A&E (E.R.) department of your tertiary care center with a three-hour history of nausea and vomiting associated with recurrent right upper quadrant pain, no longer alleviated by analgesics.

Your colleague follows her obstetric care, and pregnancy has been unremarkable to date. Routine prenatal laboratory investigations, aneuploidy screening, and second-trimester fetal morphology survey have all been unremarkable. Obstetric history is significant for gestational diabetes mellitus in her second pregnancy, which resolved postpartum. She had two uncomplicated term vaginal deliveries. There are no obstetric complaints. As requested by the urgent care team, you attend to assist in the care of this patient.

LEARNING OBJECTIVES

1. Take a focused history, and verbalize essentials of a physical examination related to biliary diseases in the prenatal period
2. Recognize risk factors for new-onset biliary diseases in the antenatal period
3. Counsel on maternal-fetal complications related to biliary diseases
4. Identify safe diagnostic interventions in the antenatal evaluation of biliary diseases
5. Discuss conservative and surgical options for biliary diseases in pregnancy, including timing of endoscopic retrograde cholangiopancreatogram (ERCP)

SUGGESTED READINGS

1. Brown KE, Hirshberg JS, Conner SN. Gallbladder and biliary disease in pregnancy. *Clin Obstet Gynecol.* 2020;63(1):211–225.
2. Cain MA, Ellis J, Vengrove MA, et al. Gallstone and severe hypertriglyceride-induced pancreatitis in pregnancy. *Obstet Gynecol Surv.* 2015;70(9):577–583.
3. Date RS, Kaushal M, Ramesh A. A review of the management of gallstone disease and its complications in pregnancy. *Am J Surg.* 2008;196(4):599–608.
4. Hedström J, Nilsson J, Andersson R, et al. Changing management of gallstone-related disease in pregnancy – a retrospective cohort analysis. *Scand J Gastroenterol.* 2017;52(9): 1016–1021.

5. Ibiebele I, Schnitzler M, Nippita T, et al. Outcomes of gallstone disease during pregnancy: a population-based data linkage study. *Paediatr Perinat Epidemiol.* 2017;31(6):522–530.
6. Konduk BT, Bayraktar O. Efficacy and safety of endoscopic retrograde cholangiopancreatography in pregnancy: A high-volume study with long-term follow-up. *Turk J Gastroenterol.* 2019;30(9):811–816.
7. Shah JN, Bhat YM, Hamerski CM, et al. Feasibility of nonradiation EUS-based ERCP in patients with uncomplicated choledocholithiasis (with video). *Gastrointest Endosc.* 2016;84(5):764–769.
8. Vohra S, Holt EW, Bhat YM, et al. Successful single-session endosonography-based endoscopic retrograde cholangiopancreatography without fluoroscopy in pregnant patients with suspected choledocholithiasis: a case series. *J Hepatobiliary Pancreat Sci.* 2014;21(2): 93–97.

POINTS

1. In relation to the gastrointestinal presentation, what aspects of a focused history would you want to know? *(1 point each)*

Max 10

Details of the pain:
☐ Pattern (*i.e., colicky/constant*)
☐ Onset in relation to meals
☐ Recent intake of a fatty meal
☐ Radiations to the back, shoulder, chest
☐ Aggravating/alleviating factors
☐ Prior similar episodes, including any investigations, medical or surgical procedures
☐ Medications received since presentation to hospital and analgesics ingested at home

Associated manifestations:
☐ Fever
☐ Details of vomitus (*i.e., bilious, hematemesis, amount and frequency*)
☐ Lower gastrointestinal (*i.e., bloating, pain, diarrhea*) or renal manifestations

Personal and family history:
☐ Gallstones, hepatic disease, gastroesophageal reflux disease, or peptic ulcers

Social history and allergies:
☐ Smoking, alcohol consumption, and intravenous drug use
☐ Recent travel
☐ Allergies

The patient received an intravenous antiemetic and intramuscular analgesic by the urgent care team, allowing her to converse, albeit in a fetal position. She describes a constant pain that started one hour after having a fatty meal. The pain lasted four hours and remained localized to the right upper quadrant. She had symptomatic relief with acetaminophen (*i.e.,* paracetamol) at home. Nausea and nonbilious vomiting later developed, with recurrence of pain. She has no lower gastrointestinal or urinary complaints. The patient does not smoke or drink alcohol while pregnant; she only takes daily prenatal vitamins. You learn of a remote similar episode where investigations revealed gallstones. Conservative treatment was successful, and she has remained asymptomatic for the past two years.

At presentation, the patient is afebrile, normotensive, and hemodynamically stable. Fetal viability is ascertained. She clearly has an obese habitus, with a documented prepregnancy BMI of 36 kg/m². The urgent care physician elicited a positive Murphy's sign, and later called you and the gastroenterology team to assist in her care.

2.	Identify the most probable diagnosis, and four non-pregnancy-related differential diagnoses for this gravida's presentation. *(1 point each, unless specified)*	Max 6

Most probable diagnosis:
- ☐ Cholelithiasis *(2 points)*

Differential diagnoses:
- ☐ Choledocholithiasis
- ☐ Cholecystitis
- ☐ Gastroesophageal reflux disease
- ☐ Peptic ulcer disease
- ☐ Hepatitis
- ☐ Appendicitis
- ☐ Right lobe pneumonia

3.	Indicate five investigations most specific to the diagnostic assessment of the clinical presentation. *(1 point per main bullet, unless specified)*	5

- ☐ Abdominal ultrasound *(2 points)*
- ☐ CBC/FBC *(primarily for leukocyte count)*
- ☐ ALT, AST, total bilirubin, alkaline phosphatase
  - ○ *Transaminases and total bilirubin should remain within normal nonpregnant values*
- ☐ Amylase and lipase
  - ○ *Generally, remain within normal limits, although slight gestational increases may occur*

Abdominal ultrasound shows many small gallstones with presence of sludge. There is no dilation of the common biliary duct. Laboratory tests are unremarkable.

In your discussion with the gastroenterology team, you concur that the presumptive diagnosis is cholelithiasis with self-limited biliary colic. The patient is anxious about fetal risks of biliary colic and curious why the gallstones caused colic.

4.	Counsel the patient regarding obstetric risks with biliary colic.	1

- ☐ Reassurance: no associated fetal morbidity or preterm delivery

5.	Explain the mechanism by which gallstones cause symptomatic colic.	1

- ☐ Gallbladder contraction due to temporary stone impaction at the cystic duct

6. Discuss the ideal therapeutic approach for this patient's biliary colic. *(1 point each)*   Max 5

☐ Conservative management, with close gastroenterology follow-up, and planned postpartum cholecystectomy
☐ Consultation with general surgery team prior to discharge
☐ Inform the patient that recurrence is common in pregnancy, ranging from 40% to 90%
☐ Advise avoidance of fatty meals
☐ Reassure the patient that in case of severe or refractory symptoms, laparoscopic cholecystectomy can be safely performed across trimesters *(preferable in the second trimester)*

After several hours of observation, during which the patient received intravenous hydration, analgesics, and antiemetics, she is discharged in stable condition with planned conservative management. The patient is encouraged to consider cholecystectomy after delivery. Appropriate multidisciplinary follow-up appointments are made.

You use this opportunity to address your obstetric trainee's inquiries about gallstone disease in pregnancy.

7. What is the predominant type of gallstones in pregnancy?   1

☐ Cholesterol stones

8. Identify the two main mechanisms for bile formation in pregnancy. *(1 point each)*   2

☐ Increased lithogenicity of bile due to estrogen-mediated increased cholesterol secretion and progesterone-mediated decreased bile acid secretion
☐ Progesterone-mediated decreased gallbladder motility

9. Elicit risk factors for cholelithiasis that may or may not relate to this patient's pregnancy. *(1 point each)*   Max 5

☐ Prepregnancy obesity, or increased gestational weight gain
☐ Multiparity
☐ Gestational changes in hormones
☐ Insulin resistance
☐ Hypertension
☐ High fat diet
☐ Oral contraceptive use
☐ Genetic background

At 26 weeks' gestation, the patient returns for urgent care with similar symptoms; right upper quadrant pain is not improving with oral analgesics at home. The patient appears distressed and is vomiting. The epigastrium is tender without rebound. She is febrile at 38.3°C with leukocytosis at 18.2×10^9/L. Transaminases, bilirubin, lipase, and amylase are normal. Abdominal ultrasound shows gallstones with a distended gallbladder with a wall thickness above 5 mm and pericholecystic fluid. The diameter of the common bile duct is normal. The imaging technologist elicits a Murphy's sign.

Gestational diabetes mellitus (GDM) was diagnosed at 25 weeks' gestation, diet-controlled (GDM-A1) to date. She has no obstetrical complaints at presentation and the fetal status is normal.

10. What is the most probable diagnosis?   1

☐ Acute cholecystitis

The patient's husband asks whether additional testing is required prior to entertaining this diagnosis.

11. In liaison with the gastroenterology team, address her partner's inquiry regarding the need   1
for further diagnostic investigations.

☐ No further testing required in presence of the classic triad for acute cholecystitis:
  ○ Persistent right upper quadrant pain
  ○ Clinical features on examination
  ○ Laboratory and abdominal imaging signs

Special note:
Neither MRI nor magnetic resonance cholangiopancreatogram (MRCP) will provide additional information; endoscopic retrograde cholangiopancreatogram (ERCP) is not required in work-up of cholecystitis

Your trainee asks you about the differences in pathophysiology between this entity and that of biliary colic at prior presentation.

12. Differentiate between the mechanism leading to acute cholecystitis relative to   2
gallstone-induced colic.

☐ Stone impaction in the cystic duct resulting in chronic obstruction leads to the acute infection, compared to transient obstruction resulting in biliary colic

13-A. Indicate maternal-fetal risks associated with acute cholecystitis to consider in patient counseling, particularly with suboptimal management. *(1 point each)*   5

Maternal: *(max 3)*
☐ Gallbladder necrosis, empyema, gangrene, perforation, and increased risk of malignancy
☐ Sepsis
☐ Cholangitis
☐ Pancreatitis
☐ Mortality

Fetal:
☐ Preterm labor with/without preterm birth; the risk of prematurity associated with cholecystectomy in the first and second trimesters is comparable to the general obstetric population, at 5%–10%
☐ Intrauterine fetal demise (IUFD) *[5%–10% with conservative treatment, and <5% with surgery]*

13-B. In addition to hospitalization, what are important elements of clinical management for the gravida's acute cholecystitis? *(1 point each)*   6

☐ Maintain an initial nil-per-os status
☐ Provide symptom-control with analgesia and antiemetics; intravenous opioids are preferred over nonsteroidal anti-inflammatory agents in a prenatal patient
☐ Initiate intravenous fluid hydration
☐ Initiate broad-spectrum antibiotics; options include, but are not limited to: *(1 point for any one subbullet)*
   ○ Intravenous ampicillin 3 g every six hours
   ○ Intravenous piperacillin-tazobactam 3.375 IV every six hours
   ○ Intravenous ceftriaxone 1 g once daily, or another third-generation cephalosporin
☐ Request early surgical consultation at admission, recognizing the need to consider cholecystectomy based on improved maternal morbidity and fetal morbidity[†] and mortality, increased risk of recurrence with conservative treatment; reassure the patient she is currently in the ideal second-trimester period for surgical intervention
☐ Obtain an obstetric ultrasound for fetal growth biometry

Special note:
† Conservative management incurs up to 30% risk of prematurity

After consultation with the general surgeon, the patient provides consent for a laparoscopic cholecystectomy with possible laparotomy and Cesarean section.

14. Address preoperative and intraoperative <u>obstetric</u> considerations for the planned surgical procedure at 26 weeks' gestation. *(1 point each unless specified)*

Max 6

☐ Consideration for fetal pulmonary corticosteroids, and instigate an insulin-sliding scale based on GDM *(2 points)*
☐ Consideration for magnesium sulfate fetal neuroprotection
☐ Presurgical neonatology consultation
☐ Maintain a maternal left lateral decubitus position intraoperatively
☐ Use the open technique for umbilical port insertion to minimize high intraperitoneal pressures
☐ Limit use of electrocautery proximal to the uterus
☐ Obtain fetal cardiotocographic monitoring pre- and postoperatively

Laparoscopic cholecystectomy is performed without intraoperative or postoperative complications. By postoperative day 6, the patient is asymptomatic and is discharged with normal laboratory investigations.

Two weeks later, during a prenatal follow-up at 28 weeks' gestation, the patient reports upper abdominal discomfort and mentions that her husband thought her eyes were slightly yellow. The fetus is active, and she denies uterine contractions or other obstetric complaints. Promptly, you order an obstetrical and abdominal ultrasound and send the patient to the hospital's obstetrical emergency assessment unit.

Abdominal ultrasound shows dilation of the common bile duct at 9 mm *(i.e., abnormal being >6 mm)*. Fetal assessment is normal. Laboratory investigations reveal the following:

		Normal
Leukocytes	12.3×10^9/L	$5–18 \times 10^9$/L
Platelets	180×10^9/L	$150–400 \times 10^9$/L
AST	95 IU/L	6–35 IU/L
ALT	190 IU/L	6–45 IU/L
Total bilirubin	77 umol/L (4.5 mg/dL)	5.1–20.5 umol/L (0.3–1.2 mg/dL)
Direct bilirubin	60 umol/L (3.5 mg/dL)	<5.1 umol/L (0.3 mg/dL)
Amylase	75 U/L	30–110 U/L
Lipase	10 U/L	0–160 U/L

Within several hours, a nurse notifies you that the patient's oral temperature is 38.5°C and she has shaking chills. The general surgical team has been similarly notified.

15. Share with your obstetric trainee your main differential diagnoses as you promptly attend to the care of this patient. *(1 point each)*   Max 2

☐ Choledocholithiasis evolving to ascending cholangitis due to a small stone, missed at surgery, that is causing obstruction of the common duct
☐ Iatrogenic postcholecystectomy biliary stricture after recent surgery
☐ Papillary stenosis due to papillitis from prolonged periods of sludge and stones
☐ Rarely, vital illnesses such as cytomegalovirus (CMV) or human immunodeficiency virus (HIV)

16. Biliary stasis that occurs in cholangitis predisposes to bacterial infections, requiring adequate coverage with intravenous broad-spectrum antibiotics. Enumerate the most implicated organisms. *(1 point each)*   Max 4

☐ *Escherichia coli* (25%)
☐ *Klebsiella* species (15%)
☐ *Enterococcus* species (15%)
☐ *Streptococcus* (10%)
☐ *Enterobacter* (5%–10%)
☐ Anaerobes: *Clostridium perfringens/Bacteroides fragilis*

17. Indicate the safest diagnostic modalities for cholangitis in the antenatal management of this patient.   1

☐ MRI/MRCP *(can confirm stones or strictures in the common bile duct)*

The MRI/MRCP shows intra- and extrahepatic biliary dilation with the common bile duct measuring 10 mm, without strictures or stones. She remains febrile and normotensive with mild maternal tachycardia at 110 bpm. Laboratory investigations are significant for a serum total bilirubin of 145 umol/l (8.5 mg/dL) and leukocyte count of 19.7×10^9/L. The gastroenterologist is closely involved in her care.

18. As discussed with the gastroenterologist, what is the next best step in the management of this patient?   1

☐ Endoscopic ultrasound/ERCP, with sphincterotomy and biliary drainage
　○ *Pre- and postprocedure fetal cardiotocography*
　○ *Fetal shielding and limited procedure duration result in low rates of maternal/fetal morbidity*

The endoscopist finds a single small 3-mm stone at the distal common bile duct, close to the major papilla. Sphincterotomy is performed and the stone is extracted. The biliary tree is drained, and lavage is performed with physiologic solution. No stent is placed. The patient responds well to treatment and is later discharged with oral antibiotics.

---

19. Explain why the MRCP did not detect the stone seen at ERCP. *(1 point each)*   2

☐ MRCP has limited accuracy (40%–75%) in detecting small stones (<5 mm)
☐ Stones may sometimes pass, only leaving behind residual dilation, detected with high accuracy by MRCP

At 30^{+4} weeks' gestation, the patient presents to hospital with severe epigastric pain radiating to her back. She is normotensive, without symptoms suggestive of preeclamptic syndromes. Urine protein is normal. Laboratory investigations are only significant for increased amylase and lipase levels at 850 U/L *(normal 30–110 U/L)* and 1500 U/L *(normal 0–160 U/L)*, respectively. Hemoglobin, coagulation function tests, and transaminases are unremarkable. Abdominal and fetal ultrasounds are normal.

---

20. What is the most probable diagnosis? *(1 point each)*   2

☐ Post-ERCP acute pancreatitis
  ○ *Most frequent complication after ERCP/sphincterotomy (3%–8%)*

The patient continues to refrain from alcoholic beverages in fear of fetal alcohol syndrome. The gastroenterologist concurs that her presentation is *most likely* a complication of the ERCP, although medical causes of acute pancreatitis should be assessed.

---

21. Which laboratory tests would be most valuable in establishing the cause of acute   2
pancreatitis? *(1 point each)*

☐ Serum triglycerides
☐ Serum cholesterol

Investigations reveal:

• Serum triglycerides 14 mmol/L (1240 mg/dL)
• Serum cholesterol 9.0 mmol/L (351 mg/dL)

Family history is negative for dyslipidemia.

22. Discuss the management for the patient's severe hypertriglyceridemia-induced acute pancreatitis. Multidisciplinary teams are involved in her care. *(1 point each unless specified)*   8

☐ Admission with conservative management
☐ Intravenous hydration and analgesia
☐ Maintain nil-per-os status for several days
☐ Consideration for total parenteral nutrition
☐ At least daily fetal cardiotocographic monitoring
☐ Triglyceride levels should be lowered, with reassuring safety data for: *(**either subbullet for 3 points**)*
  ○ Lipopheresis or therapeutic plasma exchange *(treatment of choice; up to 70% decrease in triglyceride levels after one treatment session)*
  ○ Omega-3 fatty acid supplementation *(30% decrease in triglycerides)*

With lowering of serum triglycerides and resolution of acute pancreatitis, the remainder of pregnancy is unremarkable. Spontaneous labor occurs at term and a healthy female infant is born.

SPECIAL SCENARIO

23. If the patient initially presented with acute cholecystitis at 34 weeks' gestation, with otherwise stable maternal-fetal status, would your management considerations have differed from that proposed to the patient at the 25 weeks' episode? *(1 point for either response)*   1

☐ Medical or conservative management is preferred with third-trimester disease due to the technical difficulty imposed by the gravid uterus and increased risk of prematurity (up to 25%)
☐ Cholecystectomy would have been recommended at least six weeks postpartum

TOTAL: **80**

CHAPTER 45

Pregnancy after Liver Transplantation

Neha Agrawal, Amira El-Messidi, and Maged Peter Ghali

A 29-year-old primigravida is a recipient of a liver transplant. She is referred by her primary care provider to your high-risk obstetrics clinic for consultation and prenatal care of a spontaneous intrauterine singleton pregnancy at 12^{+0} weeks' gestation by dating sonogram. The patient takes prenatal vitamins and has no obstetric complaints.

LEARNING OBJECTIVES

1. Elicit salient points on prenatal history of a liver transplant recipient, identifying common comorbidities, while recognizing disease-related factors that may predict poor obstetric outcome
2. Develop a diagnostic differential for abnormal serum hepatic investigations, and promote safe diagnostic testing and therapeutic management in pregnancy
3. Encourage adherence to immunosuppressive agents with reassuring safety profile in pregnancy
4. Detail counseling on obstetric morbidity with a liver transplant, appreciating that pregnancy itself does not contribute to deteriorating allograft function
5. Discuss postpartum considerations for liver organ recipients

SUGGESTED READINGS

1. Blume C, Pischke S, von Versen-Höynck F, et al. Pregnancies in liver and kidney transplant recipients: a review of the current literature and recommendation. *Best Pract Res Clin Obstet Gynaecol.* 2014 Nov;28(8):1123–1136.
2. Jabiry-Zieniewicz Z, Dabrowski FA, Pietrzak B, et al. Pregnancy in the liver transplant recipient. *Liver Transpl.* 2016 Oct;22(10):1408–1417.
3. Marson EJ, Kamarajah SK, Dyson JK, et al. Pregnancy outcomes in women with liver transplants: systematic review and meta-analysis. *HPB (Oxford).* 2020 Aug;22(8):1102–1111.
4. National Guideline Alliance (UK). *Intrapartum Care for Women with Existing Medical Conditions or Obstetric Complications and Their Babies.* London: National Institute for Health and Care Excellence (UK); 2019.
5. Parhar KS, Gibson PS, Coffin CS. Pregnancy following liver transplantation: review of outcomes and recommendations for management. *Can J Gastroenterol.* 2012;26(9):621–626.
6. Rahim MN, Long L, Penna L, et al. Pregnancy in liver transplantation. *Liver Transpl.* 2020 Apr;26(4):564–581.
7. Ramirez CB, Doria C. Pregnancy after liver transplantation. *Best Pract Res Clin Obstet Gynaecol.* 2014 Nov;28(8):1137–1145.

8. UK medical eligibility criteria for contraceptive use, 2016; amended Sept 2019. Available at www.fsrh.org. Accessed September 29, 2020.

9. Women in Hepatology Group; Italian Association for the Study of the Liver (AISF). AISF position paper on liver transplantation and pregnancy: Women in Hepatology Group, Italian Association for the Study of the Liver (AISF). *Dig Liver Dis*. 2016 Aug;48(8):860–868.

10. Zullo F, Saccone G, Donnarumma L, et al. Pregnancy after liver transplantation: a case series and review of the literature. *J Matern Fetal Neonatal Med*. 2019 Oct;21:1–8.

POINTS

1. With respect to the liver transplant, what aspects of a focused history would you want to know? *(1 point each)*	Max 15

Details of the liver transplant:
☐ Indication for transplantation
☐ Interval of time since the transplant surgery
☐ Live or cadaveric donor
☐ History of posttransplant complications *(e.g., cellular rejection)*, or need of other surgeries
☐ Name and contact of treating hepatologist

Comorbidities:
☐ Hypertension or diabetes mellitus *(including treatment, complications, and disease-control)*
☐ Chronic renal disease *(proteinuria, serum creatinine)*

Medications: *(given the patient takes prenatal vitamins)*
☐ Corticosteroids
☐ Maintenance immunosuppressant agents

Routine health maintenance:
☐ Time since the most recent Papanicolaou smear *(higher risk for cervical malignancy)*
☐ Vaccination status *(e.g., influenza, hepatitis A and B, pneumococcus, tetanus)*
☐ Allergies

Social and sexual history:
☐ Intravenous drug use/needle sharing *(hepatitis B and C, HIV)*
☐ Alcohol consumption (including duration and quantity), smoking
☐ Multiple sexual partners
☐ History of genital infections
☐ Recent travel history

You learned that the patient had a cadaveric liver transplant at the age of six years for biliary atresia and has been generally healthy since. Surgery was performed at the Children's Hospital affiliated with your tertiary center. She has not experienced graft rejection and does not have hypertension or diabetes mellitus. She takes oral tacrolimus 1 mg twice daily and prednisone 5 mg daily. The patient was on mycophenolate mofetil (MMF) until eight months ago when it was discontinued by her transplant hepatologist. Although she is compliant with medical care, she missed the preconception consultation scheduled with you due to a family emergency. Up to 12 weeks after discontinuing MMF, she maintained dual-contraception with male condoms and progesterone-only oral agents, as advised by her transplant hepatologist. The patient is in a monogamous relationship with her husband of seven years. She does not recall the timing of her last cervical smear, although she ascertains she has no history of cervical dysplasia. Her vaccinations are up to date. She has not traveled recently.

The patient intends to abstain from alcoholic beverages during pregnancy; she has never used illicit drugs. Outside of pregnancy, she consumes a maximum of one to two glasses/week of wine. She tries to exercise regularly and maintains a healthy diet.

On examination, she is afebrile, normotensive with a normal pulse rate; fetal viability is ascertained. Her BMI is 31 kg/m^2. You have discussed aspects of *routine* prenatal care.

2. Indicate the recommended baseline prenatal investigations in relation to the liver transplant and other medical considerations for this patient. *(1 point each)*

Max 12

Hematologic:
- ☐ Full/complete blood count (FBC/CBC)
- ☐ Serum ferritin

Liver enzymes: *(assessment of graft injury)*
- ☐ Serum ALT, AST, GGT

Liver function tests: *(assessment of graft dysfunction)*
- ☐ Serum bilirubin, INR[†]

Renal status:
- ☐ Proteinuria (*e.g.*, urine protein/creatinine ratio)
- ☐ Serum creatinine
- ☐ Urinalysis and culture

Infection screening:
- ☐ CMV PCR *(occurs in up to 25% of transplant recipients on combined immunosuppressants)*
- ☐ Toxoplasma serology
- ☐ HIV antigen/antibody (fourth-generation testing)
- ☐ HBV: HBsAg, HBsAb, HBcAb
- ☐ HCV: Hepatitis C antibody

Pelvic investigations:
- ☐ Cervical smear, unless performed within three months of pregnancy
- ☐ Cervicovaginal cultures

Metabolic risks:[‡]
- ☐ Glycosylated hemoglobin (HbA1c) and/or fasting serum glucose

Immunosuppressant agents:
- ☐ Serum tacrolimus levels

Special notes:
† Serum albumin levels have limited value in assessment of liver function during pregnancy
‡ Although hyperlipidemia may occur in relation to tacrolimus and obesity, total serum cholesterol and triglyceride levels have limited value in baseline screening given maintenance of a healthy lifestyle is part of routine prenatal care; lipid-lowering agents are contraindicated in pregnancy

The patient agrees to perform the suggested investigations. Meanwhile, she expresses concern regarding the effects of her liver transplant on pregnancy. Although her hepatologist discussed antenatal immunosuppressant treatment with her, and she understands the importance of continued therapy, she is worried about potential fetal effects.

---

3. Discuss the <u>fetal</u> risks associated with her current immunosuppressive regimen.   Max 5
(*1 point each*)

Tacrolimus: (*a calcineurin inhibitor*)
☐ No proven teratogenicity
☐ Transient neonatal renal insufficiency (hyperkalemia), with spontaneous resolution

Prednisone:
☐ Preterm prelabor rupture of membranes (PPROM)
☐ Fetal growth restriction (FGR) and low birthweight (LBW)
☐ Neonatal adrenal suppression or infections
☐ *Theoretical* risk of fetal cleft palate; no demonstrated teratogenicity[†]

Special note:
† (1) *Refer to* Hviid A, Mølgaard-Nielsen D. *CMAJ.* 2011 Apr;183(7):796–804; (2) Skuladottir H et al. *Birth Defects Res A Clin Mol Teratol.* 2014; 100:499–506; (3) US-FDA supports no evidence of human teratogenicity

---

Your trainee recalls having patients on antenatal azathioprine therapy, an alternative immunosuppressant agent, and wonders why the treating hepatologist might have preferred tacrolimus over azathioprine.

---

4. Which side effect, particular to azathioprine, is obviated by use of a calcineurin inhibitor?   1

☐ Myelosuppression

---

5. Indicate features to discuss with regard to medical and obstetric risks associated with liver   Max 5
transplantation. (*1 point each*)

Medical aspects:
☐ Increased risk of nephrotoxicity, which generally improves with dose-reduction of tacrolimus
☐ Increased risk of new or worsening hypertension or preeclampsia (but <u>not</u> eclampsia)
☐ Increased risk of urinary tract infections associated with use of immunosuppressant agents
☐ Reassurance that liver transplantation is not associated with maternal or fetal mortality

Obstetric risks:
☐ Early pregnancy loss in up to 20% of patients
☐ Gestational diabetes mellitus (GDM), ranging from 0% to 38%
☐ Preterm delivery, likely attributed to preeclampsia
☐ Postpartum hemorrhage and blood transfusions
☐ Cesarean delivery, ranging from 20% to 100%

6. Address the patient's concern as to whether pregnancy may incite rejection of her liver transplant.

☐ Stable allograft function is not affected by pregnancy itself; rates of organ rejection are relatively low, at 0%–20%

1

Your trainee finds your structured approach and evidence-based counseling invaluable, although inquires why the patient is at risk for GDM and hypertension.

7. What are three <u>possible</u> risk factors for gestational diabetes mellitus or hypertensive diseases in pregnancy for this patient? *(1 point each)*

3

☐ Obesity
☐ Tacrolimus[†]
☐ Chronic oral steroids

Special note:
† Tacrolimus-based immunosuppression is associated with lower rates of hypertension compared with cyclosporin regimens

At 14 weeks' gestation, her gastroenterologist communicates that baseline investigations are all normal to date and tacrolimus is therapeutic; the patient has been informed that her obstetric course is favorable. Continued interdisciplinary care is planned.

8. Further to the summative evaluation by her hepatologist, teach your obstetric trainee factors used to predict optimal obstetric outcome for this patient with a liver transplant. *(1 point each)*

Max 5

☐ Long transplant-to-pregnancy interval of at least 12–24 months
☐ Absence of hypertension or diabetes mellitus
☐ Normal serum creatinine (<1–1.2 mg/dL)
☐ Minimal proteinuria
☐ Absence of prior graft rejection in the preceding year
☐ Low doses of maintenance immunosuppressive agents
☐ Use of immunosuppressive agents with a good safety profile, with discontinuation of teratogenic agents such as mycophenolate mofetil

9. Subsequent to investigations requested at the initial prenatal visit, outline your antenatal management plan for this liver transplant recipient, in collaboration with the hepatologist. *(1 point each)*

Max 8

☐ Anticipate frequent multidisciplinary antenatal evaluations

☐ Consideration for calcium and vitamin D supplementation, mainly due to chronic steroid therapy

☐ Early treatment of anemia, common to pregnant-transplant patients

☐ Arrange for serial serum tacrolimus levels; the typical frequency of testing is every 12 weeks, although monthly testing may be reasonable due to increased volume of distribution, renal clearance, and lipophilicity of the drug

☐ Serial serum and urine investigations at least every trimester

☐ Serial vaginal cultures at least every trimester

☐ Screening for gestational diabetes mellitus at 24–28 weeks' gestation

☐ Consideration for repeat CMV PCR in the second and third trimesters based on risk of reactivation

☐ Offer early nutritional consultation, based on obesity and risk of gestational diabetes mellitus

☐ Encourage early reporting of symptoms possibly related to hypertensive diseases of pregnancy

☐ Plan serial fetal growth biometry in the second and third trimesters

☐ Plan weekly fetal monitoring in the third trimester (*e.g.,* nonstress test, biophysical profile)

Special note:
Prophylactic antenatal thromboprophylaxis is generally not required solely for prior liver transplantation

Pregnancy remained unremarkable until 26 weeks' gestation; the patient screened negative for gestational diabetes mellitus. Routine serial hepatic and renal investigations reveal the following:

		Normal range
ALT	68 U/L	6–32 IU/L**
AST	55 U/L	11–29 IU/L**
GGT	74	5–43 IU/L**
Total bilirubin	12.1 umol/L	3–13 umol/L**
INR	1.0	0.9–1.0
Creatinine	88 umol/L (1 mg/dL)	44–64 umol/L**
UPCR	28 mg/mmol	<30 mg/mmol (265 mg/g)

** *Pregnancy reference ranges: from Girling J.C. et al. Br J Obstet Gynecol 1997; 104:246–250 and Nelson-Piercy, C. Handbook of obstetric medicine. 5th ed. London (UK): Informa Healthcare; 2015*

10-A. Indicate five <u>non-pregnancy</u>-related hepatic conditions that can account for the increased liver enzymes. *(1 point each)*

Max 5

☐ Autoimmune hepatitis
☐ Nonalcoholic fatty liver disease
☐ Budd-Chiari syndrome
☐ Allograft rejection
☐ Viral hepatitis
☐ Focal lesions of the biliary tree
☐ Portal vein thrombosis

10-B. Identify the investigations you anticipate would be recommended by her hepatologist in assessment of the above diagnostic possibilities. *(1 point each)*

Max 5

☐ Repeat HAV and HCV antibodies, and ensure persistent immunity to HBV
☐ Autoantibodies panel‡
☐ Abdominal ultrasound with vascular study
☐ Tacrolimus level
☐ Lipid profile
☐ Fasting serum glucose and/or HbA1c

Special note:
‡ *ANA, antismooth muscle antibodies, anti-liver-cytosol liver antibody-1 (ALC-1), anti-liver-kidney-microsome-1 antibodies (ALKM-1)*

Abdominal ultrasound requested by her transplant hepatologist reveals mild hepatomegaly with hepatic steatosis; hepatic vasculature is patent with normal Doppler velocimetry.

Results of serum investigations show:

		Normal range
Triglycerides	250 mg/dL (2.82 mmol/L)	<150 mg/dL (<1.7 mmol/L)
Serum cholesterol	150 mg/dL (3.9 mmol/L)	<170 mg/dL (4.4 mmol/L)
HbA1c	5.5%	<6.0%
Virology panel	normal	
Autoimmune antibodies panel	negative	

11. What are your top two differential diagnoses at this time? *(1 point each)*

2

☐ Nonalcoholic fatty liver disease
☐ Graft rejection *(generally due to discontinuation, decreasing doses of immunosuppressant agents, or inadequate dose-adjustments in pregnancy)*

The patient is now 27 weeks' gestation. The hepatologist calls you to discuss two possible diagnostic tools in the evaluation of this gravida.

12. Indicate the safest, next best step in the diagnostic evaluation of this obstetric patient.   1

☐ Liver biopsy

Special note:
Noninvasive techniques that provide information about the extent of liver fibrosis include transient elastography (TE) and fibrosure; TE was previously contraindicated in pregnancy but is now considered safe. Nevertheless, liver stiffness increases in pregnancy due to increased blood flow; interpretation of fibroscan is unreliable and should generally be avoided. Fibrosure does not provide definitive diagnosis

After counseling the patient regarding the safety of percutaneous liver biopsy in pregnancy, she provides informed consent. The biopsy shows 30% steatosis, ballooning degeneration, and fibrous portal expansion; there is no cholestasis, bile duct loss, endotheliitis, or liver cirrhosis. Pathologist's interpretation is consistent with nonalcoholic steatohepatitis (NASH) <u>without</u> rejection.

The gastroenterologist has informed the patient of the biopsy findings and management plan until delivery.

Now at 28 weeks' gestation, the patient sees you for a prenatal visit. Blood pressure and urinalysis are normal. She reports regular fetal activity and recent sonography showed normal growth velocity along the 13th percentile and normal amniotic fluid volume. The patient seems overwhelmed by the new findings of NASH; she asks you to review aspects of her forthcoming prenatal care.

13. Outline your counseling and prenatal management of NASH. *(1 point each)*   Max 2

☐ Explain that clinical features of NASH are often absent in pregnancy; diagnostic evaluation is often initiated by abnormal liver enzymes/function tests
☐ Arrange consultation, or follow-up, with a nutritionist
☐ Reassure the patient that NASH does **not** increase her risk of developing acute fatty liver of pregnancy (AFLP)[†]

Special note:
† <u>Macro</u>vascular steatosis is seen with NASH; <u>micro</u>vascular steatosis occurs with AFLP

Blood pressure remains normal and she follows the advised diet and exercise regimen. Serial laboratory investigations remain stable and her tacrolimus required increasing dose-adjustments at 29 weeks' gestation. Fetal well-being is regularly ascertained.

The patient presents for a prenatal visit at 35 weeks' gestation.

14. Discuss your recommended timing and mode of delivery, including important management considerations for this patient. *(1 point each)*

☐ Aim for delivery at term; preterm delivery is guided by maternal-fetal status
☐ Plan for vaginal delivery, with Cesarean section being reserved for obstetric indications
☐ Anticipate postpartum hemorrhage (PPH) and arrange for blood products' availability

Steroid stress doses in labor:[‡] *(based on need for chronic oral steroids ≥5 mg daily for more than three weeks)*
☐ Continue regular oral steroid dose, **and**
☐ Add IV or IM hydrocortisone 50–100 mg every six hours until six hours after vaginal delivery

Special note:
‡ *Refer to* NICE 2019 Guidelines for Intrapartum Complex Care. National Guideline Alliance (UK). Intrapartum care for women with existing medical conditions or obstetric complications and their babies. London: National Institute for Health and Care Excellence (UK); 2019 Mar. PMID: 31194308.

5

As you call to notify the anesthesiologist and allied professionals in the birthing unit regarding your patient's delivery considerations, your trainee is researching the internet to understand the basis for the risks of bleeding.

15. Facilitate your trainee's understanding of the basis for postpartum hemorrhage among liver transplant recipients. *(1 point each)*

☐ Operative risk, in case of Cesarean delivery
☐ Thrombocytopenia induced by immunosuppressants
☐ Coagulopathy, primarily due to preeclampsia

3

Spontaneous labor and vaginal delivery occur at 35^{+6} weeks' gestation. Active management of the third stage of labor is performed, aiding to obviate a postpartum hemorrhage. A vigorous male is born, with birthweight 2300 g.

On day 1 postpartum, your trainee notifies you that physical examination is significant for bilateral swelling of the lower extremities and significant abdominal distension. The patient is normotensive and only complains of right upper quadrant pain. Dose-adjustment of tacrolimus was initiated postpartum, and serum levels are therapeutic. Laboratory derangements include:

- ALT 1545 IU/L
- AST 1400 IU/L

Having assessed the patient, the hepatology team help coordinate urgent transfer to an intensive care setting, given the possibility of impending hepatic failure. An urgent abdominal ultrasound with vascular studies shows hepatomegaly, massive ascites, and absence of flow in the hepatic vein. The radiologist's interpretation is consistent with Budd-Chiari syndrome.

16. Based on the hepatologist's counseling, identify therapeutic options in the acute treatment of this postpartum patient. *(1 point each)*   Max 3

- ☐ Anticoagulation *(i.e., low molecular weight heparin)*
- ☐ Transjugular intrahepatic portosystemic shunt (TIPS)
- ☐ Thrombophilic investigations to identify procoagulant states
- ☐ Repeat liver transplantation

The TIPS procedure is performed and the patient recovers. Upon discharge, she continues close follow-up with her hepatologist and presents to you at eight weeks postpartum for an elective visit. She has now resumed pregestational oral prednisone 5 mg and tacrolimus 1 mg twice daily. Although her hepatologist reassured her regarding lactation, she asks you to readdress the safety of breastfeeding while on her immunosuppressive agents.

17. Outline important postpartum considerations to discuss at this postpartum visit in a liver transplant recipient, post TIPS procedure. *(1 point each)*   9

General maternal-fetal well-being:
- ☐ Screen for postpartum depression and continue to offer psychosocial support services, particularly in the context of chronic steroid treatment and complications during pregnancy
- ☐ Reassure the patient that breastfeeding is safe with continued use of low-dose corticosteroids and tacrolimus; monitoring of tacrolimus drug levels in the infant will be required

Contraceptive options:
- ☐ There is no ideal method for contraception among liver transplant recipients
- ☐ Barrier agents are safe for use among liver transplant recipients; beware of the risk of urinary infections due to diaphragm use
- ☐ Progesterone-only agents are safe for use, as advantages outweigh theoretical or proven risks among organ-recipients *(UK and US Medical Eligibility Criteria for Contraceptive Use, 2016)*
- ☐ There is an existing controversy[‡] regarding use of intrauterine contraception; while it may be the ideal contraceptive option for a transplant recipient, beware of possibly increased risk of infections or reduced efficacy among immunosuppressed patients due to decreased anti-inflammatory environment in utero
- ☐ Beyond lactation, exercise caution with use of estrogen-containing hormonal contraceptives in liver transplant recipients and beware of metabolic interactions with immunosuppressants
- ☐ Consideration for sterilization if completed childbearing

Pregnancy post-TIPS:
- ☐ Limited available data to guide counseling; the reduction in portal hypertension after TIPS procedure should be beneficial for pregnancy hemodynamics. Portal hypertension is associated with maternal mortality (2%–10%) and maternal-fetal morbidity

Special note:

‡ American Society of Transplantation does not recommend IUDs as first-line agents among transplant recipients; however, this modality is recommended by UK and US Medical Eligibility Criteria for Contraceptive Use, 2016 as advantages outweigh theoretical or proven risks with continuation of use

TOTAL: **90**

CHAPTER 46

Pregnancy after Renal Transplantation

Tiina Podymow, Amira El-Messidi, and Michelle Hladunewich

A 38-year-old primigravida is a recipient of a renal transplant. She is referred by her primary care provider for consultation and prenatal care of a spontaneous pregnancy at 10 weeks' gestation by dating sonogram. She takes prenatal vitamins and has no obstetric complaints.

LEARNING OBJECTIVES

1. Elicit salient points on prenatal history, and identify important baseline investigations related to the renal allograft, maintaining continued collaboration with nephrologists in the perinatal care of renal transplant recipients
2. Counsel patients on renal transplant–associated features and related comorbidities that may predict a favorable obstetric outcome
3. Understand the teratogenicity associated with specific immunosuppressants while encouraging adherence to others with reassuring perinatal safety to optimize maternal-fetal outcomes
4. Anticipate medical and obstetric risks with a renal allograft, and outline appropriate management
5. Appreciate and address nongestational causes of worsening renal allograft function
6. Recognize that mode of delivery among renal transplant recipients depends on obstetric indications, albeit with increased rates of Cesarean section, where surgical and medical particularities are required

SUGGESTED READINGS

1. Bramham K. Pregnancy in renal transplant recipients and donors. *Semin Nephrol.* 2017;37(4):370–377.
2. Chandra A, Midtvedt K, Åsberg A, et al. Immunosuppression and reproductive health after kidney transplantation. *Transplantation.* 2019;103(11):e325–e333.
3. Hladunewich MA, Melamed N, Bramham K. Pregnancy across the spectrum of chronic kidney disease. *Kidney Int.* 2016;89(5):995–1007.
4. Hui D, Hladunewich MA. Chronic kidney disease and pregnancy. *Obstet Gynecol.* 2019;133(6):1182–1194.
5. McKay DB, Josephson MA, Armenti VT, et al. Reproduction and transplantation: report on the AST Consensus Conference on Reproductive Issues and Transplantation. *Am J Transplant.* 2005;5(7):1592–1599.
6. Shah S, Venkatesan RL, Gupta A, et al. Pregnancy outcomes in women with kidney transplant: Metaanalysis and systematic review. *BMC Nephrol.* 2019;20(1):24.

7. Wiles K, Chappell L, Clark K, et al. Clinical practice guideline on pregnancy and renal disease. *BMC Nephrol.* 2019;20(1):401.

POINTS

1. With respect to her renal transplant, what aspects of a focused history are most relevant?   Max 25
(1 point per main bullet, unless specified)

Renal transplant details:
☐ Indication for transplantation
    ○ Anticipate genetics consultation depending on etiology (*e.g.*, polycystic kidney disease) ***(2 points)***
☐ Interval of time since the transplant surgery
☐ Live or cadaveric donor
☐ History of posttransplant complications including rejection or need of other surgeries, especially within the past year
☐ Stability and level of graft function/results of most recent investigations
☐ Obtain operative report of the renal transplant procedure (*primarily to ascertain location of the allograft and ureter should Cesarean delivery be required*)
☐ Name and contact of treating nephrologist

Comorbidities/complications:
☐ Hypertension ***(additional 1 point per subbullet)***
    ○ Determine the baseline/prepregnancy blood pressure (BP) and review her home recordings
    ○ Secondary end-organ dysfunction (*i.e., ocular, cardio-neurovascular*)
☐ History of diabetes mellitus and glycemic control
☐ Occurrence and frequency of urinary tract infections, or other infections within the past year
☐ Anemia (including current/prior treatments)

Medications:
☐ Corticosteroids
☐ Inhibitors of the renin angiotensin system (*angiotensin-converting enzyme inhibitors [ACEi] and angiotensin II receptor blockers*)
☐ Antihypertensive agents
☐ Maintenance immunosuppressive agents (*e.g., tacrolimus, cyclosporin, mycophenolate mofetil [MMF]*)

Systemic symptoms:
☐ Headaches
☐ Peripheral edema
☐ Symptoms of urinary tract infections or other infections
☐ Symptoms of graft rejection/dysfunction (*e.g., fever, abdominal pain, oliguria*)

Routine health maintenance:
☐ Vaccination status (*e.g., influenza, hepatitis A and B, pneumococcus, tetanus, COVID-19*)
☐ Cigarette smoking, alcohol consumption, recreational drug use
☐ Diet and exercise activity; weight maintenance
☐ Allergies

You learn the patient had a cadaveric renal transplant four years ago for membranous nephropathy, with stable graft function on tacrolimus, MMF, and perindopril; she has not experienced episodes of rejection. She has chronic hypertension, well controlled on nifedipine. There have not been any urinary nor other infections in the recent past. Blood sugar values have remained normal posttransplantation.

In anticipation of desired pregnancy, her nephrologist discontinued MMF and replaced it with azathioprine.[§] Since her transplant, and for six weeks after replacing MMF, she maintained use of a copper-IUD and male condoms, as her nephrologist advised reliable contraception.

The patient maintains a healthy lifestyle and is in a monogamous relationship with her husband of eight years. Her vaccinations are up to date. She has no intent of having alcoholic beverages during pregnancy and does not smoke nor use recreational drugs. There are no drug allergies.

On exam, her body habitus, blood pressure, and pulse are normal; the fetus is viable. You have already discussed aspects of *routine* prenatal care.

Special note:
§ Testing to ensure normal TPMT (thiopurine methyltransferase) enzyme activity is required prior to initiating thiopurines

---

2. As you open your institution's electronic records, which baseline prenatal investigations would you expect were requested by her nephrologist in relation to her transplant and comorbidities? *(1 point each bullet)*   Max 10

Hematologic: *(baseline and serial)*
☐ CBC/FBC
☐ Serum ferritin

Renal tests and immunosuppressant status: *(baseline and serial)*
☐ Serum creatinine, electrolytes
☐ Serum tacrolimus level[‡]
☐ Urinalysis
☐ Urine culture
☐ Spot urine protein/creatinine or microalbumin/creatinine ratio

Infection screening:
☐ CMV PCR *(infection occurs in up to 25% of transplant recipients on combined immunosuppressants, with a higher risk in the first year post renal transplant)*
☐ HIV antibody/antigen (fourth-generation) testing
☐ HBV and HCV testing (*i.e.*, HBsAg, HBsAb, HBcAb, HCV antibody)

Metabolic risks:
☐ HbA1c and/or fasting glucose, or oral glucose tolerance test (OGTT) – *(baseline and serial)*

Hepatic markers:
☐ Serum AST, ALT, LDH, uric acid, bilirubin

Special note:
Renal imaging is not indicated
‡ Although hyperlipidemia may occur with tacrolimus therapy, total serum cholesterol and triglyceride levels have limited value in baseline screening; lipid-lowering agents are contraindicated in pregnancy, maintenance of a healthy prenatal lifestyle is encouraged

You note the following baseline, prepregnancy results:

		Normal **
Serum creatinine	112 µmol/L (1.27 mg/dL)	35–62 µmol/L (0.4–0.7 mg/dL)
Proteinuria	0.4 g/g (0.4 g/24 hours equivalent)	<0.3 g/g
Hemoglobin	100 g/L	110–140 g/L
Mean corpuscular volume	78 µm^3	80–99 µm^3
Ferritin	5 µg/L (0.5 µg/dL)	6–130 µg/L (0.6–13 µg/dL)

** Not adjusted to pregnancies with renal allograft

Although her nephrologist discussed antenatal immunosuppressant treatment with her, and she understands the importance of continued therapy, the patient is worried about possible fetal risks. Meanwhile, you take this opportunity to address your trainee's queries regarding investigations and management of gestational anemia among transplant patients.

3. Further to the provided hematological results, which additional markers might you expect with iron-deficiency anemia? *(1 point each)* — Max 3

☐ Increased levels of transferrin protein
☐ Low transferrin saturation (<20%)
☐ Hypochromia
☐ Low reticulocyte count

Special note:
Serum iron level is not reliable; confounded by daily variations

4. With reference to <u>fetal</u> risks, detail why mycophenolate mofetil was replaced for azathioprine preconceptionally and indicate pregnancy recommendations specific to mycophenolate. — 6

Mycophenolate mofetil – preconception recommendations: *(1 point per bullet for 2 points)*
☐ Ideally discontinued ≥6 weeks preconception; UK guidelines *(Suggested Reading 7)* recommend discontinuation ≥12 weeks preconception
  ○ Inadvertent use periconceptionally or during pregnancy requires referral to a high-risk obstetrics expert for individualized discussion and management)
☐ Reliable contraception is strongly advised up to six weeks post discontinuation

Fetal risks: *(1 point each; max 4)*
☐ Risk of early pregnancy loss
☐ 'Mycophenolate embryopathy' *(i.e., craniofacial defects of the eyes, ears, lip/palate)*
☐ Neural tube defects (NTDs)
☐ Cardiac anomalies *(i.e., atrio-ventricular septal defects)*
☐ Esophageal atresia
☐ Defects of the hand digits

Special note:
Refer to Chapter 42 for fetal/neonatal risks of azathioprine, and to Chapter 45 for fetal risks of tacrolimus

The patient is interested in fetal aneuploidy screening. She read about cell-free DNA (cfDNA), understands results are quicker and comparable to standard integrated prenatal screening (IPS); the patient asks you for cfDNA testing.

---

5. Provide your recommendations for prenatal aneuploidy screening among renal transplant   5
    recipients, if different from the general population.

☐ *Currently*, cfDNA aneuploidy screening is not reliable in patients with renal allografts
    given existing DNA from kidney donors

As planned by her nephrologist, the patient will maintain antenatal immunosuppression with tacrolimus and azathioprine and continue nifedipine for blood pressure control. Although excited about the pregnancy, she is concerned whether her transplant status will have a negative impact on her pregnancy outcome.

---

6. Facilitate the patient's understanding of her anticipated pregnancy outcome with reference   8
    to specific renal transplant prognostic factors. *(1 point for main bullet and per subbullet)*

☐ Reassure the patient of her overall good renal prognosis, given the following factors:
    ○ Timing of her pregnancy is more than one year after renal transplantation *(rates of long-
      term graft loss are also low as conception occurred more than two years posttransplant)*
    ○ Absence of graft rejection during the previous year
    ○ Absence of current/recent fetotoxic infections (*e.g.,* CMV)
    ○ Adequate interval to conception since discontinuation of teratogenic/fetotoxic agents
    ○ Minimal/well-controlled hypertension
    ○ Stable graft function, implied by baseline serum creatinine <133 µmol/L (1.5 mg/dL)[‡]
      with minimal to no proteinuria
    ○ Maintenance dosing of immunosuppressants

Special note:
[‡] Patients with higher baseline serum creatinine risk losing graft function during the
    antenatal or immediate postpartum period

---

7. Address her concern as to whether pregnancy may incite rejection of her kidney   1
    transplant.

☐ Stable renal allograft function is generally not affected by pregnancy itself, with risks of
    acute rejection <5%

The patient appreciates your reassurance that conception occurred at a favorable period post-transplant and that renal function is unlikely to deteriorate as a result of pregnancy. She still recalls the nephrologist's discussion of her ACEi agent during pregnancy[†]; she has already purchased a home BP monitoring device and recalls the triggers upon which to seek urgent care[††]. She understands the importance of continued collaboration with her nephrologist and other health professionals; she plans to remain adherent to management plans.

Special note:
Refer to Chapter 47 for (i)[†]fetal risks and prenatal management of ACEi agents, and (ii)[††]blood pressure management recommendations for patient with chronic renal insufficiency

---

8. Further to discussing the anticipated graft prognosis, outline your discussion of the <u>maternal</u> risks with a renal allograft. *(1 point per main bullet)* — Max 10

☐ Anemia *(oral, ± IV iron; erythropoietin treatment is not required in this case)*
☐ Vitamin D deficiency
   ○ *Routine prenatal supplementation*
☐ New or superimposed preeclampsia on chronic hypertension (or other hypertensive syndromes)
   ○ Initiate LDASA 150–162 mg nightly as prophylaxis, starting <16 weeks' gestation; supplementary calcium may be considered
   ○ Encourage early reporting of signs/symptoms, including weight gain >1 kg/week or BP >140/90 mmHg
☐ CMV reactivation
☐ Gestational diabetes mellitus (GDM)
   ○ Prednisone and tacrolimus-associated risks of GDM (~8%)
   ○ Early oral glucose tolerance test (OGTT)
   ○ Early nutritional consultation
☐ Nephrotoxicity *(generally improves by decreasing the dose of tacrolimus)*
☐ Graft rejection
☐ Urinary tract infections
   ○ Augmented risks related to immunosuppressant treatment
   ○ Monthly urine cultures are advised
☐ Increasing proteinuria (levels may also remain stable)
   ○ Augmented risks related to hyperfiltration and discontinuation of ACEi/angiotensin receptor blocker
   ○ Reassure the patient that minimally increased proteinuria is generally nonpathologic *(significant increases warrant nephrologist evaluation)*
☐ Low threshold for elective hospitalizations
☐ Iatrogenic preterm delivery
   ○ *Mostly due to comorbidities rather than spontaneous preterm labor*
☐ Risk of Cesarean delivery, although reserved for obstetric indications

Special notes: (a) Maternal mortality is not increased from renal transplantation;
   (b) No heightened baseline risk of venous thromboembolism in this patient unless other risk factors exist

Refer to Chapter 47, Question 8 for obstetric counseling and management of patient with chronic renal dysfunction

9. Indicate <u>fetal</u> morbidities among renal transplant recipients. *(1 point each)*   Max 3

☐ Prematurity
☐ Fetal growth restriction (FGR) or low birthweight
  ○ Arrange serial fetal growth sonograms in the second and third trimesters
☐ IUFD *(higher than general population risk <1%)*
☐ Reassure the patient that early/spontaneous pregnancy loss is generally associated with comorbidities or immunosuppression (i.e., MMF), rather than renal allograft itself

Special note:
By age five years, children born to renal transplant recipients have reached comparable milestones as general population

The patient remains on tacrolimus and azathioprine with regular serum monitoring and dose-adjustments of tacrolimus according to her nephrologist. Blood pressure is maintained ≤140/90[†] mmHg on nifedipine 30 mg daily. Fetal morphology and amniotic fluid volume at 20 weeks' gestation are normal, with biometry at the 30th percentile; her cervix is long and closed. Serial glucose testing is normal. The patient does not have any obstetric complaints.

At 24 weeks' gestation, her routine monthly self-voided urine culture is positive for *E. coli* at 10^8 cfu/mL, with wide sensitivity analysis. The patient is afebrile, asymptomatic and not tender in the costovertebral angle. Your obstetric trainee recognizes the renal-protective effects of treating asymptomatic bacteriuria in pregnancy, particularly for renal transplant recipients, although he or she wonders if there are obstetric benefits to treatment.

Special note:
† No universal consensus on optimal BP among prenatal renal transplant recipients; UK guideline *(Suggested Reading 7)* recommends target BP ≤135/85 mmHg in pregnancies with chronic renal disease

10. Address your trainee's inquiry regarding the obstetric risks associated with asymptomatic bacteriuria. *(1 point each)*   2

☐ Preterm birth (PTB)
☐ Low birthweight

11. At this gestational age of 24 weeks, name three possible <u>oral</u> antibiotics to treat her *E. coli* urinary infection. *(1 point each)*   3

☐ Nitrofurantoin[†§]
☐ Amoxicillin[‡]
☐ Cephalexin
☐ Trimethoprim-sulfamethoxazole[†]

Special notes:
† Preferred avoidance in first and late third trimesters, or earlier if anticipated risk of preterm delivery
§ Avoid if eGFR <45 mL/min or in patients with G6PD deficiency
‡ Avoid clavulin after mid gestation *(neonatal necrotizing enterocolitis)*

A follow-up urine culture performed one week after completion of treatment shows successful eradication of the bacteria.[‡]

Thereafter, pregnancy progresses unremarkably until 28 weeks' gestation when the patient presents to the obstetric emergency assessment unit with home BP elevation to 140/84 mmHg, despite adherent use of nifedipine. The patient is asymptomatic and fetal cardiotocography monitoring is normal. Her fetal sonogram performed two days ago showed normal biometry, UA Doppler and amniotic fluid volume; fetal growth velocity is appropriate.

Urgent laboratory investigations are performed; your obstetric trainee tells you the following:

- Serum creatinine rose to 155 µmol/L (1.75 mg/dL)
- AST/ALT, platelets, random serum glucose are normal
- Uric acid is 360 µmol/L (1.75 mg/dL) [normal second-trimester value is 143–292 µmol/L; 2.4–4.9 mg/dL]
- Urine protein rose to 1.25 g/g

Her nephrologist has been informed and will attend to the patient shortly. Meanwhile, your trainee seems convinced the patient is developing preeclampsia/HELLP syndrome.

Special note:
‡ Consideration for continued prophylaxis against urinary tract infections after one episode in women with chronic renal disease on immunosuppressive agents

---

12. Indicate four <u>non-pregnancy</u>-related causes that may account for the acute rise in serum creatinine. *(1 point each)*   4

☐ Tacrolimus toxicity
☐ Prerenal (hypovolemic) acute kidney injury
☐ Acute pyelonephritis
☐ Obstruction, related to the transplant
☐ Renal allograft rejection

Special note:
Recurrence of patient's native renal disease, membranous nephropathy, is not likely

---

The patient is admitted for further investigations and monitoring. Serum tacrolimus level was supra-therapeutic; dose-adjustments made by her nephrologist restabilized serum creatinine at 122 µmol/L (1.38 mg/dL). Oral labetalol 200 mg twice daily was added to maintain BP <140/90 mmHg. After brief hospitalization, she is discharged on dual antihypertensive treatment and immunosuppressants; arrangements for clinical follow-up and serial investigations are made.

Although pleased that renal allograft rejection has not occurred, you find your obstetric trainee surfing the internet for clinical features and diagnosis of rejection.

13. Elicit clinical signs/symptoms that may raise concern of acute rejection in a pregnant renal allograft recipient. *(1 point each)*

Max 3

☐ Mostly asymptomatic presentation, detected upon routine investigations
☐ Fever
☐ Abdominal pain/graft tenderness
☐ Oliguria

14. Indicate the confirmatory test for renal allograft rejection, generally only performed in pregnancy when results will alter management.

1

☐ Ultrasound-guided renal biopsy *(unless clinically contraindicated)*

At 33 weeks' gestation, routine testing shows a rise in serum creatinine to 168 μmol/L (1.9 mg/dL) with proteinuria at 3.5 g/g. Her calcineurin inhibitor is therapeutic and hematologic and hepatic markers are stable. At presentation, her BP is 145/77 mmHg and she is asymptomatic; urine culture does not show recurrent infection. Comprehensive investigations performed in conjunction with her nephrologist, including kidney biopsy, reveal acute allograft rejection[§]; treatment will be started. Prophylactic low-dose aspirin has been discontinued. Fetal activity remains reassuring, cardiotocography (CTG) tracing is normal and the patient does not have obstetric complaints.

At hospitalization, the nephrologist adjusts the tacrolimus dose to target higher therapeutic levels and IV methylprednisolone once daily is started for five days, followed by oral prednisone 40 mg daily to be tapered over five to six weeks.

Special note:
§ Although hypertensives syndromes of pregnancy are more likely to manifest in this renal allograft patient relative to graft rejection, the presentation is as such for academic purposes; refer to Chapter 47 for clinical presentation of preeclampsia and challenges in diagnosis among patients with underlying renal insufficiency and hypertension

15. Considering the risks of corticosteroids, outline your counseling and management of potential <u>maternal</u> complications. *(1 point each)*

Max 4

☐ Inform the patient of the potential need to augment antihypertensive treatments
☐ Monitoring of glycemia and higher risks of GDM
☐ Offer psychosocial support services if psychiatric disturbances occur
☐ Beware of increased infectious complications, including vaginal candidiasis
☐ Discuss the risk of preterm prelabor rupture of membranes (PPROM)
  ○ *this may be considered a maternal or fetal complication of oral corticosteroids*

Special note:
*Refer to Chapter 45 for **fetal** effects of maternal corticosteroids*

The patient is discharged after one week of hospitalization; she responded well to empiric therapy for acute renal rejection and serum creatinine stabilized at 128 µmol/L (1.45 mg/dL). Apart from augmenting oral labetalol to 200 mg four-times daily and nifedipine to 30 mg twice daily, she has not experienced other side effects from corticosteroids. Fetal biometry, growth velocity, Doppler assessment, and amniotic fluid volume were normal prior to discharge.

At 36^{+1} weeks' gestation, obstetric sonography reveals footling breech presentation with biometry on the 9th percentile from prior 25th–30th percentile curves; amniotic fluid volume is also decreased for gestational age and UA Doppler shows intermittently absent end-diastolic velocity. Clinically, history is nonsuggestive of PPROM and she is otherwise asymptomatic. Fetal activity has been normal at home. Her BP is stable at 132/85 mmHg and she continues to take both oral antihypertensive agents and immunosuppressants and is tapering off prednisone every five days as instructed by her nephrologist. Urgent laboratory investigations confirm a normal platelet count and coagulation function. Fetal CTG monitoring shows recurrent variable decelerations and persistent minimal variability; there are no uterine contractions.

16. As you are a senior obstetric surgeon and maternal-fetal medicine expert, detail your   Max 10
    management of this patient. *(1 point per main bullet and subbullet)*

☐ Admission to the birthing center
☐ Maintain continuous electronic fetal monitoring
☐ Keep nil per os for anticipated Cesarean delivery
☐ Initiate judicious IV crystalloid hydration (close monitoring of urine output)
☐ Urgent multidisciplinary collaboration for Cesarean delivery *(i.e., nephrology, neonatology, anesthesiology, and allied medical professionals)*
☐ Counsel and consent the patient for Cesarean delivery given obstetric indications
☐ Consideration for reviewing the transplant operative report to anticipate location of the renal allograft and ureter, or locate using bedside sonography
☐ Consideration for blood product availability if bleeding is anticipated
☐ Continue immunosuppressant treatment intrapartum and postpartum, and titer antihypertensives

At planned Cesarean delivery:
☐ Steroid stress doses are required at Cesarean delivery *(based on the need for chronic oral steroid dose of ≥ 5 mg daily for more than three weeks)*[‡]
   ○ Continue her oral steroid dose, **and**
   ○ Give IV hydrocortisone 100 mg when starting anesthesia and 50–100 mg IV/IM at six hours postpartum
☐ Caution with low-transverse skin incisions; may consider vertical skin incision in view of possible pelvic location of renal allograft
☐ Recommend avoidance of developing a bladder flap *(risks injury to the transplanted ureter)*

Special note:
This patient does not require magnesium sulfate for fetal neuroprotection and has no indications for eclampsia prophylaxis; given urgent delivery, intramuscular corticosteroids for fetal lung maturity is not timely

‡ NICE 2019 Guidelines for Intrapartum Complex Care, National Guideline Alliance (UK). Intrapartum care for women with existing medical conditions or obstetric complications and their babies. London: National Institute for Health and Care Excellence (UK); 2019 Mar. PMID: 31194308.

A live male neonate weighing 2180 g is delivered by standard breech maneuvers at Cesarean section. The newborn is taken to the NICU for care. Surgery was uneventful with average blood loss.

Postpartum BP is maintained ≤130/85 mmHg with oral agents; analgesia and lower extremity edema are managed as standard for patients with renal dysfunction *(see Chapter 47, Questions 14 and 15)*. Prior to discharge, enalapril is restarted by her nephrologist given stable renal function *(see Chapter 47, Question 13)* and she has been reassured regarding breastfeeding with her anti-hypertensives, low-dose oral steroids, tacrolimus, and azathioprine *(see Chapters 38, 42, and 45)*.

Prior to discharge, you provide contraceptive counseling and recommendations related to chronic renal insufficiency *(see Chapter 47, Question 16)*.

You later receive a telephone call from a colleague in a remote center seeking your obstetric advice for the prenatal care of a 30-year-old renal transplant donor who remains healthy six years postdonation to her sister.

---

17. Provide your best practice recommendations for prenatal risks, *if any*, among pregnancies with history of renal transplant <u>donation</u>. *(1 point each)*   2

☐ Inform the colleague that renal donation is associated with increased risk of preeclampsia or gestational hypertension, although the absolute risk is small

☐ Suggest early prenatal prophylaxis *(e.g.,* LDASA) and close monitoring of clinical manifestations of preeclampsia

Special note:
No increased rates of low birthweight or preterm delivery (PTD) among renal donors

TOTAL: **100**

CHAPTER 47

Chronic Renal Insufficiency in Pregnancy

Tiina Podymow, Amira El-Messidi, and Michelle Hladunewich

A 33-year-old primigravida at eight weeks' gestation by dating sonography is referred by her primary care provider to your high-risk obstetrics unit for chronic kidney disease. She takes perindopril 8 mg daily. The patient does not have any obstetric complaints.

LEARNING OBJECTIVES

1. Demonstrate an understanding of the antenatal and postnatal effects on maternal renal function in the context of moderately severe chronic kidney disease (CKD), and provide detailed counseling on perinatal complications

2. Recognize that the significant association between CKD and preeclampsia warrants timely prophylaxis and that diagnosing preeclampsia may prove challenging among CKD patients with baseline, prepregnancy proteinuria and hypertension

3. Identify that deteriorating renal function near term may trigger delivery, with or without preeclampsia or blood pressure changes, although on its own, nephrotic range proteinuria >3 g/g typically does not necessitate delivery

4. Know the blood pressure targets in pregnancy complicated by CKD, and provide safe guidance on the use of angiotensin-converting enzyme inhibitors (ACEi) in women with compelling renal indications

5. Appreciate the importance of multidisciplinary collaboration in caring for the obstetric-CKD patient

SUGGESTED READINGS

1. Gonzalez Suarez ML, Kattah A, Grande JP, et al. Renal Disorders in Pregnancy: Core Curriculum 2019. *Am J Kidney Dis.* 2019;73(1):119–130. [Correction in Am J Kidney Dis. 2019 Jun;73(6):897]

2. Hladunewich MA, Melamed N, Bramham K. Pregnancy across the spectrum of chronic kidney disease. *Kidney Int.* 2016;89(5):995–1007

3. Hui D, Hladunewich MA. Chronic kidney disease and pregnancy. *Obstet Gynecol* 2019; 133: 1182–1194

4. Piccoli GB, Cabiddu G, Attini R, et al. Risk of Adverse Pregnancy Outcomes in Women with CKD. *J Am Soc Nephrol.* 2015 Aug;26(8):2011–2022.

5. Imbasciati E, Gregorini G, Cabiddu G, et al. Pregnancy in CKD stages 3 to 5: fetal and maternal outcomes. *Am J Kidney Dis.* 2007;49(6):753–762.

6. Jones DC, Hayslett JP. Outcome of pregnancy in women with moderate or severe renal insufficiency. *N Engl J Med.* 1996;335(4):226–232.

7. Wiles K, Chappell L, Clark K, et al. Clinical practice guideline on pregnancy and renal disease. *BMC Nephrol.* 2019;20(1):401.

	POINTS
1. With regard to CKD, which aspects of a focused history would you want to know? *(1 point per main bullet and subbullet)*	Max 20

General disease-related details:
- ☐ Ascertain the type of CKD based on renal biopsy
- ☐ Interval of time since initial diagnosis
- ☐ Names and contacts of treating nephrologist

Disease-related complications/comorbidities:
- ☐ Hypertension
  - ○ Determine the baseline/prepregnancy blood pressure (BP) and review her home recordings
  - ○ Current treatment, particularly current or recent use of ACEi/angiotensin receptor blocking agents
  - ○ Secondary end-organ dysfunction *(i.e., ocular, cardio-neurovascular)*
- ☐ Proteinuria
  - ○ Quantification of prepregnancy proteinuria *(i.e., urine protein/creatinine ratio)*
- ☐ Renal dysfunction
  - ○ Prepregnancy serum creatinine, and determine stability of renal function
  - ○ Elucidate treatment history, including use of corticosteroids or mycophenolate mofetil (MMF)
- ☐ Occurrence and frequency of urinary tract infections
- ☐ Presence of autoimmune diseases with renal manifestations *(e.g., diabetes or SLE)*
- ☐ Anemia (including current/prior treatments)

Presence of disease-related symptoms:
- ☐ Headaches
- ☐ Peripheral edema
- ☐ Gross hematuria (current or prior)

Pregnancy particularities related to CKD:
- ☐ Mode of conception *(i.e., spontaneous or assisted reproduction)*

Social factors and routine health maintenance:
- ☐ Smoking, alcohol consumption, recreational drug use
- ☐ Vaccination status *(e.g., influenza, hepatitis A and B, pneumococcus, tetanus)*
- ☐ Allergies

Family history:
- ☐ Renal disease
- ☐ Hypertension
- ☐ Diabetes mellitus
- ☐ Preeclampsia among first-degree relatives

You learn that eight years ago, the patient presented with edema and hypertension; she was also found to have microscopic hematuria and 5 g/g (equivalent to g/d) proteinuria. Following a renal biopsy and a diagnosis of IgA nephropathy, she was treated with prednisone for six months, which achieved partial remission. The patient has residual hypertension, proteinuria and renal dysfunction which are well controlled by the single-agent perindopril; she is not diabetic. Her home BP is 120/80 mmHg and she has no edema nor headaches; she does not experience gross hematuria nor urinary tract infections. The patient is adherent to her medications and nephrology follow-up. Renal investigations have been stable for the past five years and most prepregnancy results revealed the following:

		Normal
Serum creatinine	159.16 µmol/L (1.80 mg/dL)	46.86–61.01 µmol/L (0.53–0.69 mg/dL) **
Estimated GFR [eGFR]	40 ml/min	
Urine protein/creatinine ratio	1.5 g/g (1.5 g/24 hours equivalent)	<0.3 g/g
Urinalysis	Microscopic hematuria	

** *Harel Z, McArthur E, Hladunewich M, et al. Serum Creatinine Levels Before, During, and After Pregnancy. JAMA. 2019;321(2):205–207.*

After she and her husband of 10 years endured numerous years of subfertility and investigations, conception occurred spontaneously.

2. In teaching your obstetric trainee, <u>detail</u> four hormonal *or* physiological derangements possibly accounting for sub/infertility among women with nondialysis CKD.
   (1 point each)

4

- ☐ Absence of the lutenizing hormone surge
- ☐ Low levels of estradiol and progesterone
- ☐ Hyperprolactinemia
- ☐ Menstrual irregularities
- ☐ Sexual dysfunction

3. Explain the importance of sonographic pregnancy dating among women with chronic renal insufficiency.   2

☐ Serum β-hCG undergoes renal excretion; serum β-hCG tests may be falsely positive among women with advanced/end stage renal disease

4. With regard to her chronic renal insufficiency, which investigations would you consider at this first prenatal visit? *(1 point each)*   4

☐ Renal function: serum creatinine *(baseline and serial)*
☐ Baseline preeclampsia serum investigations
☐ Urinalysis and urine protein/creatinine or albumin/creatinine ratio *(baseline and serial)*
☐ Urine culture *(assess presence of asymptomatic bacteriuria and urinary tract infections)*

Special note:
renal imaging is NOT indicated

Test results demonstrate both an increased serum creatinine to 168 μmol/L (1.9 mg/dl), and urine protein/creatinine ratio to 2 g/g (equivalent to 2-g/24-hour collection), with urinalysis showing persistent 2+ microscopic hematuria. Urine culture is negative.

The patient's appointment with her nephrologist is in two days; you call him/her and learn that findings are relatively stable without indication of disease flare.

5. In collaboration with her nephrologist, provide counseling and management of the patient's ACEi agent. *(1 point each, unless specified)*   5

☐ Continuation of this patient's ACEi at least to conception for management of proteinuric renal disease would have been recommended in prepregnancy counseling
☐ Discontinuation of ACEi agents is required prior to 12 weeks' gestation
☐ First-trimester exposure is not associated with an increased risk of major malformations compared with other antihypertensive agents
☐ Exposure in later trimesters is associated with fetal abnormalities including *(1 point per subbullet; max 2)*
    ○ Renal dysgenesis
    ○ Potter's sequence
    ○ Hypocalvaria

6. Indicate the target blood pressure in prenatal care of patients with chronic renal insufficiency and specify directives for home monitoring, *if any. (1 point each)*

  Max 2

☐ Aim for BP ≤140/90 mmHg *(Safe outpatient antihypertensive agents include labetalol, methyldopa, nifedipine, and hydralazine in standard dosages)*
☐ Advise home BP monitoring for titration of medication
☐ Daily BP measurements are recommended at ≥20 weeks' gestation as a preeclampsia monitoring strategy *(patient should be aware to present to hospital if BP ≥160/110 mmHg)*

7. In general terms, outline anticipated changes in renal function among prenatal patients with chronic renal insufficiency, and indicate those pertaining to this patient. *(1 point per bullet)*

  Max 7

General changes in maternal renal function with CKD:
☐ Among women with renal insufficiency and normal baseline serum creatinine, pregnancy generally does not have an adverse effect on underlying renal disease
☐ The worse the pregestational renal insufficiency, the greater the risk of antenatal renal function deterioration
☐ Preconception preserved serum creatinine <123 μmol/L (<1.4 mg/dL) [stage 1 or 2 CKD] tends to remain stable in the antenatal and postnatal periods *(permanent decline in renal function is seen in 0%–10% of patients)*
☐ Among women with more advanced preconception serum creatinine >177 μmol/L (>2.90 mg/dL) [stage 4–5 CKD], ~65% experience renal function decline and ~20% require dialysis by the time of delivery (without postpartum recovery in renal function)

Projected changes in this patient's renal function:
☐ With her baseline serum creatinine between 123–168 μmol/L (1.4–1.9 mg/dL) [stage 3 CKD], the risk of antenatal renal function decline and permanent postpartum decline is ~40%–50%
☐ Having a baseline proteinuria >1 g/g increases her risk of renal function decline

Proteinuric change:
☐ May remain stable, or increase from baseline, by the end of pregnancy *(due to discontinuation of ACEi/angiotensin receptor blocking agents and hyperfiltration)*
☐ Increasing proteinuria does not tend to represent pathology, although significant increases require investigation

8. In addition to informing the patient of the effects of pregnancy on moderate renal dysfunction, address important aspects of obstetric counseling and management. *(1 point per main bullet)*

Maternal: *(Max 9 points)*
☐ Early initiation of multidisciplinary care, including planned delivery in a tertiary-care center and consultation with the neonatology team
☐ Inform the patient of increased risks of hypertensive disorders of pregnancy *(i.e., gestational hypertension, preeclampsia, HELLP syndrome)*
☐ Initiate prophylaxis with LDASA 150–162 mg nightly, started before 16 weeks and calcium supplementation *(if inadequate dietary intake or absorption)*
  ○ *Preeclampsia develops in 30%–40% of women with renal insufficiency and proteinuria*
  ○ *Risk of preeclampsia is magnified by chronic hypertension*
☐ Encourage early reporting of headache, peripheral edema, visual changes, or abdominal pain
☐ Risk of early pregnancy loss is increased
☐ Inform the patient of increased risk of spontaneous or iatrogenic preterm birth (PTB)
  ○ *>50% of women with moderate to advanced CKD*
☐ Early treatment of maternal anemia *(e.g., oral iron or erythropoietin supplementation)*
☐ Serial serum and urine investigations *(individualized frequency)*
☐ Discuss the lower threshold for elective hospitalizations due to complications related to renal insufficiency *(e.g., uncontrolled hypertension, suspected preeclampsia, deteriorating renal function anticipating delivery, or obstetric manifestations of maternal renal disease)*
☐ Plan for vaginal delivery at 37 weeks, if possible (Cesarean section is reserved for obstetric indications)

Fetal: *(Max 3 points)*
☐ Teratogenicity is related to treatment agents and timing of exposure, rather than to renal insufficiency itself
☐ Prematurity
☐ Fetal growth restriction (FGR) or suboptimal growth velocities; low birthweight (LBW)
☐ Plan serial obstetric ultrasounds for fetal growth, Doppler assessment, and amniotic fluid volume
☐ IUFD/neonatal mortality

The patient's ACEi is discontinued prior to 12 weeks' gestation, and methyldopa and nifedipine are initiated, with appropriate blood pressure control. She remains compliant with the planned antenatal protocol. Routine aneuploidy screening, fetal morphology scan, and serial obstetric imaging are normal. She has not developed gestational diabetes.

At 32^{+2} weeks' gestation, the patient reports to your emergency obstetric assessment unit with a one-day history of frontal headache, pedal edema and a recent home BP of 152/94 mmHg. Antihypertensive agents have been titrated during pregnancy and she now takes methyldopa

500 mg twice daily and nifedipine 30 mg daily. The patient reports fetal activity and has no obstetric complaints. Obstetric ultrasound performed three days ago showed fetal biometry on the 30th percentile, with normal umbilical artery Doppler and amniotic fluid volume.

Her initial BP at presentation to hospital was 154/96 mmHg, improving to 140/84 mmHg with receipt of an additional dose of nifedipine 30 mg; her headache resolved without further treatment. Routine cardiotocography (CTG) monitoring shows an appropriate fetal tracing without uterine activity.

Your trainee calls you with results of her current investigations:

- Serum creatinine is 177 μmol/L (2.0 mg/dl)
- Serum uric acid is 397 μmol/L (4.5 mg/dl) [*normal: 150–350 μmol/L; 1.7–4.0 mg/dL*]
- Urine protein is at 4 g/g (4 g/d equivalent)

Transaminases, CBC, LDH, and coagulation profile are within normal limits.

Your trainee suggests the patient has preterm preeclampsia, although he or she recognizes that worsening of baseline renal dysfunction and underlying proteinuria impose challenges in diagnosis.

---

9. Which principal elements related to diagnosis or management of superimposed preeclampsia with chronic renal insufficiency, should your trainee appreciate? (*1 point per main bullet, unless specified*)

Max 10

Blood pressure:
☐ Well-controlled (*or easy to control*) blood pressure is reassuring
☐ Uncontrolled BP or BP ≥160/110 mmHg serves as an important sign of preeclampsia

Serum investigations:
☐ Unique to preeclampsia, an increased sFLT-1/PlGF ratio or decreased PlGF adds diagnostic value for preeclampsia (*2 points*)
☐ Laboratory derangements including thrombocytopenia, abnormal transaminases, increased indirect bilirubin and hemolysis are suggestive of preeclampsia relative to worsening CKD alone
　○ Uric acid is commonly elevated with underlying renal dysfunction (*limited clinical utility in this population*)

Proteinuria:
☐ Isolated increasing proteinuria is **not** a trigger for delivery in the absence of fetal or maternal indications (*4 points*)

Symptoms:
☐ Neurologic and right upper quadrant abdominal pain are suggestive of preeclampsia syndromes (*2 points*)

10. After discussing the patient's clinical status with her nephrologist, outline your proposed plan of management. *(1 point each)*   Max 7

☐ Admission for close expectant management
☐ Assessment of BP parameters at least three times daily, titrating the selected antihypertensive agent(s) to target BP<140/90 mmHg
☐ At least daily serum laboratory testing of preeclampsia panel
☐ At least daily fetal monitoring (*e.g.,* electronic CTG monitoring)
☐ Individualized frequency of fetal ultrasound assessments
☐ Consideration for corticosteroids for fetal lung maturity
☐ Neonatology consultation, if not done prior
☐ Continued multidisciplinary care, including close collaboration with her nephrologist for monitoring of renal function and BP management

Special note:
Anticoagulation thromboprophylaxis (*e.g.,* LMWH) is not required for this patient; for consideration in patients with nephrotic syndrome when serum albumin is <30 g/L (3.0 g/dL)

The patient remains stable during the first two weeks of hospital admission; blood pressure is maintained with oral methyldopa 500 mg three times daily and nifedipine 30 mg twice daily until 34^{+2} weeks when additional labetalol 200 mg twice daily is required.

By 35^{+3} weeks' gestation, serial serum creatinine increased to 220 μmol/L (2.6 mg/dl) and urine protein is now 6 g/g (6 g/d equivalent). Liver function testing and platelets are normal. Blood pressure has now risen to 160/90 mmHg despite three agents. The patient complains of increasing pedal and leg edema, without headache, visual changes, epigastric pains, nor generalized unwellness. She noticed decreased frequency of urination over the past 36 hours. The CTG remains normal and obstetric sonography is unremarkable; the fetus is in the cephalic presentation.

11. In collaboration with her nephrologist, identify your next step in management of this patient?   1

☐ Counseling for induction of labor

Cervical ripening proceeds uneventfully and in labor, the patient receives an epidural and oxytocin augmentation. Despite three oral antihypertensives and adequate pain control, her intrapartum BP remains increased at ~158/105 mmHg. The patient is not bleeding and the CTG remains normal. She responds well to two doses of hydralazine 5 mg IV, given at a 20-minute interval.[†]

Special note:
† Among women with chronic renal insufficiency, there is no preferential antihypertensive agent to treat obstetric hypertensive emergencies (*for additional options, see Chapter 38*)

12. In initiating magnesium sulfate for eclampsia prophylaxis, specify your management particular to this patient with moderate renal dysfunction. *(1 point each)*	2

☐ Decreased magnesium sulfate bolus dose and slower hourly infusion rate is advisable (*e.g.,* 2 g IV bolus instead of 4 g, and 1 g/hr infusion rate)

☐ Serum magnesium levels should be followed *(in addition to the recommended clinical assessment for signs of magnesium toxicity among patients without underlying renal disease)*

At 35^{+4} weeks, the patient has an uncomplicated spontaneous delivery of a healthy preterm male neonate, admitted to the NICU for observation. She intends to breastfeed.

On day 1 postpartum, her blood pressure is 150/94 mmHg and serum creatinine decreased to 210 µmol/L (2.38 mg/dL). Shortly after the nephrologist's ward visit, the patient says she forgot to inquire about ways to decrease leg edema, which is a nuisance for her.

13. In collaboration with her nephrologist, outline the management steps involved in the peripartum care of this patient, with regard to blood pressure management and resumption of the ACEi with lactation. *(1 point per main bullet and subbullet)*	Max 4

☐ Discontinue IV magnesium sulfate prophylaxis at 24 hours postpartum

☐ Resume antepartum antihypertensive agents *(patient's three agents are safe with breastfeeding)*

☐ Target postpartum BP is ≤130/85 mmHg

☐ Consider resumption of an ACEi with a reassuring safety profile in breastfeeding once serum creatinine has stabilized[§]

 ○ Enalapril, captopril, and quinapril are the preferred ACEi in breastfeeding; all have been shown to be absent in breast milk *(collaboration with nephrologist is advised)*

Special note:

§ Angiotensin receptor blocking agents are not recommended in breastfeeding due to insufficient safety evidence

14. Provide therapeutic options for postpartum lower extremity edema among patients with chronic renal insufficiency. *(1 point each)*	3

☐ Compressive stockings

☐ Low salt diet

☐ Diuretic agent *(e.g., low dose oral or IV furosemide)*, can be considered if peripheral edema is prominent

15. Indicate a particularity, *if any*, in the postpartum analgesic care of patients with CKD.   5

☐ Nonsteroidal anti-inflammatories (NSAIDs) are contraindicated
  ○ *Opioids and acetaminophen/paracetamol are safe analgesic options*

Special note:
Indomethacin is similarly avoided in acute preterm labor, regardless of gestational age

By postpartum day 5, the patient is ready for discharge; on triple antihypertensive therapy. Her serum creatinine stabilized at 210 μmol/L (2.4 mg/dL) and low-dose oral enalapril 2.5 mg twice daily was prescribed. Leg edema diminished with two doses of a diuretic agent.[‡] Follow-up with her nephrologist is planned in 10 days.

Special note:
[‡] Monitor for electrolytes aberrations

16. With respect to chronic renal insufficiency, what are important elements to discuss   Max 7
with your patient prior to discharge and/or at the routine postpartum visit?
(1 point per main bullet)

Renal dysfunction and future care:
☐ Inform the patient that her serum creatinine at delivery-discharge signifies loss of renal function, which may be permanent
☐ Future preconceptional counseling is crucial given the strong likelihood of dialysis-dependency in subsequent pregnancy
☐ Encourage long-term follow-up with the nephrologist for management of CKD and BP control

Lactation:
☐ Reassure the patient regarding use of ACEi and her antihypertensive agents are safe *(i.e., methyldopa, nifedipine, labetalol)*

Contraceptive issues related to chronic renal insufficiency:
☐ Estrogen-containing contraceptives should be avoided in patients with hypertension, advanced CKD and proteinuria
☐ Depot medroxyprogesterone acetate (DMPA) is not recommended in women with low bone mineral density
  ○ *i.e., increased risk of osteopenia in patients with chronic renal insufficiency, on corticosteroids or calcineurin inhibitors*
☐ Progestin-only pill is safe, without restrictions in use, but must be taken at a consistent time daily for full effect
☐ Long-acting reversible contraceptives (LARCs) are safe, without restrictions in use
  ○ *i.e., IUDs (with or without levonorgestrel impregnation), or progesterone-only implant*
☐ Sterilization procedure for the patient or partner is suitable

TOTAL: 95

CHAPTER 48

Dialysis in Pregnancy

Tiina Podymow, Amira El-Messidi, and Michelle Hladunewich

A 33-year-old primigravida on thrice weekly hemodialysis while awaiting renal transplantation is referred by her nephrologist to your high-risk obstetric unit. Given irregular menstrual cycles, she did a home urine pregnancy test after three months of amenorrhea. Yesterday, she was pleasantly surprised with dating sonography confirming a single viable intrauterine fetus at 11^{+1} weeks' gestation. The request for consultation ensures that her nephrologist, nutritionist, and other allied members in dialysis care will follow her pregnancy with you.

LEARNING OBJECTIVES

1. Take a focused history for a prenatal patient on hemodialysis, and identify important investigations related to dialysis in pregnancy
2. Discuss noninvasive options and recognize caveats of fetal aneuploidy screening for particular tests in patients on chronic dialysis
3. Appreciate the importance of multidisciplinary collaboration in caring for the pregnant patient on long-term dialysis, recognizing essentials of medical management of dialysis
4. Provide detailed counseling and manage common obstetric complications among patients on long-term dialysis
5. Recognize and manage particularities in the intrapartum care of a preterm patient on dialysis with obstetric complications requiring prompt delivery

SUGGESTED READINGS

1. Cabiddu G, Castellino S, Gernone G, et al. Best practices on pregnancy on dialysis: the Italian Study Group on Kidney and Pregnancy. *J Nephrol.* 2015;28(3):279–288.
2. Hladunewich MA, Hou S, Odutayo A, et al. Intensive hemodialysis associates with improved pregnancy outcomes: a Canadian and United States cohort comparison. *J Am Soc Nephrol.* 2014;25(5):1103–1109.
3. Hoffman M, Sibai B. Dialysis in pregnancy: role of the underlying cause of renal failure on peripartum outcomes. *Am J Perinatol.* 2020;37(6):570–576.
4. Piccoli GB, Minelli F, Versino E, et al. Pregnancy in dialysis patients in the new millennium: a systematic review and meta-regression analysis correlating dialysis schedules and pregnancy outcomes. *Nephrol Dial Transplant.* 2016;31(11):1915–1934.

5. Tangren J, Nadel M, Hladunewich MA. Pregnancy and end-stage renal disease. *Blood Purif.* 2018;45(1–3):194–200.
6. Wiles K, Chappell L, Clark K, et al. Clinical practice guideline on pregnancy and renal disease. *BMC Nephrol.* 2019;20(1):401.
7. Wiles K, de Oliveira L. Dialysis in pregnancy. *Best Pract Res Clin Obstet Gynaecol.* 2019; 57:33–46.

	POINTS
1. With regard to hemodialysis, which aspects of a focused history would you want to know? *(1 point per main bullet, unless specified)*	Max 25

General disease-related details:

☐ Determine whether the underlying renal pathology is of primary renal origin or secondary systemic disease (*e.g., diabetes or SLE*)

☐ Anticipate genetic consultation depending on etiology of renal failure

☐ Duration of time on hemodialysis (*e.g., months, years*)

☐ Record names and contacts of treating team (*e.g., nephrologist, nutritionist, dialysis nurse*)

Disease-related complications/comorbidities:

☐ Renal dysfunction and treatment: *(1 point per subbullet)*
  ○ Urine output volume to assess residual renal function
  ○ Current dialysis intensity (hours/week)
  ○ Type of vascular access for dialysis and anticoagulant used
  ○ List of vitamin or mineral supplements with particular assessment of folic acid dose

☐ Frequency of urinary tract infections, if any

☐ Hypertension *(1 point per subbullet)*
  ○ Current/recent treatment, particularly ACEi/angiotensin receptor blocking agents (teratogenic), or nonpreferred antihypertensive agents during gestation (*e.g., atenolol*)
  ○ Average BP recordings on dialysis and at home
  ○ Secondary end-organ dysfunction (*i.e., ocular, cardio-neurovascular*)

☐ Anemia (including current/prior treatments)

Presence of disease-related symptoms:

☐ Headaches

☐ Peripheral edema

☐ Current symptoms of a urinary tract infection

Pertinent pregnancy symptoms:

☐ Nausea/vomiting

☐ Vaginal bleeding

☐ Abdominal cramps

Social factors and routine health maintenance:
- ☐ Supportive partner ± family
- ☐ Cigarette smoking, alcohol consumption, recreational drug use
- ☐ Dietary care, particularly to ascertain adequate daily antenatal protein intake with prenatal dialysis
- ☐ Vaccination status *(e.g., influenza, hepatitis A and B, pneumococcus, tetanus, COVID-19)*
- ☐ Allergies

Family history:
- ☐ Renal disease; relatives on dialysis
- ☐ Hypertension
- ☐ Preeclampsia among first-degree relatives

For the past three years, the patient has been on hemodialysis for hereditary nephritis. She has an arteriovenous fistula, maintained by tinzaparin. She informs you that upon confirmed conception, her nephrologist adjusted some medications and reassured her of the safety of other maintenance treatments. Recent treatment modifications made by her treating physician are being uploaded to your hospital's electronic system; meanwhile, you find the list of antecedent treatments among which include:

- perindopril 8 mg daily
- atenolol 50 mg daily
- amlodipine 10 mg daily
- darbopoetin injections *(erythropoiesis-stimulating agent)*
- calcitriol supplementation
- calcium carbonate and sevelamer *(phosphate binders)*
- dialysis multivitamins

The patient informs you her blood pressure (BP) is well controlled during dialysis; she does not monitor her home-BP. Despite recent light-headedness, she does not have headaches nor peripheral edema. Her urine output is ~500 mL/d, and she had one urinary tract infection since initiation of dialysis.

Since confirmation of pregnancy, the nutritionist increased her daily dietary protein intake as required among dialyzed pregnancies. The patient does not have any pregnancy-related symptoms or complications. She is in a monogamous relationship with her husband of 10 years; social history is otherwise unremarkable, vaccinations are up to date, and she has no allergies.

2. In reviewing recent investigations requested by her nephrologist, <u>detail</u> the most relevant   15
   baseline tests you would find in relation to dialysis in pregnancy. *(1 point each)*

Serum: (Note that there is no need to follow serial creatinine levels)
☐ CBC/FBC
☐ Sodium
☐ Potassium
☐ Calcium
☐ Albumin
☐ Phosphate
☐ Blood urea nitrogen
☐ Bicarbonate
☐ Random glucose
☐ Parathyroid hormone
☐ Hepatic markers (AST, ALT, LDH, GGT, bilirubin, INR)
☐ Iron studies *(ferritin, iron, total iron binding capacity, percent transferrin saturation)*

<u>Urine:</u> (Note that there may be no urine)
☐ Urinalysis
☐ Culture and sensitivity analyses
☐ Spot urine protein/creatinine or albumin/creatinine ratio (a baseline value may assist in
   the later diagnosis of preecclampsia)

<u>Special note:</u>
Renal imaging is not indicated

3. Which of the long-term treatment agents do you anticipate her nephrologist discontinued   3
   (or substituted) due to either fetal safety *or* decreased physiological need among dialyzed
   patients? *(1 point each)*

☐ Perindopril
☐ Atenolol
☐ Sevelamer

The patient brought her updated list of tablets; indeed, her nephrologist replaced perindopril and
atenolol for labetalol, and discontinued sevelamer. Your obstetric trainee recalls the teratogenic
effects of ACEi but is curious if management recommendations in this dialysis patient differ from
women with chronic kidney disease not requiring dialysis·[†]

<u>Special note:</u>
† *Refer to Chapter 47 for fetal risks ACEi agents*

4. Discuss the periconceptional management of ACEi in dialysis versus nondialysis patients. *(1 point each)*

2

☐ Dialysis patients may discontinue ACEi preconceptionally given only marginal benefit
☐ Nondialysis patients with chronic kidney disease and proteinuria may continue ACEi until pregnancy is confirmed (nephroprotection), so long as treatment is discontinued prior to 12 weeks' gestation

5. Address why atenolol and sevelamer were discontinued in pregnancy.

4

Atenolol: *(1 point each; max 3)*
☐ Low birthweight
☐ Neonatal bradycardia
☐ Neonatal hypoglycemia
☐ Not recommended in pregnancy or breastfeeding

Sevelamer: *(1 point for either bullet)*
☐ Irregular ossification of fetal bones (animal studies); although not contraindicated in humans
☐ Unnecessary treatment in pregnancy due to increased intensity of dialysis

Special note:
Amlodipine can be safely continued in pregnancy and breastfeeding; some experts prefer replacement for another calcium channel blocker (*e.g.,* nifedipine) with greater safety data

Although a desired pregnancy, the patient is interested in noninvasive tests for fetal aneuploidy screening, primarily to make necessary sociomedical arrangements prior to delivery, if necessary.

6. With regard to dialysis, elaborate on considerations for fetal aneuploidy screening. *(1 point per main bullet)*

3

☐ Noninvasive cfDNA (cell-free fetal DNA) tests are feasible, with risk of insufficient fetal fraction (*i.e.,* <4%) due to dialysis filtration
☐ Maternal age and first-trimester fetal ultrasound markers [*e.g.,* nuchal translucency (NT), nasal bone, tricuspid regurgitation, ductus venosus Doppler] are not impacted by dialysis
☐ First-trimester biomarkers (ß-hCG, PAPP-A) are unreliable in dialysis patients; results of integrated prenatal testing (IPS) should be interpreted with caution
    ○ Serum ß-hCG is inversely correlated with creatinine clearance
    ○ PAPP-A is higher due to end-stage renal disease and with anticoagulation to maintain patency of her dialysis port

7. In collaboration with her renal care team, discuss the essentials of <u>medical</u>   Max 12
    management for dialysis during this patient's antenatal period. *(1 point per main
    bullet, unless specified)*

Nutritional factors:
- ☐ Dialysis is an indication for higher-dose folic acid supplementation (5 mg/d) *(4 points)*
- ☐ Inform the patient to continue dialysis vitamins
- ☐ Vitamin D supplementation if parathyroid hormone levels are increased on serial monthly investigations
- ☐ Ensure daily protein intake of 1.5–1.8 mg/kg, in addition to 20 g daily for fetal development
- ☐ Allow unrestricted dietary phosphate intake, although may need supplementation in the dialysate
- ☐ Close monitoring of her dry weight

Dialysis care:
- ☐ Based on expert consensus, advise target BP <140/90 mmHg postdialysis
- ☐ Avoid intradialytic hypotension (*i.e.*, BP <120/70 mmHg) to maintain uteroplacental perfusion
- ☐ Inform the patient that increased frequency and/or duration of dialysis during pregnancy, ideally to 36 hours/week, improves maternal-fetal adverse outcomes
    - ○ *Maternal benefits:* BP control and nutritional care
    - ○ *Fetal benefits:* improved growth, amniotic fluid volume control, and gestational age at delivery
- ☐ Frequency/duration of dialysis is targeted to keep serum urea low, at ~10–16 mmol/L (28–45 mg/dL)
- ☐ Routine antenatal anticoagulation (*e.g.*, LMWH), primarily to maintain patency of her arteriovenous fistula
- ☐ Address the need to keep antenatal serum hemoglobin at 100–110 g/L (10–11 g/dL), usually with oral or weekly IV iron at dialysis and increasing erythropoietin/darbopoetin dosage
    - ○ Higher doses of erythropoietin stimulating agent is needed due to increased erythropoietin resistance in pregnancy and rise in intravascular volume
    - ○ Iron supplementation is crucial to accommodate increasing fetal demands
    - ○ Aim to avoid blood transfusions
- ☐ Electrolyte adjustments of the dialysis bath (by the nephrologist):
    - ○ Target bicarbonate ~30 mEq/L to avoid metabolic acidosis
    - ○ Target potassium at 3–4 mEq/L, adjusted to the serum levels
    - ○ Keep magnesium and calcium at ~1.5 mmol/L
- ☐ Low threshold for hospitalization for medical or obstetric complications

8. Discuss important aspects in counseling the pregnant dialysis patient with regard to obstetric risks and/or antenatal management. *(1 point per main bullet, unless specified)* — Max 11

□ Reassure the patient that dialysis or renal insufficiency is not teratogenic
  ○ *Teratogenicity is mostly related to treatment agents and timing of exposure*
□ Increased rates of early pregnancy loss
□ Risk of cervical incompetence is increased among pregnant women on dialysis **(additional 1 point per subbullet)**
  ○ Serial transvaginal cervical length assessments starting 16 weeks *(individualized frequency and duration)*
  ○ Consideration for cerclage and/or daily vaginal progesterone[‡]
□ Detailed second-trimester fetal morphology survey, with transvaginal cervical length
□ Risks of fetal growth restriction (FGR), suboptimal growth velocity, abnormal Doppler parameters and amniotic fluid volume derangements require serial obstetric sonography in the second and third trimesters (individualized frequency)
  ○ Polyhydramnios prompts an increase in dialysis dose <u>or</u> an increase in ultrafiltration volume (consider weekly amniotic fluid volume assessment starting 26 weeks)
□ Monitor for new or superimposed preeclampsia on chronic hypertension, or other hypertensive syndromes[§] **(additional 1 point per subbullet)**
  ○ Consider prophylactic LDASA150–162 mg nightly, started before 16 weeks' gestation *(no data on effectiveness in dialysis population)*
  ○ Recommend frequent CBC and hepatic markers starting 26 weeks' gestation (monitor for signs of HELLP syndrome; clinical presentation is confounded among dialyzed patients)
□ Prematurity is common, secondary to obstetric or medical complications among pregnant women on dialysis
□ Ideally, plan vaginal delivery in a tertiary center at ~37 weeks' gestation (Cesarean section is reserved for obstetric indications)
  ○ Avoid spontaneous labor as dialysis patients are routinely anticoagulated
□ NICU admission
□ IUFD/neonatal death

Special notes:
§ *Refer to* Chapter 8 for clinical/sonographic indications, and progesterone regimens
‡ *Refer to* Chapter 47, Question 9, on challenges and means to identify preeclampsia with underlying hypertension and renal disease

Attentive to your counseling, your obstetric trainee is curious about the mechanisms for polyhydramnios among dialyzed patients, and whether it differs from that with pregestational diabetes. He or she recalls that maternal or fetal hyperglycemia are believed to contribute to fetal polyuria among diabetic patients.

9. Explain the most likely mechanism for polyhydramnios among dialyzed patients *without* underlying diabetes. *(1 point each)*

☐ Increased blood urea nitrogen levels resulting in fetal diuresis (sonographic marker that may guide dialysis-intensity)
☐ Inadequate fluid ultrafiltration on dialysis

Max 1

10. If fetal growth and markers of well-being remain reassuring throughout gestation, and the patient delivers at term, justify your initial request for neonatology consultation.

☐ Neonatal osmotic diuresis may occur in the early postnatal period *(correlates with maternal urea level at delivery)*

3

First-trimester ultrasound reveals normal fetal morphology and aneuploidy markers; results of noninvasive cfDNA also show low risk for common aneuploidies. At 20 weeks' gestation, fetal morphology scan is normal, and the cervix is 28 mm long on transvaginal assessment. Her nephrologist has arranged for 36 hours/week of dialysis, and her pretreatment urea remains low, at a mean of 7 mmol/L (20 mg/dL).

At 22 weeks' gestation, transvaginal cervical length is 14 mm; there is a funnel without presence of sludge/biofilm. Viability is ascertained. The cervix is 2 cm dilated on pelvic examination. She is asymptomatic. You arrange for admission and the patient consents to Macdonald cerclage upon assuring absence of genitourinary infections.

At admission, your obstetric trainee signs the preprinted orders for cervical incompetence at previable gestations, admitted for planned rescue cerclage. Shortly thereafter, you are called by the patient's nurse.

11. With regard to management options prior to rescue cerclage, what do you anticipate is the nurse's concern with the signed preprinted admission protocol?

☐ Indomethacin administration *(generally considered to decrease amniotic fluid volume prior to surgery)* is <u>contraindicated</u> in this patient with chronic renal disease and hypertension

3

Special note:
Refer to Chapter 8

A Macdonald cerclage is placed without complications and the patient continues nightly vaginal progesterone, also avoiding sexual intercourse. The patient remains stable and the funnel resolves, possibly with dialysis-guided amniotic fluid control.

At 26 weeks' gestation, the patient presents to the obstetric emergency assessment unit with a frontal headache and home BP at 150/95 mmHg; she is otherwise asymptomatic and reports normal fetal activity. Her antihypertensive agents include methyldopa 250 mg twice daily and nifedipine 30 mg daily. Upon presentation, fetal cardiotocographic (CTG) monitoring is appropriate for gestational age; there are no uterine contractions on the CTG. With an additional dose of nifedipine 30 mg, her BP improves to 140/84 mmHg. Fetal biometry is on the 30th percentile with adequate growth velocity, normal umbilical artery (UA) Doppler and normal amniotic fluid volume. The patient is admitted for maternal and fetal monitoring. Her routine screening test for gestational diabetes (GDM) was normal last week.

The nephrologist will soon attend to the patient with you.

12. Identify which laboratory investigations are <u>unreliable</u> in identifying preeclampsia in a pregnant dialysis patient. *(1 point each)*

3

☐ Serum uric acid (increased in patients with renal dysfunction)
☐ Serum creatinine (due to removal by hemodialysis)
☐ Spot urine protein/creatinine ratio (patients may not have urine output)

Special note:
Refer to Chapter 47 for clinical factors and laboratory markers potentially useful in differentiating between preeclampsia vs. worsening of underlying renal disease and/or chronic hypertension

During the one-month course of admission, stepwise adjustments of her antihypertensive agents are required to maintain BP <140/90 mmHg, with continued collaboration from her nephrologist. The patient is maintained on three antihypertensive agents (methyldopa, nifedipine, and labetalol), and dialysis continues six days/week. She receives betamethasone for fetal lung maturity. Fetal monitoring is performed twice to thrice daily and CTG tracings remain normal; fetal growth scans are also unremarkable. Routine prenatal acellular pertussis vaccination is administered and vaginal-rectal GBS swab at admission was positive.

At 30^{+2} weeks' gestation, her nurse urgently notifies you that the patient's BP is 160/100 mmHg despite antihypertensive agents; the patient complains of scotomas and epigastric pain. She recently completed dialysis seven hours ago. Relative to her laboratory investigations 24 hours ago, her hepatic transaminases have doubled, and platelet count shows a relative decline from 260×10^9/L to 105×10^9/L, with recent serum anti-Xa concentration at 0.4 U/mL. Fetal CTG monitoring is normal; bedside sonography confirms persistent cephalic presentation.

13. What is your <u>next best step</u> in management of this patient?   1

☐ Induction of labor

---

14. After counseling and in collaboration with her nephrologist, the patient is transferred to   Max 7
the birthing center for acute care. Her BP remains increased. <u>Detail</u> the intrapartum steps
in management of this patient. *(1 point per main bullet)*

☐ Continuous electronic fetal monitoring
☐ Initiate standard management for obstetric hypertensive emergencies regardless of the
serum creatinine level
  ○ Preferred agents have rapid onset, short duration, and can be titrated
  ○ No preferential agent: Choices include hydralazine or labetalol IV, oral short-acting
  nifedipine[†]
☐ Magnesium sulfate for eclampsia prophylaxis and fetal neuroprotection *(i.e., 30 weeks'
gestation)* at a half-bolus dose and typically a lower (half-infusion rate) or <u>no</u> continuous
infusions among patients on dialysis, with close monitoring of serum levels and clinical
signs of toxicity
  ○ Maintain serum magnesium levels at 4–7 mEq/L or 5–9 mg/dL
  ○ Magnesium toxicity is treated by urgent dialysis *(contrary to standard calcium gluconate
  antidote treatment)*
☐ Early anesthesiology consultation, particularly with recent anticoagulant administrations
☐ Protamine sulfate by slow IV infusion may partially reverse LMWH (~60%)
  ○ Give protamine sulfate 1 mg for every 100 anti-factor Xa units of tinzaparin; maximum
  single dose is 50 mg
☐ Ensure neonatology team is available at delivery
☐ Removal of the Macdonald cerclage; mode of induction depends on obstetrical assessment
☐ Penicillin G IV for her positive GBS vaginal-rectal swab within the past five weeks
  ○ This patient on hemodialysis may receive standard intrapartum dosing:[‡] *(i.e., penicillin
  G 5 million units IV initial dose, then 2.5 million units IV every four hours until delivery)*
☐ Anticipate risk of postpartum hemorrhage (PPH) if only partial reversal of anticoagulation
is achieved

Special notes:
† *Refer to* Question 33 in Chapter 38 for treatment regimens
‡ For hemodialysis patients, antibiotic dosing generally requires close monitoring of
pharmacologic response, signs of adverse reactions, and possible assessment of drug
concentrations in relation to trough

The patient has an uncomplicated spontaneous vaginal delivery of a healthy preterm neonate. At
two hours postpartum, her BP is 150/94 mmHg.

15. With respect to her dialysis and associated comorbidities, what are important postpartum considerations in the management of this patient prior to discharge? *(1 point per main bullet)*   Max 7

General maternal-fetal well-being:
- [ ] Screen for postpartum depression, especially given complicated antenatal course and chronic disease, and continue to offer psychosocial support services
- [ ] Reassure the patient that breastfeeding is safe with dialysis

Dialysis-related care:
- [ ] Arrange for close outpatient follow-up with her nephrologist for management of chronic kidney disease and comorbidities
- [ ] Postpartum, she may resume her regular three-times-weekly dialysis schedule, although extra sessions may be necessary to manage edema
- [ ] Target postpartum BP is $\leq$130/85 mmHg
- [ ] Continue her oral antihypertensives during the postpartum period *(dose-adjustments as necessary)*
- [ ] In collaboration with her nephrologist, reinitiate an ACEi
  - *e.g.,* enalapril, captopril, and quinapril have reassuring lactation-safety profiles
- [ ] Transplant reassessment, as pregnancy is a sensitizing event that may impact renal transplantations

Contraception: *(individualized discussion)*
- [ ] Safe and effective reversible options include progestin-only pill, IUDs (with or without levonorgestrel impregnation), and implants
- [ ] Estrogen-containing contraceptives should be avoided in patients with advanced CKD, hypertension, and proteinuria
- [ ] Depot medroxyprogesterone acetate (DMPA) impacts bone health (not recommended in this patient)

TOTAL: **100**

SECTION 8

Connective Tissue Disorders in Pregnancy

Systemic Lupus Erythematosus and Antiphospholipid Antibody Syndrome in Pregnancy

Oseme Etomi and Catherine Nelson-Piercy

A 28-year-old nulligravida is referred by her primary care provider to your high-risk obstetrics clinic for preconception counseling for known systemic lupus erythematosus (SLE).

Special note: Although pregnant women with SLE have increased rates of concomitant medical and obstetric morbidities, including but not limited to hypertension, diabetes, mental health issues, fetal growth restriction, preterm labor, and therapeutics common to other conditions, the case scenario avoids overlap of content addressed in other chapters. Readers are encouraged to complement subject matter where clinically required.

LEARNING OBJECTIVES

1. Take a focused history from a patient with SLE, recognizing features and risk factors that can affect maternal-fetal outcome
2. Appreciate the effects of pregnancy on SLE-associated complications and effects of disease activity on obstetric risk
3. Understand essentials of therapeutic management for SLE during pregnancy and breastfeeding
4. Demonstrate an approach to investigating potential SLE flares in pregnancy
5. Plan and manage antepartum, intrapartum, and postpartum care of a patient with SLE, recognizing the importance of continued multidisciplinary collaboration

SUGGESTED READINGS

1. Andreoli L, Bertsias GK, Agmon-Levin N, et al. EULAR recommendations for women's health and the management of family planning, assisted reproduction, pregnancy and menopause in patients with systemic lupus erythematosus and/or antiphospholipid syndrome. *Ann Rheum Dis.* 2017;76(3):476–485.
2. Do SC, Druzin ML. Systemic lupus erythematosus in pregnancy: high risk, high reward. *Curr Opin Obstet Gynecol.* 2019;31(2):120–126.
3. Flint J, Panchal S, Hurrell A, et al. BSR and BHPR guideline on prescribing drugs in pregnancy and breastfeeding-Part I: standard and biologic disease modifying anti-rheumatic drugs and corticosteroids. *Rheumatology (Oxford).* 2016;55(9):1693–1697.
4. Giles I, Yee CS, Gordon C. Stratifying management of rheumatic disease for pregnancy and breastfeeding. *Nat Rev Rheumatol.* 2019;15(7):391–402.
5. Knight CL, Nelson-Piercy C. Management of systemic lupus erythematosus during pregnancy: challenges and solutions. *Open Access Rheumatol.* 2017;9:37–53.

6. Lazzaroni MG, Dall'Ara F, Fredi M, et al. A comprehensive review of the clinical approach to pregnancy and systemic lupus erythematosus. *J Autoimmun.* 2016;74:106–117.

7. Nahal SK, Selmi C, Gershwin ME. Safety issues and recommendations for successful pregnancy outcome in systemic lupus erythematosus. *J Autoimmun.* 2018;93:16–23.

8. *Nelson-Piercy's Handbook of Obstetric Medicine*, 6th ed. London: Taylor and Francis; 2020.

9. Petri M. Pregnancy and systemic lupus erythematosus. *Best Pract Res Clin Obstet Gynaecol.* 2020;64:24–30.

10. Sammaritano LR, Bermas BL, Chakravarty EE, et al. 2020 American College of Rheumatology guideline for the management of reproductive health in rheumatic and musculoskeletal diseases. *Arthritis Rheumatol.* 2020;72(4):529–556.

POINTS

1. With regard to SLE, which aspects of a focused history would you want to know?   Max 30
   (1 point per main bullet unless specified; points indicated per section)

General disease-related details:
(5 points)
☐ Age at diagnosis or disease duration
☐ Inquire how diagnosis was established
☐ Time-interval since the last flare, frequency of flares and known triggers (*e.g., ultraviolet light for skin flares*)
☐ Determine the patient's common symptoms/pattern of flares, where relevant
☐ Name and contact of treating rheumatologist

Current/prior SLE-associated clinical manifestations:
(max 4 points)
☐ *Dermatologic:* alopecia, malar rash, discoid rash, photosensitivity
☐ *Neurologic:* seizures, psychosis
☐ *Oral:* Painless ulcers in the oral or nasopharyngeal cavity
☐ *Hematologic:* hemolytic anemia, leukopenia [$<4 \times 10^9$/L], lymphopenia [$<1.5 \times 10^9$/L], thrombocytopenia [$<100 \times 10^9$/L]
☐ *Cardiopulmonary:* pulmonary arterial hypertension, pleuritis, pericarditis
☐ *Renal:* lupus nephritis, proteinuria, cellular casts
☐ *Musculoskeletal:* nonerosive arthritis

SLE-associated immunologic features[§§]:
(2 points for each of first 3 bullets; max 7)
(Known to the patient, or inquire about test results, if available)
☐ Anti-Ro and anti-La antibody status
☐ Antiphospholipid antibodies *[lupus anticoagulant, anticardiolipin antibodies, anti-ß2 glycoprotein-I antibodies]*
☐ Complement levels (*i.e.,* C3, C4)
☐ Anti-double-stranded DNA (dsDNA)

Disease-related comorbidities:
(4 points)
☐ Current/prior venous thromboembolism
☐ Chronic hypertension
☐ Chronic renal disease

☐ Other autoimmune diseases (*e.g., type* 1 *diabetes mellitus, hypothyroidism/antithyroid antibodies, immune thrombocytopenic purpura [ITP]*)

Gynecologic features most relevant to SLE ± immunosuppressive treatment:
(max 3 points)
☐ Inquire about potentially undisclosed early pregnancy losses
☐ Current contraceptive method, if any
☐ Menstrual cycle regularity/last menstrual period
  ○ *Lupus nephritis, disease-associated end-stage renal disease, or certain pharmacologic agents may cause amenorrhea*
☐ Inquire about cervical cytology screening and/or human papillomavirus (HPV) immunization
  ○ *Women with SLE have higher risk of cervical dysplasia (though not cervical cancer), vaginal and vulvar cancers, likely associated with HPV infection (EULAR recommendations[1])*
  ○ *Increased vigilance for cervical dysplasia with exposure to immunosuppressive drugs*

Current/prior pharmacologic agents used in treatment of SLE, clinical response and side effects:
(3 points)
☐ **Therapies generally <u>not</u> compatible with pregnancy:** mycophenolate mofetil (MMF)[†], warfarin[††], methotrexate[°], cyclophosphamide[#], leflunomide
☐ **Therapies compatible with pregnancy:** hydroxychloroquine, corticosteroids[§], tacrolimus[§], azathioprine[°], cyclosporin A, nonsteroidal anti-inflammatory agents (NSAIDs) *[limited to <32 weeks' gestation]*
☐ Allergies

Social features and routine health maintenance:
(2 points)
☐ Smoking, alcohol consumption, or recreational drugs
☐ Vaccination status (*e.g.*, pneumococcus, meningococcus, influenza, COVID-19)
  ○ *Live viral vaccines are avoided with immunosuppressant treatment and in pregnancy*

Family history:
(2 points)
☐ SLE or other autoimmune morbidities
☐ Antiphospholipid syndrome

Special notes:
§§ Antinuclear antibody (ANA) and anti-Smith antibodies are part of the laboratory diagnostic criteria for SLE, but would not contribute to preconception counseling
† *Refer to* Question 4 in Chapter 46 for discussion on pregnancy recommendations and fetal risks associated with MMF
†† *Refer to* Questions 5 and 6 in Chapter 31
° *Refer to* Question 2 in Chapter 42 for discussion on fetal/neonatal risks and pregnancy recommendations with methotrexate and azathioprine therapies
Refer to Question 10 in Chapter 70 and Question 18 in Chapter 73 for antenatal considerations for therapeutic treatment with cyclophosphamide
§ *Refer to* Question 3 in Chapter 45 for fetal risks of tacrolimus and prednisone; refer to Question 15 in Chapter 46 for discussion of maternal risks of prednisone

You learn that the patient was diagnosed five years ago when she presented with lethargy, arthralgias, hair loss, and a photosensitive rash, accompanied by hematologic derangements and immunologic markers including increased ANA and anti-dsDNA titers, as well as hypocomplementemia. She shares with you results of investigations appropriately confirming diagnostic confirmation of triple positive antiphospholipid antibodies for which she remains asymptomatic *(i.e., meets laboratory criteria but not clinical antiphospholipid syndrome)*, as well as recently positive anti-Ro/La status, with markedly high anti-Ro titers.[†] The patient does not have any comorbid medical diseases.

She developed lupus nephritis three years ago, for which she received a short course of oral prednisolone and MMF; disease was well controlled on MMF thereafter. As her rheumatologist advised reliable contraception, she used the levonorgesterol intrauterine system (LNG-IUS) and male condoms. In anticipation of a desired pregnancy, MMF was substituted for a disease-modifying antirheumatic drug compatible with pregnancy; meanwhile, LNG-IUS was maintained for a six-week overlap period. She currently relies on the male condom and indicates her menstrual cycles are regular.

Her last nonrenal SLE flare, involving the joints and skin, was eight months ago. The patient maintains a healthy lifestyle and is in a monogamous relationship with her husband of four years. Her vaccinations are up to date. She does not drink alcohol, smoke, or use recreational drugs. There are no drug allergies. Family history is noncontributory.

On examination, her body habitus, blood pressure and pulse are normal.

Special note:
† The greater the anti-Ro titers, the greater the risk of heart block *(Suggested Reading 9)*

2. With respect to SLE disease and in collaboration with her rheumatologist, which <u>additional investigations</u> would contribute to preconception counseling of this patient? *(1 point each)*	Max 7

Imaging:[†]
☐ Echocardiogram

Serum:[§]
☐ Full/complete blood count (FBC/CBC)
☐ Erythrocyte sedimentation rate and C-reactive protein
☐ Creatinine
☐ Bilirubin and INR *(liver function tests)*
☐ AST, ALT, GGT *(liver transaminases)*
☐ Consideration for HbA1c *(with prolonged steroid use or other risk factors)*
☐ Consideration for 25-hydroxy-vitamin D levels *(with prolonged steroid use or other risk factors)*

Urine:
☐ Random protein/creatinine ratio
☐ Urinalysis with urine sediment

Special notes:

† Chest X-ray, pulmonary function testing, or chest CT scan would be considered with a history of respiratory involvement

§ There is no indication to repeat this patient's positive anti-Ro/La or antiphospholipid antibodies *(American College of Rheumatology Guideline[10])*

---

3. Inform the patient of potential fetal/neonatal risks of anti-Ro/La antibodies, while teaching your trainee of underlying pathophysiology. *(1 point each)*

Max 4

Neonatal lupus syndrome:

☐ Congenital heart block *(primary incidence is ~2%)[†]*

☐ Neonatal cutaneous lupus syndrome *(primary incidence is ~5%)[†]*

☐ Hepatic and hematologic disease (rare)

Pathophysiology:

Congenital heart block

☐ Placental active transport of maternal autoantibodies results in endomyocardial fibrosis, calcification, and macrophage/giant cells infiltration of the atrioventricular node, destroying the Purkinje system and resulting in a fixed fetal bradycardia of 60–80 bpm most commonly at 16–28 weeks

Neonatal cutaneous lupus syndrome

☐ Maternal autoantibodies persisting in the neonate for up to six months of age may cause temporary inflammatory lesions on the face and scalp, typically provoked by ultraviolet exposure within two weeks of life, resolving spontaneously and without consequences

Special note:

† Rarely do both conditions occur in the same fetus/neonate

---

4. For academic interest,[†] provide a biological rationale explaining to your trainee why <u>most</u> fetuses of mothers with anti-Ro/La antibodies <u>do not</u> manifest congenital heart block.

4

☐ Anti-Ro exists in two molecular sizes (52 kDa and 60 kDa) with the former [smaller molecule] being capable of transplacental transfer

    ○ *Anti-La itself rarely causes heart block*

Special note:

† Distinguishing anti-Ro subtypes is not routinely performed in the clinical setting at this time

5. Address the adverse <u>obstetric</u> outcomes associated with the patient's high-risk antiphospholipid antibody profile, namely triple positivity,[†] that you may discuss in patient counseling. *(1 point each)*

Max 4

Maternal:
- ☐ (Pre)-eclampsia/HELLP syndrome
- ☐ Arterial and/or venous thromboembolism
- ☐ Recurrent early pregnancy loss <10 weeks' gestation

Fetal-placental:[‡]
- ☐ Fetal growth restriction (FGR) or low birthweight
- ☐ Placental abruption
- ☐ Intrauterine fetal demise (IUFD)/stillbirth of a morphologically normal fetus at ≥10 weeks' gestation

Special notes:
- † High-risk autoantibody profile also includes moderate-high titers or lupus anticoagulant in particular
- ‡ Risk of preterm prelabor rupture of membranes (PPROM) is associated with SLE disease, and not the presence of antiphospholipid antibodies

6. Outline additional <u>maternal</u> risks of SLE disease not addressed above. *(1 point each)*

Max 3

- ☐ Disease flares, mostly in the second half of pregnancy and postpartum
- ☐ Gestational diabetes mellitus, especially with need for prednisone ≥10 mg daily
- ☐ Preterm birth
- ☐ Emergency Cesarean delivery
- ☐ Infections *(related to immunosuppression)*
- ☐ Blood transfusions
- ☐ Mortality *(e.g., mostly due to active lupus or secondary infections)*

The patient shares results of recently completed tests, showing inactive disease in the various organ systems, namely with urine protein/creatinine ratio <50 mg/mmol and normal renal function *(EULAR recommendations[1])* Although her rheumatologist discussed the safety of azathioprine° in pregnancy, and she understands the importance of continued antenatal therapy, the patient inquires about potential adjunctive pharmacologic treatment that may modify disease-associated adverse outcomes. She informed you that her rheumatologist also counseled her to initiate folate-containing prenatal vitamins, minimize (and where possible, discontinue) preconception NSAID use.

Special note:
° Refer to Question 2 in Chapter 42 for discussion on fetal/neonatal risks and pregnancy recommendations with azathioprine

7. Highlight to your obstetric trainee the fundamental investigation performed by the rheumatologist to ensure substitution of MMF for azathioprine is safe.   1

☐ Testing to ensure normal TPMT *(thiopurine methyltransferase)* enzyme activity for drug metabolism; low enzyme levels can result in fatal myelosuppression

Special note:
This question serves to reinforce the learning point provided in the clinical description after Question 1 in Chapter 42

8. Explain to your obstetric trainee the biological rationale for considering discontinuation of NSAIDs in the periconception period.   2

☐ Inhibition of cyclooxygenase-dependent ovulation can result in infertility due to development of 'luteinized unruptured follicle syndrome'

9. In addition to continued azathioprine therapy in a future pregnancy, address the patient's inquiry regarding the role of adjunctive pharmacologic agents in modifying SLE and/or autoantibody-associated morbidity.   Max 7
    (1 point per main bullet, unless indicated; max points specified where relevant)

Hydroxychloroquine: *(max 4 points)*
☐ Initiation of hydroxychloroquine 400 mg[††] daily either prepregnancy or as soon as possible <16 weeks' gestation and continued throughout the antenatal period for its multiple benefits and favorable features: ***(additional point per subbullet)***
    ○ *(a)* reduced risk of SLE flares
    ○ *(b)* decreased occurrence/recurrence of congenital heart block
    ○ *(c)* reduced risk of thrombosis from antiphospholipid antibodies
    ○ *(d)* apparent decreased risk of preterm birth and preeclampsia
    ○ *(e)* no increased risk of congenital anomalies or adverse obstetric outcomes

Preeclampsia prophylaxis:[†]
☐ Nightly LDASA started prior to 16 weeks' gestation is recommended for preeclampsia prophylaxis[†] based on presence of SLE disease or positive antiphospholipid antibodies
    ○ *LDASA dose recommendations of 75–162 mg varies by international jurisdiction*
☐ Calcium supplementation 1.2–2.5 g elemental calcium per day in women with low calcium intake (*i.e.,* Less than 600–800 mg/d or fewer than four servings per day)
    ○ *Calcium supplementation is recommended by the ISSHP and SOGC guidelines, however, ACOG does not endorse calcium supplementation for preeclampsia prophylaxis (refer to Chapter 38)*

Heparin or low molecular weight heparin (LMWH):
☐ Inform the patient that while heparin or LMWH is ***not*** generally required for positive antiphospholipid antibodies only, individualized considerations may depend on her triple positivity status or in the presence of a strongly positive lupus anticoagulant result[$]

○ *Prophylactic and therapeutic heparin/LMWH would be advocated with obstetric and thrombotic antiphospholipid syndrome, respectively*

Adjunctive treatment:

☐ Daily vitamin D 1000 IU is recommended during the antenatal period and until end of lactation for women with SLE[#] *(routine prenatal vitamins generally contain only vitamin D 400–600 IU)*

Special notes:

†† Dose reductions may be needed with renal impairment; beware of retinal toxicity with doses >5 mg/kg

† Autoimmune disease is a major risk factor warranting LDASA for preeclampsia prophylaxis; refer to Questions 6 and 11 in Chapter 38

§ Need for artificial reproductive technology may also impact clinical decision-making for LMWH prophylaxis in the context of positive antiphospholipid antibodies alone

\# Fischer-Betz R, Specker C. Pregnancy in systemic lupus erythematosus and antiphospholipid syndrome. *Best Pract Res Clin Rheumatol.* 2017;31(3):397–414.

Your obstetric trainee recalls learning of several drugs associated with a lupus-like syndrome, manifested by antihistone antibody positivity. Reassuringly, you highlight that such agents do not provoke SLE flares among women with known disease.

10. List three etiologies for <u>drug-induced lupus</u> among patients <u>not</u> affected by SLE.   Max 3
    (1 point each)

☐ Alpha-methyldopa
☐ Diltiazem
☐ Hydralazine
☐ Isoniazid
☐ Minocycline
☐ Phenytoin
☐ Phentoin
☐ Procainamide
☐ Quinidine

The patient understands that while her obstetric care will require multidisciplinary collaboration in a high-risk unit given known lupus nephritis and autoantibodies-associated risks, not all pregnant women having SLE are considered to have a 'high-risk' pregnancy.[†] She appreciates your evidence-based counseling and intends to comply with the designated pharmacologic management.

Special note:

† Refer to Cauldwell M, Nelson-Piercy C. Maternal and fetal complications of systemic lupus erythematosus. *The Obstetrician and Gynaecologist* 2012;14:167–174.

11. Complementary to pharmacologic treatment, provide additional important elements of your preconception counseling and outline the antenatal care plan in collaboration with the rheumatologist/obstetric medicine physician.   Max 8
(1 point per main bullet; max points specified per section)

Maternal: *(max 4)*

☐ Reassure the patient that quiescent disease, including stable lupus nephritis, for more than six months are important for favorable obstetric outcomes

☐ Inform the patient that pregnancy does not seem to endanger long-term renal function where baseline creatinine is within normal after prior lupus nephritis *(the higher the baseline creatinine, the greater the risk of deterioration)*

☐ Where SLE is stable, plan (at least) monthly clinical visits up to 28 weeks, bimonthly until 34 weeks, and weekly thereafter, to document presence or absence of flare or preeclampsia symptoms, blood pressure control, presence of significant proteinuria *(see 'Fetal' section below)*

☐ Arrange routine laboratory assessment of disease activity at least once per trimester
    ○ *i.e.,* CBC/FBC, creatinine, urinalysis and assessment of urinary sediment, and random urine protein/creatinine ratio, dsDNA[§] and complement levels[§]

☐ Inform the patient that more frequent assessments with/without hospitalization will depend on disease activity or onset of comorbidities

☐ Counsel the patient that route of delivery is based on obstetric indications (*i.e.,* aim for vaginal delivery)

☐ Individualized considerations for consultation with affiliated health care providers (*e.g.,* anesthesiologist, neonatologist, perinatal mental health experts)

Fetal: *(max 4)*

☐ Inform the patient that her offspring has a lifetime estimate of 3% for developing SLE[†]

☐ Plan routine ultrasonographic screening in the first and second trimesters (with maternal uterine artery Doppler)

☐ Arrange for fetal echocardiogram as of ~16–18 weeks' gestation *(anti-Ro/La positivity)*
    ○ *Serial assessments from 16 weeks to 26–32 weeks without history of prior heart block*
    ○ *Weekly assessments if prior obstetric history of heart block*
    ○ *Congenital heart block rarely occurs after 26–28 weeks; fetal heart rate auscultation remains warranted*

☐ Where initial fetal echocardiogram is normal, arrange for fetal heart rate auscultation every one to two weeks (between gestational weeks 20–28) in the antenatal clinic for detection of heart block

☐ Monthly fetal sonographic surveillance in the second and third trimesters (*e.g.,* growth biometry, amniotic fluid volume, and fetal Doppler interrogation where required[‡])
    ○ *Individualized considerations in the third trimester for additional fetal monitoring, such as nonstress tests or biophysical profile*

Special notes:

§ SLE can be serologically active yet clinically quiescent; consideration for close monitoring for risk of flares

† Kuo CF, Grainge MJ, Valdes AM, et al. Familial Aggregation of Systemic Lupus Erythematosus and Coaggregation of Autoimmune Diseases in Affected Families. *JAMA Intern Med.* 2015;175(9):1518–1526.

‡ Refer to Chapter 9

12. Alert your trainee about SLE-associated morbidities where conception or continuation   Max 8
    of pregnancy may pose heightened risks to maternal well-being, thereby advising
    postponement or avoidance of pregnancy would be contemplated. *(1 point each)*

Postponement of pregnancy:
☐ Severe SLE flare within the past six months *(e.g., lupus nephritis, cerebritis, pneumonitis)*
☐ Current need for prednisone ≥10 mg daily to achieve disease control
☐ Need for treatment with teratogenic agent(s) for disease control
☐ Uncontrolled hypertension

Preferred avoidance of pregnancy:
☐ Pulmonary hypertension
☐ Moderate-severe heart failure *(i.e.,* left ventricular ejection fraction <40%)
☐ Severe valvulopathy
☐ Severe restrictive lung disease (forced vital capacity <1 L or <50% predicted)/alveolar
  damage
☐ Stage 4 or 5 chronic renal disease
☐ Stroke within the past six months

Special note:
Although not relevant to this case scenario, (a) prior severe early-onset (<28 weeks)
preeclampsia-HELLP syndrome despite both aspirin and heparin therapy, and (b)
antiphospholipid syndrome with prior thrombosis while on anticoagulation would also
warrant careful consideration prior to future pregnancy

SCENARIO A
SLE with laboratory evidence of antiphospholipid antibodies only
By four months after this consultation, the patient conceives spontaneously. She remained in
remission at conception, well controlled on azathioprine and hydroxychloroquine. In view of
SLE-associated morbidities, you follow her antenatal care as a high-risk obstetrician, according
to the established antenatal care plan and in collaboration with her rheumatologist/obstetric
medicine physician.

13. Elaborate on <u>physiologic changes of pregnancy</u> that may pose challenges in assessment   7
    of SLE disease activity. *(1 point each)*

Clinical: *(max 4)*
☐ Fatigue/lethargy
☐ Physiologic dyspnea
☐ Palpitations
☐ Malar and palmar erythema; chloasma

- ☐ Neuropathies
- ☐ Mild arthralgia
- ☐ Mild edema
- ☐ Telogen effluvium *(postpartum hair loss)*

Laboratory: *(max 3)*
- ☐ Hypercoagulability *(increases prothrombotic risk)*
- ☐ Gestational anemia and thrombocytopenia
- ☐ Increased intravascular volume *(may worsen cardiac or renal function)*
- ☐ Increased glomerular filtration rate *(increases proteinuria)*
- ☐ Increased maternal-fetal calcium demands *(may impact presence or risk of osteoporosis)*
- ☐ Increased erythrocyte sedimentation rate up to 70 mm/hr
- ☐ Increased complement concentrations *(a fall in levels may be clinically important, despite within 'normal' ranges)*

Maternal-fetal progress remains unremarkable until a follow-up fetal echocardiogram at 20 weeks' gestation reveals a second-degree heart block. Fetal biometry, morphology, and amniotic fluid volume are normal.

14. Document the treatment recommended by the fetal cardiologist, recognizing that benefit of this therapy remains unproven.[†]

1

- ☐ Initiate maternal dexamethasone 4 mg daily *(for first- or second-degree heart block[‡])*

Special notes:
[†] Contrary to proven benefit of hydroxychloroquine *(see Question 9 above)* in prevention of primary or recurrent congenital heart block among patients with anti-Ro/La antibodies
[‡] Dexamethasone is not recommended for third-degree (complete) heart block

At the 26-weeks' gestation clinical visit, the patient reports a 10-day history of increasing early morning stiffness lasting one hour, hair loss, oral ulcers, generalized body aches and pains, and a low-grade fever ~37.7°C orally. She also noticed new-onset headaches and upper abdominal discomfort, without aggravating or alleviating factors. The patient has remained adherent to her medical treatment plan and serial laboratory investigations have been unremarkable to date. She has no other medical or obstetric complaints and fetal activity has been normal.

The patient converses well and does not appear in acute distress. A low-grade fever is confirmed, blood pressure is 140/90 mmHg, pulse is 103 bpm, and fetal viability is ascertained. A rheumatologist/obstetric medicine physician will attend shortly to assist you in the care of the patient.

15. In affiliation with the medical expert, outline comprehensive <u>maternal investigations</u>   18
to address your differential diagnosis. *(1 point each)*

Serum:[‡]
- ☐ CBC/FBC
- ☐ C-reactive protein *(suggestive feature of infection)*
- ☐ Ferritin and iron studies
- ☐ AST, ALT
- ☐ Lactate dehydrogenase (LDH)
- ☐ Urate or uric acid *(controversial)*
- ☐ Complement C3, C4, CH50 levels
- ☐ dsDNA
- ☐ sFlt-1/PlGF ratio
- ☐ Blood cultures[†]
- ☐ Troponin and brain natriuretic peptide [BNP] *(i.e., useful surrogate markers of cardiac involvement)*

Urine:
- ☐ Urinalysis and assessment for sediment
- ☐ Random protein/creatinine ratio
- ☐ Urine culture[†]

Imaging:
- ☐ Electrocardiogram (ECG)
- ☐ Chest X-ray

Other:
- ☐ Blood film *(i.e., signs of hemolysis)*
- ☐ Other screening tests for infections *(e.g., H. influenza, CMV, Epstein-Barr virus)*[†]

Special notes:
[†] Complete septic work-up should always be performed for suspected lupus flares due to greater risk of infectious morbidity and mortality
[‡] Although erythrocyte sedimentation rate is increased in pregnancy due to hepatic production of fibrinogen, the *trend* in erythrocyte sedimentation rate relative to baseline may be valuable

---

16. Among the investigations performed, highlight the <u>laboratory derangements</u>[†] that would   Max 4
be most characteristic of a lupus flare over preeclampsia. *(1 point each)*

- ☐ Decrease in baseline complement levels by ≥25%[‡]
- ☐ Increased dsDNA titers *(marker of lupus nephritis)*
- ☐ Leukopenia, lymphopenia

☐ Normal hepatic transaminases

☐ Active urinary sediment/red cell casts

☐ Hematuria

Special notes:

† Renal biopsy is the only confirmatory investigation to differentiate a flare of lupus nephritis from preeclampsia; procedural morbidity makes it an option of last resort, when clinical management will depend on results of tissue sampling

‡ Absolute values may remain within normal limits due to natural increases in hepatic production during pregnancy

With laboratory investigations being compatible with a lupus flare, the patient is counseled regarding initiation of corticosteroids.† Monitoring for maternal-fetal risks of prednisone treatment, including risk of gestational diabetes mellitus (GDM), is arranged and a gradual weaning period is planned over six weeks. Azathioprine, as tolerated, is increased by the rheumatologist/ obstetric medicine physician to a maximum of 2.5 mg/kg/d.

By 33 weeks' gestation, the patient has discontinued corticosteroids, without associated complications. Her blood pressure spontaneously normalized relative to the initial presentation at 26 weeks' gestation. Fetal echocardiographic findings remain stable, for which dexamethasone is continued until delivery.

Special note:

† Refer to Question 3 in Chapter 45 and Question 15 in Chapter 46 for discussion on fetal and maternal aspects of counseling with regard to maternal use of corticosteroids; refer to Questions 14 and 16 in respective chapters for management of stress doses in vaginal and Cesarean delivery, respectively

17. Discuss the planned timing and mode of delivery for <u>this</u> patient, assuming an unremarkable late third trimester.

    1

☐ Plan a term elective Cesarean section given fetal heart block due to inability to reliably monitor fetal cardiotocography in labor

18. After an uncomplicated Cesarean section at term, what are important postpartum considerations to discuss, either prior to discharge or at the routine postpartum visit in relation to SLE disease?

General maternal-fetal well-being: *(1 point each; 3 points)*
☐ Screen for postpartum depression and continue to offer psychosocial support services
☐ Inform the patient of the ~16%–18% recurrence rate of congenital heart block given a previously affected child
☐ Encourage repeat future preconception counseling *(i.e., fewer maternal-fetal complications and higher pregnancy success rates)*

Thromboprophylaxis: *(1 point)*
☐ Consideration for pharmacologic prophylaxis *(i.e., LMWH)* for seven days[$] given antiphospholipid antibodies and operative delivery, in the absence of indications for longer postpartum administration

SLE disease control and breastfeeding recommendations: *(1 point per main and subbullet; 5 points)*
☐ Reassure her of the safety of azathioprine, hydroxychloroquine, LMWH (or coumadin where needed) with breastfeeding
☐ Inform the patient that resumption of NSAIDs treatment for flare symptoms is safe while breastfeeding, provided absence of renal impairment
☐ Encourage reporting of flare symptoms, that may appear particularly in first four months postpartum *(Suggested Reading 4)*
☐ Ensure arrangements are made for maternal outpatient follow-up in the rheumatologist/ obstetric medicine clinic at four to six weeks postpartum *(case-based interval)* to detect and manage any lupus complications and ensure appropriate return to rheumatology outpatient care
  ○ Plan interval laboratory testing postpartum *(i.e., CBC/FBC, creatinine, urea/electrolytes, liver function tests and transaminases, complement levels, anti-dsDNA titer, erythrocyte sedimentation rate, C-reactive protein)*

Contraceptive recommendations: *(1 point per main bullet; max 3)*
☐ Inform the patient that in view of known antiphospholipid antibodies, all guidance recommendations advise against use of estrogen-containing contraceptives due to increased risk of thrombosis
  ○ *Estrogen-containing contraceptives may be deemed safe in the absence of antiphospholipid antibodies (category 2), moderate-severe active SLE [including lupus nephritis], or other associated morbidity obviating use of combined hormonal contraception*
☐ Copper intrauterine device is safe in the presence of antiphospholipid antibodies and while on immunosuppressive therapy; exercise caution in the presence of severe thrombocytopenia with SLE disease
☐ No restrictions on use of barrier methods although they are the least effective agents; reinforce that unintended pregnancy may post an increased health risk with known SLE
☐ International guidance recommendations[†] vary with regard to progesterone-based contraceptives *(i.e., DMPA, LNG-IUS, progestin implants, and progestin-oral contraceptives); consultation with local practice recommendations is advised*

☐ Options for emergency contraception are available to patients with SLE regardless of antiphospholipid antibody status

Special notes:

§ Royal College of Gynaecologists, Reducing the risk of venous thromboembolism during pregnancy and the puerperium, Green-Top Guideline No. 37a (2015)

† UK and US Medical Eligibility Criteria (MEC) for Contraceptive Use, 2016; UK-MEC amended September 2019, US-MEC updated 2020

SCENARIO B

This is a continuation of the clinical scenario after Question 12

SLE with antiphospholipid syndrome

By four months after this consultation, the patient conceives spontaneously. She remained in remission at conception, well controlled on azathioprine, hydroxychloroquine and low dose aspirin. In view of SLE-associated morbidities, you follow her antenatal care as a high-risk obstetrician, according to the established antenatal care plan and in collaboration with her rheumatologist/obstetric medicine physician.

Maternal-fetal progress remains unremarkable based on the established care plan at preconception consultation; fetal morphology sonogram and echocardiogram appeared normal. At 28 weeks' gestation, fetal growth biometry starts to demonstrate suboptimal growth velocity with onset of FGR and abnormal umbilical artery Doppler parameters by 32 weeks' gestation.† Concurrently, the patient develops symptoms and laboratory manifestations of preeclampsia, clearly distinguished from a lupus flare. Delivery is necessary at 33^{+3} weeks' gestation for obstetric indications.

Special note:

† Refer to Chapter 9

19. Provide critical aspects of counseling and subsequent management recommendations, most specific to her obstetric complications. *(1 point per main bullet)*

Max 3

Counseling:

☐ Inform the patient of confirmation of obstetric antiphospholipid syndrome; future risk of thrombotic or catastrophic antiphospholipid syndrome warrants close follow-up

Management recommendations:

☐ Postpartum prophylactic-dose heparin (usually LMWH) is recommended for six weeks' duration for obstetric antiphospholipid syndrome

☐ In future pregnancy, both LDASA and prophylactic-dose anticoagulation are recommended throughout pregnancy and for six weeks postpartum
  ○ *LMWH is started upon confirmation of a viable intrauterine pregnancy (Suggested Reading 8)*

☐ Maintain treatment with hydroxychloroquine during the antenatal period to reduce risks of adverse pregnancy outcomes

20. In teaching your obstetric trainee, elaborate on the diagnostic features that would   3
constitute 'catastrophic antiphospholipid syndrome' with known antiphospholipid
antibodies. *(1 point each)*

☐ Small vessel thromboses in three or more organs within seven days
☐ Exclusion of other causations for thromboses, such as thrombotic thrombocytopenic
purpura (TTP)
☐ Histological confirmation (*i.e.*, biopsy) of at least one vascular occlusion

TOTAL: **130**

CHAPTER 50

Marfan Syndrome in Pregnancy

Marwa Salman

A 28-year-old nulligravida with Marfan syndrome is referred to your tertiary center's high-risk obstetric unit for preconceptional counseling. She has no other medical issues.

LEARNING OBJECTIVES

1. Take a focused history in the preconception assessment of a patient with Marfan syndrome, and be able to identify disease-related characteristics where pregnancy may not be recommended
2. Understand the genetic basis of Marfan syndrome, and address prenatal testing options among spontaneous conceptions
3. Demonstrate the ability to plan and manage the antepartum, intrapartum, and postpartum care of a Marfan syndrome patient, recognizing the importance of a pregnancy heart team
4. Maintain a raised suspicion for aortic dissection in the postpartum period

SUGGESTED READINGS

1. Boodhwani M, Andelfinger G, Leipsic J, et al. Canadian Cardiovascular Society position statement on the management of thoracic aortic disease. *Can J Cardiol.* 2014;30(6):577–589.
2. Curry RA, Gelson E, Swan L, et al. Marfan syndrome and pregnancy: maternal and neonatal outcomes. *BJOG.* 2014;121(5):610–617.
3. Goland S, Elkayam U. Pregnancy and Marfan syndrome. *Ann Cardiothoracic Surg* 2017; 6: 642–653.
4. Hiratzka LF, Bakris GL, Beckman JA, et al. 2010 ACCF/AHA/AATS/ACR/ASA/SCA/SCAI/ SIR/STS/SVM Guidelines for the diagnosis and management of patients with thoracic aortic disease: Executive summary: A report of the American College of Cardiology Foundation/ American Heart Association Task Force on Practice Guidelines, American Association for Thoracic Surgery, American College of Radiology, American Stroke Association, Society of Cardiovascular Anesthesiologists, Society for Cardiovascular Angiography and Interventions, Society of Interventional Radiology, Society of Thoracic Surgeons, and Society for Vascular Medicine. *Anesth Analg.* 2010;111(2):279–315.
5. Lim JCE, Cauldwell M, Patel RR, et al. Management of Marfan syndrome during pregnancy: a real world experience from a Joint Cardiac Obstetric Service. *Int J Cardiol.* 2017; 243:180–184.

6. Monteiro R, Salman M, Montiero S, et al. (eds.). Aortic dissection. Chapter 96 in *Analgesia, Anaesthesia and Pregnancy*. Cambridge: Cambridge University Press; 2019.

7. Naud K, Horne G, Van den Hof M. A woman with Marfan syndrome in pregnancy: managing high vascular risk with multidisciplinary care. *J Obstet Gynaecol Can.* 2015; 37(8):724–727.

8. Prendes C, Mani K. Pregnancy and aortic dissection. Eur J Vas Endovas Surg; in press.

9. Regitz-Zagrosek V, Roos-Hesselink JW, Bauersachs J, et al. 2018 ESC Guidelines for the management of cardiovascular diseases during pregnancy. *Eur Heart J.* 2018; 39(34): 3165–3241.

10. van Hagen IM, Roos-Hesselink JW. Aorta pathology and pregnancy. *Best Pract Res Clin Obstet Gynaecol.* 2014; 28(4):537–550.

POINTS

1. With regard to Marfan syndrome, which aspects on history would you want to know?   Max 20
   (1 point per main bullet)

Cardiac symptoms and manifestations:
☐ Functional status assessment to determine her NYHA classification
☐ Most recent aortic root dilation and rate of growth
☐ Prior aortic aneurysm, rupture, or dissection
☐ Aortic regurgitation
☐ Mitral valve prolapse
☐ Arrhythmias
☐ Hypertension
☐ Congestive heart failure

Noncardiac comorbidity:
☐ Prior spontaneous pneumothorax
☐ Dural ectasia
☐ Scoliosis
☐ Lens dislocations

Surgical history:
☐ Prior aortic root replacement or repair of aortic dissection
   ○ *Risk of dissection remains despite aortic root replacement or repaired aortic dissection*

Medications and contraception:
☐ ß-blocker agent
☐ Angiotensin-receptor blocker (losartan)
☐ Current method of contraception (*if any*)

Social features and routine health maintenance:
☐ Cigarette smoking, chronic alcohol consumption, and illicit drug use
☐ Dietary habits, weight control
☐ Exercise habits

Family history:
☐ Aortic dissection or other inherited cardiac conditions
☐ Identified disease-causing mutation of the *FBN 1* gene in the patient or family members

The patient tolerates ordinary physical activity without shortness of breath or angina. Apart from hypermobile joints and one incident of lens dislocation, she has not experienced major morbidity related to her connective tissue condition. Last year, her echocardiogram showed moderate enlargement of the aortic root diameter at 41 mm, which has remained stable for three years, without valvular regurgitation nor arrhythmia. She takes oral metoprolol and losartan daily as prophylaxis to reduce the rate of aortic dilation.

The patient has had a copper-IUD for four years, and now wishes to remove it in anticipation of a planned pregnancy. Menstrual cycles are regular, and she has not priorly tried to conceive. Remaining compliant with her medical care, she mentions occasional use of the male condom for dual contraception. She does not smoke, drink, and has a healthy lifestyle.

Her brother and father have Marfan syndrome, neither of whom have experienced an aortic dissection. Her father underwent aortic root replacement at the age of 34 years for dilation, and he remains well for over 20 years. There is no family history of sudden death.

2. Which baseline, preconceptional diagnostic imaging would be performed by her cardiologist and rheumatologist? *(1 point per bullet, unless specified)*	Max 6

☐ Baseline transthoracic echocardiogram *(2 points)*
☐ CT/MRI of the entire aorta *(2 points)*
☐ Cardiac MRI
☐ Cardiopulmonary exercise testing
☐ Lumbar spine MRI or ultrasound *(identify ductal ectasia/scoliosis)*

3. With respect to her stated noncardiac manifestations of Marfan syndrome, which additional investigation might be considered in the preconceptional period?	1

☐ Slit light examination *(for ectopia lentis)*

As you were recommending baseline investigations prior to providing clearance and counseling for conception, the patient shares with you reports of tests she recently completed. You read her cardiologist's note specifying persistent mWHO (modified WHO) Class III with an unchanged aortic root dilation at 41 mm; no other significant findings on imaging modalities are noted and her exercise testing is normal. Her rheumatologist reassured her that the dural ectasia detected on lumbar MRI is common to Marfan patients (90%), for which anesthesiologists should be informed.

4. Discuss important elements of your preconceptional counseling and evidence-based <u>antenatal</u> management with respect to Marfan syndrome. *(1 point per main bullet)*   Max 22

Genetics aspects:
☐ Inform patient of autosomal dominant inheritance
☐ Prenatal testing (CVS or amniocentesis) is feasible with a known mutation in the *FBN 1* gene
☐ Discuss potential alternatives to pregnancy *(i.e., adoption, surrogacy, gestational carrier)*
☐ Offer genetic counseling

Management of her medications:
☐ Advise continuation of ß-blocker throughout pregnancy
☐ Recommend discontinuation of the angiotensin receptor blocking agent, either prior to conception or once pregnant

Maternal cardiac risks and management:
☐ Strict blood pressure (BP) control is recommended (<140/90 mmHg)
☐ Encourage continued avoidance of smoking and alcohol consumption
☐ Maintain healthy body weight and dietary habits
☐ Educate the patient on symptoms of aortic dissection:
  ○ *Severe abrupt chest or back pain, described as tearing, stabbing or sharp pain*
☐ Inform the patient that the risk for aortic dissection (1%–10%) is dependent on aortic size
  ○ *Women with Marfan syndrome whose aortic root is <40 mm still have an approximate 1% risk of aortic dissection*
  ○ *Dissection occurs most often in the last trimester (50%) or early postpartum period (33%)*
☐ Discuss the controversial effect of pregnancy on aortic dilation, ranging from no significant growth to reported growth ≥3 mm, with partial postpartum improvement
☐ Mention risks of new-onset arrhythmias, mitral regurgitation, or heart failure
☐ Maternal echocardiography every 4–12 weeks throughout pregnancy and six months postpartum in women with ascending aortic dilation *(monitoring interval is individualized)*
☐ Consideration for natriuretic peptide levels at ~20 weeks' gestation
  ○ *N-terminal pro-BNP >128 pg/mL may be predictive of events in later pregnancy*
☐ Multidisciplinary care by a 'pregnancy heart team' *(introduced by European Society of Cardiology 2018 – Suggested Reading 9)*
  ○ *Essential consultants include a cardiologist, obstetrician, and anesthesiologist; additional experts' involvement is case based*
☐ Frequent clinical visits and low threshold for hospital admission
☐ Delivery in a tertiary center with access to cardiac surgery and a NICU

Obstetric risks and management:
☐ Early spontaneous pregnancy loss
☐ FGR: *Serial fetal growth biometry in the second and third trimesters*
☐ Cervical insufficiency: *Consideration of sonographic cervical assessment*
☐ PPROM *(maternal connective tissue laxity)* and PTD
☐ Rare neonatal risks associated with maternal use of a ß-blocker: *Consideration for 48-hour postnatal monitoring for neonatal bradycardia, hypoglycemia, or respiratory depression*
☐ Neonatal mortality
☐ Neonatology consultation is required when fetal viability is reached

The patient appreciates your counseling and wishes to comply with management recommendations by the pregnancy heart team. Recognizing her cardiac risk may change during the course of pregnancy, with updated assessment required at each prenatal visit, she is eager to know when she would require cardiac surgery during pregnancy.

---

5. Address the patient's inquiry regarding the indications for cardiac surgery during   3
    pregnancy. *(1 point per main bullet)*

    ☐ Aorta diameter becomes >45 mm
    ☐ Rapidly increasing aortic diameter
    ☐ Stanford type A aortic dissection *(surgical emergency during pregnancy)*
      ○ *Dissection of the ascending, arch and descending aorta*

    Special note:
    Conservative treatment is recommended for uncomplicated Stanford type B aortic dissection in pregnancy *(i.e., arch and descending)*, with strict BP control

---

After the consultation visit, you inform your trainee of the existing variations among societal recommendations for elective aortic repair prior to conception.

---

6. Outline situations where pregnancy would not be recommended prior to considering   1
    aortic root replacement in Marfan syndrome. *(1 point for any societal recommendation,*
    depending upon jurisdiction)

    ESC Guidelines 2018:
    ☐ Pregnancy is contraindicated with an aortic root diameter >45 mm *(mWHO Class IV)*
    ☐ Pregnancy is contraindicated with current or prior aortic dissection
    ☐ Elective repair should be considered with an aortic root diameter at 40–45 mm, in
      consideration with factors including:
      ○ Family history of dissection
      ○ Rate of aortic growth (>5 mm/year)

    Canadian Cardiovascular Society 2014:
    ☐ Pregnancy is contraindicated with an ascending aorta >45 mm *(relatively contraindicated*
      if >40 mm)
    ☐ Elective repair is recommended with an aortic root diameter at 41– 45 mm
      (preconception)

    ACC/AHA/AATS 2010:
    ☐ Elective repair is reasonable with an aortic diameter >40 mm (preconception)

You trainee recalls your mentioning that pregnancy has a variable effect on the progression of aortic disease, although does not comprehend the basis for this.

7. Identify one physiological mechanism by which pregnancy may contribute to further aortic dilation.

1

☐ Hemodynamic stress and increased blood volume
☐ Hormonal factors leading to structural changes in the aortic wall

The patient subsequently starts prenatal vitamins, has her IUD removed, and performs monthly urine pregnancy tests. She conceives a singleton within four months. As arranged by her cardiologist, losartan has been discontinued, maintaining metoprolol treatment during pregnancy. Blood pressure is well controlled without additional therapy.

As a high-risk obstetrician with expertise in managing women with heart disease, you follow her antenatal care, with the established management as outlined preconceptionally. The patient remains stable throughout her antenatal course, and aortic root diameter is unchanged from 41 mm. She does not experience obstetric morbidity.

At 35^{+6} weeks' gestation, fetal biometry is on the 15% percentile with maintained growth velocity, amniotic fluid volume and UA Doppler velocimetry. Although you previously reviewed her intrapartum care, she is wondering if planned timing of delivery is required.

8. With focus on this patient's connective tissue condition and cardiac status, detail your counseling and management of her <u>intrapartum</u> care. *(1 point per main bullet)*

Max 6

☐ Vaginal delivery is feasible with an aortic diameter of 40–45 mm, although elective Cesarean delivery may also be considered *(ESC 2018)*[‡]
  ○ *Cesarean delivery is recommended (possibly preterm) with aortic diameter >45 mm, progressive dilation during pregnancy, prior aortic dissection, or with very poor left ventricular function*
☐ Induction of labour should be considered by 40 weeks in women with cardiac disease *(ESC 2018)*[§]
  ○ *Options include mechanical means, misoprostol (prostaglandin E1), or dinoprostone (prostaglandin E2); judicious use of fluid balance with IV oxytocin is suggested*
☐ Continuous cardiotocography monitoring
☐ Labor in the lateral decubitus position *(avoids aortocaval compression)*
☐ Considerations for delayed pushing in the second stage of labor
☐ Elective assisted vaginal delivery *(with an ascending aortic diameter at 40–45 mm)*
☐ If Cesarean section is required or planned, retention sutures *(i.e., deep tension sutures)* should be considered
☐ Anesthesiologist assessment given the patient's dural sac dilation (risk of inadequate regional analgesia and dural puncture)
  ○ *Ideally, initial consultation earlier in pregnancy is preferred*
  ○ *In the absence of dural ectasia, early epidural is recommended primarily to avoid BP spikes that can induce dissection*
☐ Invasive monitoring during labor and delivery may be required
☐ Continue ß-blocker agent peripartum

Special notes:

‡ Consideration for Cesarean delivery with an aortic diameter >40 mm *(Canadian Society for Cardiology 2014)*

§ No cardiac indication for antibiotic prophylaxis unless prior valve replacement or endocarditis

Spontaneous labor occurs at 36^{+2} weeks' gestation. Close monitoring of the mother and fetus occurs in a cardiac setting and all required multidisciplinary members are involved during the labor and delivery process. With informed consent, a healthy newborn is delivered by an elective vacuum-assisted vaginal delivery. As arranged, neonatal monitoring for 48 hours is performed given preceding maternal ß-blockade.

9. What are important <u>postpartum</u> considerations for this patient? *(1 point per bullet)*   Max 8

☐ Ensure available equipment in case of postpartum hemorrhage (PPH)

☐ Slow IV oxytocin infusion (2 U over 10 minutes immediately after delivery), followed by 12 mU/min for four hours *(ESC 2018)*

☐ **Avoid** ergometrine for treatment of PPH in women with aortic disease

☐ Active management of the third stage of labor; maintain careful cord traction to avoid inherent risk of uterine inversion *(tissue laxity)*

☐ Maternal cardiac monitoring for 24–48 hours postpartum *(physiologic hemodynamic changes may precipitate heart failure)*

☐ Consideration for maternal echocardiography prior to discharge; regular assessment thereafter until six months postpartum

☐ Continued oral ß-blockade therapy, and strict BP control (<140/90 mmHg)

☐ Robust follow-up arrangements upon discharge *(given high risk of dissection postpartum)*

☐ Encourage early ambulation

☐ Breastfeeding is encouraged with metoprolol treatment

Two weeks postpartum, the patient presents to obstetric emergency unit with acute shortness of breath and a two-hour history of sharp chest pain radiating to her upper back. Her BP is 185/111 mmHg. Chest X-ray shows the following:

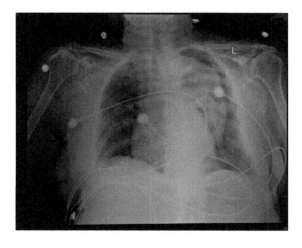

Figure 50.1

Image retrieved from: http://health-fts.blogspot.com/2012/01/aortic-dissection.html.

There is no association between this case scenario and this patient's image. Image used for educational purposes only.

10. Considering your most probable diagnosis, indicate five clinical signs that may be elicited in this patient. *(1 point each)*

☐ Unequal pulses
☐ Systolic BP limb differential >20 mmHg
☐ Focal neuropathy
☐ Murmur suggesting aortic regurgitation
☐ Syncope

5

11. What is the most likely diagnosis?

☐ Aortic dissection

1

Until arrival of the cardiac surgeons, the emergency room team and anesthesiologist on-duty assist you in stabilizing the patient. Intravenous labetalol drip is started to achieve tight control of her BP and reduce sheer stress; analgesia is also administered.

12. In addition to routine hematology and biochemistry investigations, indicate four other required diagnostic tests in the work-up of this patient. *(1 point each)*

☐ Transthoracic echocardiography
☐ CT angiography
☐ ECG
☐ Serum troponin
☐ Serum D-dimers

Max 4

Investigations show a large aortic dissection and the patient is promptly taken for emergency surgery. Meanwhile, you ensure her husband is informed of the situation and arrange for support services.

The patient survives surgery and does well in the recovery period.

Now 10 weeks postpartum, she presents to see you for her postpartum visit.

13. What are the most important <u>obstetric aspects</u> to discuss during this postpartum visit? *(1 point per main bullet)*

☐ Pregnancy is <u>not</u> recommended given history of aortic dissection
  ○ If conception occurs, discussion of early termination is warranted
  ○ With continued pregnancy, Cesarean delivery should be considered
☐ Reliable, safe contraception is strongly recommended *(combined hormonal contraception is contraindicated)*

2

TOTAL: 80

Hematologic Conditions in Pregnancy

CHAPTER 51

Sickle Cell Anemia in Pregnancy

Amira El-Messidi and Alan D. Cameron

A 29-year-old primigravida with sickle cell anemia (SCA) is referred by her primary care provider to your tertiary center's high-risk obstetrics unit for prenatal care of a sonographically confirmed single viable intrauterine pregnancy at 8^{+2} weeks' gestation. She has no obstetric complaints.

LEARNING OBJECTIVES

1. Take a focused prenatal history from a patient with SCA, recognizing fundamental aspects of inherited hemoglobinopathies and providing appropriate counseling and management
2. Discuss the effects of pregnancy on SCA-related complications as well as the effects of disease on obstetric risks
3. Appreciate the importance of timely and adequate analgesia for acute pain episodes, including other antenatal management considerations
4. Understand indications and risks of transfusion protocols for the obstetric patient with SCA
5. Demonstrate the ability to manage antepartum, intrapartum, and postpartum care of a patient with SCA to optimize outcomes, recognizing the importance of continued multidisciplinary care

SUGGESTED READINGS

1. ACOG Committee on Obstetrics. ACOG Practice Bulletin No. 78: hemoglobinopathies in pregnancy. *Obstet Gynecol.* 2007;109(1):229–237.
2. Boga C, Ozdogu H. Pregnancy and sickle cell disease: A review of the current literature. *Crit Rev Oncol Hematol.* 2016;98:364–374.
3. Eissa AA, tuck SM. Sickle cell disease and β-thalassemia major in pregnancy. *The Obstetrician and Gynaecologist* 2013;15:71–78.
4. Ezihe-Ejiofor A, Jackson J. Peripartum considerations in sickle cell disease. *Curr Opin Anaesthesiol.* 2021;34(3):212–217.
5. Green-Top Guideline. *Management of Sickle Cell Disease in Pregnancy.* London: Royal College of Obstetricians and Gynaecologists; 2011.
6. Howard J, Oteng-Ntim E. The obstetric management of sickle cell disease. *Best Pract Res Clin Obstet Gynaecol.* 2012;26(1):25–36.
7. Okusanya BO, Oladapo OT. Prophylactic versus selective blood transfusion for sickle cell disease in pregnancy. *Cochrane Database Syst Rev.* 2016;12(12):CD010378.

8. Oteng-Ntim E, Meeks D, Seed PT, et al. Adverse maternal and perinatal outcomes in pregnant women with sickle cell disease: systematic review and meta-analysis. *Blood*. 2015;125(21): 3316–3325.

9. Patil V, Ratnayake G, Fastovets G. Clinical 'pearls' of maternal critical care Part 2: sickle-cell disease in pregnancy. *Curr Opin Anaesthesiol*. 2017;30(3):326–334.

10. Smith-Whitley K. Complications in pregnant women with sickle cell disease. *Hematology Am Soc Hematol Educ Program*. 2019;2019(1):359–366.

POINTS

1. With respect to SCA, what aspects of a focused history would you want to know? *(1 point per main bullet unless specified; points indicated per section)*   30

General disease-related details: *(max 3)*
☐ Determine the type of hemoglobinopathy *[i.e., homozygous (Hb SS), or compound heterozygous (Hb SC, Hb S-β thalassemia, others)]*
☐ Record name(s) and contact information of hematologic care provider/team
☐ Need for hospitalizations, ICU (ITU) admissions secondary to SCA
☐ Duration of time since last SCA-related complication, if any

Current clinical manifestations that may be associated with SCA: *(max 6)*
☐ Fever or signs/symptoms of infection
☐ Chest pain, tightness, shortness of breath
☐ Nighttime symptoms/awakenings, use of pulse oximetry or nocturnal oxygen supplementation
☐ Dysuria, hematuria
☐ Abdominal pains or other gastrointestinal symptoms
☐ Bony aches and pains
☐ Symptoms of venous thromboembolism (VTE)
☐ Symptoms related to depression and/or anxiety

History of comorbidities associated with SCA: *(max 6)*
☐ *Neurologic: e.g.,* Cerebral vein thrombosis, stroke, transient ischemic attacks, seizures, cranial nerve palsy, Moyamoya disease
☐ *Ophthalmologic: e.g.,* Retinopathy, visual field changes
☐ *Hematologic and immune: e.g.,* VTE, hypertension, blood or exchange transfusions, splenic sequestration/auto-infarction, sensitization to red cell antigens, chronic infections such as hepatitis or HIV
☐ *Cardio-pulmonary: e.g.,* Pulmonary hypertension, cardiomyopathy, high-output heart failure, acute chest syndrome, pneumonia
☐ *Gastrointestinal: e.g.,* Cholelithiasis, mesenteric thrombosis
☐ *Renal: e.g.,* Sickle-nephropathy, pyelonephritis/urinary tract infection, papillary necrosis, renal medullary carcinoma
☐ *Musculoskeletal: e.g.,* Leg ulcers, osteomyelitis,$ avascular necrosis of the humerus or femur
☐ *Psychiatric: e.g.,* Depression and/or anxiety
☐ *Narcotic dependence*

Social factors[†] and routine health maintenance: *(5)*

☐ Cigarette smoking, alcohol consumption, or illicit drug use
  ○ *May precipitate sickle cell crisis as well as SCA-associated obstetric complications*
☐ Vaccination of encapsulated organisms *(1 point per subbullet for 3 points total)*
  ○ *Meningococcal vaccine (single dose, as part of primary vaccination)*
  ○ *H. influenza type B (single dose, as part of primary vaccination)*
  ○ *Polyvalent pneumococcal (every five years)*
☐ Other vaccinations (*e.g.*, hepatitis B, pertussis, COVID-19, yearly influenza vaccine)

(i) Treatments compatible with pregnancy: *(5)*

☐ Assess whether the patient commenced preconception high-dose folic acid (~4–5 mg)[‡]
☐ Determine if chronic opioid analgesia is required for pain management
☐ Inquire whether she requires chronic prophylactic blood transfusions
☐ Use of oral/parenteral iron therapy *(with low ferritin)*
☐ Drug allergies *(especially to penicillin or erythromycin)*

(ii) Treatments generally not compatible with pregnancy: *(max 3)*

☐ Hydroxycarbamide (hydroxyurea)
☐ Iron chelating agents (*e.g.*, deferasirox, deferoxamine, deferiprone)
☐ Angiotensin-converting enzyme inhibitors (ACE*i*) or angiotensin receptor blockers
☐ Warfarin
☐ Nonsteroidal anti-inflammatory drugs (NSAIDS) (*e.g.*, ibuprofen, diclofenac)
  ○ *NSAIDs are not recommended before 12 weeks and after 28–30 weeks' gestation, and only with medical guidance in the second trimester*

Family history: *(1)*

☐ Assess for hemoglobinopathy-related pregnancy complications among affected family members (or the patient herself if multiparous)

Male partner: *(max 1)*

☐ Determine if his hemoglobin genotype status is known *(if his genetic screen is unknown, the partner's ethnicity helps determine his carrier status and fetal risk calculation for SCA)*
☐ Consanguinity

Special notes:

§ Salmonella osteomyelitis is essentially pathognomonic of SCA
† Ethnicity is noncontributory with known disease status
‡ Largely by expert consensus opinion (ACOG[1]); folic acid should be taken in the form of a multivitamin containing vitamin B12 (refer to Chapter 13)

The patient and her husband provide you with laboratory evidence of her homozygous Hb SS status and his being hemoglobin AS. She has a history of infrequent acute pain while receiving hydroxyurea which was discontinued by her hematologist for desired pregnancy planning given its known teratogenicity in animals. For three months after discontinuing hydroxyurea, she maintained use of a copper-IUD and condoms, to allow for a 'wash-out period.' High-dose folic acid (5 mg daily) was initiated preconception and vaccination status updated. She does not take other medications, has no drug allergies, and social habits are unremarkable. The patient is currently clinically asymptomatic. Although a preconception consultation was planned with you, as an expert in maternal-fetal medicine, the patient could not attend due to a family emergency.

She recalls a remote temporary unilateral retinal vaso-occlusive event; she received several red cell transfusions over the years based on acute clinical indication, without delayed hemolytic transfusion reactions. The patient has not required long-term opioid analgesia. She recalls painful vaso-occlusive episodes in association with premenstrual hormonal changes. Two years ago, she was hospitalized for pneumococcal sepsis. She has not experienced other disease-related morbidities.

The patient is concerned as her sister, with whom she shares the same hemoglobin genotype, had a recent complicated pregnancy due to SCA-associated morbidities.

On examination, you note the patient converses well and maintains an oxygen saturation of 98%. Her body mass index (BMI) is 21 kg/m^2, blood pressure is 110/70 mmHg, and she is afebrile with normal pulse and respiratory rates. You confirm embryonic heart rate by bedside sonography.

Special note:
It is prudent to discontinue hydroxyurea three months preconception (Refer to Pregnancy, contraception and fertility. In: Standards for the Clinical Care of Adults with Sickle Cell Disease in the UK, 2008. p.59)

2. In collaboration with her hematologist, detail the recommended <u>baseline</u> prenatal   Max 10
    <u>investigations most significant to SCA</u>, anticipating overlap with routine prenatal tests.
    (1 point each)

Serum tests:
☐ Blood type and antibody screen *(increased risk of alloantibodies given prior transfusions)*
☐ Full/complete blood count (FBC/CBC)
☐ Reticulocyte count
☐ Serum ferritin
☐ Hemoglobin electrophoresis *(not to confirm the known hemoglobinopathy, but to determine the level of Hb S)*
☐ Hepatic markers: AST, ALT, LDH, uric acid, and bilirubin
☐ Serum creatinine
☐ Infection screening: HIV; hepatitis A, B and C[†]; rubella antibody titer; syphilis screening; consideration for tuberculosis skin test

Urine tests:
☐ Urinalysis
☐ Urine culture (including consideration for chlamydia/gonorrhea testing)
☐ Spot urine protein/creatinine or microalbumin/creatinine ratio

Special note:
† The risk of hepatitis C virus infection is higher with SCA than among the general population, related to international variations in transfusion practices

3. Address the couple's inquiry regarding their offspring's risk of SCA and indicate options for prenatal testing, if indicated. *(1 point each)*   3

- ☐ For this homozygous Hb SS mother and heterozygous Hb AS father, offspring have a 50% risk of Hb SS disease and 50% risk of being asymptomatic Hb AS carriers
- ☐ Options for prenatal genetic diagnosis include chorionic villous sampling (CVS) and amniocentesis
- ☐ Inform the couple that noninvasive cell-free DNA (cfDNA) testing for autosomal recessive conditions remains investigational

Special note:
Refer to Question 10 in Chapter 13 for discussion on risks associated with mid-trimester amniocentesis, Question 10 in Chapter 6 for risks associated with early amniocentesis, and to Question 10 and 11 in Chapter 64 for discussion on chorionic villous sampling

The couple appreciates your comprehensive discussion on risks and benefits of options for invasive prenatal diagnosis. Albeit generally low rates of procedure-related complications for either CVS or amniocentesis among experienced providers, they opt to defer testing to the postnatal period, as fetal diagnosis will not influence their gestational plans. You thereby intend to provide evidence-based counseling of the effects of SCA on the prenatal course, as well as disease adversities associated with pregnancy.

4. Present a structured outline of the effects of maternal SCA on <u>obstetric complications</u> which you may discuss with the patient. *(1 point each; max specified per section)*   8

Maternal: *(max 4)*
- ☐ Early pregnancy loss
- ☐ Preterm labor
- ☐ Gestational hypertension, preeclampsia, or eclampsia
- ☐ Alloimmunization
- ☐ Antepartum bleeding[†]
- ☐ Cesarean delivery *(related to increased maternal-fetal complication rates)*
- ☐ Postpartum infections
- ☐ Mortality

Fetal-placental: *(max 4)*
- ☐ Fetal growth restriction (FGR)/low birthweight
- ☐ Iatrogenic or spontaneous prematurity
- ☐ Hemolytic disease of the fetus and newborn
- ☐ Placental abruption
- ☐ Abnormal fetal cardiotocography (CTG) tracing
- ☐ Intrauterine fetal death (IUFD)

Special note:
† Controversial risk of postpartum hemorrhage

5. With reference to the <u>pathophysiology</u> of SCA, explain the mechanisms for fetal-placental complications, *regardless* of concurrent hypertensive syndromes of pregnancy. *(1 point each)*

    Max 2

☐ Sickling cells adhere to vascular endothelium, leading to intravascular occlusion and placental infarction
☐ Hyperviscosity
☐ Maternal chronic hemolytic anemia[†]

Special note:
†   Life span of a sickle cell is ~17 days, which is approximately seven times less than a normal red blood (120 days)]

---

6. With reference to <u>physiology</u>, address the patient's concern regarding fetal risks of in utero sickling events.

    2

☐ Fetal Hb F protects the fetus (and neonate) from sickling events, which occur when Hb F is replaced by Hb S production at 3–12 months of age

Special note:
Hb F (α_2, γ_2) is the primary fetal hemoglobin at 12–24 weeks' gestation; production of Hb F decreases in the third trimester as β-chain production necessary for Hb A (α_2, β_2) begins

---

7. Indicate sickle cell disease-associated maternal complications. *(1 point per main bullet)*

    Max 10

☐ Acute exacerbations, or worsening steady state, of chronic hemolytic anemia[†]
☐ Acute painful vaso-occlusive episodes or actual sickle cell crises[‡]
    ○ *Acute pain episodes occur in 30%–50% of pregnancies, as well as during labor and delivery; symptoms are more common with SS than SC genotypes*
☐ Acute chest syndrome
☐ Systemic inflammatory response syndrome
☐ Transfusions and transfusion reactions or alloimmunization
☐ Infections (*e.g.*, meningitis, pulmonary, symptomatic or asymptomatic urinary tract, puerperal sepsis)
☐ Pulmonary embolism/deep venous thrombosis (PE/DVT), or bone marrow embolism
☐ Neurological manifestations (*i.e.*, ischemic or hemorrhagic stroke, cerebral vein thrombosis, seizures)
☐ Retinal disease *(patient also has an antecedent history thereof)*
☐ Pulmonary hypertension
☐ Cardiomyopathy
☐ Acute onset or worsening of renal disease
☐ Acute onset or worsening of hepatic dysfunction
☐ Mortality *(greater risk with SS than SC genotypes, and in lower-resource settings)*

Special notes:

† Patients with SCA are **not** commonly iron deficient

‡ Although the term 'sickle cell crisis' is still used by many providers, the preferred terminology is painful episodes because not all patients are in true crisis; furthermore, pain should not be allowed to progress to the point of a 'crisis' for receipt of appropriate analgesia

You inform the patient that obstetric care of women with SCA is best suited to a multidisciplinary setting with combined excellence in maternal-fetal medicine, hematology, transfusion medicine, adult and neonatal intensive care. Encouraged that interdisciplinary management decreases disease-related adverse events,† the patient indicates her intent to remain compliant with planned management.

Special note:

† Refer to de Montalembert M, Deneux-Tharaux C. Pregnancy in sickle cell disease is at very high risk. *Blood.* 2015;125(21):3216–3217.

8. Maintaining multidisciplinary collaboration, provide the patient with comprehensive counseling and antenatal management plan most specific to SCA, assuming an uncomplicated pregnancy. *(1 point each; max specified per section)*   24

Maternal management:

Consultations {unless recently performed}:† (max 6)

☐ Genetics *(further discussion on fetal risk of inheritance and variability of sickle cell phenotype)*

☐ Ophthalmology *(assess for proliferative sickle retinopathy, which may progress during gestation)*

☐ Respirology *(pulmonary function test assessment)*

☐ Cardiology *(maternal echocardiogram)*

☐ Dietician *(patients with SCA are reported to be at risk of dietary deficiencies including vitamins and minerals)*

☐ Anesthesiology *(discussion in the second or third trimester to plan intrapartum analgesia)*

☐ Neonatology *(infant care given maternal disease-associated risks, including need for postnatal diagnostic testing)*

☐ Consideration for social worker or perinatal mental health expert involvement *(individualized)*

Prophylactic measures and treatments: (9 points)

☐ Continuation of daily high-dose folic acid 4–5 mg throughout pregnancy is recommended

☐ Provide iron-free prenatal vitamins, unless iron deficient

☐ Early treatment of nausea and vomiting of pregnancy is advised to prevent dehydration/ stress-induced sickle cell crisis

☐ Recommend avoidance of stress, cold temperatures or hypoxic environments as these may precipitate sickle cell crisis

☐ Low-dose aspirin 75–162 mg taken nightly as preeclampsia prophylaxis, starting at 12 weeks and continuing throughout pregnancy *(RCOG[5])*; otherwise, initiate prior to 16 weeks' gestation[‡]
  ○ *Although there is no evidence for the role of low-dose aspirin in pregnant women with SCA, it is used for its benefits for preeclampsia prophylaxis among high-risk women*
☐ Penicillin V 250 mg orally twice daily [or erythromycin in case of penicillin allergy] is recommended throughout gestation, particularly given the patient's prior pneumococcal sepsis
  ○ *In England, penicillin prophylaxis is routinely recommended due to functional hyposplenism (Suggested Reading 6); otherwise, international practice variations exist*
☐ Consideration for daily use of compression stockings; encourage mobilization and hydration
☐ Inform the patient that outpatient thromboprophylaxis would be advised with concurrent risk factors
☐ Inform the patient that universal antenatal prophylactic blood/exchange transfusions are not recommended

Prenatal visits: *(3 points)*
☐ Anticipate frequent interdisciplinary prenatal visits *(individualize frequency as appropriate)*
☐ Monitoring for hypertension every two to four weeks is advised *(Suggested Reading 10)*
☐ Encourage early reporting of signs/symptoms of hypertensive syndromes of pregnancy, vaso-occlusive crises, VTE, infection, preterm labor, or decreased fetal activity in the third trimester

Serial laboratory studies: *(max 4)*
☐ CBC/FBC with reticulocyte count (monthly, or at least every trimester)
☐ Serum iron and ferritin (monthly, or at least every trimester)
☐ Urinalysis (each antenatal visit) *RCOG[5]*
☐ Urine culture and sensitivity analysis (monthly) *RCOG[5]*
☐ Urine screening for proteinuria (monthly) *(Suggested Reading 10)*
☐ Repeat screening for red cell antibodies in mid-gestation and at delivery-admission

Fetal management: *(2 points)*
☐ After routine first-trimester sonogram (*i.e.*, 11^{+0}–13^{+6} weeks) plan second-trimester biometry and morphology ultrasound (*e.g.*, 18–20 weeks) followed by monthly assessment of fetal growth biometry *(or more frequent, as clinically indicated)* to screen for fetal growth restriction (FGR)
☐ Provide greater fetal surveillance (*e.g.*, CTG monitoring or biophysical profile) for subjectively reduced fetal movements

Special notes:
† Maternal-fetal medicine referral, as implied in this case scenario, would otherwise be warranted if beyond one's expertise
‡ Refer to Question 6 in Chapter 38

9. Although no dose-recommendation studies have been performed among women with SCA, rationalize why expert consensus recommends higher dose folic acid relative to routine prenatal care.

1

☐ SCA is associated with a state of chronic hemolysis, where folic acid is needed for increased hematopoiesis.

While counseling the patient, your obstetric trainee attentively noted your mention that routine exchange transfusions in pregnancy are not advised due to excess maternal risk, similarly noting that universal prophylactic blood transfusions at regular intervals have not been shown to improve obstetric outcomes. You highlight that insufficient evidence exists to recommend prophylactic transfusion rather than standard care transfusion for pregnant patients with SCA *(Suggested Reading 7)*. Interestingly, you allude to a preliminary study suggesting nocturnal oxygen supplementation may decrease antenatal need for red cell transfusions in women with SCA.[‡]

After this initial prenatal visit, you take the opportunity to discuss with your trainee features of transfusion in pregnant women with SCA.

Special note:
‡ Ribeil JA, Labopin M, Stanislas A, et al. Transfusion-related adverse events are decreased in pregnant women with sickle cell disease by a change in policy from systematic transfusion to prophylactic oxygen therapy at home: A retrospective survey by the international sickle cell disease observatory. *Am J Hematol.* 2018;93(6):794–802.

10. Elaborate on <u>risks of routine red cell transfusions</u> in obstetric patients with SCA. *(1 point each)*

Max 2

☐ Precipitation of an acute painful episode or sickle cell crisis (especially with hematocrit >35%)
☐ Immediate or delayed transfusion reactions
☐ Red cell alloimmunization *(donor blood is often from people of different ethnic origin than the patient)*
☐ Transfusion-related iron-overload organ damage
☐ Transfusion-transmitted infection

11. Identify clinical situations where the hematologist may have recommended <u>prophylactic</u> transfusion at <u>regular intervals</u> throughout pregnancy. *(1 point per main bullet)*   4

Prophylactic transfusion:
- ☐ History of severe SCA-related complications before the current pregnancy, or in previous pregnancies, if any[‡]
  - ○ *Aims to reduce recurrent pain episodes, incidence of acute chest syndrome, or other disease-related comorbidities*
- ☐ Additional features of high-risk pregnancy (*e.g.*, other comorbidities, medical conditions or nephropathy)[‡]
- ☐ Onset of SCA-related complications during the current pregnancy[‡] (*e.g.*, if exchange transfusion is required during pregnancy or >1 simple transfusion)
- ☐ Twin pregnancies (*RCOG*[5] *and Suggested Reading 10*)

Special note:
‡   Chou ST, Alsawas M, Fasano RM, et al. American Society of Hematology 2020 guidelines for sickle cell disease: transfusion support. *Blood Adv.* 2020;4(2):327–355

In combination with her hematologist, you reassure the patient that baseline laboratory investigations were normal. First-trimester assessment of her eyes, heart, and lungs did not reveal disease comorbidity. Maternal-fetal progress is unremarkable, and the patient remains adherent to the management plan.

During your on-call duty, the patient presents to the obstetric emergency assessment unit at 30^{+3} weeks' gestation with a two-day history of sharp, throbbing pains in her legs and proximal arms since her recent return from a weekend trip where she accompanied her husband in support of his downhill ski competition. She recalls her symptoms were preceded by two days of paresthesia and dull aches at these bony sites. Paracetamol (acetaminophen) did not provide symptomatic relief. Despite resting and attempting oral hydration, she had brief vomiting and diarrhea after a chef-made fruit drink during the trip. You recall the patient is now on day 5 of 10 oral second-generation cephalosporin treatment for a urinary tract infection detected on routine antenatal screening prior to her trip. The urinary bacterial infection was resistant to penicillin V, which the patient continues to take as prophylaxis for functional hyposplenism and history of pneumococcal infection. She has no obstetric complaints and fetal activity has been normal.

A hematologist has been notified and will promptly attend to assist you in the care of this patient.

12. State the <u>initial</u> essential aspects of your focused physical examination. *(1 point each)*   15

General appearance:
- ☐ Apparent shortness of breath/ability to provide complete sentences
- ☐ Distress from bodily pains and ability to walk without apparent hip pain
- ☐ Markers of dehydration, including dry mucous membranes and skin turgor

Vital signs:†
- ☐ Blood pressure (BP)
- ☐ Respiratory rate
- ☐ Pulse rate
- ☐ Oxygen saturation by pulse oximetry
- ☐ Temperature

Abdominal examination:
- ☐ Flank or costovertebral angle tenderness *(i.e., renal complications associated with infection)*
- ☐ Uterine tenderness

Lower extremities:
- ☐ Joint swelling
- ☐ Localized tenderness of the thighs, tibial bones, or calves *(considering risk of DVT and veno-occlusive disease)*
- ☐ Differential swelling, warmth, or pitting edema *(considering risk of DVT and heart failure)*
- ☐ Leg ulcers *(vaso-occlusive skin manifestations, typically of the medial and lateral malleoli)*

Fetal assessment:
- ☐ CTG for fetal heart rate and uterine activity

Special note:
† Perform cardiopulmonary examination where clinically indicated

The patient converses without distress; you notice she exerts gentle massage-like pressure on her arms and legs in attempt to soothe her pains. Her oral mucosa appears dry. Vital signs reveal the following:

- BP 90/60 mmHg
- Respiratory rate 12 breaths/min
- Pulse rate 100 bpm
- Oxygen saturation 98% on room air
- Oral temperature 37.0°C (98.6°F)

Her abdomen is soft and nontender; there is no costovertebral angle tenderness. The patient's legs appear normal without marked swelling, pitting edema or ulceration. Fetal CTG tracing is normal and uterine quiescence is ascertained.

In collaboration with the hematologist, comprehensive investigations are in progress.

---

13. Based on her clinical presentation and findings on examination, what is the <u>most probable</u> diagnosis?   1

- ☐ Acute painful vaso-occlusive episode

14. Identify the patient's precipitating factors for an acute vaso-occlusive pain episode. *(1 point each)*

Max 5

☐ Pregnancy
☐ Active urinary tract infection
☐ Dehydration *(i.e., vomiting and diarrhea, dry oral mucosa, tachycardia, hypotension)*
☐ Exposure to cold ambient temperature
☐ Exposure to high altitudes *(i.e., lower oxygen environment)*
☐ Stress

You highlight to your obstetric trainee that timely and adequate analgesia is fundamental in the setting of vaso-occlusive pain; normal laboratory results should not be used to justify withholding or titrating the dose of pain medications to which the patient responds well. In fact, as your trainee is a native of the U.K., you indicate that UK Standards require patients with acute SCA-related pain to receive initial analgesia within 30 minutes of presentation and pain should be well controlled by one hour.[†] You teach your trainee that in the absence of randomized trials addressing the efficacy and safety of interventions for treating antenatal pain episodes related to SCA, management is largely based on a standard approach.[‡]

Special notes:
[†] (a) Standards for the Clinical Care of Adults with Sickle Cell Disease in the UK. Sickle Cell Society 2008. www.sicklecellsociety, and (b) Rees DC, Olujohungbe AD, Parker NE et al. Guidelines for the management of acute painful crisis in sickle cell disease. *Br J Haematol.* 2003; 120: 744–752. British Committee for Standards in Haematology, General Haematology Task Force by the Sickle Cell Working Party.
[‡] Martí-Carvajal AJ, Peña-Martí GE, Comunián-Carrasco G, Martí-Peña AJ. Interventions for treating painful sickle cell crisis during pregnancy. *Cochrane Database Syst Rev.* 2009;2009(1): CD006786. Published 2009 Jan 21.

15. In liaison with the hematologist, outline a structured, comprehensive approach to management of this obstetric patient's vaso-occlusive pain episode. *(1 point per main bullet)*

Max 15

General aspects of maternal care:
☐ Hospitalization in a patient-monitored setting
☐ Administer oxygen *only* if saturation becomes <95% or drops >3% from baseline
    ○ *Do not administer oxygen as a routine measure given the risk of rebound sickling with its discontinuation*
☐ Serial assessment of other vital signs, with thorough evaluation of any abnormality such as fever, tachypnea, hypertension, marked or persistent tachycardia
☐ Keep the patient warm (*e.g.*, warm blankets, adjust room temperature)
☐ Provide, and encourage use of incentive spirometry during hospitalization as a measure to prevent acute chest syndrome

☐ Consideration for social worker or perinatal mental health expert involvement *(individualized)*

Analgesia and related side effects:

☐ Consider consultation with pain management services or an anesthesiologist (*e.g.*, patient-controlled analgesia system)

☐ Administer opioid analgesia, preferably with morphine or hydromorphone (parenteral or oral); oral codeine or acetaminophen (paracetamol) may also be considered

   ○ *Meperidine (pethidine) is not recommended in first-line treatment of vaso-occlusive pain crises among patients with SCA due to the risk of seizures associated with its metabolite, normeperidine*

   ○ *Preferred avoidance of nonsteroidal anti-inflammatory analgesics at this gestational age*

   ○ *If respiratory rate is <10/min, omit maintenance opioid analgesia and administer naloxone (RCOG[5])*

☐ Provide antiemetics, laxatives, and antihistamines to treat side effects of opioids

Hydration:

☐ Initiate fluid hydration with a goal of 60 mL/kg/24 hours, either intravenously (warm fluid) or orally, where possible

   ○ *Correct electrolyte imbalances, noting that patients in crisis lose more urinary sodium*

Antibiotics:

☐ Continue treatment of her urinary tract infection and penicillin V antenatal prophylaxis

☐ Administer broad-spectrum antibiotics in the event of fever, acute chest symptoms, or evidence of other infection

Anticoagulation:

☐ Initiate standard regimen of low molecular weight heparin (LMWH) for thromboprophylaxis during hospitalization

☐ Encourage ambulation

☐ Provide sequential pneumatic compression devices

Fetal management:

☐ Arrange for regular fetal CTG tracings during hospital admission *(individualized frequency)*, recognizing that maternal opioid use may interfere with nonstress testing/fetal heart rate tracing *(transient suppression of fetal movement and reduced baseline fetal heart rate variability)*

☐ Obtain sonography for assessment of fetal growth and well-being

☐ Consideration for fetal pulmonary corticosteroids

☐ Request neonatology consultation during maternal hospitalization, alerting experts to maternal need of opioid analgesia *(risk of neonatal withdrawal)* and the need to perform newborn testing given she had declined prenatal diagnosis

Special note:

This patient does not require transfusion at this time (see Question 16)

With management of this acute painful episode already initiated, results of *selected* investigations reveal the following:

White blood cell count	$15.0 \times 10^3/mm^3$
Hemoglobin concentration	7.8 g/dL (78 g/L) – *You note this is similar to her baseline level*
Hematocrit	36%
Reticulocyte count	1%
Platelet concentration	$350 \times 10^9/L$

16. What do you anticipate the hematologist would advise with regard to recommending blood transfusion for this obstetric patient with an acute painful vaso-occlusive episode?   1

☐ There is no indication for blood transfusion in this patient
  ○ *Note that neither an acute painful episode nor vaso-occlusive crisis are absolute indications for transfusion*

17. Inform your obstetric trainee of clinical situations where <u>on-demand blood transfusion or exchange transfusion</u> would be considered in the context of SCA. *(1 point each)*   Max 5

On-demand transfusion:
☐ Hemoglobin concentration <6 or 7 g/dL (60 or 70 g/L) or hematocrit <25%
☐ Acute exacerbation of anemia with illness [*i.e.*, decrease in hemoglobin by 2 g/dL (20 g/L)]
☐ Symptomatic/orthostatic anemia
☐ Acute exacerbation of steady-state anemia, possibly related to iron-deficiency, renal disease, or increased hemolysis
☐ Acute chest syndrome
☐ Congestive heart failure due to anemia
☐ Acute stroke[†]
☐ Multiorgan failure
☐ Preoperatively [aim for a hemoglobin concentration ≥10–12 g/dL (100–120 g/L) and Hb S <35%–40%]
☐ Preeclampsia that does not improve as expected after delivery

Special notes:
[†] Thrombolysis is **not** helpful to treat sickle stroke

The patient is discharged after five days of hospitalization; she responded well to the outlined management and is currently using nonopioid analgesia, including acetaminophen (paracetamol) and warm pads, on an as-needed basis. Fetal sonography, performed during hospital admission, showed growth biometry on the 15th percentile, with appropriate growth velocity, and normal amniotic fluid volume. Fetal CTG tracings have been normal. A repeat mid-stream urine culture (*i.e.*, test-of-cure) is arranged for one week after completion of treatment. She will maintain penicillin V prophylaxis for functional hyposplenism. Thromboprophylaxis is discontinued upon discharge and with resolution of the acute pain episode.

Pregnancy thereafter progresses well. Although intrapartum management has been serially updated during the antepartum period, you review delivery plans with her at the 36 weeks' visit. She remains normotensive, fetal presentation is cephalic with stable sonographic findings, and the patient does not have medical or obstetric complaints. You have just performed the group B streptococcus (GBS) vaginal-rectal swab for which routine care is anticipated.

---

18. Outline pertinent aspects of <u>intrapartum</u> management considerations with regard to this patient with SCA. (*1 point per main bullet*)   Max 12

☐ Plan for delivery at 38–40 weeks' gestation, unless complications arise
☐ Aim for vaginal delivery, with Cesarean section is reserved for obstetric indications[†]
   ○ *Consideration for prophylactic blood transfusion where Cesarean delivery is planned to avoid precipitating an acute pain episode due to blood loss*
☐ Continued liaison with the hematology team involved in her care, ensuring delivery in a tertiary-care center with adequate blood bank services
☐ Repeat red cell antibody screen upon labor admission
☐ Continuous electronic fetal heart rate monitoring
   ○ *Note increased rates of stillbirth, placental abruption, and compromised placental reserve in a parturient with SCA*
☐ Encourage early and adequate labor analgesia (*no contraindications to mode of labor analgesia*)
   ○ *If Cesarean delivery is required, avoidance of general anesthesia is preferred*
☐ Ensure adequate hydration in labor, using a fluid balance chart to prevent fluid overload
☐ Keep the patient warm (*e.g.*, warm fluid, blankets, adjust room temperature)
☐ Maintain continuous maternal pulse oximetry; (a) administer oxygen supplementation if saturation is below 95% and (b) obtain an arterial blood gas analysis
☐ Maintain a low threshold for initiating intrapartum antibiotics with evidence, or high clinical suspicion, of infection
☐ Maintain a low threshold for assisted second stage
☐ Obtain umbilical cord blood specimen at the time of delivery to assess for hemoglobinopathy in the neonate
☐ Active management of the third stage of labor is advised to reduce the risk of postpartum hemorrhage
☐ Include the neonatology team at delivery and convey the need for diagnostic testing for SCA

Special note:
† Cesarean delivery may be preferable if a patient had a hip replacement for avascular necrosis

Spontaneous labor ensues at 39^{+4} weeks' gestation where she receives early epidural analgesia. A vigorous male weighing 2400 g[†] is delivered with vacuum-assistance to avoid a prolonged second stage. Repair of a second-degree laceration was unremarkable.

On postpartum day 1, you visit the patient and review postpartum care focused on SCA. You had already informed her she *may* remain in hospital for approximately three days during which fluid and electrolyte balances will be maintained and hematologic parameters followed daily *(Suggested Reading 2)*. Neonatal tests are in progress to determine the infant's genotype. Incidentally, the couple is curious about future pregnancy considerations to eliminate risk of possibly affected offspring.

Special note:

† ~30% of newborns of mothers with SCA have low birthweight (*i.e.*, <2500 g)

19. Given a successful vaginal delivery, what are important <u>postpartum</u> considerations to discuss, either prior to discharge or at the routine postpartum visit in relation to maternal SCA? *(1 point per main bullet)*   13

Prevention of postpartum acute pain episodes:
- ☐ Encourage pulmonary support with use of incentive spirometry, at least prior to discharge
  - ○ *Continuous positive airway pressure support may occasionally be required*
- ☐ Encourage adequate analgesia, hydration, ambulation, rest, and family support to decrease precipitating acute pain episodes or sickle cell crises
- ☐ Encourage early reporting of symptoms related to postpartum endometritis such as fever, abnormal vaginal discharge, or abdominal pain given risk of precipitating an acute pain episode or sickle cell crisis
- ☐ Inform the patient not to reinitiate the long-term disease-modifying drug (*i.e.*, hydroxyurea) without collaborating with her hematologist *(reinitiation is generally only considered after completion of breastfeeding)*

Thromboprophylaxis:[‡] *(2)*
- ☐ International practice variations exist regarding routine postpartum thromboprophylaxis among women with SCA **who deliver vaginally**; examples of recommendations include:
  - ○ *RCOG[5]* suggest LMWH prophylaxis during postpartum hospitalization and for seven days after discharge

  OR

  - ○ *ACOG[1]* supports LMWH prophylaxis after vaginal delivery in women with additional risk factors
- ☐ Antithrombotic stockings are recommended in the puerperium

Contraceptive recommendations for hormonal and intrauterine methods:[†] *(2)*
- ☐ Category 1 (no restrictions) for progestin-only methods including levonorgesterol intrauterine system, implant, DMPA, and progestin-only oral contraceptives
  - ○ DMPA *may* reduce the frequency and severity of painful episodes
- ☐ Category 2 (advantages of use generally outweigh theoretical or proven risks) for combined hormonal contraceptive methods and copper-intrauterine device

General maternal-fetal well-being:

☐ Encourage breastfeeding

☐ Screen for postpartum depression and continue to offer psychosocial support services

☐ Recommend long-term liaison with a dietician to promote adequate intake of vitamins and minerals

☐ Arrange for maternal outpatient follow-up with a hematologist and for postpartum obstetric care

☐ Advise future preconception counseling

Special notes:

‡ If this patient required a Cesarean delivery, or has other risk factors, such as advanced maternal age, obesity, or preeclampsia, thromboprophylaxis would be recommended for six weeks' duration

† Indicated recommendations are based on UK and US Medical Eligibility Criteria (MEC) for Contraceptive Use, 2016; UK-MEC amended September 2019, US-MEC updated 2020

---

20. Address their inquiry on considerations for future modes of conception that would ensure absence of SCA-affected offspring. *(1 point per main bullet)*   Max 2

☐ Plan in vitro fertilization to allow for preimplantation genetic diagnosis, selecting this couple's heterozygous Hb AS (*i.e.*, sickle cell trait) embryos; such offspring would not demonstrate hematological abnormalities and are essentially asymptomatic unless hypoxic or very dehydrated although gestational complications associated with maternal SCA remain

    ○ *Should their current fetus be affected with SCA, future HLA-typing of an unaffected embryo that is HLA identical to the affected offspring can allow consideration for stem cell transplantation of this sibling*

☐ Use of a donor oocyte from a female without hemoglobinopathy (*i.e.*, Hb AA) and this heterozygous male's sperm would imply that 50% of embryos would have the sickle cell trait and 50% would be unaffected, with persistent maternal-fetal risks of pregnancy complications associated with maternal SCA

☐ Surrogacy where the surrogate, who does not have the hemoglobinopathy, undergoes intrauterine insemination of this male's heterozygous sperm (or donor); this obviates an affected offspring and gestational complications associated with maternal SCA

☐ Adoption

TOTAL: 165

CHAPTER 52

Inherited Thrombophilia and Venous Thromboembolism in Pregnancy

Amira El-Messidi and Audrey-Ann Labrecque

A 28-year-old nulligravida with known factor V Leiden mutation is referred by her primary care provider to your hospital center's high-risk obstetrics unit for preconception counseling.

LEARNING OBJECTIVES

1. Take a focused preconception history from a patient with heterozygous factor V Leiden mutation, and provide counseling for prevention of a primary venous thromboembolism (VTE) related to pregnancy
2. Understand the pathophysiology of inherited thrombophilias
3. Recognize signs and symptoms of deep venous thrombosis (DVT) and pulmonary embolism (PE) in the antenatal period, and develop a differential diagnosis of acute lower leg pain in pregnancy
4. Detail investigations for acute DVT and PE in pregnancy, recognizing the importance of multidisciplinary collaboration and appreciating international variations in professional guideline recommendations
5. Present evidence-based regimens for anticoagulation in the perinatal period, and formulate a safe plan for delivery while on therapeutic anticoagulation

SUGGESTED READINGS

1. American College of Obstetricians and Gynecologists' Committee on Practice Bulletins–Obstetrics. ACOG Practice Bulletin No. 197: Inherited thrombophilias in pregnancy. *Obstet Gynecol.* 2018;132(1):e18–e34. [Correction in Obstet Gynecol. 2018 Oct;132(4):1069]
2. American College of Obstetricians and Gynecologists' Committee on Practice Bulletins—Obstetrics. ACOG Practice Bulletin No. 196: Thromboembolism in Pregnancy. *Obstet Gynecol.* 2018;132(1):e1–e17. [Correction in Obstet Gynecol. 2018 Oct;132(4):1068]

3. Bates SM, Rajasekhar A, Middeldorp S, et al. American Society of Hematology 2018 guidelines for management of venous thromboembolism: venous thromboembolism in the context of pregnancy. *Blood Adv.* 2018;2(22):3317–3359.

4. Chan WS, Rey E, Kent NE, et al. Venous thromboembolism and antithrombotic therapy in pregnancy. *J Obstet Gynaecol Can.* 2014;36(6):527–553.

5. Cohen SL, Feizullayeva C, McCandlish JA, et al. Comparison of international societal guidelines for the diagnosis of suspected pulmonary embolism during pregnancy. *Lancet Haematol.* 2020;7(3):e247–e258.

6. Horlocker TT, Vandermeuelen E, Kopp SL, et al. Regional anesthesia in the patient receiving antithrombotic or thrombolytic therapy: American Society of Regional Anesthesia and Pain Medicine Evidence-Based Guidelines (Fourth Edition). *Reg Anesth Pain Med.* 2018;43(3):263–309. [Correction in Reg Anesth Pain Med. 2018 Jul;43(5):566]

7. Konstantinides SV, Meyer G, Becattini C, et al. 2019 ESC Guidelines for the diagnosis and management of acute pulmonary embolism developed in collaboration with the European Respiratory Society (ERS): The Task Force for the diagnosis and management of acute pulmonary embolism of the European Society of Cardiology (ESC). *Eur Respir J.* 2019;54(3):1901647.

8. Leffert L, Butwick A, Carvalho B, et al. The Society for Obstetric Anesthesia and Perinatology Consensus Statement on the anesthetic management of pregnant and postpartum women receiving thromboprophylaxis or higher dose anticoagulants. *Anesth Analg.* 2018;126(3): 928–944.

9. (a) Royal College of Obstetricians and Gynaecologists, Green-Top Guideline No. 37a. Reducing the risk of venous thromboembolism during pregnancy and the puerperium. April 2015. Available at www.rcog.org.uk/en/guidelines-research-services/guidelines/ gtg37a/. Accessed March 19, 2021.

   (b) Royal College of Obstetricians and Gynaecologists, Green-Top Guideline No. 37b. Thrombotic disease in pregnancy and the puerperium: acute management. April 2015. Available at www.rcog.org.uk/en/guidelines-research-services/guidelines/gtg37b/. Accessed March 19, 2021.

10. van der Pol LM, Tromeur C, Bistervels IM, et al. Pregnancy-adapted YEARS algorithm for diagnosis of suspected pulmonary embolism. *N Engl J Med.* 2019;380(12):1139–1149.

1. With regard to her factor V Leiden mutation, which aspects of a focused history would   Max 15
   you like to know? *(1 point each)*

Medical details related to the factor V Leiden diagnosis:
☐ Ascertain the patient's zygosity
☐ Personal history of VTE (unprovoked, provoked, estrogen-related)
   ○ *Surgical history would be included as a potential source of provoked VTE*
☐ First-degree family history of VTE
☐ Family history of factor V Leiden and/or other inherited thrombophilia

Preexisting medical factors for pregnancy-related VTE:[§] *(max 5)*
☐ Obesity (*i.e.*, BMI $\geq$30 kg/m^2)
☐ Cardiac disease (*e.g.*, hypertension, atrial fibrillation, heart failure within prior three
   months)
☐ Autoimmune disease (*e.g.*, diabetes mellitus, active systemic lupus erythematosus)
☐ Hematologic (*e.g.*, sickle cell disease, need for frequent blood transfusions)
☐ Infections (*e.g.*, HIV, pneumonia, and urinary tract infection)
☐ Nephrotic syndrome
☐ Active inflammatory bowel disease or inflammatory arthropathy
☐ Large venous varicosities (*e.g.*, symptomatic, above-knee, associated with edema/phlebitis,
   or known to be $\leq$5 cm of the deep venous system or affecting $\geq$5 cm of the vein)
☐ Active malignancy/chemotherapy treatment

Social history:
☐ Occupation/physical activity as a marker of immobility (*e.g., driver, frequent air travel*)
☐ Cigarette smoking
☐ Alcohol consumption
☐ IV drug use

Medications and allergies:
☐ Current or past use of estrogen-containing hormonal contraception
☐ Allergies (particularly to anticoagulants including a history of heparin-induced
   thrombocytopenia, if pertinent history of use)

Special note:
§ Other maternal-specific risk factors, not pertinent to this case scenario include advanced
   maternal age ($\geq$35 years), multiparity ($\geq$3), or acquired thrombophilia

You learn the patient was diagnosed with a heterozygous factor V Leiden mutation at age 16 years during testing for inherited thrombophilia after her older sister's unprovoked pulmonary embolism (PE). Family history is otherwise negative for VTE or other inherited thrombophilia. The patient has neither experienced a VTE nor used combined hormonal contraceptives. For the past eight years, she has used the levonorgestrel-releasing IUD (LNG-IUD) without complications; she plans to discontinue it in the upcoming months, anticipating conception with her husband. As a computer administrator, she describes a mostly sedentary lifestyle, although she attempts to practice yoga for one hour/week. She does not smoke, drink alcohol, or use illicit drugs.

On examination, the patient is normotensive, weighs 72 kg with a BMI of 29.5 kg/m^2. She does not have prominent varicosities.

2. Provide evidence-based aspects to discuss in preconception counseling for prevention of first VTE event in a patient with heterozygous factor V Leiden mutation whose sister had a prior PE. Detail one possible LMWH regimen, where indicated

Max 10

Antepartum:[†] *(1 point per main bullet and if specified for subbullets; max 5)*
- ☐ Highlight the importance of multidisciplinary collaboration with an obstetric physicians/ hematologist during the antepartum and postpartum period
- ☐ Pharmacologic thromboprophylaxis is <u>not</u> recommended
  - ○ *Only slightly higher risk of VTE in pregnancy (15/1000 deliveries) than that conferred by her thrombophilia alone (5–12/1000 deliveries)*
  - ○ *If this patient had a prior VTE, her recurrence risk would be ~10% in pregnancy and antepartum prophylaxis recommended*
- ☐ Initiation of thromboprophylaxis may be warranted based on additional risk factors *(RCOG)*
- ☐ Inform the patient that a substantial portion of thromboembolic events happen in the first trimester; early instigation of preventative mechanisms is crucial *(add 1 point per subbullet)*
  - ○ Advise adequate hydration and mobilization
  - ○ Graduated compression stockings should be considered during high-risk periods (*e.g.*, long-distance travel of more than four hours or hospitalization)
- ☐ Reinforce personal and clinical vigilance for signs and symptoms of VTE

Postpartum: *(1 point per subbullet and 3 points for providing one regimen; max 5)*
- ☐ *Controversial* management options among societal guidelines *(individualized discussion)*

Options include:
- ○ No thromboprophylaxis (due to lack of strong evidence for postpartum prophylaxis to prevent a VTE *(ASH[3], SOGC[4] without an additional risk factor)*

OR
- ○ Subcutaneous low molecular weight heparin (LMWH)[‡] thromboprophylaxis for six weeks** based on risk factor combinations

Options:
- ▪ Enoxaparin 40 mg once daily or 30 mg twice daily
- ▪ Dalteparin 5000 U once daily
- ▪ Tinzaparin 4500 U once daily

Special notes:
† If this patient with low-risk thrombophilia had a previous VTE, both antepartum and postpartum thromboprophylaxis would have been recommended
‡ Thromboprophylaxis is started no sooner than four hours after neuraxial catheter removal provided she has full neurological recovery and no evidence of active bleeding
** Short-term postpartum anticoagulation for 10 days would not be appropriate in this setting in view of her sister's history of VTE *(RCOG[9])*

3. In addition to heterozygous factor V Leiden, identify three inherited thrombophilias where antepartum antithrombotic prophylaxis is not recommended to prevent a first VTE, regardless of family history. *(1 point each)*   3

Additional low-risk thrombophilias:
☐ Heterozygous prothrombin gene mutation G20210A
☐ Protein C deficiency
☐ Protein S deficiency

Recognizing the importance of multidisciplinary care, the patient inquires about the obstetric features that may prompt consideration for thromboprophylaxis.

4. Counsel the patient on obstetric-specific and transient risk factors warranting consideration for perinatal thromboprophylaxis. You inform her that practice variations exist regarding the number of risk factors required for initiation of thromboprophylaxis. *(1 point per main bullet; max points specified per section)*   15

Obstetric-specific VTE risk factors: *(max 10)*
☐ In vitro fertilization/assisted reproductive technology
☐ Multiple gestation
☐ Strict antepartum bedrest or hospitalization for three or more days
  ○ *SOGC[4] recommends prophylactic thromboprophylaxis with bedrest of seven or more days*
☐ Preeclampsia in current pregnancy
☐ Preterm delivery in current pregnancy – postpartum prophylaxis
☐ Fetal growth restriction (FGR) – postpartum prophylaxis *(SOGC[4])*
☐ Preterm prelabor rupture of membranes (PPROM) – postpartum prophylaxis *(SOGC)*
☐ Placental abruption – postpartum prophylaxis *(SOGC)*
☐ Placenta previa – postpartum prophylaxis *(SOGC)*
☐ Prolonged labor (>24 hours)
☐ Emergency/unplanned Cesarean section
☐ Elective Cesarean section
☐ Mid-cavity/rotational forceps delivery
☐ Obstetric hemorrhage >1000 mL or need for blood product replacement
☐ Postpartum infection requiring IV antibiotics or hospitalization
☐ Stillbirth in current pregnancy

Transient risk factors for VTE: *(max 5)*
☐ Ovarian hyperstimulation syndrome [OHSS] *(transient risk factor by RCOG)*
  ○ *Women with OHSS are particularly prone to upper body VTE*
☐ Hyperemesis gravidarum *(transient risk factor by RCOG)*
☐ Nonobstetric surgery during pregnancy or puerperium (except immediate perineal repair)
☐ Systemic infection *(pregnancy or puerperium)*
☐ Immobility *(pregnancy or puerperium)*
☐ Dehydration *(pregnancy or puerperium)*
☐ Long-distance travel more than four hours *(pregnancy or puerperium)*

You explain that the overall absolute risk of VTE in pregnancy is ~1/1000 deliveries, with equal absolute incidence during the antepartum and postpartum periods, although the shorter post-partum period results in a higher *daily* thrombotic risk than antepartum.

You take note to elaborate on the pathophysiology and pathogenesis of pregnancy-associated VTE with your obstetric trainee after this consultation visit.

---

5. <u>Detail</u> the principal <u>mechanisms</u> contributing to pregnancy-associated VTE which you would teach your trainee. *(1 point per main and subbullet)*   Max 6

Virchow's triad:
- ☐ Venous stasis in the lower extremities
  - ○ Uterine compression
  - ○ Compression of the left iliac vein by the right iliac artery
  - ○ Hormonally induced venous dilation, leading to valvular incompetence and blood pooling
- ☐ Endothelial injury, particularly at instrumental vaginal delivery or Cesarean section
- ☐ Hypercoagulability
  - ○ Increased procoagulant factors (*i.e., Factors II, V, VII, VIII, IX, X, XII and VWF*)
  - ○ Decreased natural anticoagulants (*i.e., protein S, increased activated protein C resistance*)
  - ○ Fibrinolysis inhibition (*i.e., decreased tissue plasminogen activator (tPA), and increased platelet activator inhibitor-1 and placental-derived platelet activator inhibitor-2*)

You later present a schematic sketch of the anticoagulation pathway to reinforce an understanding of aberrations with inherited thrombophilia. You highlight that '*all thrombophilias are not created equal,*' with different thrombogenic potential guiding treatment.

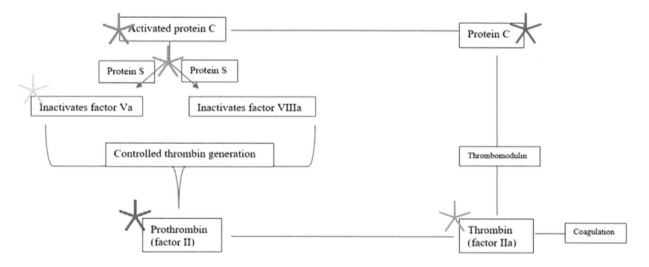

Figure 52.1

✶ signs represent thrombophilias interrupting the anticoagulant pathway (Adapted from: Seligsohn U, Lubetsky A. Genetic susceptibility to venous thrombosis. *N Engl J Med.* 2001;344 (16):1222–1231 and Williams Obstetrics, 24th edition, figure 52–1, page 1030)

6-A. Identify the 'star' symbol <u>and explain</u> the thrombophilic aberration representing   1
the *only mutation* where *increased* circulating levels of substrate result in
prothrombotic activity.

✶ Prothrombin G20210A polymorphism
  ○ Missense point mutation causes a *g*uanine to *a*denine nucleotide switch at the
    202010 position leads to increased gene translation

6-B. Identify the 'star' symbol rendering the substrate refractory to proteolysis by activated   1
protein C.

✶ Factor V Leiden mutation

---

7. List three mutations or assay abnormalities <u>not</u> recommended in thrombophilia screening.   Max 3
(1 point each)

☐ Methylenetetrahydrofolate reductase polymorphism (C677T, A1298C)
☐ Serum testing for increased homocysteine levels
☐ Factor VIII level *(nonstandardized assays and unknown prenatal interpretation)*
☐ Platelet activator inhibitor-1 polymorphism

---

8. Identify inherited thrombophilias warranting <u>both</u> antepartum and postpartum   4
thromboprophylaxis to prevent a first VTE in the context of a positive family history.
(1 point each)

High-risk inherited thrombophilias:
☐ Antithrombin deficiency *(homozygous form is always lethal)*
☐ Homozygous factor V Leiden mutation
☐ Homozygous prothrombin gene mutation G20210A
☐ Compound heterozygous factor V Leiden/prothrombin gene mutation

---

SCENARIO A

Eight months later, during your obstetrics call duty at a tertiary center, the patient, now 32^{+4} weeks' gestation by early dating sonography, presents to the obstetrics emergency assessment unit with a three-day history of groin pain with progressive swelling of her entire left leg. Occasionally, she has flank pain radiating to the buttocks. There are no obstetric complaints; fetal viability is ascertained at presentation. There is no history of trauma or immobility.

You have been following her antenatal care according to the management plan established during the preconception visit. Maternal-fetal aspects of prenatal care have been unremarkable to date.

9. Verbalize essentials of your focused physical examination. *(1 point per main bullet)*   Max 10

Vital signs and general appearance:
- ☐ Observe for general signs of discomfort related to dyspnea or pain
- ☐ Blood pressure
- ☐ Pulse *(assess for tachycardia)*
- ☐ Oxygen saturation
- ☐ Respiratory rate *(assess for tachypnea)*
- ☐ Temperature *(may demonstrate a mild/low-grade fever)*

Cardio-pulmonary system:
- ☐ Jugular venous distention
- ☐ Auscultation of the heart and lung
  - ○ Air entry, wheezing, right-sided heave, accentuated second heart sound (S2)

Lower extremity assessment:
- ☐ Difference of ≥2 cm among calf circumferences *(measured 10 cm below the tibial tuberosity)*
- ☐ Erythema
- ☐ Warmth
- ☐ Localized tenderness to the deep vein system
- ☐ Assess for lower extremity pulses

Vital signs and cardiopulmonary assessment are normal, and although she is in no acute distress, she is limping with a visibly swollen left leg[†] that is 4 cm larger than the contralateral calf and tenderness at the mid-thigh. The skin is of normal touch and color.

You notify the obstetric physician who will promptly attend to the patient. Meanwhile, your obstetric trainee is doing an on-line literature search for possible causes to explain the presentation.

Special note:
† Case scenario is structured to highlight (a) the predilection (70%–90%) for left-sided DVT in pregnancy, most commonly in proximal/pelvic veins, and (b) studies have demonstrated that risk of antenatal VTE is highest in the third trimester *(RCOG[9a])*

10. Facilitate your trainee's learning by providing <u>structured approach</u> to the diagnostic possibilities for her presentation. *(1 point each)*   Max 5

Vascular:
- ☐ DVT
- ☐ Superficial venous thrombosis (thrombophlebitis)
- ☐ Chronic venous insufficiency
- ☐ Popliteal venous or arterial aneurysm
- ☐ Lymphedema
- ☐ Cutaneous vasculitis

Soft tissue:
- ☐ Cellulitis
- ☐ Baker's cyst

Musculoskeletal:
- ☐ Ruptured/strained muscle or tendon
- ☐ Knee joint injury

11. In collaboration with the obstetric physician, identify two clinical presentations of large proximal DVT that would require urgent treatment and consideration for vascular intervention. *(1 point each)*   2

- ☐ 'Phlegmasia alba dolens' (painful white leg)
- ☐ 'Phlegmasia caerulea dolens' (painful blue leg)

12. What is the next <u>preferred,</u>[†] <u>most specific</u> test in the diagnostic evaluation of this patient? *(1 point each)*   2

SOGC:
- ☐ Compression ultrasound along the entire venous system from the femoral to the popliteal vein
- ☐ Doppler studies should be performed at the level of the iliac vein to ensure patency to flow

Special notes:
(a)[†] Magnetic resonance venography (MRV) is *rarely* used as an initial investigation
(b) Serum tests may show leukocytosis and increased C-reactive protein, but do not have a 'diagnostic' role

Given the heightened clinical suspicion, normal serum investigations performed upon presentation, and in the absence of contraindications, empiric[§] LMWH anticoagulation is given while awaiting imaging confirmation.

The radiologist informs you there is no evidence of thrombosis in the common femoral vein, femoral vein, or popliteal, with appropriate compressibility on Doppler interrogation. However, assessment of the common iliac vein and external iliac vein is suboptimal due to the gravid uterus.

You mention to teach your trainee that predictive scoring systems[†] have not been validated in prospective pregnant populations for gestationally associated DVT.

Special notes:

§ Recommended by ESC[7], RCOG[9b], GTH[13], ASTH-SOMANZ[14], and not by the remaining three societal guidelines *(Suggested Readings 3, 11, 12)*

† 'LEFt' rule *{i.e.,* Chan WS, Lee A, Spencer FA, et al. Predicting deep venous thrombosis in pregnancy: out in 'LEFt' field? [published correction appears in Ann Intern Med. 2009 Oct 6;151 (7):516]. *Ann Intern Med.* 2009;151(2):85–92}, and the modified Wells Score in pregnancy {O'Connor C, Moriarty J, Walsh J, Murray J, Coulter-Smith S, Boyd W. The application of a clinical risk stratification score may reduce unnecessary investigations for pulmonary embolism in pregnancy. *J Matern Fetal Neonatal Med.* 2011;24(12):1461–1464.}

---

13. Rationalize the findings on compression ultrasound and indicate your subsequent diagnostic plan. *(1 point each)*   2

☐ Compression ultrasound of the proximal veins is less sensitive for pelvic vein thrombosis *(more commonly encountered in pregnancy)* and calf vein thrombosis *(less common)*
☐ Given a 'high clinical suspicion'[‡] for iliac vein thrombosis, the next best management is pelvic magnetic resonance imaging (MRI)

Special note:
‡ If clinical suspicion were low to moderate, recommended management would be serial compression ultrasounds in three and seven days

---

MRI confirms a left iliac vein thrombus, for which therapeutic anticoagulation will be recommended.

---

14. What are <u>nonpharmacologic</u> strategies you would include in counseling with regard to acute DVT? *(1 point per main bullet)*   3

(RCOG[9b])
☐ Leg elevation
☐ Early ambulation/mobilisation
☐ Graduated elastic compression stocking
    ○ *reduces pain and edema, with unclear role in prevention of postthrombotic syndrome*

---

15. In collaboration with the obstetric internist/hematologist, list <u>serum investigations</u> performed in anticipation of requiring anticoagulation. *(1 point each)*   4

☐ CBC/FBC
☐ Coagulation screen
☐ Renal function tests (creatinine, urea, electrolytes)
☐ Liver function tests

16. Indicate situations, which may or may not pertain to this patient, where use of LMWH would be contraindicated or caution exercised. *(1 point each)*   Max 6

☐ Known bleeding disorder
☐ Active perinatal bleeding or increased risk of obstetric hemorrhage
☐ Serum platelet count $<75 \times 10^9/L$
☐ Heparin-induced thrombocytopenia *(from RCOG [9a], Section 10)*
☐ Severe renal disease (glomerular filtration rate <30 mL/min/1.73 m^2)
☐ Severe liver disease (prothrombin time above normal or known varices)
☐ Uncontrolled hypertension (systolic blood pressure >200 mmHg or diastolic blood pressure >120 mmHg)
☐ Acute ischemic or hemorrhagic stroke within the previous four weeks

SCENARIO B

Supplementary Suggested Readings *(most relevant to this section)*:

11. Bajc M, Neilly JB, Miniati M, Schuemichen C, Meignan M, Jonson B. **EANM** guidelines for ventilation/perfusion scintigraphy: Part 2. Algorithms and clinical considerations for diagnosis of pulmonary emboli with V/P(SPECT) and MDCT. *Eur J Nucl Med Mol Imaging.* 2009;36(9):1528–1538.

12. Leung AN, Bull TM, Jaeschke R, et al. American Thoracic Society documents: an official American Thoracic Society/Society of Thoracic Radiology Clinical Practice Guideline–Evaluation of Suspected Pulmonary Embolism in Pregnancy. *Radiology.* 2012;262 (2):635–646. **[ATS]**

13. Linnemann B, Bauersachs R, Rott H, et al. Diagnosis of pregnancy-associated venous thromboembolism – position paper of the Working Group in Women's Health of the Society of Thrombosis and Haemostasis (**GTH**). *Vasa.* 2016;45(2):87–101. doi:10.1024/0301–1526/a000503

14. McLintock C, Brighton T, Chunilal S, et al. Recommendations for the diagnosis and treatment of deep venous thrombosis and pulmonary embolism in pregnancy and the postpartum period. *Aust N Z J Obstet Gynaecol.* 2012;52(1):14–22. **[ASTH-SOMANZ]**

Eight months later, during your obstetrics call duty at a tertiary center, the patient, now 32^{+4} weeks' gestation by early dating sonography, presents to the obstetrics emergency assessment unit with a four-hour history of increasing breathlessness on exertion and pleuritic chest pain; she recently coughed up a streak of blood, which she has not experienced before. She has *no signs or symptoms of lower extremity DVT.*[‡] Fetal viability was ascertained at presentation. Vital signs and cardiopulmonary assessment are normal.

You have been following her antenatal care according to the management plan established during the preconception visit. Maternal-fetal aspects of prenatal care have been unremarkable to date.

Special note:

‡   Where PE is suspected in the presence of DVT symptoms, a compression ultrasound would obviate maternal-fetal radiation

17. Although nonspecific, elicit signs and symptoms that may raise suspicion for pregnancy-associated pulmonary embolism in this patient with a known inherited thrombophilia. *(1 point each)*

Max 6

Symptoms:
☐ Acute dyspnea
☐ Pleuritic chest pain
☐ Hemoptysis
☐ Palpitations
☐ New-onset cough

Signs:
☐ Tachycardia
☐ Tachypnea
☐ Hypoxia
☐ Hypotension
☐ Fever

18. What is your most probable diagnosis?

1

☐ Pulmonary embolism (PE)

Special note:
Risk stratification varies by international societal guideline from high/low *(RCOG[9b])*, low/nonlow *(SOGC[4])*, high/nonhigh *(ESC[7], ATS[12], GTH[13], ASTH-SOMAZ[14])*; only EANM[11] does not recommend risk stratification

You alert your trainee that among seven international medical society guidelines,[§] there are different proposed algorithms for investigations of suspected PE in pregnancy, with existing controversies regarding the *best* performance order of diagnostic modalities. Recently, in 2019, the pregnancy adapted YEARS algorithm *(Suggested Reading 10)* has been validated as a prediction tool in combination with serum D-dimer levels and lower extremity ultrasound. The most recent societal guideline *(European Society of Cardiology[7])* endorses the concept of clinical prediction tools, without indicating which tools to use. Meanwhile, other societal guidelines do not recommend use of clinical prediction tools to determine the status of PE in pregnancy *(SOGC[4], RCOG[9b], ATS[12], GTH[13], ASTH-SOMAZ[14])*, or do not discuss this topic *(EANM[11])*.

Special note:
§ *Suggested Readings 4, 7, 9b, 11–14*

19. Indicate the three <u>clinical prediction criteria</u> used in the pregnancy adapted YEARS algorithm. *(1 point each)*

3

☐ Clinical signs of DVT
☐ Hemoptysis
☐ PE as the most likely diagnosis

20. Discuss the concept, limitations and potential value of D-dimers in the diagnostic work-up of suspected PE in pregnancy. *(1 point each)*   3

D-dimers:
☐ D-dimers are the breakdown products of cross-linked fibrin, commonly elevated in pregnancy due to hypercoagulability

Limitations:
☐ Levels normally increase throughout pregnancy, thereby increasing the probability of false positives (low positive predictive value)

Potential value:
☐ D-dimers may be valuable when negative (<500 ng/mL) as many pregnant women will already have an elevated D-dimer concentration, although solitary testing in the absence of a validated clinical prediction rule in pregnancy is not advised for diagnostic evaluation of PE in pregnancy

Special note:
Laboratory D-dimer testing is only recommended by GTH[13] and not high-risk patients in the ESC guideline[7]; all five other international society guidelines do not recommend use of D-dimer testing (SOGC[4], RCOG[9b], EANM[11], ATS[12], ASTH-SOMANZ[14])

In accordance with your practice and the most probable diagnosis, the patient consents to empirical[§] treatment before imaging studies.

Special note:
§ Recommended by ESC[7], RCOG[9b], GTH[13], ASTH-SOMANZ[14], and not by the remaining three societal guidelines *(Suggested Readings 3, 11, 12)*

21. Although neither sensitive nor specific for PE, identify why chest radiography[†] is recommended by some societal guidelines[§] prior to advanced imaging modalities for suspected PE in pregnancy among patients at increased risk. *(1 point per main bullet)*   2

☐ Abnormal chest X-ray promotes consideration for alternative causes of chest symptoms, such as pneumonia, pneumothorax, or lobar collapse
   ○ *Radiologic findings with pulmonary infarction may include Hampton's hump (wedge-shaped opacity in the lung periphery), Westermark sign (decreased vascularity), atelectasis, effusion, or pulmonary edema*
☐ Chest X-ray may guide the choice of advanced imaging, with a normal/negative chest X-ray being followed by V/Q scan and abnormal/positive chest X-ray being followed by computed tomographic pulmonary angiography

Special notes:
† Refer to Chapter 73 for discussion on fetal exposure to ionizing radiation for chest X-ray
§ Recommended by ESC[7], RCOG[9b], ATS[12], GTH[13], ASTH-SOMANZ[14], and not by the remaining two societal guidelines *(Suggested Readings 4, 11)*

22. Indicate the two advanced imaging modalities used to diagnose PE in pregnancy, noting that the initial choice may depend on performance of chest radiography, local practice, and resources. *(1 point each)*

2

☐ Lung scintigraphy (ventilation/perfusion [V/Q] scan)
☐ Computed tomographic pulmonary angiography

23. Outline the principal technical aspects involved in V/Q scans and indicate maternal-fetal risks to discuss with the patient. *(1 point each)*

Max 7

Technical aspects:
☐ Ventilation (V): Involves inhalation of Tc-99m DTPA[†] (*i.e.*, a nebulized radioisotope)
☐ Ventilation scan is performed when perfusion scan is abnormal to minimize radiation exposure in pregnancy
☐ Perfusion (Q – *quotient*): Involves injection of Tc-99m MAA[‡]

Fetal risks with V/Q scan:[§]
☐ Estimated fetal radiation exposure from the ***ventilation lung scan (V)*** is 0.10–0.30 mGy, which is far below the 50 mGy (5 rad) threshold associated with fetal radiation complications
☐ Estimated fetal radiation exposure from ***perfusion lung scan*** with Tc-99m MAA is 0.02–0.20 mGy (***low-dose*** protocol) or 0.20–0.60 mGy (***high-dose*** protocol)

Maternal risks with V/Q scan:[§]
☐ Estimated radiation exposure to breast tissue from the ***ventilation lung scan (V)*** is <0.01 mGy
☐ Estimated radiation exposure to breast tissue from the ***perfusion lung scan*** with Tc-99m MAA is 0.16–0.5 mGy (***low-dose*** protocol) or 1.2 mGy (***high-dose*** protocol)

Special notes:
† DTPA= diethylene-triamine-pentaacetate
‡ MAA=microaggregated albumin
§ *Suggested Reading 7, table 12*

After extensive counseling, and in collaboration with the obstetric physician, a chest X-ray was deemed unnecessary; her V/Q scan results are indeterminate. You teach your trainee that recent meta-analysis[†] found an average prevalence of indeterminate results of 14%, with rates of up to 40%, for V/Q scans in pregnancy.

Special note:
† Tromeur C, van der Pol LM, Le Roux PY, et al. Computed tomography pulmonary angiography *versus* ventilation-perfusion lung scanning for diagnosing pulmonary embolism during pregnancy: a systematic review and meta-analysis. *Haematologica.* 2019;104(1):176–188.

24. What is your <u>next best</u> diagnostic test in evaluation of this patient?   1

☐ Computed tomographic pulmonary angiography

25. Discuss important aspects of counseling for computed tomographic pulmonary   Max 2
angiography and <u>elaborate</u> on its effect on maternal breast cancer. *(1 point per main bullet)*

Fetal:§
☐ Provide reassurance that estimated fetal radiation exposure is 0.05–0.5 mGy

Maternal:§
☐ Provide reassurance that modern computed tomographic pulmonary angiography techniques
have a negligible effect on the lifetime risk of maternal cancer, based on available data
  ○ *computed tomographic pulmonary angiography increases the lifetime risk of cancer by a*
    factor of 1.003–1.004
  ○ *Estimated radiation exposure to breast tissue is 3–10 mGy*
  ○ *Modern computed tomographic pulmonary angiography imaging techniques may expose*
    breast tissue to median doses as low as 3–4 mGy
☐ Indicate that CT technology has evolved, reducing radiation exposure without
compromising image quality

  Technical changes include:
  ○ *Reduced anatomical coverage of the scan*
  ○ *Reduced kilovoltage*
  ○ *Reduced contrast-monitoring component*
  ○ *Iterative reconstruction techniques*

Special note:
§ *Suggested Reading 7*

With a normal renal function and absence of contrast allergies, the patient provides informed
consent for computed tomographic pulmonary angiography.

The radiologist informs you of an abnormal opacification of the right interlobar pulmonary artery,
without other significant abnormalities.

There have not been any changes in the patient's hemodynamic status. She is returning to the
obstetric emergency assessment unit for subsequent management.

26-A. What is the treatment of choice for PE in pregnancy?   1

☐ LMWH is the treatment of choice for PE during pregnancy

26-B. List four advantages of LMWH over unfractionated heparin (UFH). *(1 point each)*   Max 4

Advantages of LMWH over UFH:†
☐ More predictable pharmacokinetic profile
☐ Fewer bleeding complication (*e.g., lower risk of heparin-induced thrombocytopenia*)
☐ Lower risk osteoporotic fractures (*0.04% vs 2%*) and loss of bone mineral density

☐ Dose-dependent clearance
☐ Longer half-life
☐ Low requirement for monitoring
☐ Less costly *(international variations may exist)*

Special note:
† UFH is preferred with severe renal insufficiency (creatinine clearance <30 mL/min) due to its combined hepatic and renal metabolism, or where option for rapid reversal of anticoagulation is important

27. In collaboration with the obstetric physician/hematologist, indicate important aspects of management and <u>preferred</u> treatment of pregnancy-associated VTE. *(1 point per main bullet, unless specified)*

Max 10

☐ Immediate initiation of therapeutic anticoagulation to decrease maternal mortality to <1%
☐ Therapeutic anticoagulation is recommended for a minimum of three months with acute VTE in pregnancy, with continued anticoagulation for remainder of pregnancy and for at least six weeks postpartum
  ○ *Given 32^{+4} weeks' gestation, this patient would require continued therapeutic anticoagulation until at least several weeks postpartum*
☐ Consideration for early antenatal obstetric anesthesia consultation

Options for therapeutic subcutaneous LMWH:†

(any regimen for 3 points {i.e., drug, dose, and frequency are 1 point each})
☐ Enoxaparin 1 mg/kg every 12 hours
☐ Enoxaparin 1.5 mg/kg once daily
☐ Enoxaparin 80 mg every 12 hours [body weight 70–89 kg]
☐ Enoxaparin 120 mg once daily [body weight 70–89 kg]
☐ Dalteparin 8000 IU every 12 hours [body weight 70–89 kg]
☐ Dalteparin 16,000 IU once daily [body weight 70–89 kg]
☐ Dalteparin 100 U/kg every 12 hours
☐ Dalteparin 200 U/kg once daily
☐ Tinzaparin 175 U/kg once daily

Therapeutic monitoring:
☐ Serum anti-Xa levels are of uncertain clinical benefit for monitoring of therapeutic LMWH based on a predictable pharmacokinetic profile, limitations in assays, and lack of evidence for optimal serum levels *(ASH 2018, ESC 2019, RCOG 2015: Suggested Readings 3, 7, 9)*
  ○ Routine therapeutic monitoring may be reserved for specific high-risk circumstances such as recurrent VTE, renal impairment, antithrombin deficiency and extremes of body weight [<50 kg and ≥90 kg]

Potential side effects of LMWH include, but are not limited to:

(1 point each; max 3. Other responses may be accepted)
☐ Injection-site bruising or hematomas
☐ Antepartum/postpartum bleeding
☐ Major skin reaction or allergy

- ☐ Elevated liver enzymes
- ☐ Decreased bone mineral density at therapeutic doses
- ☐ Heparin induced thrombocytopenia *{rare}*

Special note:
† International guidance variations exist; revision of local practice recommendations is suggested

The patient plans to be adherent with treatment and compliant with multidisciplinary care. She is concerned about labor analgesia and inquired about delivery plans, assuming pregnancy progresses well.

28. Discuss important elements of <u>delivery and postpartum</u> management in the context of therapeutic anticoagulation. She plans to breastfeed. *(1 point per main bullet)*   Max 6

- ☐ Consideration for elective induction of labor, with Cesarean section being reserved for obstetric indications *(case-based decision for timing of delivery)*
- ☐ Possible conversion to UFH at ~36–37 weeks (or earlier if preterm delivery is anticipated)
  - ○ *The purpose of conversion has less to do with risk of maternal bleeding at delivery, but rather the risk of spinal hematoma from neuraxial analgesia if reverting anticoagulation is inadequate*
- ☐ Ensure availability of blood product replacement
- ☐ In collaboration with an obstetric anesthesiologist, inform the patient that ≥24 hours should have elapsed since the last injection of LMWH before insertion of a spinal or epidural needle
- ☐ Postpartum reinitiation of *therapeutic LMWH* **≥24 hours** after the regional analgesia and **≥4 hours** after removal of the epidural catheter, provided the risk of postpartum bleeding is not increased and there has not been a blood/traumatic epidural
- ☐ Early notification of the obstetric anesthesiologist if the patient is unable to straight-leg raise at four hours from the last dose of epidural/spinal anesthetic‡
- ☐ Keep pneumatic compression devices until the patient is ambulatory and anticoagulation therapy restarted
- ☐ Options for postpartum anticoagulant therapy include heparins or oral vitamin K antagonist therapy *(i.e., warfarin)*§
  - ○ *For bridging therapy to warfarin, co-treatment with therapeutic heparin for at least five days until the international normalized ratio (INR) is therapeutic at 2.0–3.0 for two consecutive days to avoid warfarin's initial anti–protein C effect (i.e., paradoxical thrombosis and skin necrosis)*

Special notes:
‡ *Refer to* Yentis SM, Lucas DN, Brigante L, et al. Safety guideline: neurological monitoring associated with obstetric neuraxial block 2020: A joint guideline by the Association of Anaesthetists and the Obstetric Anaesthetists' Association. *Anaesthesia.* 2020;75(7): 913–919.
§ Direct oral anticoagulants should not be used in pregnancy or breastfeeding

With multidisciplinary collaboration, pregnancy progresses well, and the patient is switched to subcutaneous UFH† 15,000 U twice daily at 36⁺⁰ weeks' gestation.

The patient presents at 36^{+4} weeks' gestation in vigorous labor after recent spontaneous rupture of amniotic membranes; distressed with labor pains, she requests analgesia. Fetal cardiotocography tracing is normal and there is no vaginal bleeding. The patient indicates her last dose of subcutaneous UFH was 1.5 hours ago. Her INR is therapeutic. Experts affiliated in her care have been notified.

You teach your trainee that although use of protamine sulfate can fully reverse UFH, its use in pregnancy to facilitate neuraxial anesthesia has not been studied (SOAP[8]).

Special note:

† Conversion to UFH allows for more complete reversal of anticoagulation; protamine sulfate reverses anti-IIa fraction of LMWH without full reversal of the anti-Xa effect.

Although in clinical practice, LMWH twice daily would have been practical, the option of UFH was selected for *educational* purposes, with reference to Question 29.

---

29. If IV protamine sulfate were to be used upon hospital admission, explain how to calculate the amount of protamine sulfate required for reversal of UFH. *(1 point each)*   2

☐ Full neutralization requires 1 mg protamine sulfate per 100 U *residual* circulating heparin
☐ With a half-life of heparin of ~45 minutes, residual UFH is ~3750 U at 1.5 hours after injection, requiring 37.5 mg protamine sulfate

---

With acute reversal of anticoagulation and normal aPTT, the patient receives epidural analgesia. Labor proceeds uneventfully and a vigorous male is delivered spontaneously with appropriate birthweight for gestational age, normal umbilical cord blood gas values and normal Apgar scores.

The patient opted for postpartum warfarin treatment to avoid the nuisance of injections, knowing the importance of close follow-up for therapeutic drug monitoring. She has been informed that warfarin is safe with breastfeeding. After appropriate bridging of therapy and outpatient follow-ups arranged, you review her queries on contraceptive methods prior to discharge.

---

30. Outline features specific to contraceptive recommendations for this patient during the period of continued anticoagulation and thereafter. *(1 point each)*   Max 3

☐ Safe modalities include LNG-intrauterine system, progestin implants, DMPA, and progestin-oral contraceptives
☐ Although safe, copper-IUD is suboptimal *while on* anticoagulation due to increased vaginal bleeding and anemia; use after completion of anticoagulation could be offered
☐ All estrogen-containing contraceptives are contraindicated for patients with current/prior VTE
☐ Barrier methods (male or female condoms) can be offered

          TOTAL: 145

CHAPTER 53

Thrombotic Thrombocytopenic Purpura in Pregnancy

Paula D. James and Laura M. Gaudet

During your call duty, a *healthy* 32-year-old primigravida at 22^{+3} weeks' gestation, confirmed by first-trimester sonography, presents to the obstetrics emergency assessment unit of your hospital center with new-onset, asymptomatic port-wine-colored urine with chills and an oral temperature of 39.1°C at home; she also notes a two-day history of headache, now accompanied by visual changes. Your obstetric trainee informs you that clinical history is not suggestive of an infectious etiology, although comprehensive investigations are pending. She has no obstetric complaints, and fetal viability was ascertained upon presentation. Routine prenatal laboratory investigations, aneuploidy screening, and fetal morphology survey were unremarkable. The laboratory urgently notifies you that the platelet concentration is $12 \times 10^9/L$, confirmed on manual count; other requested laboratory tests are in progress.

Special note: *Although clinical presentations of thrombotic thrombocytopenic purpura (TTP) may be more 'subtle' than presented, the case scenario is designed for academic purposes, while avoiding overlap of content addressed in other chapters, including the differential diagnosis of thrombocytopenia in pregnancy. Readers are encouraged to complement subject matter where clinically required.*

LEARNING OBJECTIVES

1. Take a focused history from a prenatal patient presenting with cardinal features of thrombotic microangiopathy, demonstrating the ability to formulate a structured differential diagnosis of pregnancy-specific and non-pregnancy-related etiologies
2. Recognize laboratory derangements in TTP, including differential features from HELLP syndrome or preeclampsia
3. Initiate urgent multidisciplinary care for a prenatal patient with clinical and laboratory manifestations most consistent with TTP disease

4. Understand obstetrically relevant differences between acquired and congenital forms of TTP, fundamental to prenatal management and future preconception counseling
5. Appreciate the pathophysiology of TTP disease and the role of designated treatments

SUGGESTED READINGS

1. Battinelli EM. TTP and pregnancy. *Blood.* 2014;123(11):1624–1625.
2. Fyfe-Brown A, Clarke G, Nerenberg K, et al. Management of pregnancy-associated thrombotic thrombocytopenia purpura. *AJP Rep.* 2013;3(1):45–50.
3. Jiang Y, McIntosh JJ, Reese JA, et al. Pregnancy outcomes following recovery from acquired thrombotic thrombocytopenic purpura. *Blood.* 2014;123(11):1674–1680.
4. Keiser SD, Boyd KW, Rehberg JF, et al. A high LDH to AST ratio helps to differentiate pregnancy-associated thrombotic thrombocytopenic purpura (TTP) from HELLP syndrome. *J Matern Fetal Neonatal Med.* 2012;25(7):1059–1063.
5. Pourrat O, Coudroy R, Pierre F. Differentiation between severe HELLP syndrome and thrombotic microangiopathy, thrombotic thrombocytopenic purpura and other imitators. *Eur J Obstet Gynecol Reprod Biol.* 2015;189:68–72.
6. Savignano C, Rinaldi C, De Angelis V. Pregnancy associated thrombotic thrombocytopenic purpura: Practical issues for patient management. *Transfus Apher Sci.* 2015;53(3):262–268.
7. Scully M, Thomas M, Underwood M, et al. Thrombotic thrombocytopenic purpura and pregnancy: presentation, management, and subsequent pregnancy outcomes. *Blood.* 2014;124(2):211–219.
8. Vesely SK. Life after acquired thrombotic thrombocytopenic purpura: morbidity, mortality, and risks during pregnancy. *J Thromb Haemost.* 2015;13(Suppl 1):S216–S222.
9. von Auer C, von Krogh AS, Kremer Hovinga JA, et al. Current insights into thrombotic microangiopathies: thrombotic thrombocytopenic purpura and pregnancy. *Thromb Res.* 2015;135(Suppl 1):S30–S33.
10. Zheng XL, Vesely SK, Cataland SR, et al. ISTH guidelines for treatment of thrombotic thrombocytopenic purpura. *J Thromb Haemost.* 2020;18(10):2496–2502.

1. Which <u>additional</u> aspects of a focused history would you inquire about, either from your obstetric trainee or the patient? *(1 point each)*

Clinical signs/symptoms:[†]
☐ Nausea and/or vomiting
☐ Convulsions, confusion, or manifestations of stroke
☐ Epigastric and/or right upper quadrant pain
☐ New-onset rash, including its pattern
☐ Suspected oliguria, relative to standard urinary frequency in pregnancy
☐ Bloody diarrhea

Medications:
☐ Anticoagulants
☐ Recent antibiotic treatments, or use of other pharmacologic agents
☐ Inquire whether the patient is a Jehovah witness
☐ Allergies

Social features:
☐ Cigarette smoking, chronic alcohol abuse, or illicit drug use
☐ Ethnicity *(TTP is more common among non-Hispanic black race)*

Family history:
☐ Upshaw-Shulman syndrome (*i.e.,* congenital TTP) or other hereditary microangiopathies
☐ Autoimmune diseases

Special note:
†   Assessment for a source of infection related to fever and urinary manifestations would have been required in the absence of being specified in the clinical stem: '. . .*clinical history is not suggestive of an infectious etiology*. . .'

You learn that clinical history is only significant for a nonpruritic rash on both her lower legs, without inciting or alleviating factors. She takes no medications apart from routine prenatal vitamins and is not opposed to transfusion of blood products, although there have not been indications to date. She leads a healthy lifestyle and has no allergies. Family history appears noncontributory, although she has not recently contacted relatives in her African country of birth.

The patient's oral temperature is currently 38.9°C and pulse is 110 bpm; other vital signs are normal. Neurologic, cardiorespiratory and abdominal examinations are normal, without costo-vertebral angle tenderness. Numerous petechiae are evident on both lower extremities.

2. Apart from the platelet concentration, <u>explain</u> to your trainee which other features are of particular interest on full/complete blood count (FBC/CBC) as you consider a differential diagnosis. *(2 points each)*

Max 8

FBC/CBC Parameter	Rationale
☐ Leucocyte count	Leucocytosis beyond gestational range may be a marker of infection or acute fatty liver of pregnancy (AFLP)
☐ Hemoglobin concentration	Anemia (wide differential; potential need of replacement/transfusion)
☐ Reticulocyte count	Reticulocytosis suggests accelerated red cell destruction
☐ Lymphocyte count	Lymphopenia may be marker of autoimmune disease, infection, or malignancy
☐ Blood smear	Schistocytes, including triangular and helmet cells

Her hemoglobin concentration is 70 g/L (7.0 g/dL); reticulocytosis is noted and peripheral blood smear demonstrates numerous schistocytes, including burr and helmet cells. The lymphocyte count and leucocyte concentration are within normal for gestation. You take this opportunity to review potential etiologies for, or association with, such laboratory findings while recognizing the working diagnosis in the absence of other causations.

3. <u>Specify</u> the patient's hematological disorder on blood smear.

2

☐ Microangiopathic hemolytic anemia

4. Contemplate diagnostic considerations or risk factors for microangiopathic hemolytic anemia and thrombocytopenia with your obstetric trainee. *(1 point each)*

Max 6

Conditions specific to, or associated with, pregnancy:
☐ Acquired pregnancy-associated TTP
☐ HELLP syndrome
☐ Acute fatty liver of pregnancy (AFLP)

Conditions not specific to pregnancy:
☐ Hemolytic uremic syndrome
☐ Disseminated intravascular coagulation (DIC)
☐ Rheumatologic diseases, such as systemic lupus erythematosus (SLE) or antiphospholipid antibody syndrome
☐ Severe hypertension
☐ Infections, such as human immunodeficiency virus (HIV) or bacterial endocarditis
☐ Systemic malignancy
☐ Drug-induced manifestations after stem cell transplantation

5. In the absence of non-pregnancy-related conditions, highlight the patient's clinical and laboratory features consistent with the most probable diagnosis. *(1 point each)*   4

Four of five 'pentad' criteria of TTP:
- ☐ Severe thrombocytopenia *(i.e., 12 × 10⁹/L)*
- ☐ Hemolytic anemia *(i.e., schistocytes on peripheral blood smear, reticulocytosis, 'port wine' colored urine)*
- ☐ Fever
- ☐ Neurologic abnormalities *(i.e., headaches and visual changes)*

Special note:
Laboratory evidence of acute kidney injury is yet unavailable in this clinical scenario

You teach your trainee that the complete 'pentad,' with its associated increased maternal mortality rate, is now rarely encountered as diligent awareness and prompt initiation of therapy have improved maternal outcomes. You also alert your trainee that microangiopathic hemolytic anemia and severe thrombocytopenia in a priorly healthy patient may be sufficient to establish the acquired form of the disorder, as other components of the pentad may not yet be present.

A hematologist will attend to assist you in prompt management of this patient.

6. With reference to pathophysiology, explain why severe thrombocytopenia and microangiopathic hemolytic anemia form the principal manifestations of TTP. *(1 point each)*   2

- ☐ Thrombi formed by interaction of platelets with unprocessed Von Willebrand factor (VWF) multimers[†] in microvasculature result in thrombocytopenia
- ☐ Red blood cell fragmentation or shearing results from their passing through small vessels containing platelet-rich thrombi

Special note:
† Formation results from deficient ADAMTS13 enzyme

7. Among other requested maternal investigations, outline <u>laboratory results</u> that would be most compatible with TTP, realizing that not all may manifest in a given patient. *(1 point each)*   10

- ☐ Severely reduced ADAMTS-13[†] protease activity to <10% with inhibitor testing *(positive in acquired TTP)* or genetic studies *(enzymatic mutation in hereditary TTP)*
- ☐ Reduced serum haptoglobin
- ☐ Negative direct and indirect antiglobulin (Coombs') test[‡]
- ☐ Normal coagulation function *(i.e., PT, aPTT, INR)*
- ☐ Elevated indirect/unconjugated bilirubin
- ☐ Markedly elevated lactate dehydrogenase (LDH)[§]
- ☐ Elevated LDH/AST ratio >22.12 (or 25:1)
- ☐ Normal to minimally elevated hepatic transaminases (AST, ALT)
- ☐ Normal to minimally elevated serum creatinine
- ☐ Physiologic amount of proteinuria in pregnancy

Special notes:

† ADAMTS-13 represents '*A D*isintegrin *A*nd *M*etalloprotease with a *T*hrombo*S*pondin type 1 motif, member *13*, primarily produced by hepatocytes with minor amounts made by vascular endothelium

‡ Confirms that red cell hemolysis is of mechanical origin, not an autoimmune process

§ Manifestation of hemolysis and systemic ischemia

As multiple hepatic biomarkers further consolidate the working diagnosis, you collaborate with the hematologist in patient counseling and management. Your obstetric trainee appreciates that while severely deficient protease activity (<10%) and detection of its serum inhibitor would be confirmatory of disease in the absence of an alternate etiology, the challenges in testing, inherent delays in results, and imperfect sensitivity and specificity preclude it from decision-making regarding treatment of this life-threatening condition. You highlight the existing controversy in establishing a TTP diagnosis among patients whose ADAMTS-13 activity level is ≥10% with a compatible clinical presentation.

8. In collaboration with the hematologist, discuss important aspects of patient counseling regarding medical and obstetric considerations. *(1 point per main and subbullet)*   Max 10

Medical management:

☐ Inform the patient of the seriousness of the most likely diagnosis, TTP
  ○ Maternal mortality without treatment being ~50%, decreasing to 25% with treatment
  ○ Multiorgan damage and risk of long-term dysfunction *(see Question 15)*

☐ Explain the need for urgent and aggressive initiation of plasma exchange with fresh frozen plasma§/plasmapheresis

☐ Acknowledge the potential need for red blood cell transfusion to optimize maternal and utero-placental oxygenation *(i.e., in contrast to platelet transfusion; see Question 11)*

☐ (Where required), address the need for urgent transfer of care to a hospital center with expertise in maternal-fetal medicine and hematology

Obstetric considerations:

☐ Inform the patient that delivery does not cure the condition

☐ Timing and mode of delivery is based on clinical indications, including gestational age, treatment response, and fetal well-being

☐ Reassure the patient that the fetus/newborn is not affected by thrombocytopenia with maternal TTP

☐ Mention that stillbirth rate decreased with modern treatment from 69% to 45%†

☐ Antenatal consultations with anesthesiology and neonatology are warranted

Special notes:

† Martin JN Jr, Bailey AP, Rehberg JF, Owens MT, Keiser SD, May WL. Thrombotic thrombocytopenic purpura in 166 pregnancies: 1955–2006. *Am J Obstet Gynecol* 2008;199:98–104.

§ Different replacement solutions, similar to fresh frozen plasma exist with all being effective in TTP as they contain normal amounts of ADAMTS-13; solvent/detergent-treated plasma offers several advantages in the context of pregnancy *(refer to Suggested Reading 6)*

9. Given the high morbidity and mortality rates associated with untreated TTP, address a patient inquiry regarding potential ancillary therapy. *(1 point per main bullet)*   Max 2

- ☐ Corticosteroids
  - ○ *reserved for acquired form of TTP; contributes to inhibition of anti-ADAMTS-13 antibody formation*
- ☐ Caplacizumab
  - ○ *anti–Von Willebrand factor monoclonal antibody*
- ☐ Rituximab[†]
  - ○ *antineoplastic monoclonal antibody*
- ☐ Splenectomy for refractory TTP

Special note:
† Refer to Question 19 in Chapter 73

10. Explain to your trainee why you did not mention platelet transfusion as ancillary treatment for TTP, recognizing an indication for administration. *(1 point each)*   2

- ☐ Platelet transfusion may result of increased thrombus formation
- ☐ Current recommendations are that platelet transfusion should only be used to prevent or manage life-threatening hemorrhage *(Suggested Reading 2)*

The patient appreciates your counseling and provides consent for plasmapheresis, which will be arranged by the hematologist. She is grateful that your hospital center offers advanced medical and obstetric care; a maternal-fetal medicine expert will collaborate in prenatal care. Understanding that the disorder may have presented in nonpregnant states, the patient is curious whether pregnancy lowered the threshold for disease onset.

11. Provide rationale for the association, or lack thereof, between pregnancy and onset of TTP. *(1 point each)*   3

Reasons why TTP is 10-times more common in pregnancy than the general population:
- ☐ Physiologic decrease of ADAMTS13 protease activity due to increased gestational levels of VWF
- ☐ Hypercoagulable state of pregnancy
- ☐ Synergistic features of TTP and preeclampsia/HELLP syndrome

Large volume daily plasma exchange is commenced, continuing for 48 hours after the platelet count rose to $>150 \times 10^9$/L and LDH levels improved; remission was achieved after 23 days. This was not surprising, having later received pretreatment ADAMTS-13 protease level being 6% with high levels of anti-ADAMTS-13 IgG autoantibodies. Hemoglobin concentration improves with treatment of hemolysis. In the early days of therapy, fetal viability was regularly ascertained by Doptone; this was converted to cardiotocography (CTG) upon fetal viability.

12. Discuss with your trainee the <u>obstetric</u> relevance of differentiating acquired from congenital TTP based on presence of ADAMTS-13 inhibitor antibody or genetic mutation of the protease itself, respectively. *(1 point each)*

Max 3

☐ Corticosteroids are only required for acquired disease to promote suppression of autoantibody formation

☐ Acquired TTP is treated with plasma exchange therapy to remove ADAMTS-13 inhibitor and replenish normal protease enzyme

☐ Congenital TTP requires serial antenatal plasma infusion, continued until six weeks postpartum; this is due to the high risk of fetal loss and relapsing TTP *(Suggested Reading 7 and ISTH[10])*

☐ Family study would be indicated in congenital TTP to identify siblings or relatives with ADAMTS-13 mutations *(Suggested Reading 13)*

13. Outline why plasma <u>exchange</u> is preferable to plasma <u>infusion</u> as therapeutic intervention for *acquired[†]* TTP. *(1 point each)*

4

☐ Plasma exchange allows for removal of ADAMTS-13 inhibitor (autoantibody)
☐ Improved survival rates[‡]
☐ Improved remission rates[‡]
☐ Increased volume of administered plasma

Special notes:

† Plasma infusion is generally adequate for *hereditary* TTP as it supplies ADAMTS13 to compensate for the genetically mutated enzyme

‡ Refer to Michael M, Elliott EJ, Ridley GF, Hodson EM, Craig JC. Interventions for haemolytic uraemic syndrome and thrombotic thrombocytopenic purpura. *Cochrane Database Syst Rev.* 2009;2009(1):CD003595

At 35^{+4} weeks' gestation, the patient presents to the obstetrics emergency assessment unit feeling unwell and complaining of a headache and epigastric pain. There are no obstetric complaints. Blood pressure is 150/100 mmHg on two measurements, oxygen saturation is 97%, and her temperature is 38.3°C orally. Neurological examination is normal. Her extremities are covered with purpura and petechiae. A urine sample is port-wine colored, similar to her initial presentation, with new 3+ proteinuria on dipstick. The CTG monitor ascertains uterine quiescence and a normal fetal heart tracing. Antihypertensive treatment will be initiated.

Recalling that preeclampsia/HELLP syndrome can occur in 17% of gravidas with TTP *(Suggested Reading 2)* timely multidisciplinary collaboration is arranged in attempt to establish the etiology of her presentation, crucial to planning medical and obstetric management.

14. Outline features that *may contribute* to a diagnosis of TTP relapse relative to preeclampsia or HELLP syndrome. *(1 point each)*

Max 10

Clinical:
☐ Petechiae/purpura
☐ Fever
☐ Absence of acute weight gain and body swelling/edema

Investigations:[†]
☐ Evidence of microangiopathic hemolytic anemia on peripheral blood smear
☐ Gross hemoglobinuria
☐ Increased LDH/AST ratio >22.12 (or 25:1)
☐ ADAMTS-13 protease activity at <10%
☐ Normal coagulation function, without signs of DIC
☐ Normal sFlt-1/PlGF ratio *(increased in preeclampsia)*
☐ Sonographic absence of signs suggestive of uteroplacental insufficiency, such as oligohydramnios, FGR/suboptimal growth velocity, or abnormal umbilical artery Doppler velocimetry

Management:
☐ Corticosteroids do not result in rapid resolution (within 8–12 hours) of severe thrombocytopenia[‡]
☐ Positive response to plasmapheresis
☐ Failure to improve after delivery

Special notes:
† Histological evidence is both invasive and impractical as thrombocytopenia encountered in most patients prohibits renal biopsy

‡ Martin JN Jr, Bailey AP, Rehberg JF, Owens MT, Keiser SD, May WL. Thrombotic thrombocytopenic purpura in 166 pregnancies: 1955–2006. *Am J Obstet Gynecol* 2008;199:98–104.

With investigations favoring relapsing TTP, plasma exchange is commenced, guided by her blood pressure, urine output and fetal heart rate tracing on cardiotocography. On the second day of therapy, fetal heart tracing demonstrated absent variability and recurrent deep variable decelerations unresponsive to intrauterine resuscitation. An urgent Cesarean section was necessary under general anesthesia as platelet count had only increased from 9×10^9/L to 43×10^9/L. Platelet and red cell transfusions were required intraoperatively to manage surgical site bleeding. Plasmapheresis resumed postoperatively. The patient was initially managed in a high-dependency unit, followed by routine postnatal wards where she remained for five days.

Prior to hospital discharge, the patient voices appreciation for the medical and psychological care provided. Despite a difficult prenatal course, she is already contemplating a future pregnancy. In the meantime, she understands that only non-estrogen-containing contraceptive methods would be offered due to the risk of recurrent acquired-TTP with combined oral contraception.

15. Counsel the patient on future pregnancy considerations regarding <u>acquired</u> TTP.   Max 8
   (1 point each)

□ Address the need for prenatal care in a high-risk center, under care of maternal-fetal medicine and hematology experts

□ Risk of recurrent TTP in future pregnancy is 45% with acquired pregnancy-associated TTP[†]

□ Mention that most pregnancies, with appropriate management, results in live births

□ Close clinical follow-up and diligence for onset of possible signs/symptoms of TTP relapse

□ Increased risk of preeclampsia, even in the absence of recurrent episodes of TTP in future pregnancy *(Suggested Reading 3)*

□ Preconception assessment of ADAMTS-13 levels and anti-ADAMTS-13 antibodies

□ Prophylactic treatment is recommended for asymptomatic patients with low plasma ADAMTS-13 activity (*e.g.*, <30 U/dL or <30% of normal) due to risk of poor maternal-infant outcomes; limited evidence exists on effect of available regimens *(ISTH guidelines[10])*

□ Individualized decision-making regarding frequency of monitoring of ADAMTS-13 activity; recommend monitoring at the onset of pregnancy and at least every trimester if values remain normal *(Suggested Readings 6, 7)*

□ Antenatal monitoring of platelet count, LDH, haptoglobin and evidence of microangiopathic hemolysis at least monthly

□ Serial fetal sonographic assessment for growth biometry and Doppler velocimetry for placental function

Special notes:

Little supporting evidence for *routine* prophylaxis with low molecular weight heparin (LMWH) or low dose aspirin in prevention of TTP recurrences in the absence of a history of venous thromboembolism (VTE) with platelet count remaining $>50 \times 10^9$/L

† Vesely SK, Li X, McMinn JR, Terrell DR. George JN. Pregnancy outcomes after recovery from thrombotic thrombocytopenic purpura-hemolytic uremic syndrome. *Transfusion.* 2004;44(8):1149–1158.

† Recurrence rate is up to 92% with congenital TTP

---

16. Address the patient's inquiry regarding <u>long-term complications</u> associated with TTP.   Max 4
   (1 point each)

□ Transfusion-associated morbidities (*e.g.*, infections, atypical antibodies)

□ Relapse of TTP

□ Chronic hypertension

□ Renal disease requiring dialysis or transplantation

□ Systemic lupus erythematosus (SLE)

□ Major depression

□ Cognitive deficits

□ Mortality

TOTAL: **90**

CHAPTER 54

Thrombocytopenia in Pregnancy

Amira El-Messidi, Marwa Salman, and Anita Banerjee

During your obstetric call duty in a tertiary hospital center, you receive a telephone call from a colleague at an external center for an incidental isolated platelet count of 69×10^9/L in a 22-year-old primigravida with a singleton pregnancy at 24^{+3} weeks' gestation by early dating sonography. The full/complete blood count (FBC/CBC) was performed to follow up on iron-deficiency anemia. Fetal activity is normal.

LEARNING OBJECTIVES

1. Collaborate with an obstetric care provider inquiring about incidental thrombocytopenia in an obstetric patient
2. Initiate laboratory investigations for newly identified thrombocytopenia in pregnancy, recognizing etiologies that may or may not relate to pregnancy
3. Appreciate the indications and treatments for probable immune thrombocytopenic purpura (ITP) in the antenatal period with continued multidisciplinary collaboration
4. Detail comprehensive aspects of intrapartum and postpartum care of an obstetric patient with thrombocytopenia

SUGGESTED READINGS

1. ACOG Practice Bulletin No. 207: Thrombocytopenia in pregnancy. *Obstet Gynecol.* 2019;133(3):e181–e193.
2. Baucom AM, Kuller JA, Dotters-Katz S. Immune thrombocytopenic purpura in pregnancy. *Obstet Gynecol Surv.* 2019;74(8):490–496.
3. Care A, Pavord S, Knight M, et al. Severe primary autoimmune thrombocytopenia in pregnancy: a national cohort study. *BJOG.* 2018;125(5):604–612.
4. Cines DB, Levine LD. Thrombocytopenia in pregnancy. *Hematology Am Soc Hematol Educ Program.* 2017;2017(1):144–151.
5. Fogerty AE. Thrombocytopenia in pregnancy: approach to diagnosis and management. *Semin Thromb Hemost.* 2020;46(3):256–263.
6. Gernsheimer T, James AH, Stasi R. How I treat thrombocytopenia. *Blood* 2013;121(1): 38–47.
7. Eslick R, McLintock C. Managing ITP and thrombocytopenia in pregnancy. *Platelets.* 2020;31(3):300–306.

8. Goldman BG, Hehir MP, Yambasu S, et al. The presentation and management of platelet disorders in pregnancy. *Eur J Haematol.* 2018;100(6):560–566.
9. Pishko AM, Levine LD, Cines DB. Thrombocytopenia in pregnancy: Diagnosis and approach to management. *Blood Rev.* 2020;40:100638.
10. Provan D, Arnold DM, Bussel JB, et al. Updated international consensus report on the investigation and management of primary immune thrombocytopenia. *Blood Adv.* 2019;3(22):3780–3817.

POINTS

1. What aspects of a focused history would you inquire about in <u>telephone conversation</u> with the obstetric provider? *(1 point each; max points indicted where required)*

Max 25

Features related to the laboratory result:
- ☐ Determine the trend in platelet count relative to routine prenatal testing and values prior to pregnancy, if available
- ☐ Ascertain if the result is validated on repeat FBC/CBC or by manual count
- ☐ Assess the severity of anemia relative to the stage of pregnancy

Features associated with obstetric care:
- ☐ Results of routine prenatal virology tests [*i.e.,* HIV, HBV, and HCV] and result of other virology screening, if testing was indicated [*e.g.,* CMV, parvovirus B19]
- ☐ Signs or symptoms of hypertensive diseases (preeclampsia/HELLP syndrome)
- ☐ Signs or symptoms of acute fatty liver of pregnancy (AFLP)
- ☐ Signs or symptoms of venous thromboembolism in pregnancy
- ☐ Current/recent vaginal bleeding, gingival bleeding, or epistaxis

Medical, surgical and gynecologic histories: *(max 5)*
- ☐ Ascertain there are no undisclosed early pregnancy losses or therapeutic terminations
- ☐ Prior blood product transfusions
- ☐ Thyroid dysfunction
- ☐ Liver disease
- ☐ Systemic infections (*e.g., H. pylori,* Shiga-toxin mediated hemolytic uremic syndrome, malaria)
- ☐ Known history or symptoms of autoimmune disease (*e.g.,* systemic lupus erythematosus [SLE], antiphospholipid antibody syndrome, rheumatoid arthritis, scleroderma)
- ☐ History of prolonged bleeding after trauma, surgical or dental procedures
- ☐ Antecedent menorrhagia
- ☐ Current/prior malignancy or transplant

Medications and allergies: *(max 3)*
- ☐ Commonly used agents in pregnancy that are known to cause thrombocytopenia (*e.g.,* heparin, penicillins, and cephalosporins), particularly if initiated in the past few weeks
- ☐ Over the counter or '*home remedy*' agents with potential anticoagulant effects
- ☐ Confirm use of folic acid containing prenatal vitamins[†]
- ☐ Recent exposure to toxin(s), including immunosuppressants

Social features and routine health maintenance: *(max 3)*
- ☐ Occupation-prone exposure to blood-borne products
- ☐ Dietary practices, primarily for risk of folate and vitamin B12 deficiencies

☐ Chronic alcohol consumption or illicit drug use
☐ Recent travel
☐ Recent vaccinations (*e.g.*, pertussis, *H. influenza*, COVID-19)
☐ High-risk sexual practices

Family history:
☐ Genetic thrombocytopenia (*e.g.*, Bernard-Soulier syndrome, Evans syndrome, Glanzmann thrombasthenia), thrombotic microangiopathy syndromes, history of excessive bleeding/bruising, or thrombocytopenic complications in pregnancy

Inquire on physical examination findings:
☐ General appearance of unwellness or skeletal deformity[§]
☐ Blood pressure and pulse
☐ Temperature[‡]
☐ Mucocutaneous bleeding, petechiae, purpura
☐ Evidence of needle track marks
☐ Evidence of eczema[§§]
☐ Hepatosplenomegaly
☐ Lymphadenopathy
☐ Fetal viability

Special notes:
[†]   Folate deficiency can result in thrombocytopenia
[§]   Absent radius can suggest thrombocytopenia-absent radium syndrome
[§§] Component of Wiskott-Aldrich syndrome
[‡]   Although a component of vital signs, focused inquiry reflects consideration of pregnancy-specific and non-pregnancy-specific etiologies

Your colleague indicates that the platelet count was reported by automated laboratory technology, which had revealed a normal value in early pregnancy. Routine prenatal virology screening was unremarkable, and the patient is HBV-immune. Her prenatal course has been unremarkable. Although now asymptomatic, she recalls occasional bleeding gums with tooth brushing and increased bruising of her arms and legs. Social history is unremarkable. As you requested, your colleague confirmed with the patient that she takes iron supplements and folic acid-containing prenatal vitamins without use of other unprescribed pharmacologic agents or medicinals. Common to her mother and sister, medical history suggests menorrhagia for which she never sought medical attention.

Your colleague reports a normal blood pressure and temperature; no abnormalities are detected on physical examination. Fetal viability has been ascertained.

2. Present your colleague with a <u>structured</u> approach for potential causes for thrombocytopenia (TCP) in pregnancy that *may or may not* relate to this patient. *(1 point each)*

Max 10

	Conditions specific to pregnancy	Conditions not specific to pregnancy
Isolated TCP	☐ Gestational TCP	☐ Primary ITP (*i.e.,* autoimmune IgG-mediated thrombocytopenia) ☐ Secondary ITP ☐ Pseudo-TCP due to platelet-agglutination induced by ethylenediaminetetraacetic acid ☐ Drug-induced TCP ☐ Type IIB Von Willebrand' disease ☐ Congenital TCP
TCP-associated systemic disorders	☐ Preeclampsia ☐ HELLP syndrome ☐ AFLP	☐ SLE ☐ Antiphospholipid syndrome ☐ Infections (*e.g.,* HIV, HBV, HCV, *H. pylori*) ☐ Thyroid dysfunction ☐ TTP ± hemolytic uremic syndrome ☐ Disseminated intravascular coagulation (DIC) ☐ Bone marrow disorders ☐ Folate and/or vitamin B12 deficiency ☐ Splenic sequestration–associated conditions (*e.g.,* hepatic disease, storage disease, portal vein thrombosis)

(Suggested Reading 6)

3. Inform your colleague of <u>laboratory investigations</u> you would <u>recommend or advise</u>   Max 8
<u>consideration for</u>[†] in evaluation of this patient, assuming repeat automated count shows
a consistent level of TCP. *(1 point per main bullet)*

☐ Peripheral blood film revision of all three cell lines: white blood cells, red blood cells, and
platelets

☐ VWD type IIB testing*
   ○ VWF: ristocetin cofactor activity [VWF: RCo] and VWF antigen; confirmatory testing
   includes ristocetin-induced platelet aggregation and genetic analysis

☐ Hemolysis labs: [reticulocyte count, lactate dehydrogenase (LDH), haptoglobin levels, total
and direct bilirubin]

☐ Liver transaminases: [aspartate aminotransferase (AST), alanine aminotransferase (ALT)]

☐ Serum creatinine and spot urine protein/creatinine ratio

☐ Coagulation screen: [prothrombin time (PT), activated partial thromboplastin time
(aPTT), fibrinogen, D-dimers]

☐ Direct antiglobulin (Coombs) test[‡]

☐ TSH, free thyroxine level, ± antithyroid antibodies

☐ Antiphospholipid antibodies: [lupus anticoagulant, anticardiolipin antibodies, ß2
glycoprotein-I antibodies]

☐ Antinuclear antibody

☐ Consideration for quantitative immunoglobulins[§]

☐ Consideration for *H. pylori* stool or antigen test

☐ Consideration for Shiga-toxin testing, where hemolytic uremic syndrome is suspected

☐ Consideration for repeat HIV and HCV testing

Special notes:

† Bone marrow examination, antiplatelet antibody testing, and thrombopoietin levels are
<u>not</u> indicated *(Suggested Reading 10)*

Comprehensive assessment of the peripheral smear ensures absence of a
thrombocytopenia associated with a microangiopathic process

* Testing is critical in the context of this patient's medical and family history

‡ Supports assessment of potential hemolysis-associated thrombocytopenia (*i.e.*, Evans
syndrome) in the setting of anemia and reticulocytosis

§ Testing may reveal underlying immunodeficiency, such as common variable immune
deficiency

In a planned timely follow-up conversation with the obstetric provider, you learn that the limited
number of platelets found on peripheral smear examination are larger than normal; there are no
signs of clumping or red cell fragmentation. Although assessment of quantitative immunoglobins
and first-tier tests for VWD are unavailable in your colleague's hospital center, all remaining
investigations for evaluation of isolated TCP in pregnancy are unremarkable.

4. What is your <u>next best recommendation</u> to the obstetric provider for management of this patient?   4

☐ Transfer to a tertiary center for multidisciplinary care by maternal-fetal medicine, hematology, transfusion medicine, anesthesiology, and neonatology

With timely transfer of the patient to the tertiary center where you practice maternal-fetal medicine, you ascertain her medical history and unchanged findings on maternal assessment. Obstetric sonography confirms normal fetal biometry without evidence of fetoplacental hemorrhagic complications; amniotic fluid volume is normal. Follow-up hematologic values are stable; results of VWD or hemolysis-associated thrombocytopenia remain pending. The patient's blood type is B-positive without atypical red blood cell antibodies. Gestational diabetes screening, performed routinely in your jurisdiction, is normal.

5. In collaboration with a hematologist, outline aspects to discuss with the patient regarding the etiology of TCP and initial management. *(1 point per main and subbullet)*   8

☐ While TCP is physiologic in pregnancy with platelet counts *mostly* $>70–80 \times 10^9$/L, gestational TCP has also been reported with platelet counts at $50–80 \times 10^9$/L *(Suggested Reading 6)*, or as low as 43×10^9/L[†] *(Suggested Reading 1)*

☐ In the absence of other diagnostic possibilities, the main differential diagnosis would be gestational TCP or primary ITP

☐ Differentiating between gestational TCP or primary ITP may only be possible postpartum, although the exact diagnosis has little bearing on antepartum and intrapartum management for the remainder of pregnancy

☐ Reassure the patient that earlier diagnosis would not have altered management in the absence of indications warranting therapeutic intervention:
  ○ Planned diagnostic or therapeutic procedure
  ○ Bleeding complications
  ○ Platelet counts <20 to 30×10^9/L[‡]

☐ In the absence of a universally accepted surveillance protocol, initiation of weekly platelet counts may be considered based on clinical reasoning until relative ascertainment of diagnosis, or need to initiate treatment

Special notes:

† *Refer to* Burrows RF, Kelton JG. Thrombocytopenia at delivery: a prospective survey of 6715 deliveries. *Am J Obstet Gynecol* 1990;162:731–4

‡ *Refer to* Rajasekhar A, Gernsheimer T, Stasi R, James AH. 2013 Clinical practice guide on thrombocytopenia in pregnancy. Washington, DC: American Society of Hematology. Available at www.hematology.org.proxy3.library.mcgill.ca/Clinicians/Guidelines-Quality/Quick-Reference.aspx, accessed September 10, 2021.

6. Respond to a patient inquiry about potential reasons for physiologic decreases in gestational platelet count, noting that an interplay of multiple mechanisms is most likely. *(1 point each)*

    Max 2

- ☐ Hemodilution from expanded plasma volume
- ☐ Increased von Willebrand factor (VWF) expression, leading to increased platelet binding and clearance
- ☐ Enhanced platelet sequestration in the placenta *(similar to splenic sequestration)*
- ☐ Pregnancy-induced antiplatelet antibody formation
- ☐ Insufficient response to thrombopoietin

Consultation with the obstetric anesthesiologist takes place during this clinical visit. Meanwhile, arrangements are made for the patient to repeat the automated platelet count in one week. She understands the importance of prompt presentation to the obstetric emergency assessment unit in the event of bleeding or new-onset systemic complains. Routine receipt of the pertussis vaccine in the context of maternal thrombocytopenia was addressed with the patient, as general benefits of vaccination outweigh risks of ecchymosis and/or bleeding.

7. Summarize considerations for <u>intrapartum anesthesia</u> as indicated in the obstetric anesthesiologist's consultation report with regard to thrombocytopenia. *(1 point each)*

    5

- ☐ As the precise platelet count needed to safely perform neuraxial analgesia is unknown, practices may depend on local guidelines and individual preferences
- ☐ Spinal epidural hematoma associated with a platelet count $\geq 70 \times 10^9$/L is likely to be very low in obstetric patients with thrombocytopenia secondary to gestational thrombocytopenia, ITP, and hypertensive disorders of pregnancy in the absence of other risk factors[†]
- ☐ Platelet transfusion is not appropriate solely to prepare for spinal anesthesia, as posttransfusion increments may be inadequate or short-lived; platelet transfusion should be reserved to treat bleeding complications or to raise platelet levels $>50 \times 10^9$/L if Cesarean delivery is required
- ☐ Collaboration with experts in hematology and maternal-fetal medicine will take place for antenatal treatment considerations, particularly in the one to two weeks prior to anticipated delivery, to maximize the platelet count for delivery considerations
- ☐ If platelet counts at delivery remain low but $>20\text{–}30 \times 10^9$/L, alternate considerations for labor analgesia would be considered

Special note:

† *Refer to* Bauer ME, Arendt K, Beilin Y, et al. The Society for Obstetric Anesthesia and Perinatology Interdisciplinary Consensus Statement on Neuraxial Procedures in Obstetric Patients With Thrombocytopenia. *Anesth Analg.* 2021;132(6):1531–1544.

Weekly automated platelet counts remain stable for two weeks, without signs or symptoms of maternal-fetal bleeding. The patient is being managed expectantly.

At 26^{+0} weeks' gestation, the patient complains of hematuria and new-onset petechial hemorrhages, evident on all extremities. She does not have obstetric complaints; the patient remains normotensive, afebrile, and the platelet count is now 52×10^9/L.[†] Comprehensive assessment is not suggestive of a thrombotic microangiopathy, urine culture is free of an infectious etiology, and fetal-placental sonography remains unremarkable. In collaboration with the hematologist, therapeutic intervention will be addressed for probable primary ITP, in the absence of alternative etiologies.

You learn that diagnostic assays for VWD were not processed due to technical factors and repeat testing will be arranged.

Special note:

[†] This case scenario highlights the importance of *clinical correlation* with laboratory platelet counts; treatment is warranted based on bleeding manifestations regardless of a designated laboratory value.

---

8. With focus on primary ITP, describe the relationship between maternal and fetal-neonatal platelet counts to address with the patient. *(1 point each)*

Max 2

☐ There is no direct way to measure fetal platelet count; maternal-fetal risks of intervention outweigh benefits

☐ The correlation between fetal and maternal platelet counts is poor; a positive maternal treatment response does not protect against newborn thrombocytopenia (despite treatments that cross placenta) and failed maternal treatment does not increase the risk of adverse neonatal outcome

☐ Among mothers with ITP, {~10% of newborns will have platelets counts $<50 \times 10^9$/L and ~5% have platelets counts $<20 \times 10^9$/L, with rare risks of severe neonatal hemorrhagic complications, particularly intracranial hemorrhage[‡] $(<1\%)$}[†]

Special notes:

[†] *Suggested Readings 1, 10, with reference to* (a) Webert KE, Mittal R, Sigouin C, Heddle NM, Kelton JG. A retrospective 11-year analysis of obstetric patients with idiopathic thrombocytopenic purpura. *Blood.* 2003;102(13):4306–4311, and (b) Loustau V, Debouverie O, Canoui-Poitrine F, Baili L, Khellaf M, Touboul C, et al. Effect of pregnancy on the course of immune thrombocytopenia: a retrospective study of 118 pregnancies in 82 women. *Br J Haematol* 2014;166:929–35.

[‡] Evidence of intracranial hemorrhage on antenatal fetal sonography is exceedingly rare among mothers with ITP; this rare finding usually occurs in the *neonatal* period, in contrast to fetal-neonatal alloimmune thrombocytopenia

9. In the absence of contraindications, outline <u>first-line</u> therapeutic options for this obstetric patient with probable primary ITP, and highlight expected disease-related response. *(1 point per main and subbullet)*   4

☐ Oral corticosteroids[†] (*e.g.,* prednisone 1 mg/kg), where this high dose could be justified in the context of the patient's hematuria, despite the general lack of proven benefit relative to lower starting doses (*e.g.,* prednisone 10–20 mg/d)
   o Initial treatment response usually occurs within 4–14 days and peaks in one to four weeks
☐ Intravenous immunoglobulin (IVIG) 1–2 g/kg delivered over two to five days
   o Initial treatment response is usually rapid, within a mean of two days of infusion, peaking within two to seven days, yet effects are often transient

Special note:
†   Refer to Question 3 in Chapter 45 for fetal risks associated with maternal corticosteroids

10. Apart from a rapid treatment response, identify <u>maternal features</u> where IVIG may be a preferred first choice to oral corticosteroids. *(1 point each)*   Max 5

☐ Hypertension or high risk thereof in pregnancy
☐ Underlying obesity or increased gestational weight gain
☐ Gestational or preexisting diabetes
☐ Mental illness/psychosis
☐ Underlying osteoporosis or increased thereof
☐ Risk of nonadherence to daily intake of corticosteroids

After comprehensive interdisciplinary discussion and informed consent, the patient agrees to remain adherent to *combination therapy* (*i.e.,* second-line treatment) with IVIG and oral corticosteroids in view of bleeding manifestations. As was discussed with the patient, she experienced primary adverse side effects, being general malaise and headache during IVIG therapy, although no active treatment was required.

Continuation of corticosteroids at the same dose for 21 days is planned *(Suggested Reading 1)*. While tapering is generally recommended thereafter, the hematologist may continue basal dose corticosteroid to maintain a stable platelet count for the remainder of pregnancy and prevent recurrent bleeding.

11. Address a patient concern regarding other treatment options that may be considered in the second trimester, third trimester, or either trimester, should she develop side effects to combination IVIG and oral corticosteroids or not respond to treatment. *(1 point each)*   **Max 4**

☐ Intravenous methylprednisolone in combination with IVIG and/or azathioprine
☐ Intravenous anti-D immunoglobulin as this patient is anti-D-positive and nonsplenectomised
☐ Rituximab°
☐ Thrombopoietin-receptor agonist *[Limited safety data in pregnancy]*
☐ Azathioprine‡ or cyclosporine *[suboptimal options in the third trimester as treatment response may take three to six months]*
☐ Splenectomy is best performed in the *second* trimester for refractory ITP

Special notes:
° Refer to Question 19 in Chapter 73
‡ Refer to Question 42 in Chapter 42 for discussion on fetal/neonatal risks and pregnancy recommendations with azathioprine therapy

You mention to your obstetric trainee that use of other therapies for ITP, including vinca alkaloids, cyclophosphamide, danazol, and mycophenolate mofetil are contraindicated in pregnancy.

Having heard of evidence, albeit limited, for effectiveness of anti-D immunoglobulin in raising maternal platelet count in the second and third trimesters, in addition to reassuring maternal-fetal tolerance, your obstetric trainee contemplates why it is among *third-line* options for ITP in pregnancy, despite being used for routine prophylaxis against rhesus isoimmunization among D-negative mothers.

12. Explain the morbidities associated with anti-D immunoglobulin, limiting use to refractory ITP in pregnancy.   **5**

☐ Contrary to prophylactic anti-D immunoglobulin for anti-D prophylaxis, treatment for ITP in pregnancy requires high-dose intravenous administration (50–75 ug/kg) whereby antibodies can cross placenta and lead to neonatal anemia, acute hemolysis, and jaundice

The patient demonstrates a positive clinical response to combined prednisone and IVIG, as hematuria resolves within four days of initiating therapy, and systemic petechial hemorrhages stabilize. By 36 weeks' gestation, she remains on prednisone 5 mg daily and automated platelet count have stabilized over the past two weeks, currently at 75×10^9/L.

A multidisciplinary meeting is arranged to devise a maternal-fetal plan for delivery, based on which you intend to counsel the patient at the upcoming prenatal visit. The fetus has remains in the cephalic presentation and obstetric aspects of maternal-fetal care have been unremarkable.

13. Excluding analgesic care, outline maternal-fetal <u>delivery considerations</u> with probable ITP presenting in pregnancy. *(1 point per main bullet, unless specified)*   Max 10

Maternal:
☐ Plan for a mode of delivery based on obstetric indications, realizing that Cesarean delivery does not decrease the already rare risk of fetal intracranial hemorrhage among parturients with ITP
☐ Timed delivery (*e.g.,* induction of labor at 38–39 weeks' gestation) based on the trajectory of the platelet fall, maternal bleeding or placental abruption; consideration for an expert's availability for potential postpartum hemorrhage (PPH)
☐ Arrange for corticosteroid stress doses in labor[†]
☐ Ensure availability of blood products in case of bleeding complications
☐ Consider the availability of tranexamic acid[#]
☐ Early notification of the obstetric anesthesiologist upon delivery admission and ensure the neonatology team attends delivery
☐ Avoid an episiotomy, where possible
☐ Plan for active management of the third stage of labor
☐ Avoid intramuscular injections (*e.g.,* uterotonics, analgesics)
☐ Avoid postpartum nonsteroidal anti-inflammatory agents (NSAIDs) if platelet count is $<70 \times 10^9$/L due to increased risk of hemorrhagic complications

Fetal:
☐ Maintain continuous electronic fetal monitoring in labor
☐ Avoid intrapartum procedures that increase fetal hemorrhagic risks: *(1 point per subbullet; max 3)*
   ○ Fetal scalp electrodes
   ○ Fetal scalp sampling
   ○ Vacuum-assisted delivery
   ○ Midcavity rotational forceps delivery[§]
☐ At delivery, collect an umbilical cord blood sample by *venipuncture* (*i.e.,* rather than drainage) for platelet count for dual advantages: (a) determine the need for immediate neonatal therapy[‡] and (b) obviating pseudo-thrombocytopenia in neonates due to difficulties in obtaining unclotted blood

Special notes:
† Refer to Question 14 in Chapter 45 for corticosteroid dosing at planned vaginal delivery, and Question 16 in Chapter 46 for dosing at Cesarean delivery, as per NICE guideline recommendations: National Institute for Health and Care Excellence (NICE) Guideline 121: Intrapartum care for women with existing medical conditions or obstetric complications and their babies. 2019. Available at www.nice.org.uk/guidance/ng121, accessed May 18, 2021.
# Refer to Question 6 in Chapter 22 for adverse effects of tranexamic acid
§ Low outlet forceps can be used: fetal hemorrhagic risk is lower relative to vacuum or rotational forceps
‡ Where cord sampling is not performed, peripheral blood sampling of the neonate is possible, with avoidance of heel-prick as clot formation is common and may result in pseudo-thrombocytopenia

Spontaneous labor and vaginal delivery ensue at 38^{+4} weeks' gestation where intrapartum care proceeds according to the care plan. Atony-induced PPH responded well to tranexamic acid.

Routine vitamin K injection, as well as elective circumcision, of the male newborn will be withheld until the infant's platelet count is known to be normal.

Umbilical cord platelet count is later reported to be normal, at $>100 \times 10^9$/L, and the neonatologist informs the patient that no further tests are required.

14. With focus on the patient's antenatal morbidities, what are important postpartum considerations to discuss prior to discharge and/or at the routine outpatient clinical visit, pending results of follow-up platelet count? *(1 point per main bullet; max points specified where required)*

Max 8

General maternal-fetal well-being:
- ☐ Encourage breastfeeding/pumping[†]
- ☐ Screen for postpartum depressions and continue to offer psychosocial support
- ☐ Encourage future preconception counseling
- ☐ Reassure the patient that a normal neonatal platelet count is favorable for future siblings' risk of thrombocytopenia

Thrombocytopenia:
- ☐ Taper the intrapartum corticosteroid stress dose, aiming to discontinue treatment for subsequent assessment of platelet count, maintaining interdisciplinary care
- ☐ Postpartum thromboprophylaxis should be considered for a patient with ITP whose platelet count is stably $>50 \times 10^9$/L and has additional thrombotic risk factors *(Suggested Reading 10)*

Contraceptive recommendations: *(max 3)*
- ☐ Levonorgesterol intrauterine system (LNG-IUS) may be useful for this patient if severe isolated thrombocytopenia persists and with a probable history of menorrhagia
- ☐ Estrogen-containing contraceptives, progesterone-only oral contraceptives and progesterone implants are safe for this patient with isolated thrombocytopenia
- ☐ Initiation of depo-medroxyprogesterone acetate (DMPA) should be done with caution if severe thrombocytopenia persists due to increased amounts/erratic patterns of bleeding and its irreversibility for 11–13 weeks after administration
- ☐ Initiation of copper intrauterine device (IUD) should be done with caution if severe thrombocytopenia persists due to increased vaginal bleeding and anemia
- ☐ Barrier methods can be offered

Special note:
† Although neonatal platelet count is normal in this case scenario, persistent neonatal thrombocytopenia for more than one week could be secondary to antiplatelet antibodies in breast milk, where intermittently holding-off breastfeeding could be advised

TOTAL: **100**

On day 2 postpartum, outstanding test results confirm VWD type IIB. You take this opportunity to highlight to your obstetric trainee that thrombocytopenia may first appear during pregnancy and be misdiagnosed as ITP, emphasizing the importance of a comprehensive personal and family history that guides testing. Phenotypic manifestation of VWD type IIB is also consistent with the incident PPH and response to antifibrinolytic therapy.

The hematologist explained the increased risk of delayed PPH over the ensuing six weeks, where antifibrinolytic therapy will be continued for two to six weeks and VWF replaced for three to seven days postpartum to maintain levels >50%.

Endocrine Disorders in Pregnancy

CHAPTER 55

Thyroid Disease in Pregnancy

Michael A. Tsoukas, Ji Wei Yang, and Amira El-Messidi

A 29-year-old primigravida is referred by her primary care provider to your tertiary center's high-risk obstetrics unit for preconception counseling for known Graves' disease.

Special note: *International jurisdictions vary with regard to availability of methimazole or carbimazole. This chapter reflects doses of methimazole, as carbimazole, the pro-drug derivative, is metabolized in full to methimazole. Doses of carbimazole are ~40% higher than doses of methimazole.*

LEARNING OBJECTIVES

1. Take a focused history from a patient with Graves' disease, and provide appropriate counseling for optimal timing of conception to reduce morbidities of overt hyperthyroidism in pregnancy
2. Present a structured approach to differentiate Graves' disease from other etiologies of hyperthyroidism, including thyroiditis
3. Provide counseling on therapeutic options for hyperthyroidism in the preconception period, develop an interdisciplinary antenatal plan, and recognize principles in emergency management of maternal thyroid dysfunction
4. Reflect on physiologic changes of pregnancy to outline clinical manifestations and plan treatment of hypothyroidism in pregnancy

SUGGESTED READINGS

1. Alexander EK, Pearce EN, Brent GA, et al. 2017. Guidelines of the American Thyroid Association for the diagnosis and management of thyroid disease during pregnancy and the postpartum. *Thyroid.* 2017;27(3):315–389. [Correction in Thyroid. 2017 Sep;27(9):1212]
2. Illouz F, Luton D, Polak M, et al. Graves' disease and pregnancy. *Ann Endocrinol (Paris).* 2018;79(6):636–646.
3. Spencer L, Bubner T, Bain E, et al. Screening and subsequent management for thyroid dysfunction pre-pregnancy and during pregnancy for improving maternal and infant health. Cochrane Database Syst Rev. 2015;(9):CD011263.
4. Okosieme OE, Khan I, Taylor PN. Preconception management of thyroid dysfunction. *Clin Endocrinol (Oxf).* 2018;89(3):269–279.
5. PN, Lazarus JH. Hypothyroidism in pregnancy. *Endocrinol Metab Clin North Am.* 2019;48(3):547–556.

6.   Thyroid disease in pregnancy: ACOG Practice Bulletin No. 223. *Obstet Gynecol.* 2020;135(6): e261–e274.

7.   Wright HV, Williams DJ. Thyrotoxicosis in pregnancy. *Fetal and Maternal Medicine Review* 2013; 24:2 108–128.

POINTS

1.   With regard to Graves' disease, what aspects of a focused history would you want to know? *(1 point each; max points indicated where required)*   Max 25

General disease-related details:
☐   Age at diagnosis or disease duration
☐   Inquire how diagnosis was established
☐   Name and contact of treating endocrinologist

Current/prior symptoms of hyperthyroidism: *(max 10)*

General or neurometabolic	☐ Fatigue ☐ Insomnia ☐ Irritability or emotional lability ☐ Increased perspiration/heat intolerance ☐ Decreased concentration ☐ Tremor ☐ Menstrual cycle irregularity (amenorrhea/oligomenorrhea)
Ophthalmologic:	☐ Retro-orbital pressure/pain ☐ Diplopia ☐ Redness/inflammation/grittiness
Cardiopulmonary:	☐ Palpitations ☐ Dizziness ☐ Dyspnea
Dermatologic:	☐ Hair loss ☐ Dermopathy/pretibial myxedema ☐ Brittle nails
Gastrointestinal:	☐ Diarrhea/loose stools

Most recent laboratory features:
☐   Thyroid stimulating hormone (TSH)
☐   Free thyroxine (T4) and total triiodothyronine (T3)
☐   Thyroid receptor antibody (TRAb) levels
☐   Thyroid peroxidase antibody (anti-TPO) levels

Disease-related comorbidities:

☐ Presence of other autoimmune diseases (*e.g.,* diabetes mellitus, Addison's disease, SLE, pernicious anemia)

☐ Anemia (normocytic, microcytic, or macrocytic)

☐ Chronic hypertension

Gynecologic features most relevant to Graves' disease ± medical treatment:

☐ Inquire about potentially undisclosed early pregnancy losses or history of subfertility

☐ Current contraceptive method, if any

☐ Menstrual cycle regularity/last menstrual period (LMP)

Medications and treatments, clinical response, and side effects:

☐ Thionamides: methimazole (or its pro-drug derivative, carbimazole), propylthiouracil

☐ Definitive treatment with radioiodine or thyroidectomy

☐ Determine if prenatal vitamins have been initiated

☐ Allergies

Social features and routine health maintenance:

☐ Cigarette smoking,[†] alcohol consumption, or recreational drugs

☐ Vaccination status

Family history:

☐ Autoimmune thyroid or nonthyroid diseases

Special note:

† Graves' disease has been frequently associated with smoking (*Suggested Reading 9*)

You learn that the patient was diagnosed nine months ago when she presented with tremors, anxiety, excessive perspiration, and weight loss despite a good appetite, accompanied by biochemical thyroid dysfunction and thyroid receptor antibodies (TRAb) at >5-times the upper reference for the assay. Based on comprehensive considerations for management options, treatment was initiated with oral carbimazole (methimazole) 40 mg daily for six weeks' duration, followed by weaning to a current maintenance dose of 5 mg daily; she has only experienced minor side effects.

Recent testing revealed:

		Nonpregnant normal values
Free T4	16.5 pmol/L (1.3 ng/dL)	10.3–21.9 pmol/L (0.8–1.7 ng/dL)
TSH	0.8 mU/L	0.34–4.25 mU/L
TRAb	15 U/L	0–5 U/L

The patient is currently asymptomatic and does not have any comorbid medical diseases.

Although she initially anticipated conception alongside stabilization of Graves' disease, the patient has been compliant with the endocrinologist's recommendations to postpone pregnancy until a 'stable euthyroid state' has been achieved. She now wishes to discontinue progesterone-only pill and condoms (*i.e.,* dual contraception). She maintains a healthy lifestyle and is in a monogamous relationship with her husband of four years. Vaccinations are up to date. She does not drink alcohol, smoke, or use recreational drugs. One of her sisters has Hashimoto's thyroiditis and another was just diagnosed with hyperthyroid manifestations of thyroiditis at two months postpartum on routine screening for women with type 1 diabetes mellitus. The patient has no drug allergies.

2. Assuming the patient's laboratory set is the first to reveal a normal hormonal profile since initiation of treatment, clarify the recommendation for timing conception after a 'stable euthyroid state' has been achieved. *(1 point each)*   3

□ Two sets of thyroid function tests within the reference range
and
□ Serum tests performed at least one month apart
and
□ No changes in therapy between tests

3. Justify the endocrinologist's recommendation to defer pregnancy until a 'stable euthyroid state' is achieved by discussing maternal-fetal risks of overt maternal hyperthyroidism, independent of drug-associated adverse effects. *(1 point each)*   10

Maternal: *(max 5)*	Fetal-neonatal: *(max 5)*
□ Early pregnancy loss	□ Goiter *(the earliest sonographic signs of fetal thyroid dysfunction)*
□ Preterm labor	□ Craniosynostosis and advanced bone age
□ Gestational hypertension and preeclampsia	□ Tachycardia
□ Placental abruption	□ Polyhydramnios *(due to goiter-induced hyperextension of the fetal neck)* with/without hydrops
□ Arrhythmia	□ Fetal growth restriction (FGR) or low birthweight
□ Congestive heart failure	□ Stillbirth
□ Thyroid storm	□ Complications of prematurity
□ Postpartum flare of Graves' disease	□ Neonatal thyrotoxicosis *(particularly with increased third trimester TRAb levels)* with/without secondary neonatal hypothyroidism[†]
	□ Central congenital hypothyroidism *(rare with Graves' disease, estimated risk at 1:35,000 pregnancies)*[‡]

Special notes:

[†] Via neonatal hyperthyroidism-induced suppression of neonatal pituitary TSH secretion
[‡] *Refer to* Kempers MJ, van Tijn DA, van Trotsenburg AS, de Vijlder JJ, Wiedijk BM, Vulsma T. Central congenital hypothyroidism due to gestational hyperthyroidism: detection where prevention failed. *J Clin Endocrinol Metab.* 2003;88(12):5851–5857.

4. Given the patient's risk of postpartum disease flare, she expresses concern that her sister's current hyperthyroid phase may be underlying Graves' disease. Discuss features that would favor a hyperthyroid phase of postpartum thyroiditis relative to Graves' disease. *(1 point each)*

Max 4

Timing	☐ Onset of the hyperthyroid phase within three months postpartum suggests postpartum thyroiditis; Graves' disease would more commonly present after 6 months postpartum
Clinical manifestations	☐ Signs and symptoms more specific to Graves' disease are absent in postpartum thyroiditis (*e.g.,* ophthalmopathy, pretibial myxedema, and goitre/ significant thyroid enlargement)
Diagnostic investigations	☐ Radioiodine uptake is low in postpartum thyroiditis, yet increased in Graves' disease ☐ Sonographic imaging of the thyroid gland may show decreased vascular flow in postpartum thyroiditis
Immunological features	☐ Levels of TRAb are normal or undetected in postpartum thyroiditis
Hormonal features	☐ Serum T4 tends to be disproportionately elevated beyond T3 in a destructive process causing thyrotoxicosis; the reverse is more common in thyrotoxicosis caused by direct thyroid hyperactivity

On examination, body habitus, physical appearance, blood pressure and pulse are normal. Physical features of thyrotoxicosis are absent, as confirmed by the endocrinologist. You read the clinical note indicating that while exposure to antithyroid drugs during the first trimester would best be obviated, clinical guidance prefers propylthiouracil over methimazole; treatment would best be switched[†] as early as possible and until 16 weeks' gestation (*ATA[1]*).

After comprehensive discussion with the endocrinologist, methimazole 5 mg daily will be converted to propylthiouracil 50 mg twice daily using a dose-ratio of 20:1[†] propylthiouracil: methimazole (*ATA[1], ACOG[7]*) upon achieving a stable euthyroid state. Meanwhile, she will maintain use of contraception.

Special note:
† From a practical standpoint, maintenance doses of an antithyroid drug need not be switched prior to or during pregnancy

5. <u>Detail</u> why propylthiouracil is preferred to methimazole in the first trimester, where treatment is clinically indicated.   8

☐ Although teratogenic effects occur with similar incidence among both thionamide drugs, at 2%–4% of children exposed in early pregnancy *(ATA[1])*, birth defects associated with propylthiouracil appear less severe[†] than with methimazole *(4 points)*

Methimazole/carbimazole embryotoxicity: *(1 point each; max 4)*
☐ Aplasia cutis
☐ Facial dysmorphism
☐ Ocular defects
☐ Ventricular septal defects
☐ Esophageal atresia with/without tracheoesophageal fistula
☐ Abdominal wall defects *(e.g., omphalocele and gastroschisis)*
☐ Choanal atresia
☐ Urinary tract anomalies

Special note:
† Propylthiouracil-associated anomalies are primarily face/neck cysts, and urinary tract abnormalities (in males)

6. Inform your trainee why methimazole is preferred to propylthiouracil, where treatment is clinically indicated after 16 weeks' gestation.   1

☐ Propylthiouracil-associated maternal hepatotoxicity

7. Review with the patient critical signs/symptoms for which urgent drug discontinuation and seeking of medical care would be warranted, while explaining to your trainee clinical monitoring thereof, if any. *(1 point each)*   4

Propylthiouracil-induced hepatotoxicity: *[~1/1000]*
☐ *Critical signs/symptoms*: malaise, weakness, nausea and vomiting, jaundice, dark urine or pale stools
☐ *Monitoring*:Testing of hepatic enzymes during administration of propylthiouracil may be considered, with an understanding that serial monitoring has not been shown to be effective in prevention of fulminant of propylthiouracil-induced hepatotoxicity; reviewing concurrent pharmacologic agents ingested by the patient to preferably avoid other hepatotoxic drugs should be considered

Agranulocytosis with either antithyroid agent: *[~0.1%]*
☐ *Critical signs/symptoms*: Fever, sore throat, skin eruptions, general malaise
☐ *Monitoring*: Antithyroid related agranulocytosis is an acute idiosyncratic reaction (no apparent dose–response relationship) where serial leukocyte counts for clinical monitoring are not helpful

With an understanding that all treatment options for Graves' disease were appropriately entertained at initial diagnosis, your obstetric trainee inquires about considerations for definitive treatment. The patient thereby takes this opportunity to summarize that thionamide treatment or surgery were deemed preferable to radioiodine therapy based on her clinical profile and personal obstetric preferences.

8. Rationalize why surgery may have been an appropriate alternative to thionamides, while radioiodine would have been the least favored treatment of this patient. *(1 point each)*

Max 6

Benefits of thyroidectomy for *this* patient:
☐ Gradual remission of the high levels of autoimmunity (*i.e.*, TRAb at five times the upper-normal range) present at diagnosis
☐ A stable euthyroid state easily achieved on replacement thyroxine therapy
☐ Obstetric features of thionamide treatments would have been obviated

Caveats of radioiodine therapy for *this* patient:
☐ Post-^{131}I therapy, serum TRAb levels tend to increase and take many months to disappear
☐ Treatment with ^{131}I requires a negative pregnancy be documented within 48 hours of therapy
☐ Reliable contraception posttreatment would be advised; pregnancy should be avoided for six months and until a stable euthyroid state is achieved after radioiodine ablation to ensure treatment success and allow initiation of thyroxine replacement therapy
☐ Fetal-neonatal monitoring for thyrotoxicosis would still be indicated after a euthyroid state has been achieved due to antithyroid antibodies crossing placenta

9. Although the patient opted against elective surgical intervention for Graves' disease, address her inquiry on indications for thyroidectomy during pregnancy, noting overlap with indications among nonpregnant individuals. *(1 point each)*

Max 3

☐ Situations posing significant risk to the mother or fetus, such as dysphagia or stridor
☐ Known or suspected malignant nodule(s)
☐ Severe adverse reactions prohibiting continued thionamides, such as agranulocytosis
☐ Nonadherence to treatment or follow-up
☐ Uncontrolled thyrotoxicosis despite high (or maximum) doses of thionamide drug

This consultation visit is briefly interrupted by an emergency telephone call from a colleague at an external center: after a patient with prior tubal sterilization recently received therapeutic ^{131}I for treatment of hyperthyroidism, an inadvertent single intrauterine pregnancy at nine weeks' gestation was discovered on sonography for pelvic pain. You reinforce the importance of pregnancy testing of patients who may, albeit rarely, be pregnant.

10. With focus on receipt of therapeutic ^{131}I in the first trimester, provide your colleague with evidence-based management counseling and recommendations as the patient may desire pregnancy continuation; an urgent referral for consultation in your high-risk obstetrics unit will be arranged. *(1 point each)*

4

☐ Although the fetal thyroid does not appear to be damaged from inadvertent ^{131}I prior to 12 weeks' gestation, the main fetal risk is related to the whole-body radiation dose due to indirect exposure to gamma emissions from ^{131}I in the maternal bladder (~50–100 mGy/MBq of administered dose)

☐ Maternal hydration and frequent voiding should be encouraged to increase excretion of iodine

☐ Monitoring of the fetus and neonate for signs of hypothyroidism is advisable after radioiodine exposure in the first (or second) trimesters

☐ Individualized considerations for termination of pregnancy; limited data suggests normal outcomes with first-trimester exposure to radioiodine

After your telephone conversation, the patient attending for preconception consultation appreciates that obstetric care will require multidisciplinary collaboration in a high-risk unit, particularly with increased antithyroid antibodies and/or need for continued thionamide treatment. She intends to comply with the designated antenatal management.

11. Outline important elements of focused antenatal management of this patient if conception were to occur on maintenance propylthiouracil therapy with persistently increased TRAb levels for the specific assay. *(1 point each)*

Max 8

Maternal:

☐ Maintain affiliation with experts in endocrinology or obstetric medicine; individualized consideration for consultation with perinatal mental health experts

☐ Monitor thyroid function tests monthly; increase frequency of monitoring (*e.g.*, every two weeks) when converting from propylthiouracil to methimazole after 16 weeks' gestation

☐ Aim to keep the total T4 and free T4 values at or just above the pregnancy-specific upper-normal limit to avoid fetal hypothyroidism and goiter (*this usually requires dose-reduction in the second half of pregnancy*)

☐ With elevated TRAb levels at (pre)-conception, repeat measurements at 18–22 weeks and 30–34 weeks' gestation to evaluate the need for neonatal and postnatal monitoring

☐ Inform the patient that frequency of clinical assessments with/without hospitalization will depend on disease activity, treatment-related complications, or onset of comorbidities

☐ Reinforce the importance of compliance with postpartum serum thyroid function tests at individualized frequency of testing planned by the endocrinologist

☐ Counsel the patient that timing and route of delivery is based on obstetric indications (*i.e.*, aim for a term vaginal delivery)

Fetal-neonatal:

☐ Plan sonographic surveillance in the first and second trimesters for thionamide-related embryo-fetal toxicity

☐ Plan serial sonographic assessments (*e.g.*, monthly) after 20 weeks' gestation when the fetus would typically manifest signs of hyperthyroidism [*cross-placental transfer of TRAb occurs ≥20 weeks' gestation*] (*see Question 3*)

☐ Auscultate the fetal heart rate at obstetric antenatal visits for risks of fetal demise and tachycardia

☐ Arrange for neonatology consultation in the second or third trimester

☐ Collect umbilical cord blood at delivery for TRAb levels

12. Address your trainee's inquiry regarding why maternal total T4 and free T4 values should be maintained at or just above the pregnancy-specific upper-normal limit.

1

☐ All thionamide drugs tend to be more potent on the fetal thyroid than in the maternal thyroid; a maternal euthyroid state risks iatrogenic fetal goiter and hypothyroidism

Four months after this consultation, in vitro fertilization with intracytoplasmic sperm injection is performed for male-factor infertility, leading to a viable intrauterine singleton. As a high-risk obstetrician, you plan to follow her obstetric care, according to the established antenatal plan and in collaboration with her endocrinologist/obstetric medicine physician. Prior to the first prenatal visit, you review the patient's thyroid profile during controlled ovarian hyperstimulation.

13. Illustrate to your obstetric trainee how hormonal manipulations from controlled ovarian hyperstimulation may alter thyroid function. (*1 point each*)

2

☐ Administration of human chorionic gonadotropin (hCG) can directly stimulate thyroidal TSH receptors, leading to increased thyroid hormone and subsequent decreases in TSH (*i.e.*, hCG-mediated hyperthyroidism/gestational [biochemical] thyrotoxicosis)

☐ Supraphysiologic rise in serum estradiol levels increases thyroxine binding globulin which binds thyroid hormones and reduces free serum concentrations; a feedback mechanism increases serum TSH levels

Although the most recent thyroid profile shows a 'stable euthyroid state' with persistently increased serum TRAb levels, your obstetric trainee informs you the patient is experiencing symptoms of thyrotoxicosis. She is normotensive and physical features particular to thyrotoxicosis are absent. Her endocrinologist has continued propylthiouracil at maintenance dose.

14. Elicit clinical manifestations of hyperthyroidism that overlap with those of euthyroid pregnant women. *(1 point each)*

Max 4

☐ Fatigue and lethargy
☐ Heat intolerance
☐ Malar and palmar erythema
☐ Palpitations, tachycardia
☐ Physiologic dyspnea
☐ Emotional lability
☐ Minimal goiter in regions of iodine sufficiency
☐ Hair loss

Special note:
Refer to Question 15 in Chapter 4 for features differentiating between gestational (biochemical) thyrotoxicosis (*i.e.,* hCG-mediated hyperthyroidism) and thyroid gland-induced dysfunction

Pregnancy progresses well until 29^{+3} weeks' gestation when the patient is hospitalized for close observation of new-onset preeclampsia requiring initiation of oral labetalol 200 mg twice daily. She responds well to the first dose of labetalol; all other vital signs are normal at admission. There are no adverse maternal-fetal features of preeclampsia.

During your call duty on the evening of admission, the patient's oral temperature is now 40.5°C, blood pressure is 190/93 mmHg at one hour after receipt of labetalol, and pulse is 135 bpm. She remains nonhypoxic yet appears confused, restless, and diaphoretic. You notice her hands trembling at her bedside. Cardiotocography shows fetal tachycardia at 170 bpm with decreased variability; there are no fetal decelerations and uterine quiescence is maintained. Although comprehensive laboratory investigations have been requested, you promptly alert interdisciplinary experts and recognize the importance of initiating therapy based on the most suspected diagnosis. You alert your trainee that while laboratory results will likely be consistent with hyperthyroidism (*i.e.,* increased free T4, free T3, and depressed TSH), values do not always correlate with the severity of the hypermetabolic state. The patient will be transferred to the intensive care unit (ICU) or birthing center.

15-A. State the most probable diagnosis.

1

☐ Thyroid storm

15-B. Pending investigations, identify the most evident precipitating cause for thyroid storm.

1

☐ Preeclampsia

16. Highlight to your obstetric trainee the <u>principal goals</u> of management of thyroid storm. *(1 point each)*

6

Thyroid storm – goals of management:
- ☐ Reduce the synthesis and release of thyroid hormone
- ☐ Block the peripheral conversion of T4 to T3
- ☐ Block the systemic actions of thyroid hormone
- ☐ Reduce thyroid hormone from the circulation and increase the concentration of thyroxine-binding globulin
- ☐ Treat complications and manifestations of thyroid storm
- ☐ Identify and treat potential precipitating conditions

Special note:
Refer to Foley MR, Strong TH Jr, Garite TJ (Ed). Obstetric intensive care manual, 4th edition. McGraw Hill Education; 2014.

17. Reflecting upon the principal goals of therapy, outline <u>conventional pharmacologic and adjunctive agents</u> for management of the patient's thyroid storm, in the absence of thyrotoxic heart failure. *(1 point per main bullet)*

9

- ☐ Propylthiouracil given orally or via nasogastric tube
  - ○ Decreases the synthesis of thyroid hormone by inhibiting iodination of tyrosine, as well as blocking of peripheral conversion of T4 to T3
- ☐ Iodine administration, in the form of sodium iodide, saturated solution of potassium iodide, Lugol's iodine or lithium carbonate, started one to two hours *after* propylthiouracil has been given
  - ○ Block the release of preformed thyroid hormone
- ☐ High-dose corticosteroids, started with initiation of treatment (*e.g.,* dexamethasone,[†] hydrocortisone, or prednisone)
  - ○ Block the release of preformed thyroid hormone *(as iodide)*
  - ○ Block the peripheral conversion of T4 to T3 *(as propylthiouracil)*
- ☐ ß-adrenergic blocking agents (may continue the patient's antihypertensive agent)
  - ○ Controls the patient's tachycardia and hypertension
- ☐ Phenobarbital
  - ○ Controls the patient's restlessness
- ☐ (Cold) intravenous fluid and electrolyte replacement
- ☐ Antipyretic agent, such as acetaminophen or paracetamol
- ☐ Cooling blankets and control room temperature accordingly
- ☐ Provide oxygenation if maternal saturation becomes <94%–95%

Special note:
† Treatment regimen generally involves intravenous or intramuscular dexamethasone at 2 mg every 6 hours for four doses; this differs from regimen used for fetal pulmonary maturation, being intramuscular dexamethasone at 6 mg every 12 hours for four doses

18. Describe why iodine must only be started *after* propylthiouracil in treatment of thyroid storm.

☐ Iodine initially increases the synthesis of thyroid hormone; blocking production with thionamide therapy is important before inhibiting hormone release

Continuous electronic fetal monitoring is maintained during correction of the thyroid storm. You reassure the treating team that intervention on behalf of the fetus is not warranted until maternal status has been stabilized. As anticipated, fetal tachycardia and decreased variability normalize with resolution of the maternal hypermetabolic state. Based on interdisciplinary agreement, fetal pulmonary corticosteroids and magnesium sulfate (fetal neuroprotection and eclampsia prophylaxis) were administered during treatment of the thyroid storm.

The patient subsequently developed HELLP syndrome, requiring delivery at 30^{+4} weeks' gestation. As umbilical cord blood TRAb levels were increased, the newborn will be monitored for clinical and laboratory manifestations of thyroid dysfunction. The patient is reassured that should Graves' disease flare postpartum requiring reintroduction of methimazole, she may continue to breastfeed with up to 15 mg/d.

You later meet the patient's sister at 16 weeks' gestation while covering your colleague's clinic. Given her history of Hashimoto's thyroiditis, you learn she had adjusted the dose of levothyroxine as soon as pregnancy was suspected, as advised in preconception counseling; once-daily dosing was thereby increased by an additional two tablets weekly (*i.e., a 29% increase*) to mimic gestational physiology and obviate maternal hypothyroidism in the first trimester (*ATA[1]*).[†] While reviewing recent serial laboratory investigations, you note TSH increased from normal at <2.5 mU/L to 4.2 mU/L over the past month. She has no discriminatory symptoms of thyroid dysfunction in pregnancy yet complains of signs and symptoms common to normal pregnancy. There are no obstetric complaints.

Special note:
† Another option is to increase daily levothyroxine by ~25%–30% (*ATA[1]*).

19. With regard to a focused history, elicit clinical manifestations of hypothyroidism that overlap with those of euthyroid pregnant women. (*1 point each*)

☐ Fatigue and lethargy
☐ Decreased concentration
☐ Weight gain and edema
☐ Minimal goiter in regions of iodine sufficiency
☐ Paresthesias and carpal tunnel syndrome
☐ Muscle cramps
☐ Hair loss
☐ Constipation
☐ Abdominal distension
☐ Amenorrhea

The patient is keen to correct the recent suboptimal thyroid control, knowing this decreases risks of adverse perinatal outcomes associated with overt hypothyroidism. Concerned about the risk of neonatal hypothyroidism associated with thyroid inhibitory antibodies, you reassure her that, unlike the risk of neonatal thyrotoxicosis with thyroid-stimulating antibodies (TRAb) in Graves' disease, the risk fetal hypothyroidism with maternal Hashimoto's thyroiditis is rare, at 1: 180,000 newborns *(ACOG[6])*.

20. Explore potential causes of suboptimal control of hypothyroidism in this obstetric patient and address a query to convert to triiodothyronine (T3) treatment to obtain a euthyroid state. *(1 point each)*	4

☐ Determine patient adherence to therapy
☐ Inquire about nausea and/or vomiting (*i.e.,* decreased absorption)
☐ Verify the timing of thyroxine intake; ingestion concurrent with proton pump inhibitors or prenatal vitamins containing calcium or iron decreases absorption of thyroxine
☐ Explain to the patient that T3-containing preparations should be *avoided* in pregnancy as the fetal central nervous system is relatively impermeable to T3; fetal T3 derives from maternal T4 actively transported into the fetal brain

21. Refer to the physiological changes of pregnancy to elaborate to your trainee on factors accounting for increased T4 needs in pregnancy. *(1 point each)*	Max 4

☐ Reduced absorption of thyroid hormone associated with iron-containing prenatal vitamins or nausea/vomiting
☐ Transplacental transfer of T4 necessary for fetal neurological development *(particularly until the fetal thyroid becomes functional at ~12 weeks' gestation)*
☐ Placental deiodinase activity metabolises T4
☐ Weight gain and increased volume of distribution
☐ Increased thyroxin-binding globulin concentration

TOTAL: 115

CHAPTER 56

Gestational Diabetes Mellitus

Amira El-Messidi and Alan D. Cameron

A healthy 38-year-old secundigravida presents for a first prenatal visit after sonography at your hospital center just dated a spontaneous intrauterine pregnancy at 12^{+4} weeks' gestation. Early fetal morphology and sonographic screening markers for aneuploidy are unremarkable. You learn that she and her husband just moved to the country. Five years ago, she had gestational diabetes mellitus (GDM) and delivered vaginally. The patient has no obstetric complaints and has been taking folate-containing prenatal vitamins. She does not drink alcohol, smoke cigarettes, or use any recreational substances.

Special note: _In this case scenario, 'diabetes' implies 'diabetes mellitus.'_

LEARNING OBJECTIVES

1. Take a focused history with prior GDM, eliciting risk factors that warrant testing prior to or early in subsequent pregnancy
2. Detail an approach to establishing a GDM diagnosis, appreciating international practice variations
3. Provide principles of dietary and exercise counseling, identifying the need for pharmacologic therapy based on glycemic targets
4. Appreciate short-term and long-term morbidities associated with GDM
5. Present comprehensive intrapartum and postpartum management plans for a patient with GDM

SUGGESTED READINGS

Selected Guidelines or Recommendations from Policy Makers

1. ACOG Practice Bulletin No. 190: gestational diabetes mellitus. _Obstet Gynecol._ 2018;131(2): e49–e64.
2. American Diabetes Association. Management of diabetes in pregnancy: standards of medical care in diabetes – 2021. _Diabetes Care._ 2021;44(Suppl 1):S200–S210.
3. (a) Berger H, Gagnon R, Sermer M. Guideline No. 393 – diabetes in pregnancy. _J Obstet Gynaecol Can._ 2019;41(12):1814–1825. [Correction in J Obstet Gynaecol Can. 2020 Oct;42(10):1288]
   (b) Diabetes Canada Clinical Practice Guidelines Expert Committee, Feig DS, Berger H, et al. Diabetes and pregnancy. _Can J Diabetes._ 2018;42(Suppl 1):S255–S282. [Correction in Can J Diabetes. 2018 Jun;42(3):337]

4. Diagnostic criteria and classification of hyperglycaemia first detected in pregnancy: a World Health Organization Guideline. *Diabetes Res Clin Pract.* 2014;103(3):341–363.

5. Duarte-Gardea MO, Gonzales-Pacheco DM, Reader DM, et al. Academy of Nutrition and Dietetics gestational diabetes evidence-based nutrition practice guideline. *J Acad Nutr Diet.* 2018;118(9):1719–1742.

6. (a) <u>FIGO</u>: Hod M, Kapur A, Sacks DA, et al. The International Federation of Gynecology and Obstetrics (FIGO) Initiative on gestational diabetes mellitus: a pragmatic guide for diagnosis, management, and care. *Int J Gynaecol Obstet.* 2015;131(Suppl 3):S173–S211.

   (b) <u>FIGO</u>: McIntyre HD, Oats JJN, Kihara AB, et al. Update on diagnosis of hyperglycemia in pregnancy and gestational diabetes mellitus from FIGO's Pregnancy and Non-Communicable Diseases Committee. *Int J Gynaecol Obstet.* 2021;154(2):189–194.

7. National Institute for Health and Care Excellence (NICE). Diabetes in pregnancy: management from preconception to the postnatal period; NICE guideline. February 25, 2015. Available at www.nice.org.uk/guidance/ng3. Accessed July 18, 2021.

8. Scottish Intercollegiate Guidelines Network (SIGN). Management of diabetes, a national clinical guideline. March 2010, updates November 2017. Available at www.sign.ac.uk/assets/sign116.pdf. Accessed July 18, 2021.

9. Society of Maternal-Fetal Medicine (SMFM) Publications Committee. SMFM Statement: pharmacological treatment of gestational diabetes. *Am J Obstet Gynecol.* 2018;218(5):B2–B4.

10. US Preventive Services Task Force, Davidson KW, Barry MJ, et al. Screening for gestational diabetes: US Preventive Services Task Force recommendation statement. *JAMA.* 2021;326(6):531–538.

Adjunctive Readings

11. Dickens LT, Thomas CC. Updates in gestational diabetes prevalence, treatment, and health policy. *Curr Diab Rep.* 2019;19(6):33.

12. Egan AM, Dow ML, Vella A. A review of the pathophysiology and management of diabetes in pregnancy. *Mayo Clin Proc.* 2020;95(12):2734–2746.

13. Johns EC, Denison FC, Norman JE, et al. Gestational diabetes mellitus: mechanisms, treatment, and complications. *Trends Endocrinol Metab.* 2018;29(11):743–754.

14. Lende M, Rijhsinghani A. Gestational diabetes: overview with emphasis on medical management. *Int J Environ Res Public Health.* 2020;17(24):9573.

15. Mussa J, Meltzer S, Bond R, et al. Trends in national Canadian guideline recommendations for the screening and diagnosis of gestational diabetes mellitus over the years: a scoping review. *Int J Environ Res Public Health.* 2021;18(4):1454.

16. Saravanan P, Diabetes in Pregnancy Working Group. Maternal Medicine Clinical Study Group, Royal College of Obstetricians and Gynaecologists, UK. Gestational diabetes: opportunities for improving maternal and child health. *Lancet Diabetes Endocrinol.* 2020;8(9):793–800.

17. Thayer SM, Lo JO, Caughey AB. Gestational diabetes: importance of follow-up screening for the benefit of long-term health. *Obstet Gynecol Clin North Am.* 2020;47(3):383–396.

18. Tieu J, McPhee AJ, Crowther CA, et al. Screening for gestational diabetes mellitus based on different risk profiles and settings for improving maternal and infant health. *Cochrane Database Syst Rev.* 2017;8(8):CD007222.

19. Zhang M, Zhou Y, Zhong J, et al. Current guidelines on the management of gestational diabetes mellitus: a content analysis and appraisal. *BMC Pregnancy Childbirth.* 2019;19(1):200.

1. With regard to prior GDM, what aspects of a focused history would you want to know? *(1 point per main bullet, unless specified)*

Past obstetric history:

Maternal
- ☐ (Approximate) gestational age at GDM diagnosis
- ☐ Determine the White's classification
  - ○ *i.e.,* dietary control (GDM-A_1) or pharmacologic therapy (GDM-A_2)
- ☐ Prepregnancy weight
- ☐ (Approximate) gestational weight gain
- ☐ Onset of hypertensive syndromes of pregnancy
- ☐ Gestational age at delivery
- ☐ Establish whether labor was induced for purposes of GDM care
- ☐ Ascertain whether glucose testing was performed at least six weeks postpartum
- ☐ Breastfeeding

Fetal-neonatal
- ☐ Inquire about sonographic features of glycemic control (*e.g.*, polyhydramnios, large-for-gestational age biometry and/or fetal growth velocity)
- ☐ Infant features: *(1 point per subbullet; max 2)*
  - ○ Birth trauma (*i.e.*, shoulder dystocia, brachial plexus palsy, infant fractures, extensive maternal laceration)
  - ○ Need for operative vaginal delivery
  - ○ Birthweight *(may/may not be consistent with sonographic estimated fetal weight)*
  - ○ Need for NICU admission for glycemia-related complication

Medications related to prior GDM care or current risk of diabetes:
- ☐ Determine the type of insulin used, any complications or adverse reactions
- ☐ Use of oral hypoglycemic agents (*e.g.*, metformin, glibenclamide [glyburide]), any complications or adverse reactions
- ☐ Chronic corticosteroid use

Clinical features or lifestyle practices:
- ☐ Known history of polycystic ovarian syndrome
- ☐ Current symptoms of polydipsia or polyuria
- ☐ Dietary and exercise regimes
- ☐ Determine whether glycosylated hemoglobin (HbA1c) has been measured for yearly screening of diabetes mellitus since last pregnancy

Social and family history:
- ☐ High risk race or ethnicity (*e.g.*, African American, Latino, Native American, Aboriginal, Asian American, Pacific Islander, Middle Eastern)
- ☐ First-degree relatives with diabetes

You learn that the patient of mixed South Asian and Middle Eastern ethnicity, had diet controlled GDM initially detected at 24 weeks' gestation. Prior to her first pregnancy, she was obese and recalls gaining excess gestational weight yet has since engaged in a healthy diet and regular exercise regime, improving her body mass index (BMI) from 31.2 kg/m^2 to 26.2 kg/m^2, as most recently calculated. She notes improvement in clinical markers associated with insulin resistance, including regular menstrual cycles, which facilitated this spontaneous conception.

The patient recalls that fetal sonographic evaluations were deemed normal, although the actual birthweight of 4100 grams was 15% greater than the last sonographic estimate prior to spontaneous labor at 39^{+5} weeks' gestation. Delivery was complicated by shoulder dystocia, without maternal-fetal complications. The patient missed postpartum GDM testing.

Motivated to continue healthy lifestyle practices, she inquires about means for early detection of hyperglycemia, recalling a continuous spectrum of adverse maternal-fetal outcomes. You take this opportunity to highlight that the optimal screening test prior to 24 weeks' gestation is unclear; obstetric care providers' selection may depend on jurisdictional practices. You intend to later alert your trainee that while early diagnosis and treatment of GDM reduces *short-term fetal-neonatal morbidities*, there is currently no evidence to support prevention of *long-term adverse outcomes* in offspring.

2. Address her inquiry regarding an approximate risk of recurrent GDM and elicit features that may increase this patient's a priori risk. *(1 point each)*   8

☐ There is a 40% risk of recurrence based on prior GDM§

Clinical:[#]
☐ Prior adverse outcomes related to GDM *(i.e., shoulder dystocia and neonatal metabolic derangements)*
☐ Features of insulin resistance
☐ BMI >25 kg/m^2[†] *(ACOG[1])*
☐ Infant's birthweight >4000 g[‡] *(ACOG[1])*

Demographic:
☐ Age >35 years *(SOGC[3a])*
☐ High-risk ethnic origin *(i.e., South Asian and Middle Eastern)*
☐ First-degree family history of diabetes

Special notes:
§ Getahun D, Fassett MJ, Jacobsen SJ. Gestational diabetes: risk of recurrence in subsequent pregnancies. Am J Obstet Gynecol 2010;203:467.e1
\# Additional risk factors <u>not</u> specific to this case scenario include physical inactivity, repeated glycosuria, hypertension/cardiovascular disease, hyperlipidemia, impaired glucose tolerance, impaired fasting glucose or HbA1c ≥5.7% on prior testing, corticosteroid use, multiple pregnancy, and prior stillbirth
† *SOGC* [3a], *NICE*[7], *SIGN*[8] define a BMI >30 kg/m^2
‡ *NICE*[7], *SIGN*[8] recommend a birthweight ≥4500 g

Early glycemic testing is normal, and the patient continues to engage in healthy lifestyle practices. She understands the need for repeat testing at 24–28 weeks' gestation.[§]

Special note:
§ Period of significantly increasing insulin resistance *(see Question 5)*

3. Appreciating the lack of an ideal approach, discuss an accepted practice regimen with its glycemic targets to consider at 24–28 weeks' gestation.

(7 points for any societal recommended testing regime; other practices may be acceptable)

Guideline	Glucose load	Fasting blood glucose	1-hour post prandial plasma glucose	2-hour post prandial plasma glucose	3-hour post prandial plasma glucose
☐ NICE[7]	75-g, 2-hour oral glucose tolerance test (OGTT)[†]	<5.6 mmol/L (100 mg/dL)	——————	<7.8 mmol/L (140 mg/dL)	
☐ SOGC[3a] and DiabetesCanada[3b] Preferred screening and diagnostic two-step approach					
	Screening 50-g, 1-hour glucose challenge test (GCT)[§]		<7.8 mmol/L [GDM if ≥11.1 mmol/L]		
	If plasma glucose is 7.8–11.0 mmol/L, do the OGTT				
	75-g, 2-hour OGTT[†]	<5.3 mmol/L (95 mg/dL)	10.6 mmol/L (191 mg/dL)	9.0 mmol/L (162 mg/dL)	
☐ SOGC[3a] and Diabetes Canada[3b]: Alternative approach, ○ International Association of Diabetes and Pregnancy Study Group (IADPSG) criteria ○ Endorsed by ADA[2,‡] FIGO[6a], SIGN[8]					
	75-g, 2-hour OGTT[†]	<92 mg/dL (5.1 mmol/L)	<180 mg/dL (10.0 mmol/L)	<153 mg/dL (8.5 mmol/L)	
☐ ACOG[1] and ADA[2‡]	Screening 50-g, 1-hour GCT[§]	———	<130–140 mg/dl (7.2–7.8 mmol/L) [institutional thresholds vary]	———	———

(cont.)

Guideline	Glucose load	Fasting blood glucose	1-hour post prandial plasma glucose	2-hour post prandial plasma glucose	3-hour post prandial plasma glucose
		FOLLOWED BY: Diagnostic 100-g, 3-hour oral glucose tolerance test (OGTT)			
	Target #A	<95 mg/dL (5.3 mmol/L)	<180 mg/dL (10.0 mmol/L)	<155 mg/dL (8.6 mmol/L)	<140 mg/dL (7.8 mmol/L)
	Target #B	<105 mg/dL (5.8 mmol/L)	<190 mg/dL (10.6 mmol/L)	<165 mg/dL (9.2 mmol/L)	<145 mg/dL (8.0 mmol/L)
☐ WHO[4] *Testing may be done at any time*	75-g, 2-hour OGTT	<92–125 mg/dL (5.1–6.9 mmol/L)	<180 mg/dL (10.0 mmol/L)	<153–199 mg/dL (8.5–11.0 mmol/L)	

Special notes:

§   Not recommended by NICE[7]

†   Abnormal result requires ≥1 abnormal value

‡   American Diabetes Association. Classification and Diagnosis of Diabetes. Diabetes Care 2017;40(Suppl. 1):S11-S24

#A and #B   Carpenter and Coustan (plasma or serum level) and National Diabetes Data Group (plasma level), respectively; abnormal results require ≥2 abnormal values

You had planned a chosen diagnostic test be performed early in the 24–28 weeks' window and the patient had booked the test for 24^{+3} weeks' gestation. However, she presented at 3:00 AM with threatened preterm labor two days prior to her test; a course of betamethasone was initiated for fetal pulmonary maturity, among other management. You visit the patient during her brief hospitalization where she requests consideration for having the GDM test prior to discharge. She is grateful that the threatened preterm labor has resolved.

4.   Specify your recommended timing of GDM testing based on the patient's clinical course.   1

☐   GDM testing should be delayed at least seven days after administration of betamethasone

Special note:

This applies to *both* screening and diagnostic tests

The patient undertakes the designated glycemic test at 25^{+6} weeks' gestation, which is consistent with GDM. You alert your obstetric trainee that while certain jurisdictions recommend measurement of HbA1c at a GDM diagnosis *(NICE[7])*, this would not be adjunctive to the diagnostic evaluation of this patient, as her glycemic testing in early pregnancy ensured absence of type 2 diabetes. Prior to patient counseling, you take this opportunity to discuss the pathophysiology of GDM with your obstetric trainee, recognizing that complex mechanisms consisting of environmental, and (epi)genetic factors occur over time.

5. In teaching your trainee, provide an overview of pathophysiology that leads to maternal   6
    GDM. *(1 point per main bullet, unless specified)*

[A] ß-cell dysfunction:[§]
☐ Decreased ability to sense blood glucose concentration or release appropriate insulin in response due to chronic fuel excel (*i.e.,* glucotoxicity) and prolonged, excessive insulin production that exhausts cells over time

[B] Contributor factors to chronic insulin resistance:
☐ Increased maternal and placental hormonal production *(1 point per subbullet; max 4)*
  ○ Human placental lactogen
  ○ Progesterone
  ○ Growth hormone
  ○ Cortisol
  ○ Prolactin
☐ Increased maternal caloric intake and body weight

Special note:
§   *Refer to* Plows JF, Stanley JL, Baker PN, Reynolds CM, Vickers MH. The Pathophysiology of Gestational Diabetes Mellitus. *Int J Mol Sci.* 2018;19(11):3342.

You inform the patient of the glycemic test results and reassure her that recent second-trimester sonogram revealed normal fetal growth, morphology, and amniotic fluid (liquor) volume. She understands the need for good glycemic control to optimise pregnancy outcome; multidisciplinary care will be coordinated in your hospital center's specialized clinic.

6. Inform your obstetric trainee of overall goals of medical nutritional therapy in the care of   Max 3
    GDM. *(1 point each)*

☐ Achieve normoglycemia
☐ Achieve adequate maternal weight gain in relation to BMI
☐ Contribute to fetal well-being by achieving or maintaining appropriate fetal biometry, growth velocity, and amniotic fluid volume
☐ Prevent ketosis

7. Provide the patient with general recommendations on caloric and carbohydrate intake, allotment and distribution for management of GDM until comprehensive meal plans are developed with the nutritionist. *(1 point per main bullet)*

Calories:
- [ ] Being overweight (*i.e.*, BMI 26.2 kg/m^2), the patient's caloric intake would average 25 kcal/kg/d
- [ ] Calories are divided into three meals and two to four snacks daily
  - ○ *Rationale:* Lower likelihood of postprandial glucose fluctuations and distribute daily carbohydrate intake

Carbohydrate:
- [ ] Advise switch from high to low glycemic index foods (NICE[7]); complex carbohydrates are recommended over simple carbohydrates
  - ○ *Rationale:* Lower likelihood of postprandial hyperglycemia, slower digestion, and may reduce insulin resistance
- [ ] Constitutes ~30%–40% of calories, ensuring absence of ketonuria *(with remaining distributed as ~20% protein and ~40% fat)*

8. Present a structured outline of short-term <u>maternal-fetal</u> morbidities that have been associated with GDM, when poorly controlled. *(1 point each)*

Maternal	Fetal-neonatal
Antepartum	☐ Polyhydramnios
☐ Preeclampsia, gestational hypertension	☐ Large-for-gestational age/macrosomia
☐ Urinary tract infections	☐ Hypertrophic cardiomyopathy
☐ Preterm labor	☐ Shoulder dystocia
☐ Anxiety, depression	☐ Birth injury
	☐ Prematurity
Intrapartum or postpartum	☐ Delayed pulmonary maturity; respiratory distress syndrome
☐ Labor dystocia	☐ Stillbirth or neonatal death
☐ Operative delivery (instrumental vaginal or Cesarean)	☐ Neonatal hypoglycemia, hypocalcemia, polycythemia, hyperbilirubinemia
☐ Postpartum infection	
☐ Postpartum hemorrhage	
☐ Failure to initiate or maintain breastfeeding	

9. Alert your trainee of long-term risks among offspring of women with GDM, with an understanding that antenatal disease control may not mitigate the morbidities.
    (1 point each)

                                                                                Max 3

☐ Childhood obesity or excess abdominal adiposity
☐ Type 2 diabetes
☐ Hypertension
☐ Female offspring are more likely to have GDM in their pregnancies

The initial visit at the multidisciplinary specialized clinic is arranged in a timely fashion. With a fasting plasma glucose at 5.1 mmol/L (90 mg/dL) on the morning of consultation, she is provided with a personalized dietary regime, instructed to perform blood glucose monitoring several times daily, and encouraged to engage in 30 minutes of moderate-intensity aerobic exercise at least four days/week or at least 150 minutes/week. She recalls being informed that 30 minutes of physical activity may decrease glucose levels by up to 1.3 mmol/L (23 mg/dL).[§] Walking is also encouraged for 15–30 minutes after each meal, prior to testing postprandial glucose. Reassuringly, she has not developed contraindications to exercise in pregnancy and obstetric progress is otherwise unremarkable.

Special note:
§ *Refer to* Avery MD, Walker AJ. Acute effect of exercise on blood glucose and insulin levels in women with gestational diabetes. *J Matern Fetal Med.* 2001;10(1):52–58.

10. Document <u>maternal-fetal targets</u> with lifestyle interventions for management of GDM.

    (1 point for either maternal target; 1 point for fetal target)

                                                                                Max 2

Maternal: *(Achieving glycemic targets while avoiding hypoglycemia is paramount)*
☐ Option A: ACOG[1], ADA[2], SOGC[3a], Diabetes Canada[3b], NICE[7]

Units: mmol/L (mg/dL)

○ Fasting	<5.3 (95)
○ 1-hour postprandial[§]	<7.8 (140)
○ 2-hour postprandial[§]	<6.4 (115) *for NICE[7]* <6.7 (120) *for ACOG[1], ADA[2], SOGC[3a], Diabetes Canada[3b], FIGO[6a]*

☐ Option B: SIGN[8]

Units: mmol/L (mg/dL)

○ Fasting	<5.5 (99)
○ 2-hour postprandial	<7.0 (126) at ≤35 weeks <8.0 (144) at >35 weeks

Fetal:

☐ Sonographically normal amniotic fluid volume, fetal abdominal circumference <75th percentile and EFW <90th percentile

Special note:

§ Either one- or two-hour glucose testing after meals may be done without evidence of superiority with either approach

For eight weeks' duration, the patient progresses well on medical nutritional therapy and an exercise regime that includes daily walks post meals. The frequency of blood glucose monitoring was decreased to two to three times daily. In view of her previous obstetric history, monthly fetal sonographic assessment is arranged for biometry, growth velocity and amniotic fluid volume. You alert your trainee, however, of otherwise wide variations in antenatal fetal surveillance protocols for women with well-controlled GDM-A1 in the absence of high-quality evidence to guide practice patterns.

At the 32 weeks' prenatal visit, the patient shares her logs of fasting and one-hour postprandial glucose values over the past week, with the prior week's results being similar. She has remained adherent to the nonpharmacological regimen. Recent fetal sonography was unremarkable. The patient has no obstetric complaints.

Units: mmol/L (mg/dL)

date	*Fasting*	*Breakfast*	*Lunch*	*Dinner*
1	6.1 (110)		7.9 (142)	
2		6.9 (124)		6.3 (118)
3	6.4 (115)		7.4 (133)	
4		7.2 (130)		6.0 (108)
5	7.0 (126)		7.3 (131)	
Today	7.2 (130)			

11. Based on your impression of her glycemic log, <u>specify</u> your <u>single most significant</u>   2
management.

- ☐ Advise *immediate insulin* treatment *at bedtime* due to fasting hyperglycemia
  - ○ Intermediate-acting insulin (neutral protamine Hagedorn [NPH]) is preferred

Special note:
An oral antihyperglycemic agent would not provide timely management of this patient's fasting hyperglycemia; some guidelines *(FIGO[6a], NICE[7], SIGN[8], SMFM[9])* consider oral antihyperglycemic agents, namely metformin or glibenclamide (glyburide), potential initial pharmacologic treatments for women with GDM who have postprandial hyperglycemia with normal fasting glucose, especially at <30 weeks' gestation *(FIGO[6a])*; combined insulin and an oral antihyperglycemic agent may also be considered. Refer to Chapter 58 for obstetric considerations with use of oral antihyperglycemic agents.

Insulin therapy achieves glycemic control over the remainder of pregnancy, with dose adjustments being made regularly based on capillary glucose levels. Her total daily needs of insulin have not exceeded 15 U by 36 weeks' gestation. She has been counseled to rotate injection sites within the same body area to avoid cutaneous amyloidosis *(NICE[7])*. Fetal sonography at 36 week's gestation shows a cephalic presentation, estimated fetal weight is 3000 g with appropriate growth velocity and amniotic fluid volume. Having collaborated with colleagues in the GDM clinic, you plan to discuss delivery management at this 36 weeks' prenatal visit.

12. Detail essentials of <u>intrapartum and early postpartum</u> management regarding insulin-   Max 10
requiring gestational diabetes (*i.e.,* GDM-A2) and this patient's obstetric history.
(*1 point per main bullet*)

Intrapartum:
- ☐ Delivery is recommended at 39[+0] to 39[+6] weeks with well-controlled GDM-A2[†]
- ☐ Aim for vaginal delivery unless obstetric indications require Cesarean delivery
- ☐ Inform the patient and alert delivery personnel about risk of (recurrent) shoulder dystocia, even without suspected macrosomia
- ☐ Home insulin regimen may continue prior to planned induction of labor
- ☐ Inform the patient to anticipate decreased insulin needs in labor due to decreased oral intake and increased energy requirements in labor
- ☐ Capillary blood glucose is monitored hourly in labor; intravenous dextrose solution with variable rate insulin infusion (*i.e.,* 'sliding scale') is used to maintain blood glucose at 4–7 mmol/L (72–126 mg/dL), if required
  - ○ *Maintaining intrapartum euglycemia is particularly important to decrease risks of neonatal hypoglycemia*
- ☐ Maintain continuous electronic fetal heart monitoring in active labor
- ☐ Inform the neonatology team of the delivery admission

Early postpartum:
- ☐ Discontinue all pharmacologic treatment because insulin sensitivity rapidly increases following placental delivery

☐ Monitor maternal blood glucose prior to hospital discharge

☐ Encourage breastfeeding and explain its *benefits* in relation to GDM: *(1 additional point per subbullet)*

    ○ Long-term risk of type 2 diabetes among women and offspring

    ○ Neonatal hypoglycemia

    ○ Childhood obesity

    ○ Postpartum weight loss

Special note:

† If this patient had remained well-controlled GDM-A1 without other complications, delivery would be recommended by 40 weeks' gestation *(SOGC[3a])* or from 39^{+0} to 40^{+6} weeks' gestation *(ACOG[1], NICE[7])*

The patient had an uncomplicated induction of labor and spontaneous vaginal delivery at 39^{+5} weeks' gestation. Early initiation of breastfeeding was implemented. Serial newborn blood glucose testing and monitoring for other potential metabolic complications is being performed.

13. With focus on GDM-A2, what are important postpartum considerations to discuss or arrange prior to hospital discharge and/or at the routine outpatient clinical visit? *(1 point per main bullet, unless specified)*

Max 10

General maternal-fetal well-being:

☐ Promote maintenance of breastfeeding for at least six months, and consider readdressing its long-term maternal-child benefits; individualized consideration for lactation consultation

☐ Screen for postpartum depression and continue to offer psychosocial support

    ○ *Depression is more common among women with gestational (and pregestational diabetes) than in unaffected women*

☐ Encourage healthy lifestyle practices, particularly regarding diet, aerobic exercise, gestational weight loss, and achieving a normal BMI; reinforce continued avoidance of smoking and alcohol (ab)use

Contraceptive recommendations:

☐ Counseling about spacing pregnancies is important for women with GDM to maximize health between pregnancies; this also reduces risk of subsequent GDM or diabetes in future pregnancy *(FIGO[6a])*

☐ There are no restrictions to contraceptive recommendations for *history of* GDM; however, disease transition to diabetes requires counseling accordingly‡

Medical care and counseling after GDM:

☐ Review symptoms of hyperglycemia with the patient *(NICE[7])*

☐ Inform the patient that up to 70% of women develop diabetes (predominately type 2) later in life, with actual rate being influenced by risk factors

☐ Facilitate return to her primary care physician

☐ Encourage preconception counseling, even with resolved GDM

[Jurisdictional variations exist, as outlined; other practices may be deemed acceptable] (5 points for any accepted practice)

ACOG[1], ADA[2]

☐ Plan a 75-g, two-hour oral glucose tolerance test (OGTT) at 4–12 weeks postpartum[†] to identify diabetes, impaired fasting glucose, or impaired glucose tolerance
　○ *An isolated fasting plasma glucose is not recommended as it lacks sensitivity for detecting other forms of abnormal glucose metabolism*

☐ Counsel the patient that repeat testing is warranted every one to three years if her postpartum screening test results are normal, although testing more frequent testing is advised based on her medical and demographic risk factors; yearly testing is recommended for impaired fasting glucose and/or impaired glucose tolerance

SOGC[3a]

☐ Plan a 75-g, two-hour oral glucose tolerance test (OGTT) between six weeks and six months postpartum, including assessment of HbA1c

☐ Reinforce the importance of repeating an OGTT prior to a future pregnancy if current GDM resolves

FIGO[6a]

☐ Plan a 75-g OGTT at 6–12 weeks postpartum

☐ No clear guidance on type of subsequent surveillance tests, frequency, or duration of monitoring

NICE[7]

☐ Plan a fasting plasma glucose at 6–13 weeks postpartum
　○ *Routine OGTT is not routinely offered*
　○ *Fasting plasma glucose ≥7 mmol/L is then confirmed with HbA1c; if HbA1c is ≥48 mmol/mol (i.e., ≥6.5%), the patient is diagnosed with type 2 diabetes*

☐ Counsel the patient that annual HbA1c is offered with normal or impaired fasting glucose

☐ If postpartum fasting plasma glucose is not performed, HbA1c may be done at >13 weeks postpartum

SIGN[8]

☐ Plan for a minimum of fasting glucose and perform a 75-g, two-hour OGTT if clinically indicated

☐ Counsel the patient that annual fasting glucose or HbA1c is recommended thereafter

Special notes:

[†] *Refer to* Metzger BE, Buchanan TA, Coustan DR, de Leiva A, Dunger DB, Hadden DR, et al. Summary and recommendations of the Fifth International Workshop-Conference on Gestational Diabetes Mellitus [published erratum appears in Diabetes Care 2007;30:3154]. Diabetes Care 2007;30 Suppl 2:S251–60

[‡] *Refer to* Question 15 in Chapter 58, addressing contraceptive recommendations

TOTAL:　　**85**

CHAPTER 57

Pregestational Type 1 Diabetes Mellitus

Melissa-Rosina Pasqua, Amira El-Messidi, and Natasha Garfield

During your call duty, a 25-year-old primigravida with a 12-year history of type I diabetes mellitus (T1DM) at 26^{+1} weeks' gestation by early sonographic dating of an unplanned pregnancy is accompanied by her husband to the obstetric emergency assessment unit at 4:00 AM for a three-hour history of nausea followed by recurrent nonbilious vomiting. Despite the lack of oral intake since her standard bedtime snack, her husband indicates the patient passed urine at least five times over the last hour, as he assisted her due to drowsiness and visual blurring.

You had met the patient in the multidisciplinary diabetes clinic, where you reported a normal fetal morphology sonogram at 20 weeks' gestation and ensured results of the fetal echocardiogram were similarly unremarkable. The patient has been compliant with routine prenatal care provided by your colleague. Prior to pregnancy, she required replacement of multiple daily doses of subcutaneous insulin by a continuous subcutaneous insulin infusion (insulin pump therapy) due to persistent hypoglycemic unawareness.

The patient is alert, though lethargic, unable to remain engaged in conversation. While diaphoretic, her oral mucosa appears dry. Vital signs reveal she is afebrile, blood pressure is 95/63 mmHg with a pulse rate at 110 bpm, and respiratory rate is 22 breaths/min, with normal oxygen saturation at 97% on room air. As you review the cardiotocographic (CTG) tracing, urgent maternal bedside and laboratory investigations are being performed upon your request.

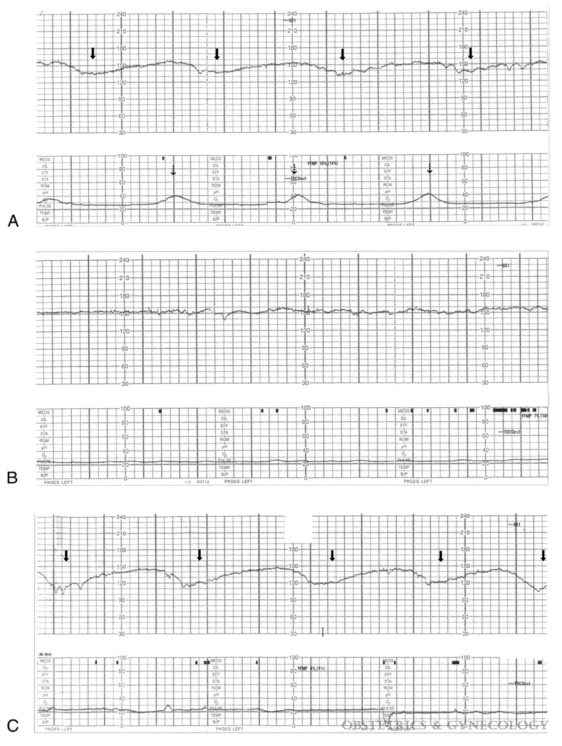

Figure 57.1

With permission: Figure 2, panel A from Sibai BM, Viteri OA. Diabetic ketoacidosis in pregnancy. Obstet Gynecol. 2014;123(1): 167–178.

There is no association between the source of the maternal-fetal tracing and this case scenario. Image used for educational purposes only.

Special note: To avoid content overlap, readers are encouraged to refer to Chapter 58 for aspects related but not limited to preconception counseling and pharmacologic recommendations, glycemic care during maternal administration of fetal pulmonary corticosteroids, and routine management considerations in pregnancy and postpartum.

LEARNING OBJECTIVES

1. Demonstrate vigilance in recognizing clinical features and results of investigations suggestive of diabetic ketoacidosis (DKA) in pregnancy
2. Appreciate precipitating factors and physiological features for DKA in pregnancy
3. Provide counseling on perinatal complications of DKA, recognizing potential metabolic mechanisms for fetal adversity
4. Illustrate a detailed understanding of guiding principles in management of the obstetric patient with DKA
5. Counsel an obstetric patient with T1DM on evidence-based advantages of real-time continuous glucose monitoring, and appreciate basic principles involved in intrapartum and postpartum management of continuous subcutaneous insulin infusion with continued interdisciplinary collaboration

SUGGESTED READINGS

1. American College of Obstetricians and Gynecologists' Committee on Practice Bulletins – Obstetrics. ACOG Practice Bulletin No. 201: pregestational diabetes mellitus. *Obstet Gynecol.* 2018;132(6):e228–e248.
2. American Diabetes Association. 14. Management of diabetes in pregnancy: standards of medical care in diabetes – 2021. *Diabetes Care.* 2021;44(Suppl 1):S200–S210.
3. Alexopoulos AS, Blair R, Peters AL. Management of preexisting diabetes in pregnancy: a review. *JAMA.* 2019;321(18):1811–1819.
4. Diabetes Canada Clinical Practice Guidelines Expert Committee, Feig DS, Berger H, et al. Diabetes and pregnancy. *Can J Diabetes.* 2018;42(Suppl 1):S255–S282. [Correction in Can J Diabetes. 2018 Jun;42(3):337]
5. Joint British Diabetes Societies for Inpatient Care (JBDS-IP). Management of glycaemic control in pregnant women with diabetes on obstetric wards and delivery units. May 2017. Available at https://abcd.care/sites/abcd.care/files/resources/JBDS_Pregnancy_201017.pdf. Accessed September 6, 2021.
6. McCance DR, Casey C. Type 1 diabetes in pregnancy. *Endocrinol Metab Clin North Am.* 2019;48(3):495–509.
7. Mohan M, Baagar KAM, Lindow S. Management of diabetic ketoacidosis in pregnancy. *The Obstetrician and Gynaecologist* 2017;19:655–662.
8. National Institute for Health and Care Excellence (NICE). Diabetes in pregnancy: management from preconception to the postnatal period; NICE guideline. February 25, 2015. Available at www.nice.org.uk/guidance/ng3. Accessed July 18, 2021.
9. Scottish Intercollegiate Guidelines Network (SIGN). Management of diabetes, a national clinical guideline. March 2010, updates November 2017. Available at www.sign.ac.uk/assets/sign116.pdf. Accessed July 18, 2021.
10. Sibai BM, Viteri OA. Diabetic ketoacidosis in pregnancy. *Obstet Gynecol.* 2014;123(1):167–178.

1. Outline the <u>maternal laboratory derangements</u> that would be most consistent with the working diagnosis, pending knowledge of underlying cause(s). *(1 point each)*

Max 6

Laboratory findings of diabetic ketoacidosis in pregnancy:
- ☐ Ketonemia or significant ketonuria (*i.e.,* >2+ on standard urine keto-sticks)
- ☐ Arterial or venous pH ≤7.30
- ☐ Anion gap >12 mEq/L
- ☐ Base deficit ≥4 mEq/L
- ☐ Serum bicarbonate <15 mEq/L (mmol/L)
- ☐ Osmolality >290 mOsm/kg
- ☐ Pseudo-normal serum potassium level
- ☐ Increased serum blood urea nitrogen and creatinine
- ☐ Euglycemia or hyperglycemia

2. Identify *potential* precipitating factors for this medical emergency, noting current limitations in obtaining a focused history. *(1 point each)*

Max 5

- ☐ Protracted vomiting/hyperemesis gravidarum
- ☐ Local or systemic infection
- ☐ Insulin pump failure
- ☐ Inadequate monitoring of glycemic levels and adherence to therapy
- ☐ Medications including current/recent administration of corticosteroids or ß-sympathomimetics
- ☐ Diabetic gastroparesis

3. Explain how the <u>physiological changes of pregnancy</u> could instigate this medical emergency in a patient with preexisting diabetes, in the absence of precipitating etiology. *(1 point per main bullet and subbullet)*

6

- ☐ Respiratory alkalosis
  - ○ Renal excretion of bicarbonate increases in compensation for respiratory alkalosis; this limits the capacity of bicarbonate to buffer ketoacids, thereby promoting DKA at lower glucose levels in pregnancy relative to nonpregnant states
- ☐ Hormonal-induced insulin resistance (*i.e.,* counterregulatory hormones)
  - ○ Human placental lactogen, human placental growth hormone, cortisol, progesterone, prolactin[†]
- ☐ Accelerated starvation
  - ○ Nausea and vomiting/hyperemesis gravidarum or poor nutritional intake promote lipolysis, hepatic ketogenesis, and hepatic glucose production through gluconeogenesis and glycogenolysis

Special note:
† Refer to Question 5 (Section B) in Chapter 56

A nurse promptly alerts you the insulin pump's battery is nonfunctional and capillary blood glucose level is 19 mmol/L (342 mg/dL). Meanwhile, a team member is concerned about the possibility for urgent delivery based on the CTG tracing.

4.	Recognizing this emergency, identify a fundamental concept of <u>fetal management</u> at this time.	5
☐	Intervention for fetal well-being is not warranted until stabilization of the acute maternal condition has been achieved, or maternal-fetal status continues to deteriorate despite appropriate therapeutic interventions	

5.	Describe features of potential concern on the CTG tracing. *(1 point each)*	3
☐	Late fetal heart decelerations	
☐	Minimal variability	
☐	Uterine contractions	

Despite pronounced hyperglycemia, with complementary clinical signs and symptoms, you indicate that pregnant women with diabetes have an increased propensity to progress rapidly, and at lower glycemic levels, into DKA relative to nonpregnant states, thereby making this a *supportive* feature, rather than *absolute* requirement for diagnosis.

In briefing the couple on the seriousness of this condition and its most likely precipitating factor, you highlight investigations are underway to assess for co-etiologies. The patient understands that interdisciplinary care has been initiated.

6.	Albeit not pathognomonic, elicit her signs and symptoms you mentioned in discussion with experts in adult medicine (*e.g.*, endocrinology, critical care) who will assist in devising a therapeutic plan. *(1 point each)*	Max 8

Signs	Symptoms
☐ Hypotension	☐ Nausea and vomiting
☐ Tachycardia	☐ Drowsiness
☐ Tachypnea	☐ Blurred vision
☐ Dehydration (*dry oral mucosa*)	☐ Polyuria
☐ Abnormal fetal heart tracing and presence of uterine contractions	☐ Lethargy

7. What are additional signs and symptoms of DKA *not* otherwise featured in this patient's presentation to later teach your trainee? *(1 point each)*   Max 3

☐ Kussmaul breathing ('fruity breath' odor)/hyperventilation
☐ Polydipsia
☐ Muscle weakness or leg cramps
☐ Abdominal pain *(due to the presence of ketones)*
☐ Shock
☐ Coma, altered sensorium, disorientation

Selected results of requested blood tests reveal the following:

		Normal
Plasma glucose	20 mmol/L (355 mg/dL)	<11.1 mmol/L (200 mg/dL) random
Leukocyte count	13.3 × 10⁹/L, unremarkable differential	5.6–14.8 3 × 10⁹/L
ALT	30 IU/L	2–33 IU/L
AST	30 IU/L	3–33 IU/L
Sodium	127 mEq/L	129–149 mEq/L
Chloride	95 mEq/L	97–109 mEq/L
Potassium	4.1 mEq/L	3.5–5.5 mEq/L
Bicarbonate	11 mmol/L	>15 mmol/L
Anion gap: $[Na^+]-[Cl^- + HCO3^-]$	15 mEq/L	≤12 mEq/L
Creatinine	75 umol/L (0.85 mg/dL)	35.37–70.74 umol/L (0.4–0.8 mg/dL)
Venous pH	7.15	>7.30
Effective serum osmolality*	261.7 mOsm/kg	276–289 mOsm/kg
3-ß-hydroxybutyrate (by point-of-care capillary ketone testing)	4.5 mmol/L	<0.42 mmol/L
Urine acetoacetate	>3+	

* Effective serum osmolality (mOsm/kg) = {2[measured Na(mEq/L)] + [glucose (mg/dL)]/18}

Large-bore intravenous access site has been secured and a bladder catheter inserted; at this gestational age, continuous CTG monitoring will be maintained during correction of DKA in the intensive care/treatment unit (ICU/ITU).

8. During patient transfer to the ICU/ITU, address her husband's inquiry regarding potential maternal-perinatal complications of DKA. *(1 point each)* — Max 6

Maternal adverse events:
- ☐ Cerebral edema
- ☐ Adult respiratory distress syndrome
- ☐ Cardiac arrhythmias or ischemia
- ☐ Acute renal failure
- ☐ Mortality *(<1%, with early recognition and appropriate treatment)*

Perinatal complications:
- ☐ Preterm delivery (iatrogenic or preterm labor)
- ☐ Fetal/neonatal hypoxia-related complications; fetal brain injury associated with 3-ß-hydroxybutyrate and lactate
- ☐ Intrauterine fetal demise *(9%–36%)*

9. Regarding the fetoplacental complications you discussed, elaborate to your obstetric trainee the metabolic mechanisms for fetal complications. *(1 point each)* — Max 2

- ☐ Massive osmotic diuresis, dehydration, and volume depletion can decrease uteroplacental perfusion
- ☐ Hypophosphatemia will decrease 2,3-diphosphoglycerate, thereby increasing maternal red blood cell affinity for oxygen which can result in fetal hypoxia
- ☐ Maternal hypokalemia can lead to fatal arrhythmias for the mother and/or fetus
- ☐ Fetal hyperinsulinemia stimulates oxidative metabolism which requires oxygen

As the pharmacologic treatment plan is being devised with multidisciplinary collaboration, you explain to your trainee that correction of acidemia takes much longer than correction of hyperglycemia even though metabolic derangements are treated simultaneously.

10. Outline six <u>guiding principles</u> for management of the obstetric patient with DKA. *(1 point each)* — 6

- ☐ Intravenous volume replacement *(deficit is usually ~100 mL/kg maternal body weight)*
- ☐ Intravenous insulin therapy
- ☐ Correction of acidosis and electrolyte disturbances
- ☐ Evaluation for potential need of bicarbonate administration (pH ≤7.0)
- ☐ Identification and treatment of any precipitating factors
- ☐ Intensive maternal-fetal monitoring of treatment response

11. Based on the guiding principles, summarize to your trainee the <u>metabolic targets</u> that will guide the treatment protocol, and the defining <u>criteria for resolution</u> of DKA. *(1 point each)*

Max 6

Metabolic targets:[§]
- ☐ Lower the capillary glucose by 3 mmol/L/hr (54 mg/dL/hr)
- ☐ Maintain serum potassium at 4–5 mEq/L[†]
- ☐ Increase venous bicarbonate by 3 mmol/L/hr

Resolution criteria:
- ☐ Capillary ketone level (*i.e.*, 3-ß-hydroxybutyrate) <0.6 mmol/L[‡]
- ☐ Blood glucose <11.1 mmol/L (200 mg/dL)
- ☐ Bicarbonate ≥15 mEq/L
- ☐ pH >7.3
- ☐ Anion gap ≤12 mEq/L

Special notes:
§   The practice of monitoring 3-ß-hydroxybutyrate levels varies by international jurisdiction
†   Ensure urine output is ≥50 mL/hr as a marker of adequate hydration
‡   Level of ketonuria does not mark resolution due to continued excretion of urinary acetoacetate formed from metabolism of 3-ß-hydroxybutyrate

12. With an understanding that close clinical and biochemical monitoring guide treatment response, summarize *essential aspects* for <u>pharmacologic</u> management of an obstetric patient with DKA. *(1 point per main bullet)*

12

Intravenous fluids:
- ☐ Start with isotonic (0.9%) sodium chloride infusion, administering 1–2 L in the first hour
- ☐ Aim for a total fluid replacement of 4–6 L in the first 12 hours, 75% of the fluid deficit in the first 24 hours, and total volume replacement by 48 hours of treatment
- ☐ When blood[†] glucose level is <14 mmol/L (250 mg/dL), add 5%–10% dextrose and consider replacing normal saline with 0.45% normal saline, depending on serum electrolytes and hemodynamic response

Intravenous insulin and potassium: *(the following regimen represents an example of an accepted protocol; variations may exist based on institutional practices)*
- ☐ Use regular insulin starting at a fixed rate of 0.1 U/kg/hr *(not to exceed 15 U/hr)*
  - ○ a bolus dose of 0.1 U/kg is not required unless there is a delay in initiation of treatment
- ☐ Adjust insulin infusion rate according to rate of decline in blood[†] glucose level
- ☐ When glucose level is ≤14 mmol/L (250 mg/dL), decrease insulin infusion to 0.05 U/kg/hr
- ☐ Noting that ongoing insulin and fluid therapy can risk hypokalemia, initiate potassium repletion regardless of the patient's apparently normal levels[‡] (*i.e.*, 4.1 mEq/L) to maintain serum potassium at 4–5 mEq/L

Bicarbonate and phosphate: *(Controversial need for replacement)*
- ☐ Consider bicarbonate replacement in severe acidosis (*i.e.*, pH <7.0), cardiac dysfunction, sepsis or shock
- ☐ Phosphate replacement is only indicated if serum level is <0.32 mmol/L (1 mg/dL)

Additional pharmacologic agents:
- ☐ Provide antiemetic treatment, as required
- ☐ Consideration for thromboprophylaxis *(particularly during dehydration, hospitalization, and until resolution of DKA precipitating factor(s) that may contribute to the risk of thrombosis)*

Special note:
- † Serum or plasma glucose
- ‡ There is a *total* potassium deficit

13. Explain the controversy surrounding bicarbonate administration with regard to fetal well-being.

2

- ☐ Profound alkalosis can inhibit compensatory hyperventilation needed to washout excess carbon dioxide, thereby decreasing fetal oxygenation

Maternal serial laboratory markers show gradual improvement using the designated treatment protocol, simultaneous to normalization of maternal-fetal features on CTG monitoring within six hours *(range four to eight hours*†*)* of commencing therapy. Reassuringly, preliminary results do not show a precipitating etiology beyond insulin pump failure. Glycosylated hemoglobin is stable relative to last assessment four to six weeks ago at 6.5%, an improvement relative to disease control in early pregnancy when HbA1c was 7.3% (56.3 mmol/mol).

With symptom resolution and ability to tolerate oral intake, the subcutaneous insulin pump is reinitiated after a period of overlap (*e.g.*, approximately two hours) with intravenous therapy. Prenatal vitamins are restarted, as well as low-dose aspirin for preeclampsia prophylaxis. Based on routine early prenatal thyroid stimulating hormone (TSH) screening for women with T1DM, the patient has not required hormone replacement in pregnancy.

During this hospital admission, you arrange for ophthalmologic reassessment as the patient missed the third-trimester follow-up; long-standing retinal microaneurysms and intraretinal dot-blot hemorrhages showed slight progression from early to midgestation. Reassuringly, she did not manifest retinal neovascularization, vitreous hemorrhage, or fibrosis.

Special note:
† *Refer to* Hagay ZJ, Weissman A, Laurie S, Insler V. Reversal of fetal distress following intensive treatment of maternal diabetic ketoacidosis. Am J Perinatol 1994;11:430–2.

14. Further to decreasing the episodes of severe hypoglycemia by instigating insulin pump therapy prior to pregnancy, describe the underlined evidence-based advantages of continuous glucose monitoring pump relative to finger-prick testing for a gravida with T1DM. *(1 point each)*

Max 5

Maternal:
- ☐ Mildly improved HbA1c values at 34 weeks' gestation[§]
- ☐ Decreased time spent with hyperglycemia[§]
- ☐ Longer time spent in the target glycemic range[§]
- ☐ Less glycemic variability at 34 weeks' gestation[§]

Fetal/neonatal:
- ☐ Lower incidence of macrosomic infants[§]
- ☐ Fewer intensive care admissions lasting >24 hours, and one-day shorter hospital stay[§]
- ☐ Lower risk of neonatal hypoglycemia[§]

Special note:
§   *Refer to* Feig DS, Donovan LE, Corcoy R, et al. Continuous glucose monitoring in pregnant women with type 1 diabetes (CONCEPTT): a multicentre international randomised controlled trial [published correction appears in Lancet. 2017 Nov 25;390(10110):2346]. *Lancet.* 2017;390(10110):2347–2359.

15. Address the patient's apparent 'self-guilt' regarding the progression of diabetic retinopathy in pregnancy. *(1 point each)*

Max 3

Contributors to progression of diabetic retinopathy in pregnancy:[§†]
- ☐ Inform her that pregnancy itself is an independent risk factor for worsening of diabetic retinopathy
- ☐ Highlight that the duration of diabetes is a known contributor to the rate of progress of retinopathy during pregnancy; as the patient has had T1DM for 10–19 years, the rate of progression in pregnancy is ~10%[‡]
- ☐ Presence of long-standing retinopathy and level of disease at the beginning of pregnancy are independent risk factors for progression in pregnancy
- ☐ Reassure the patient that optimized glycemic control in pregnancy *(i.e., her HbA1c improved from 7.3% [56.3 mmol/mol] to 6.5% [47.5 mmol/mol])* offers maternal-fetal benefits that outweigh the short-term risks of progression in diabetic retinopathy

Special notes:
§   While chronic hypertension and/or preeclampsia can promote progression of diabetic retinopathy in pregnancy, such features are not relevant to this case scenario
†   *Refer to* Morrison JL, Hodgson LA, Lim LL, Al-Qureshi S. Diabetic retinopathy in pregnancy: a review. *Clin Exp Ophthalmol.* 2016;44(4):321–334.
‡   *Refer to* Temple RC, Aldridge VA, Sampson MJ, Greenwood RH, Heyburn PJ, Glenn A. Impact of pregnancy on the progression of diabetic retinopathy in type 1 diabetes. *Diabet Med.* 2001;18(7):573–577.

The remainder of pregnancy is unremarkable; maternal glycemic control remains appropriate on continuous subcutaneous insulin infusion and fetal surveillance modalities reveals persistent cephalic presentation, normal biometry, growth velocity and amniotic fluid volume. Apart from mild progression of diabetic retinopathy, she does not experience other maternal complications associated with preexisting diabetes such as preeclampsia, preterm labor, or nephropathy.

At 36^{+2} weeks' gestation, you counsel the patient according to the agreed-upon interdisciplinary recommendations for delivery management.

16. Counsel the patient on delivery considerations with T1DM complicated by diabetic retinopathy, with focus on antenatal use of continuous subcutaneous insulin infusion. *(1 point per main bullet unless specified)*

Max 6

☐ Reassure the patient that vaginal delivery is *not* contraindicated with diabetic retinopathy
  ○ *Although the risk of Valsalva-induced retinal bleeding in the context of active proliferative retinopathy with neovascularization is a concern, there is no evidence proving benefit to elective Cesarean delivery*
☐ If maternal-fetal markers of glycemic control remain satisfactory delivery, without indications for earlier delivery, plan delivery at 37^{+0} to 38^{+6} *(NICE[8])* or 39^{+0} to 39^{+6} weeks' gestation *(SMFM,[§] ACOG*)*
☐ Provided a Cesarean section is not required, encourage the patient to keep the insulin pump in place on basal settings to allow safe transition to the postnatal regimen
  ○ *Insulin pump should be removed for a Cesarean section due to use of diathermy*
☐ Inform the patient she may continue to use her insulin infusion pump whilst in labor, using correction boluses and/or temporary basal rate changes to maintain optimal glycaemic control
☐ Alert the patient that capillary glucose tests are more accurate during labor and delivery
☐ Aim for an intraoperative glycemia target of 4.0 and 7.0 mmol/L [*i.e.,* 72–126 mg/dL] *(Diabetes Canada[4], JBDS-IP[5], NICE[8])*
☐ Plan for conversion to variable rate intravenous insulin infusion in labor if any of the following situations: *(JBDS-IP[5])*

  (1 point per subbullet; max 2)
  ○ Inability or lack of the desire to manage her own insulin needs
  ○ Blood glucose is >7 mmol/L on two separate occasions
  ○ Ketonuria ≥2+ on dipstick or ketonemia >1.5 mmol/L

Special notes:
§ Hameed AB, Combs CA. Society for Maternal-Fetal Medicine Special Statement: Updated checklist for antepartum care of pregestational diabetes mellitus. *Am J Obstet Gynecol.* 2020;223(5):B2-B5
* American College of Obstetricians and Gynecologists' Committee on Obstetric Practice, Society for Maternal-Fetal Medicine. Medically Indicated Late-Preterm and Early-Term Deliveries: ACOG Committee Opinion, No. 831. *Obstet Gynecol.* 2021;138(1):e35-e39

Spontaneous labor at 38^{+4} week's gestation leads to an uncomplicated vaginal delivery of a newborn with birthweight 3600 g. Intrapartum, conversion to intravenous insulin infusion was necessary. The neonatology team, present at delivery, is performing principal newborn assessment for infants of mothers with preexisting diabetes, including possible undiagnosed antenatal malformations. The patient intends to commence breastfeeding shortly thereafter.

Postpartum, the insulin pump is reconnected for one hour prior to discontinuation of insulin infusion once the patient indicated the ability to manage her own pump. Based on the care plan arranged by the endocrinologist, basal rates will be reduced to 0.5 U/hr (*i.e.,* at least 50% reduction), insulin-to-carbohydrate ratio changed to one unit to 15 g, and insulin sensitivity increased to 4 mmol/L *(JBDS-IP[5])*. Although aware that postpartum blood glucose targets will now increase to 6–10 mmol/L, the patient contemplates its necessity.

---

17. Provide the patient with the rationale for relaxing postpartum blood glucose targets.   Max 2
   (1 point each)

Emphasis is on avoidance of maternal hypoglycemia:
- ☐ Breastfeeding-associated hypoglycemia
- ☐ Increased insulin sensitivity that starts immediately after delivery of the placenta[†]
- ☐ Decreased oral and carbohydrate intake relative to the antenatal period

Special note:
†   Refer to Question 14 in Chapter 58; cortisol, prolactin, and progesterone are less responsible for postpartum changes in insulin needs

---

Prior to hospital discharge, you ensure that critical aspects of postpartum care of women with preexisting diabetes have been addressed.[†]

Special note:
† Refer to Question 15 in Chapter 58, with focus on the following sections: general maternal well-being, breastfeeding, and contraceptive recommendations

---

18. Reinforce to your obstetric trainee the importance of a particular laboratory test to be   2
   assessed postpartum among women with T1DM relative to T2DM.

- ☐ Thyroid stimulating hormone (TSH) level is recommended to screen for postpartum thyroiditis between two and six months postpartum, depending on international practice recommendations

---

The patient presents for the routine interdisciplinary visit at six weeks' postpartum, complaining of frequent diaphoresis, palpitations, and mild anxiety. Glycemic control has been appropriate and routine postpartum screening does not suggest a depressive illness. The patient continues to breastfeed, and family members remain supportive of her and the newborn's well-being.

The patient is afebrile, blood pressure is 130/80 mmHg, and pulse is 110 bpm. There is no apparent goiter on examination although a hand tremor is evident at rest. The following are resulted among other investigations performed in collaboration with the endocrinologist:

		Normal
TSH	0.01 mIU/L	0.4–4.4 mIU/mL
Free thyroxine	35.90 pmol/L	8.00–18.00 pmol/L
TSH-receptor antibody	Absent	

19. Based on the most probable diagnosis, counsel the patient and devise an appropriate management plan in collaboration with the endocrinologist. *(1 point each)*   Max 2

☐ Explain that in the absence of TSH-receptor antibody to suggest Graves' disease, her symptoms are most probably attributed to postpartum thyroiditis, common to ~25% of women with T1DM

☐ Offer treatment based on symptomatic control (*e.g.,* beta-blocker for tachycardia)

☐ Inform her that antithyroid treatment is not warranted as recovery from the thyrotoxic phase is expected by ~4–6 months postpartum; she may revert to being euthyroid or enter a hypothyroid phase, most commonly transient for 6–12 months

TOTAL: **90**

CHAPTER 58

Pregestational Type 2 Diabetes Mellitus

Amira El-Messidi, Melissa-Rosina Pasqua, and Natasha Garfield

A 37-year-old G1P1 with a three-year history of type 2 diabetes mellitus (T2DM) is referred by her primary care provider to your high-risk obstetrics clinic for preconception counseling. Six years ago, she delivered her son at another hospital center.

LEARNING OBJECTIVES

1. Take a focused history, identifying obstetric and nonobstetric morbidities for preconception counseling of a multiparous patient with T2DM
2. Appreciate the importance of interdisciplinary collaboration for necessary pharmacologic adjustments among women with T2DM throughout the gestational spectrum
3. Provide counseling on fetal benefits of optimal prepregnancy and antenatal glycemic control
4. Present a comprehensive evidence-based scheme for maternal-fetal management for the antenatal period, including the ability to adjust insulin needs for women receiving fetal pulmonary corticosteroids
5. Relate clinical management considerations to maternal-fetal (patho)physiology with preexisting diabetes mellitus

SUGGESTED READINGS

1. American College of Obstetricians and Gynecologists' Committee on Practice Bulletins – Obstetrics. ACOG Practice Bulletin No. 201: pregestational diabetes mellitus. *Obstet Gynecol.* 2018;132(6):e228–e248.
2. American Diabetes Association. 14. Management of diabetes in pregnancy: standards of medical care in diabetes – 2021. *Diabetes Care.* 2021;44(Suppl 1):S200–S210.
3. Alexopoulos AS, Blair R, Peters AL. Management of preexisting diabetes in pregnancy: a review. *JAMA.* 2019;321(18):1811–1819.
4. (a) Berger H, Gagnon R, Sermer M. Guideline No. 393 – diabetes in pregnancy. *J Obstet Gynaecol Can.* 2019;41(12):1814–1825. [Correction in J Obstet Gynaecol Can. 2020 Oct;42(10):1288]

    (b) Diabetes Canada Clinical Practice Guidelines Expert Committee, Feig DS, Berger H, et al. Diabetes and pregnancy. *Can J Diabetes.* 2018;42(Suppl 1):S255–S282. [Correction in Can J Diabetes. 2018 Jun;42(3):337]
5. Egan AM, Dow ML, Vella A. A review of the pathophysiology and management of diabetes in pregnancy. *Mayo Clin Proc.* 2020;95(12):2734–2746.

6. Hameed AB, Combs CA. Society for Maternal-Fetal Medicine Special Statement: updated checklist for antepartum care of pregestational diabetes mellitus. *Am J Obstet Gynecol.* 2020;223(5):B2–B5.
7. Kapur A, McIntyre HD, Hod M. Type 2 diabetes in pregnancy. *Endocrinol Metab Clin North Am.* 2019;48(3):511–531.
8. National Institute for Health and Care Excellence (NICE). Diabetes in pregnancy: management from preconception to the postnatal period; NICE guideline. February 25, 2015. Available at www.nice.org.uk/guidance/ng3. Accessed July 18, 2021.
9. Scottish Intercollegiate Guidelines Network (SIGN). Management of diabetes, a national clinical guideline. March 2010, updates November 2017. Available at www.sign.ac.uk/assets/sign116.pdf. Accessed July 18, 2021.

POINTS

1. With focus on T2DM, what aspects of a focused history would you want to know?   30
   (1 point per main bullet unless specified; max points indicated where required)

General disease-related details:
☐ Determine the circumstances related to diagnosis: *(2 points)*
   ○ 1. Postpartum screening after gestational diabetes mellitus (GDM)
   ○ 2. Symptoms of hyper/hypoglycemia
   ○ 3. Diabetes-associated complications or comorbidities
   ○ 4. Medical conditions associated with onset of diabetes *(e.g., medications [chronic glucocorticoid use, second-generation atypical antipsychotics], cystic fibrosis, hereditary hemochromatosis, hormone-secreting tumors [glucagonomas])*
☐ Name and contact of treating endocrinologist *(if different from the referring primary provider)*

Disease-related complications/comorbidities: *(max 5)*

Microvascular complications
☐ Retinopathy
☐ Neuropathy
☐ Nephropathy

Macrovascular complications
☐ Ischemic heart disease
☐ Cerebrovascular disease
☐ Peripheral vascular disease

Comorbidities
☐ Hypertension
☐ Dyslipidemia
☐ Nonalcoholic steatohepatitis
☐ Chronic/long-standing infections
☐ Obstructive sleep apnea

Glycemic control:
☐ Inquire about known hemoglobinopathy *(e.g., Hb SS)* where HbA1c would not be reliable
☐ Identify the most recent HbA1c value

□ Determine frequency and mechanism of checking blood glucose values (*e.g., fingerpick vs. continuous glucose monitoring*)
□ Inquire about values of blood glucose readings

Current/prior pharmacologic agents for T2DM and comorbidities, including clinical response and side effects/adverse reactions: *(max 3)*
□ Oral or injectable antihyperglycemic agents
□ Determine the type of insulin and treatment protocol
□ Angiotensin receptor inhibitor (ACEi), angiotensin receptor blocker, statins or nonpreferred antihypertensive agents during pregnancy (*e.g.*, atenolol)
□ Allergies

Obstetric history: *(max 8)*
□ Determine if GDM screening was performed (*antenatal, and postnatal where required*), and whether pharmacologic therapy was needed
□ Inquire about postpartum weight gain (particularly if pregnancy was complicated by GDM)
□ Assess for onset of hypertensive diseases of pregnancy, particularly <32 weeks' gestation
□ Assess for antenatal diabetes-associated fetal complications (*e.g.*, congenital malformations related to undiagnosed T2DM, polyhydramnios, large-for-gestational-age biometry)
□ Gestational age at delivery
□ Mode of labor and delivery (*i.e.*, spontaneous/induced, vaginal/operative vaginal/ Cesarean)
□ Birth trauma (*i.e.*, shoulder dystocia, brachial plexus injury, infant fractures, extensive maternal lacerations)
□ Birthweight
□ Occurrence of early postpartum metabolic complications associated with in utero hyperglycemia

Gynecologic features related to T2DM:
□ Current/prior mode of contraception, if any
□ Menstrual cycle details (*e.g.*, last menses, cycle regularity)
□ Inquire about known polycystic ovarian syndrome
□ Assess for potentially undisclosed early pregnancy losses, particularly since diagnosis of T2DM

Social history and general health maintenance:
□ Cigarette smoking, (chronic) alcohol consumption, illicit substance use (*e.g.*, cocaine, amphetamines)
□ Dietary and exercise regimens
□ Vaccinations (*e.g.*, COVID-19, rubella, hepatitis B, influenza, pertussis, others if applicable)

You learn that the patient developed T2DM on annual screening after having abnormal post-partum fasting glucose secondary to GDM.[†] She recalls large for gestational age fetal biometry starting at 32 weeks' gestation when insulin was started. Labor was induced at 38^{+4} weeks' gestation due to rapidly decreasing insulin needs at term, with an uncomplicated delivery of a newborn weighting 3690 g at birth, 15% lower than the last sonographic estimate prior to delivery. Neonatal correction of GDM-associated metabolic derangements were required, during which she continued to breastfeed.

Although aerobic exercise and medical nutrition helped her lose excess weight gained during pregnancy (current BMI 24.5 kg/m²), her primary care provider drew attention to an inherently increased risk of T2DM based on demographic features, family history, and known long-standing polycystic ovarian syndrome. She does not smoke, drink alcohol, or use illicit substances. The patient is unsure if her vaccinations are up to date.

Apart from hypertension and dyslipidemia diagnosed simultaneously with T2DM, she has not experienced other comorbidities. The patient informs you her last HbA1c was 7.9% (62.8 mmol/mol). She monitors her fasting blood glucose by fingerpick twice to thrice weekly, with readings consistently between 7.0 mmol/L (126 mg/dL) and 11.4 mmol/L (205 mg/dL). Her long-term treatment regimen to which she remains adherent includes:

- Metformin 1000 mg orally twice daily
- Empagliflozin 25 mg orally daily *[i.e., sodium glucose cotransporter 2 (SGLT2) inhibitor]*
- Semaglutide 1 mg subcutaneously weekly *[i.e., glucagon like peptide-1 receptor agonist (GLP-1RA)]*
- Rosuvastatin 10 mg orally daily
- Ramipril 5 mg orally daily
- Oral iron supplements for iron-deficiency anemia
- Levonorgesterol intrauterine system (LNG-IUS)

Understanding the importance of maintaining an optimal weight, aerobic exercise, and nutritional plan, she inquires about her pharmacologic regimen prior to and during pregnancy.

Special note:
† Refer to Question 13 in Chapter 56 for various jurisdictional recommendations for postpartum and later screening practices for diagnosing T2DM after GDM.

---

2. Provide evidence-based <u>preconception pharmacologic</u> counseling for this patient with T2DM, with an understanding that therapeutic modifications will be made with multidisciplinary collaboration. *(1 point per main bullet, max points specified where required)*

Max 10

Antihyperglycemic agents:
☐ Given T2DM and polycystic ovarian syndrome, continuation of metformin may be considered for its fertility benefits *(Diabetes Canada[4b])*
☐ Reassure the patient that use of metformin in the first trimester has not been proven to increase risks of early pregnancy loss or congenital anomalies
☐ In early pregnancy, metformin may be discontinued in favor of insulin given lack of long-term neonatal safety data as well as placental transfer
☐ Nonmetformin antihyperglycemic agents namely the SGLT-1 inhibitor and GLP-1RA should be discontinued ideally three months prior to conception because of lack of safety data; agents are replaced by insulin, provided for both basal needs and meals

Insulin therapy and monitoring of glycemic control:
☐ Reassure the patient that insulin is nonteratogenic
☐ Glucose testing should be increased to three to four times daily

☐ Glycemic targets should aim to achieve glucose control as close to normal as possible; the preconception HbA1c target is $\leq$7%[†] (53 mmol/mol[‡]) preferably $\leq$6.5% (43 mmol/mol), if this can be achieved without significant hypoglycemia
  ○ *Two consecutively normal HbA1c values measured at a three-month interval preconception improve pregnancy outcomes when maintained antenatally (Suggested Reading 8)*

Contraceptive agent:
☐ Educate the patient that current removal of the LNG-IUS is **not** advised until target glycemic control is achieved and required pharmacologic adjustments have been made

ACEi and statin agents:
☐ Discontinuation of the ACEi is advised *prior to* conception in the absence of chronic renal insufficiency*; replace with antihypertensive agent(s) with reassuring safety profiles in pregnancy *(e.g., labetalol, methyldopa, nifedipine, hydralazine)*
☐ Provide patient education: while statin therapy should be discontinued in most women planning to conceive, get pregnant, or breastfeed, policy makers' consideration (Food and Drug Act; July 2021) for continued therapy is accepted for women at very high risk of antenatal cardiovascular events (individualized risk assessment)

Folic acid recommendations: *(max 1)*
[Controversial advisories]
☐ Dietary supplementation with at least folic acid 400 ug preconception *(ACOG[1], ADA[2], Diabetes Canada[4b])*; commencement of folic acid intake varies from one to three months preconception
☐ Doses up to 5 mg daily started prepregnancy and continued until 12 weeks' gestation have also been recommended[§] to reduce risks of fetal neural tube defects *(NICE[8], SIGN[9])*

Vaccinations:
☐ Encourage comprehensive revision of immunization status prior to conception

Special notes:
[†] Units as a percentage as per the Diabetes Control and Complications Trial (DCCT)
[‡] Units as mmol/mol as per the International Federation of Clinical Chemistry (IFCC), facilitating comparison in international studies; preferred unit by NICE[8]
[*] Refer to Question 5 in Chapter 47 for ACEi recommendations specific to women with renal disease and fetal teratogenic effects
[§] Benefits on fetal risks of neural tube defects are theoretical; there are no intervention trials to support folic acid doses >1 mg for women with preexisting diabetes mellitus *(Diabetes Canada[4b])*

The patient appreciates the importance of an interprofessional diabetes health care team, both prior to conception and during pregnancy, for nonpharmacologic and pharmacologic management of T2DM and associated maternal-fetal risks. She recalls her primary care provider reviewed disease-related adverse effects on maternal[†] and neonatal[‡] outcomes, requesting your expertise in addressing *fetal* risks and management in consultation.

Special notes:
[†] and [‡] Refer to the clinical description after Question 15 in Chapter 57 and refer to the table in Question 8 in Chapter 56, respectively

3. Counsel the patient on <u>fetal benefits</u> of achieving optimal glycosylated hemoglobin levels prior to, and during, pregnancy. *(1 point each)*

Max 4

Decreased risks of:
☐ Early spontaneous pregnancy loss
☐ Congenital anomalies *(direct correlation with HbA1c levels)*
☐ Macrosomia
☐ Stillbirth
☐ Neonatal death

4. Inform the patient on your plan for <u>fetal investigations</u> in the context of preexisting diabetes mellitus, making note to explain your recommendations or considerations to the trainee based on fetal risk of adverse outcomes, particularly where glycemic control is suboptimal.

6

(1 point per description of proposed assessment modality in each trimester, where relevant)

	First trimester	Second trimester, at 18–20 weeks' gestation	Third trimester
Sonography	○ Viability ○ Accurate pregnancy dating, particularly given the risk of menstrual irregularity ○ Neural tube defects, particularly anencephaly and holoprosencephaly	○ Biometry ○ Amniotic fluid volume ○ Cardiac and noncardiac malformations, such as open spina bifida, orofacial clefts, renal agenesis, ectopic kidney, sacral agenesis/caudal dysplasia	○ Serial growth biometry and velocity for risk of large-for-gestational-age biometry or fetal growth restriction ○ Individualized considerations for fetal Doppler velocimetry ○ Amniotic fluid volume, preferably based on the deepest vertical pocket relative to four-quadrant fluid index
Fetal echocardiography		*e.g.,* ○ Ventricular septal defects ○ Complex lesions, including transposition of	

(cont.)

	First trimester	Second trimester, at 18–20 weeks' gestation	Third trimester
		the great arteries, double-outlet right ventricle, tricuspid atresia, and truncus arteriosus ○ Hypertrophic cardiomyopathy	
Modalities for fetal surveillance [*e.g.,* nonstress test, (modified) biophysical profile, or combinations thereof]			○ Generally started at ~32 weeks in the absence of complications as the risk of stillbirth is higher at all gestations >32 weeks among women with preexisting diabetes[†] ○ No known preferred modality or frequency of surveillance
Aneuploidy screening	○ Consideration for noninvasive cell-free DNA screening; second-trimester maternal serum biomarkers (*i.e.,* alpha-fetoprotein, unconjugated estriol and inhibin A) require laboratory adjustment as values are lower in women with preexisting diabetes than nondiabetic population		

Special note:

† Holman N, Bell R, Murphy H, Maresh M. Women with pre-gestational diabetes have a higher risk of stillbirth at all gestations after 32 weeks. *Diabet Med.* 2014;31(9):1129–1132.

You take note to later inform your trainee that while sacral agenesis/caudal dysplasia is *most characteristic* of diabetic embryopathy, its occurrence in nondiabetic pregnancies highlights that the defect is *not pathognomonic* for maternal preexisting diabetes.

On physical examination, you confirm a normal BMI and blood pressure is 125/70 mmHg. You learn that on recent assessment of her lower extremities, her primary care provider reassured her of normal sensation and perfusion.

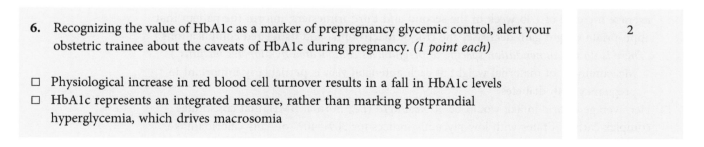

5. With focus on this patient with T2DM, list the preconception <u>investigations</u> you would consider, in affiliation with interprofessional experts. *(1 point each)*   6

Serum:
- ☐ HbA1c
- ☐ Full/complete blood count (FBC/CBC) and ferritin *[particularly with known baseline anemia]*
- ☐ Creatinine

Urine:
- ☐ Spot (random) urine protein/creatinine ratio or albumin/creatinine ratio

Other:
- ☐ Electrocardiogram, based on her age ≥35 years and cardiac risk factors *(SMFM[6])*
- ☐ Ophthalmology consultation for fundoscopic examination *(assess for retinopathy or maculopathy)*

Results of requested investigations reveal a normal electrocardiogram and absence of diabetic nephropathy; routine prenatal tests performed simultaneously are unremarkable. Retinal examination was normal. The patient attended the specialized diabetic care clinic in your high-risk hospital center where pharmacologic modifications were made and nutritional guidance provided; simultaneously, she engaged in an exercise program.

Ten months later, the patient is now referred to you at 8^{+2} weeks' gestation by dating sonography. She takes 20 U subcutaneous NPH insulin nightly as the basal dose, accompanied by three bolus doses of lispro insulin directly before mealtimes (10 U at breakfast, 8 U at lunch and 8 U at supper), labetalol, folic acid, and iron supplementation. Metformin was discontinued upon confirmation of a viable intrauterine pregnancy. Combined pharmacologic modifications and nonpharmacologic interventions had improved her glycosylated hemoglobin to 6.4% within five months of your last consultation. The LNG-IUS was removed thereafter, leading to spontaneous conception within three months. Prepregnancy BMI remained normal at 23.5 kg/m^2.

6. Recognizing the value of HbA1c as a marker of prepregnancy glycemic control, alert your obstetric trainee about the caveats of HbA1c during pregnancy. *(1 point each)*   2

- ☐ Physiological increase in red blood cell turnover results in a fall in HbA1c levels
- ☐ HbA1c represents an integrated measure, rather than marking postprandial hyperglycemia, which drives macrosomia

7. In relation to T2DM, outline <u>maternal</u> aspects of antenatal counseling and management you would address in the early prenatal visits with this patient. *(1 point per main bullet, unless specified)*

Max 15

Prenatal care:
- ☐ (Continued) multidisciplinary care in the specialized 'combined obstetric/diabetes clinic,' in addition to routine prenatal care
- ☐ Reinforce the importance of compliance with clinical visits and adherence to management

Glycemic goals in pregnancy:
- ☐ Encourage multiple daily self-glucose monitoring (*e.g.*, fasting, pre and one-hour post meals, bedtime, and if feels unwell)
- ☐ Alert the patient to target glycemic values *where achievable without causing problematic hypoglycemia*

(2 points for either recommendation; other jurisdictional values may be accepted)

		Fasting	1-hour postprandial	2-hour postprandial	Before bed
☐	*[ACOG[1], ADA[2], Diabetes Canada[4b], NICE[7]]‡*	<5.3 (95)	<7.8 (140)	<6.4 (115) *for NICE[7]* or <6.7 (120) *for ACOG[1], ADA[2], Diabetes Canada[4b]*	———————
☐	*SIGN[9]*	4–6 (72–108)	<8 (144)	<7 (126)	>6 (108)

Units: mmol/L (mg/dL)

Nausea and vomiting in pregnancy ± hyperemesis gravidarum:
- ☐ Maintain a low threshold to prevent or manage symptoms common to early pregnancy due to the risk of provoking diabetic ketoacidosis *(refer to Chapter 4)*

Nonpharmacologic interventions:
- ☐ Based on the patient's normal prepregnancy BMI of at 23.5 kg/m^2 with a singleton gestation, recommended total gestational weight gain is 25–35 lb (~11–15 kg),[†] with an average increase of 1 lb/week in the second and third trimesters; inform the patient that appropriate weight gain decreases the risk of macrosomia and its related complications *(There is no recommendation specific to pregnancies complicated by diabetes mellitus[†])*
  - ○ Measurement of maternal weight at each antenatal visit is particularly important in pregnancy with diabetes
- ☐ Her average caloric intake would be 30 kcal/kg/d (*i.e.*, normal BMI), that constitutes complex carbohydrates with low-glycemic indices for 30%–40% of daily caloric intake, ~20% protein and ~40% fat, with serial monitoring for ketonuria
- ☐ Encourage continued engagement in ~150 minutes/week of moderate-intensity exercise over a minimum of four days, where tolerated and in the absence of contraindications[§]

Pharmacologic management:

☐ Address the upcoming physiological decrease in insulin needs until ~16 weeks' gestation, after which insulin requirements normally increase significantly until late gestation; dose adjustments generally require an endocrinologist's expertise

Chronic hypertension:

☐ Titrate antihypertensive treatment to target blood pressure (BP) at 110–135/85 mmHg with preexisting diabetes to reduce risks of hypertensive complications in pregnancy and minimize suboptimal fetal growth *(ADA[2])*

☐ Home BP monitoring *(individualized frequency)*

☐ Encourage early reporting of symptoms or signs suggestive of hypertensive disease

☐ Initiate low dose aspirin ~81–162 mg/d *(dosing varies by jurisdiction)*, taken nightly starting before 16 weeks' gestation until delivery or diagnosis of preeclampsia
   ○ *Delayed initiation up to 28 weeks' gestation offers some benefit for preeclampsia prophylaxis*

☐ Maintain a low-salt diet *(given chronic hypertension)*

☐ Calcium supplementation 1.2–2.5 g elemental calcium per day in women with low calcium intake *(i.e., <600–800 mg/d or <4 daily servings)* [#]

Other morbidities-specific counseling:

☐ Repeat retinal evaluation in early pregnancy is warranted as her prior was more than six months ago *(NICE[7])*

☐ Encourage early reporting of symptoms or signs suggestive of: *(1 point per subbullet)*
   ○ Preterm labor *(refer to Chapter 7)*
   ○ Local or systemic infection *(decreases threshold for diabetic ketoacidosis)*

Overview of delivery planning:

☐ Aim for vaginal delivery, with Cesarean section being reserved for obstetric indications

☐ If maternal-fetal markers of glycemic control are satisfactory, without fetal growth restriction, superimposed preeclampsia or other vascular complication, delivery would be advised at 37^{+0} to 38^{+6} *(NICE[7])* or 39^{+0} to 39^{+6} weeks' gestation *(SMFM[6], ACOG*)*
   ○ *Earlier delivery is based on individual considerations*

Special notes:

[†] Institute of Medicine (now, 'National Academy of Medicine'): Weight gain during pregnancy: reexamining the guidelines. National Academy of Sciences. 28 May 2009; endorsed by the American College of Obstetricians and Gynecologists. ACOG Committee opinion no. 548: weight gain during pregnancy. *Obstet Gynecol.* 2013;121(1):210–212.

[§] Davies GAL, Wolfe LA, Mottola MF, MacKinnon C. No. 129-Exercise in Pregnancy and the Postpartum Period. *J Obstet Gynaecol Can.* 2018;40(2):e58-e65.

[‡] Target capillary plasma glucose values among women with preexisting diabetes are consistent with target values among women with GDM; *refer to* Question 10 in Chapter 56

[#] With reference to *Suggested Reading 6* in Chapter 38; calcium supplementation is recommended by ISSHP and SOGC guidelines, however, ACOG does not endorse calcium supplementation for preeclampsia prevention

[*] American College of Obstetricians and Gynecologists' Committee on Obstetric Practice, Society for Maternal-Fetal Medicine. Medically Indicated Late-Preterm and Early-Term Deliveries: ACOG Committee Opinion, No. 831. *Obstet Gynecol.* 2021;138(1):e35-e39

8. The patient understands that maintaining her exercise regime is fundamental to optimizing glycemic control and general cardiovascular health.

Max 5

In relation to diabetes-associated obstetric morbidities, elaborate on her understanding of evidence-based benefits of exercise in pregnancy. *(1 point each)*

Exercise benefits for diabetes-associated obstetric morbidities:
☐ Preeclampsia and other hypertensive disorders of pregnancy
☐ Extremes of fetal weight (macrosomia/fetal growth restriction)
☐ Excessive gestational weight gain
☐ Preterm birth
☐ Cesarean delivery
☐ Operative vaginal delivery
☐ Postpartum depression

Special note:
Refer to Davies GAL, Wolfe LA, Mottola MF, MacKinnon C. No. 129-Exercise in Pregnancy and the Postpartum Period. *J Obstet Gynaecol Can.* 2018;40(2):e58-e65

Pregnancy progresses well until 26^{+5} weeks' gestation when the patient presents to the obstetric emergency assessment unit with threatened preterm labor, requiring initiation of a course of betamethasone for fetal pulmonary maturity, among other management. While the endocrinology care team is occupied with a medical emergency, you use this opportunity to review with your obstetric trainee the general scheme for insulin adjustments at this time. Upon your request, the patient shares with you her most recent insulin dosing schedule over the past three days, as appropriate for the glycemic readings:

date	Fasting (Lispro, Humalog®)	Before Lunch (Lispro, Humalog®)	Before Dinner (Lispro, Humalog®)	Bedtime (Neutral Protamine Hagedorn insulin [NPH], Novolin® N)
1	18	18	16	24
2	20	18	18	26
Yesterday	20	20	20	30

9. While explaining the outline of your evidence-based protocol, calculate the planned insulin dose adjustments after receipt of the first of two betamethasone doses for fetal pulmonary maturity. You alert your trainee that individual adaptations of a respective insulin dose will be based on actual blood glucose levels. *(1 point each)*

Max 4

☐ Insulin dose-increments are relative to the insulin doses on the day before the first dose of glucocorticoid (*i.e.*, 20, 20, 20, 30)

	Lispro (Humalog®)	NPH (Novolin® N)
Insulin doses used for adjustment	20, 20, 20	30
☐ At day 1, the night insulin dose was increased by 25%	20, 20, 20	38
☐ At days 2 and 3, all insulin doses were increased by 40%	28, 28, 28	42
☐ At day 4, all insulin doses were increased by 20%	24, 24, 24	36
☐ At day 5, all insulin doses were increased by 10%–20%	22, 22, 22	33
At days 6 and 7, the insulin dose was gradually reduced to its level before glucocorticoid treatment		

Special note:

Refer to Diabetes Canada[4b]

With resolution of preterm labor and normal maternal-fetal status, the patient is discharged from hospital within five days of admission, having resumed her standard insulin schedule.

She remains compliant with multidisciplinary follow-up and adherent to treatment. By 33^{+1} weeks' gestation, the patient is pleased to have maintained appropriate glycemic control, although she feels dismayed by large-for-gestational age fetal abdominal circumference, overall biometry >95th percentile and an accelerated growth velocity over the past month. The sonographic report indicates image quality is appropriate for biometric assessment.

10. With reference to pathophysiology, explain the onset of 'diabetic fetopathy' in the context of appropriate maternal glycemic control. *(1 point each, or any appropriate explanation thereof)*   4

Petersen 'hyperglycemia-hyperinsulinemia' hypothesis' and the 'fetal glucose steal' syndrome:
- ☐ Based on the concentration of maternal glucose, transplacental transfer occurs by facilitated diffusion along the concentration gradient
- ☐ Fetal hyperglycemia leads to fetal hyperinsulinemia, increasing glucose use and lowering fetal glycemia; this promotes further maternal-fetal transplacental transport
- ☐ Persistently high glucose efflux from the maternal compartment continues, leading to an apparent (near) normal glycemic index
- ☐ Continued influx of glucose into the fetal compartment stimulates triacylglycerol formation and excess fetal adiposity

By 37^{+5} weeks' gestation, the patient reports, to the antepartum clinic with decreasing insulin requirements, indeed calculated to have decreased by 7% over the past week. Comprehensive maternal-fetal evaluation is otherwise only remarkable for an estimated fetal weight of 4580 g and a deepest maximal vertical fluid pocket at 10.5 cm. Fetal presentation remains cephalic.[§]

Your obstetric trainee recalls you teaching about placental hormones that contribute to the physiological increases in antenatal insulin resistance[†] and is now researching for potential causes for the patient's decreasing insulin needs.

Special notes:
§ Performance of the fetal biophysical profile varies internationally.
† Refer to Question 5 (Section B) in Chapter 56

11. Address the significance, if any, of decreasing insulin requirements in pregnancy and propose clinical management considerations thereof. *(1 point each)*   Max 4

Significance of decreasing insulin needs in pregnancy:
- ☐ Unconfirmed impact: studies show contrasting results
- ☐ Placental insufficiency is a hypothesized etiology
- ☐ Onset (or worsening) of renal function leading to decreased insulin excretion

Management considerations:
- ☐ Serum creatinine testing
- ☐ Comprehensive assessment of fetal well-being, considering other risks for perinatal mortality (*e.g.,* maternal and gestational age, glycemic control, comorbidities)

12. Close maternal-fetal surveillance is arranged with interdisciplinary collaboration. Expecting delivery within the week, present an <u>obstetric consideration</u> regarding the mode of delivery.

☐ Prophylactic Cesarean section **may be considered** where the estimated fetal weight is ≥4500 g in pregnancies with preexisting [or gestational] diabetes *(ACOG[1], RCOG[†])*

Special note:

† Royal College of Obstetricians and Gynaecologists. Shoulder dystocia. Green Top guideline No. 42. 2nd ed. March 2012. Available at www.rcog.org.uk/en/guidelines-research-services/guidelines/gtg42/, accessed March 5, 2021.

After an informed consent process on risks and benefits of delivery modalities, an elective Cesarean section[†] is agreed-upon; intraoperative glycemia will be closely monitored to remain within target of 4.0 and 7.0 mmol/L [*i.e., 72–126 mg/dL*] *(Diabetes Canada[4b], NICE[7])*. The postoperative insulin regimen, as devised by the endocrinologist, specifies dose adjustments to take effect immediately postpartum, whereby insulin requirements will be decreased by 30%–50% of antepartum doses.

You review the neonatologist's consultation note, indicating potential risks for which the newborn of this mother with T2DM will be closely monitored.[‡]

Special notes:

† Refer to Question 16 in Chapter 57 for glycemic control during induction of labor and vaginal delivery.

‡ Refer to Questions 8 and 9 in Chapter 56 for short- and long-term neonatal morbidities, respectively, associated with poorly controlled diabetes in pregnancy.

13. What are the benefits of maintaining intraoperative euglycemia in a parturient with preexisting diabetes that you would address with your obstetric trainee? *(1 point each)*

Decreased risk of:

☐ Neonatal hypoglycemia
☐ Cesarean wound infection
☐ Maternal-neonatal metabolic complications

Max 2

14. With reference to maternal and placental hormones that contribute to insulin resistance,[†]   2
identify the ones whose circulating levels drop most significantly after delivery of the
placenta, accounting for rapid increases in insulin sensitivity. *(1 point each)*

☐ Human placental lactogen
☐ Human placental growth hormone

Special note:
†   Refer to Question 5 (Section B) in Chapter 56; cortisol, prolactin, and progesterone are less
responsible for postpartum changes in insulin needs

An *urgent* Cesarean section is required at 38^{+1} weeks' gestation for an abnormal fetal heart
cardiotocographic tracing during surveillance arranged for decreasing insulin requirements.
Your trainee remarks that while preoperative prophylactic antibiotics are routine, pharmacologic
administration is particularly important for this patient to mitigate risks of postoperative
infectious morbidity. Surgery is uncomplicated and maternal glycemia is maintained at target
values with intravenous insulin. A macrosomic infant is delivered with birthweight consistent with
the sonographic estimate. The neonatology team, present at delivery, is performing principal
newborn assessment for infants of mothers with preexisting diabetes, including possible undiagnosed antenatal malformations.

15. Discuss aspects of <u>postpartum</u> care and management of this patient with T2DM.   Max 10
(1 point per main bullet)

General maternal well-being:
☐ Screen for postpartum depression and continue to offer psychosocial support services
☐ Encourage healthy lifestyle practices (*e.g.,* diet, exercise, loss of gestational weight gain,
continued avoidance of smoking and alcohol [ab]use)
☐ Facilitate return to her primary care physician

Pharmacologic thromboprophylaxis:
☐ The patient's risk factors for venous thromboembolism include an emergency Cesarean
section, hypertension, and T2DM (*i.e.,* autoimmunity); individualized considerations for
the type and number of risk factors required to meet the threshold for pharmacologic
thromboprophylaxis of practice guidelines

Breastfeeding:
☐ Breastfeeding should be strongly encouraged for maternal-child benefits among women
with preexisting (or gestational) diabetes[†]
☐ Reassure the patient that delayed lactation tends to occur in women with preexisting
diabetes; milk supply can be lower and nursing difficulties more common relative to
women without diabetes, warranting consideration for lactation consultation
☐ Provide patient education on risks of maternal hypoglycemia with breastfeeding, and
promote intake of an additional ~500 kcal/d *(as this patient is nonobese)* from
prepregnancy caloric intake; maintain close monitoring of glycemic logs

Oral antihyperglycemics during breastfeeding:

☐ Resumption of the patient's metformin can be considered during breastfeeding as infant exposure is below the 10% 'level of concern'; inform the patient to remain diligent for signs of child hypoglycemia
  ○ *Only metformin, glibenclamide [glyburide], and insulin are accepted during breastfeeding; human safety data for her prior agents (i.e., SGLT2 inhibitors and GLP-1RA, among others) remains lacking*

Resumption of ACEi (*i.e.*, ramipril) during breastfeeding:

☐ While ramipril is not recommended during breastfeeding, agents including enalapril, captopril, and quinapril are the preferred ACEi in breastfeeding given absent breast milk excretion

Contraceptive recommendations:

☐ Support (repeat) reliable contraception with timed pregnancy to optimize preconception glycemic control and comorbidities to mitigate the risk of congenital anomalies and adverse outcomes for pregnancy and preexisting diabetes
☐ There are no restrictions on use of the copper intrauterine device (IUD) with insulin/non-insulin-dependent diabetes with/without micro/macrovascular disease
☐ All progesterone-only methods are considered safe *(category 2)* for women with preexisting diabetes *(UK-MEC)*[‡]; however, risk of depot medroxyprogesterone acetate (DMPA) may outweigh its advantages *(category 3)* among women with diabetic micro/macrovascular disease *(US-MEC)*[‡]
☐ Combined oral contraceptive agents would not be recommended for this patient with comorbid hypertension *(category 3 or 4, depending on the presence of vascular disease and blood pressure control)*; however, in the absence of diabetic micro/macrovascular disease, estrogen-containing oral contraceptive would otherwise be deemed safe *(category 2)*

Special notes:

[†] Refer to Question 13 in Chapter 56
[‡] UK and US Medical Eligibility Criteria (MEC) for Contraceptive Use, 2016; UK-MEC amended September 2019, US-MEC updated 2020

TOTAL: **105**

Infectious Conditions in Pregnancy

CHAPTER 59

Cytomegalovirus Infection in Pregnancy

Amira El-Messidi and Eva Suarthana

A healthy 23-year-old G2P1 presents for prenatal care at 12^{+0} weeks' gestation by dating ultrasound. Her last pregnancy was cared for by your colleague, who is currently away. Pregnancy was uncomplicated, and she had a spontaneous vaginal delivery at term. You learn from the antenatal notes that the patient had a flu-like illness in early pregnancy; investigations were unremarkable, and symptoms resolved with supportive care. She tells you her healthy two-year-old son has been attending daycare since six months of age and is meeting his developmental milestones.

LEARNING OBJECTIVES

1. Appreciate the essential criteria for a universal screening test, and recognize risk factors for cytomegalovirus (CMV) infection that may justify universal testing
2. Interpret results of maternal CMV serology, and understand the accuracy of diagnostic tests involved in defining primary maternal infection and congenital CMV infection
3. Highlight evolving therapies for prevention or treatment of congenital CMV infection
4. Detect fetal sonographic manifestations of CMV infection, and understand the limitations in predicting postnatal outcome
5. Acknowledge long-term sequelae of congenital CMV infection, not limited to symptomatic neonates at birth

SUGGESTED READINGS

1. Bartlett AW, Hamilton ST, Shand AW, et al. Fetal therapies for cytomegalovirus: what we tell prospective parents. Prenat Diagn. 2020;1–12.
2. Boucoiran I, Yudin M, Poliquin V, et al. Guideline No. 420: cytomegalovirus infection in pregnancy. *J Obstet Gynaecol Can.* 2021;43(7):893–908. [Correction in J Obstet Gynaecol Can. 2021 Oct 11]
3. Bonita R, Beaglehole R, Kjellström T. *Basic Epidemiology.* 2nd ed. Geneva: WHO; 2016.
4. Gaur P, Ffrench-Constant S, Kachramanoglou C, et al. Is it not time for international guidelines to combat congenital cytomegalovirus infection? a review of central nervous system manifestations. *Clin Radiol.* 2020;75(8): 644.
5. Kagan KO, Hamprecht K. Cytomegalovirus infection in pregnancy. *Arch Gynecol Obstet.* 2017;296(1):15–26.

6. Khalil A, Heath P, Jones C, et al. Congenital cytomegalovirus infection: update on treatment: Scientific Impact Paper No. 56. *BJOG.* 2018;125(1):e1–e11.

7. Lazzarotto T, Blázquez-Gamero D, Delforge ML, et al. Congenital cytomegalovirus infection: a narrative review of the issues in screening and management from a panel of European experts. *Front Pediatr.* 2020;8:13.

8. Leruez-Ville M, Ville Y. Fetal cytomegalovirus infection. *Best Pract Res Clin Obstetr Gynaecol* 2017;38:97–107.

9. Rawlinson WD, Boppana SB, Fowler KB, et al. Congenital cytomegalovirus infection in pregnancy and the neonate: consensus recommendations for prevention, diagnosis, and therapy. *Lancet Infect Dis.* 2017;17(6):e177–e188.

10. Society for Maternal-Fetal Medicine (SMFM), Hughes BL, Gyamfi-Bannerman C. Diagnosis and antenatal management of congenital cytomegalovirus infection. *Am J Obstet Gynecol.* 2016;214(6):B5–B11.

POINTS

1. During this first prenatal visit, you recognize the patient was last seronegative for CMV and take this opportunity to discuss modes of transmission and educate her on hygienic measures to prevent primary maternal CMV infection. You inform your obstetric trainee you would have provided similar advice for prevention of maternal reinfection. *(1 point each)*

Max 5

Modes of transmission:
- ☐ Inform the patient that the *principal mechanism* of infection is through exposure to young children who become infected by droplet contact from other children
- ☐ Other modes of transmission include genital secretions, saliva, urine, leukocyte-containing cellular blood products, transplacental, intrapartum, or breastfeeding

Preventative measures:
- ☐ Advise handwashing with soap and water after child handling (*i.e.,* changing diapers, feeding, bathing, handling dirty laundry, wiping secretions)
- ☐ Avoid sharing food, eating utensils, and towels with children
- ☐ Avoid sleeping in the same bed as children
- ☐ Avoid mucosal contact with children

The patient appreciates your counseling, although she is concerned about adherence as she, her husband and son are temporarily living in a three-bedroom apartment with family members who also have young children.

2. State risk factors for maternal CMV infection, which *may or may not* relate to this patient. *(1 point each)*

Max 7

- ☐ Exposure to infective children/adults
- ☐ Low socioeconomic status
- ☐ Birth in developing countries
- ☐ Multiparity
- ☐ Young maternal age at first pregnancy

☐ Recipients of blood transfusions
☐ Childcare workers
☐ Prior abnormal cervical cytology
☐ Multiple sexual partners
☐ Sexually transmitted infections

You inform the patient that although routine prenatal screening for CMV is not universally recommended, you advise serological assessment based on her risk factors.

3. With regard to the WHO criteria for a screening program, explain why universal CMV screening is not recommended. *(1 point each)*

Max 4

Unmet criteria of a screening test:
☐ Difficulty in predicting sequelae
☐ Assays lack consistently high sensitivity and specificity
☐ Lack of early intervention to prevent transmission
☐ Insufficient cost-effectiveness data
☐ Risk of harm from screening due to inappropriate termination of pregnancies and increased parental anxiety

Serology shows CMV IgG + and IgM +. All other investigations, including first-trimester sonography are normal. Upon your request, the patient presents at 14 weeks' gestation for counseling and management.

4. Which alternative test may establish a maternal CMV infection?

1

☐ Blood or urine CMV DNA PCR

5. Explain to the patient the results of her CMV serology. *(1 point each)*

Max 5

☐ Explain that CMV seroconversion has occurred since her last pregnancy

Possible explanations for IgG and IgM positive serologies:
☐ Primary infection
☐ Distant infection as IgM can remain positive at low levels for 12–18 months after primary infection
☐ False-positive IgM based on standard enzyme-linked immunoassay testing due to detection of IgM from nonspecific polyclonal stimulation of the immune system
☐ Cross-reactivity of IgM with other antiherpes virus' IgM *(e.g., Epstein-Barr virus)*
☐ Reactivation of latent virus in the salivary glands based on seroconversion after her last screening; CMV IgM levels can increase in nonprimary infections

6-A. What is your <u>next best</u> test?   1

☐ CMV IgG avidity

6-B. How would you explain 'avidity testing' to the patient? (** *implies required response:*   2
1 point each)

☐ ** In primary infections, antibodies have lower avidity (*'affinity'*) for viral antigens than those produced in a nonprimary response
☐ ** Combining CMV IgM + and low avidity IgG (<30%) strongly suggests a primary infection in the prior three- to four-month period
☐ Low-moderate avidity antibodies remain for ~16–18 weeks after primary infections
☐ Avidity rises with time such that a high IgG avidity result of >60% suggests a distant infection or reactivation

The laboratory of the tertiary-care center where you work reports CMV IgG avidity at 20%. The patient is now 15 weeks' gestation. Referrals for multidisciplinary consultation have been instigated.

7. Discuss the principal elements of counseling and fetal diagnostic testing.   Max 6
(** *implies required response: 1 point per main bullet*)

☐ **Maternal primary infection most probably occurred in the first trimester, or periconceptional period
☐ **The likelihood of CMV transmission to the fetus increases proportionally with gestational age, but disease is most severe with first-trimester infections; the risk of long-term infant sequelae is inversely proportional to gestational age when congenital CMV infection was acquired
☐ **Most fetal infections (~99%) occur with maternal primary infections
☐ **Based on her results, the likelihood of congenital CMV infection is 30%–40%
  ○ Of infected fetuses, the majority (~90%) are asymptomatic at birth, with 8%–15% of these neonates developing long-term sequelae (*mainly unilateral or bilateral sensorineural hearing loss*)
    ▪ *Sensorineural hearing loss is mostly a consequence of first-trimester infections as inner ear structures and sensory cells form within the first 12 weeks of development*
  ○ Of the 10% of symptomatic neonates at birth, 40%–60% may have permanent sequelae
☐ Reassure the patient that breastfeeding is considered safe with CMV infection acquired during pregnancy

Fetal diagnosis:
☐ **Amniocentesis for CMV DNA PCR is recommended to confirm fetal infection (*viral culture is disfavored because results may take up to six weeks*)
  ○ Specificity of a positive amniotic fluid PCR is 100% and sensitivity of a negative result ranges from 45% to 93% based on timing of at least eight weeks[†] from maternal infection

- ○ *Controversial:* Quantification of amniotic fluid CMV DNA count $\geq 10^3$ genome equivalents/mL of amniotic fluid may confirm infection
- ○ *Controversial:* CMV DNA count $\geq 10^5$ genome equivalents/mL of amniotic fluid may predict severity of congenital CMV
- □ **Ultrasound screening for fetal manifestations is recommended at approximately two- to four-week intervals, recognizing that findings are not specific for congenital CMV disease
- □ *Controversial:* fetal blood markers (*e.g.,* platelet count, beta-2 microglobulin, and CMV IgM)

Special note:

† *Refer to* Enders M, Daiminger A, Exler S, Ertan K, Enders G, Bald R. Prenatal diagnosis of congenital cytomegalovirus infection in 115 cases: a 5 years' single center experience. *Prenat Diagn.* 2017;37(4):389–398.

8-A. What is meant by the 'sensitivity' of a test?　1

- □ The ability of a test to classify persons *with* the disease as positive

8-B. What is meant by the 'specificity' of a test?　1

- □ The ability to classify persons *without* the disease as negative

You decide to read a paper about the ability of ultrasound to detect fetal manifestations of CMV infection. Authors studied 100 pregnant women with CMV infection, of which half had sonographic CMV manifestations. The study reported the following results:

	Congenital CMV infection	Healthy fetuses
Ultrasound manifestations	25	0
Normal imaging	25	50

9-A. Based on the results of this study, what is the sensitivity and specificity of ultrasound as a screening test? *(1 point each)*　2

- □ Sensitivity: a/(a + c) = 25/(25 + 25) = 50%
- □ Specificity: d/(b + d) = 50/(0 + 50) = 100%

9-B. According to the study, what is the overall accuracy of ultrasound manifestations in correctly identifying congenitally infected fetuses?　2

- □ Accuracy = (a + d)/(a + b + c + d) = 75/100 = 75%

10. Address a patient inquiry about therapies that have been studied for prevention or treatment of fetal CMV infection and provide your best practice recommendations. *(** implies required response: 1 point each)*

☐ ****CMV hyperimmune globulin (CMV-HIG):**
  ○ *Theoretical mechanism of action*: Administration of high avidity IgG preparations during early stages of primary infections when avidity is low may prevent transplacental viral transmission or decrease the severity of postnatal infections
  ○ ****High-quality evidence recommends against use of CMV-HIG for <u>prevention</u> of congenital CMV infection among women with primary infection
  ○ ****Insufficient evidence exists to recommend CMV-HIG for <u>treatment</u> of congenital CMV infection to reduce sequelae in infected fetuses
☐ ****Oral antiviral therapy (valacyclovir):**
  ○ *Rationale*: Reduction of maternal viremia limits transplacental transmission
  ○ ****Limited data supports oral valacyclovir 2 g four times daily (total 8 g/d) in <u>prevention</u> of congenital CMV among patients with first-trimester primary infections
  ○ ****Valacyclovir for the <u>treatment</u> of congenital CMV infected fetuses shows plausibility, but remains under investigation
    ▪ *Valacyclovir is converted to acyclovir by hepatic first-pass metabolism*
    ▪ *Valacyclovir has greater bioavailability (55%) than acyclovir (10%–20%)*
☐ ****The preconception live-attenuated vaccine is not recommended based on limited efficacy; hygienic measures alone are at least of equal benefit

7

In a hypothetical simulation clinical trial of 100 women with CMV infection, half received valacyclovir treatment and half received placebo. Transplacental transmission of CMV occurred in 20 women who took the treatment drug and 30 women who received placebo.

11-A. Calculate the ratio of disease risk between the treated and the untreated population. *(1 point per step)*

3

☐ Risk of CMV transmission among the valacyclovir group: 20/50 = 40%
☐ Risk of CMV transmission among the placebo group: 30/50 = 60%
☐ Relative risk = 40%/60% = 0.67

11-B. If the p-value was 0.024, explain the meaning of this relative risk.

1

☐ Relative risk of 0.67 implies that the treatment drug was ***significantly*** protective against transplacental transmission of CMV infection among pregnant women

After thorough counseling at 15 weeks' gestation, the patient opts for fetal diagnostic testing within a week as she feels it may alleviate anxiety and help prepare the couple for possible neonatal disease. She confirms that irrespective of laboratory or findings on fetal imaging, pregnancy termination is not an option for the couple.

You take this opportunity to inform your trainee that while traditional recommendations were to arrange for amniocentesis after 21 weeks' gestation and at least six weeks from suspected maternal infection, contemporary evidence suggests only a minimum of eight weeks have elapsed after suspected maternal infection.[†]

Amniotic fluid CMV PCR is positive with a quantification of 10^4 genome equivalents/mL. Allied professionals have been informed. As priorly discussed with the patient, you proceed to arrange for serial sonography.

Special note:
† *Refer to* Enders M, Daiminger A, Exler S, Ertan K, Enders G, Bald R. Prenatal diagnosis of congenital cytomegalovirus infection in 115 cases: a 5 years' single center experience. *Prenat Diagn.* 2017;37(4):389–398

12. Inform the patient on the likelihood of developing fetal sonographic abnormalities based on confirmed maternal primary infection and congenital CMV infection.   1

☐ ~15%

You review a study that examined the ability of ultrasound to differentiate fetuses with and without CMV-associated abnormalities. The reported area under the receiver operating curve was 0.6.

13. Explain to your trainee the meaning of an area under the receiver operating curve of 0.6.   2

☐ Area under the receiver operating curve of 0.6 implies that there is a 60% chance that the model will be able to discriminate between fetuses with sonographic abnormalities and those with a normal scan

Special note:
Area under the receiver operating curve can range from 0.5 (no test discriminative ability) to 1.0 (ideal test with 100% sensitivity and 100% specificity)

Fetal sonography remains unremarkable until 24 weeks' gestation, when biometry decreased from the 16th to the 8th percentile and echogenic bowel is noted. Fetal Doppler interrogation is normal, and amniotic fluid volume is appropriate. Cerebral imaging reveals the following:

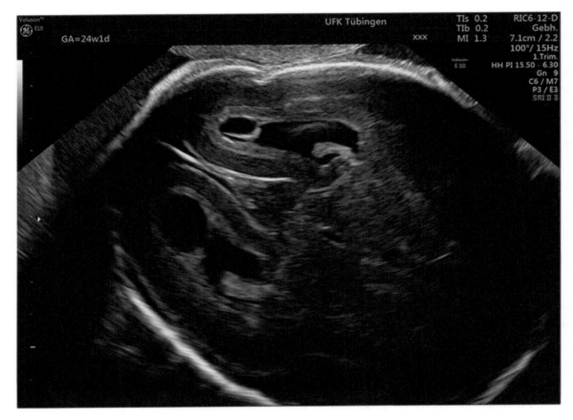

Figure 59.1

With permission: *"Cytomegalovirus infection in pregnancy"*, *Arch Gynecol Obstet 2017, vol 296:15–26 (Figure 1).*

There is no association between this case scenario and this patient's image. Image used for educational purposes only.

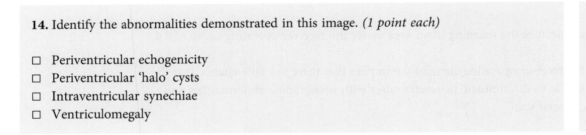

14. Identify the abnormalities demonstrated in this image. *(1 point each)*   4

☐ Periventricular echogenicity
☐ Periventricular 'halo' cysts
☐ Intraventricular synechiae
☐ Ventriculomegaly

15. Which other fetal ultrasound abnormalities, not portrayed in the above image, may be associated with congenital CMV? *(1 point each)*

Max 10

Cerebral	Cardiac	Abdominopelvic	Other
☐ Choroid plexus cysts ☐ Hydrocephalus ☐ Microcephaly ☐ Periventricular calcifications ☐ Porencephaly ☐ Cerebellar hypoplasia ☐ Megacisterna magna	☐ Cardiomegaly ☐ Pericardial effusions ☐ Calcifications	☐ Echogenic bowel ☐ Intrahepatic calcifications ☐ Ascites ☐ Splenomegaly ☐ Pelvic cysts ☐ Hepatomegaly (left liver lobe >40 mm)	☐ Fetal growth restriction (FGR) ☐ Nonimmune hydrops ☐ Intrauterine fetal death (IUFD) ☐ Either placentomegaly or small placenta ☐ Amniotic fluid abnormalities (more commonly 'oligohydramnios' due to viral-mediated tissue damage in fetal kidneys)

16. Pending neonatology consultation, address the patient's concern regarding the chance of CMV disease manifestations at birth based on existing sonographic manifestations. *(1 point each)*

4

☐ With confirmed amniotic fluid PCR and ultrasound findings, the chance of a symptomatic neonate is ~78% *(not 100%)*

☐ Fetal ultrasound abnormalities may change or disappear during pregnancy

☐ Ultrasound does not detect all manifestations of congenital CMV inclusion disease

☐ A normal fetal ultrasound would not have excluded the risk of neurological damage

17. Inform her of the potentially adjunctive value of <u>fetal MRI</u> in assessment of congenital CMV infection.

2

☐ This fetus is *infected* (by amniocentesis PCR) and *affected* (ultrasound abnormalities), limiting added value of MRI in this scenario; MRI may be adjunctive in the absence of sonographic fetal manifestations of CMV disease or as an asset to assess abnormal myelation and gyration

Special note:
While standard use of MRI is controversial, it may facilitate evaluation of certain intracranial abnormalities including lissencephaly, polymicrogyria, white matter injury, or lenticulostriate vasculopathy in the basal ganglia

18. What are long-term sequelae of congenital CMV infections? *(1 point each)*

Max 6

Auditory	Ocular	Central nervous system
☐ Sensorineural hearing loss	☐ Chorioretinitis	☐ Seizures
	☐ Optic atrophy	☐ Delays in cognitive function, learning and language
	☐ Central vision blindness	
	☐ Cataracts	

Fetal growth velocity remains adequate and sonographic manifestations stable until term.

At 38 weeks' gestation, spontaneous labor ensues, and the patient has an uncomplicated vaginal delivery of a neonate weighing 2450 g; postnatal assessment is ongoing in the neonatal intensive care unit (NICU). You intend to request assessment of the placenta for virology and histology.

19. Inform your obstetric trainee how a congenital CMV diagnosis will be confirmed postnatally. *(2 points for main bullet)*

2

☐ Testing for CMV DNA PCR in neonatal urine or saliva within the first 21 days of life to differentiate congenital versus postnatal CMV acquisition, via delivery or breastfeeding
  o If the 21-day window is missed, the dried blood spot obtained routinely from neonates may be tested *(nonconfirmatory; lower sensitivity at 82%)*
  o Neonatal testing for congenital CMV infection is required even with evidence of fetal infection by amniocentesis

On day 1 of life, neonatal salivary CMV PCR is positive. In addition to being growth restricted, comprehensive investigations reveal unilateral sensorineural hearing loss above 21 decibels, intracerebral calcifications, thrombocytopenia, and petechiae. The NICU team confirms moderate to severe symptomatic congenital CMV disease.

20. Outline the recommended pharmacologic treatment of this neonate, explaining its purpose to the mother.

2

☐ Oral valganciclovir started within the first month of life and continued for six months is recommended to slow the progression of hearing loss and improve long-term neurodevelopmental outcome

Special note:
Recommended dose administration is 16 mg/kg/dose twice daily; follow-up of neutrophil count and hepatic transaminases is required until completion of treatment

21. What is the pathophysiological basis of petechiae seen in congenital CMV disease?

2

☐ Cutaneous extramedullary hematopoiesis ('blueberry muffin sign')

22. *Assuming* this congenitally infected neonate had a birthweight of 3000 g and was otherwise asymptomatic apart from isolated sensorineural hearing loss, what would be the recommended antiviral therapy, if any?

2

☐ Antiviral therapy would <u>not</u> be routinely recommended (*European consensus and United States/Australian recommendations*)
  ○ Nonstatistically significant improvement in hearing and long-term developmental outcomes

23. Identify the most common causes for long-term mortality, quoted at 5%–30%, among severely affected infants with CMV disease. *(1 point each)*

Max 2

☐ Disseminated intravascular coagulation
☐ Hepatic failure
☐ Bacterial superinfection

You intend to address future pregnancy considerations following the most recent pregnancy affected by congenital CMV infection.

24. Highlight important aspects to address in counseling after a congenital CMV-affected pregnancy. *(1 point each)*

3

☐ Inform the patient that the risk of reactivating endogenous latent virus or reinfection by exogenous virus is far lower, at 0.5%–1.5%, than risks for primary infection, although congenital sequelae are comparable to those of primary infection
☐ Inform the patient that serologic screening for CMV reactivation or reinfection is not useful
☐ Encourage continuation of hygienic measures

TOTAL: **90**

CHAPTER 60

Hepatitis B and C Virus Infections in Pregnancy

Amira El-Messidi and Maged Peter Ghali

You are seeing a new patient in consultation for transfer of care to your high-risk obstetrics unit at a tertiary center. She is a 27-year-old primigravida at 14^{+3} weeks' gestation with an incidentally positive surface antigen to the hepatitis B virus (HBsAg) on routine prenatal testing. A copy of the original laboratory report has been provided to you. Although detailed serological investigations were performed, results are not available. The patient is aware of the results. Referral to a hepatologist has also been instigated. The patient's first-trimester sonogram and aneuploidy screen were unremarkable. She has no obstetric complaints.

LEARNING OBJECTIVES

1. Take a focused history, and verbalize essentials of the physical examination for incidental HBV infection on prenatal screening
2. Interpret HBV serology, and counsel on various combinations
3. Provide detailed counseling and management of obstetric risks related to maternal HBV or HCV infection, and understand the hepatic markers guiding antenatal treatment of chronic HBV infection
4. Troubleshoot special situations involving invasive diagnostic procedures and percutaneous exposure to HBV-contaminated blood
5. Recognize the rationale for evolving recommendations related to routine maternal HCV screening

SUGGESTED READINGS

Hepatitis B

1. Castillo E, Murphy K, van Schalkwyk J. No. 342 – hepatitis B and pregnancy. *J Obstet Gynaecol Can.* 2017 Mar;39(3):181–190.
2. CDC guidance for evaluating health-care personnel for hepatitis B virus protection and for administering postexposure management. *MMWR Recomm Reports* 2013; 62(RR-10):1–19.

3. European Association for the Study of the Liver. EASL 2017 clinical practice guidelines on the management of hepatitis B virus infection. *J Hepatol.* 2017 Aug;67(2):370–398.

4. Gagnon A, Davies G, Wilson RD. Genetics Committee. Prenatal invasive procedures in women with hepatitis B, hepatitis C, and/or human immunodeficiency virus infections. *J Obstet Gynecol Can* 2014;36: 648–653.

5. National Institute for Health and Care Excellence. Hepatitis B (chronic): diagnosis and management of chronic hepatitis B in children, young people and adults. Clinical guideline 165. 2013. Available at http://guidance.nice.org.uk/CG165. Accessed April 22, 2022.

6. Schillie S, Vellozzi C, Reingold A, et al. Prevention of hepatitis B virus infection in the united States: recommendations of the Advisory Committee on Immunization Practices. *MMWR Recomm Rep.* 2018 Jan 12;67(1):1–31.

7. Society for Maternal-Fetal Medicine (SMFM), Dionne-Odom J, Tita AT, Silverman NS. No. 38: Hepatitis B in pregnancy screening, treatment, and prevention of vertical transmission. *Am J Obstet Gynecol.* 2016 Jan;214(1):6–14.

8. Terrault NA, Lok ASF, McMahon BJ, et al. Update on prevention, diagnosis, and treatment of chronic hepatitis B: AASLD 2018 hepatitis B guidance. *Hepatology.* 2018 Apr;67(4): 1560–1599.

9. World Health Organization. Prevention of mother-to-child transmission of hepatitis B virus: guidelines on antiviral prophylaxis in pregnancy, 2020 Jul. PMID: 32833415.

Hepatitis C

1. ACOG Practice Advisory: Routine hepatitis C virus screening in pregnant individuals. May 2021. Available at www.acog.org/clinical/clinical-guidance/practice-advisory/articles/2021/05/routine-hepatitis-c-virus-screening-in-pregnant-individuals. Accessed October 26, 2021.

2. Havens PL, Anderson JR. Updated CDC recommendations for universal hepatitis C virus screening among adults and pregnant women: implications for clinical practice. *JAMA.* 2020 Jun 9;323(22):2258–2259.

3. Hepatitis C guidance: recommendations for testing, managing, and treating hepatitis C virus. American Association for the Study of Liver Diseases and the Infectious Diseases Society of America (AASLD-IDSA). Available at www.hcvguidelines.org/sites/default/files/full-guidance-pdf/AASLD-IDSA_HCVGuidance_January_21_2021.pdf. Accessed October 26, 2021.

4. Jhaveri R, Broder T, Bhattacharya D, et al. Universal screening of pregnant women for hepatitis C: the time is now. *Clin Infect Dis.* 2018 Oct 30;67(10):1493–1497.

5. Schillie S, Wester C, Osborne M, et al. CDC recommendations for hepatitis C screening among adults – United States, 2020. *MMWR Recomm Rep.* 2020 Apr 10;69(2):1–17.

6. Society for Maternal-Fetal Medicine (SMFM). Dotters-Katz SK, Kuller JA, Hughes BL. Society for Maternal-Fetal Medicine Consult Series No. 56: Hepatitis C in pregnancy-updated guidelines: Replaces Consult No. 43, November 2017. *Am J Obstet Gynecol.* 2021;225(3): B8–B18.

7. US Preventive Services Task Force Recommendation Statement. Screening for Hepatitis C Virus Infection in Adolescents and Adults. *JAMA* 2020;323(10):970–975.

1. What aspects of a focused history would you want to know? *(1 point each)*

HBV-related hepatic manifestations:
- ☐ Jaundice
- ☐ Upper abdominal pain
- ☐ Rapid increase in abdominal girth
- ☐ Dark urine/pale stools
- ☐ Unexplained fatigue/loss of appetite

HBV-related extrahepatic manifestations:
- ☐ Current or recent fever
- ☐ Arthralgias
- ☐ Peripheral neuropathy
- ☐ Renal disease
- ☐ Nausea/vomiting, malaise, skin changes *(symptoms overlap with pregnancy)*

Comorbidities and medical history:
- ☐ Evaluate if/when HBsAg was previously reported negative
- ☐ Dyslipidemia, nonalcoholic fatty liver, diabetes, or hypertension
- ☐ Receipt of blood transfusions, or prior surgeries
- ☐ Prenatal results of hepatitis C, HIV, and syphilis testing
- ☐ Prior hepatitis A vaccination
- ☐ Medications and allergies

Social history:
- ☐ Occupation *(particularly for risk of acquisition of blood-borne pathogens)*
- ☐ Country of birth where hepatitis B is endemic
- ☐ Ethnicity – especially Asian and African origin *(affects disease progression and risk of hepatocellular carcinoma)*
- ☐ Alcohol consumption (including duration and quantity), smoking
- ☐ Intravenous drug use/tattoos/acupuncture
- ☐ Prior incarceration
- ☐ Recent travel history

Sexual history:
- ☐ Current or prior multiple sexual partners
- ☐ History of HPV vaccination, cervical dysplasia, and results of latest Papanicolaou smear
- ☐ Prior STIs

Family history:
- ☐ Hepatitis B status/vaccinations of her sexual partner and household contacts
- ☐ Hepatitis B status of her siblings and parents *(identifies likely vertical transmission and useful in assessing likely natural history in the patient)*
- ☐ Hepatobiliary disease: fibrosis, cirrhosis, hepatocellular carcinoma

The patient and her husband of four years moved to the city from a nearby town 18 months ago and she has not needed to seek health care services prior to conception. She cannot recall when her hepatitis B immunity status was last verified, but she received all routine childhood vaccinations in accordance with jurisdictional protocols. She and her husband temporarily reside with her sister and partner. The patient does not know the immune status of her household contacts.

Currently unemployed, she was an office administrative assistant. To her knowledge, she has always been healthy. Her medical, social, and family histories are noncontributory. The patient does not smoke, use recreational drugs, and has not consumed alcohol since conception. She only takes prenatal vitamins, which she tolerates. She hands you the results of her prenatal screening results for HIV, hepatitis C and syphilis, which are all negative.

You document a normal blood pressure and pulse; fetal viability is ascertained.

The patient's initial consultation with the hepatologist is arranged for next week.

---

2. Outline aspects of a focused physical examination with respect to the patient's hepatitis infection. *(1 point each)*

Max 9

General characteristics or findings:
- ☐ Temperature *(fever may occur with acute infection)*
- ☐ BMI
- ☐ Assess for confusion/signs of encephalopathy in conversation
- ☐ Asterixis/liver flap
- ☐ Jaundice and/or scleral icterus

Cutaneous and musculoskeletal:
- ☐ Needle tracks/tattoos
- ☐ Clubbing or presence of Terry's or Muehrcke's nails
- ☐ Lower extremity edema *(an uncommon manifestation of pregnancy at this gestational period)*
- ☐ Spider angiomas, palmar erythema

Abdomen:
- ☐ Hepatosplenomegaly
- ☐ Right upper quadrant tenderness
- ☐ Palpable liver mass *(for hepatocellular carcinoma)*
- ☐ Cruveilhier-Baumgarten murmur *(heard at the abdominal wall in the region of the portocaval system)*
- ☐ Ascites
- ☐ Caput medusa

Pelvic exam:
- ☐ Lesions or signs of possible infection *(consideration for urine or cervicovaginal cultures for chlamydia/gonorrhea if not recently performed)*

The patient is of normal body habitus and physical examination is unremarkable. You inform her that further testing is necessary to determine whether she has an acute or chronic HBV infection.

3-A. In addition to HBsAg, and given documented absent HCV or HIV infections, which further investigations would you initiate in assessment of her hepatitis B infection? *(1 point each)*

Max 9

Serum tests:
- ☐ HBV DNA PCR (viral load)
- ☐ HBeAg
- ☐ Anti-HBe
- ☐ Anti-HBs
- ☐ Anti-HBc IgG and IgM
- ☐ Hepatitis D virus antibody
- ☐ Hepatitis A antibody
- ☐ Liver enzymes: ALT, AST, GGT
- ☐ Liver function tests: albumin, bilirubin, prothrombin time
- ☐ CBC/FBC *(platelets serve as a surrogate marker for portal hypertension)*

Imaging:
- ☐ Hepatic ultrasound *(for masses, signs of cirrhosis or portal hypertension)*

Special note:
Although hepatic evaluation is required in the diagnostic work-up of hepatitis, hepatologist may defer to the postpartum period; liver biopsy is safe in pregnancy. Liver elastography was previously contraindicated in pregnancy but is now considered safe. Nevertheless, liver stiffness increases in pregnancy due to increased blood flow, and so fibroscan cannot be reliably interpreted, and should generally be avoided.

3-B. Counsel the patient on recommended, or required, health measures with HBV infection. *(1 point each)*

Max 6

- ☐ Inform the patient of the need to adhere to local regulations for public health reporting of chronic hepatitis B infections *(jurisdictional policies may vary)*
- ☐ Determine HBV immune status of household contacts and her sexual partner
- ☐ Recommend barrier protection during sexual intercourse until her husband's immune status is known
- ☐ Recommend hepatitis A vaccination, *unless immune*
- ☐ Exercise caution in use of over-the-counter medication or herbals among women with chronic HBV
- ☐ Refrain from consuming alcohol in pregnancy and beyond (hepatotoxicity)
- ☐ Avoid sharing toothbrushes or razor blades; may share food and utensils
- ☐ Cover breached skin
- ☐ Use bleach solutions to clean her blood spills

The patient's consultation visit with the hepatologist is arranged for 15^{+5} weeks' gestation. Anxiously, she presents to your office a day prior to discuss results of her investigations. Hepatic ultrasound did not reveal any masses, fibrosis, or portal hypertension, and the gallbladder appeared normal. Serological results reveal:

HBV DNA PCR/viral load[‡]	75,000 IU/mL
HBeAg	positive
Anti-HBe	negative
Anti-HBs	negative
Anti-HBc IgG	positive
Anti-HBc IgM	negative
ALT	55 IU/L (normal: 6–32 IU/L) *

* *Pregnancy reference range from Girling J.C et al. Br J Obstet Gynecol 1997; 104:246–250*

Special note:

‡ WHO recommends HBV DNA be expressed as IU/mL; conversion requires dividing copies/mL by 5 to obtain IU/mL

4. What is your <u>most specific</u> diagnosis?   2

☐ Chronic HBV infection with high infectivity/replication

As you are about to counsel the patient, you receive a call from a physician requesting your expertise in interpretation and management of your patient's three household contacts. All parties consented to disclosure of their laboratory results with you, and none have known health issues.

Patient's sister:

Serum β-hCG**	positive
HBsAg	negative
Anti-HBc	negative
Anti-HBs	negative

** *Test performed based on clinical suspicion*

Patient's partner

HBsAg	negative
Anti-HBc	positive
Anti-HBs	positive

Sister's partner

HBsAg	negative
Anti-HBc	negative
Anti-HBs	Low-positive, <10 IU/L

5. For each household contact, interpret the serology results and indicate your recommended management for your colleague. *(1 point each)*

Patient's sister (pregnant): *(max 3 points)*
- ☐ Susceptible to HBV infection
- ☐ Advise vaccine series[†] *(especially given positive household contact from her sister)*
- ☐ Reassure of safety and efficacy of vaccination throughout gestation
- ☐ Repeat testing of HBsAg in later pregnancy (one to two months after last dose of vaccine)

Patient's partner:
- ☐ Immune due to natural infection/reassurance

Sister's partner:
- ☐ Evidence of prior vaccination with naturally waning immunity over time *(or incomplete receipt of vaccination series)*
- ☐ Booster doses may be considered for a health care worker at risk of exposure to infectious material or in immunocompromised states

Special note:
- † Estimated incidence of anaphylaxis among HBV vaccine recipients is 1.1 per million vaccine doses; contraindicated among yeast-sensitive persons *(Suggested Reading 6, ACIP 2018)*

Your colleague is appreciative of your expertise and indicates both the patient's sister and partner agree to start HBV vaccination series today. The sister, in particular, is reassured to learn of the safety of vaccination during pregnancy.

6. Discuss your counseling and <u>antenatal</u> management of your patient, realizing that care will ensue in conjunction with her hepatologist. *(1 point per main bullet)*

Effects of pregnancy on the natural history of chronic HBV:
- ☐ Pregnancy is not known to alter the course of infection
- ☐ Serial follow-up of HBV DNA and liver biochemistry *(approximately every three months)*
  - ○ To determine the need for antiviral treatment and monitoring signs of hepatitis flares *(i.e., more than a two- to threefold rise in ALT, which already is elevated beyond the reference range)*
- ☐ Inform the patient that chronic HBV infection may flare postpartum in ~25% of women (close monitoring by the hepatologist is necessary)

Effects of chronic HBV on pregnancy:
- ☐ Reassure the patient that neither HBV infection nor treatment with tenofovir disoproxil fumarate affects pregnancy outcome unless existing cirrhosis or advanced liver disease[†]
- ☐ Neither HBV nor treatment with tenofovir disoproxil fumarate is associated with congenital anomalies
  - ○ *Tenofovir disoproxil fumarate is the preferred agent due to its safety, potency, and low rates of drug resistance*
- ☐ Mother-to-child HBV transmission may occur in utero, intrapartum, or postpartum; most commonly intrapartum
  - ○ *Risks of child transmission decrease from >90% to <10% with appropriate neonatal postexposure prophylaxis (within 12 hours of delivery)*
- ☐ Mode and timing of delivery depend on obstetric indications; Cesarean section does not prevent vertical transmission

Special note:

† If this patient were to have cirrhosis, perinatal risks would be increased (*e.g.,* fetal risks include FGR, PTD, IUFD; maternal risks include abruption, hypertension, liver failure, variceal bleeding, perinatal hemorrhage, mortality)

Although the patient appreciates your detailed counseling, she is most concerned about the risks of perinatal transmission.

7. List factors related to the <u>biology</u> of HBV that increase the risk of perinatal transmission. *(1 point each)*   Max 3

☐ Maternal HBeAg status
☐ HBV DNA viral load
☐ Treatment-resistant virus
☐ HBV genotype

Subsequent to the hepatologist's encounter with the patient, he or she calls to inform you of the plan agreed upon with the patient: hepatic biochemistry will be repeated in three months to assess the need for treatment initiation.

8-A. Indicate the three principal hepatic markers you anticipate would be most valuable to guide the hepatologists' decision to initiate antenatal treatment for chronic HBV infection? *(1 point each)*   3

☐ HBV DNA PCR
☐ ALT
☐ HBeAg status

8-B. If this patient were to require antiviral therapy in pregnancy, specify the benefits of therapy. *(1 point each)*   Max 3

☐ Decrease mother-to-child transmission
☐ Induction of HBeAg loss *(preferably with anti-HBe seroconversion)*
☐ Maternal health: improve survival and quality of life by preventing disease progression, including HBV-associated extrahepatic manifestations
☐ ALT normalisation

Pregnancy progresses well: fetal morphology survey at 20 weeks' gestation is normal, GDM testing is negative and the patient receives routine pertussis vaccination. She remains clinically asymptomatic from HBV infection and has no obstetric complications.

Coincidentally, you receive a telephone call from the obstetrics ultrasound unit; a colleague asks whether he or she can perform an amniocentesis for a patient with chronic HBV infection who is currently 17 weeks' gestation, referred from an affiliated hospital, with a fetal exomphalos. Your colleague confirms that the patient would consider pregnancy termination if aneuploidy is found.

9. Provide advice and guidance on invasive prenatal testing among women with chronic HBV infection. *(1 point per main bullet)*

☐ Diagnostic invasive obstetrical procedures should not be withheld as the risk of fetal hepatitis B infection from obstetrical procedures is generally low; the risk of in utero transmission is increased among highly viremic women at >200, 000 IU/mL
☐ Attempt nonplacental needle entry
☐ Aim for single-entry procedure
☐ Use a small gauge needle

Max 3

After your telephone call with your colleague, you are notified that as a technician was drawing your patient's routine blood sample at 27 weeks' gestation, he or she had a needlestick injury. Unfortunately, this individual is unimmunized, holding antecedent preference against routine vaccinations. The technician promptly washed his or her hands with soap and water*. He or she will present to the Infection Control Center of your hospital.

Special note:
* Use of antiseptics is not contraindicated, although has not been shown to reduce HBV transmission *(CDC 2018)*

10-A. Approximate the risk of contracting HBV and the risk of clinical hepatitis from percutaneous exposure to this patient. *(1 point each)*

2

HBsAg- and HBeAg-positive source (*i.e.,* the patient):
☐ Risk of serologic HBV infection: 37%–62% *(CDC 2013)*
☐ Risk of clinical hepatitis: 22%–31% *(CDC 2013)*

10-B. Specify your management recommendations for the unvaccinated health professional's exposure to your patient's blood. *(1 point per main bullet)*

3

☐ Recommend postexposure prophylaxis with HBV vaccine <u>and</u> HBIG* within 24 hours of exposure
  ○ *Limited evidence suggests that the maximum interval after exposure is preferably within 7 days for percutaneous exposures (and 14 days for sexual exposures)*
  ○ *Accelerated vaccine schedule (0, 7, 21–30 days followed by a booster at 12 months) is optional when rapid immune response is preferred*
☐ Prevaccination anti-HBc testing, without delaying postexposure prophylaxis
☐ Postvaccination response status testing of anti-HBs at least six months after HBIG administration
☐ Advise refraining from body-fluid donation during the follow-up period, although no modification in sexual practice or avoidance of conception is needed

Special note:
* HBIG: Standard dose is 0.06 mL/kg; patient consent is required for receipt of human plasma product *(jurisdictional protocols may vary)*

The technician immediately agreed to receiving prophylaxis, fearing viral infection.

Meanwhile, your patient calls the office concerned about the results of her investigations. Her hepatic tests show the following:

At 27 weeks' gestation

HBV DNA PCR/viral load	275,000 IU/mL
HBeAg	positive
Anti-HBe	negative
ALT	70 IU/L

Given her laboratory results and as the patient is 26–28 weeks' gestation, the patient has been counseled by her hepatologist to start oral tenofovir disoproxil fumarate[†] 300 mg daily. Serum creatinine was ascertained to be normal prior to initiating antiviral therapy.

Special notes:

AASLD 2018 recommends antiviral treatment to reduce perinatal transmission in HBsAg-positive women with an HBV DNA >200, 000 IU/mL; treatment may further reduce mother-to-child transmission by up to 70%

AASLD recommends against antiviral therapy to reduce perinatal transmission with HBV DNA ≤200,000 IU/mL

NICE 2013: Tenofovir is indicated to reduce perinatal transmission with HBV DNA >10^7 IU/mL

[†] Newer formulation, tenofovir alafenamide, has not been extensively studied in pregnancy

She remains compliant with treatment and serial testing of biomarkers. Repeat liver biomarkers reveal the following:

At 34 weeks' gestation

HBV DNA PCR/viral load	9167 IU/mL
HBeAg	negative
Anti-HBe	positive
ALT	35 IU/L

11. Describe her treatment response. *(1 point each)*   3

- ☐ Virological response to treatment
- ☐ Decreased infectivity/serological conversion to anti-HBe
- ☐ Normalization of ALT

Reassured of her treatment response, the patient remains compliant. At her 36-weeks visit, she recalls you indicated a term, vaginal delivery is the goal; she now asks about special considerations for intrapartum and neonatal care in the context of her hepatitis infection.

---

12. For this <u>HBsAg-positive</u> patient, counsel her on risks of mother-to-child transmission and discuss intrapartum and postpartum management, accordingly. *(1 point per main bullet)*

Max 8

- ☐ Avoid intrapartum invasive fetal procedures, *if possible*
- ☐ Avoid episiotomy, *if possible*
- ☐ Inform patient of inability to donate umbilical cord blood to public banking systems
- ☐ Alert delivery room and nursery staff to administer neonatal intramuscular HBV vaccine and hepatitis B immunoglobulin (HBIG) within 12 hours of birth
  - ○ *Only monovalent HBV vaccine should be used at less than six weeks of life*
- ☐ Explain the importance of completing the infant's hepatitis B vaccine series, and having postvaccination testing at age 9–12 months *(anti-HBs and HBsAg)*[‡]
- ☐ Individualized input from her long-term treating expert is necessary to address postpartum tenofovir treatment *(generally discontinued at birth to three months postpartum)*
- ☐ Breastfeeding is **not** contraindicated among untreated women or on tenofovir disoproxil fumarate-based therapy (EASL 2107)
  - ○ *(AASLD 2018; ACIP 2018; SOGC 2013)*: May initiate breastfeeding before neonatal vaccination
  - ○ *(SMFM 2016)*: As long as the infant receives immunoprophylaxis at birth
- ☐ Advise to guard against bleeding from cracked nipples
- ☐ For viral hepatitis: No restrictions exist for modes of contraception among women with chronic infections or with mild-compensated cirrhosis without complications *(UK-MEC 2016, amended September 2019)*

Special note:
‡ Infant anti-HBc testing is not recommended because passively acquired maternal anti-HBc may be detected in infants of HBsAg-positive mothers up to age 24 months *(Suggested Reading 6)*

Three weeks later, you are seeing a healthy prenatal patient in early pregnancy, referred for isolated hepatitis C antibody identified on routine prenatal tests. She had provided voluntarily consent for HCV screening. Comprehensive investigations for other infections are negative; immunity to hepatitis A and B is ascertained. Her history and physical examination are unremarkable.

As a scientist who researched this infection prior to seeing you, she learned that societal recommendations recently shifted from risk-based screening to routine prenatal HCV screening.

13. Recognizing evolving international practice standards, discuss the rationale for routine HCV prenatal screening.[†] *(1 point each)*

Max 6

☐ Risk-based screening is inconsistent among obstetric care providers, thereby missing HCV cases

☐ Patients may not have risk factors for testing, or may withhold risky current/prior lifestyle behaviors

☐ Pregnancy offers a unique opportunity to seek consistent care, allowing assessment of liver disease status and facilitating linkage to specialist care; long-term treatment initiated after pregnancy would ultimately improve life-expectancy

☐ Knowledge of HCV positivity may guide obstetric management to decrease mother-to-child transmission

☐ Possible changes in risky lifestyle behaviors and guide partners to testing/treatment

☐ Postnatal screening of exposed infants and treatment of infected children

☐ Universal HCV screening is cost-effective until the prevalence of HCV drops below 0.03%[‡]

Special notes:
[†] Universal prenatal HCV screening is advocated by the AASLD-IDSA 2021, USPTF 2020 and CDC 2020 (except where prevalence of HCV infection is <0.1%) and ACOG Practice Advisory, endorsed by SMFM 2021
[‡] *Refer to* Chaillon A, Rand EB, Reau N, Martin NK. Cost-effectiveness of Universal Hepatitis C Virus Screening of Pregnant Women in the United States. *Clin Infect Dis.* 2019;69(11):1888–1895.

The patient is convinced of the benefits of universal prenatal HCV testing. She is curious if her results confirm a hepatitis C infection.

14. Identify the <u>next best test</u> to confirm hepatitis C infection once anti-HCV antibody has been detected in the patient.

1

☐ Quantitative HCV RNA PCR; qualitative HCV RNA PCR is an acceptable alternative

Until the result of her confirmatory HCV RNA test is available, she has concerns regarding the relationship between pregnancy and HCV infection, if infection is found.

15-A. Counsel the patient on the impact of pregnancy on HCV infection. *(1 point each)*

Max 2

☐ Pregnancy itself does not worsen the prognosis of chronic HCV; immunomodulation and plasma volume lead to naturally decreasing ALT level during pregnancy

☐ Spontaneous clearance of HCV RNA can occur postpartum, likely due to immunotolerance mechanisms during pregnancy

☐ Until data is available for safety and efficacy for antenatal use of direct-acting antivirals, treatment of HCV infection will be evaluated postpartum; delays in treatment until the postpartum period has not been shown to worsen outcome

15-B. Specify your discussion of obstetric risks and management if HCV infection is confirmed in this patient. *(1 point each)*

Max 5

☐ Pregnancy with maternal HCV infection is generally well tolerated; adverse perinatal outcomes are primarily associated with advanced liver disease or potential confounders among infected women

☐ Risk of obstetric cholestasis among mothers with HCV infection requires clinical screening of symptoms

☐ Vertical transmission with HCV mono-infection is ~5.8%

☐ Preferred avoidance of internal fetal monitoring, early artificial rupture of membranes, and episiotomy in labor with HCV-positive women

☐ Mode and timing of delivery depend on obstetric indications

☐ Breastfeeding is not discouraged

The patient's HCV RNA is confirmed to be negative on serial testing. Reinfection with HCV (different strains) has not occurred. She realizes that although a caveat of screening was anxiety and feeling stigmatized about possibly harbouring HCV, she appreciates the net benefits of testing.

16. Outline the implications of confirmed anti-HCV antibody in the absence of viral antigen. *(1 point each)*

3

☐ Natural viral clearance of acute infection occurred in this patient (15%–45% of patients)

☐ Reassure that vertical transmission is not a risk among anti-HCV-antibody-positive and undetectable HCV RNA patients at delivery

☐ Inform the patient that anti-HCV antibody will remain detectable on future testing; risk reduction strategies should be implemented to protect against different strains

TOTAL: 105

CHAPTER 61

Herpes Simplex Virus Infection in Pregnancy

Amira El-Messidi

A 23-year-old primigravida is referred for consultation at 21^{+5} weeks' gestation with a new onset of genital lesions. Her referring physician informs you that she has no history of genital herpes and that her obstetric progress has been unremarkable. All routine prenatal screening tests and investigations have been normal. She has no obstetric complaints and indicates the fetus is active.

LEARNING OBJECTIVES

1. Take a focused history of genital lesions in pregnancy, and identify tests that would confirm clinical suspicion of genital herpes
2. Detail counseling and antenatal management of primary genital herpes, including treatment of recurrence and suppression
3. Recognize the emotional burden implicated with genital herpes, and understand the importance of the provider's counseling and community-available resources
4. Appreciate variations in recommendations of international professional societies for delivery management of various clinical scenarios, including recurrent genital or nongenital herpes and prolonged ruptured membranes
5. Understand essentials of newborn care related to maternal herpes simplex virus (HSV), and be familiar with features of neonatal herpes
6. Acknowledge preferred delivery management with third-trimester primary or nonprimary first episodes of genital herpes, and be able to troubleshoot plans under urgent situations

SUGGESTED READINGS

1. American College of Obstetricians and Gynecologists' Committee on Practice Bulletins – Obstetrics. Management of genital herpes in pregnancy: ACOG Practice Bulletin, No. 220. *Obstet Gynecol.* 2020;135(5):e193–e202.
2. Canadian guidelines on sexually transmitted infections – management and treatment of specific infections – genital herpes simplex virus (HSV) infections. Available at www.canada .ca/en/public-health/services/infectious-diseases/sexual-health-sexually-transmitted-infections/canadian-guidelines/sexually-transmitted-infections/canadian-guidelines-sexually-transmitted-infections-32.html. Accessed August 27, 2020.
3. Centers for Disease Control and Prevention. Sexually transmitted diseases treatment guidelines, 2015. Available at www.cdc.gov/std/tg2015/genital-ulcers.htm. Accessed August 29, 2020.

4. Feltner C, Grodensky C, Ebel C, et al. serologic screening for genital herpes: an updated evidence report and systematic review for the US Preventive Services Task Force. *JAMA.* 2016;316(23):2531–2543.

5. Foley E, Clarke E, Beckett VA, et al. Guideline: management of genital herpes in pregnancy. R Coll Obstet Gynaecol 2014. Available at www.rcog.org.uk/globalassets/documents/guidelines/management-genital-herpes.pdf. Accessed August 27, 2020.

6. Hollier LM, Wendel GD. Third trimester antiviral prophylaxis for preventing maternal genital herpes simplex virus (HSV) recurrences and neonatal infection. Cochrane Database Syst Rev. 2008;(1):CD004946.

7. Lee R, Nair M. Diagnosis and treatment of herpes simplex 1 virus infection in pregnancy. *Obstet Med.* 2017;10(2):58–60.

8. Money DM, Steben M. No. 208 – guidelines for the management of herpes simplex virus in pregnancy. *J Obstet Gynaecol Can.* 2017;39(8): e199–e205.

9. Patel R, Kennedy OJ, Clarke E, et al. 2017 European guidelines for the management of genital herpes. *Int J STD AIDS.* 2017;28(14):1366–1379.

10. Stephenson-Famy A, Gardella C. Herpes simplex virus infection during pregnancy. *Obstet Gynecol Clin North Am.* 2014;41(4):601–614.

POINTS

1. What elements of a focused history would you want to know? *(1 point each)*	Max 17

Details of the lesions:
- ☐ Establish time of onset and changes in appearance
- ☐ Characteristics *(i.e., raised/flat, ulcerated, size, texture, crusted, peeling or exfoliating, dry/serosanguinous secretions)*
- ☐ Distribution *(i.e., vulvar, vaginal, anal, buttocks, thighs)*
- ☐ Associated pain or pruritis
- ☐ Determine if treatment, prescribed or over-the-counter, was attempted

Associated systems:
- ☐ Flu-like symptoms *(i.e., fever, malaise, cough, sore throat, nausea/vomiting)*
- ☐ Headaches, visual changes, seizures
- ☐ Systemic rash, particularly on the palms and soles
- ☐ Dysuria
- ☐ Dyschezia or anal pain/bleeding

Medical history:
- ☐ Systemic or immunosuppressive condition *(e.g., Crohn's, Behcet's disease)*
- ☐ Drug allergy or hypersensitivity *(i.e., condoms, sanitary agents)*

Gynecologic and sexual history:
- ☐ Prior STIs
- ☐ Recent HIV status
- ☐ Date of last cervical cytology smear *(i.e., Papanicolaou smear)* and history of abnormalities, including condyloma
- ☐ Perineal hygiene *(i.e., soap, perfumed products, colored undergarments, douching, or epilation)*
- ☐ Use of sexual toys
- ☐ Number of current (and lifetime) sexual partners

Social history:
- ☐ Occupation *(i.e., exchanging sex for money)*
- ☐ Substance-use *(i.e., cigarette smoking, alcohol, recreational drugs)*

Partner:
- ☐ Presence of similar lesions or symptoms
- ☐ History of genital infections
- ☐ HIV status, if known

The patient works as an administrative agent. She has been in a monogamous relationship for two years and recalls having three partners over the past five years. She is healthy and does not smoke cigarettes or drink alcohol while pregnant. There is no history of recreational drug use. She has no allergies and has not changed her perineal hygiene. Her Papanicolaou smear in early pregnancy, was normal. Her HIV test was recently negative.

Six days ago, she felt malaise which she attributed to pregnancy. She then developed painful, unilateral, localized vulvar vesicles two days later. She does not recall genital burning or pruritis prior to onset of the lesions. The lesions are dry. She has not tried anything for symptom-control, for fear of affecting her pregnancy. The patient reports dysuria coinciding with the lesions. Her partner had a genital herpes infection five years ago, which she was informed of now, as he has not had recurrences.

On examination, the patient does not appear distressed though prefers to lay reclined to relieve the pain. She is afebrile and does not have a nongenital rash. There is no cervical lymphadenopathy, however ipsilateral inguinal notes are palpable. Tender, coalescing vesicles on an erythematous base are noted. Sterile speculum examination does not reveal lesions or abnormalities. Obstetrical assessment is normal.

2. What are the available serologic and virologic tests that would identify your most probable diagnosis?

          5

Viral identification tests from the lesions: *(1 point each; max 3)*
- ☐ PCR *(gold standard)*
- ☐ Viral culture
- ☐ Immunofluorescent staining[†]
- ☐ Enzyme immunoassay[†]
- ☐ Papanicolaou staining[†]
- ☐ Tzanck smear[†]

Serology testing of the patient and partner:
- ☐ HSV-1 and HSV-2 IgG antibodies[‡] *(2 points)*

Special notes:
- † *No longer recommended; reserved for resource limited settings*
- ‡ *IgM antibodies should not be tested, being nonspecific and results may be positive with recurrences*

3. Describe your technique in collecting the viral swabs from the lesions. *(1 point each)*   2

☐ Vesicles should be unroofed with a needle or sterile blade
☐ Swabs taken from the base of the lesions

Shortly, the microbiologist calls you for a positive real-time PCR for HSV-2. Urinalysis is normal.

4. Discuss your counseling and management at this time. *(1 point per main bullet,*   Max 10
   unless specified)

☐ Inform the patient of active genital herpes, and start empiric treatment for primary
   infection *(treatment is required with high clinical suspicion, prior to the availability of viral
   tests)*[†]: *(1 point for main bullet and 1 point for any of the following)*
   ○ Valacyclovir 1 g orally, twice daily for 7–10 days, or
   ○ Acyclovir 200 mg orally five times daily for 7–10 days, or
   ○ Acyclovir 400 mg orally three times daily for 7– 10 days
☐ Reassure the patient of no known teratogenicity from the antivirals
☐ Explain that serum drug monitoring is not required
☐ Mention the very rare risk of drug intolerance/allergic reactions
☐ Inform the patient of the course of infection *(usually self-limiting)* with periods of
   subclinical shedding or exacerbations *(i.e., reactivation of latent virus in local sensory
   ganglia)*
☐ Discuss her most commonly acquired source being asymptomatic shedding
☐ Advise abstinence from genital or orogenital sexual activity until complete healing
☐ Recommend adequate handwashing after perineal hygiene, and avoid sharing towels
☐ Offer analgesics and recommend sitz baths
☐ Reassure the patient of very rare risk of congenital anomalies from HSV in pregnancy
☐ Inform the patient that if delivery does not ensue within six weeks, expectant management
   is planned with anticipated vaginal delivery if no recurrent infection or prodromal
   symptoms at time of delivery
   ○ *Low risk of neonatal infection from vaginal delivery if only asymptomatic shedding of
      HSV (0.04%)*
   ○ *High risk of neonatal infection from vaginal delivery with active/recent primary (40%) or
      nonprimary first episode (30%)*
☐ Consider providing open prescriptions for recurrences and encourage patient to start
   treatment with onset of prodromal symptoms or early when lesions appear (within 12–24
   hours). Treatment options for recurrence include: *(any one of the following; 1 point)*
   ○ Valacyclovir 1 g orally for five days, or
   ○ Valacyclovir 500 mg orally twice daily for three days, or
   ○ Acyclovir 200 mg orally five times daily for five days, or
   ○ Acyclovir 400 mg orally three times daily for five days, or
   ○ Acyclovir 800 mg orally twice daily for five days, or
   ○ Acyclovir 800 mg orally three times daily for two days
☐ Advise on suppressive treatment at 36 weeks until labor onset *(reduces asymptomatic
   shedding, recurrence in labor, and Cesarean delivery)*[‡]: *(any one of the following; 1 point)*

- Valacyclovir 500 mg orally twice daily, or
- Acyclovir 400 mg orally three times daily, or
- Acyclovir 200 mg orally four times daily

Special notes:
† Treatment may be extended as necessary; topical antiviral therapy has minimal clinical benefit and is discouraged
‡ Benefit of suppressive treatment for risk of neonatal herpes is uncertain

Your trainee hears you mention that risk of transplacental transmission is very rare relative to intrapartum infection.

5. What is the rationale for the low risk of congenital HSV infection?   1

☐ Transplacental maternal IgG antibody provides passive fetal immunity

6. What is the mechanism of action for the antiviral agents approved in treatment or prevention of antenatal HSV infections? *(1 point for main bullet)*   1

☐ Acyclovir is a nucleoside analogue that enters infected cells to block DNA replication through the inhibition of viral thymidine kinase
    - Valacyclovir is a prodrug that is converted to acyclovir through rapid hepatic metabolism†

Special note:
† Refer to Question 10 in Chapter 59

The patient is safely discharged with a prescription for treatment and analgesic options. The lesions start crusting by day 9. She is maintaining healthy hygiene and returns for follow-up in two weeks. The fetus is active, and she has no obstetric complaints.

You received results of her serologies: HSV-1- and HSV-2 IgG-negative. Other investigations at initial assessment are unremarkable. Her partner's testing shows HSV-1- and HSV-2 IgG-positive; he is HIV-negative.

7. What is her specific diagnosis?   1

☐ Primary genital HSV-2 infection

8. Regarding her serology, what is the next step that may contribute to your delivery management?   1

☐ Repeat HSV-2 IgG in several weeks *(seroconversion before labor decreases neonatal HSV transmission and morbidity)*

At 25^{+3} weeks, the patient feels genital burning and mild pruritis lasting 1.5 days. She recalls your advice that this may be a recurrence and starts your prescribed three-day course of valacyclovir. Although she develops mild localized labial lesions, she copes well with oral treatment at home.

During a routine prenatal visit the following week, she informs you of this event, mentioning that she has been cautious with genital hygiene and used condoms before her recent episode; she wonders if she 'did something wrong' to cause recurrence.

---

9. Address the patient's concerns and list <u>general risk factors</u> for recurrent genital or oral HSV infections. *(1 point each)*

Max 6

- ☐ Alleviate self-blame and reinforce the natural history of HSV
  - ○ *Average recurrence rates decrease yearly by ~0.8 outbreaks per year, irrespective of the initial rates of outbreaks*
- ☐ Male latex condoms may decrease transmission by 50% from infected men to women, but effectiveness is limited by the location of lesions
- ☐ Advise against orogenital sexual practices given her risk of HSV-1 infection *(i.e., nonprimary infection)*
- ☐ Consider providing patient education resources

Risk factors: *(any three factors)*
- ☐ Immunosuppression
- ☐ Menstrual cycle/hormonal changes
- ☐ Tissue trauma/emotional stress
- ☐ Surgery
- ☐ Extreme temperatures
- ☐ Ultraviolet light

---

10. She asks you about the mode of delivery if a recurrent genital infection were to be present in labor. Address her inquiry.

2

- ☐ Risk of neonatal infection from vaginal delivery during an HSV recurrence ranges from 0% to 5% *(1 point)*
- ☐ Individualized doctor-patient discussion is warranted; international recommendations vary: *(1 point for either subbullet, based on jurisdiction)*
  - ○ *RCOG[5]: Vaginal delivery should be offered given low risk of neonatal herpes with recurrence at delivery, although Cesarean delivery may be considered*
  - ○ *ACOG[1] and SOGC[8]: Cesarean delivery is indicated with recurrence or prodrome at delivery due to potentially serious neonatal disease*

At 27^{+1} weeks, she presents with confirmed PPROM. Routine maternal investigations for PPROM are requested. Fetal presentation is cephalic and obstetrical status is stable. Fetal monitoring is appropriate and there are no contractions. Sonography shows normal fetal biometry and growth velocity with a low-normal amniotic fluid volume, compatible with PPROM. There is a 2 × 2 cm amniotic fluid pocket.

The patient denies prodromal symptoms or genital lesions.

11. She is informed of planed admission and recommended obstetric management for PPROM. Address the current management plan with focus on prior genital herpes infections. *(1 point per main bullet)*	Max 3

☐ Expectant management as risks of prematurity outweigh ascending in utero infection
☐ Thorough genital and speculum examination for herpetic lesions
   ○ If active lesions occur in the setting of PPROM, IV acyclovir may decrease the viral burden and duration of infection
☐ Start suppressive treatment
☐ If recurrent genital HSV develops during expectant management of PPROM, individualized discussion for later mode of delivery is advised
   ○ Benefit of Cesarean delivery may be reduced with more than four hours of membrane rupture
   ○ Studies have not established an *absence* of neonatal benefit from operative delivery nor a *protective* effect with prolonged ruptured membranes and active genital herpes
☐ Neonatology consultation during admission

She remains stable until 35^{+6} weeks when labor commences. Fetal status is normal. She has not had prodromal symptoms or recurrent infection. She has been on daily antiviral prophylaxis.

12. Indicate critical aspects of your labor management regarding her history of antenatal genital herpesvirus. *(1 point each)*	4

☐ Repeat thorough examination of the perineum, anus, and speculum assessment
☐ Preferred avoidance of instrumental delivery *(i.e., forceps, vacuum)*
☐ Preferred avoidance of invasive procedures *(i.e., fetal scalp electrodes/blood sampling)*
☐ Neonatology team notification for newborn examination

The patient is keen for vaginal delivery. Perineal and speculum examinations are clear of lesions. Several herpetic lesions are found on her lateral left buttock.

13. Advise on mode of delivery.	2

☐ Individualized discussion is advised in the setting of nongenital lesions on the back, thighs or buttocks; international recommendation vary:
   ○ ACOG[1]: *Cesarean delivery is not recommended if only nongenital lesions are present; an occlusive dressing is advised*
   ○ SOGC[8]: *Cesarean delivery is recommended*

After discussion with the patient and multidisciplinary consultation, you proceed with vaginal delivery; lesions are covered with a dressing. She has a spontaneous delivery of a vigorous male neonate.

Neonatal examination and investigations are normal. The infant will be followed by the pediatric infectious disease team for possibility of late manifestations appearing in 10–30 days.

14. Indicate which features on pediatric assessment may indicate neonatal herpes. *(1 point each)*   3

☐ Skin, eye, and mouth disease, with a vesicular rash being most common *(0% mortality; <2% morbidity with antiviral treatment)*
☐ Central nervous system *(4%–15% mortality; ~70% morbidity)*: bulging fontanelles, seizures, encephalitis, irritability, temperature instability, tremors, or poor feeding
☐ Disseminated disease *(30%–90% mortality; 17% have long-term neurological sequelae)*

Special note:
Neonatal HSV implies clinical findings at >48 hours of life; overlapping manifestations are common

After delivery, you hear the pediatrics consultant teach a trainee that although rates of maternal HSV-2 have decreased, some epidemiological studies found stable prevalence of neonatal herpes.

15. Provide a rationale for this discordant relationship.   1

☐ Increasing rates of HSV-1 through orogenital contact or inadvertent self-inoculation

The patient is breastfeeding.

16. Facilitate her understanding of newborn care with antenatal genital herpes. *(1 point each)*   Max 3

☐ Adequate handwashing before handling the infant if lesions are present anywhere on her, or caretakers,' body *(~10% of neonatal herpes is acquired through family members)*
☐ Advise against maternal or caretakers' oral contact with the infant, even in the absence of active lesions *(possibility for asymptomatic shedding)*
☐ Breastfeeding is only contraindicated with active breast lesions
☐ Continue breastfeeding if antiviral treatment is needed for orogenital herpes

SCENARIO B
The above patient had an unremarkable antenatal course until 30 weeks' gestation when she presents with a first episode of genital herpes. Treatment is given with no recurrence for the remaining pregnancy.

17-A. When would you start suppressive treatment? 1

☐ Suppressive therapy to continue immediately after treatment of the first episode

17-B. Indicate your evidence-based mode for delivery. 1

☐ Cesarean delivery is recommended for third-trimester onset of primary or nonprimary first episodes of genital herpes

17-C. Identify two reasons for this delivery recommendation. *(1 point each)* 2

☐ Greater viral concentration and longer duration of shedding
☐ Absence of maternal type-specific antibodies *(seroconversion may take 90 days)*

SCENARIO C

With third-trimester first episode of genital herpes, the patient is treated, and an elective Cesarean delivery is planned at term. However, she presents in advanced labor with intact membranes and vaginal delivery is deemed unavoidable.

18. Indicate <u>critical aspects</u> of your obstetric management in this situation. 4

☐ Consideration for IV acyclovir
☐ Delay or avoid amniotomy
☐ Avoid fetal invasive procedures
☐ Inform neonatology/pediatric infectious disease teams

TOTAL: 70

CHAPTER 62

Human Immunodeficiency Virus Infection in Pregnancy

Erica Hardy and Amira El-Messidi

A new patient presents for consultation and transfer of care to your high-risk obstetrics unit at a tertiary center. She is a healthy 22-year-old primigravida at 14^{+3} weeks' gestation with an incidentally positive test for human immunodeficiency virus (HIV) on routine prenatal testing. A copy of the original laboratory report has been provided to you. The patient is aware of the results. Referral to a virologist has also been instigated. Her first-trimester sonogram and aneuploidy screen were unremarkable. She has no obstetric complaints.

LEARNING OBJECTIVES

1. Take a focused history for a new prenatal diagnosis of HIV, and demonstrate the ability to initiate investigations required in continued multidisciplinary care
2. Provide detailed counseling on the maternal-fetal importance of antepartum combined antiretroviral therapy, recognizing common frameworks of therapy in pregnancy
3. Comprehensively counsel and plan the antepartum, intrapartum, and postpartum care of women with HIV infection, continuously aiming to reduce the stigma associated with pregnancy and HIV
4. Utilize virology-specific information to formulate evidence-based recommendations and counseling on timing and mode of delivery
5. Troubleshoot special obstetrical situations involving invasive diagnostic procedures and labor management of HIV-positive women, possibly untreated or with high viremia

SUGGESTED READINGS

1. American College of Obstetricians and Gynecologists' Committee on Practice Bulletins–Gynecology. Practice Bulletin No. 167: Gynecologic care for women and adolescents with human immunodeficiency virus. *Obstet Gynecol*. 2016;128(4):e89–e110.
2. Bailey H, Zash R, Rasi V, et al. HIV treatment in pregnancy. *Lancet HIV*. 2018;5(8):e457–e467.
3. Centers for Disease Control and Prevention, Association of Public Health Laboratories. Laboratory testing for the diagnosis of HIV infection: updated recommendations. Atlanta (GA), Silver Spring (MD). CDC, APHL; 2014. Available at http://stacks.cdc.gov/view/cdc/ 23447. Accessed November 8, 2020.
4. Committee on Obstetric Practice; HIV Expert Work Group. ACOG Committee Opinion No. 751: labor and delivery management of women with human immunodeficiency virus infection. *Obstet Gynecol*. 2018;132(3):e131–e137.

5. Floridia M, Masuelli G, Meloni A, et al. Amniocentesis and chorionic villus sampling in HIV-infected pregnant women: a multicentre case series. *BJOG*. 2017;124(8):1218–1223.

6. Gibson KS, Toner LE. Society for Maternal-Fetal Medicine (SMFM) Special Statement: Updated checklists for pregnancy management in persons with HIV. *Am J Obstet Gynecol*. 2020;223(5):B6–B11.

7. Gilleece DY, Tariq DS, Bamford DA, et al. British HIV Association guidelines for the management of HIV in pregnancy and postpartum 2018. *HIV Med*. 2019;20(Suppl 3):s2–s85. Available at www.bhiva.org/pregnancy-guidelines. Accessed October 22, 2020.

8. Irshad U, Mahdy H, Tonismae T. HIV In Pregnancy. In *StatPearls*. Treasure Island, FL: StatPearls Publishing; 2020.

9. Loutfy M, Kennedy VL, Poliquin V, et al. No. 354 – Canadian HIV pregnancy planning guidelines. *J Obstet Gynaecol Can*. 2018;40(1):94–114.

10. Panel on Treatment of Pregnant Women with HIV Infection and Prevention of Perinatal Transmission. Recommendations for the use of antiretroviral drugs in pregnant women with HIV infection and interventions to reduce perinatal HIV transmission in the United States. Available at https://clinicalinfo.hiv.gov/sites/default/files/guidelines/documents/Peri_Recommendations.pdf. Accessed November 7, 2020.

POINTS

1. What aspects of a focused history would you want to know? *(1 point each)*

Max 20

Comorbidities and medical history:
☐ Evaluate if/when HIV was previously reported negative
☐ Receipt of blood transfusions, or prior surgeries
☐ Prenatal results of hepatitis B, C, syphilis, chlamydia, and gonorrhea testing
☐ Assess for updated vaccinations *(including HPV and COVID-19)*
☐ Current or prior opportunistic infections *(e.g., toxoplasmosis, TB, pneumocystis pneumonia)*

Social history:
☐ Place of birth or having lived in a country where HIV is endemic
☐ Current housing/socioeconomic status
☐ Occupation *(particularly for risk of blood-borne pathogens or risk of transmission to others)*
☐ Prior needlestick injuries
☐ Intravenous or intranasal recreational drug use/tattoos/acupuncture/shared needles
☐ Alcohol consumption, smoking
☐ Prior incarceration

Medications:
☐ Use of opiates or over-the-counter agents

Sexual history:
☐ Current and prior lifetime sexual partners
☐ History of coercive sexual activity
☐ History of exchanging sex for money
☐ Prior partner with known HIV positivity
☐ Results of latest Papanicolaou smear and history of cervical dysplasia
☐ Prior STIs *(including HSV, trichomonas, chlamydia, gonorrhea, syphilis*

Partner:
☐ HIV status, if known
☐ History of IV drug use
☐ Updated vaccination status, if known

Originally from a country where HIV is endemic, the patient immigrated to your country six months ago and was sponsored by her husband. Currently unemployed, she was a teacher in her native country. Her husband is her only lifetime sexual partner and the couple are in a monogamous relationship, although the patient is uncertain of his sexual past. She does not believe he had recent HIV testing. Just prior to immigration, she tested negative for HIV. The patient does not smoke, use recreational drugs, and has not consumed alcohol since conception. She only takes prenatal vitamins which she tolerates.

The patient is of normal habitus without lymphadenopathy, signs of wasting, needle tracks, rash or oral thrush. You document a normal blood pressure, pulse, and temperature; fetal viability is ascertained.

You decide to initiate investigations in preparation for her consultation with the virologist. Meanwhile, your obstetric trainee is interested in the evolution of HIV testing, now involving a fourth-generation assay, rather than conventional algorithms testing for HIV antibodies.

2. Discuss the advantages of current HIV screening using the fourth-generation   Max 2
    immunoassay. *(1 point each)*

    ☐ Allows detection of *acute* HIV infections that would be missed by antibody tests alone
    ☐ Quick turnaround of results *(expedites treatment initiation)*
    ☐ HIV antibody-antigen combination tests and subsequent nucleic acid testing, where
       needed, improves HIV detection rate compared to conventional antibody testing
    ☐ Allows for diagnostic distinction between HIV-1 and HIV-2 infections

3. Outline additional investigations required in evaluation and subsequent management of   Max 15
    her new HIV diagnosis. *(1 point per main bullet)*

HIV virology-related tests:
☐ HIV RNA viral load
☐ Antiretroviral drug resistance (genotype) panel
   ○ *Performed when viral load is above the threshold for resistance testing*
     (i.e., >500– 1000 copies/ml)
☐ CD4 T-lymphocyte[‡] cell count and percentage
   ○ *Start prophylaxis for opportunistic infections with CD4 counts <200 copies/mL*
   ○ *CD4 percentage remains stable due to pregnancy alone; CD4 counts naturally decline,*
     although are used to monitor treatment response

Serum tests:

- ☐ CBC/FBC with differential
- ☐ Creatinine and electrolytes
- ☐ Hepatic transaminases and function tests
- ☐ Toxoplasmosis serology (IgG)[§]
- ☐ G6PD and HLA-B* 5701
  - ○ *With G6PD deficiency, trimethoprim/sulfamethoxazole cannot be used for Pneumocystis jirovecci prophylaxis/treatment*
  - ○ *HLA-B* 5701- positive allele obviates use of abacavir; risk of hypersensitivity*
- ☐ Hepatitis A total antibody
  - ○ *If not immune, the patient will require vaccination*
- ☐ Hepatitis B serology (HBsAg, HBsAb, HBcAb)
  - ○ *If not immune, the patient will require vaccination*
  - ○ *A chronic hepatitis B infection will have implications in selection of antiretroviral medications whereby the chosen regimen for treatment of HIV infection will include two agents that are active against hepatitis B infection)*
  - ○ *If chronic maternal hepatitis B infection is detected, the infant will require prophylaxis with an initial hepatitis B vaccine dose and HBIG at birth*
- ☐ Hepatitis C antibody
- ☐ Syphilis screening *(either conventional or reverse screening algorithm)* **

Other investigations:

- ☐ Testing for latent TB (tuberculin skin test [TST] or interferon gamma-release assay [IGRA])[†]
- ☐ Cervical cytology with/without HPV testing depending on age of the patient (HPV testing is not recommended for patients with HIV <30 years of age)
- ☐ Screening for Trichomonas vaginalis; in case of infection, retest three months posttreatment[#]
- ☐ Urine screening for chlamydia/gonorrhea
- ☐ Urinalysis *(required prior to potential initiation of tenofovir-based regimens)*

Special notes:

‡   T-lymphocyte Cluster of Differentiation 4

§   CMV serology is not indicated in routine testing for HIV in pregnancy

**   Refer to Chapter 65

†   Refer to Chapter 36

Trichomonas vaginalis in HIV-positive women increases the risk of vertical and horizontal transmission of HIV; *refer to* Workowski KA, Bachmann LH, Chan PA, et al. Sexually Transmitted Infections Treatment Guidelines, 2021. *MMWR Recomm Rep.* 2021;70(4): 1–187. Published 2021 Jul 23.

4. Until results of investigations are available, counsel the patient on social health measures with HIV infection. *(1 point each)*

☐ Discuss partner notification (interpersonally or via partner services programs)
☐ Offer HIV testing of the partner and recommend updating vaccinations, *if necessary*
☐ Recommend condom use during sexual intercourse to decrease risk of HIV transmission to a sexual partner, and avoid intercourse if body fluids are visibly contaminated with blood
☐ Discuss consideration for partner's preexposure prophylaxis, if seronegative
☐ Avoid sharing toothbrushes or razor blades; may share food and utensils
☐ Cover breached skin
☐ Use bleached solutions to clean her blood spills
☐ Inform the patient that public health reporting of HIV infection may be required by jurisdictional policies *(consult local legal counsel, while providing continued patient reassurance of confidential proceedings)*

Max 5

5. Discuss the indications for HIV testing in pregnancy. *(1 point each)*

☐ Universal screening among early routine prenatal investigations
☐ Repeat screening in the third trimester in cases where risk factors for infection persist, or women who develop signs/symptoms consistent with acute HIV infection
☐ Encourage partner screening where HIV status is unknown

3

The patient would appreciate linkage with local HIV partner notification programs to support her in the disclosure process.

Meanwhile, she is concerned about the detrimental interactions between pregnancy and HIV infection.

6. Address the patient's concern regarding the impact of pregnancy on her HIV infection.

☐ Reassuringly, pregnancy does not impact the course or severity of infection

1

7. Excluding effects of antiretroviral therapy, indicate <u>maternal</u> perinatal morbidities with HIV infection to mention in counseling. *(1 point each)*

☐ Chorioamnionitis
☐ Postpartum endometritis
☐ Wound infections

3

8. Discuss adverse birth outcomes with <u>untreated</u> HIV infection in pregnancy. *(1 point per main bullet)* 4

☐ Preterm birth (PTB)
☐ Low birthweight
☐ Stillbirth/ intrauterine fetal death (IUFD)
☐ Baseline risk of mother-to-child transmission (MTCT) of 20%–25%
   ○ Rate of transmission decreases to <2% with combined antiretroviral therapy and current care recommendations

9. Identify fetal/neonatal risks associated with HIV <u>antiretrovirals</u> accepted, or recommended, for antenatal use. *(1 point per main bullet)* 3

☐ NTDs with periconceptional exposure to dolutegravir (DTG)
   ○ Controversy regarding high-dose folic acid supplementation with use of DTG:
      ■ *BHIVA 2020: Folic acid 5 mg daily is advised until 12 weeks' gestation*
      ■ *Guidelines (Suggested Reading 10): No established link between DTG and impaired folate metabolism; no evidence that added supplementation prevents DTG-associated NTDs*
☐ Prematurity *(controversial association with protease inhibitor-based regimens)*
☐ Possible risk of low birthweight

Special note:
Evidence suggests no increased NTDs among infants exposed to efavirenz *[Ford N et al. AIDS 2014;28(suppl 2): S123–31]*

Investigations reveal an HIV viral load of 34,500 copies/ml with a CD4 count at 538 cells/mm^3. Apart from a hemoglobin of 10 g/dL *(normal pregnancy = 11–14)*, the remainder of her test results are unremarkable. She does not have latent TB or antibodies to HAV. Oral iron supplementation will be started.[†]

The patient encounters the virologist at 14^{+6} weeks' gestation who later calls to discuss the care plan with you.

Special note:
† Regarding HIV, maternal anemia increases MTCT of infection

10. In collaboration with the virologist, detail the <u>antepartum maternal</u> management of her HIV infection. *(1 point per main bullet, unless specified)* Max 17

Treatment-related care plan:
☐ Begin a combined antiretroviral therapy regimen as soon as possible, especially given patient is in the second trimester
   ○ Earlier viral suppression in pregnancy lowers HIV-MTCT
   ○ Controversy regarding timing the initiation of combined antiretroviral therapy:
      ■ *SMFM 2020 (Suggested Reading 6) and United States guidelines by the Department of Health and Human Services (Suggested Reading 10): initiate treatment as soon as possible among pregnant women*

- *BHIVA 2020 (Suggested Reading 7): recommended gestational age at which treatment is started depends on viral load (first-trimester initiation is with viral load >100,000 copies/mL and/or with CD4 count <200 cells/mm³); otherwise early second-trimester initiation is preferred*
  - Controversy regarding initiation of combined antiretroviral therapy relative to drug-resistance genotype evaluation:
    - *SMFM 2020 (Suggested Reading 6) and United States guidelines by the Department of Health and Human Services (Suggested Reading 10): Advises not to wait for genotype results*
    - *BHIVA 2020: Advises awaiting results of resistance testing for women not already taking antiretroviral therapy, except for third-trimester presentations*
- ☐ Reassure the patient that the rate of virologic control (*i.e.,* suppression) with combined antiretroviral therapy is not affected by pregnancy
- ☐ Preferred options for combined antiretroviral therapy regimens: *(1 point per subbullet)*
  - i. 2 nucleoside reverse transcriptase inhibitors + integrase inhibitor, *or*
  - ii. 2 nucleoside reverse transcriptase inhibitors + protease inhibitor, *or*
  - iii. 2 nucleoside reverse transcriptase inhibitors + non-nucleoside reverse transcriptase inhibitor *(primarily an alternative first-line regimen in resource-limited settings)*
- ☐ Emphasize the importance of 100% adherence to combined antiretroviral treatment regimen at every patient visit
  - Missed doses provide opportunities for developing drug resistance
  - Failed HIV suppression increases risks of MTCT
- ☐ Encourage lifelong treatment for HIV, including postpartum continuation of treatment as planned with her virologist
- ☐ Encourage early notification of treatment-related side effects or intolerance (including nausea/vomiting)
- ☐ Viral load at two to four weeks after initiating (or changing) combined antiretroviral regimens
  - Viremia should decrease by one to two logs after initiating treatment
  - Suppression should occur by a mean of 20 weeks after initiating treatment
- ☐ Subsequent suggested frequency of serial viral load testing may vary:
  - *SMFM 2020 (Suggested Reading 6) and United States guidelines by the Department of Health and Human Services (Suggested Reading 10): Monthly HIV viral load until undetectable, then every one to three months thereafter, including close to delivery (34–36 weeks in order to plan for mode of delivery).*
  - *BHIVA 2020: Viral load at least once every three months, at 36 weeks, and at delivery*
- ☐ Inform the patient that unless vaginal delivery is contraindicated for obstetrical factors, viral load at 34–36 weeks' gestation will guide mode of delivery
- ☐ Serial CD4 count frequency will vary based on local resources and guidelines, one option is every three months and at delivery
  - *SMFM 2020: May assess at six-month intervals for patients with undetectable viral load and CD4 count >200 copies/mL*
- ☐ Serial serum hematologic, renal, hepatic, metabolic testing *(monitoring of combined antiretroviral regimen toxicity)*
- ☐ Consideration for early screening for gestational diabetes mellitus with protease-based combined antiretroviral regimens
- ☐ Consideration for sonographic fetal growth monitoring; *individualized frequency*
  - *Risk of suboptimal fetal growth with some combined antiretroviral regimens*
- ☐ Neonatology/pediatric virology consultation to plan newborn's care plan

Health maintenance:

☐ Vaccinate for HAV, influenza, pneumococcus, and pertussis *(patient is immune to HBV)*; ensure receipt of COVID-19 vaccination

☐ Repeat third-trimester screening for syphilis, gonorrhea, and chlamydia *(e.g.,* at 28–34 weeks' gestation)

☐ Ensure access to psychosocial support services especially given a new diagnosis of HIV *(Encourage and support treatment adherence)*

☐ Access to evaluation of domestic violence and perinatal mental health

☐ Recommend delivery in a tertiary center or facility with access to pediatric care

☐ Prepare the patient that breastfeeding is not recommended among women with HIV in resource-rich nations, irrespective of an undetectable viral load

☐ Continued evaluation for onset of opportunistic infections

Her treating virologist will initiate tenofovir disoproxil fumarate-emtricitabine, forming the 2-nucleoside backbone, and darunavir/ritonavir as the protease inhibitor component. The patient starts treatment at 15^{+0} weeks; genotype results later show appropriate viral sensitivity. Repeat viral load two weeks later shown a rise to 50,000 copies/mL.

Special note:

Guidelines for choice of combined antiretroviral therapy in pregnancy in *resource-limited* settings are provided by the WHO, available on its website

11. Identify four goals of combined antiretroviral therapy during pregnancy. *(1 point each)* | 4

☐ Maintain the patient's health
☐ Restore her immune system
☐ Suppress viral replication
☐ Diminish risks of vertical transmission

12. Address why two nucleoside reverse transcriptase inhibitors form the backbone of combined antiretroviral therapy among antiretroviral-naïve women. | 1

☐ High rate of transplacental transfer optimizes preexposure prophylaxis

13. Outline general interventions or considerations for this patient where combined antiretroviral therapy appears to fail in viral suppression despite resistance analysis. *(1 point each)* | 3

☐ Review treatment adherence, exploring potential confounders or drug interactions with concomitant medications
☐ Consider therapeutic drug monitoring, if available
☐ Consider intensifying/optimizing treatment regimen with input from virologist

Realizing that nausea may account for the rise in viral load, antiemetics are provided and subsequent viral load analyses demonstrate appropriately decreasing trends.

Fetal morphology survey at 21 weeks' gestation is normal and early GDM testing, performed at 24 weeks' gestation, is negative. She receives routine acellular pertussis vaccination *(e.g., Tdap – tetanus, diphtheria, acellular pertussis vaccine)*. The patient has not experienced obstetrical complications.

At 29 weeks' gestation, low-detectable levels are seen at 65 copies/mL. Along with the virologist, you remain optimistic for undetectable viral levels prior to delivery. Your obstetrics trainee suggests that risks of perinatal transmission remain consistent throughout the gestational period.

---

14. Clarify your trainee's misconceptions, *if any*, by indicating the gestational period conferring the greatest risk of perinatal HIV transmission.

☐ Intrapartum period entails the greatest risk of perinatal HIV *(up to 40% of MTCT)*

Special note:
Antepartum period is associated with 10%–25% of perinatal transmissions; breastfeeding accounts for ~14% of transmissions, although may be ~40% in low-income countries with limited access to infant formula

	1

Coincidentally, you receive an external call from a colleague requesting management advice for an HIV-positive patient requiring urgent therapeutic amnioreduction. Although results of her viral load are not yet available, combined antiretroviral therapy will be started as soon as possible.

---

15. In collaboration with a virologist, provide recommendations where an urgent invasive fetal procedure is required in an HIV infected patient who is not yet on treatment with detectable viral load. *(1 point per main bullet)*

Treatment recommendations:
☐ Single-dose oral nevirapine 200 mg should be given two to four hours prior to the invasive prenatal procedure
☐ Commence an integrase-inhibitor containing combined antiretroviral therapy regimen *(i.e., raltegravir)*
  ○ *Achieves rapid viral load reduction*

Procedural advice:
☐ Avoid transplacental needle entry
☐ Single entry technique

	4

Your patient's pregnancy progresses well, and she continues to practice 100% adherence to her combined antiretroviral therapy regimen, without any missed doses. At 36 weeks' gestation, her viral load is undetectable according to your practice policies, at <50 copies/mL[†] and her CD4 count is 350 cells/mm³. The fetus is in a complete breech presentation with growth biometry on the 33rd percentile and normal amniotic fluid volume. The patient has no obstetrical contraindications to an external cephalic version. Although she prefers a vaginal delivery, the patient will comply with your best practice recommendations.

Special note:
† Level at which viral load is deemed undetectable varies from <20–50 copies/mL by jurisdictional guidelines; individualized delivery decision-making based on local protocol is advised

16. In collaboration with her virologist, indicate your recommendations for the mode of delivery. *(1 point per main bullet)*   2

☐ External cephalic version may be offered as the plasma viral load is <50 HIV RNA copies/mL *(BHIVA 2020)*

☐ Vaginal delivery may be offered given a suppressed viral load, unless obstetrically contraindicated

   ○ *Controversy exists regarding level of viremia at which vaginal delivery is permissible:*

     ▪ United States guidelines by the Department of Health and Human Services *(Suggested Reading 10)*: ≤1000 copies/mL

     ▪ SMFM 2020: <1000 copies/mL

     ▪ BHIVA 2020: <50 copies/mL

   ○ Where Cesarean delivery is required for obstetrical reasons in women with suppressed viral load, suggest delivery at ≥39 weeks

   ○ Where Cesarean delivery is advised solely for prevention of vertical HIV transmission, suggest delivery at 38–39 weeks' gestation

Special note:
Respect patient autonomy in deciding on route of delivery; ensure informed consent

With informed consent, an external cephalic version is performed and the fetus successfully turns to a cephalic presentation. A multidisciplinary discussion occurs among treating team members regarding delivery and postnatal management.

17. Outline essentials of <u>labor and delivery</u> management with regard to her HIV infection. *(1 point per main bullet)*   Max 11

☐ Ensure appropriate protective equipment for all personnel; maintain universal body fluid precautions

☐ Continue her combined antiretroviral regimen in labor and postpartum

☐ No indication for additional intrapartum intravenous zidovudine for this patient[§]

☐ No association between duration of ruptured membranes and risk of perinatal transmission as the patient is virally suppressed

☐ Maintain a low threshold to treat intrapartum fever

☐ Avoid internal monitoring, such as scalp electrodes or intrauterine pressure catheters, if possible

   ○ *Regardless of viral suppression status*

☐ Avoid instrumental vaginal delivery, if possible

   ○ *Regardless of viral suppression status*

☐ Avoid episiotomy, if possible

☐ Wash off maternal fluid from the newborn as soon as possible after delivery, and prior to newborn vaccinations and vitamin K injection

☐ Use bulb-suction to remove maternal fluid from the newborn as soon as possible

☐ Avoid ergotamines, if possible *(patient takes a protease-inhibitor regimen)*

☐ Ensure pediatric virology experts have arranged a pathway for neonatal prophylaxis as soon as possible, but no later than within 12 hours of delivery

Special notes:

§ Intravenous zidovudine is indicated for laboring women with unknown viral load, or for women with viral load ≥1000 copies/mL; treatment may be considered at lower detectable levels (*i.e.*, 50–1000 copies/mL)

Indications for intrapartum intravenous zidovudine are not affected by documented zidovudine resistance

Spontaneous labor ensues at 39^{+4} weeks' gestation; the patient receives appropriate intrapartum HIV treatment and delivery management. She has an uncomplicated vaginal delivery of a vigorous neonate. Reassuringly, the newborn's initial HIV test is negative. Empiric neonatal oral zidovudine is started soon after delivery and follow-up arranged with a pediatric virology expert.

After delivery, you find your trainee taking notes to consolidate elements of the obstetrical care plan that contributed to this preferred neonatal outcome.

18. Elicit current care recommendations contributing to decreased MTCT of HIV. *(1 point per main bullet)*   5

 □ Universal HIV testing in pregnancy
 □ Antenatal combined antiretroviral therapy leading to undetectable viral load
 □ Antiretroviral prophylaxis in the infant
 □ Elective Cesarean delivery based on viral load at ~36 weeks
 □ Avoidance of breastfeeding

You visit the patient on postpartum day 1 and find her formula feeding the newborn. You sense that abstinence from breastfeeding is distressing her; she also complains of pain related to engorgement. After the stress she endured this pregnancy, she cannot remember your antenatal counseling of safe contraceptives.

19. In relation to HIV, address important <u>postpartum</u> issues to discuss with, and plan for, this patient. *(1 point each, max points specified per section)*   Max 14

General well-being and HIV infection care: *(max 9)*
 □ Encourage continuation of combined antiretroviral therapy (*based on consultation with her virologist*)
 □ Provide continued psychosocial support services, either within the medical system or available community resources
 □ Screening for, and treatment of, postpartum depression
 □ May administer MMR vaccine, if indicated for rubella nonimmunity, given the patient's CD4 count is >200 cells/mm³ (*otherwise, exercise caution with live-viral vaccinations among HIV-positive individuals*)
 □ Counsel the patient on preexposure prophylaxis for her partner if they are serodiscordant and if her HIV viral load is not suppressed

☐ Arrange for routine postpartum obstetrical follow-up

☐ Arrange for Papanicolaou cervical cytology screening *(particularly important for women living with HIV)*

☐ Encourage adherence with long-term follow-up with primary care provider and virologist

☐ Support completion of neonatal postexposure prophylaxis and pediatric care follow-up

☐ Recommend future preconceptional counseling

Contraceptive particularities for this HIV patient with CD4 count $\geq$200 cells/mm^3: *(max 2)*

☐ Dual contraception is ideal; stress importance of condoms with HIV infection

☐ Avoid use of diaphragms or nonoxyl-9 spermicides

☐ No restrictions for use of combined hormonal contraceptives, however, potential drug-drug interactions between hormonal contraceptives and antiretroviral therapy may lead to failed contraception; *individualized assessment is required*[§]

☐ IUDs are an option to be considered (US-MEC, category 1 and UK-MEC, category 2)[§†]

Breastfeeding considerations [medical and social]: *(max 3)*

☐ Arrange for free formula as breastfeeding is contraindicated for the infant's health *(jurisdictional variations exist)*

☐ Beware of possible psychological repercussions to the patient for whom lactation is contraindicated; provide support services

☐ Consideration for cabergoline to suppress lactation *(BHIVA 2020)*
   ○ *Off-label use for HIV-positive women*

☐ Inform the patient about the earlier return of ovulation in absence of breastfeeding

Special notes:

§ UK and US Medical Eligibility Criteria (MEC) for Contraceptive Use, 2016; UK-MEC revised September 2019, US-MEC amended 2020

† Contraceptive recommendations for IUDs differ for CD4 counts <200 cells/mm^3; refer to the UK or US-MEC

The following week, an ambulance presents with a recent immigrant who is clearly in labor and appears to be at term; cervical dilation is 9 cm with ruptured chorioamniotic membranes. Cardiotocography is normal. There is no record of prenatal care. Using opt-out screening, the patient's 'rapid HIV test' is reactive.[‡]

Your trainee calls you concerned; the team cannot access the HIV treatment protocol for such situations and the virologist has yet to call back. Multidisciplinary members including neonatology and anesthesiology are present for delivery.

Special note:

‡ Reactive rapid HIV test is not definitive, although immediate initiation of antiretroviral prophylaxis for mother and neonate is recommended until confirmatory results are available

20. Given unknown treatment of HIV in this term-laboring patient, which <u>oral</u> antiviral agent should this patient receive <u>as soon as possible</u>?

☐ Nevirapine *(200 mg once)*

Special note:
Women should commence combined antiretroviral therapy in general, containing an integrase inhibitor due to its utility in rapidly lowering the viral load; intravenous zidovudine is required for the duration of labor

TOTAL: 120

CHAPTER 63

Parvovirus B19 Infection in Pregnancy

Amira El-Messidi and Marie-France Lachapelle

You are on obstetrics call duty at a community hospital center, where a 30-year-old G2P1 elementary schoolteacher presents concerned, after receiving notification during this spring week holiday, that there is an outbreak of 'slapped cheek syndrome' among the children. The patient is at 16^{+3} weeks' gestation by dating sonography performed by her primary care provider; first-trimester fetal morphology was normal with a low risk of aneuploidy. Three years ago, she had a healthy pregnancy and term vaginal delivery of her son, who currently attends daycare. The patient does not have any obstetric complaints.

LEARNING OBJECTIVES

1. Take a focused history for prenatal exposure to parvovirus B19 infection, and initiate timely assessment of maternal serologies
2. Interpret parvovirus B19 serology, and arrange for subsequent testing where appropriate
3. Recognize the importance of early referral to maternal-fetal medicine experts and a tertiary center with expertise in intrauterine transfusion when maternal parvovirus B19 infection is confirmed
4. Counsel on risks of adverse obstetric outcomes, and demonstrate an understanding of therapeutic interventions for parvovirus B19 infection
5. Appreciate sonographic manifestations of hydrops fetalis, promptly recognizing potentially life-threatening related maternal manifestations

SUGGESTED READINGS

1. Attwood LO, Holmes NE, Hui L. Identification and management of congenital parvovirus B19 infection. *Prenat Diagn*. 2020;40(13):1722–1731.
2. Bascietto F, Liberati M, Murgano D, et al. Outcome of fetuses with congenital parvovirus B19 infection: systematic review and meta-analysis. *Ultrasound Obstet Gynecol*. 2018;52(5): 569–576.
3. Bhide A, Acharya G, Bilardo CM, et al. ISUOG practice guidelines: use of Doppler ultrasonography in obstetrics. *Ultrasound Obstet Gynecol*. 2013;41(2):233–239.
4. Brennand J, Cameron A. Fetal anaemia: diagnosis and management. *Best Pract Res Clin Obstet Gynaecol*. 2008;22(1):15–29.
5. Crane J, Mundle W, Boucoiran I. Maternal Fetal Medicine Committee. Parvovirus B19 infection in pregnancy. *J Obstet Gynaecol Can*. 2014;36(12):1107–1116.

6. Désilets V, De Bie I, Audibert F. No. 363 – Investigation and management of non-immune fetal hydrops. *J Obstet Gynaecol Can.* 2018;40(8):1077–1090.
7. Khalil A, Sotiriadis A, Chaoui R, et al. ISUOG Practice Guidelines: role of ultrasound in congenital infection. *Ultrasound Obstet Gynecol.* 2020;56(1):128–151.
8. Lamont RF, Sobel JD, Vaisbuch E, et al. Parvovirus B19 infection in human pregnancy. *BJOG.* 2011;118(2):175–186.
9. Public Health England. 2019. Guidance on the investigations, diagnosis and management of viral illness or exposure to viral rash illness in pregnancy. Available at www.gov.uk/government/publications/viral-rash-in-pregnancy. Accessed February 18, 2021.
10. Society for Maternal-Fetal Medicine (SMFM), Norton ME, Chauhan SP, Dashe JS. Society for maternal-fetal medicine (SMFM) clinical guideline No. 7: nonimmune hydrops fetalis. *Am J Obstet Gynecol.* 2015;212(2):127–139.

POINTS

1. Given the etiology of *'slapped cheek syndrome,'* what elements of a focused history would you want to know? *(1 point per main bullet)* — Max 8

Clinical manifestations with parvovirus B19 infection:
- ☐ Recent prodromal illness including fever, headache, pharyngitis, nausea/vomiting
- ☐ Symmetric polyarthralgia, mostly of the hands, wrists ankles, and knees
  - ○ *May be the only manifestation in pregnant women (most common adult symptom)*
  - ○ *Immune-mediated, with onset coinciding with appearance of IgM antibodies*
  - ○ *Arthropathy may last up to several months*
- ☐ Current/recent rash and description of its pattern (erythema infectiosum)
  - ○ *Typical rash is maculopapular, reticular, lattice, or lace-like*
  - ○ *Rash may be on the face and/or trunk and extremities*
  - ○ *Immune-mediated, with onset coinciding with appearance of IgM antibodies*
  - ○ *Onset of the rash or arthropathy generally marks the end of infectivity*
- ☐ Fatigue/palor
  - ○ *May suggest anemia or aplastic crisis*
- ☐ Shortness of breath/chest pain
  - ○ *May suggest myocarditis*

Details of her exposure:
- ☐ Determine when the patient was exposed to children with confirmed parvovirus B19 infection
- ☐ Determine if her son has symptoms of erythema infectiosum

Medical history most relevant to possible parvovirus B19 infection:
- ☐ HIV infection or other associated immunodeficiencies *(risk of severe chronic anemia)*
- ☐ Hematological conditions, such as sickle cell disease, thalassemia, autoimmune hemolytic anemia, hereditary spherocytosis, or pyruvate kinase deficiency
  - ○ *more likely to develop transient aplastic crisis*
- ☐ Recent transfusion of blood or blood products

Special note:
Clinical history of her immune status to parvovirus B19 is only contributory when laboratory evidence is available; otherwise, confirmatory testing is warranted based on exposure and/or symptoms

You learn that the patient is healthy with unremarkable routine prenatal investigations. She has been feeling well. Her weeklong holiday for spring break commenced three days ago, prior to which she has been in close contact with children now confirmed to have erythema infectiosum. She recalls her son having a two-day history of low-grade fever followed by an intermittent nonpruritic rash ~10 days ago; his symptoms resolved spontaneously and were presumed to be common illnesses among daycare children.

The patient appears well with normal vital signs.[†] Physical examination is unremarkable, and fetal viability is ascertained by Doptone.

Special note:
† Vital signs include blood pressure, pulse, temperature, respiratory rate and oxygen saturation

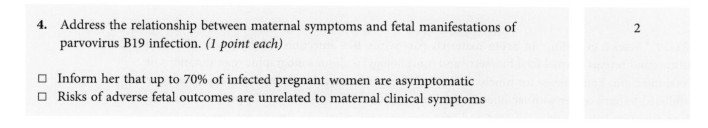

2. Indicate the <u>next best</u> diagnostic investigation for this patient?   2

☐ Obtain parvovirus B19 IgG and IgM serology

As your obstetric trainee has an interest in the evolution of medicine, you take a brief opportunity to address the interesting history and nomenclature of parvovirus B19.

3. Explain why parvovirus B19 is synonymous with 'fifth disease' and indicate the   2
significance of its 'B19' nomenclature. *(1 point each)*

☐ Parvovirus B19 was presumed to be the next classic childhood exanthem after measles, scarlet fever, rubella, and 'fourth disease'/Dukes' disease
☐ A novel antigen was discovered in 'Panel B, Sample 19'of the laboratory testing kit while screening blood donations for hepatitis B in 1975
   ○ *Parvoviruses had a known property of morphological and serological similarity to the hepatitis B antigen*

You inform the patient that serology results are expected within several days. Meanwhile, she *believes* that her absence of clinical symptoms implies lower risk of infection. She asks for your recommendations on risk prevention in this 'window of opportunity,' prior to potential onset of symptoms, as she recalls her sister receiving varicella zoster immunoglobulin (VZIG) shortly upon exposure to an affected child.

4. Address the relationship between maternal symptoms and fetal manifestations of   2
parvovirus B19 infection. *(1 point each)*

☐ Inform her that up to 70% of infected pregnant women are asymptomatic
☐ Risks of adverse fetal outcomes are unrelated to maternal clinical symptoms

5. Provide evidence-based advice on prophylactic interventions to decrease maternal-fetal infection after potential exposure to parvovirus B19 infection. *(1 point each)*

☐ Lack of prophylactic interventions to decrease risks of infection after possible exposure
☐ Lack of evidence to support preventative leave for pregnant women susceptible to parvovirus B19 infection; the risk of acquiring infection through the workplace (*e.g.*, the school where she works) is *less than* through household contacts (*e.g.*, her son or other personal contacts)

Max 1

Within four days, at 17^{+0} weeks' gestation, enzyme-linked immunoassay (ELISA) shows presence of parvovirus IgM without IgG antibodies. As the patient's primary care provider is now on vacation, she presents to your clinic, as requested, for counseling and management.

6. Based on the patient's laboratory findings, provide your <u>most accurate</u> interpretation of her investigations, and indicate your next step in the diagnostic evaluation. *(1 point each)*

Parvovirus IgG-negative and IgM-positive serologies:
☐ Very recent infection, or
☐ False-positive IgM result[†]

Next best diagnostic step:
☐ Repeat parvovirus B19 IgG and IgM in one to two weeks

Special note:
[†] Although IgM may remain positive for four to six months after acute infection, the IgG would be expected to be positive; as such, prolonged positive IgM would not explain this scenario

3

7. Address her inquiry on results of repeat serology that would confirm an acute parvovirus B19 infection and the immediate subsequent step in management. *(1 point per main bullet)*

☐ Appearance of IgG antibody at repeat serology confirms an acute infection
  ○ *IgG appears a few days after IgM antibody and persists indefinitely*
  ○ *Failure to detect IgM antibody would indicate an initial false-positive result*
☐ Referral to a maternal-fetal medicine expert and a tertiary center with expertise in intrauterine transfusion

2

At 19^{+4} weeks' gestation, an acute maternal parvovirus B19 infection is confirmed. Obstetric ultrasound reveals normal fetal biometry and morphology, without sonographic manifestations of fetal infection. You arrange for timely transfer of care to a maternal-fetal medicine expert in your affiliated tertiary center with facilities for fetal transfusions. Prior to referral, the patient is curious how she may have become infected and asks you to detail what you foresee for her care in the tertiary center.

8. Inform the patient of all modes of transmission for parvovirus B19 and indicate her probable source(s) of infection. *(1 point each)*

Modes of transmission:
- ☐ Respiratory droplets from infected contacts
- ☐ Blood/product transmission
- ☐ Transplacental passage

Patient's sources of infection:
- ☐ Either her home contacts (*e.g.*, son) **OR** occupational contacts at school

4

9. Outline important aspects of your counseling on <u>fetal</u> effects of parvovirus B19 infection. *(1 point per main bullet)*

- ☐ Reassure the patient that parvovirus is not teratogenic
- ☐ Inform the patient that parvovirus B19 does not cause fetal growth restriction (FGR)
- ☐ Maternal infection is associated with a 25%–30% risk of fetal transmission
- ☐ Majority (~90%) of *in*fected fetuses are not *aff*ected
- ☐ Risk of early pregnancy loss is dependent on gestational age at infection
  - ○ ~15% prior to 20 weeks' gestation, decreasing to 0.5%–2% in later pregnancy
- ☐ Fetal anemia
- ☐ Myocarditis
  - ○ *Myocarditis leading to severe dilated cardiomyopathy may require a heart transplant*
- ☐ Thrombocytopenia
- ☐ Hydrops fetalis (2%–3%)
- ☐ Hydropic or nonhydropic IUFD
  - ○ *Risk of IUFD decreases with advancing gestational age at infection, from ~15% at 13–20 weeks' gestation to ~6% with infections after 20 weeks' gestation*

Max 8

You now take note of your intent to teach your obstetric trainee the biological basis for fetal anemia due to parvovirus B19 infection, after this clinical encounter.

10. Highlight essential elements to teach your trainee regarding the biological explanation for fetal anemia due to parvovirus B19. *(1 point per main bullet)*

- ☐ Parvovirus B19 has affinity for the <u>P-antigen</u>, which is a glycolipid (globoside) receptor present in trophoblast, erythroid progenitor cells, and myocardium
  - ○ *Virus mainly affects fetal bone marrow, but may also impact extramedullary hematopoiesis in the liver and spleen*
- ☐ <u>Cytotoxic apoptosis</u> prevents erythropoiesis, which induces an aplastic crisis
  - ○ *S-phase cycle of DNA mitosis is especially vulnerable to parvovirus B19 infection*

2

You inform the patient that rates of fetal complications are greater with first- or second-trimester infections than later in pregnancy. Your trainee takes note to later research the physiological basis for this phenomenon.

11. What is the biological rationale that underscores the greater fetal risks from parvovirus B19 infection in the first half of pregnancy? *(2 points per main bullet)*

4

☐ P-antigen receptor is highly expressed in the first and second trimesters, allowing for greater transplacental transmission of parvovirus B19; the receptor is virtually nonexistent in the third trimester
☐ A >30-fold increase in second-trimester red blood cell mass with concomitant reduction in red blood cell life span to 45–70 days makes the fetus vulnerable to insult in erythropoiesis
   ○ *The need for a large number of red blood cells is decreased in the third trimester, and life span is increased*

12. Outline the <u>details of obstetric management</u> for acute parvovirus B19 infection anticipated by the maternal-fetal medicine expert. *(1 point per main bullet)*

5

☐ Fetal sonographic surveillance every 1–2 weeks for 8–12 weeks' duration from the time of seroconversion for risk of anemia, ascites or hydrops fetalis
   ○ *Sonographic surveillance should start no later than four weeks after maternal seroconversion or onset of illness*
   ○ *Fetal adverse outcome in the absence of sequelae by 12 weeks of sonographic monitoring is highly unlikely*
☐ Use MCA-PSV (middle cerebral artery – peak systolic velocity) >1.5 MoM (multiples of the median) to assess for fetal anemia
   ○ *Sensitivity of 94% and specificity of 93% for detecting anemia in parvovirus B19 infected fetuses*
☐ Intrauterine red blood cell transfusion may be performed until 34–35 weeks' gestation *(individualized assessment)*, after which delivery is advocated; presence of platelets at time of transfusion is prudent
   ○ *Nonhydropic fetuses usually need only one transfusion*
☐ Early neonatology consultation
☐ Consideration for fetal pulmonary corticosteroids with/without magnesium sulfate for neuroprotection for intrauterine transfusions after the threshold of viability

The patient contemplates whether amniocentesis for confirmation of fetal infection can potentially avoid weekly surveillance. Your obstetric trainee starts by informing her that invasive testing is only indicated when the procedure is being performed for therapeutic interventions of fetal anemia or hydrops.

13. Provide evidence-based explanations why amniocentesis for <u>diagnostic</u> considerations with acute parvovirus B19 infection is not standard of care. *(1 point each)*   3

 ☐   Likelihood of coexisting thrombocytopenia
 ☐   Viral DNA may be detected intermittently in amniotic fluid (~days 4–14 of infection)
 ☐   Fetal IgM antibodies are only produced as of ~22 weeks' gestation, and occasionally later (false-negative results)

The patient appreciates your medical expertise and evidence-based care; she is reassured that you will follow up on the progress on her obstetric care. Initial consultation with the maternal-fetal medicine expert is arranged for next week.

Realizing that technical factors[†] are involved in accurate MCA Doppler acquisition, you find your obstetric trainee surfing the internet on elements that contribute to false elevations in PSV readings. Your trainee is impressed by how MCA-PSV is valuable for ascertainment of fetal anemia in various clinical scenarios.

Special note:
† Refer to Chapter 10 for discussion on technical aspects of MCA measurement

14. Facilitate your trainee's learning by indicating contributing factors to false-positive MCA-PSV assessments. *(1 point each)*   Max 5

 ☐   Improper technique
 ☐   Fetal behavioral states *(e.g., breathing, movement, heart rate accelerations)*
 ☐   Uterine contractions
 ☐   Advanced gestational age
 ☐   Prior intrauterine transfusions
 ☐   Abnormal placentation
 ☐   Fetal growth restriction (FGR)

15. Identify additional clinical scenarios where MCA-PSV may be valuable for diagnosis of fetal anemic states. *(1 point each)*   Max 3

 ☐   Rhesus alloimmunization
 ☐   Massive feto-maternal hemorrhage
 ☐   Homozygous alpha-thalassemia
 ☐   Fetal anemia secondary to fetal or placental tumor *(e.g., chorioangioma)*
 ☐   Twin–twin transfusion syndrome with a fetal demise in one twin

At 25 weeks' gestation, the maternal-fetal medicine expert informs you that reliable fetal MCA-PSV is now >1.5 MoM without ascites. The patient has consented for cordocentesis and possible intrauterine transfusion; neonatology consultation and a course of fetal pulmonary corticosteroids are in progress.

16. Identify essential factors required to determine the volume of fetal red blood cell transfusion. *(1 point each)*   5

- ☐ Estimated fetal weight
- ☐ Donor pretransfusion hemoglobin/hematocrit
- ☐ Fetal pretransfusion hemoglobin/hematocrit
- ☐ Target hemoglobin/hematocrit
- ☐ Fetoplacental blood volume

Special note:
Refer to Chapter 10 for discussion on intrauterine transfusion techniques, preparations, and procedure-related complications

You later learn that the patient required one intrauterine transfusion, following which pregnancy progressed unremarkably to term and she had a spontaneous vaginal delivery of a healthy newborn.

17. Summarize important aspects of maternal counseling regarding long-term neurological outcome of offspring after in utero parvovirus B19 infection. *(1 point each)*   Max 1

- ☐ Neurologic outcome is favorable based on infection itself without *significant* anemia
- ☐ Hydrops fetalis may be associated with a 10% risk of neurodevelopmental abnormalities

SCENARIO B
The maternal-fetal medicine expert to whom you referred the patient notifies you of her progress: at 20^{+0} weeks' gestation, the patient left town for an urgent family matter. Just prior to her trip, the fetal morphology scan was normal and there were no manifestations of parvovirus B19. Throughout her three-week trip, she did not have any fetal surveillance.

Now at 23^{+2} weeks' gestation, fetal MCA-PSV is at 1.9 MoM. Your colleague shares the current sonographic images with you and your obstetric trainee:

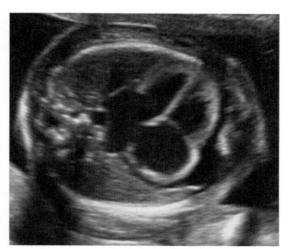

Figure 63.1

With permission: Figure 6, panel B from suggested reading #7 – Khalil A et al. Ultrasound Obstet Gynecol. 2020;56(1): 128–151.

There is no association between the patient's image and this case scenario. Image used for educational purposes only.

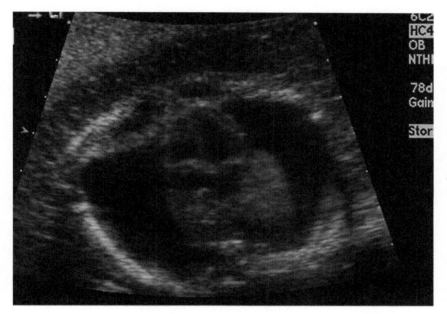

Figure 63.2

With permission: Figure 1, panel B from suggested reading #10 – Norton ME, et al. Am J Obstet Gynecol. 2015;212(2): 127–139.

There is no association between the patient's image and this case scenario. Image used for educational purposes only.

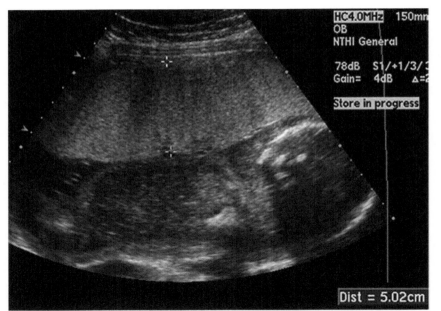

Figure 63.3

With permission: Figure 1, panel C from suggested reading #10 – Norton ME, et al. Am J Obstet Gynecol. 2015;212(2): 127–139.

There is no association between the patient's image and this case scenario. Image used for educational purposes only.

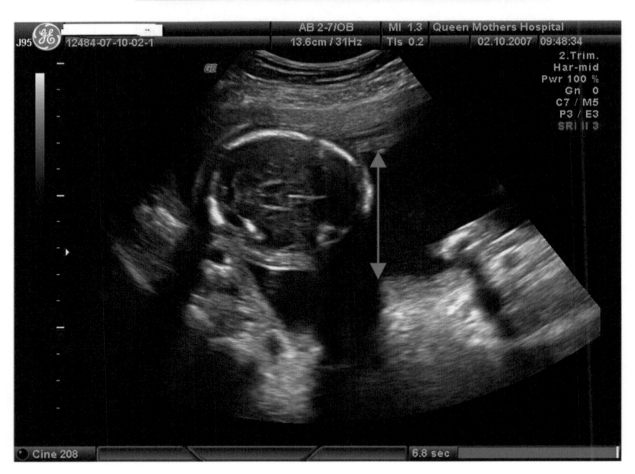

Figure 63.4

Image is courtesy of Professor Alan D. Cameron

There is no association between the patient's image and this case scenario. Image used for educational purposes only.

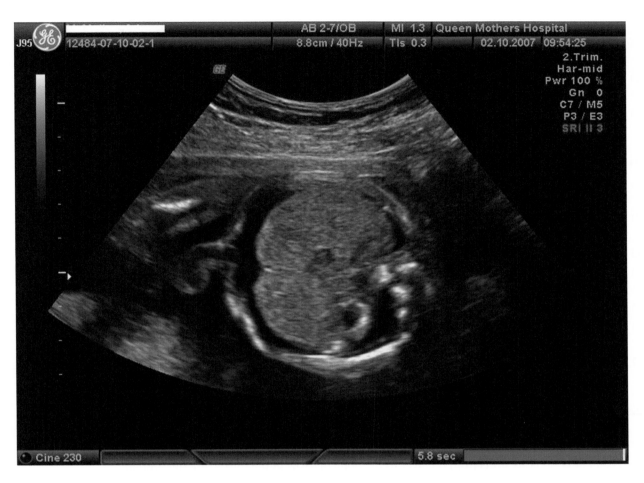

Figure 63.5

Image is courtesy of Professor Alan D. Cameron

There is no association between the patient's image and this case scenario. Image used for educational purposes only.

The patient has not had any obstetric complaints and there is no history of trauma.

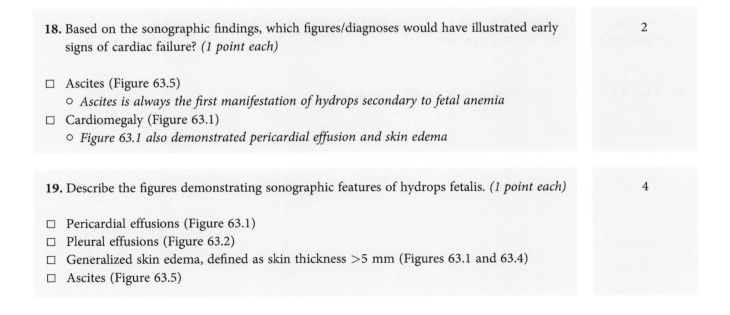

18. Based on the sonographic findings, which figures/diagnoses would have illustrated early   2
signs of cardiac failure? *(1 point each)*

☐ Ascites (Figure 63.5)
   ○ *Ascites is always the first manifestation of hydrops secondary to fetal anemia*
☐ Cardiomegaly (Figure 63.1)
   ○ *Figure 63.1 also demonstrated pericardial effusion and skin edema*

19. Describe the figures demonstrating sonographic features of hydrops fetalis. *(1 point each)*   4

☐ Pericardial effusions (Figure 63.1)
☐ Pleural effusions (Figure 63.2)
☐ Generalized skin edema, defined as skin thickness >5 mm (Figures 63.1 and 63.4)
☐ Ascites (Figure 63.5)

20. Identify the image panels showing <u>associated</u> findings with hydrops. *(1 point each)*   2

☐ Placental thickening (Figure 63.3)
  ○ *≥4 cm in the second trimester and ≥6 cm in third trimester*
☐ Polyhydramnios (Figure 63.4)

21. Outline the natural history of parvovirus-associated hydrops to your obstetric trainee. *(1 point per pain bullet)*   Max 4

☐ Hydrops occurs at a median of three weeks after primary infection and the majority develop by the eighth week after maternal infection
☐ Peak incidence between 17–24 weeks, depending on gestational age at infection
☐ Rate of spontaneous resolution may be ~**30%** and may occur from one to seven weeks after infection
☐ Risk of IUFD is ~**30%**
☐ Therapeutic intervention (or delivery based on gestational age) is indicated
  ○ ~**30%** of hydropic fetuses will need ≥2 transfusions
☐ Hydrops usually resolves within six weeks of intrauterine blood transfusion

22. Your trainee is surprised to learn that unlike unremitting, progressive anemia of rhesus disease, anemia due to parvovirus has potential to resolve spontaneously. Explain why.   1

☐ Fetal hematopoiesis shifts from the liver to the bone marrow in the third trimester and life span of red blood cells increases

She is now admitted to hospital on continuous electronic cardiotocography (CTG) monitoring with arrangements underway for intrauterine transfusion. Fetal monitoring is appropriate for gestational age; there is no representation of anemia.

The patient's blood group is B-positive without atypical antibodies. The maternal-fetal medicine expert informs you that although parvovirus B19 is the most probable etiological infection for this nonimmune hydrops, other agents are possible.

23. What is the CTG tracing most consistent with fetal anemia?   1

☐ Sinusoidal waveform

24. List five other <u>pathogens</u> associated with nonimmune fetal hydrops. *(1 point each)*   Max 5

- ☐ Cytomegalovirus
- ☐ Herpes simplex virus type 1/human herpesvirus 6 and 7
- ☐ Rubella
- ☐ Coxsackievirus
- ☐ Varicella zoster virus
- ☐ Treponema pallidum
- ☐ Toxoplasma gondii
- ☐ Trypanosoma cruzi (Chagas disease)
- ☐ Adenovirus
- ☐ Respiratory syncytial virus
- ☐ Congenital lymphocytic choriomeningitis virus
- ☐ Leptospirosis

25. Provide your trainee with four general <u>mechanisms</u> through which infectious pathogens contribute to nonimmune hydrops. *(1 point each)*   4

- ☐ Anemia
- ☐ Anoxia
- ☐ Endothelial cell damage and increased capillary permeability
- ☐ Myocarditis

Prior to the fetal intrauterine transfusion, the patient's blood pressure became 162/112 mmHg; she complained of a new-onset headache, visual disturbances and epigastric pain. Requiring 2 L oxygen by nasal prongs, pulmonary edema was suspected on clinical examination, and confirmed by bedside chest radiography. Over the past few hours, her face, arm and legs have become notably swollen. Laboratory investigations are consistent with the clinical diagnosis. Immediate maternal treatment is initiated.

26. What is the most accurate diagnosis?   2

- ☐ Mirror syndrome

                                              TOTAL: 85

CHAPTER 64

Rubella in Pregnancy

Amira El-Messidi

A healthy 27-year-old G1P0 at 10^{+3} weeks' gestation, confirmed by sonography two days ago, presents for prenatal care. She arrived last month from overseas and currently lives with her sister and nephew, who has been home from daycare with German measles.

LEARNING OBJECTIVES

1. Take a focused history, and recognize essentials of a focused physical examination for prenatal exposure to rubella
2. Formulate a differential diagnosis, and recognize the importance of comprehensive investigations in establishing the infection at stake
3. Counsel on prenatal risks and management options for maternal rubella infection
4. Illustrate an understanding of counseling for chorionic villous sampling
5. Discuss the mechanisms for prevention of congenital rubella syndrome

SUGGESTED READINGS

1. Alfirevic Z, Navaratnam K, Mujezinovic F. Amniocentesis and chorionic villus sampling for prenatal diagnosis. *Cochrane Database Syst Rev* 2017; 9:CD003252.
2. Banatvala JE, Brown DW. Rubella. *Lancet.* 2004;363(9415):1127–1137.
3. Boucoiran I, Castillo E. Rubella in pregnancy. *J Obstet Gynaecol Can.* 2018; 40(12):1646–1656
4. Khalil A, Sotiriadis A, Chaoui R, et al. ISUOG Practice Guidelines: role of ultrasound in congenital infection. *Ultrasound Obstet Gynecol.* 2020;56(1):128–151.
5. McLean HQ, Fiebelkorn AP, Temte JL, et al. Prevention of measles, rubella, congenital rubella syndrome, and mumps, 2013: summary recommendations of the Advisory Committee on Immunization Practices (ACIP). *MMWR Recomm Rep.* 2013;62(RR-04):1–34. [Correction in MMWR Recomm Rep. 2015 Mar 13;64(9):259]
6. Mujezinovic F, Alfirevic Z. Procedure-related complications of amniocentesis and chorionic villous sampling: a systematic review. *Obstet Gynecol.* 2007;110(3):687–694. [Correction in Obstet Gynecol. 2008 Mar;111(3):779]
7. National Advisory Committee on Immunization. Blood products, human immune globulin and timing of immunization. Part 1 – key immunization information. In *Canada Immunization Guide Ottawa.* Government of Canada; 2013. Available at www.canada.ca/en/public-health/services/publications/healthy-living/canadian-immunization-guide-part-1-key-immunization-

information/page-11-blood-products-human-immune-globulin-timing-immunization
.html#p1c10t1. Accessed on August 25, 2020.

8. White SJ, Boldt KL, Holditch SJ, et al. Measles, mumps, and rubella. *Clin Obstet Gynecol.*
2012;55(2):550–559.

9. Yazigi A, De Pecoulas AE, Vauloup-Fellous C, et al. Fetal and neonatal abnormalities due to
congenital rubella syndrome: a review of literature. *J Matern Fetal Neonatal Med.* 2017;30(3):
274–278.

POINTS

1. What would you ask on focused history regarding rubella exposure? *(1 point per main bullet)*

Max 5

Nonspecific symptoms associated with rubella:
- ☐ Recent symptoms of a minor upper respiratory infection
  - ○ *Low-grade fever, sore throat, malaise, cough, coryza*
- ☐ History of a rash and description of its pattern
  - ○ *Typical rash associated with rubella is erythematous and maculopapular (scarlatiniform), occasionally mildly pruritic*
  - ○ *Characteristically, the rash starts on the face with rapid spread to the trunk and extremities, and resolves in the order of appearance*
- ☐ Symmetric polyarthralgia or polyarthritis of the hands, knees, wrists, and ankles
  - ○ *Typical onset is approximately one week after the rash*
- ☐ Symptoms of viral conjunctivitis (*e.g., watery/mucoserous discharge, burning, or sandy/gritty feeling of an eye*)

Medical history:
- ☐ Vaccination/immunization history

Nephew:
- ☐ When and how was he diagnosed
- ☐ Establish whether his vaccinations are updated

You learn that the patient is recovering from a sore throat and fever. She still has a mild rash that started four days ago, though the patient says it is improving. She had no joint pains. The patient has no record of, nor does she recall, her immunization status.

Her nephew's rubella infection was confirmed this week by his pediatrician. He had missed his prior routine vaccination visit.

2. Indicate aspects of a focused physical exam? *(1 point each)*

Max 3

- ☐ Vital signs (must specify temperature)
- ☐ Cervical lymphadenopathy
- ☐ Oral cavity: Forcheimer spots (petechiae on the soft palate) may precede or accompany the rash
- ☐ Skin: assess for presence and distribution of a rash

On examination, oral temperature is 37.8°C; blood pressure, pulse, oxygen saturation, and respiratory rate are normal. Cervical lymph nodes are slightly tender on palpation. You note evidence of a faint maculopapular rash on her lower legs.

---

3. List four infections that may account for the patient's symptoms and clinical findings. *(1 point each) [the following is a general guide; other responses not listed below may be accepted]*   **Max 4**

☐ Rubella
☐ Parvovirus B19
☐ Measles
☐ Human herpesvirus 6 and 7
☐ Scarlet fever (Group A streptococcus)
☐ Mononucleosis (Epstein-Barr virus)
☐ Arboviruses (Zika, West Nile virus, Chikungunya, Dengue)

---

4. Outline your recommended investigations for the clinical assessment of this patient. *(1 point each)*   **Max 10**

☐ Rubella IgG and IgM antibodies
☐ Measles IgG antibody
☐ Parvovirus B19 IgG and IgM antibodies
☐ Cytomegalovirus IgG and IgM antibodies
☐ Toxoplasma IgG and IgM antibodies
☐ HepBsAg and Anti-HepBs antibody
☐ HIV antibody-antigen (*i.e.,* fourth-generation testing)
☐ Syphilis testing (conventional or reverse algorithm screening)
☐ Viral culture from blood, urine, throat (or cerebrospinal fluid, *if clinically indicated*)
☐ CBC/FBC
☐ Hepatic transaminases (ALT, AST) and serum creatinine (*i.e.,* to assess for possible hepatitis or hemolytic-uremic syndrome, which are rare manifestations with rubella infection)

Rubella titers are positive for IgM and negative for IgG antibodies. Other serologic investigations are unremarkable.

Her blood group is O negative; there are no atypical antibodies detected.

---

5. Interpret the results of the patient's rubella serologies?   **1**

☐ Nonconfirmatory for primary infection given the high false-positive rate of IgM (15%–50%)
   o *False-positive rubella IgM may occur in Rh-positive patients, or with parvovirus infection, heterophile antibodies for infectious mononucleosis, long-term persistence after vaccination, and presence of antiphospholipid or other autoantibodies*

6. Elaborate on subsequent options in the diagnostic evaluation of maternal rubella in this patient. *(1 point each)*   3

☐ Repeat serologies in two to three weeks, where IgG seroconversion would confirm primary infection

☐ Viral cultures or nucleic acid amplification tests of the throat or body fluids *(may remain positive up to two weeks after the onset of the rash)*

☐ Rubella IgG avidity *(low avidity indicates recent infection)*

A throat culture is positive for rubella virus. Upon your request, she presents to your clinic to discuss the results and subsequent care.

7. Discuss important elements to include in counseling and management of the patient at this time. *(2 points for each main bullet)*   Max 8

☐ Explain this is a recent/acute rubella viral infection

☐ Discuss the high rate of fetal infection, being ~80%–90% with first-trimester maternal infection

    o *Rates of fetal infection decrease with gestational age at maternal infection: 55%–60% with infection at 12–16 weeks, and 30%–40% at 16–20 weeks, rising again in the third trimester to almost 100% for fetal exposures after 36 weeks*

☐ Inform the patient that the risk of an <u>infected</u> fetus being <u>affected</u> approximates 85%–90% with first-trimester infections

    o *Risk of congenital defects is 20%–35% for infections occurring at 12–16 weeks, with minimal to no risk of congenital defects when primary maternal infections occur after 20 weeks*

☐ In addition to defects associated with congenital rubella syndrome, prenatal risks of spontaneous abortion and stillbirth are increased

☐ Termination of pregnancy should be offered to this patient given early prenatal infection *(especially with infections prior to 16 weeks)*

☐ Consideration for referral to a high-risk obstetrics team

The patient understands her obstetric risks, and she indicates that termination is not an option for her. You thereby inform her that colleagues in the high-risk obstetrics unit of your tertiary center will be providing prenatal care thereafter. Upon referral, the patient is seen at 12^{+3} for subsequent care.

Before leaving your clinic, the patient is curious as to how she contacted the infection, which she recognizes was most likely via her nephew.

8. How is the rubella virus transmitted?   1

☐ Droplet contact from nasopharyngeal secretions lead to viral replication in the lymph nodes of the upper respiratory tract, followed by hematogenous dissemination

9. Under the care of high-risk unit, which fetal diagnostic procedure might the patient be offered now?

☐ Chorionic villous sampling (CVS)

Special note:
The ideal time for amniocentesis is ≥6 weeks after maternal rubella infection and >18–20 weeks' gestation

1

Although the patient is adamant that a positive CVS result will not affect her decision to continue pregnancy, she wants to maximize her information during the antenatal period to help arrange for future medical and psychosocial support systems.

In preparation for the CVS, an ultrasound is performed during her visit at 12^{+3} weeks' gestation.

10. What are the sonographic features that should be examined preceding CVS? *(1 point each)*

☐ Fetal viability (and number)
☐ Screen for fetal structural anomalies
☐ Placental location

3

Ultrasound shows a single, viable fetus corresponding to gestational age, without detectable anomalies to date. Fundal placentation is noted. A transabdominal CVS is planned.

11. Discuss the important aspects to include in the planning and consent process for this patient's CVS? *(1 point per main bullet)*

☐ Administer Rh immunoglobulin *(patient is Rh-negative)* for risk of feto-maternal hemorrhage
☐ Fetal loss rate may approximate 1% within one month of the procedure
  ○ *Randomized trials suggest higher rate of pregnancy loss with CVS compared to amniocentesis, although rates of transabdominal CVS and amniocentesis appear to be similar*
  ○ *For this patient, given a transabdominal procedure is planned, the predictors of fetal loss would depend on the number of attempts and operator skill*
☐ Maternal tissue contamination resulting in false-positive fetal rubella PCR
☐ Risk of sampling failure being 4.8% *(relative to 1.6% at amniocentesis)*
☐ Low risk of limb-reduction defects or oromandibular hypogenesis when procedure is performed >10 weeks' gestation
☐ Resumption of normal activity is possible postprocedure, although most experts recommend avoidance of sexual and strenuous activity for 24–48 hours
☐ Although small amounts of vaginal spotting may be normal, patients should be encouraged to report persistent or heavy bleeding, pain, rupture of membranes, or signs of infection

7

Special note:
CVS-associated risk of confined placental mosaicism would not be applicable to this patient

The patient has an uncomplicated procedure with an uneventful recovery.

Results of the CVS later reveal rubella-specific PCR.

12. Outline aspects of prenatal management that you anticipate will be arranged by the high-risk obstetrical unit. *(1 point each)*	Max 4

☐ Detailed second-trimester morphology scan
☐ Serial fetal sonography *(there is no consensus on the ideal frequency of fetal monitoring; a case-based approach is required)*
☐ Fetal echocardiography
☐ Neonatology consultation
☐ Delivery in a tertiary-care center

13. Indicate six prenatal sonographic features of rubella for which this fetus would be monitored. <u>Be specific</u> *(1 point each)*	Max 6

Cardiac	Cerebral	Ocular	Other:
☐ Ventricular septal defects	☐ Microcephaly	☐ Microphthalmia	☐ Fetal growth restriction (FGR)
☐ Pulmonary stenosis	☐ Ventriculomegaly	☐ Cataracts	☐ Amniotic fluid abnormalities
	☐ Periventricular calcifications		☐ Hepatosplenomegaly

<u>Special note:</u>
All sonographic features are nonspecific for congenital rubella infection

14. Identify the only known obstetric sequelae that could result if this patient were to become infected with rubella in the third trimester.	2

☐ Fetal growth restriction

The patient delivers a growth restricted fetus at 34 weeks' gestation with signs of congenital rubella syndrome. She inquires about the need for future prenatal testing for rubella serology.

15. What would be your recommended management regarding prenatal screening for rubella in her future pregnancies, and why?

4

☐ Rubella serology would <u>not</u> be indicated because this patient already had a confirmed infection which leads to natural immunity. For patients with history of immunity from natural infection, postpartum vaccination is not warranted even when serum rubella IgG antibody is not detected or if titer is low.
  ○ *Reinfection in the context of prior immunity results in <5% risk of fetal infection and 8% risk of congenital defects, limited to the first trimester*

16. List six postnatal features of congenital rubella syndrome *which you did not mention among the prenatal characteristics in Question 13? (1 point each)*

Max 6

Cardiac: (10-20%)	☐ Patent ductus arteriosus ☐ Pulmonary stenosis
Central nervous system: (10-25%)	☐ Microcephaly ☐ Meningoencephalitis
Ocular: (19%)	☐ Sensorineural hearing loss *(unilateral or bilateral)*
Ophthalmic: (10-25%)	☐ Retinopathy ☐ Chorioretinitis ☐ Cataracts *(unilateral or bilateral)* ☐ Microphthalmia ☐ Pigmentary and congenital glaucoma
Other	☐ "Blueberry muffin" syndrome– *thrombocytopenia* ☐ Hepatosplenomegaly ☐ Jaundice ☐ Radiolucent bone disease ☐ Purpura

Over the next few weeks, you see the patient in the hospital while the baby is in the NICU. She has been forgetting to ask the neonatologist whether there may be any future effects of rubella that may only become apparent as her baby grows up.

17. Identify late manifestations of congenital rubella syndrome which the pediatricians would be discussing with the patient? *(1 point each)*

    ☐ Type 1 diabetes mellitus
    ☐ Thyroiditis
    ☐ Growth hormone deficit
    ☐ Behavioral disorder
    ☐ Progressive panencephalitis
    ☐ Intellectual disability
    ☐ Autism

Max 6

The patient mentions that her sister panicked and got the MMR vaccine as soon as her son and sister became infected, unknowing she was in the early weeks of a pregnancy.

18. If the sister were to have seen you for advice after inadvertent rubella vaccination, what would have been your recommendations for the management of her pregnancy?

    ☐ Routine care: *there have been no reports of congenital rubella syndrome in offspring of women inadvertently vaccinated early pregnancy*

1

Special note:
Women who receive the rubella vaccine are advised to avoid pregnancy for 28 days following vaccination

After your encounter with a prenatal case of rubella, you decide to freshen your knowledge on ways to decrease congenital rubella syndrome on a population level.

19. Outline five recommendations in prevention of congenital rubella syndrome. *(1 point each)*

    ☐ Universal infant vaccination
    ☐ MMR for catch-up vaccination or as a two-dose regimen
    ☐ Ensure girls are immune before child-bearing age and assess the immunity among women of child-bearing age, and vaccinate accordingly
    ☐ Screen for antibody status of pregnant women with no vaccination record or evidence of past immunity *(Note: In the UK, routine prenatal rubella immunity testing has recently been discontinued)*
    ☐ Immunize postpartum nonimmune women before hospital-discharge (but not if they have documented 1 MMR vaccine before)
    ☐ Screen all health care workers
    ☐ Immunize all immigrant and refugee women
    ☐ For nonimmune pregnant women, encourage (1) handwashing, (2) avoid contact with individuals with viral-like illnesses, and (3) avoid travel to endemic areas

Max 5

BONUS Questions

20. A healthy, primiparous Rh-negative patient delivers an Rh-positive infant. There is no record of rubella immunity and no proof of immunization, as she immigrated from overseas. What would be the *ideal* plan of management in this situation?   5

☐ Administer Rh immunoglobulin postpartum

☐ Delay postpartum MMR (or MMRV) vaccination by three to six months for patient receiving immunoglobulin-containing preparations or blood products during pregnancy or in the peripartum period

21. What is the rationale for the two-dose MMR (or MMRV) vaccination regimen in children?   5

☐ To protect against measles, mumps, and varicella – <u>not</u> rubella, because a single dose of the vaccine is all that is required for protection against rubella

TOTAL: 90

CHAPTER 65

Syphilis in Pregnancy

Amira El-Messidi and Erica Hardy

A 23-year-old primigravida is referred to your high-risk obstetrics clinic at 17^{+3} weeks' gestation for a reactive VDRL test on routine prenatal screening. Although her appointment with you is in two days, she presents urgently to your office for new-onset tongue lesions and a rash. She had an early dating sonography, and aneuploidy screening was unremarkable. She takes prenatal vitamins and has no obstetric complaints.

LEARNING OBJECTIVES

1. Maintain a high index of suspicion for syphilis in pregnancy despite nonspecific clinical manifestations, recognizing the importance of universal routine prenatal screening, and understand which patients should be rescreened in the third trimester
2. Interpret traditional or new reverse syphilis screening algorithms
3. Understand and troubleshoot pregnancy particularities involved in treating syphilis, appreciating the importance of continued multidisciplinary care for maternal and fetal health
4. Elicit and treat clinical manifestations at various stages of syphilis
5. Detail counseling of maternal-fetal risks, and identify antenatal features possibly associated with congenital syphilis

SUGGESTED READINGS

1. Adhikari EH. Syphilis in pregnancy. *Obstet Gynecol.* 2020 May;135(5):1121–1135.
2. Centers for Disease Control and Prevention. Syphilis (Treponema pallidum) 2018 case definition. Available at wwwn.cdc.gov/nndss/conditions/syphilis/case-definition/2018/. Accessed October 17, 2020.
3. Ghanem KG, Ram S, Rice PA. The modern epidemic of syphilis. *N Engl J Med.* 2020 Feb 27;382(9):845–854.
4. Janier M, Unemo M, Dupin N, Tiplica GS, Potočnik M, Patel R, 2020 European guideline on the management of syphilis. *J Eur Acad Dermatol Venereol.* 2021 Mar;35(3):574–588.
5. Kingston M, Fifer H, French P, et al. Amendment to the UK guidelines on the management of syphilis 2015: Management of syphilis in pregnant women. *Int J STD AIDS.* 2019 Nov;30(13):1344–1345.
6. Public Health Agency of Canada. Canadian guidelines on sexually transmitted infections: management and treatment of specific infections – syphilis. Available at www.canada.ca/en/public-health/services/infectious-diseases/sexual-health-sexually-transmitted-infections/canadian-guidelines/syphilis.html. Accessed October 14, 2020.

7. Trinh T, Leal AF, Mello MB, et al. Syphilis management in pregnancy: a review of guideline recommendations from countries around the world. *Sex Reprod Health Matters.* 2019 Dec;27(1):69–82.
8. UK Standards for Microbiology Investigations. Syphilis Serology. *Virology* 2016; 44(2.1).
9. WHO. *Guideline on Syphilis Screening and Treatment for Pregnant Women.* Geneva: World Health Organization; 2017.
10. Workowski KA, Bolan GA, Centers for Disease Control and Prevention. Sexually transmitted diseases treatment guidelines, 2015. *MMWR Recomm Rep.* 2015 Jun 5;64(RR-03):1–137. [Erratum in MMWR Recomm Rep. 2015 Aug 28;64(33):924]

POINTS

1. What aspects of a focused history, or results of particular routine prenatal investigations, would you want to know?

30

General: *(1 point each)*
☐ Evaluate for a history of previously diagnosed and/or treated for syphilis *(particularly the treatment regimen)*
☐ Request her quantitative VDRL titer before and after treatment *(correlates with disease activity and used to follow treatment response)*‡
☐ Prenatal serum screening results for HIV, hepatitis B and C, and urogenital nucleic acid testing for chlamydia/gonorrhea

Past medical/family history:
☐ Systemic or immunosuppressive conditions *(e.g., SLE or HIV)* *(1 point)*

Details of oral, and possibly genital, lesions: *(1 point each; max 5)*
☐ Characteristics of oral lesions *(e.g., painful, ulcerative, vesicular, location)*
☐ Establish if a primary event or recurrence
☐ Associated speech or respiratory difficulty, sore throat, cough, nausea/vomiting
☐ Any history of preceding medication which could raise suspicion of drug allergy/hypersensitivity reaction
☐ Recollection of recent genital or extragenital ulcer in patient or partner, either treated or spontaneously resolved *(primary syphilis)*
☐ Presence of an active genital lesion *(raised or flat papules with gray exudate may be seen with secondary syphilis)*
☐ Presence of condyloma latum *(soft, verrucous plaque; highly contagious; may be seen in secondary syphilis)*

Description of the rash and other systemic manifestations: *(1 point each unless specified)*
☐ Appearance, distribution, and characteristics *(variable presentations; syphilis is a 'great imitator')*
  ○ Rash on the palms and/or soles *(3 points)*
☐ Inquire about symptoms or signs of neurologic/ophthalmic/otic disease *(3 points)*

□ Inquire about cervical or inguinal lymphadenopathy
□ Associated flu-like or other systemic symptoms (*i.e., fever, malaise, arthralgia*)
□ Patchy alopecia

Allergies:
□ Particularly to penicillin, including reactions *(4 points)*

Sexual history: *(1 point each; max 2)*
□ Prior sexually transmitted infections (STIs)
□ Results of last cervical cytology smear (*i.e.*, Papanicolaou smear) and history of abnormalities, including condylomas
□ Current or prior multiple sexual partners (including history of male sexual partner who has sex with men, or a history of a partner with HIV)

Social history: *(1 point per main bullet; max 3)*
□ Other STI risk history (*i.e., history of exchange of sex for money or goods*)
□ Recent immigrant from an endemic region for syphilis; unstable housing
□ Substance-use (*i.e., smoking, alcohol, recreational drugs*)
  ○ *Crack cocaine has been associated with syphilis infection*
□ Recent travel

Partner: *(1 point each)*
□ Prior or active genital lesions/infections or unexplained systemic complaints
□ HIV status, if known

Special note:
‡ Nontreponemal titers are not interchangeable between different tests, and ideally the same lab should be used

A city-native without recent travel, she attends a local college. Pregnancy was planned with her monogamous partner of two years. She recalls six partners over the past five years. Generally healthy, she does not smoke and now abstains from social alcohol consumption in pregnancy. There is no history of recreational drug use. She describes a remote urticarial reaction with amoxicillin which resolved upon discontinuation of the drug. Recent Papanicolaou smear, serological and genital screening for gonorrhea and chlamydia were normal; the VDRL titer was 1:64 at 12 weeks' gestation. Four years ago, she was treated for a *C. trachomatis* infection, without recurrence. Her partner has not voiced any local or systemic complaints and his HIV status is unknown to her.

Her symptoms started acutely, and this nonpruritic rash is spreading. History does not suggest an allergy. With your guidance, she remembers a brief episode of a vulvar ulcer two months ago. As the lesion was not painful, and she was suffering with hyperemesis gravidarum at the time, she did not seek medical attention. Clinical history is negative for neurologic or ophthalmic issues.

On examination, you note a maculopapular erythematous rash of her trunk and soles *(see figures)*. The oral mucous patches do not impact her breathing. You find bilateral inguinal lymphadenopathy, without concomitant genital lesions. The remainder of her examination, including a detailed neurologic examination, is unremarkable and obstetrical assessment is normal.

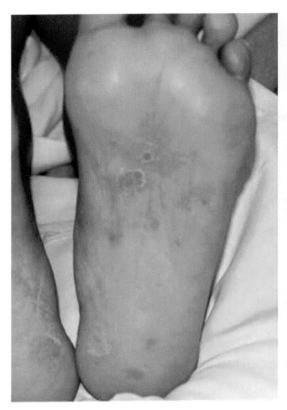
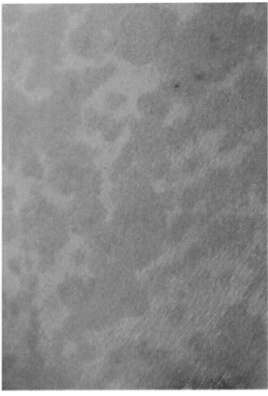

Figure 65.1 and 65.2

With permission: "Obstet Gynecol 2020; 135:1121–35." Figure 3, panel B & D.

There is no association between this case scenario and this patient's image. Images used for educational purposes only.

Although biologic false-positive nontreponemal sera usually have low antibody titers (≤1:4), you use this opportunity to benefit your obstetric trainee.[†]

Special note:
† Nontreponemal tests include VDRL, rapid plasma reagin (RPR), or rarely, TRUST (toluidine red unheated serum test); rapid point-of-care testing can be used if access to high-quality laboratory screening is limited or at delivery for women without routine antenatal syphilis testing

2. Provide a structured differential diagnosis for a positive VDRL result. *[the following is a guide; other responses may be acceptable] (1 point each)*

Max 6

Infectious *(max 4 points)*	**Noninfectious** *(max 2 points)*
☐ Syphilis	☐ Connective tissue disorders
☐ Other TORCH infections: CMV, toxoplasmosis, HSV	☐ Lymphoproliferative disorders
☐ TB	☐ IV drug use
☐ Viral hepatitis	☐ Advanced malignancy
☐ Leprosy	☐ Pregnancy
☐ Lyme disease	
☐ Measles, mumps, varicella (infections or immunizations)	
☐ Vaccinia	
☐ Malaria	
☐ Chancroid	
☐ Lymphogranuloma venereum	
☐ Mycoplasma/pneumococcal pneumonia	
☐ Bacterial endocarditis	

Aside from this educational briefing, you diagnose her condition and initiate discussion on counseling and management. You request confirmatory testing.

3. List three <u>serologic</u> treponemal tests. *(1 point each)*

Max 3

☐ *T. pallidum* Enzyme immunoassay (TP-EIA)
☐ Chemiluminescence immunoassay (CLIA)
☐ Treponema pallidum particle agglutination assay (TP-PA)
☐ Microhemagglutination assay (MHA-TP)
☐ Indirect fluorescent-antibody (fluorescent treponemal antibody absorption test [FTA-ABS])‡

Special note:
Different treponemal tests detect antibodies to different antigens on *T. pallidum*; nontreponemal tests detect nonspecific antibodies to cardiolipin on *T. pallidum's* cell membrane
‡ becoming obsolete

As these antibody tests are foreign to your trainee, he or she surfs the internet and learns of new, automated, syphilis-screening algorithms.

4. If this patient had initial reverse algorithm screening, outline the sequence of tests confirming a syphilis infection.

☐ Treponemal specific test, *then,* reflexive nontreponemal test (quantitative VDRL or RPR)
  ○ *With nonreactive reflexive VDRL, a confirmatory treponemal specific test (TP-PA is recommended for this step) different from the first and preferably in same sample, is done*

Your trainee seems confused regarding the need for reflexive nontreponemal testing, regardless of a positive specific serology.

5. Explain four purposes of nontreponemal testing after an initial positive specific test used in the reverse algorithm. *(1 point each)*

☐ Treponemal test is associated with high false-positive rates; individual use is not advised
☐ Nontreponemal titer identifies active syphilis while specific tests mostly remain positive lifelong, even after treatment
☐ Nontreponemal titers monitor response to treatment
☐ Nontreponemal titers at delivery are needed for comparison with neonatal titers

6. Discuss the <u>maternal</u> aspects of counseling and management of her syphilis infection. *(1 point per main bullet)*

☐ Indicate your clinical suspicion of secondary syphilis
☐ Explain the most common route of infection (*i.e.,* open lesions with treponemal organisms)
☐ Discuss the highly contagious nature of her oral lesions *(and genital lesions, if present)*
  ○ *Risk of sexual transmission is ~50%–60%*
  ○ *Sexual transmission occurs **only** in the presence of mucocutaneous lesions, and is uncommon after the first year*
☐ Nontreponemal titer (*e.g.,* VDRL) must be obtained on day 1 of treatment; baseline titer serves to monitor treatment response (*additionally, long interval elapsed from this patient's initial test*)
☐ Referral for penicillin desensitization
☐ Intramuscular benzathine penicillin G 2.4 million units as a single dose (first line)
  ○ Some experts recommend repeating treatment in one week, based on efficacy and altered pharmacokinetics in pregnancy
  ○ Intramuscular procaine penicillin G is second line**
  ○ *WHO 2017 (Suggested Reading 9): Caution with azithromycin, erythromycin, or ceftriaxone as they treat the mother without reliably treating the fetus*[†]
☐ Reassure the patient that penicillin effectively decreases, but does not eliminate, vertical transmission, adverse obstetric outcome, and maternal disease
☐ Abstinence from sexual contact for seven days posttreatment *(Suggested Reading 6)*
☐ Advise for sexual partner postexposure prophylaxis regardless of testing
  ○ For secondary syphilis, the patient's sexual contacts within six months of her symptoms' onset, require evaluation *(Suggested Readings 6, 10);* contact tracing may be extended up to two years *(Suggested Reading 4)*

□ Inform the patient that public health reporting of syphilis infections is required *(jurisdictional policies may vary)*

□ Frequency of monitoring nontreponemal titer posttreatment may be individualized or vary by jurisdiction *(e.g., monthly or every three months)*
  ○ *Titer needed at delivery to compare with neonate's titer*

□ Inform her that most individuals (85%) with positive treponemal tests remain so lifelong despite successful treatment

□ Forecast symptom resolution within a few weeks of adequate syphilotherapy *(resolution without treatment that may take up to six months)*

□ Reassure patient that the course of syphilis infection is not altered by pregnancy

□ Repeat STI screening tests in the third trimester are recommended for any patient with an STI diagnosed in pregnancy or in another high-risk group or with high-risk features for STI acquisition *(e.g., new partner, multiple sexual partners, inconsistent condom use)* (in this case, patient also had remote chlamydia)

□ Delivery in a tertiary center is preferred:
  ○ Neonatal examination and serial pediatric care
  ○ Pathology of the placenta/umbilical cord

□ Mode and timing of delivery depend on obstetric indications

Special notes:
** Inadvertent IV procaine can cause acute psychiatric reaction (Hoigné syndrome)
† Where access to penicillin is limited or desensitization is not possible

7. Outline your counseling of the <u>fetal</u> risks and management to discuss with the patient.

Max 7

Risks: *(1 point per main bullet; max 4)*
□ Pregnancy loss previability
□ Vertical transmission/congenital infection
  ○ 50%–60% with secondary syphilis, decreasing to 1%–2% *despite* adequate maternal treatment
  ○ Two-thirds of liveborns are asymptomatic at birth
  ○ Early (age less than two years) or late congenital syphilis[‡]
□ Nonimmune hydrops
□ Prematurity
□ Low birthweight *(neonatal)*
□ IUFD or neonatal mortality

Management: *(1 point per main bullet)*
□ Arrange for serial sonographic monitoring after the routine morphology scan *(case-based frequency of monitoring)*
  ○ *Abnormalities rarely appear before 20 weeks' gestation due to fetal immunologic immaturity*
□ Consideration for diagnostic testing by amniocentesis
□ Arrange for neonatology consultation

Special note:
‡ Clinical manifestations of late congenital syphilis are stigmata induced by early lesions or chronic inflammation

Pretreatment VDRL titer has increased to 1:128 and her TP-PA is reactive. An infectious disease expert will co-follow the patient.

Inpatient desensitization therapy was successful at 17^{+5} weeks' gestation, and the patient received syphilotherapy. She was informed to seek care should a febrile reaction or other side effects manifest.

Fetal morphology scan at 20 weeks' gestation was normal. Invasive testing was declined; she agreed to fetal sonographic follow-up. Her symptoms resolve within a few weeks of treatment and although serial VDRL titer shows an initial acceptable response (a fourfold decline in titer), a fourfold rise is found on subsequent testing by 35 weeks' gestation.[†] Repeat HIV testing is negative and she remains asymptomatic. The infectious disease expert informed her that treatment failure may be a sign of unrecognized neurologic infection (asymptomatic neurosyphilis); lumbar puncture is being considered. If her cerebrospinal fluid evaluation and neurologic exam rules out neurologic syphilis, she needs retreatment with three-times-weekly injections of her initial treatment.

Unfortunately, although syphilotherapy is effective against mother-to-child transmission with treatment <28 weeks' gestation, fetal sonography at 35 weeks shows the following:

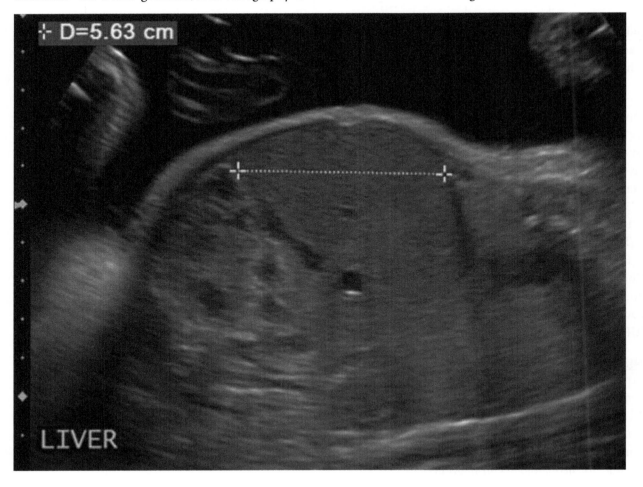

Figure 65.3

With permission: "Obstet Gynecol 2020; 135:1121–35". Figure 7

There is no association between this case scenario and this patient's image. Image used for educational purposes only.

Special note:

† Unless symptomatic, treatment failure or reinfection requires fourfold rise in nontreponemal titer for more than two weeks

---

8. Describe this sonographic finding. 1

☐ Hepatomegaly (left lobe >40 mm)

Special note:

Often the first feature to appear and last to resolve after maternal syphilis treatment

---

9. Although not specific to congenital syphilis, indicate five other sonographic risks to this fetus. *(1 point each)* 5

☐ Placentomegaly
☐ Polyhydramnios
☐ Anemia (requires MCA-PSV assessment)
☐ Ascites/hydrops
☐ IUFD

---

10. Detail specific clinical arrangements and counseling for syphilotherapy at this time. *(1 point for each main and subbullet)* 4

☐ Consideration for inpatient treatment given fetal viability
☐ Inform the patient of fetal and maternal side effects, typically within 24 hours of treatment:†
  ○ *Fetal:* Abnormal cardiotocography, decreased movement
  ○ *Maternal:* Preterm labor, fever, hypotension, headache, rash, myalgia, pharyngitis

Special note:

† Jarisch-Herxheimer reaction can be mistaken for penicillin-allergy; European guideline *(Suggested Reading 4)* recommends prednisolone for prevention of Jarisch-Herxheimer reaction while other guidelines *(Suggested Readings 6, 9, 10)* suggest antipyretics and supportive care only

---

Fetal sonographic monitoring suggests congenital syphilis, without overt anemia or hydrops. Nontreponemal VDRL titers decrease after retreatment and repeat third-trimester STI screening is negative. Her obstetrical course is otherwise unremarkable.

Spontaneous labor and uncomplicated vaginal delivery ensue at 39^{+3} weeks' gestation; the neonatology team is present at delivery. Prior to requesting histopathologic assessment, you examine the placental unit.

11. Describe three *gross* placental characteristics with syphilitic infections. *(1 point each)*	3

☐ Large
☐ Pale
☐ Hydropic

Special note:
Findings are more common in **un**treated maternal syphilis

12. Although infrequently used, inform your trainee of <u>direct</u> spirochete detection technologies. *(1 point each)*	Max 2

☐ Immunohistochemistry
☐ PCR
☐ Darkfield microscopy *(gold standard for definitive diagnosis)*
☐ Direct fluorescent antibody *(obsolete; Suggested Reading 4)*
☐ Rabbit infectivity testing *(research purposes)*

Special note:
Direct-detection methods require clinical lesions, placental, or autopsy tissues

Several hours later, you visit the NICU where aqueous crystalline penicillin G has been started. The neonatologist illustrates features of early congenital syphilis.

Feeling unlucky, the patient recalls your mentioning that treatment of her antenatal infection could reduce the risk of congenital syphilis by up to 98%. To provide support, you think of confounders for vertical transmission.

13. Discuss the risk factors for congenital syphilis despite maternal treatment. Factors *may or may not* relate to this patient. *(1 point each)*	Max 3

☐ Early-stage infection (primary, secondary, or early latent)[†]
☐ Higher antibody titers at delivery than pretreatment
☐ Delivery within 30 days of initiating treatment
☐ Inadequate maternal treatment
☐ Prematurity

Special note:
† CDC 2018 revised 'early latent syphilis' to 'syphilis, early nonprimary nonsecondary' and 'late latent syphilis' to 'unknown duration or late syphilis'

Three weeks later, a physician from a remote town calls you for treatment advice for a 50-year-old new immigrant presenting for fertility counseling with ovum donation; the physician finds cutaneous nodules and granulomatous lesions of her mucous membranes; her husband confirms remote syphilis. Her HIV test is negative. There are no other significant comorbidities or drug allergies. The physician is awaiting the infectious disease expert's assistance.

14. Given the likely attributing cause of this patient's findings, which two other <u>organ systems</u> would you advise your colleague to investigate? *(2 points each)*

    4

☐ Cardiac *(aortitis, aneurysms, regurgitation)*
    ○ *Chest X-ray shows linear aortic calcifications*
☐ Central nervous system *(lumbar puncture to assess for neurosyphilis)*

15. If serum VDRL and TP-PA are reactive with a negative lumbar puncture, indicate your treatment recommendations for this patient's syphilitic infection.

    2

<u>Tertiary syphilis:</u>
☐ Benzathine penicillin G 2.4 million units as three consecutive weekly intramuscular doses

<u>Special note:</u>
Both clinical and laboratory criteria are required to confirm neurosyphilis

Upon request, your colleague updates you that uncontaminated cerebrospinal fluid sampling showed a reactive VDRL[†] and the neurologist found her pupils to be small, fixed, and nonreactive to light. The patient will be transferred to a near-by center for neurological monitoring and treatment. Public health services are informed.

<u>Special note:</u>
† Unlike serum, RPR testing in cerebrospinal fluid is **not** recommended; positive cerebrospinal fluid treponemal specific tests may have false-positive implications as IgG antibodies cross the blood-brain barrier; only negative results are helpful

16-A. Characterize this patient's ocular manifestation of syphilis.

    1

☐ Argyll-Robertson pupil

16-B. List three other clinical features of neurosyphilis. *(1 point each)*

    Max 3

☐ General paresis, dementia, seizures, various psychiatric syndromes
☐ Syphilitic meningitis
☐ Cranial nerve dysfunction
☐ Stroke-syndrome
☐ Tabes dorsalis

17. Anticipate the syphilitic treatment, including posology, this patient requires. *(2 points for either regimen)*

2

Neurosyphilis:
☐ Aqueous crystalline penicillin G 4 million units IV every four hours for 10–14 days

OR
☐ Penicillin G procaine 2.4 million units one intramuscular daily dose **and** oral probenecid 500 mg four times daily, both for 10–14 days *(outpatient; compliance required)*

Special note:
May consider treatment regimen of late latent syphilis after completion of neurosyphilis treatment for comparable total duration of therapy *(CDC Guideline 2015, Suggested Reading 10)*

TOTAL: **95**

CHAPTER 66

Toxoplasmosis in Pregnancy

Amira El-Messidi

You are seeing a healthy 28-year-old primigravida for her second prenatal visit. She is currently at 14 weeks' gestation and works at an accounting firm. All routine prenatal laboratory investigations as well as first-trimester fetal anatomy and aneuploidy screenings are unremarkable. Incidentally, she tells you her friend is away for the summer, leaving her to care for two cats.

LEARNING OBJECTIVES

1. Understand the modes of transmission for *T. gondii* in pregnancy, and counsel on hygienic measures to lower the risk of primary infection among pregnant women
2. Detail an understanding of various combinations of maternal *T. gondii* serology results, and appreciate confirmatory tests required to establish acute maternal and congenital infections
3. Understand the treatment involved in fetal prophylaxis, depending on gestational age at the time of acute maternal infection
4. Recognize the circumstances and therapy involved in fetal treatment of congenital toxoplasmosis
5. Identify caveats of early neonatal *T. gondii* serology, and summarize essentials of neonatal treatment
6. Acknowledge long-term sequelae of congenital toxoplasmosis, not limited to symptomatic neonates at birth

SUGGESTED READINGS

1. Berghella, V. *Maternal-Fetal Evidence-Based Guidelines*. Boca Raton, FL: CRC Press; 2017.
2. Centers for Disease Control and Prevention. Available at www.cdc.gov/parasites/toxoplasmosis/. Accessed July 26, 2020.
3. Montoya JG, Liesenfeld O. Toxoplasmosis. *Lancet* 2004;36:1965–1976.
4. Montoya JG, Remington JS. Management of Toxoplasma gondii infection during pregnancy. *Clinical Infectious Diseases* 2008;47(4):554–566.
5. Paquet C, Yudin MH. No. 285 – toxoplasmosis in pregnancy: prevention, screening, and treatment. *J Obstet Gynaecol Can.* 2018;40(8):e687–e693.
6. Petersen E. Toxoplasmosis. *Semin Fetal Neonatal Med.* 2007;12(3):214–223.

7. Saso A, Bamford A, Grewal K, et al. Fifteen-minute consultation: management of the infant born to a mother with toxoplasmosis in pregnancy. Arch Dis Child Educ Pract Ed 2020.

8. Villard O, Cimon B, L'Ollivier C, et al. Serological diagnosis of Toxoplasma gondii infection: recommendations from the French National Reference Center for Toxoplasmosis. *Diagn Microbiol Infect Dis.* 2016;84(1):22–33.

POINTS

1. You realize this is a prime opportunity to inform the patient how to best care for the cats in order to decrease her risks of acquiring toxoplasmosis. Discuss specific hygienic recommendations for prenatal cat-handing. *(1 point each)*

Max 3

☐ Disinfect emptied cat-litter box with near boiling water for five minutes before refilling
☐ Wear gloves when in contact with potentially contaminated cat feces (litter or gardening)
☐ Domesticate the cats and provide them cooked, preserved, or dry foods
☐ Change litter every 24 hours (oocysts require at least one day to become infective after deposition)

The patient appreciates your advice and is curious if there are any additional recommendations in prevention of primary T. gondii infection.

2. Elaborate on other lifestyle measures in your counseling. *(1 point each)*

Max 5

☐ Cook meat to 'well done' or to at least 67°C/153°F
☐ Freezing meat to at least −20°C/−4°F (kills T. gondii cysts)
☐ Clean surfaces and utensils used in handling raw meat
☐ Avoid consumption of raw eggs or raw milk
☐ Wash fruits and vegetables
☐ Avoid drinking potentially contaminated water

The following week, at 15 weeks' gestation, the patient calls your office as she has been home for two days with malaise and low-grade fever at 38.3°C. She recalls your advice about caring for the cats and she is worried she became infected.

She presents to your office upon your request, late in the day, after all prenatal patients have been seen. She is afebrile and physical examination is normal. The fetus is viable, and there are no obstetric complaints. You send her for serologic testing.

You receive her results the following week: *T. gondii* ELISA IgG and IgM antibodies are positive, all other laboratory tests are unremarkable. The patient presents to your office for counseling. She tells you she fully recovered from her brief mild illness. Expert consultations are being arranged.

3. Discuss her serology results and outline your subsequent management. *(1 point for each main bullet, unless specified)*
Max 6

☐ Explain to the patient that possibilities for toxoplasma IgG and IgM positive antibodies include: *(1 point for each subbullet)*
- Acute infection
- False-positive IgM (up to 60%)
- Distant infection *(T. gondii specific IgM can remain detectable up to two years after infection in some highly specific assays)*

☐ Do NOT recommend termination of pregnancy at this time, given high false-positive rate of IgM: *confirmatory testing is required*

☐ Empiric Spiramycin 1 g (3 million U) orally every eight hours without food, should be started with this first positive serum screen
- To be continued until delivery if amniocentesis PCR is negative and no fetal ultrasound markers develop
- May be started in women suspected of acquired infection <18 weeks' gestation

☐ Confirmatory testing is required at a reference laboratory. *(1 point for one testing option)*
- *Options:*
  - IgG avidity test *(high avidity implies distant infection, but low avidity is not a reliable indicator of recent infection)*
  - Sabin-Feldman dye test (total IgG)
  - Indirect fluorescent antibody test
  - Differential agglutination (AC/HS) test
  - IgG titer analysis
  - *T. gondii*-specific nucleic acid amplification tests (e.g PCR) in body fluids

4. What is the goal of treatment with spiramycin?
2

☐ Fetal prophylaxis (spiramycin concentrates in placental tissue to reduce rates of vertical transmission by ~60%)

With the patient's IgG and IgM positive serologies, your hospital's laboratory sends the sample for avidity testing.

Being concerned for the patient's risk of acute toxoplasmosis in pregnancy, you call for results several days later and are told testing is not yet finalized but 'T. gondii avidity is low.'

5. What is the implication of this low avidity result, if any? *(2 points for main bullet)*
2

☐ As an independent confirmatory test, low toxoplasma avidity is <u>nonconclusive</u> of an acute infection
- Rise in avidity may be delayed 3–12 months from infection
- Avidity testing is used in conjunction with the agglutination test *(or other confirmatory T. gondii test)*

In view of low avidity, the laboratory assesses the AC/HS pattern (differential agglutination test), which yields an 'acute pattern,' consistent with a recently acquired infection.

---

6. The patient presents to your office at 17 weeks' gestation. Discuss your counseling and management. *(1 point for each main bullet)*   3

☐ Explain the confirmation of acute maternal toxoplasmosis, likely acquired in early gestation
  ○ First-trimester maternal infection has a 10%–30% risk of congenital infection *(30%–60% risk of congenital infection with second-trimester infection, and 70%–90% with third-trimester infection)*
☐ Severity of fetal/neonatal disease is greatest with first-trimester maternal infection (~60%)
  ○ Note that frequency of transmission and severity of disease have an inverse correlation
☐ Discussion of possible termination of pregnancy *(given confirmatory maternal T. gondii infection in early pregnancy and associated highest risk for fetal disease)*
  ○ Option of termination varies by country and gestational age

---

7. If her toxoplasma IgG and IgM serologies were to be repeated, what would be the expected trend given the patient's current diagnosis of acute *T. gondii* infection?   1

☐ Fourfold rise in IgG titers *(some laboratories accept threefold rise in IgG titers)*

Having been counseled by you as well as other experts regarding her acute *T. gondii* infection, the patient opts to continue pregnancy. Expert consultants will continue follow-up during the course of pregnancy.

---

8. Although the patient realizes delivery is probably several months away, she is curious if an elective Cesarean delivery could decrease the risk or severity of congenital toxoplasmosis. Provide evidence-based recommendations. *(1 point for main bullet)*   1

☐ Aim for vaginal delivery at term, unless obstetrically indicated
  ○ Mode of delivery is not influenced by maternal infection
  ○ Cesarean section does not decrease risk of congenital infection

---

9. The patient is curious about the future possibility of breastfeeding. Address her inquiry on transmission of the parasite through breastfeeding.   1

☐ Encourage breastfeeding *(studies have not confirmed transmission of the parasite through breast milk)*

10. With confirmed acute maternal *T. gondii* infection, what are the next best steps in the management of this patient? *(1 point for each main bullet and subbullet)*   3

☐ Recommend fetal diagnostic testing with amniocentesis
  ○ Amniocentesis is ideally performed after 18 weeks' gestation and more than 4 weeks from the maternal infection *(specificity and positive predictive value of amniotic fluid PCR is almost 100%, with sensitivity at 70%–80%, depending on gestational age of infection and with the target gene tested)*
☐ Arrange monthly fetal ultrasounds to assess for manifestations of toxoplasmosis

At 18^{+6} weeks' gestation, sonography does not reveal signs of congenital toxoplasmosis. Amniocentesis PCR is positive for the parasite.

11. What is the most commonly tested target gene in amniotic fluid PCR?   1

☐ B1 gene (35 copies)

12. With confirmed fetal toxoplasma infection, what is the subsequent management of this patient? *(1 point per bullet: drug dosages are indicated for interest)*   6

☐ Switch spiramycin to the following triple therapy, continued until term:
☐ Pyrimethamine 50 mg orally twice-daily for two days, then 50 mg orally daily, *plus*
☐ Sulfadiazine 75 mg/kg/d orally in two divided doses (maximum 4 g/d) for two days, then 100 mg/kg/d orally in two divided doses (maximum 4 g/d), *and*
☐ Folinic acid 10–20 mg orally daily during therapy, and for one week after completion of pyrimethamine treatment
  ○ *Folic acid* should not be used as a substitute for *folinic acid*
  ○ Folinic acid serves to protect against the hematologic toxicity of pyrimethamine
☐ Counsel the patient that congenital infection may increase her risk of miscarriage, PTB (preterm birth), FGR (fetal growth restriction), or IUFD
☐ Inform the patient that among fetuses with amniotic fluid toxoplasma PCR positivity, 70%–80% remain only serologically positive (subclinical infection) and the remaining 20%–30% develop fetal manifestations or childhood illness, despite antenatal treatment

The patient understands her fetus is *infected* with toxoplasma, and she continues serial ultrasound surveillance for possible emerging disease manifestations (ie: *affected* fetus).

13. Indicate eight features on sonography that may suggest congenital toxoplasmosis.   Max 8
    (1 point each)

Central nervous system	Abdominal	Other:
☐ Microcephaly	☐ Hepatomegaly	☐ FGR
☐ Intracranial calcifications	☐ Intrahepatic calcifications	☐ Pleuro-pericardial effusions
☐ Ventriculomegaly	☐ Echogenic bowel	☐ Hydrops
☐ Hydrocephalus	☐ Ascites	☐ Placentomegaly
		☐ IUFD *(5%, 2%, and 0% with first, second, and third trimester infection, respectively)*

Special note:

All ultrasound features are nonspecific

Upon return from her friend's summer vacation, the patient returns the cats and updates her friend on her pregnancy. The cat owner is a healthy 30-year-old nulligravida who just started preconception prenatal vitamins. Concerned after what happened to your patient, the cat owner undergoes tests for toxoplasmosis and results confirm a recent infection. She is referred for expert consultation.

14. What is the recommended approach for recently acquired *T. gondii* infection in the   1
    preconception period?

☐ Delay conception for six months from the date the acute infection is diagnosed

At 26 weeks' gestation, fetal ultrasound demonstrates normal growth biometry, with new unilateral ventriculomegaly at 13 mm with intracranial calcifications and echogenic bowel. Prior fetal imaging, including the morphology scan, was normal. All investigations that may be associated with such new-onset fetal findings are negative.

Subsequent fetal imaging is stable until 38 weeks' gestation when the patient has spontaneous labor and an uncomplicated vaginal delivery in your tertiary-care center, with necessary personnel present at birth.

With the newborn in the NICU, you come across your patient in hospital several days after her delivery-discharge. She is pleased to share with you that the junior pediatrics trainee just informed her that the child tested negative for *T. gondii* IgM and IgA antibodies. The patient is due to meet the consultant neonatologist in several hours to discuss these results and subsequent management.

15. What are the implications of negative *T. gondii* serology in the first few days of life for this neonate? *(1 point for main bullet)*   1

☐ The newborn's negative *T. gondii*-specific IgM and IgA is *nonconclusive*
  ○ 40%–50% of congenitally infected infants will have negative serology in the first month of life, especially with maternal antenatal treatment or if neonatal treatment was started soon after birth

16. Until neonatal toxoplasmosis serology is repeated in several weeks, which diagnostic test may confirm congenital infection?   1

☐ Nucleic acid amplification test (PCR) on neonatal body fluids (cerebrospinal fluid, blood, or urine)

17. What is the 'classic tetrad' of neonatal toxoplasmosis? *(1 point each)*   4

☐ Chorioretinitis *(periods of remission and exacerbation, with permanent impairment in the affected eye)*
☐ Hydrocephalus
☐ Convulsions
☐ Intracranial calcifications

Special note:
None are pathognomonic (signs mimic presentations with other pathogens)

Thorough neonatal physical examination and investigations confirm end-organ disease related to toxoplasmosis.

18. Discuss essentials of postnatal drug therapy in congenital toxoplasmosis. *(1 point each)*   2

☐ One-year treatment with pyrimethamine + sulfadiazine + folinic acid *(international variations in treatment duration)*
☐ Add corticosteroids when cerebrospinal fluid protein is ≥1 g/dL or with chorioretinitis

19. If this neonate with congenital toxoplasmosis were *asymptomatic* at birth, what would be an essential aspect of maternal counseling for the long-term care of the child? *(1 point each)*   Max 4

Long-term sequelae:
☐ Seizures
☐ Learning disabilities
☐ Motor deficits
☐ Deafness
☐ Chorioretinitis/retinal scarring/blindness

20. Postnatally, your patient is concerned about her risk of recurrent toxoplasmosis infection in future pregnancies. How would you counsel her?

☐ Reassurance: transmission of congenital toxoplasmosis occurs during a current pregnancy (*cases of second congenital infections of siblings are unique to immunocompromised mothers, such as HIV-positive status or patients on long-term steroids*)

Assuming you counseled this healthy patient on hygiene measures against toxoplasmosis during her prenatal visit at 14 weeks' gestation, indicate your best practice management in the following situations:

Scenario A: Serial toxoplasma serology showed conversion to IgG and IgM positivity at 29 weeks' gestation.

☐ Treatment recommendations favor starting pyrimethamine + sulfadiazine + folinic acid (*not spiramycin*) when acute maternal infection is ***suspected or confirmed*** at ≥18 weeks' gestation, due to the high probability of fetal infection
  ○ Late maternal infection (third trimester) usually results in asymptomatic offspring, with risk of long-term sequelae

Scenario B: Initial toxoplasma serology was negative for IgG and IgM.

☐ Serological surveillance in pregnancy (*absence of IgG and IgM antibodies rules out recent infection in at least seven days in the absence of contamination/exposure within one month*)

Scenario C: Initial toxoplasma serology was IgG-positive and IgM-negative.

☐ No serological follow-up required (*immunity is assumed to protect the fetus from any reinfection in immunocompetent patients*)
  ○ International variations exist: some advisories recommend repeat serology in three weeks to track potential increases in IgG

Scenario D: Initial toxoplasma serology was IgG-negative and IgM-positive?

☐ Specificity of IgM result requires confirmation two weeks later by a reference method using a different technique (*risk of false-positive IgM or nonspecific antibodies*)

TOTAL: 60

1

1

1

1

1

CHAPTER 67

Varicella in Pregnancy

Amira El-Messidi

A healthy 27-year-old G2P1 patient immigrated from Barbados last week. Her first appointment with you is in two days. She calls your office now concerned about her pregnancy, as her three-year-old son has chickenpox. She is currently at 15^{+2} weeks' gestation by early dating sonography, which she had in her native country; routine prenatal investigations and aneuploidy screen were normal. Recent HIV testing was negative. She had a prior healthy pregnancy and term vaginal delivery.

Your nurse assistant tells you the patient has no obstetric complaints but is very anxious given the highly contagious nature of this infection. You promptly call back the patient.

LEARNING OBJECTIVES

1. Take a focused history for prenatal exposure to varicella infection, and provide timely investigations and prophylaxis of susceptible pregnant women
2. Understand the maternal and neonatal indications for varicella zoster immunoglobulin (VZIG) postexposure prophylaxis, and counsel women requiring administration
3. Become familiar with treatment and management of maternal chickenpox and varicella pneumonia, while recognizing the importance of multidisciplinary care
4. Communicate safety measures required by potentially infectious pregnant women and those with active disease to protect vulnerable contacts, including considering delays in delivery when risk for the neonate is critical
5. Provide counseling and management of fetal risks with varicella zoster virus infection, and detect sonographic manifestations of disease
6. Illustrate the ability to time postpartum varicella vaccination for women who required antepartum VZIG without having developed disease, and address related lactation concerns

SUGGESTED READINGS

1. Amirthalingam G, Brown K, Ramsay M. Updated guidelines on postexposure prophylaxis (PEP) for varicella/shingles. Public Health England, June 2019.
2. An Advisory Committee Statement (ACS) National Advisory Committee on Immunization (NACI). Updated recommendations for the use of varicella zoster immune globulin (VarIg) for the prevention of varicella in at-risk patients. Public Health Agency of Canada, June 2016. Available at www.canada.ca/en/public-health/services/publications/healthy-living/

updated-recommendations-use-varicella-zoster-immune-globulin-varig-prevention-varicella-risk-patients.html. Accessed September 13, 2020.

3. Centers for Disease Control and Prevention (CDC). Updated recommendations for use of VariZIG- United States, 2013. *MMWR Morb Mortal Wkly Rep* 2013; 62(28):574–576.

4. Center for Disease Control and Prevention (CDC). Varicella: epidemiology and prevention of vaccine-preventable diseases. In *The Pink Book: Course Textbook*, 13th ed. Available at www.cdc.gov/vaccines/pubs/pinkbook/varicella.html. Accessed September 13, 2020.

5. Hayward K, Cline A, Stephens A, et al. Management of herpes zoster (shingles) during pregnancy. *J Obstet Gynaecol.* 2018;38(7):887–894.

6. Mandelbrot L. Fetal varicella – diagnosis, management, and outcome. *Prenat Diagn.* 2012;32(6):511–518.

7. Rafael, TJ. Varicella. Chapter 51 in Berghella V, ed. *Maternal-Fetal Evidence Based Guidelines.* Boca Raton, FL: CRC Press; 2017.

8. Royal College of Obstetricians and Gynaecologists. Chickenpox in pregnancy. Green-Top Guideline No. 13, 2015. Available at www.rcog.org.uk/globalassets/documents/guidelines/gtg13.pdf. Accessed September 13, 2020.

9. Shrim A, Koren G, Yudin MH, et al. No. 274 – management of varicella infection (chickenpox) in pregnancy. *J Obstet Gynaecol Can.* 2018 Aug;40(8):e652–e657.

10. Varicella. Chapter 34 in *The Green Book*. Public Health England, June 2019.

POINTS

1. In your telephone conversation with the patient, which information would you ask in a focused history? *(1 point per main bullet)*

Max 10

Medical history:
☐ Remote varicella infection or vaccination
☐ Establish whether prior testing was performed for varicella serology *(e.g., during last pregnancy)*
☐ Ascertain patient agrees to the receipt of blood products, should VZIG be required

Details of primary varicella exanthem:
☐ Flu-like symptoms *(i.e., fever, malaise)*
☐ Presence and description of a rash
  ○ *Typical rash with varicella is initially maculopapular, followed by appearance of vesicles that later crust and disappear, possibly leaving scars*
  ○ *Approximate quantity of vesicles and distribution, if present*

Symptoms of varicella-pneumonia:
☐ Cough, dyspnea, chest pain

Social history:
☐ Cigarette smoking
☐ Immune status of exposed household contacts, or symptoms, if present

Son:
☐ When and how was he diagnosed
☐ Time of onset of his lesions
☐ Contact source *(i.e., daycare or family members)*
☐ Establish whether his vaccinations are updated

The patient does not recall having chickenpox and cannot find her vaccination records. She does not smoke. The only blood product she had was the routine Rh immunoglobulin last pregnancy.

Over the telephone, she tells you she is breathing comfortably and does not have a rash. She lives with her son and husband in a temporary residence. Her husband confirms having chickenpox remotely.

Her son developed several random vesicular skin lesions yesterday, further spreading today. Varicella infection was confirmed today by an urgent care physician. Ever since, the patient is worried and asks if she can come urgently to your clinic.

2. How would you best advise the patient over your telephone call and plan timely management? *(1 point per main bullet)*	Max 4

☐ With no history of infection or known immunity, she may be infectious to vulnerable pregnant women *(most pregnant women are unknowingly immune; a lower proportion of immigrants from tropical countries are immune to varicella)*
☐ Urgent quantitative assay for varicella IgG (<100 mIU/ml denotes susceptibility)
☐ Inform the patient that if nonimmune status, prophylactic VZIG is indicated, ideally within 72–96 hours of exposure, and up to 10 days postexposure
  ○ *Limited evidence on effectiveness of oral antiviral agents for postexposure prophylaxis, especially before 20 weeks' gestation*
☐ If serologic confirmation will not available in a timely fashion, VZIG postexposure prophylaxis is preferred
☐ Vaccination is contraindicated in pregnancy

Special note:
VZIG is also known as VariZIG™

You arrange for her serology testing. The laboratory assures you results will be timely, expected in 24 hours. Recognizing limited access to VZIG, appropriate patient compliance, and given she is within the ideal window from exposure, plans are made to reassess the following day. The urgent care team reported a normal physical examination and ascertained fetal viability.

The following day, at 15^{+3} weeks' gestation, varicella-IgG antibodies are resulted negative.

The patient attends to hospital as planned and you see her in the E.R (A&E).

3. Discuss important elements in counseling and management of this patient. *(1 point per main bullet)*   6

☐ Inform her of susceptibility to varicella
☐ Explain the rationale for VZIG postexposure prophylaxis:
   ○ *Reduce the risk of, or attenuates, maternal infection*
   ○ **Theoretical** *reduction in risk of fetal infection*
☐ Obtain informed consent for administration of a blood product (VZIG)
☐ Mention adverse effects of VZIG:
   ○ *Headache, pain or erythema at injection site*
   ○ *Anaphylaxis is very rare, <0.1%*
☐ Inform the patient that the booked prenatal visit the following day needs rearrangement to avoid exposing pregnant women; the patient is potentially infectious up to 28 days after receiving VZIG *(prophylaxis may prolong incubation of the virus for one week)*
☐ Encourage reporting of symptoms or signs of infection

4. Specify your prescription for VZIG.   1

☐ Intramuscular VZIG 125 IU/10 kg for a maximum of 625 IU (5 vials)

Having attended your meeting with the patient, your trainee is curious whether this context is unique for recommending VZIG prophylaxis.

5. Apart from VZIG administration to susceptible pregnant women, which other perinatal situations warrant VZIG prophylaxis? *(1 point each)*   Max 2

Recommendations for neonatal VZIG:
☐ Maternal varicella develops five days before to two days after delivery[§]
   ○ *Delivery in this period is associated with up to 30% risk of neonatal varicella and 5% neonatal mortality*
☐ Neonatal exposure to an infected household contact within the first seven days of life, if the mother is nonimmune to varicella
☐ Hospitalized premature neonates born at ≥28 weeks' gestation whose mothers are nonimmune to varicella zoster virus
☐ Hospitalized premature neonates born at <28 weeks' gestation or with birthweight ≤1 kg, regardless of maternal immune status

Special note:
§ *RCOG: Neonatal VZIG is recommended for mothers with varicella within the period seven days before to seven days after delivery*

The patient presented to your office for her booked first prenatal visit at the end of the day, once all patients had left the clinic. She has no side effects of VZIG, and physical exam is normal, and the fetus is viable. The remainder of her clinical visit is unremarkable.

Two days later, at 15^{+5} weeks' gestation, the patient calls your office upon returning from an urgent care unit where a diagnosis of chickenpox was clinically established. Laboratory investigations have been requested.

There are no obstetric complaints and viability was confirmed.

---

6. Although clinical diagnosis of varicella is valid, indicate two <u>possible</u> confirmatory investigations for maternal varicella. *(1 point each)*

Max 2

☐ PCR testing for varicella DNA from the base of a vesicle *(rapid testing)*
☐ Antigen testing of the vesicles by immunofluorescence
☐ Viral culture *(not recommended due to poor sensitivity and slow growth)*

Special note:
Controversial value of serology in diagnosing primary maternal varicella; varying sensitivity/ specificity of assays and cross-reactivity with other herpesviruses

---

7. Anticipate how the urgent care physician counseled the patient on <u>maternal</u> treatment and management of chickenpox. *(1 point per main bullet, unless specified)*

Max 10

☐ Advise isolation from other pregnant women *(i.e., avoid presenting to the hospital's obstetric assessment unit, or during prenatal clinics)*
  ○ Infectious period starts two days before the rash until all vesicles are crusted
☐ Inform patient that the rash lasts 7–10 days
☐ Oral acyclovir 800 mg five times daily for seven days, started within 24 hours of the rash[†]
  (1 point for main bullet and each subbullet)
  ○ Reassure the patient of no known teratogenicity with acyclovir
  ○ Explain that serum drug monitoring is not required
  ○ Mention most commonly reported side effects of acyclovir, and very rare risk of drug intolerance/allergic reactions
  ○ *VZIG has no therapeutic effect once lesions develop*
☐ Maintain hygiene to prevent bacterial superinfection from lesions *(i.e., increased erythema, warmth, purulence)*
☐ Supportive care:
  ○ Oral hydration
  ○ Medication: antihistaminic/antipyretic agents
☐ Advise to present to hospital immediately *(away from pregnant women)* if new-onset symptoms suggest a complicated varicella infection, including:
  ○ Pneumonia
  ○ Hepatitis
  ○ Encephalitis *(e.g., headache, photophobia)*
☐ Multidisciplinary consultations *(e.g., high-risk obstetrics, virology)*

Special note:
† Oral valacyclovir 1 g three times daily for seven days is an alternative to acyclovir

You call the patient, ensuring a comprehensive understanding of chickenpox and its treatment. You inform her she will be meeting experts for maternal and fetal care given varicella during pregnancy. She eagerly asks you for information regarding the fetal risks and care involved until she meets your colleagues.

8. Outline the counseling of <u>fetal</u> risks and anticipate the high-risk obstetrics team's fetal aspects of management for maternal varicella. *(1 point per main bullet)*	Max 5

☐ Risk of fetal transmission is 8% (*i.e., in*fection) when primary maternal varicella occurs before 20 weeks' gestation
   o Most of these *infected* fetuses remain *unaffected*
☐ Overall risk of an *aff*ected fetus is 2% when maternal infections occur between 13 and 20 weeks' gestation *(greatest risk period for fetal varicella syndrome)*
☐ Detailed fetal morphology scan is recommended at least 5 weeks from maternal infection *(i.e., 20 weeks' gestation for this patient)*
☐ Offer amniocentesis for PCR of varicella zoster virus DNA at five weeks after infection and after skin lesions have completely healed
   o *Normal ultrasound with positive amniotic fluid PCR requires serial fetal imaging; persistent normal fetal scan suggests low likelihood of congenital pathology*
☐ Serial fetal sonography *(individualized frequency)*
☐ Termination of pregnancy may be offered with primary varicella, especially prior to 20 weeks' gestation *(international variations)*
☐ Delivery in a tertiary-center with a neonatologist present at birth

At 16^{+2} weeks' gestation, the patient calls the obstetric emergency unit with a new-onset cough and shortness of breath. She is unable to complete full sentences. As the obstetrician on-call, you speak with the patient and suspect varicella pneumonia. Plans are made for admission under isolation and you update the virology and high-risk obstetrics teams.

Until the patient arrives, you take this opportunity to discuss varicella pneumonia with your trainee.

9. Apart from the typical timing exemplified by this patient, list four other maternal risk factors for varicella pneumonia. *(1 point each)*	Max 4

☐ Cigarette smoking
☐ Second half of pregnancy
☐ Immunosuppression *(including steroid requirements in the past three months)*
☐ Chronic lung disease
☐ Household contact with varicella infection
☐ Dense rash (>100 skin lesions) with or without mucosal lesions

At presentation, the patient appears dyspneic with a respiratory rate of 28 breaths/min. She is febrile at 39.2°C, diaphoretic, and her pulse rate is 113 bpm. Oxygen saturation is 93% on room air. Bilateral crackles are noted on exam and chest X-ray reveals bilateral peribronchial infiltrations. Serum hematology and routine cultures are performed. Fetal viability is confirmed and there are no obstetric symptoms. She is counseled and admitted to the ICU.

10. In addition to serial investigations during her hospital stay, specify <u>medical treatments</u> the patient requires with respect to her presentation. *(1 point each)*

5

☐ Maintain oxygen saturation ≥95%; mechanical ventilation as needed
☐ Acyclovir 10–15 mg/kg IV every 8 hours for 7–10 days *(within 72 hours of symptoms)*
☐ Broad-spectrum IV antibiotics
☐ Judicious use of IV fluid hydration
☐ Analgesia *(IM, IV, or oral if tolerated)*

After a two-week hospital stay, the patient recovers from varicella pneumonia and is safely discharged with outpatient care arranged. Fetal viability was confirmed periodically during admission and prior to discharge.

At 20-weeks' gestation, she presents for the fetal morphology scan in the high-risk obstetrics unit of your tertiary center. Among other features, the following is noted:

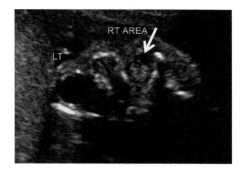

Figure 67.1

With permission from "Ultrasonographic prenatal imaging of fetal ocular and orbital abnormalities. Survey of Opthalmology 2018;63: 745–763. Figure 8A.

There is no association between this case scenario and this patient's image. Image used for educational purposes only.

11. What is being demonstrated by this sonographic image?

1

☐ Microphthalmia (right side)

12. Indicate 15 other features of fetal <u>or</u> postnatal abnormalities associated with varicella infection. *(1 point each)*

Max 15

Cutaneous and musculoskeletal:
- ☐ Dermatomal skin scarring *(most common)*
- ☐ Limb hypoplasia *(may be asymmetric)*
- ☐ Rudimentary digits
- ☐ Disseminated vesicular lesions

Neurological:
- ☐ Microcephaly
- ☐ Ventriculomegaly
- ☐ Porencephaly
- ☐ Cortical atrophy
- ☐ Seizures
- ☐ Intellectual delay
- ☐ Horner syndrome
- ☐ Diaphragmatic paralysis
- ☐ Bladder/bowel sphincteric dysfunction

Ocular:
- ☐ Chorioretinitis
- ☐ Congenital cataracts
- ☐ Optic atrophy

Gastrointestinal:
- ☐ Intrahepatic echogenic foci
- ☐ Atresia and stenosis
- ☐ Esophageal dilation and reflex

Genitourinary:
- ☐ Hydronephrosis/hydroureter
- ☐ Cryptorchidism

Other:
- ☐ FGR
- ☐ Hydrops
- ☐ IUFD

Ultrasound shows several fetal abnormalities and amniocentesis reveals varicella DNA on PCR. Termination of pregnancy is not an option for her. Serial fetal sonographic assessments are planned and consultation with the neonatologist is arranged.

The remainder of pregnancy is complicated by sonographic signs of fetal varicella syndrome, Spontaneous delivery occurs at 36 weeks' gestation and the affected neonate is admitted to the NICU for investigations and treatment.

13. Three years later, the patient conceives and presents at 31 weeks' gestation with dermatomal vesicles. She started oral acyclovir. How would you counsel her regarding fetal risks?

1

☐ Reassurance: the fetus is protected by passive transfer of maternal IgG antibodies

SCENARIO B

With varicella nonimmunity and exposure at 30 weeks' gestation, a patient receives VZIG prophylaxis and pregnancy continues uneventfully. She delivers a healthy newborn at 38 weeks' gestation.

14. Outline your considerations for her postpartum care with respect to prenatal varicella exposure. *(4 points for main bullet)*

4

☐ Arrange for varicella vaccination at three months postpartum[§]
   ○ *Safe with lactation*
   ○ *Delay conception for one month after vaccination*
   ○ *Termination of pregnancy is* not *recommended with inadvertent preconception or antenatal vaccination*

Special note:
§ Varicella vaccine should be given at least five months after VZIG administration as a two-dose schedule four to eight weeks apart

SCENARIO C

A colleague calls you for advice on timing of delivery: a patient at 39 weeks' gestation has an elective repeat Cesarean delivery today. She developed chickenpox two days ago and is on oral treatment. Your colleague wonders if delivery can proceed as planned.

15-A: What are your recommendations for timing this patient's delivery?

1

☐ Delay this patient's elective Cesarean section by three days *(if possible)*
   ○ *Delivery is ideally delayed for five days after onset of symptoms to allow passive transfer of IgG*[§]
   ○ *Thrombocytopenia or hepatitis may cause hemorrhage and/or coagulopathy if delivery is performed during viremia*

Special note:
§ *RCOG recommends awaiting seven days between rash's onset and delivery*

15-B: While you are on the telephone, your colleague asks if the patient can breastfeed.   Max 2
   (1 point each)

☐ Women with varicella infections should breastfeed if desired and well enough to do so
   (RCOG)
☐ Express milk from the affected breast; milk can be fed to newborn who is receiving VZIG
   and/or acyclovir
☐ Isolate newborn until mother's lesions have crusted

BONUS

A patient with primary varicella infection at 31 weeks' gestation receives appropriate treatment
and pregnancy progresses thereafter without complications. She was reassured of the negligible
risk of fetal varcella syndrome being <1/1000.

16. What is a possible delayed complication among infants who were infected with varicella   2
   zoster virus in utero but were asymptomatic at birth?

☐ Herpes zoster *(usually within the first two years of life)*

                                                                          TOTAL: 75

CHAPTER 68

Zika Virus Infection in Pregnancy

Anne-Maude Morency and Amira El-Messidi

CASE 1

A 32-year-old healthy primigravida at 13^{+2} weeks' gestation is referred by her primary care provider for urgent consultation at your high-risk obstetrics clinic. Four days ago, at the first prenatal visit, she reported feeling 'unwell' for a few days upon returning from an urgent family trip to a country with a Zika virus outbreak. By the time of initial prenatal visit, the patient had recovered from her illness; examination was unremarkable. First-trimester dating sonography was concordant with menstrual dates, and fetal morphology appeared normal, with a low risk of aneuploidy. Results of routine prenatal investigations are normal. The patient does not work, has healthy social habits, and takes only prenatal vitamins. She has not experienced nausea, vomiting, abdominal cramps, or vaginal bleeding. In very early gestation, she required emergent medical treatment for an allergic reaction after inadvertent exposure to a neighbor's cat.

CASE 2

A 32-year-old healthy primigravida at 13^{+2} weeks' gestation is referred by her primary care provider for urgent consultation at your high-risk obstetrics clinic. Four days ago, at the first prenatal visit, this company executive inquired about the frequency of antenatal care visits for uncomplicated pregnancies, given her obligatory weekly trips to a country with a Zika virus outbreak. She has been clinically well, and examination was unremarkable. First-trimester dating sonography was concordant with menstrual dates, and fetal morphology appeared normal, with a low risk of aneuploidy. Results of routine prenatal investigations are normal. The patient has healthy social habits and takes only prenatal vitamins. She does not have obstetrical complaints.

LEARNING OBJECTIVES

1. Take a focused prenatal history from both symptomatic and asymptomatic patients with exposure to a Zika virus–endemic area

2. Understand maternal and fetal investigations, including their advantages and caveats, in confirming Zika virus infection

3. Understand Zika virus–associated adverse pregnancy outcomes, and provide prenatal counseling and evidence-based recommendations

4. Illustrate a detailed understanding of Zika virus–associated fetal anomalies, and be able to recognize abnormalities on fetal sonography

5. Appreciate different international professional standards to define fetal microcephaly, and identify criteria most consistent for Zika virus etiology

SUGGESTED READINGS

1. Khalil A, Sotiriadis A, Chaoui R, et al. ISUOG practice guidelines: role of ultrasound in congenital infection. *Ultrasound Obstet Gynecol.* 2020;56(1):128–151.

2. Lin KW, Kraemer JD, Piltch-Loeb R, et al. The complex interpretation and management of Zika virus test results. *J Am Board Fam Med.* 2018;31(6):924–930.

3. Management of patients in the context of Zika virus: ACOG COMMITTEE OPINION, No. 784. *Obstet Gynecol.* 2019;134(3):e64–e70.

4. Oduyebo T, Polen KD, Walke HT, et al. Centers for Disease Control (CDC). Update: interim guidance for health care providers caring for pregnant women with possible Zika virus exposure — United States (including U.S. territories), July 2017. MMWR Morb Mortal Wkly Rep 2017;66:781–793.

5. Pomar L, Musso D, Malinger G, et al. Zika virus during pregnancy: from maternal exposure to congenital Zika virus syndrome. *Prenat Diagn.* 2019;39(6):420–430.

6. (a) Royal College of Obstetricians and Gynaecologists (RCOG)/Royal College of Midwives (RCM)/Public Health England (PHE)/Health Protection Scotland (HPS): Clinical guidelines on Zika virus infection and pregnancy. June 2016; last updated February 2019.

   (b) Royal College of Obstetricians and Gynaecologists (RCOG)/Royal College of Midwives (RCM)/Health Protection Scotland (HPS). Zika virus: algorithm for assessing pregnant women with a history of travel during pregnancy. PHE publications gateway No. GW-187; v10 published February 2019.

   (c) Public Health England (PHE) publications gateway No. 2015662. Mosquito bite avoidance for travellers; August 2017, version 3.

7. Sayres L, Hughes BL. Contemporary understanding of Ebola and Zika virus in pregnancy. *Clin Perinatol.* 2020;47(4):835–846.

8. Society for Maternal-Fetal Medicine (SMFM) Publications Committee. Ultrasound screening for fetal microcephaly following Zika virus exposure. *Am J Obstet Gynecol.* 2016 Jun;214(6): B2–4.

9. (a) World Health Organization (WHO). Pregnancy management in the context of Zika virus infection. 2016. Available at www.who.int/publications/i/item/pregnancy-management-in-the-context-of-zika-virus-infection. Accessed February 11, 2021.

   (b) World Health Organization. Emergencies preparedness, response: psychosocial support for pregnant women and for families with microcephaly and other neurological complications in the context of Zika virus: interim guidance for health-care providers. Available at http://who.int/csr/resources/publications/zika/psychosocial-support/en/. Accessed on February 15, 2021.

10. Zorrilla CD, García García I, García Fragoso L, et al. Zika virus infection in pregnancy: maternal, fetal, and neonatal considerations. *J Infect Dis.* 2017;216(suppl_10):S891–S896.

CASE 1
(Symptomatic pregnant woman)

1. With regard to risk of Zika virus infection, what aspects of a <u>focused</u> history do you want to know? (*1 point per main bullet; points specified per section*)

10

Zika virus exposure history: (5)
☐ Specify the dates of the outward and return journeys (before and/or during this pregnancy)
  ○ *Important to ascertain whether exposure occurred before the current pregnancy*
☐ Specify the dates of illness onset and resolution
☐ Determine travel history of her male sexual partner, whether he resides in the endemic area and history of unprotected sexual relations
  ○ *Sexual transmission of Zika virus is unique among the flaviviruses (e.g., dengue, West Nile, yellow fever viruses)*
☐ Assess whether patient or her sexual partner recalls mosquito bite(s) while in the endemic area (*i.e.*, the type of travel)
☐ Ensure absence of prior laboratory confirmation of infection before or during pregnancy:
  ○ By either nucleic acid testing (NAT) or serology [positive/equivocal Zika virus or dengue IgM and Zika virus plaque reduction neutralization test (PRNT) ≥10 and dengue PRNT <10]
    ▪ *Additional Zika virus testing would not be recommended*

Nonspecific clinical manifestations possibly suggestive of Zika virus disease:[§] *(max 5)*
Systemic:
☐ Maculopapular rash (occasionally pruritic); pattern of the rash may be in a *descending* fashion
☐ Fever
☐ Lymphadenopathy

Neurologic:
☐ Headache
☐ Guillain-Barré syndrome

Ocular:
☐ Conjunctivitis (*e.g.*, watery discharge, burning, gritty feeling)
☐ Retro-orbital pain

Musculoskeletal:
☐ Myalgia/arthralgia/arthritis
☐ Lower back pain

Special note:
§ WHO[9] defines a **suspected** case as a person with a rash and/or fever and at least one of arthralgia, arthritis, or conjunctivitis

You learn that the patient and her husband returned from their five-week trip at 10^{+1} weeks' gestation. Within the past two weeks, specifically at 11^{+4} weeks, she had low-grade fever, body aches, and a pruritic rash that responded well to topical calamine lotion and menthol based aqueous agents. Symptoms otherwise resolved spontaneously after three to four days, and she did not feel the need to report for medical care. Her husband has been feeling well, and the couple engaged in unprotected sex during a camping trip. She ascertains never being diagnosed with a Zika virus infection.

Based on your clinical concern, you coordinate a consultation with a perinatal-virology expert. During your telephone conversation, your colleague indicates that the type of test performed and timing relative to Zika virus exposure depend on individual countries and public health guidance; changes in disease prevalence, testing techniques and interpretation of results evolved during the course of the epidemic.

2. Based on your telephone conversation with the perinatal virologist, specify investigations, ideally performed as soon as possible[†] in a recently symptomatic pregnant woman with 'possible Zika exposure'.[‡] *(1 point each)*

☐ Serum Zika virus nucleic acid testing (NAT)

AND

☐ Urine Zika virus NAT
   o *Generally, urine has an expanded window of Zika virus RNA detection compared to serum*
   o *United Kingdom's Rare and Important Pathogens Laboratory (RIPL) recommends urine testing where patient was symptomatic within 21 days ago*

AND

☐ Serum Zika virus IgM enzyme-linked immunoassay (ELISA)[§]
   o *Zika virus IgG testing is not widely available: testing is performed in the United Kingdom's Rare and Important Pathogens Laboratory (RIPL); testing is not performed by guidance provided by WHO or United States' CDC*

Special notes:
† The CDC[4] recommends testing through 12 weeks after symptom onset to allow for longer period of NAT-confirmed diagnosis of Zika virus infection in some pregnant women – this may be due to active replication in the feto-placental unit; the UK guidelines[6] recommends testing current/previously symptomatic pregnant women within two weeks of leaving an area at-risk or sexual contact with a male partner who traveled to an area at moderate to high risk within the past three months

‡ 'Possible Zika virus exposure' is defined as (i) travel to, or residence in, an area with risk for mosquito-borne Zika virus transmission; or (ii) sex with a partner without a condom who traveled to or resides in an area with risk for mosquito-borne Zika virus transmission *(Suggested Reading 4)*

§ Immunofluorescence may also be used for IgM detection (WHO[9])

3

In collaboration with the perinatal virologist, the patient presents upon request, five days after primary consultation, for counseling and management of her Zika virus panel:

Serum NAT	Urine NAT	IgM
Positive	Negative	Negative

3. Highlight to your trainee general advantages and caveats of Zika NAT. *(1 point each)*

Advantages:
- ☐ Rare cross-reactivity with other flaviviruses
- ☐ High specificity rates (a positive NAT result usually confirms acute Zika infection)

Caveats:
- ☐ Negative NAT result does not exclude Zika virus infection as viremia is temporary
  - ○ *Viremia usually lasts for two weeks after symptom onset, although pregnant women's serum may have prolonged detection >60 days after symptom onset and for several weeks after symptom resolution*

3

4. Based on the patient's clinical history and laboratory findings, provide the <u>most accurate</u> interpretation of her investigations, and explain your rationale.

- ☐ <u>Suggestive</u> of acute Zika virus infection *(2 points)*
  - ○ *Note that this is based on the CDC[4]; U.K guidelines[6] interpret the detection of Zika virus RNA in any sample as diagnostic of infection*

Explanation: (1 point each)
- ☐ Confirmation of acute infection requires two positive NAT results, or one positive NAT and presence of Zika IgM antibodies
- ☐ Small risk of false positive with only one NAT

4

5. In collaboration with the expert during this multidisciplinary encounter, counsel the patient on subsequent management for diagnostic confirmation of an acute Zika virus infection. *(1 point per main bullet)*
*{**This question is provided for academic interest and is based on the CDC[4] algorithm; readers following the U.K guidelines[6] may consider this patient infected with Zika virus}*

- ☐ Repeat testing on the original serum specimen
  - ○ *A positive repeat serum NAT confirms an acute infection*
- ☐ A negative repeat serum NAT requires serum IgM testing in at least two weeks from her initial specimen collection date[§]
  - ○ *A positive repeat IgM is interpreted as evidence of an acute Zika virus infection*
  - ○ *Persistently negative IgM is interpreted as absence of Zika infection (advise routine prenatal care)*

Special note:
§ Repeat serum IgM would also be indicated in at least two weeks for another patient if exposure or symptom onset was within two weeks prior

2

At 14[+3] weeks' gestation, confirmatory testing shows evidence of maternal acute Zika virus infection based on appearance of IgM antibodies. The patient is expected shortly for prenatal counseling and management.

Meanwhile, you take this opportunity to teach your obstetric trainee on aspects of laboratory tests and interpretations where Zika virus infection is suspected.

6. Illustrate to your obstetric trainee the limitations of interpreting Zika virus IgM antibody results. *(1 point each)*   3

□ False-negative result if testing is performed before development of IgM antibodies or after they have waned
□ False-positive result due to 8%–40% risk of cross-over with other flaviviruses (*e.g.,* Dengue virus, West Nile virus, yellow fever virus)
  ○ *Risk of IgM cross-reactivity depends on where you traveled/lived, or vaccination against related flaviviruses*
□ Limited value in timing infection as IgM antibodies may last longer than 12 weeks

You present your trainee with the **assumption** that this pregnant patient's initial investigations revealed IgM antibodies in the absence of serum or urine NAT, as illustrated:

Serum NAT	Urine NAT	IgM
Negative	Negative	Positive

7. In this scenario, explain to your trainee the next best laboratory test, highlighting results that would confirm Zika virus infection. You reinforce that in this circumstance, timing of infection would be unknown. *(1 point per main bullet)*   2

Next best laboratory test:
□ Plaque reduction neutralization test (PRNT) for Zika and Dengue viruses
  ○ *Measures virus-specific neutralizing antibody titers*

Zika virus infection: *(either bullet for 1 point)*
□ *[CDC [4]]:* Zika virus PRNT titer ≥10 <u>AND</u> Dengue virus PRNT <10
□ *[WHO [9]]:* Zika virus PRNT titer ≥20 <u>AND</u> titer ratio ≥4 compared with other flaviviruses

Special note:
PRNT confirmation may take up to four weeks for results; test may not be recommended in certain areas of residence; referral to local recommendations is advised

Your trainee appreciates you facilitating the complex interpretation of Zika virus investigations; he or she intends to expand on learning using your proposed resources.

As a maternal-fetal medicine expert, you ensure adequate time to counsel the patient on acute maternal Zika virus infection; you intend to discuss subsequent prenatal care and options for pregnancy management. Having considered your advice, she presents accompanied by her husband.

8. With acute maternal Zika virus infection, inform the couple of potential adverse pregnancy outcomes and outline your counseling of prenatal management. *(1 point per main bullet; points specified per section)*

12

Zika-associated adverse pregnancy outcomes: *(max 4)*
☐ Early pregnancy loss
☐ Congenital anomalies, with characteristic neurotropism *(see Question 10)*
☐ Fetal growth restriction (FGR)
☐ Preterm birth *(Controversial association)*
☐ IUFD *(via placental vascular injury, or infarction)*
   ○ Unlike other perinatal infections, Zika virus does <u>not</u> cause a placental inflammatory response

Prenatal counseling and management: *(max 8)*
☐ Inform the patient of the lack of treatment or vaccine to prevent congenital infection or mitigate sequelae of Zika virus infection during pregnancy or in the neonate
☐ Discuss the apparent lack of association between presence or severity of infection (*e.g.*, symptom status, severity, viral load), or co-existing antibodies to flaviviruses and infant outcome
   ○ *i.e.*, the risk of congenital disabilities may be <u>independent</u> of the presence or absence of maternal symptoms *(ISUOG[1])*
☐ Mention that estimated risk of congenital Zika virus syndrome is 5%–10%, which is largely consistent across studies globally *(ACOG[3])*
☐ Consideration for termination of pregnancy *(international variations in cultural and jurisdictional policies)*
☐ Inform that patient that the risk for vertical transmission exists throughout pregnancy, with greatest risk of serious fetal/newborn sequelae with first- and early second-trimester infection (third-trimester infection may also lead to fetal/neonatal Zika disease)
☐ Arrange for an early detailed fetal morphology scan for congenital anomalies, particularly neuroanatomy (*e.g.*, at 16–18 weeks' gestation)
   ○ Fetal sonographic manifestations of Zika virus may appear *as early as* two weeks after maternal infection; insufficient data on *optimal timing* between exposure and initial sonographic screening in pregnant women with Zika virus infection
☐ Arrange for serial fetal ultrasounds (*e.g.*, every three to four weeks) for monitoring of growth biometry and development of Zika-associated anomalies
   ○ Insufficient data on *optimal frequency* of sonographic screening in pregnant women with Zika virus infection
   ○ Serial antenatal and postnatal follow-up until at least until 12 months of age is recommended *(ISUOG[1])*
      ▪ *Children (~2%) with severe neurodevelopmental delay related to Zika virus infection had normal neuroimaging at birth*
   ○ Fetal MRI may be considered, where available, as a complementary tool to neurosonography to facilitate assessment of gyration, migration disorders, increased cerebrospinal fluid, and cortical development; MRI may be adjunctive where findings may alter prenatal management
   ○ *No consensus statements, guidelines, or best practice recommendations exist for antepartum fetal surveillance [cardiotocography or biophysical profile (BPP)] for Zika-infected fetuses*

☐ Early antenatal neonatology consultation ± pediatric neurology expert
☐ Ensure delivery is planned in a hospital center with adequate maternal-fetal-neonatal medical services, and psychosocial care facilities for the patient and her family
☐ Plan for vaginal delivery *(Cesarean section is reserved for obstetrical indications)*

9. Address your trainee's interest regarding *behavioral differences* in biometry with asymmetric FGR associated with placental insufficiency relative to Zika virus infection. *(1 point each)*

2

Asymmetric FGR:
☐ Head-sparing with placental insufficiency
☐ Femur-sparing with fetal Zika infection syndrome

The couple appreciates your nondirective[†] counseling and evidence-based care plan and offer of psychosocial support services in this anxiety-provoking period. They had searched the internet for '*possible Zika virus–associated birth defects*' and have been acquainted with the considerable list of abnormalities. Although your local regulations promote patient preferences for pregnancy decisions, the patient is early in gestation and knowing that postnatal neurodevelopmental abnormalities may appear despite normal fetal imaging, the couple inform you that termination of pregnancy is not an option to them.

As her husband is pursuing a degree in neuroscience, he is interested in a detailed presentation of cerebral findings in offspring with congenital Zika syndrome. You highlight to your attendant obstetric trainee that you may have initially provided a general overview of abnormalities in this situation, where risk of multiple complex congenital anomalies exists.

Special note:
† Nondirective counseling is advocated by the WHO[9] to allow patient(s) the fully informed choice regarding subsequent steps in pregnancy management.

10. With focus on the <u>brain/head,</u> identify abnormalities featured with Zika virus disease. *(1 point each)*

Max 10

☐ Microcephaly
☐ Collapse of the skull/overlapping sutures
☐ Redundant scalp skin *(secondary to microcephaly)*
☐ Cortical atrophy/microencephaly
☐ Cortical and white matter abnormalities *(e.g.,* agyria, pachygyria, polymicrogyria, lissencephaly)
☐ Intracranial calcifications *(secondary to focal necrosis);* may be localized to any part of the brain *[predilection for cortex, basal ganglia (which includes the caudate nucleus)]*
☐ Brainstem calcifications
☐ Ventriculomegaly *(often asymmetric or unilateral, suggesting focal injury)*
☐ Choroid plexus cyst

- [ ] Porencephaly
- [ ] Dys-/agenesis of the corpus callosum
- [ ] Vermian dys-/agenesis
- [ ] Cerebellar atrophy
- [ ] Megacisterna magna >95th percentile
- [ ] Blake's pouch cyst
- [ ] Brainstem/spinal cord degeneration

You highlight that fetal microcephaly will almost never be found with normal brain imaging, although brain abnormalities may be seen in Zika virus disease despite normal head circumference.

11. Elaborate on differences in standard definitions for prenatal microcephaly and discuss diagnostic considerations in fetal assessment for Zika virus disease. *(1 point per main bullet; max points specified per section)*

5

Microcephaly: *(max 3)*
- [ ] Head circumference ≥2 standard deviations (SD) below the mean for gestational age *(ISUOG[1])* or >2 SD below the mean *(CDC[4], RCOG[6], WHO[9])*
  - ○ Higher risk of brain abnormalities with head circumference ≥3SD below the mean *(ISUOG[1])*
- [ ] Isolated fetal head circumference ≥3SD below the mean for gestational age *(SMFM[8])*
  - ○ Pathologic microcephaly is considered certain when the fetal head circumference is ≥5 SD below the mean
    - ▪ Finding a sloping forehead on fetal profile view raises index of suspicion for pathologic microcephaly
- [ ] Head circumference ≥3SD below the mean for gestational age *(SOGC)[†]*
- [ ] Head circumference <3rd percentile *(CDC[4])* or <2.5th percentile *(RCOG[6])*
  - ○ *Percentile charts have been proposed given their use in the pediatric population*

Prenatal considerations in head circumference with Zika virus: *(2)*
- [ ] Microcephaly is not commonly seen early in the spectrum of Zika virus–associated anomalies; detection may require 15–24 weeks from onset on maternal symptoms
- [ ] Microcephaly associated with congenital Zika infection may be absent at birth, but develop within the first year of life
  - ○ *This may be independent of fetal hydrocephalus that may mask the diagnosis of microcephaly*

Special note:
† Refer to the SOGC Practice Guideline [De Bie I, Boucoiran I. No. 380-Investigation and Management of Prenatally Identified Microcephaly. *J Obstet Gynaecol Can.* 2019;41(6): 855–861]

The couple understand that with the patient's confirmed acute Zika virus infection, a sonographic diagnosis of fetal microcephaly would *likely* be associated with this viral infection syndrome, in the absence of other suspected causes. They are curious where other situations would suggest a strong link between Zika virus and fetal microcephaly.

12. Based on the World Health Organization, elaborate on other <u>epidemiologic and molecular</u> criteria where relation of microcephaly to Zika virus infection would be most suspected. *(1 point each)*   Max 3

- ☐ Pregnant patient had common clinical manifestation of Zika virus infection and epidemiologic antenatal *'potential Zika virus exposure' (refer to definition indicated in 'Special notes' of Question 2)*
- ☐ Pregnant patient had antenatal sexual activity with an individual with confirmed Zika virus infection
- ☐ Amniotic fluid Zika virus real-time reverse transcription polymerase chain reaction (rRT-PCR)
- ☐ Fetal brain Zika PCR detection postmortem

13. Recognizing a constellation of <u>noncerebral</u> fetal/infant malformations or manifestations, provide a <u>structured</u> framework to features associated with Zika virus disease. *(1 point per main bullet)*   Max 10

Visual:[†]
- ☐ Microphthalmia
- ☐ Intraocular calcifications
- ☐ Pigmented retinopathy
- ☐ Macular scars and atrophy
- ☐ Optic-nerve abnormalities

Auditory:
- ☐ Sensorineural deafness

Neuromuscular:
- ☐ Talipes[‡]
- ☐ Congenital arthrogryposis or isolated joint contractures
  - ○ *Unique clinical finding to this congenital infection*
  - ○ *Etiology may be loss of motor neurons and/or connections motor neurons and cortex*[§]
- ☐ Neonatal/infant hypertonia with spasticity, extreme irritability, hyperreflexia, tremors, extrapyramidal symptoms, hypotonia, or mixed hypertonia-hypotonia motor dysfunction
- ☐ Neonatal/infant swallowing difficulties
- ☐ Epilepsy

Other:
- ☐ Oligohydramnios
- ☐ Craniofacial disproportion
- ☐ Failure to thrive

Special notes:
- † Ocular abnormalities may be most common clinical findings in infants of infected women [Britt WJ. *Semin Perinatol.* 2018;42(3):155–167]
- ‡ Talipes may be the *earliest* appearing sign *(CDC*[4]*)*
- § Britt WJ. *Semin Perinatol.* 2018;42(3):155–167

With your expertise in maternal-fetal medicine and antenatal sonography, you perform the detailed 20-week fetal morphology sonogram which appears normal; fetal biometry and amniotic fluid volume are also unremarkable. Although the couple will not terminate pregnancy based on development of any fetal anomalies, they would like to discuss the role of amniocentesis in confirming fetal Zika virus infection.

14. Discuss potential benefits and caveats of amniocentesis for Zika virus rRT-PCR.[†] The patient understands procedure-related risks. *(1 point each)*

4

Potential benefits of amniocentesis:
☐ Detection of Zika virus RNA in amniotic fluid is diagnostic of an *infected* fetus

Caveats of amniocentesis: (max 3)
☐ Confirming an *infected* fetus may not be predictive of an *affected* fetus
☐ Confirming fetal infection does not exclude concurrent chromosomal or other infectious etiologies
☐ Nondetection of Zika virus RNA would not definitively exclude congenital Zika virus infection as RNA may be detected transiently
☐ Optimal timing is largely unknown; recommendations suggest >20 weeks' gestation and after six to eight weeks after maternal exposure to allow time for excretion of Zika virus in fetal urine

Special note:
† rRT-PCR: real-time reverse transcription polymerase chain reaction

After comprehensive discussion, the patient opted against amniocentesis for confirmation of Zika virus infection. She will continue monthly sonographic imaging; neonatal consultation is planned for the later second or early third trimester.

Although she is early in pregnancy, the patient questions whether breastfeeding can transmit the Zika virus to the infant, assuming serial antenatal fetal sonograms remain normal and her newborn does not demonstrate disease postnatally.

15. Provide your evidence-based recommendations for breastfeeding with acute maternal Zika virus infection, assuming a normal newborn. Justify your answer. *(1 point each)*

2

☐ Encouragement of breastfeeding is advised
  ○ ACOG[3], CDC[4], RCOG[6], WHO[9]
☐ Justification: Small amount of viral transmission in breast milk has not caused infant infection or developmental complications; benefits of breastfeeding outweigh theoretical risk

Special note:
Breastfeeding is also encouraged with suspected or probable Zika virus infection or women who live in, or have traveled to, areas with Zika

Monthly fetal sonograms remain normal until 30^{+1} weeks' gestation when the following significant findings are noted:

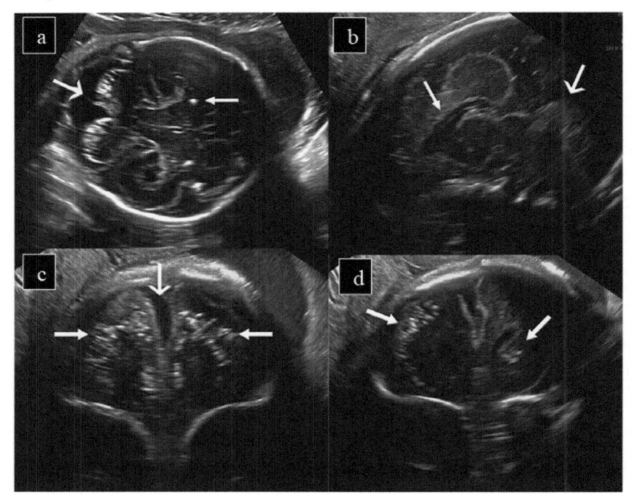

Figure 68.1

With permission: Figure 1 from Oliveira Melo AS, et al. Ultrasound Obstet Gynecol. 2016;47(1):6–7.

There is no association between the patient's images and this case scenario. Images are used for educational purposes only

After explaining relevant findings to the couple, you later recall having your obstetric trainee's presence during early antenatal discussion of fetal brain abnormalities associated with Zika virus disease. You decide to refresh your trainee's memory by encouraging him/her to identify the abnormalities.

You clarify your trainee's understanding that the term congenital Zika syndrome[‡] refers to five distinctive criteria for *postnatal phenotype* in infants and children with structural anomalies and functional disabilities.

Special note:
‡ *Refer to* Moore CA, et al. *JAMA Pediatr.* 2017;171(3):288–295.

16. For each sonographic panel, identify the fetal brain findings indicated by the arrows.   Max 5
    (1 point each)

Panel 'a' *(transabdominal axial view)*
☐ Vermian dysgenesis (large arrow)
☐ Intracerebral calcifications (small arrow)

Panel 'b' *(transvaginal sagittal view)*
☐ Corpus callosal dysgenesis (small arrow)
☐ Vermian dysgenesis (large arrow)

Panel 'c' *(coronal view)*
☐ Brain atrophy represented by widening of the interhemispheric fissure (vertical arrow)
☐ Bilateral coarse intracerebral calcifications (horizontal arrows)

Panel 'd' *(coronal view, more posteriorly than panel 'c')*
☐ Intracerebral calcifications similar to panel 'c' with caudate calcifications now presented

While following her antenatal course, you decide to read a <u>hypothetical</u> paper designed for <u>academic interest</u> on the ability of fetal sonography to predict Zika-virus related abnormalities with known acute maternal infection in a country where prevalence of Zika infection is 10%.

17. With reference to this study design, what is meant by the positive and negative predictive   2
    values (PPV and NPV, respectively) of ultrasound? *(1 point per main bullet)*

☐ PPV is the probability of fetal Zika virus infection given sonographic abnormalities
    ○ *(i.e., the probability that a condition is present given a positive test result)*
☐ NPV is the probability of a noninfected fetus with normal fetal sonography
    ○ *(i.e., the probability that the condition is absent given a negative test result)*

Authors present the following hypothetical scenario:

	Fetal Zika virus infection	
	Positive	Negative
Prenatal sonographic abnormalities	80	90
Normal sonography	20	810

18. Explain how disease prevalence is 10% in this study.   2

☐ Prevalence: $(a + c)/(a + b + c + d) = (80 + 20)/(80 + 90 + 20 + 810) = 100/1000 = 10\%$

19. Based on results presented by this study, what is the positive and negative predictive values (PPV and NPV, respectively) of ultrasound as a screening test? *(2 points each)*   4

☐ PPV: a/(a + b) = 80/(80 + 90) = 47.1%
☐ NPV: d/(c + d) = 810/(20 + 810) = 97.6%

Fetal findings remain stable on serial sonographic assessments. Growth biometry and velocity are within the 12th–15th percentiles and amniotic fluid volume remains appropriate. The remainder of prenatal care is unremarkable; the patient does not experience obstetric complications and reports normal fetal activity.

Perinatal psychosocial support services will continue during the postpartum period; you intend to screen her for postpartum depression.

The patient presents in spontaneous labor at 37^{+2} weeks' gestation and has an uneventful vaginal delivery; the neonatal care team will proceed with required investigations. Your obstetric trainee is contemplating the need for histological assessment of the placenta given known acute maternal Zika virus infection.

20. Discuss the indications for laboratory examination of the placenta (and potentially fetal tissues) for possible fetal Zika virus infection where antenatal acute maternal infection had been confirmed. *(1 point each)*   2

☐ Pregnancy loss <u>with</u> or <u>without</u> possible Zika virus–associated birth defects
☐ Infant death following live birth

Special note:
No additional diagnostic information from placental testing from live births *without* obvious Zika virus–associated birth defects at birth where acute maternal infection had been confirmed; placental assessment is also not indicated where live births suggest possible Zika virus–associated birth defects, although case-by-case consideration is warranted *(CDC[4])*

CASE 2
(Asymptomatic pregnant woman with ongoing possible Zika virus exposure)

21. For this asymptomatic pregnant patient with ongoing possible exposure[§] to a country with a Zika virus outbreak, identify most important questions on history relating to exposure. *(1 point per main bullet)*   3

☐ Possible sexual exposure before and during this pregnancy with a male partner from the country with a Zika virus outbreak, or co-travelling with her male sexual partner
☐ Type of travel/assess risk of exposure to mosquito-borne illness
☐ Prior laboratory confirmation of infection before or during this pregnancy
   ○ *Additional Zika virus testing would not be recommended*
   ○ *Previous Zika virus infection is likely to confer immunity, although limited data is available*

Special note:
§ Ongoing possible exposure includes those who reside in or travel frequently (*e.g.*, daily, weekly) to an area with mosquito transmission

You ascertain the patient never had laboratory confirmation of Zika virus infection. She has been sexually active with her husband, who occasionally travels with her. Although she mostly attends administrative meetings during her trips, the patient also inspects outdoors workers. In the absence of prenatal complications, she made an informed decision to continue travel until the early third trimester.

22-A. If laboratory screening for Zika virus is performed, identify the optimal test for this asymptomatic patient given ongoing exposure. — 2

Optimal mode for testing:
☐ Serum Zika virus NAT[†]

22-B. Rationalize your intended <u>timing</u> and <u>frequency</u> of testing, recognizing that no *optimal* recommendations exist. *(1 point per main bullet)* — 3

Proposed timing and frequency of testing:
☐ Initiate NAT at the first prenatal care visit
☐ If the first NAT is negative for Zika virus, two additional NAT are advised during pregnancy, coinciding with prenatal visits

Rationale:
☐ Proportion of fetuses/infants with Zika virus–associated birth defects is highest with first- and early second-trimester infections, although adverse outcomes have also been associated with third-trimester infections; consideration for testing every trimester *(CDC[4])*
  ○ *Optimal frequency of testing remains unspecified*

Special note:
† IgM is no longer recommended routinely for asymptomatic pregnant patients with ongoing Zika virus exposure due to prolonged persistence after infection *(CDC[4])*

23. Detail recommended measures to prevent Zika virus transmission during the antenatal period, in view on *ongoing* travel to an at-risk region. *(1 point per main bullet)*　　Max 5

Prevention of sexual transmission:
☐ Use latex condoms or abstinence throughout pregnancy, given *ongoing* exposure

Prevention of mosquito bites:
☐ Wear loose-fitted clothing with long-sleeves, tucked-in shirts, long pants/trousers, socks and shoes
☐ Light-colored clothing is preferred
☐ Wear hats with mosquito nets to protect face and neck
☐ Apply insecticide (*e.g.*, permethrin) to clothing and travel gear to provide significant protection against biting mosquitos
☐ Use insecticide-treated mosquito nets when resting/sleeping outdoors
☐ Use insect repellent day and night, indoors and outdoors, on exposed skin; DEET (N, N-diethyl-meta-toluamide) is preferred for pregnant women
　○ *50% DEET is safe and effective for pregnant/breastfeeding women*
　○ *DEET-based repellents have the longest duration of action (fewer applications)*
☐ Keep living areas well screened or use air-conditioning in closed areas

The patient appreciates your advice and the pamphlet you provided indicating the strategies discussed in prevention of Zika virus infection. She remembered that her sister and her husband were recently on vacation in a region with Zika outbreak; the couple aspires to conceive soon and have been asymptomatic.

24. Indicate your <u>preconception</u> advice for the patient's sister and her husband who recently returned from an area with risk of Zika virus transmission.　　2

☐ Delay conception for at least <u>three months</u> after return, or after the male's symptom onset (if present)

Special note:
If only the female partner traveled, delay of conception for <u>two months</u> is advised from last possible Zika virus exposure or symptom onset

TOTAL:　　105

CHAPTER 69

SARS-CoV-2 Infection in Pregnancy

Isabelle Malhamé, Rohan D'Souza, and Amira El-Messidi

A 37-year-old nulligravida with a one-year history of well-controlled essential hypertension is referred to your high-risk obstetrics clinic for preconception counseling. Recent comprehensive investigations are free of end-organ dysfunction. Maintaining a healthy lifestyle, she lost weight over the past year; her body mass index (BMI) is now 31 kg/m^2. She uses condoms for contraception and is adherent to long-acting nifedipine once daily; folic acid–containing prenatal vitamins were initiated last month.

The referring practitioner alerts you that the patient cancelled her COVID-19 vaccination appointment due to ambivalence about the vaccine in the periconception period.

Special note: *As literature on COVID-19 vaccination and effects of SARS-CoV-2 infection on maternal-fetal well-being continues to accrue, this case scenario provides principles of counseling and management up to September 30, 2021.*

LEARNING OBJECTIVES

1. Recognize the importance of contemporary evidence-based provider counseling on COVID-19 vaccination throughout the perinatal spectrum
2. Appreciate that overlap in clinical manifestations of SARS-CoV-2 infection and normal pregnancy requires clinical vigilance in evaluating the afebrile-symptomatic patient
3. Discuss the risks of SARS-CoV-2 infection on perinatal outcome as well as the effects of pregnancy on disease severity
4. Understand obstetric considerations of pharmacologic interventions commonly administered in pregnancy
5. Address obstetric-associated aspects of intrapartum and postpartum care with maternal SARS-CoV-2 infection, maintaining interdisciplinary collaboration

SUGGESTED READINGS

1. Allotey J, Stallings E, Bonet M, et al. Clinical manifestations, risk factors, and maternal and perinatal outcomes of coronavirus disease 2019 in pregnancy: living systematic review and meta-analysis. *BMJ.* 2020;370:m3320.
2. Conde-Agudelo A, Romero R. SARS-CoV-2 infection during pregnancy and risk of preeclampsia: a systematic review and meta-analysis. *Am J Obstet Gynecol.* 2021;S0002–9378(21)00795-X.

3. Di Mascio D, Buca D, Berghella V, et al. Counseling in maternal-fetal medicine: SARS-CoV-2 infection in pregnancy. *Ultrasound Obstet Gynecol.* 2021;57(5):687–697.

4. D'Souza R, Ashraf R, Rowe H, et al. Pregnancy and COVID-19: pharmacologic considerations. *Ultrasound Obstet Gynecol.* 2021;57(2):195–203.

5. Galang RR, Newton SM, Woodworth KR, et al. Risk factors for illness severity among pregnant women with confirmed severe acute respiratory syndrome coronavirus 2 infection – surveillance for emerging threats to mothers and babies network, 22 state, local, and territorial health departments, 29 March 2020–5 March 2021. *Clin Infect Dis.* 2021;73(Suppl 1):S17–S23.

6. Moore KM, Suthar MS. Comprehensive analysis of COVID-19 during pregnancy. *Biochem Biophys Res Commun.* 2021;538:180–186.

7. Royal College of Obstetricians and Gynaecologists. Coronavirus (COVID-19) infection in pregnancy; Version 14, August 25, 2021. Available at www.rcog.org.uk/coronavirus-pregnancy. Accessed September 25, 2021.

8. Shimabukuro TT, Kim SY, Myers TR, et al. Preliminary findings of mRNA Covid-19 vaccine safety in pregnant persons. *N Engl J Med.* 2021;384(24):2273–2282. [Correction in N Engl J Med. 2021 Sep 8]

9. (a) SMFM – Coronavirus (COVID-19) and pregnancy: what maternal-fetal medicine subspecialists need to know; November 23, 2020. Available at www.smfm.org/covidclinical. Accessed September 25, 2021.

    (b) SMFM – Management considerations for pregnant women with COVID-19; February 2, 2021. Available at at www.smfm.org/covidclinical. Accessed September 25, 2021.

    (c) SMFM – Provider considerations for engaging in COVID-19 vaccine counseling with pregnant and lactating patients; September 24, 2021. Available at https://www.smfm.org/covidclinical. Accessed September 25, 2021.

10. Wei SQ, Bilodeau-Bertrand M, Liu S, et al. The impact of COVID-19 on pregnancy outcomes: a systematic review and meta-analysis. *CMAJ.* 2021;193(16):E540–E548.

POINTS

1. Indicate aspects you would discuss with the patient with regard to COVID-19 vaccination in the periconception period. *(1 point each)*

Max 6

Provide reassurance on the following:

☐ There is no need to delay conception following vaccination

☐ The COVID-19 vaccine does not affect fertility

☐ There are no 'safety signals' with respect to early pregnancy loss, congenital anomalies, fetal growth restriction, preterm birth, stillbirth or neonatal death *(Suggested Reading 8)*; a pregnancy test is thereby not required prior to vaccination

☐ There are no live viral particles in vaccines, and the vaccine does not replicate to cause disease in the mother [or embryo-fetus] *(she may experience side effects related to activation of an immune response)*

☐ Either messenger RNA or adenoviral-vector vaccine(s) may be administered periconception, during pregnancy, or lactation

☐ The risk of thrombosis with thrombocytopenia syndrome (TTS)[†] reported with adenoviral-vector vaccine is minimal

☐ Side effects of vaccination are outweighed by the risk of (severe) SARS-CoV-2 infection in pregnancy and related maternal-fetal complications

- ☐ Maternal vaccine-elicited antibodies may confer fetal-neonatal protection through passive immunization
- ☐ Vaccination decreases risks of morbidity and mortality with SARS-CoV-2 infection

Special note:

† Provide reassurance that risk of TTS would not be increased even if the patient were to receive vaccination in pregnancy/postpartum despite being hypercoagulable states

She appreciates your directed counseling and inquires about maternal-fetal risks of SARS-CoV-2 infection in the event she does not receive appropriate vaccination.

2. Independent of comorbidities, inform the patient of <u>adverse maternal-fetal outcomes</u> with SARS-CoV-2 infection particularly among symptomatic, hospitalized women. *(1 point each)*

5

Maternal:

- ☐ Hospitalization and intensive treatment/care unit (ITU/ICU) admission
- ☐ COVID-pneumonia, acute respiratory distress syndrome
- ☐ Need for ventilation and extracorporeal membrane oxygenation (ECMO) support
- ☐ Acute venous and arterial thrombo-embolic disease
- ☐ Preterm birth *(primarily iatrogenic)*
- ☐ Preeclampsia, eclampsia, and HELLP syndrome
- ☐ Cesarean delivery
- ☐ Mental illness, including anxiety and depression
- ☐ Mortality

Fetal:†

- ☐ Complications of prematurity
- ☐ Stillbirth
- ☐ Possible association with small-for-gestational age newborns

Special note:

† Despite >100 million reported cases worldwide, there are no reported increases in congenital anomalies *(RCOG[7])*

After comprehensive counseling with regard to prenatal care with comorbidities, the patient plans to arrange her COVID-19 vaccination appointment. You later learn she missed this opportunity, being hospitalized with hyperemesis gravidarum at nine weeks' gestation. Prenatal care is then transferred to you, which you arrange based on evidence-based management discussed at preconception consultation. Low-dose aspirin is initiated for preeclampsia prophylaxis. Subsequent first- and second-trimester medical and obstetric care are unremarkable.

Due to unrelated delays, the patient receives the first dose of mRNA COVID-19 vaccine at 29^{+3} weeks' gestation, *simultaneously* with routine antenatal pertussis vaccination. At 30^{+0} weeks' gestation, she experiences nonspecific symptoms that she attributed to pregnancy and possibly, postvaccination immune response; the patient remained afebrile during this 48-hour period, without any obstetric complaints. With onset of a sore throat shortly thereafter, a positive reverse transcriptase polymerase chain reaction (RT-PCR) for SARS-CoV-2 was tested and reported at 30^{+3} weeks' gestation. Promptly, you conduct a telehealth session with the patient.

You brief your obstetric trainee on the importance of maintaining clinical vigilance for SARS-CoV-2 infection in afebrile-symptomatic obstetric patient.

3. Elaborate on early clinical manifestations of COVID-19 illness that overlap with symptoms common to pregnancy. *(1 point each)*	Max 3

☐ Fatigue
☐ Nasal congestion
☐ Nausea/vomiting
☐ Dyspnea

4-A. Based on her demographic and clinical history, elicit this gravida's known risk factors that may contribute to hospitalization with COVID-19 or increased severity of illness. *(1 point each)*	Max 3

☐ Chronic hypertension
☐ Obesity (BMI $\geq$30 kg/m^2)
☐ Maternal age $\geq$35 years *(i.e., 37 years old)*
☐ Being in the second or third trimester of pregnancy

4-B. Highlight to your trainee additional risk factors for severe COVID-19 illness, which may not be specific to pregnancy. *(1 point each)*	Max 5

☐ Gestational or pregestational diabetes mellitus
☐ Immunosuppressive diseases or treatments (*e.g.,* sickle cell disease, cancer, chronic obstructive lung disease, heart conditions, chronic kidney disease, organ transplant)
☐ Smoking
☐ Being a health care professional
☐ Living in areas or households of socioeconomic deprivation
☐ Being from a racialized or minoritized ethnic background

5. With focus on a positive RT-PCR for SARS-CoV-2, what aspects of a focused history would you want to know from the patient during your telehealth sessions? *(1 point each)*	Max 15

Symptom-severity of respiratory illness:
☐ Note the ability to complete sentences without gasping for air
☐ Note the patient's lucidity in conversation
☐ Note the presence of auditory wheezing
☐ Dyspnea beyond baseline pregnancy symptoms

□ Hemoptysis
□ Chest pain or pressure
□ Ability to tolerate oral intake
□ Dizziness while standing
□ Severe headache, neurological deficit, or symptoms of thromboembolism

Assessment of the patient's comorbidities:
□ Current or recent blood pressure (BP) control on home values, *if performed*
□ Current or recent glycemia

Obstetric morbidities related to respiratory illness:
□ Decrease in fetal activity
□ Uterine contractions/pressure

Social features:
□ Living arrangements/ability to self-isolate
□ Inform the patient about contact tracing
□ Recent travel

Although lucid, you note the patient speaks short sentences, coughs sporadically and you detect she is dyspneic. She avoided oral ingestion today due to persistent nausea. Remaining screening features for symptom-severity of SARS-CoV-2 infection are unremarkable; she has no obstetric complaints. The patient will provide names for contact tracing.

Upon your recommendation, she will promptly present to the isolated hospital facility for clinical assessment where a medical expert will assist you in her cardiorespiratory care.

6. With appropriate infection control practices and with interdisciplinary collaboration, state   15
   aspects of the focused physical examination. *(1 point each)*

General appearance and mental status:
□ Change in mental status during conversation relative to your recent telehealth assessment
□ Use of accessory muscles of respiration
□ Cyanosis

Vital signs:
□ BP
□ Pulse rate
□ Respiratory rate
□ Oxygenation
□ Temperature

Cardiopulmonary auscultation:
□ Prolonged expiratory phase
□ Decreased air entry
□ Extravesicular sounds (*e.g.,* crackles or wheezing)

Cardiovascular examination:
- ☐ Elevated jugular venous pressure
- ☐ Auscultate heart sounds for regularity of S1 and S2, presence of S3, S4, or pathological murmurs
- ☐ Pitting edema in the lower extremity *(although this may be physiological in pregnancy)*

Fetal well-being:
- ☐ Doptone auscultation or consideration for electronic fetal monitoring to assess for tachycardia

Further to clinical features you detected by telehealth, the patient is noted to be using accessory neck muscles of respiration. Vital signs reveal:

BP	105/65 mmHg
Pulse rate	95 bpm
Respiratory rate	22 breaths/min
Oxygen saturation	88% on room air
Temperature	37.5°C

There is decreased air entry with presence of coarse crackles at the base of both lung fields; other maternal aspects on examination are unremarkable. Cardiotocography shows a normal fetal heart tracing and uterine quiescence.

7. Recognizing that laboratory investigations may not have definitive prognostic   Max 5
   value, outline the expected trend in laboratory derangements associated with severe
   COVID-19 illness. *(1 point each)*

Increased levels:
- ☐ C-reactive protein[†] *(physiologically increased in pregnancy)*
- ☐ D-dimer *(physiologically increased in pregnancy)*
- ☐ Lactate dehydrogenase (LDH)
- ☐ Troponin T
- ☐ Ferritin
- ☐ Creatine phosphokinase

Decreased levels:
- ☐ Absolute lymphocyte count[†]

Special note:
† Most common laboratory signs of infection in pregnancy *(Suggested Reading 4)*

Oxygen supplementation at 5 L/min raises her saturation to 96% and appears to facilitate her work of breathing. With patient consent, a chest X-ray[†] shows diffuse air-space disease, consistent with COVID-19 pneumonia. While arrangements for admission are taking place, you address her concerns regarding risks of antenatal or intrapartum transmission.

Special note:

† Refer to Question 3 in Chapter 73 for counseling and considerations related to chest radiography in pregnancy

8. Counsel the patient on the risk and assessment of vertical transmission of SARS-CoV-2 infection. *(1 point each)*	3

☐ While the <u>extent</u> of vertical transmission is yet unclear, rates of hematological spread in utero and ascending infection intrapartum are generally low[†]

☐ Reassure the patient that the risk of vertical transmission is not affected by mode of delivery or delayed cord-clamping

☐ Postnatal pathologic examination of the placenta and umbilical cord blood collection for SARS-CoV-2 testing by RT-PCR will be performed to assess for congenital infection (neonatal blood may be tested within 12 hours of life if umbilical cord blood collection is not performed)

Special note:

† Estimated risk of vertical transmission is about 3.2%: *refer to* Kotlyar AM, Grechukhina O, Chen A, et al. Vertical transmission of coronavirus disease 2019: a systematic review and meta-analysis. *Am J Obstet Gynecol.* 2021;224(1):35–53.e3

9. Address your trainee's inquiry on the <u>physiological bases</u> for the rarity of SARS-CoV-2 intrauterine transmission. *(1 point each)*	2

☐ There is negligible placental transcription of angiotensin-converting enzyme II (ACE2) receptor and transmembrane serine protease 2 (TMPRSS2) required for cell entry of SARS-CoV-2 virus[†]

☐ SARS-CoV-2 viremia is transient, thereby limiting the opportunity for placental involvement

Special note:

† This contrasts with viruses (*e.g.*, CMV, Zika) whose receptors are highly expressed by human placental tissues

The patient is reassured that fetal heart tracing remains normal. You explain that as recent fetal biometry, performed in the context of medical comorbidities, was normal, subsequent sonography will be arranged approximately two weeks after hospitalization or recovery from severe illness, unless a clinical reason develops for earlier imaging. At least daily fetal cardiotocographic surveillance is planned during hospitalization. Measures for safe prone positioning[†] at this advanced gestational age will be considered among the multidisciplinary team.

Significant laboratory findings at admission include C-reactive protein at 100 mg/L and lymphopenia; platelet count, prothrombin time, creatinine, and liver biochemistries remain within normal limits.

Special note:

† *Refer to* Tolcher MC, McKinney JR, Eppes CS, et al. Prone Positioning for Pregnant Women With Hypoxemia Due to Coronavirus Disease 2019 (COVID-19). *Obstet Gynecol.* 2020;136(2):259–261.

---

10. Based on interdisciplinary discussion, summarize to your trainee the <u>first-line pharmacologic</u> management for COVID-19 pneumonia in a hospitalized patient requiring oxygen supplementation in this gravida with known hypertension and obesity. *(1 point each)*

Max 5

☐ Oxygen supplementation will be provided to maintain a saturation at ≥95%

☐ Corticosteroids[†] are appropriate given the need of oxygen therapy: the standard 48-hour regimen of dexamethasone for fetal pulmonary maturity (*i.e.,* four doses of 6 mg intramuscularly 12 hours apart) may be followed by an eight-day course of a nonfluorinated corticosteroid such as methylprednisolone, hydrocortisone, or prednisone to limit fetal exposure; continuation of dexamethasone is also accepted given the short duration of exposure

☐ Strong consideration for tocilizumab[§] *[i.e., an interleukin-6 receptor antagonist]* as a single weight-based IV infusion given the patient's C-reactive protein is ≥75 mg/L *(RCOG[7])* or if acute inflammatory reaction

☐ Anticoagulation, preferably with low molecular weight heparin (LMWH), throughout the duration of hospitalization and at least until discharge; withhold therapy with COVID-19-associated thrombocytopenia $<50 \times 10^9$/L

☐ If the patient develops COVID-19-associated thrombocytopenia, withhold prophylactic aspirin as this may increase the risk of bleeding

☐ Nifedipine may be safely continued for management of chronic hypertension

Special notes:

† With diabetes mellitus, an evidence-based protocol for insulin dose adjustments after receipt of corticosteroids is presented in Question 9 of Chapter 58.

§ Improves outcomes, including survival, among admitted patients with hypoxia and evidence of systemic inflammation

---

Although the patient has not required intubation, spontaneous preterm labor commences on day 4 of admission, corresponding to 31^{+0} weeks' gestation. Electronic fetal heart tracing is appropriate for gestation and consistent with changes associated with recent receipt of fetal pulmonary corticosteroids.[†] Prophylactic anticoagulation is withheld, and cephalic presentation is assured. The patient remains on 5 L/min of oxygen by nasal prongs.

Being less than 32 weeks' gestation, a course of tocolysis[‡] is attempted, assuring the patient of no known contraindications to NSAIDs with SARS-CoV-2 infection, yet progression in labor continues. Vaginal-rectal group B *Streptococcus* swab, tested upon admission for potential risk of preterm labor, was negative. Absence of COVID-19-associated thrombocytopenia has been ensured. Interdisciplinary members in adult and neonatal medicine been informed.

Special notes:

† Refer to Question 25 in Chapter 38 for temporary maternal-fetal effects of fetal pulmonary corticosteroids.

‡ Choice of agent may vary by jurisdiction; refer to Question 5 in Chapter 7 for evidence-based tocolytic agents.

---

11. Detail important aspects of <u>intrapartum</u> management for this patient with active   Max 8
SARS-CoV-2 infection; infection control protocols are followed. *(1 point per main and subbullet)*

Maternal care:

☐ Plan for vaginal delivery *(Cesarean section is reserved for obstetric indications)*

☐ Advise epidural as the preferred pharmacologic intrapartum analgesia for benefits particular to this patient, including:
  ○ Decreased pain and anxiety-associated cardiopulmonary strain
  ○ The potential to obviate general anesthesia in case of an emergency Cesarean section

☐ Nitrous oxide gas is safe; provide a single-patient microbiological filter *(there is no evidence that Entonox is an aerosol-generating procedure, although local practice recommendations and variations exist)*

☐ Judicious use of intravenous fluid, with hourly monitoring of input-output aiming to maintain neutral intrapartum fluid balance

☐ Maintain oxygen saturation ≥95%, avoiding oxygen administration for fetal resuscitation[†]

☐ After appropriate counseling and with patient consent, consider immediate/postplacental placement of an intrauterine device (IUD),[‡] particularly since her routine in-person postpartum visit may be delayed

Fetal-neonatal care:

☐ Maintain continuous electronic fetal heart monitoring until delivery

☐ Individualized risk assessment regarding use of magnesium sulfate in this patient given the risk of maternal respiratory muscle weakness; if administered, consider a single 4 g intravenous bolus dose to obviate risks of continued infusion

☐ Obtain umbilical cord blood to test for congenital SARS-CoV-2 infection

Special notes:

† Refer to Question 14 in Chapter 15

‡ Provide resources for initiation of other contraceptive options *prior* to hospital discharge, including DMPA injection, insertion of subdermal implants, or progesterone-oral contraception

---

Preterm labor and vaginal delivery ensue; maternal needs for oxygen supplementation range from 2 to 4 L/min. Birthweight is appropriate for gestational age, umbilical arterial cord blood pH is 7.22, and testing for congenital SARS-CoV-2 is negative by umbilical cord blood. The placenta, umbilical cord and chorioamniotic membranes have been sent for pathological assessment. The premature newborn is admitted to the neonatal intensive care unit (NICU).

12. Outline aspects of <u>in-hospital postpartum management</u> considerations for *this* patient with active SARS-CoV-2 infection; infection control protocols are followed. *(1 point each)*   10

General maternal well-being:
- ☐ Continue to offer psychosocial and social work support for recent gestational complications and prematurity
- ☐ Continue oral antihypertensive treatment (*i.e.,* nifedipine), and observe for risk of postpartum onset of hypertensive disease of pregnancy
- ☐ Plan telehealth visit(s) prior to hospital discharge, maintaining vigilance to screen for postpartum depression

Postpartum analgesic considerations:
- ☐ Reassure the patient that NSAIDs and acetaminophen/paracetamol can be used among women with COVID-19
- ☐ Exercise caution with opioid analgesia due to risk of respiratory depression

Thromboprophylaxis:
- ☐ Consider resuming LMWH postpartum for at least 10 days following hospital discharge (*RCOG[7]*)
- ☐ Encourage oral hydration and ambulation when possible

Breastfeeding:
- ☐ Reassure the patient that the risk of SARS-CoV-2 transmission via breastfeeding/pumping is exceedingly low *(pumps should be cleaned by healthy individuals)*
- ☐ Encourage the patient to wear a mask and maintain hand hygiene when in contact with the newborn; breast hygiene is encouraged, despite unproven efficacy

Contraceptive recommendations:
- ☐ If postplacental intrauterine device is deferred, offer initiation of DMPA if the patient desires reliable contraception (in-person postpartum visit may be delayed)

<u>**TOTAL:**</u>   **85**

Malignant Conditions in Pregnancy

CHAPTER 70

Breast Cancer in Pregnancy

Nathaniel Bouganim and Amira El-Messidi

A 32-year-old primigravida at 16^{+1} weeks' gestation is referred by her primary care provider to your high-risk obstetrics unit at a tertiary center for evaluation of a breast lump. Routine prenatal investigations, fetal sonography, and aneuploidy screening were normal. The patient does not have any obstetric complaints and takes only prenatal vitamins.

LEARNING OBJECTIVES

1. Elicit salient points on prenatal history, and initiate diagnostic evaluation of a breast mass in pregnancy
2. Troubleshoot misconceptions related to staging investigations, including mammography and sentinel node biopsy, in pregnancy
3. Understand the importance of multidisciplinary collaboration for counseling on maternal-fetal risks and discussion of treatment options for newly diagnosed breast cancer at various stages of pregnancy
4. Recognize recommended breast cancer treatments with reassuring safety profile in pregnancy, and appreciate the need to delay specific endocrine agents to the postpartum period
5. Formulate a safe plan for delivery of a patient with active gestational breast cancer
6. Discuss relevant postpartum aspects of care for patients with active breast cancer

SUGGESTED READINGS

1. Amant F, Deckers S, Van Calsteren K, et al. Breast cancer in pregnancy: recommendations of an international consensus meeting. *Eur J Cancer*. 2010;46(18):3158–3168.
2. Amant F, Han SN, Gziri MM, et al. Management of cancer in pregnancy. *Best Pract Res Clin Obstet Gynaecol*. 2015;29(5):741–753.
3. Azim HA Jr, Santoro L, Pavlidis N, et al. Safety of pregnancy following breast cancer diagnosis: a meta-analysis of 14 studies. *Eur J Cancer*. 2011;47(1):74–83.
4. Case AS. Pregnancy-associated breast cancer. *Clin Obstet Gynecol*. 2016;59(4):779–788.
5. Macdonald HR. Pregnancy associated breast cancer. *Breast J*. 2020;26(1):81–85.
6. Martínez MT, Bermejo B, Hernando C, et al. Breast cancer in pregnant patients: A review of the literature. *Eur J Obstet Gynecol Reprod Biol*. 2018; 230:222–227.
7. Paris I, Di Giorgio D, Carbognin L, et al. Pregnancy-associated breast cancer: a multidisciplinary approach. *Clin Breast Cancer*. 2020;S1526–8209(20):30173–30177.

8. Royal College of Obstetricians and Gynaecologists (RCOG). *Pregnancy and breast cancer. Green-Top Guideline No. 12*. London: RCOG; 2011.

9. Shachar SS, Gallagher K, McGuire K, et al. Multidisciplinary management of breast cancer during pregnancy. *Oncologist*. 2017;22(3):324–334. [Correction in Oncologist. 2018 Jun;23(6):746]

POINTS

1. What aspects of a focused history would you want to know? *(1 point each)*   Max 14

Details of the breast mass:
- ☐ Onset and change in size
- ☐ Laterality *(i.e., unilateral/bilateral)*
- ☐ Location of the mass *(i.e., axillary, relation to the nipple)*
- ☐ Pain/tenderness
- ☐ Skin or nipple changes

Systemic manifestations:
- ☐ Fever
- ☐ Night sweats
- ☐ Weight loss
- ☐ Malaise
- ☐ Bone pains

Personal medical and gynecological history:[†]
- ☐ Past use of combined hormonal contraception, and duration of use
- ☐ Hormonal assisted reproductive technology
- ☐ Past personal malignancy, breast biopsy, mammography

Family history:
- ☐ Breast or ovarian cancer
- ☐ BRCA-1 or BRCA-2 mutated oncogenes

Social history:
- ☐ Smoking and/or alcohol consumption

Special note:
- † Nulliparity and lack of prior breastfeeding would be additional risk factors to elicit on history if patient were a multigravida

Incidentally, the patient noticed a small left breast lump three weeks ago, doubling in size over two weeks.[†] She has not noted any skin changes, nipple discharge, or axillary masses. Apart from pains in her back and hip bones, which she considered to accompany general malaise of pregnancy, she has not had other systemic symptoms. The patient is heathy and does not drink alcohol or smoke. She used the copper IUD for the first five years of marriage and conceived spontaneously shortly after its discontinuation. She has never used hormonal contraception and family history is negative for breast-ovarian malignancies or oncogenes.

Examination is significant for a medial, nontender fixed lump. There are no other abnormalities on breast, nodal, or abdominal examinations. Fetal viability is ascertained.

Special note:

† Any mass present for more than two weeks warrants investigation

---

SCENARIO A

You arrange for an urgent breast ultrasound on the day of primary consultation; the radiologist notifies you of a 1.6-cm unilateral solid, vascularized mass at the 5 o'clock position of the left breast. No axillary lymphadenopathy is present.

---

2. Specify the diagnostic procedure you anticipate will be performed during her breast sonography.   1

☐ Core needle biopsy for histology (with local anesthesia)

Special note:

Fine needle aspiration may be misleading and should not be performed in pregnancy; cytological assessment may be unreliable due to gestational proliferative changes

---

Five days later, at 16^{+6} weeks' gestation, the patient's breast biopsy confirms high-grade, poorly differentiated, infiltrating ductal adenocarcinoma with estrogen, progesterone and human epidermal growth factor receptor-2 (HER-2) positivity. You arrange for an urgent meeting with the patient and her husband, in collaboration with an oncologist. Genetic consultation has been arranged. With the prospect of mammographic evaluation, the couple are concerned about fetal radiation exposure; they inquire about the possibility of MRI as a diagnostic alternative in evaluation of gestational breast cancer.

---

3. Discuss the rationale and safety of mammography during pregnancy. *(1 point per main bullet)*   3

Mammography, two views:§
☐ Serves to assess the extent of disease and evaluate the contralateral breast (sensitivity is ~86% in pregnancy)
☐ Reassure the couple that fetal radiation exposure is considered to be *'very low-dose'* *(<0.1 mGy)*, with average fetal radiation at 0.001–0.01 mGy†
☐ Fetal risks of anomalies, FGR, or pregnancy loss require at least 50 mGy (5 rads) of exposure
☐ Severe intellectual disability due to in utero radiation exposure generally requires 60–310 mGy (6–31 rads), and appears mostly at 8–15 weeks' gestation
☐ Risk of carcinogenesis with diagnostic radiation is also very small *(does not influence pregnancy management decisions)*

Special note:

§ Routine abdominal shielding should be avoided in imaging modalities where ionizing radiation does not directly expose the fetus because (1) most of the fetal dose results from internal (rather than external) scatter, and (2) automatic control can cause increased dose exposure if the shield is inadvertently in the field of view during the scan. Abdominal shielding may be considered on a case by case basis if it offers patient reassurance after appropriate counselling.

† *Guidelines for diagnostic imaging during pregnancy and lactation, ACOG Committee Opinion, Oct 2017; 130(4): e210–16*

4. Identify features of breast physiology accounting for the lower sensitivity of mammograms in pregnancy. *(1 point each)*   4

☐ Increased breast density
☐ Increased water content
☐ Greater vascularity
☐ Decreased adiposity

5. In collaboration with the oncologist, indicate the limitations of screening MRI in evaluation of gestational breast cancer. *(1 point each)*   2

☐ Fetal risks with gadolinium exposure limit the applicability of MRI in pregnancy[†]
☐ Interpretation of images may be challenging in pregnancy

Special note:
† Refer to Question 10 in Chapter 42 for discussion on safety of MRI pregnancy- and gadolinium-associated fetal risks

The couple appreciates the reassurance and evidence-based counseling regarding mammography and the patient provides consent. The oncologist informs the patient that a chest X-ray,[‡] liver ultrasound and skeletal MRI are required for staging evaluation of her gestational breast carcinoma. The oncologist specifies that evaluation of bone metastases would have been deferred to the postpartum period in the absence of her bone pains. Reassuringly, he or she indicates that skeletal MRI does not require contrast.

In the advent of uncertain MRI results, the patient's husband asks about the safety of bone scans in pregnancy.

Special note:
‡ Refer to Chapter 73 for discussion of fetal exposure to ionizing radiation from chest X-ray

6. Outline obstetric considerations with serum markers and bone scans during the prenatal evaluation of bone metastases. *(1 point per main bullet, unless specified)*   Max 4

☐ Interpretation of serum alkaline phosphatase in pregnancy is confounded by placental production, limiting its value as a marker of bone metastases
☐ Reassure the patient that a 'low dose' radionuclide bone scan is safe in pregnancy *(fetal radiation exposure can be a little as 0.08 rads relative to standard 0.19 rad for a conventional bone scan)*
☐ Precautions for reduction of fetal radiation exposure during bone scans: **(1 point per subbullet; max 3)**
  ○ Injecting a lower tracer dose *(e.g., 10 mCi rather than 20 mCi of Technitium-99m [Tc-99m] methylene diphosphonate)*
  ○ Doubling image acquisition time
  ○ Intravenous maternal hydration to promote washout of the radiopharmaceutical agent
  ○ Foley catheter/promote frequent voiding

Although the couple prefer to continue pregnancy, they intend to follow recommendations in favor of optimal maternal treatment and cure.

7. Provide important aspects of counseling on the relationship between pregnancy and active breast cancer. *(1 point each)*	3

☐ Pregnancy itself does not appear to worsen the prognosis of gestational breast cancer where *treatment delays are avoided*
☐ Excluding treatment, breast cancer does not adversely affect perinatal outcome
☐ Termination of pregnancy does not appear to provide a survival advantage with gestational breast cancer, and is based on personal preferences

8. In collaboration with the oncologist, detail the options for <u>locoregional treatment</u> of this patient's gestational breast cancer. *(1 point per main bullet)*	Max 6

Breast surgery:
☐ Reassure the patient of minimal fetal risk throughout all trimesters, and inform her that fetal viability is routinely documented pre and postsurgery
  ○ Considerations for preoperative corticosteroids for lung maturity and intraoperative fetal monitoring and where surgery is performed $\geq\sim24$ weeks' gestation
  ○ Considerations for left lateral tilt, as necessary
☐ Inform the patient of the therapeutic equivalence of breast-conserving surgery (lumpectomy with postpartum radiotherapy) or mastectomy despite pregnancy
  ○ Where breast reconstruction is needed, consider postpartum delay to adjust for antenatal physiologic alterations and avoid risks of surgical complications that would delay postoperative chemotherapy
☐ Address the safety of general anesthesia and postoperative narcotic analgesia (*consultation with an anesthesiologist*)
  ○ Consideration for postoperative uterine tocometry as analgesia may mask awareness of mild early contractions
☐ Advise thromboprophylaxis given multiple risk factors for thromboembolism, including pregnancy, malignancy and surgery

Sentinel node biopsy and/or axillary lymph node dissection:
☐ Reassure the patient that Tc-99m sulfur colloid[†] remains at the injection site and within local lymphatics, without fetal exposure

Radiotherapy:
☐ Contraindicated during pregnancy, despite fetal shielding
  ○ *Growing abdomen will inadvertently increase fetal exposure*

Special note:
† Avoid blue dyes for sentinel node mapping in pregnancy

The patient opts for breast conserving treatment during pregnancy with postoperative radiotherapy; timely arrangements have been made for preoperative surgical evaluation.

Given her tumor biology, she wishes to discuss the possible need of systemic therapy in the antepartum or postpartum period. The oncologist recommends collaborating with you for planning of concurrent doxorubicin[§] and cyclophosphamide followed by paclitaxel, in equivalent doses as nonpregnant patients and adjusted to actual weight in pregnancy.[†‡] Trastuzumab and tamoxifen can only be administered after delivery.

Special notes:
§ Maternal echocardiography is required prior to anthracycline therapy;[†]refer to Chapter 73
‡ Chemotherapy with 5-fluorouricil, doxorubicin, cyclophosphamide is an alternative regimen during pregnancy; first-trimester chemotherapy is contraindicated for breast cancer

9. Based on maternal physiology and drug pharmacokinetics, justify the need to configure chemotherapy doses to changing body surface area during pregnancy. *(1 point each)*	Max 3

- ☐ Increased blood volume
- ☐ Increased renal clearance
- ☐ Increased hepatic metabolism
- ☐ Increased amount of unbound treatment drug *(due to decreased serum albumin)*
- ☐ Fetus and amniotic fluid act as a third space, sequestering chemotherapeutics from the mother *(variations in transplacental passage among different agents)*

10. Regarding the chosen chemotherapy, discuss your counseling in relation to obstetric antenatal management and delivery considerations. *(1 point per main bullet, unless specified)*	Max 7

- ☐ Reassure the patient that risks of congenital malformations are not increased with second- or third-trimester doxorubicin, cyclophosphamide, or paclitaxel (***additional point per subbullet***)
  - ○ Perinatal adverse effects of cytotoxic chemotherapy in the second and third trimesters include fetal growth restriction (FGR), low birthweight, preterm labor, and suppression of fetal hematopoiesis
  - ○ Arrange for monthly fetal growth assessments after the routine fetal morphology survey
  - ○ Generally, reassuring long-term infant outcome after in utero exposure to chemotherapy
- ☐ In collaboration with her oncologist, continue chemotherapy until ~34–35 weeks' gestation and arrange for induction of labor in 3 weeks
  - ○ *Three-weeks treatment-delivery interval avoids the period of fetal neutropenia*
  - ○ *Cesarean section is reserved for obstetric indications*
- ☐ Where possible, avoid iatrogenic preterm delivery
  - ○ *Preterm infants cannot metabolize chemotherapy as can term infants*
- ☐ Antenatal consultation with neonatology experts
- ☐ Ensure placental examination is arranged, as for all gestational cancers irrespective of type and/or treatment

Special note:
Unrelated to chemotherapy, suggest consideration for antepartum and postpartum thromboprophylaxis given active malignancy

11. Your obstetric trainee is curious why the oncologist recommends delayed trastuzumab and tamoxifen therapy until after delivery, and whether this reduces overall treatment efficacy. *(1 point per main bullet)*

Max 4

☐ Reassure the trainee and/or patient that delaying biologic and hormonal agents to the postpartum period does ***not*** reduce treatment efficacy

Trastuzumab: *(monoclonal antibody against HER-2 protein)*
☐ Contraindicated in pregnancy[†] and breastfeeding
☐ Dose-related risks of anhydramnios/oligohydramnios or oligohydramnios-sequence *(skeletal abnormalities, pulmonary hypoplasia, and neonatal demise)*
  ○ Mechanisms for fetopathy may be due strong expression of HER-2/*neu* in renal epithelium or trastuzumab-induced inhibition of vascular endothelial growth factor (VEGF)

Tamoxifen: *(selective estrogen receptor modulator)*
☐ Contraindicated in pregnancy and breastfeeding[‡]
☐ No *specific* pattern of birth defects
  ○ Known associations with Goldenhar syndrome (oculoauriculovertebral dysplasia), Pierre–Robin sequence (small mandible, cleft palate and glossoptosis), ambiguous genitalia, and IUFD

Special notes:
† Advise against conception within seven months of trastuzumab treatment
‡ Also advise against breastfeeding for three months after discontinuation of tamoxifen

Timely comprehensive serum and radiological investigations are performed, and the patient agrees to perinatal psychosocial support services. At 17^{+5} weeks' gestation, a left-sided lumpectomy with sentinel node dissection is performed. The tumor is excised in its entirety and axillary nodes are negative.

Postoperative recovery is uneventful, and the first cycle of doxorubicin-cyclophosphamide is started six weeks later. The remainder of pregnancy proceeds uneventfully with multidisciplinary care; labor is induced at 37 weeks' gestation, corresponding to 3 weeks after chemotherapy. She has an uncomplicated vaginal delivery of a vigorous neonate weighing 2890 g.

12. Outline important postpartum considerations in the care of this patient with <u>active</u> breast cancer. *(1 point per main bullet, unless specified)*

Max 6

☐ Screen for postpartum depression and continue to offer psychosocial support; encourage maternal-neonatal bonding *(particularly given inability to breastfeed)*

☐ Consideration for bromocriptine or cabergoline for primary inhibition of milk production

☐ With postpartum continuation of chemotherapy, an interval of a few days after a vaginal delivery is advised; after an uncomplicated Cesarean section, an interval of one week is appropriate *(Suggested Reading 2)*

☐ Advise against pregnancy for at least two years after completion of treatment

☐ Contraception: *(1 point per subbullet)*
  ○ Hormonal agents (combined methods or progesterone-only) are contraindicated, ***regardless of estrogen and progesterone receptor status***
  ○ Copper IUDs, or other nonhormonal methods, are safe

☐ Reassure the patient that subsequent pregnancy in breast cancer survivors does not worsen overall survival and may confer a protective effect

SCENARIO B

During her urgent breast ultrasound at 16^{+1} weeks' gestation, the radiologist notifies you of a left-sided 5.6-cm unilateral solid, vascularized mass abutting the pectoralis muscle with ipsilateral axillary adenopathy.

Core needle biopsy is consistent with poorly differentiated infiltrating ductal adenocarcinoma, *negative* for estrogen and progesterone receptors, with HER-2-positive status. You mention to your obstetric trainee that most pregnancy-associated breast cancers are indeed negative for estrogen and progesterone receptors, which he or she finds counterintuitive.

13. Based on tumor characteristics and biology, outline management differences, *if any*, from the patient in scenario A, assuming the patient chooses pregnancy continuation. *(1 point per main bullet)*

Max 3

☐ Initiation of neoadjuvant chemotherapy for approximately six months' duration
  ○ *Similar regimens as in scenario A*
  ○ *Similar treatment-delivery interval considerations as in scenario A*

☐ Surgery postchemotherapy (*i.e.*, postpartum), followed by radiotherapy

☐ Trastuzumab is reserved for the postpartum period given HER-2 positivity

☐ Tamoxifen is not indicated in hormone-negative tumors

14. Despite increased hormone levels in pregnancy, provide a rationale for why gestational breast cancers are more commonly negative for estrogen and progesterone receptors.

5

☐ <u>Mammary</u> tissue downregulation of estrogen and progesterone receptors is among pregnancy-related breast changes; high hormonal levels during pregnancy may promote carcinomas by acting on <u>stromal</u> rather than mammary tissue

TOTAL: 65

CHAPTER 71

Cervical Cancer in Pregnancy

Oded Raban, Amira El-Messidi, and Walter H. Gotlieb

You are covering an obstetrics clinic for your colleague, who left for vacation last week. A *healthy* 32-year-old primigravida at 13^{+4} weeks' gestation called for an emergency appointment after experiencing two episodes of postcoital bleeding over the past week. She met your colleague last week at her first prenatal visit, which was unremarkable. Sonographic dating was appropriate for menstrual age, and first-trimester fetal anatomy was normal. You note that all routine prenatal serum laboratory investigations are normal with low-risk screening tests for fetal aneuploidy. Without a cervical smear in over two years, cytology was performed, and results are expected shortly.

Special note: *'Papanicolau smear,' a commonly used terminology in North America, is the equivalent of 'cervical smear test,' used in the United Kingdom.*

LEARNING OBJECTIVES

1. Elicit salient points on history of a prenatal patient with new-onset postcoital bleeding, and be able to conduct a focused physical examination, recognizing the risk of cervical carcinoma
2. Recognize the need for, and particularities with, colposcopic assessment in pregnancy
3. Collaborate with gynecologic oncologists in the diagnostic evaluation and management of various stages of cervical cancer in pregnancy
4. Participate in counseling of patients diagnosed with cervical cancer during pregnancy, recognizing critical issues for delivery recommendations

SUGGESTED READINGS

1. Amant F, Berveiller P, Boere IA, et al. Gynecologic cancers in pregnancy: guidelines based on a third international consensus meeting. *Ann Oncol.* 2019;30(10):1601–1612.
2. Beharee N, Shi Z, Wu D, et al. Diagnosis and treatment of cervical cancer in pregnant women. *Cancer Med.* 2019;8(12):5425–5430.
3. Bigelow CA, Horowitz NS, Goodman A, et al. Management and outcome of cervical cancer diagnosed in pregnancy. *Am J Obstet Gynecol.* 2017;216(3): 276.e1–276.e6.
4. Cordeiro CN, Gemignani ML. Gynecologic malignancies in pregnancy: balancing fetal risks with oncologic safety. *Obstet Gynecol Surv.* 2017;72(3):184–193.

5. de Haan J, Verheecke M, Van Calsteren K, et al. Oncological management and obstetric and neonatal outcomes for women diagnosed with cancer during pregnancy: a 20-year international cohort study of 1170 patients. *Lancet Oncol.* 2018;19(3):337–346.

6. Hecking T, Abramian A, Domröse C, et al. Individual management of cervical cancer in pregnancy. *Arch Gynecol Obstet.* 2016;293(5):931–939.

7. Hunter MI, Tewari K, Monk BJ. Cervical neoplasia in pregnancy. Part 2: current treatment of invasive disease. *Am J Obstet Gynecol.* 2008;199(1):10–18.

8. Korenaga TK, Tewari KS. Gynecologic cancer in pregnancy. *Gynecol Oncol.* 2020;157(3): 799–809.

9. Perrone AM, Bovicelli A, D'Andrilli G, et al. Cervical cancer in pregnancy: analysis of the literature and innovative approaches. *J Cell Physiol.* 2019;234(9):14975–14990.

10. Yoshihara K, Ishiguro T, Chihara M, et al. The safety and effectiveness of abdominal radical trachelectomy for early-stage cervical cancer during pregnancy. *Int J Gynecol Cancer.* 2018;28(4):782–787.

POINTS

1. With respect to her postcoital bleeding, what aspects of a <u>focused</u> history would you want to know? *(1 point each unless specified; max points indicated where applicable)*   Max 15

History related to postcoital bleeding and related manifestations: *(max 8)*
☐ Patient's Rh status *(3 points)*
☐ Description, including color and amount of bleeding
☐ Presence of lower abdominal cramps or 'fetal' tissue loss
☐ Signs or symptoms of anemia *(e.g.,* dizziness, palor, fatigue, dyspnea)
☐ Bleeding from other bodily sites
☐ History of prior postcoital bleeding, or abnormal uterine bleeding
☐ Current/recent abnormal vaginal discharge
☐ Pelvic, flank, sciatic-type pain

Gynecologic and sexual history: *(max 4)*
☐ Time interval since prior known Papanicolau smear result *(i.e.,* cervical smear test)
☐ History of cervical dysplasia or malignancy
☐ Prior HPV *(human papillomavirus)* vaccination
☐ Prior sexually transmitted infections (STIs) *(including herpes simplex virus, trichomonas, chlamydia, gonorrhea, syphilis)*
☐ Current and prior lifetime sexual partners
☐ History of exchanging sex for money *(i.e.,* prostitution)

Systemic symptoms:
☐ Fever/chills
☐ Night sweats
☐ Weight loss *(overlap with early pregnancy)*

Medications:
☐ Current use of anticoagulants

Social history:
☐ Cigarette smoking, alcohol consumption, illicit substance use

The patient describes new-onset postcoital bright red blood that filled half a sanitary napkin over several hours without accompanying abnormal discharge, abdominal, pelvic or flank pain. Localized to the vagina, bleeding does not recur spontaneously; she has never experienced similar events. You confirm her blood group is B-positive. She has not noticed fetal tissue loss, although is concerned over the well-being of her pregnancy, as she and her husband are excited with this spontaneous conception after two years of marriage. Your screening questions for systemic symptoms of anemia are negative and she has not had chills, night sweats, or weight loss. The patient does not smoke, use illicit drugs, and she discontinued social alcohol consumption since conception. Apart from prenatal vitamins, she does not take other medications or medicinals.

Prior to her Papanicolau smear (*i.e.*, cervical smear test) performed by your colleague, her previous was normal, taken four years ago. She has a remote history of abnormal cervical cytology that spontaneously normalized. She never received HPV vaccination. The patient recalls approximately five lifetime consensual sexual partners prior to marriage, and never experienced pelvic infections.

2. <u>Detail</u> your focused physical examination. *(1 point per main bullet, unless specified)*   Max 10

- □ Vital signs: blood pressure, pulse, respiratory rate, oxygen saturation, and temperature
- □ Current or most recent BMI
- □ Cardiopulmonary auscultation *(particularly for pulmonary effusions)*
- □ Nodal assessment: cervical, supraclavicular, axillary, and inguinal
- □ Abdominal mass, tenderness, organomegaly
- □ Ascertainment of fetal viability by Doptone or bedside sonography *(2 points)*
- □ Leg edema
- □ Speculum: *(1 point per subbullet)*
  - ○ Assess the cervix and vagina for source of bleeding
  - ○ Inspect for cervical dilation
  - ○ Assess for abnormal-appearing cervical discharge
- □ Vaginal-rectal assessment: *(1 point per subbullet)*
  - ○ Cervical size and mobility
  - ○ Obliteration of the vaginal fornices and parametrial involvement

The patient's body habitus and vital signs are normal. Examination is significant for an enlarged-bulky cervix, without a distinct mass. You suspect an ectropion on the anterior lip with remnant bleeding. The cervix appears closed and long. The surrounding vaginal mucosa appears normal. On bimanual vaginal-rectal examination, the cervix is mobile but irregular with normal vaginal fornices and parametria. Abdominal assessment is normal. The fetus is viable, without a subchorionic hematoma detected at bedside sonography.

Upon completion of the physical examination, your assistant informs you of the screening cervical cytology indicating high-grade squamous intraepithelial lesion (HSIL).

3. Refresh your obstetric trainee's memory of three pregnancy-associated cervical changes that may incur challenges to the suspicion or diagnosis of cervical neoplasia. *(1 point each)*

 □ Ectropion (migration of the squamocolumnar junction)
 □ Cervical decidualization
 □ Increased cervical volume *(due to hyperestrogenism)*
 □ Hypervascularity *(producing a 'blue' hue)*
 □ Stromal edema *(mostly in second and third trimesters)*
 □ (Frequent) inflammation

Max 3

4. After informing the patient of your results, and sharing your concerns, what is the immediate best next step in management?

 □ Referral to a colposcopist/gynecologic oncologist

1

The following day, at 13^{+5} weeks' gestation, colposcopy reveals an area of aceto-white epithelium on the anterior cervical lip with abnormal vessels and an irregular contour.

5. Discuss the required diagnostic procedure of choice and indicate elements of the assessment which would be deferred during colposcopic assessment in the prenatal period. *(1 point per main bullet)*

 □ *Targeted* cervical biopsies of the most suspicious lesions (random biopsies are avoided in pregnancy due to hypervascularity)
  ○ Depth of biopsy specimens is preferably <1 cm
  ○ No increased rate of early pregnancy loss or preterm delivery
 □ Endocervical curettage should <u>not</u> be performed during pregnancy
  ○ Endocervical canal can be *gently* sampled with a cytobrush

2

Within 48 hours, results of directed cervical biopsies reveal squamous cell carcinoma.

A gynecologic oncologist practicing in your tertiary center calls you to discuss the management and plan his or her consultation visit with the patient.

6. After informing the patient of the biopsy results, what is the next best step recommended by the gynecologic oncologist for this obstetric patient?

 □ Cervical conization, 'coinization,'† or cone-cerclage
  ○ *Ideally performed at 14–20 weeks' gestation*

3

Special note:
† Coinization refers to a coin-shaped specimen to limit disruption of endocervical tissue; facilitated by pregnancy-related eversion of squamocolumnar junction

7. Detail the most significant risks of conization during pregnancy, which will be disclosed during patient counseling and consent. *(1 point each)*   6

☐   Hemorrhage >500 mL *(risks of bleeding increase with gestational age and with amount of tissue removed; minimal in first trimester, ~5% in second trimester, and up to 10% in third trimester)*
☐   Miscarriage or pregnancy loss in the second trimester
☐   Preterm prelabor rupture of membranes (PPROM)
☐   Preterm labor and preterm delivery
☐   Cervical laceration at vaginal delivery
☐   Infection

SCENARIO A
(microinvasive squamous carcinoma)

After patient counseling and with consent, a conization-cerclage is performed at 14^{+3} weeks' gestation. The procedure was uncomplicated, and the patient is recovering well.

Within one week, the pathology report shows squamous cell carcinoma with 2 mm stromal invasion and absence of lymphovascular space invasion.

8. Based on the International Federation of Gynecology and Obstetrics (FIGO) 2018 staging system, identify the patient's stage and indicate recommendations for subsequent management in pregnancy in relation to malignancy. *(1 point per main bullet)*   3

☐   Stage 1A1 (microinvasive squamous carcinoma)[†]
☐   Inform the patient she is cured with no impact on her survival
    ○   *Rate of lymph node metastasis is <1% (i.e., ~0.6%)*
☐   Important prenatal considerations include compliance with follow-up and adherence to serial physical examinations (*e.g.*, monthly) and colposcopic assessment at 12 weeks postpartum
    ○   *Routine care regarding patient's cerclage[‡]*

Special notes:
[†] Conservative management is advised for this patient given microinvasive *squamous* cell pathology; however, microinvasive *adenocarcinoma* is more frequently multifocal with 'skip' lesions contributing to misleading interpretation of margin status
[‡] Refer to Chapter 8

9. Address the recommended timing and mode of delivery for microinvasive squamous carcinoma of the cervix.   1

☐   Vaginal delivery at term

SCENARIO B
(invasive squamous carcinoma)
This is a continuation of the clinical scenario after Question 7)
After patient counseling and with consent, a conization-cerclage is performed at 14^{+3} weeks' gestation. The procedure was uncomplicated, and the patient is recovering well.

At 15^{+0} weeks' gestation, the pathology report shows poorly differentiated invasive squamous cell carcinoma with 7 mm stromal invasion and positive tumor margins. A multidisciplinary meeting is arranged in the presence of the patient and her husband.

10. Excluding yourself as an obstetrician (general practice) and her gynecologic oncologist, identify four experts from interdisciplinary fields in attendance at this meeting. *(1 point each)*   4

☐ Maternal-fetal medicine
☐ Radiation oncology
☐ Medical oncology
☐ Neonatologist
☐ Psychosocial/spiritual therapist
☐ Social worker

11. Prior to the meeting, you take this opportunity to inform your obstetric trainee of general criteria for consideration in discussion of her antenatal management for invasive cervical cancer. *(1 point each)*   4

☐ Pelvic lymph node status (an important prognostic feature for cervical cancer)/overall FIGO stage
☐ Gestational age *(i.e., whether the patient is less than or over 22 weeks)*
☐ Histologic subtype *(e.g., small cell carcinoma is associated with worse prognosis)*
☐ Patient's preference for pregnancy continuation or termination

12. In collaboration with the oncology experts, inform the patient of the effect of pregnancy on the newly diagnosed cervical cancer. *(1 point each)*   Max 2

☐ Tumor characteristics and maternal survival are not adversely affected by pregnancy
☐ Reassure the patient that in fact, screening cytology performed at her first prenatal visit contributed to earlier diagnosis
☐ Stage for stage, course of disease and prognosis is comparable to nonpregnant patients if the pregnant patient receives timely standard treatment

Reassured that pregnancy will not affect the disease stage, progression, or long-term prognosis, she understands you will address the potential effects of malignancy on pregnancy once the stage of the disease is established, as this will determine options for pregnancy management.

13. Outline the <u>imaging procedures of choice</u> discussed with the patient for staging of cervical cancer in pregnancy? *(1 point each)*	2

☐ Chest X-ray[†] *(to evaluate for possible lung metastases)*
☐ MRI[‡] of the abdomen and pelvis, without gadolinium contrast

Special notes:
† Refer to Question 3 in Chapter 73 for discussion of safety and risks related to fetal exposure to ionizing radiation from chest radiography
‡ Refer to Question 10 in Chapter 42 for discussion of safety of MRI in pregnancy and gadolinium-associated fetal risks

14. In addition to the known safety profile of antenatal MRI (without gadolinium), your trainee asks you to illustrate the technical advantages of MRI in evaluating cervical cancer during pregnancy. *(1 point each)*	Max 3

☐ Allows for calculation of tumor volume
☐ Assess tumor spread to adjacent organs and lymph nodes
☐ Assess dilatation of the renal collecting system
☐ Provides excellent tissue contrast

15. Noticing the oncologist did not mention positron emission tomography (PET) for the patient's staging evaluation, address her husband's inquiry regarding its prenatal considerations. *(2 points for main bullet)*	2

PET scan:
☐ Radioactive sugar tracer, FDG (fluorine-18-fluorodeoxyglucose) is taken up by the fetus; no additive role in this patient's evaluation although not contraindicated in pregnancy
　○ When performed during pregnancy to evaluate organ function and disease spread, FDG-dose reduction to 5 mCi is advised to decrease fetal exposure *(Suggested Reading 8)*

At 15^{+2} weeks' gestation, the patient undergoes an MRI of the abdomen and pelvis which demonstrates a 1.0×1.2 cm, cervical tumor without prominent lymphadenopathy, hydroureters or suspected parametrial involvement. As planned, a follow-up multidisciplinary encounter including the patient and her supportive husband, takes place the following day.

The patient has not had obstetric complaints. Complete investigations for fetal aneuploidy screening are unremarkable. Fetal viability is ascertained. Prior to commencing the meeting, the patient voices that she aspires to continue pregnancy and is open to recommended management to optimize outcomes for the unborn child.

16. In relation to the 2018 FIGO staging system for cervical cancer, indicate the gynecologic oncologist's stated <u>critical next best step</u>, as the patient is less than 22 weeks' gestation.

Stage 1B1[†]

☐ Retroperitoneal pelvic lymph node dissection
  ○ Laparoscopy can be used, preferably up to 16 weeks' gestation, thereafter laparotomy is feasible until 22 weeks' gestation *(Suggested Reading 1)*

Special note:
† Implies *invasive cancer >5 mm deep of stromal invasion and ≤2 cm in greatest dimension*

17. Discuss how results of pelvic lymph node dissection will be valuable in management considerations for this obstetric patient. *(1 point per main bullet)*

Negative pelvic lymph node dissection:

☐ Large conization *versus* simple trachelectomy can be performed during pregnancy aiming for negative margins, with concurrent cerclage placement
  ○ *Radical* trachelectomy is **not** recommended, given increased bleeding and pregnancy loss
☐ If the patient desires to defer simple trachelectomy, neoadjuvant chemotherapy to be offered and the standard of care will be delayed until delivery knowing that this can potentially impact her prognosis
  ○ Radical hysterectomy can be performed at time of delivery or as a second procedure

Positive pelvic lymph node dissection:

☐ Pregnancy termination is advised, and subsequent standard treatment outside pregnancy
☐ If pregnancy termination is declined, neoadjuvant chemotherapy can be used during the antenatal period with postpartum chemoradiation or radical hysterectomy *(European Society of Medical Oncology [ESMO]*[§]*)*

Special note:
§ *Refer to* Peccatori FA, et al. Cancer, pregnancy and fertility: ESMO Clinical Practice Guidelines for diagnosis, treatment and follow-up. *Ann Oncol.* 2013;24 Suppl 6:vi160-vi170.

18. Your obstetric trainee recalls learning that sentinel node biopsy and axillary node dissection do not pose fetal risk at surgery for *breast* cancer during pregnancy.[†] Address his or her inquiry about recommendations for sentinel node mapping for cervical cancer.

☐ Sentinel node mapping using radioactive materials is <u>contraindicated</u> for cervical cancer in pregnancy *(Suggested Reading 1)*
  ○ Although indocyanine green is experimental, its use is safe; superiority to the blue dye has been shown in well-designed studies
  ○ Blue dye incurs risk of anaphylactic reactions

Special note:
† *Refer to* Question 8 in Chapter 70

Laparoscopic pelvic lymphadenectomy is arranged within the next few days. Principles of laparoscopy in pregnancy[‡] will be followed, and pre- and postoperative fetal viability will be documented.

Feeling 'lucky' for early detection of cervical malignancy in pregnancy, the patient is keen to know recommended management had she been diagnosed in later pregnancy. Her husband is also interested to know a schematic outline for the obstetric management while on chemotherapy in the second and third trimesters.

Special note:
[‡] *Refer to* Question 16 in Chapter 72 for discussion on risks and principles of laparoscopy during pregnancy

---

19. For her given FIGO stage 1B1 cervical cancer, describe the gynecologic oncologist's prenatal management recommendations had she surpassed 22 weeks' gestation at diagnosis. *(1 point each)*   **2**

- ☐ Neoadjuvant chemotherapy during pregnancy until delivery once fetal lung maturity is achieved
- ☐ Delayed treatment after delivery (at lung maturity), if patient declined recommended antenatal treatment knowing that this may negatively impact her prognosis

---

20. Outline two preferred neoadjuvant chemotherapeutic regimens where required for antenatal treatment of cervical cancer. *(1 point each)*   **2**

- ☐ Single agent cisplatin (75 mg/m^2 every 10–21 days)
- ☐ Platinum based combination preferably carboplatin and paclitaxel every three weeks for up to six cycles (note that cisplatin/paclitaxel is not preferred due to associated toxicity)[†]

Special note:
[†] *Refer to* Question 19 in Chapter 72 for discussion of fetal/neonatal morbidities with platinum and taxane-based regimens, including obstetric advantages of carboplatin over cisplatin

---

21. Address the husband's inquiry by providing a schematic presentation for antenatal obstetric care with focus on single agent platinum regimen in the second and third trimesters. *(1 point per main bullet)*   **3**

- ☐ Serial sonographic assessment for fetal growth and amniotic fluid volume (*individualized frequency*), particularly given risk of suboptimal growth velocity and small for gestational age newborns with platinum-based regimens
- ☐ In collaboration with her oncologist, plan to continue chemotherapy until three weeks prior to arranged Cesarean section in late-preterm period (*e.g.*, with Cesarean section at ~35–36 weeks' gestation, then last dose of chemotherapy would be ~32–33 weeks' gestation)
  - ○ *Three-week treatment-delivery interval avoids the period of fetal neutropenia and maternal anemia/neutropenia*
  - ○ *Administration of fetal pulmonary corticosteroids as per standard indications*
- ☐ Antenatal consultation with neonatology experts

Laparoscopic pelvic lymphadenectomy is performed without complications. Node status is negative for malignancy and the patient opts to continue serial close follow-up for risk of disease progression, with definitive treatment at the time of delivery. Obstetric care thereafter is unremarkable. You maintain collaborative care with her gynecologic oncologist and the patient remains compliant with follow-up.

Although details of delivery were discussed in early pregnancy, a multidisciplinary meeting is arranged in the early third trimester for comprehensive management considerations and timing of delivery.

22. Indicate essential aspects of the patient discussion regarding delivery and postpartum recommendations given invasive cervical cancer. *(1 point per main bullet)*

Max 6

☐ Joint surgical procedure: obstetrics/maternal-fetal medicine expert and oncology team
☐ Regional, neuraxial anesthesia until delivery, followed by conversion to general anesthesia for radical hysterectomy
☐ Obtain patient consent for blood products, and consider blood product availability at surgery
☐ Explain that fundal/corporeal uterine incision is necessary at delivery to avoid trauma to the lower uterine segment harboring malignant cells
☐ Inform the patient that placental examination is required for all cancers diagnosed during pregnancy, irrespective of type and/or treatment
   ○ *Metastases are less common with cervical cancer than melanoma, lymphoma, or breast cancer*
☐ Discourage breastfeeding where patient requires postpartum chemotherapy
☐ Chemotherapy can resume as early as two weeks after Cesarean section in the absence of infection

23. Address the patient's inquiry regarding planned Cesarean section by elaborating on morbidities associated with vaginal delivery for patients with invasive cervical cancer. *(1 point each)*

Max 2

☐ Cervico-vaginal laceration, leading to massive hemorrhage
☐ Metastases to the episiotomy site or perineal laceration
☐ Tumor-induced obstruction to the cervical canal

While the patient is in postoperative recovery room after an unremarkable Cesarean-hysterectomy at 36^{+0} weeks' gestation, a physician from an external center calls the gynecologic oncologist to transfer a 34-year-old primigravida at 22^{+2} weeks' gestation by sonographic dating who just presented for prenatal care, primarily for vaginal bleeding. The transferring physician visualized a 3 cm tumor located anteriorly on the cervix. Urgent MRI showed a 2 cm right external iliac lymph node, with confirmation of the cervical tumor appreciated on physical examination. Being present at the time of this telephone conversation, you collaborate in the anticipated management plan upon the patient's arrival to your tertiary center. The patient is reported to be hemodynamically stable with normal fetal morphology.

	Max 2

24. Based on her FIGO 2018 staging classification, indicate recommended patient counseling and treatment with multidisciplinary collaboration. *(1 point per main bullet)*

Stage IIIC1(r):[†]
☐ Inform the patient that data is lacking regarding expectant management; delay of treatment is **not** recommended with advanced disease
☐ Termination of pregnancy followed by chemoradiotherapy is advised
  ○ Regional variations exist in legislation for fetocide prior to termination of pregnancy
☐ While chemoradiation can be initiated with the fetus in utero in the first trimester, hysterotomy should be considered in the second trimester to reduce risk of complications (*e.g.*, hemorrhage, lacerations, disseminated intravascular coagulation) and psychological stress *(Suggested Reading 1)*

Special note:
† In current staging system, radiographically suspicious lymph nodes are depicted by an 'r' notation; stage IIIC1 and IIIC2 indicate pelvic and para-aortic lymph node involvement, respectively

After extensive counseling and involvement of psychosocial support services, the patient consents to termination of pregnancy and definitive treatment given advanced stage cervical cancer.

You find your obstetric trainee carrying out an online search for management recommendations had this patient been in early pregnancy.

	1

25. Facilitate your trainee's learning by discussing early pregnancy considerations with whole pelvic (external beam) radiotherapy.

☐ Fetal death and pregnancy loss usually occur 35–45 days following pelvic radiotherapy in the first trimester, or up to 70 days in the early second trimester (*i.e.*, <20 weeks' gestation)
  ○ In the absence of spontaneous pregnancy loss by the end of external beam radiation, hysterotomy is advised for removing products of conception

TOTAL:	85

CHAPTER 72

Adnexal Mass in Pregnancy

Ahmed Nazer, Amira El-Messidi, and Lucy Gilbert

You are seeing a patient referred by her primary care provider for consultation at your tertiary center's high-risk obstetrics unit. She is a 37-year-old primigravida currently at 13^{+2} weeks' gestation with an incidental 7-cm complex right adnexal mass detected last week on routine first-trimester sonography performed at an external center. Although the ultrasound report is not yet available to you, the consultation note confirms a singleton intrauterine pregnancy with normal fetal morphology and low risk of aneuploidy using *sonographic* markers. Routine serum prenatal investigations are only significant for iron-deficiency anemia.

LEARNING OBJECTIVES

1. Elicit salient points on history of an incidental ovarian mass on routine prenatal sonography, recognizing overlapping symptoms between physiological changes of pregnancy and ovarian cancer
2. Understand the value and limitations of various biomarkers with a potentially malignant adnexal mass in pregnancy
3. Collaborate with gynecologic oncologists in the diagnostic evaluation of suspicious adnexal mass in pregnancy, and promote principles of laparoscopic surgery to optimize maternal-fetal outcome
4. Participate in the counseling of patients diagnosed with ovarian cancer during pregnancy, supporting the use of neoadjuvant chemotherapy beyond the first trimester
5. Formulate obstetric antenatal management plans and delivery recommendations for a patient on chemotherapy for ovarian cancer

SUGGESTED READINGS

1. Amant F, Berveiller P, Boere IA, et al. Gynecologic cancers in pregnancy: guidelines based on a third international consensus meeting. *Ann Oncol.* 2019;30(10):1601–1612.
2. Ball E, Waters N, Cooper N, et al. Evidence-based guideline on laparoscopy in pregnancy: commissioned by the British Society for Gynaecological Endoscopy (BSGE) Endorsed by the Royal College of Obstetricians and Gynaecologists (RCOG). *Facts Views Vis Obgyn.* 2019;11(1):5–25. [Correction in Facts Views Vis Obgyn. 2020 Jan 24;11(3):261]

This chapter is dedicated to our beloved, talented colleague Kris Jardon, who died on January 15, 2021.

3. Blake EA, Kodama M, Yunokawa M, et al. Feto-maternal outcomes of pregnancy complicated by epithelial ovarian cancer: a systematic review of literature. *Eur J Obstet Gynecol Reprod Biol.* 2015; 186:97–105.

4. Botha M, Rajaram S, Karunaratne K. FIGO CANCER REPORT 2018. Cancer in pregnancy. *Int J Gynecol Obstet* 2018;143(Suppl. 2):137–142.

5. Canavan TP. Sonographic tips for evaluation of adnexal masses in pregnancy. *Clin Obstet Gynecol.* 2017;60(3):575–585.

6. de Haan J, Verheecke M, Van Calsteren K, et al. Oncological management and obstetric and neonatal outcomes for women diagnosed with cancer during pregnancy: a 20-year international cohort study of 1170 patients. *Lancet Oncol.* 2018;19(3):337–346.

7. Franciszek Dłuski D, Mierzyński R, Poniedziałek-Czajkowska E, et al. Ovarian cancer and pregnancy – a current problem in perinatal medicine: a comprehensive review. *Cancers (Basel).* 2020;12(12):3795.

8. Fruscio R, de Haan J, Van Calsteren K, et al. Ovarian cancer in pregnancy. *Best Pract Res Clin Obstet Gynaecol.* 2017; 41:108–117.

9. Nazer A, Czuzoj-Shulman N, Oddy L, et al. Incidence of maternal and neonatal outcomes in pregnancies complicated by ovarian masses. *Arch Gynecol Obstet.* 2015;292(5):1069–1074.

10. Pearl JP, Price RR, Tonkin AE, et al. SAGES guidelines for the use of laparoscopy during pregnancy. *Surg Endosc.* 2017;31(10):3767–3782.

POINTS

1. What aspects of a <u>focused</u> history would you want to know? *(1 point per main bullet unless indicated)*   20

Abdominal-pelvic features related to the incidental adnexal mass:
- ☐ Gastrointestinal: *(1 point per subbullet; max 2)*
  - ○ Current/recent abdominal-pelvic pain *(including location, characteristics, onset, progression, radiation, aggravating/alleviating factors)*
  - ○ Abdominal distension[§]
  - ○ Change in bowel habits, or presence of hematochezia
- ☐ Gynecologic: *(1 point per subbullet; max 6)*
  - ○ Current/recent vaginal bleeding
  - ○ Current/recent abnormal vaginal discharge[§]
  - ○ Current/recent hirsutism or virilization
  - ○ Time interval since last Papanicolaou smear, or prior cervical dysplasia
  - ○ Conception using hormone assisted reproductive technology, or history of infertility
  - ○ Clinical history or ultrasound features of endometriosis
  - ○ Known tubo-ovarian abscess(es) or pelvic inflammatory disease
  - ○ Known leiomyoma(s)
- ☐ Urinary: hematuria, dysuria

☐ Prior abdominal-pelvic surgery for any etiology, including interventions for pelvic mass (es) *(e.g., aspiration)*

☐ Past personal malignancy

Systemic features: *(max 5)*

☐ Fever/chills

☐ Night sweats

☐ Bone pains

☐ Weight loss/loss of appetite/early satiety[§]

☐ Nausea/vomiting[§]

☐ Fatigue/malaise[§]

☐ Dyspnea[§]

Current and prior medications: *(max 1)*

☐ Current use of anticoagulants

☐ Past use of combined hormonal contraception, and duration of use

Social habits:

☐ Smoking and/or alcohol consumption

Family history: *(max 2)*

☐ Breast, ovarian or bowel cancer

☐ BRCA-1, BRCA-2, or other mutated oncogenes

☐ Ethnicity

Special note:

§ Particularly where symptoms or manifestations existed prior to pregnancy

The patient tells you this is a long-desired pregnancy, which she and her husband conceived after three years of primary female infertility and two failed in vitro fertilization cycles, the last being 18 months ago. She did not use any hormonal agents for conception, and only takes prenatal vitamins. The patient is a healthy Caucasian; she does not drink alcohol or smoke. She discontinued 10-year use of combined oral contraceptives for pregnancy planning. Apart from an uninformative diagnostic laparoscopy as part of fertility investigations, she had no other surgeries. At the time of her second attempted cycle of in vitro fertilization, cervical cytology was normal; there is no history of dysplasia or pelvic infections. Family history is negative for malignancies or oncogenes.

Three months prior to conception, she developed new-onset intermittent constipation and bloating. Thereafter, despite loss of appetite, she attributed increasing abdominal girth to pregnancy and recently started wearing dresses, as clothes became uncomfortable around the waist. Apart from general malaise and hip pains, which she considered were physiological adaptations to pregnancy, she has not had other systemic symptoms.

2. Reflecting on her nonspecific features, identify clinical <u>manifestations</u> that *may or may not* be present in this patient that overlap between physiological changes of pregnancy and possible ovarian malignancy. *(1 point each)*

☐ Fatigue
☐ Anemia
☐ Nausea/vomiting
☐ Dyspnea
☐ Early satiety
☐ Bloating/increased abdominal girth
☐ Abdominal pain
☐ Constipation
☐ Back pain
☐ Urinary symptoms

Max 6

3. With focus on the patient's reason for consultation and presenting features, <u>detail</u> your focused physical examination. Fetal viability has been ascertained. *(1 point per main bullet, unless specified)*

☐ Vital signs: blood pressure, pulse, respiratory rate, oxygen saturation, and temperature
☐ Current or most recent BMI
☐ Cardiopulmonary auscultation *(particularly for effusions or pulmonary consolidations)*
☐ Breast examination *(e.g., mass, skin changes, or nipple discharge)*
☐ Nodal assessment: cervical, supraclavicular, axillary, and inguinal *(4 points)*
☐ Abdominal assessment: *(1 point per subbullet; max 4)*
  ○ General inspection for distention/abnormal contour
  ○ Auscultation of bowel sounds
  ○ Palpable mass, tenderness, guarding
  ○ Organomegaly
  ○ Ascites
☐ Pelvic and rectal assessment: *(1 point per subbullet for 3)*
  ○ Visual inspection of the vulva, vagina, and cervix
  ○ Bimanual pelvic exam, with note of cul-de-sac obliteration or nodularity
  ○ Rectovaginal exam

15

Special note:
Cervical cytology and cervico-vaginal cultures are *investigations*, although performed during the physical examination

The patient's BMI is 27 kg/m^2 and vital signs are normal. Examination is significant for a nontender ***fixed right adnexal mass*** without posterior cul-de-sac obliteration. There is no appreciable abdominal organomegaly, ascites, or any palpable lymph nodes. The remainder of the examination is unremarkable.

Given your sonographic expertise, the patient accepts your intent to perform detailed sonography at this visit. She requests confirmation of normal fetal findings *prior* to thoroughly assessing the adnexal mass. You plan to facilitate your trainee's learning upon completion of this patient's consultation visit.

4. With focus on <u>gynecologic</u> etiologies, provide your trainee with structured differential diagnoses for histopathologies of <u>fixed</u> complex adnexal masses in pregnancy. *(1 point each)*   6

Benign masses with complex features:[‡]
- ☐ Endometrioma
- ☐ Tubo-ovarian abscess/mass

Malignant ovarian masses:
- ☐ Germ cell tumors
- ☐ Sex-cord stromal tumors
- ☐ Epithelial ovarian tumors (invasive or low malignant potential)
- ☐ Metastatic tumors to the ovary

Special note:
‡ Differential diagnosis of ***nonfixed*** begin masses with complex features would include mature teratoma, corpus luteum, multiloculated cystadenoma, ectopic/heterotopic pregnancy, luteoma, hyperreactio luteinalis, necrosis or degeneration of pedunculated leiomyomas

5. While several different scoring systems have been developed to stratify the risk of malignancy in ovarian masses, their usefulness in pregnant populations requires validation. Assuming the patient's adnexal mass is of ovarian etiology, discuss sonographic features that would raise concern for malignancy, *particularly* when present in combination. *(1 point each)*   Max 7

- ☐ Size >10 cm or growth rate >3.5 cm/week
- ☐ Solid/cystic consistency
- ☐ Mass contains >10 locules
- ☐ Irregular borders of the mass
- ☐ Solid component contains dense or central vascularity
- ☐ Multiple, thick, irregular septations
- ☐ Papillary projections (*e.g.*, defined as ≥4 solid projections from cyst wall into the cavity, with each projection >3 mm in height)
- ☐ Mural nodules
- ☐ Bilaterality
- ☐ Ascites or presence of free fluid in the pelvis

You explain the findings to the patient and trainee:

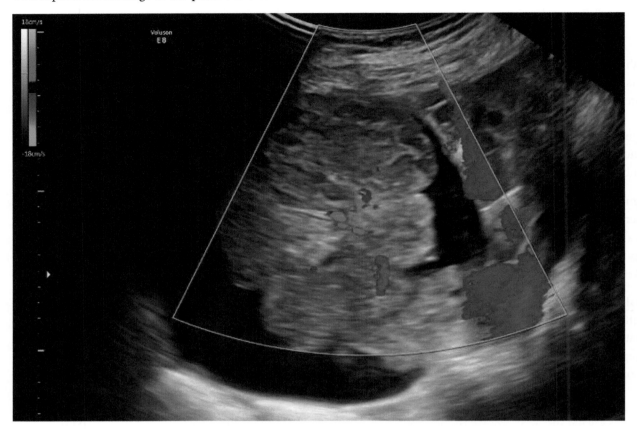

Figure 72.1

Image: Courtesy of Professor L. Gilbert

There is no association between this case scenario and this patient's image. Image used for educational purposes only.

6. What is the immediate next best step in management?   1

☐ Urgent referral to gynecologic oncology

You notify the gynecologic oncologist who will attend to the patient shortly in multidisciplinary collaboration with you. Meanwhile, the patient confirms her intent to continue pregnancy and wishes to discuss prenatal aneuploidy screening. She did the first serum component consisting of free β-hCG and PAPP-A at the time of nuchal translucency ultrasound last week and anticipates the second set of analytes screening as planned next week. You mention the caveats of specific prenatal serum markers screening in the context of an adnexal mass, and discuss others unaffected by pregnancy, remaining potentially useful in diagnosis of an ovarian malignancy.

7. Identify the maternal serum analytes, commonly used in <u>prenatal screening programs</u> for fetal aneuploidy or malformations, whose elevations may be confounded by the presence of an ovarian tumor. *(1 point each)*

□ hCG
□ Alpha-fetoprotein (AFP)
  ○ *Typically, prenatal screening levels above 2.0–2.5 multiples of the median are abnormal and warrant detailed obstetric sonographic assessment*
  ○ *Consider a potential co-existing germ cell tumor where levels of maternal serum AFP are >1000 ng/mL or >9 multiples of the median*
□ Inhibin A

Special note:
Although cancer antigen 125 (Ca 125) may also be increased, it is not a component of prenatal serum screening

3

8. Which serum tumor markers are *unaffected* by pregnancy, where increased values in the context of an ovarian mass, raises suspicion of malignancy? *(1 point each)*

□ Inhibin B
□ Lactate dehydrogenase (LDH)
□ Human epididymis protein 4 (HE4)[†]
□ Cancer antigen 19–9 (Ca 19–9)
□ Carcinoembryonic antigen (CEA)
□ Anti-Müllerian hormone (AMH)

Special note:
† HE4 is unlikely to be increased in benign conditions

Max 5

Since last week's incidental discovery of the adnexal mass, the patient did some on-line research and learned about the serum Ca 125 marker in screening for ovarian cancer. She is curious to know your evidence-based impression regarding its caveats, particularly with regard to pregnancy. You mention that while many *nongynecologic* conditions can increase Ca 125 concentrations, you will address *gynecologic* associations at this time.

9. Discuss the <u>physiologic</u> variations in Ca 125 levels during pregnancy. *(1 point per main bullet)*

□ Ca 125 levels peak in the first trimester (range 7–251 U/mL), thereafter decreasing consistently throughout pregnancy
  ○ *Between 15 weeks' gestation and delivery, markedly elevated Ca 125 (1000–10,000 U/mL) cannot be attributed to pregnancy*
□ Ca 125 peaks again within 24 hours postpartum

Special note:
Refer to Spitzer M, Kaushal N, Benjamin F. Maternal CA-125 levels in pregnancy and the puerperium. *J Reprod Med.* 1998;43(4):387–392.

2

10. Indicate six gynecologic conditions associated with increased Ca 125 levels. *(1 point each)*   Max 6

☐ Pregnancy itself
☐ Menses
☐ Endometriosis
☐ Leiomyomas
☐ Adenomyosis
☐ Functional ovarian cysts
☐ Benign ovarian tumors
☐ Ovarian hyperstimulation
☐ Pelvic inflammatory disease
☐ Meigs syndrome
☐ Epithelial ovarian/primary peritoneal/fallopian tube cancers
☐ Endometrial cancer

In collaboration with the gynecologic oncologist, the patient agrees to an MRI[†] as recommended to further characterize the clinically and sonographically evident ovarian mass, assess for peritoneal dissemination and nodal involvement. The gynecologic oncologist explains that routine chest X-ray is unnecessary, given history and physical examination are not suggestive of pulmonary disease. Comprehensive serum testing for tumor markers, hepatic, renal, and coagulation function is also arranged.

Special note:
† *Refer to Chapter 42* for discussion on safety recommendations for MRI in pregnancy and fetal risks associated with gadolinium contrast

11. As gadolinium contrast is not used in prenatal MRI examinations, identify a safe   1
substitute, most frequently used to assess for adhesions and peritoneal/intra-abdominal lesions associated with ovarian cancer in pregnancy.

☐ Pineapple juice *(Suggested Reading 1)*

12. Excluding emergent surgery, discuss three ovarian tumor consensus recommendations for   3
surgical resection in pregnancy. *(1 point per main bullet)*

☐ Persistent mass into the second trimester, ideally after 16 weeks' gestation
☐ Contain solid, mixed solid-cystic areas, or highly suspicious sonographic characteristics
☐ Diameter of the adnexal mass exceeds 10 cm
  ○ Historically, elective removal was recommended for masses >6 cm in diameter persisting after 16 weeks' gestation
  ○ Recent literature supports close observation in asymptomatic prenatal patients without concerning ultrasound features and normal tumor markers [Ca 125, LDH] *(Suggested Reading 9)*

13. Rationalize why surgery for an adnexal mass is ideally performed after 16 weeks' gestation. *(1 point per main bullet)*

☐ Organogenesis is complete, thereby minimizing risks of teratogenesis induced by medications

☐ Adnexal resection will not affect progesterone concentrations, as the placenta has replaced the hormonal functions of the corpus luteum
  ○ *With adnexectomy prior to 10–12 weeks' gestation, progesterone supplementation is advised*

☐ Majority of functional cysts would have resolved

☐ Decreased risk of pregnancy loss relative to the first trimester

☐ Increased likelihood that pregnancy losses associated with fetal abnormalities would have occurred, thereby not mistakenly attributed to surgical intervention

At 14^{+4} weeks' gestation, pelvic MRI reveals a 6.2 x 7.1 x 8.0 cm right ovarian mass of solid-cystic consistency containing papillary projections, without evidence of peritoneal carcinomatosis or local metastatic disease; a single intrauterine fetus with normal-appearing placenta is noted. Serum Ca 125 is 400 U/mL with a normal LDH level.

Timely follow-up is arranged with the gynecologic oncologist; he or she subsequently calls you to discuss the planned laparotomy at 16^{+2} weeks' gestation. At this early gestational age, brief ascertainment of fetal viability pre- and postoperatively is planned, as well as anti-D immunoglobulin for Rh-negative status. You later teach your trainee that had the patient been a candidate for laparoscopic surgery, anti-D immunoglobulin would not have been necessary as laparoscopy is not a potentially sensitizing event *(Suggested Reading 2)*.

The patient has met interdisciplinary team members including the anesthesiologist, social worker, and psychologist. She has no obstetric complaints.

14. Besides possible disease progression, what are the morbidities associated with *prolonged* delays in surgical intervention for the patient's adnexal mass? *(1 point each)*

☐ Preterm labor

☐ Labor dystocia

☐ Mass rupture and/or hemorrhage

☐ Torsion *(likelihood may decrease for masses >8 cm)*

15. You highlight to your trainee that laparotomy is preferred by the gynecologic oncologist   5
given the uterine size at this gestational age and the suspicion of malignancy.
Address the perinatal risks of laparoscopic surgery and indicate operative principles to
optimize obstetric safety for the appropriately selected patient. *(1 point each)*

Perinatal risks of laparoscopic surgery: *(max 2)*
☐ Uterine perforation with/without fetal injury
☐ Reduced uterine blood flow with increased abdominal pressure and use of carbon dioxide
☐ Surgical bleeding/tissue friability
☐ Maternal hypercapnia, fetal acidosis
☐ Venous thromboembolism[$]
☐ Portal site herniation

Principles of laparoscopy surgery during pregnancy: *(max 3)*
☐ Preferred technique is open (Hasson) introduction without a Veress needle
☐ Insertion of the first trocar at least 3–4 cm above the uterine fundus
☐ Limit surgical duration to 90–120 minutes
☐ Use low operating pressure of 10–15 mmHg
☐ Stop the flow of carbon dioxide while awaiting results of the frozen section
☐ Lateral tilt position (preferably the left-side) is advised beyond the first trimester

Special note:
[$] Consideration for intraoperative and postoperative thromboprophylaxis using pneumatic
compression devices and early postoperative ambulation in the gravid patient;
compounding risks include pregnancy, surgery, malignancy, and immobilization

As the patient is motivated for pregnancy preservation, the gynecologic oncologist informs her
that interval debulking surgery will be arranged postpartum, if required.

16. Outline the main elements of the surgical procedure that should (or may) be performed in   Max 6
evaluation of the patient's adnexal mass. *(1 point each)*

☐ Abdominal exploration for metastases, with careful inspection of the contralateral ovary
☐ Peritoneal cytology
☐ Frozen section[†]
☐ Unilateral adnexectomy, ideally avoiding spillage
☐ Infracolic omentectomy
☐ Appendectomy
☐ Pelvic-peritoneal biopsies
☐ Possible lymph node dissection

Special note:
[†] Pathologist must be made aware of her prenatal status

At laparotomy, a solid right ovarian mass is noted with a normal-appearing contralateral ovary.
Pelvic washings are performed. There is no evidence of peritoneal carcinomatosis in the upper
abdomen or omentum. Along with a right adnexectomy, removed intact in an endo-bag, a 5 mm

peritoneal nodule is resected from the right pelvic side wall. With frozen section revealing high-grade serous carcinoma, pregnancy-preserving staging is performed. The patient tolerated surgery well and postoperative recovery is unremarkable. Fetal viability is documented.

At 18 weeks' gestation, the final pathology report confirms high grade serous epithelial ovarian cancer with a malignant peritoneal nodule and cytology, consistent with FIGO stage IIb.

As her high-risk obstetrician, you attend the arranged multidisciplinary meeting with the patient, her husband and medical oncology experts.

17. Provide important aspects of the relationship between pregnancy and ovarian cancer that would be addressed at this multidisciplinary meeting with the patient. *(1 point each)*   4

☐ Pregnancy itself does not appear to worsen the prognosis of ovarian cancer compared to nonpregnant patients matched for tumor stage, grade, and histology

☐ Termination of pregnancy does not appear to provide a survival advantage with ovarian cancer in pregnancy, and is based on personal preferences

☐ As 10%–15% of ovarian cancer is associated with germline mutations, consultation with a geneticist is advised as the fetus has a 50% chance of carrier status if this patient has BRCA-1 or BRCA-2 oncogenes

☐ Reassuring safety data on combination platinum and taxane-based neoadjuvant chemotherapy when initiated after the first trimester

Using the same doses of chemotherapy as in nonpregnant patients, configured to actual pregnancy weight[§-13], the oncologist advises administration of four cycles of carboplatin and paclitaxel every 3 weeks until 35 weeks' gestation. Chemotherapy will be started two to four weeks postoperatively, in the absence of complications. The patient is aware of general perinatal adverse effects of chemotherapy used in the second and third trimesters[§-10]. Maternal side effects of chemotherapy and details of the treatment protocol are provided to the patient.

Special note:

[§-13,§-10]*Refer to Chapter 73, Questions 13 and 10, respectively*

18. As chemotherapy will only be initiated after the first trimester, address fetal/neonatal morbidities *particular* to the designated regimen and inform your trainee why carboplatin is chosen over cisplatin for antenatal treatment of epithelial ovarian cancer. *(1 point each)*   Max 3

Platinum-based agents:
☐ Small for gestational age newborns[§]
☐ Cisplatin[†] is associated with dose-dependent ototoxicity in children with in utero exposure
☐ Cisplatin[†] is associated with greater newborn nephrotoxicity than carboplatin

Taxane agents:
☐ Myelosuppression
☐ NICU admission

Special notes:
§ Recovery in early infancy-childhood is most common
† Cisplatin remains the standard of care platin agent for antenatal treatment of germ-cell malignancy

19. In addition to the effects of chemotherapy, identify <u>maternal malignancy-related</u>   Max 4
morbidities that may contribute to suboptimal fetal growth. *(1 point each)*

☐ Malnutrition
☐ Anemia
☐ Supportive medications
☐ Stress
☐ Malignancy itself

20. With focus on ovarian cancer and planned antenatal chemotherapy, outline your <u>obstetric</u>   Max 5
management and delivery recommendations, maintaining collaboration with the
oncologist. *(1 point per main bullet)*

☐ Nutritionist consultation to ensure appropriate caloric intake
☐ Subsequent to routine second-trimester fetal morphology survey, arrange for monthly/
bimonthly sonographic assessments for fetal growth and amniotic fluid volume, with
consideration for cervical length
  ○ *Where fetal growth restriction is detected, Doppler assessment is performed according to*
    standard recommendations (refer to Chapter 9)
☐ Consideration for antepartum and postpartum thromboprophylaxis
☐ Antenatal consultation with neonatology experts
☐ Continue chemotherapy until ~34–35 weeks' gestation and arrange for induction of labor
in 3 weeks (*i.e.*, from 37 weeks)
  ○ *Where possible, avoid iatrogenic prematurity; preterm infants cannot metabolize*
    chemotherapy as can term infants
☐ Reassure the patient that Cesarean section is only required for obstetric indications
☐ Ensure placental examination is arranged, as for all gestational cancers irrespective of type
and/or treatment

21. Rationalize why a three-week window is generally recommended between the last dose of   Max 3
chemotherapy and delivery. *(1 point each)*

Fetal:
☐ Decreased risk of neutropenia and drug accumulation

Maternal:
☐ Decreased risk of anemia/bleeding
☐ Decreased risk of intrapartum/postpartum infections
☐ Optimize eligibility for neuraxial anesthesia

After this consultation encounter, your obstetric trainee is curious whether antenatal adjuvant
chemotherapy may have been safely avoided with other ovarian tumor histopathologies.

22. Address your trainee's inquiry regarding particular ovarian cancers where adjuvant chemotherapy is not required. *(1 point each)*

4

☐ Epithelial ovarian cancer stage 1A, grade 1
☐ Tumors of low malignant potential
☐ Dysgerminoma stage 1
☐ Immature teratoma stage 1, grade 1

Special note:
Where chemotherapy is indicated for germ-cell cancers, BEP (bleomycin, etoposide, cisplatin) or EP is recommended after the first trimester; although evidence is limited, use of etoposide in pregnancy in combination with cisplatin with/without bleomycin appears safe *(Suggested Reading 1)*

Pregnancy progresses well, and fetal growth remains on the 10th–15th percentiles. The patient receives her last predelivery chemotherapy session at 35 weeks' gestation, and you arrange for induction of labor at 38 weeks. The neonatology team is present for delivery and you plan to grossly examine the placenta prior to histopathological assessment.

Intrapartum, the patient's husband is contemplating whether umbilical cord blood collection may be considered in the event of confirmed appropriate treatment response without residual disease at postpartum debulking surgery.

23. Troubleshoot her husband's inquiry regarding the possibility of stem cell collection from umbilical cord blood.

2

☐ Theoretical risk of contamination discourages cord blood collection for maternal or fetal therapy

24. Outline breastfeeding considerations for this patient with ovarian cancer. *(1 point each)*

2

☐ Discourage breastfeeding where patient requires chemotherapy or targeted therapy
☐ Without ongoing chemotherapy, suggest a three-week washout period from last chemotherapy administration

TOTAL: **120**

CHAPTER 73

Lymphoma and Leukemia in Pregnancy

Samantha So, Amira El-Messidi, and Elyce H. Cardonick

CASE 1

You are seeing a patient referred by her primary care provider for consultation at your tertiary center's high-risk obstetrics unit. She is a 27-year-old primigravida at 16^{+3} weeks' gestation with intermittent swelling of her arms and face that appears within several minutes of brushing her hair and resolves upon lowering her arms. First-trimester dating sonography was concordant with menstrual dates, and fetal morphology appeared normal, with a low risk of aneuploidy; apart from HIV-negative status, results of other routine baseline prenatal investigations are not yet available to you. She has not experienced abdominal cramps or vaginal bleeding. Her medications include only routine prenatal vitamins.

CASE 2

Your next patient is a healthy 22-year-old primigravida at 28^{+4} weeks' gestation with normal body habitus who presents for a routine prenatal visit. She is well known to you, and all aspects of maternal and fetal care have been normal. She reports normal fetal activity and has no obstetric complaints. Relative to last visit, she appears pale and complains of increasing fatigue; she now has prolonged gingival bleeding after brushing her teeth. Ecchymoses and petechiae are noted on her arms. Her blood pressure is 95/70 mmHg, and her pulse is 95 bpm; fetal viability is ascertained, and fundal height is 24 cm above the symphysis pubis. You send her to the hospital for urgent investigations.

LEARNING OBJECTIVES

1. Elicit salient points on prenatal history with clinical features beyond the realm of normal pregnancy, and initiate preliminary diagnostic evaluation of suspected hematologic malignancy

2. Troubleshoot misconceptions related to chest X-ray in pregnancy, while avoiding contraindicated diagnostic investigations for staging of lymphoma in pregnancy
3. Collaborate with medical oncologists to provide counseling on maternal-fetal risks, and discuss preferred management with newly diagnosed leukemia or lymphoma at various stages of pregnancy
4. Understand the principal chemotherapeutic regimens for Hodgkin's and non-Hodgkin's lymphoma at different stages of pregnancy, and monitor for related obstetric morbidities
5. Recognize situations where early termination or iatrogenic prematurity would permit optimized maternal treatment to improve survivorship
6. Promptly identify clinical manifestations of tumor lysis syndrome, recognizing it as an oncologic life-threatening complication that may be mistaken for eclampsia

SUGGESTED READINGS

1. Brenner B, Avivi I, Lishner M. Haematological cancers in pregnancy. *Lancet.* 2012;379(9815): 580–587.
2. Cardonick EH, Gringlas MB, Hunter K, et al. Development of children born to mothers with cancer during pregnancy: comparing in utero chemotherapy-exposed children with nonexposed controls. *Am J Obstet Gynecol.* 2015;212(5):658.
3. Cardonick E, Iacobucci A. Use of chemotherapy during human pregnancy. *Lancet Oncol.* 2004;5(5):283–291.
4. Cohen JB, Blum KA. Evaluation and management of lymphoma and leukemia in pregnancy. *Clin Obstet Gynecol.* 2011;54(4):556–566.
5. El-Messidi A, Patenaude V, Abenhaim HA. Incidence and outcomes of women with non-Hodgkin's lymphoma in pregnancy: a population-based study on 7.9 million births. *J Obstet Gynaecol Res.* 2015;41(4):582–589.
6. El-Messidi A, Patenaude V, Hakeem G, et al. Incidence and outcomes of women with Hodgkin's lymphoma in pregnancy: a population-based study on 7.9 million births. *J Perinat Med.* 2015;43(6):683–688.
7. Evens AM, Advani R, Press OW, et al. Lymphoma occurring during pregnancy: antenatal therapy, complications, and maternal survival in a multicenter analysis. *J Clin Oncol.* 2013;31(32):4132–4139.
8. Gurevich-Shapiro A, Avivi I. Current treatment of lymphoma in pregnancy. *Expert Rev Hematol.* 2019;12(6):449–459.
9. Lishner M, Avivi I, Apperley JF, et al. Hematologic malignancies in pregnancy: management guidelines from an international consensus meeting. *J Clin Oncol.* 2016;34(5):501–508.
10. Maggen C, Dierickx D, Lugtenburg P, et al. Obstetric and maternal outcomes in patients diagnosed with Hodgkin lymphoma during pregnancy: a multicentre, retrospective, cohort study. *Lancet Haematol.* 2019;6(11):e551–e561. [Correction in Lancet Haematol. 2020 Apr;7(4):e279]

CASE 1

1. What aspects of a <u>focused</u> history would you want to know? *(1 point per bullet)*

Details related to intermittent facial and upper extremity swelling: *(Superior vena cava syndrome)*
- ☐ Time interval since onset of her symptoms
- ☐ Chronic or intermittent dyspnea
- ☐ Fatigue/malaise
- ☐ Noted swelling of axillary or cervical lymph nodes, either painless or painful

Presence of B-symptoms:
- ☐ Fever >38.3°C
- ☐ Night sweats
- ☐ Weight loss *(>10% of her body weight in six months)*

Medical comorbidities and other systemic manifestations:
- ☐ Easy bruising
- ☐ Pruritis
- ☐ Prior malignancy
- ☐ Prior venous thromboembolism or nongestational risk factors for hypercoagulability

Social features:
- ☐ Cigarette smoking, alcohol consumption, recreational drug use

The patient, generally healthy, first noticed her symptoms early in pregnancy, although was not concerned enough to alert her physician. She was more distressed by nausea, severe fatigue, and shortness of breath, which she attributed to the first trimester. Over the past month, however, she describes increased swelling of her face and arms when she raises her arms above the horizontal, slower symptom recovery, and recent onset of chest pressure. The patient complains of insomnia due to drenching sweats. She lost 20-pounds since the beginning of pregnancy, despite maintaining a healthy diet and lifestyle. She has not noticed any nodal swelling, bruising, and did not check her temperature.

On examination, her BMI is 21 kg/m^2, a change from 25 kg/m^2 documented prepregnancy. Her blood pressure is 110/60 mmHg, pulse is 105 bpm, oxygen saturation is 97% on room air and oral temperature is 37.0°C (98.6°F). During your conversation, she appears slightly dyspneic; this becomes evident with Pemberton's sign *(bilateral arm elevation causes facial plethora)*. She does not have palpable lymphadenopathy and her skin and abdominal examinations are unremarkable. Fetal viability is ascertained.

2. Indicate your <u>preliminary</u> investigations to evaluate her clinical presentation. **8**
   (1 point each, unless specified)

Serum:
- ☐ CBC/FBC
- ☐ Ferritin
- ☐ Creatinine and electrolytes
- ☐ Hepatic transaminases and function tests (*i.e.*, AST, ALT, bilirubin, LDH, aPTT, INR)

Imaging:
- ☐ Chest X-ray, two views **(4 points)**

As you explain the need for urgent investigations, including chest X-ray, the patient expresses concern about fetal radiation effects.

3. Troubleshoot the patient's misconceptions regarding fetal exposure to ionizing radiation **Max 2**
   from chest radiography. *(1 point each)*

Chest X-ray, two views:[†§]
- ☐ Reassure the patient that fetal radiation exposure is considered to be '*very low-dose (<0.1 mGy)*, with an approximate actual dose of 0.0005–0.01 mGy
- ☐ Inform the patient that fetal risk of anomalies, fetal growth restriction (FGR), or pregnancy loss require at least 50 mGy (5 rads) of exposure
- ☐ Severe intellectual disability due to in utero radiation exposure generally requires 60–310 mGy (6–31 rads), and appears mostly at 8–15 weeks' gestation
- ☐ Risk of carcinogenesis with diagnostic radiation is also very small *(does not influence pregnancy management decisions)*

Special notes:
† *Refer to the following sources:*
   (a) Wiles R, Hankinson B, Benbow E, et al. Making decisions about radiological imaging in pregnancy. *BMJ*. 2022;377:e070486.
   (b) Tirada N, Dreizin D, Khati NJ, et al. Imaging pregnant and lactating patients. *Radiographics* 2015;35:1751–65.
   (c) American Association of Physicists in Medicine. AAPM position statement on the use of patient gonadal and fetal shielding, 2019.
   (d) British Institute of Radiology, Institute of Physics and Engineering in Medicine, Public Health England, Royal College of Radiologists, Society and College of Radiographers, the Society for Radiological Protection. Guidance on using shielding on patients for diagnostic radiology applications. 2020.
   (e) Guidelines for diagnostic imaging during pregnancy and lactation, ACOG Committee Opinion, Oct 2017;130(4):e210–16.
§ Routine abdominal shielding should be avoided in imaging modalities where ionizing radiation does not directly expose the fetus because (1) most of the fetal dose results from internal (rather than external) scatter, and (2) automatic control can cause increased dose exposure if the shield is inadvertently in the field of view during the scan. Abdominal shielding may be considered on a case by case basis if it offers patient reassurance after appropriate counselling.

The patient appreciates your reassurance and evidence-based counseling; she consents to diagnostic imaging which is performed promptly. Investigations are significant for the following:

		Normal
Chest X-ray	12-cm mediastinal mass	
Hemoglobin	7.1 g/dL (71 g/L)	10.5–14.0 g/dL (105–140 g/L)
Platelets	100 × 10⁹/L	150–400 × 10⁹/L

Remaining investigations are within normal limits.

4. After informing the patient of the results and sharing your concerns, what is the immediate next best step in management?   1

    ☐ Urgent referral to medical/hematology oncology

5. Discuss the <u>diagnostic</u> procedure of choice that you anticipate will be recommended by the oncologist.   1

    ☐ Excisional biopsy,$ under local or general anesthesia

    Special note:
    § Core biopsy or fine needle aspiration are suboptimal; greater amount of tissue can be retrieved for analysis through an excisional procedure

CASE 1
SCENARIO A
Subsequently, biopsy of the mediastinal mass is performed by the interventional radiologist without complications. You accompany your obstetric trainee where the pathologist shows you this microscopic slide, demonstrating the classic multinucleated Reed-Sternberg cells.

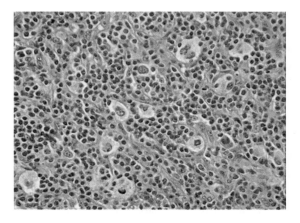

Figure 73.1

With permission: *Figure 1 from Cohen JB, Blum KA. Evaluation and management of lymphoma and leukemia in pregnancy. Clin Obstet Gynecol. 2011 Dec;54 (4):556–66.*

There is no association between the pathology slide and this case scenario. Image used for educational purposes only.

Despite the timespan since examining histology specimens, these landmark *'Reed-Sternberg'* cells resonate in your memory.

6. Identify this patient's diagnosis.

1

□ Hodgkin's lymphoma (HL)

7. What is the next best, safe test in staging of HL during pregnancy?

1

□ MRI (without contrast$^{\$}$) of the chest, abdomen and pelvis

Special notes:
Bone marrow biopsy is safe in pregnancy, but is not required in staging of classic Hodgkin's lymphoma; ultrasound is less sensitive than MRI; CT and positron emission tomography (PET) involve fetal exposure to radiation without maternal therapeutic benefit
§ Refer to Chapter 42 for safety of MRI in pregnancy and fetotoxic effects of gadolinium

As a maternal-fetal medicine expert, you continue obstetric care for the patient in collaboration with the oncology team. The MRI confirms an $8.3 \times 12.5 \times 6.0$ cm mediastinal mass with isolated hilar lymphadenopathy; no other abnormalities detected on imaging. Although her husband and family remain supportive, the patient accepts your offer of psychosocial support services.

Prior to the arranged multidisciplinary counseling, her oncologist requests pulmonary function testing and maternal echocardiography, both of which are normal.

8. With respect to potential <u>maternal</u> complications of treatment, specify why her oncologist requested pulmonary function testing and maternal echocardiography. *(1 point each)*

2

□ Bleomycin-induced pulmonary fibrosis
□ Doxorubicin (adriamycin)-associated cardiotoxicity

9. The patient is currently 16^{+6} weeks' gestation. Indicate aspects regarding the relationship between pregnancy and HL that would be addressed at the multidisciplinary meeting with the patient. *(1 point each)*

4

□ Pregnancy termination would not alter the course of disease *(i.e., outcomes of women diagnosed antenatally are not worse than nonpregnant patients of similar age)*
  ○ *Individualized patient decision*
□ Reassuring safety data on the combination-chemotherapy regimen ABVD† in the second and third trimesters *(i.e., recommended management for this patient)*
□ Inform the patient that timely treatment in pregnancy results in comparable survival outcomes to nonpregnant patients, and that HL is potentially curable
□ HL itself does not <u>directly</u> impact pregnancy outcome

Special note:
† ABVD *(adriamycin, bleomycin, vinblastine, dacarbazine).*
   More intensive regimens such as BEACOPP *(bleomycin, etoposide, doxorubicin, cyclophosphamide, vincristine, procarbazine, prednisone)* are not recommended during pregnancy due to greater fetal toxicity

10. The patient asks about <u>perinatal</u> adverse effects from combination-chemotherapy in the second and third trimesters. *(1 point each)*

Max 5

Short-term risks:
- ☐ Low birthweight
- ☐ FGR
- ☐ Preterm birth
- ☐ Preeclampsia
- ☐ IUFD[†]
- ☐ Postpartum blood transfusions

Long-term risks:[§]
- ☐ Generally reassuring data, without increased risk of adverse child neurodevelopmental dysfunction, malignancies or decreased gonadal function

Special notes:
- † May be related to underlying malignancy rather than chemotherapy
- § *Refer to* Avilés A, Neri N. Hematological malignancies and pregnancy: a final report of 84 children who received chemotherapy in utero. *Clin Lymphoma.* 2001;2(3):173–177

The patient is keen to continue pregnancy and agrees to start ABVD chemotherapy. She is curious if management may have differed with first-trimester detection of HL.

11. Outline the options for management of stable and symptomatic HL in the <u>first</u> trimester. *(1 point each)*

5

Low bulk,[‡] stable disease:
- ☐ Close observation until treatment is start in the second trimester, OR
- ☐ Termination of pregnancy

Symptomatic:
- ☐ Termination of pregnancy, OR
- ☐ Single-agent vinblastine or corticosteroids[§] as bridging therapy until ABVD therapy in the second trimester
- ☐ Combination chemotherapy after counseling on fetal risks

Special notes:
- ‡ Single node ≤10 cm of transthoracic diameter at any level of thoracic vertebrae
- § No confirmed evidence of human teratogenicity with first-trimester exposure; *refer to Chapter 45*

During the multidisciplinary meeting, the patient asks whether radiotherapy with abdominal shielding of her pregnancy would be optional, given localized chest pathology; she speculates targeted treatment may result in improved disease control.

12. Identify the indications for antenatal radiotherapy for HL and discuss maternal-fetal considerations to address in counseling. *(1 point per main bullet)*

Max 6

Indications:
- ☐ Progressive disease despite chemotherapy
- ☐ Disease that seriously threatens maternal well-being *(e.g., airway obstruction, spinal cord compression)*
- ☐ Supradiaphragmatic disease
- ☐ Noncandidates for chemotherapy

Maternal-Fetal considerations:
- ☐ Probability of childhood cancer is dose-dependent, regardless of gestational age at exposure
  - ○ Limit the whole-body fetal dose to ≤0.10 Gy (10 rad)
  - ○ Maximize the distance between the radiation field and the uterus
- ☐ Risks of severe intellectual disability and teratogenesis are greatest between 8–15 weeks' gestation
- ☐ Increased risk of late secondary maternal cancers *(e.g., breast, non-Hodgkin's lymphoma [NHL], sarcoma, lung, gastrointestinal malignancies)*
- ☐ Long-term risk of coronary artery disease secondary to radiation exposure if the heart is exposed

The patient starts ABVD chemotherapy at 17^{+0} weeks' gestation.

13. Indicate two principles of dosing chemotherapy in pregnancy.

2

- ☐ <u>Actual</u> weight in pregnancy is used to configure body surface area
- ☐ Same doses are given as nonpregnant patients

14. Discuss your obstetric management, including delivery and postpartum considerations of this HL patient. *(1 point per main bullet)*

Max 8

- ☐ Advise antepartum and postpartum thromboprophylaxis given active malignancy
- ☐ Detailed second-trimester fetal morphology survey and arrange for serial fetal growth assessments *(individualized frequency)*
- ☐ In collaboration with the oncologist, plan to continue chemotherapy until ~34–35 weeks' gestation and induce labor after a three-week interval
  - ○ *Three weeks treatment-delivery interval avoids the period of fetal neutropenia*
  - ○ *Cesarean section is reserved for obstetric indications*
- ☐ Where possible, avoid iatrogenic preterm delivery
  - ○ *Preterm infants cannot metabolize chemotherapy as can term infants*
- ☐ Antenatal consultation with neonatology experts
- ☐ Placental examination is required for all cancers diagnosed during pregnancy, irrespective of type and/or treatment
- ☐ Discourage breastfeeding where patient requires postpartum chemotherapy
- ☐ Advise two to three years of remission prior to repeat pregnancy

☐ Contraceptive particularities: *(individualized discussion)*
  ○ Combined hormonal agents are not recommended during active disease due to risks of thromboembolism; however, may be considered during long-term remission
  ○ No restrictions on use of progesterone-only preparations

Pregnancy progresses well, and fetal growth remains on the 10th–13th percentiles. She receives her last chemotherapy session at 34 weeks' gestation and induction of labor three weeks later results in an uncomplicated delivery of a vigorous newborn. You assess the placenta prior to laboratory assessment, without detected abnormalities.

After delivery, your obstetric trainee is searching the Internet, surprised to learn that if HL was newly diagnosed in the third trimester and the patient was free of life-threatening manifestations of disease, treatment could have been electively delayed until postpartum; induction of labor at 37 weeks' gestation could be considered to shorten the delay to treatment initiation.

15. What is the <u>maternal</u> advantage of deferring treatment of HL diagnosed in the third trimester to the postpartum period?

☐ Allow for full staging evaluation postpartum
  ○ *With antenatal therapy, imaging investigations postpartum are inaccurate in assigning primary stage of disease*

Special note:
A fetal advantage of deferring treatment of HL diagnosed in the third trimester to the postpartum period is to avoid fetal exposure to chemotherapy, without affecting maternal prognosis

CASE 1
SCENARIO B
(This is a continuation of the clinical scenario after Question 5)
Excisional biopsy of the mediastinal mass confirms diffuse large B-cell lymphoma, representing the most common pregnancy-associated non-Hodgkin's lymphoma (PA-NHL). B-lymphocytes are positive for CD20.

16. Which routine prenatal investigation might you first ascertain upon learning of the NHL diagnosis?

☐ HIV status

The patient undergoes an echocardiogram as treatment planning and staging MRI at 16^{+5} weeks' gestation, consistent with the chest X-ray findings. She desires to continue pregnancy.

Your obstetric trainee recalls that contrary to HL, NHL does not typically follow a contiguous spread; this can result in mistaking the primary diagnosis.

17. List four gynecological organs where primary NHL may manifest. *(1 point each)*   4

☐ Breast‡
☐ Ovaries‡
☐ Uterus
☐ Vagina

Special note:
‡ Often large and bilateral; tumors are chemo-sensitive and do not require surgical removal

18. Currently in the second trimester, identify the regimen for treatment of this patient's   5
diffuse large B-cell NHL? *(1 point per agent)*

☐ R-CHOP (rituximab, cyclophosphamide, adriamycin, oncovin, and prednisone)

Special note:
With first-trimester diagnosis, single-agent cyclophosphamide ± corticosteroids is given as
bridging therapy until the full regimen can be administered in the second trimester

19. As principles of obstetric management are similar to HL *(Question 14)*, discuss the fetal/   1
neonatal risks of adding chimeric IgG-1 antibody to the chemotherapy regimen given the
patient has B-cell disease.

☐ Rituximab causes nonclinically significant *(i.e., no increased risk of child infections)* B-cell
depletion in infants until four to six months of life; counts thereafter improve
spontaneously

At 28 weeks' gestation, the patient presents for a routine prenatal visit. Although her obstetrics
course has been unremarkable, she complains of nausea and vomiting twice daily, despite oral
metoclopramide prescribed 10 days ago after her chemotherapy cycle. She has no other symptoms.
The fetus is active and growth sonograms have been normal. Her blood pressure is normal; you
note poor weight gain over the past month.

20. List three <u>nonobstetrical</u> causes of poor maternal weight gain accompanied by nausea and   3
vomiting in this patient on combination chemotherapy. *(1 point each)*

☐ Depression
☐ Chemotherapy-induced stomatitis
☐ Suboptimal protein intake/nutritional plan
☐ Progressive disease despite chemotherapy

21-A. Specify <u>preferred</u> corticosteroids for prophylaxis of chemotherapy-induced nausea after fetal viability.   1

☐ Preferred use of prednisone, hydrocortisone, or methylprednisolone

21-B. Identify a <u>less favorable</u> corticosteroid for prophylaxis of chemotherapy-induced nausea after ~24 weeks' gestation and explain why. *(1 point per main and subbullet)*   2

☐ Decadron IV (dexamethasone)
  ○ Inherent placental transfer with associated fetal/neonatal risks of repeated doses of steroids would hamper its use for fetal lung maturation if required for spontaneous or iatrogenic prematurity; preferred use of prednisone or hydrocortisone, if needed

After seeing your patient at her prenatal visit, you receive a call to transfer a 28-year-old primigravida at 19 weeks' gestation with newly diagnosed Burkitt's lymphoma. The transferring physician has informed the patient of the highly aggressive nature of this type of NHL, and the oncology team at your tertiary center awaits her arrival.

22. Although you plan to collaborate with the oncologist, what are your general obstetric recommendations for this patient with Burkitt's lymphoma? *(1 point per main bullet)*   1

☐ Advise pregnancy termination
  ○ Treatment involves intensive chemotherapy, including intrathecal methotrexate as central nervous system prophylaxis
  ○ Rapid tumor doubling time of ~25 hours prevents expectant management
  ○ R-CHOP regimen *(see Question 18)* is ineffective for Burkitt's lymphoma and may adversely affect patient outcome

Special note:
Diagnosis of Burkitt's lymphoma in later gestation requires multidisciplinary collaboration: pregnancy management may include treatment with R-EPOCH chemotherapy, termination of pregnancy, or iatrogenic prematurity

CASE 2

The laboratory calls you urgently with results of her CBC: hemoglobin is 6.5 g/dL (65 g/L), platelets are 55×10^9/L with blasts detected. You arrange for hospitalization and a haemato-oncologist will promptly attend to the patient.

Meanwhile, fetal sonographic assessment reveals biometry on the 9th percentile, a change from the 20th percentile at the morphology scan; umbilical artery (UA) Doppler shows increased resistance with continued forward flow and the maximum vertical amniotic fluid pocket is 2.2 cm. She is kept on continuous electronic fetal monitoring in the birthing center; maternal-fetal medicine and neonatology services have been consulted.

23. In collaboration with the oncology team, identify the <u>diagnostic</u> test of choice to further evaluate the findings on CBC.

☐ Bone marrow biopsy *(safe in pregnancy)*

1

Unilateral bone marrow biopsy and aspiration reveal 70% blasts with suppressed erythropoiesis and myelopoiesis, and a slight decrease in megakaryocyte counts. Reverse transcriptase PCR testing on peripheral blood blasts is negative for the Philadelphia chromosome. While comprehensive pretreatment evaluation is being arranged by the oncologist, you present for multidisciplinary counseling of the patient.

24. Outline the recommended patient management and discuss the effects of acute lymphoblastic leukemia on pregnancy. *(1 point per main and subbullet)*

Max 10

☐ Immediate multidrug chemotherapy is mandatory, irrespective of gestational age; delays in therapy may adversely affect maternal prognosis
☐ Chemotherapy is ideally continued until ~35 weeks' gestation with induction of labor in ~3 weeks, with postpartum resumption ~1–2 weeks later
☐ Adverse perinatal outcomes are increased by virtue of acute leukemia*, unrelated to treatment:

Maternal[§]
o DIC
o Neutropenia and infections (antepartum/intrapartum/postpartum)
o Preterm labor
o Postpartum hemorrhage

Fetal/neonatal
o FGR
o Prematurity (spontaneous or iatrogenic)
o Bleeding (in utero or postnatal)
o Susceptibility to infections
o IUFD
☐ Explain that FGR found on sonography is most probably due to obstructed intervillous blood flow and nutrient exchange in the placenta by leukemic cells, and decreased fetal oxygenation

Special notes:
§ Early pregnancy termination or elective deliveries are only advised *after* induction of remission as the pregnant patient with acute leukemia is at risk of life-threatening morbidities; tocolysis should be considered to arrest spontaneous preterm labor until chemotherapy is initiated for newly diagnosed acute leukemia
* *Refer to* Catanzarite VA, Ferguson JE 2nd. Acute leukemia and pregnancy: a review of management and outcome, 1972–1982. *Obstet Gynecol Surv.* 1984;39(11):663–678.

At 29 weeks' gestation, the patient presents by ambulance to the obstetrical emergency assessment unit after her husband witnessed a grand-mal seizure lasting 30 seconds. She had two bouts of vomiting prior to the seizure and had been complaining of palpitations and decreased urination for three days since her first chemotherapy cycle.

At hospital presentation, the patient is alert and oriented although appears unwell. She does not have obstetric complaints. Fetal cardiotocographic monitoring is normal and uterine quiescence is ascertained. Her blood pressure is 100/70 mmHg, pulse is 110 bpm and oxygen saturation is 98% on room air.

The following is noted among other laboratory investigations:

		Normal
LDH (U/L)	980	<447
ALT (IU/L)	30	6–32
AST (IU/L)	33	11–30
Potassium (mmol/L)	6.4	<6.0
Phosphate (mmol/L)	2.10	<1.45
Calcium (mmol/L)	1.00	>1.75
Uric acid (umol/L)	500	<476
Creatinine (umol/L)	70	<65

Your obstetric trainee believes the patient developed eclampsia.

---

25. What is the most probable diagnosis?   4

☐ Tumor lysis syndrome

The oncologic care team has promptly attended to the patient. Treatment has been initiated and she will be transferred to a setting with cardiac monitoring.

---

26. Outline to your obstetric trainee the pathogenesis and clinical manifestations of tumor lysis syndrome. *(1 point each)*   10

Pathogenesis:
☐ Massive lysis of tumor cells within seven days of initiating cytotoxic chemotherapy, mostly with *(but not limited to)* acute lymphoblastic leukemia or high-grade lymphomas

Laboratory features:
☐ Hyperphosphatemia
☐ Hyperkalemia
☐ Hyperuricemia
☐ Hypocalcemia

Clinical manifestations:

☐ Seizures

☐ Heart failure, arrhythmias

☐ Nausea/vomiting

☐ Acute kidney injury

☐ Tetany

Special note:

Prophylactic strategies involve adequate intravenous hydration and a hypouricemic agent (allopurinol or rasburicase)

TOTAL: **100**

Miscellaneous Conditions

CHAPTER 74

Trauma in Pregnancy

Marwa Salman

A 29-year-old G1P0 at 32 weeks' gestation is brought in by ambulance to the A&E (E.R.) department in your tertiary trauma center following a road traffic accident. She was the restrained driver of a vehicle driving on an icy road at around 50 mph (80 km/h), when she lost control and had a frontal impact collision with another vehicle. She is healthy and has had an unremarkable pregnancy to date. On arrival, she is alert but appears anxious and uncomfortable. Her cervical spine is immobilized with a cervical collar and blocks, and she is on a spinal board. She complains of pains in her chest and lower abdomen. There is a bruise across her right forehead. Her vital signs show a sinus tachycardia of 115 bpm, blood pressure 87/62 mmHg, pulse oximetry 94% on room air, respiratory rate 28/min, and core temperature of 34.6°C. You are covering the birthing center and have been called urgently to the A&E department to assist in the management of this patient.

LEARNING OBJECTIVES

1. Understand the implications of blunt trauma in pregnancy for mother and fetus
2. Identify injuries in a pregnant trauma patient through systemic examination
3. Interpret clinical data that may guide the management of life-threatening conditions in maternal trauma
4. Recognize causes of maternal cardiac arrest, and demonstrate knowledge of advanced life support protocols

SUGGESTED READINGS

1. American College of Surgeons, Committee on Trauma. *Advanced Trauma Life Support®️ Student Course Manual*, 10th ed. Chicago, IL: American College of Surgeons; 2018.
2. Chu J, Johnston TA, Geoghegan J. Maternal collapse in pregnancy and the puerperium. *BJOG* 2020; 127:e14–e52.
3. Galvagno Jr SM, Nahmias JT, Young DA. Advanced trauma life support update 2019: management and support for adults and special populations. *Anesthesiol Clin* 2019; 37: 13–32.
4. Greco PS, Day LJ, Pearlman MD. Guidance for evaluation and management of blunt abdominal trauma in pregnancy. *Obstet Gynecol* 2019; 134:1343–1357.
5. Huls CK, Detlefs C. Trauma in pregnancy. *Semin Perinatol* 2018;42:13–20.

6. Jain V, Chari R, Maslovitz S. Guidelines for the management of a pregnant trauma patient. SOGC 2015. *J Obstet Gynaecol Can.* 2015;37:553–571.

7. Lipman S, Cohen S, Einav S, et al. The Society for Obstetric Anesthesia and Perinatology consensus statement on the management of cardiac arrest in pregnancy. *Anesth Analg.* 2014 May;118(5):1003–1016.

8. MacArthur B, Foley M, Gendra K, et al. Trauma in pregnancy: a comprehensive approach to the mother and fetus. *Am J Obstet Gynecol* 2019; 220: 465–468.

9. Monteiro R, Salman M, Malhotra S, et al. Trauma in pregnancy. In *Anaesthesia, Analgesia and Pregnancy*, 4th ed. Cambridge: Cambridge University Press; 2019.

10. Sakamoto J, Michels C, Eisfelder B. Trauma in pregnancy. *Em Med Clin N Am* 2019; 37: 317–338.

	POINTS
1. Based on the type of collision, what are the possible underlying mechanisms of injury in this patient? *(1 point each)* ☐ Acceleration-deceleration injury ☐ Direct impact and compression ☐ Crush injury	Max 2
2. Outline the steps required in the assessment and initial stabilization of this patient during the Primary Survey. *(1 point each, unless specified)* ☐ Establish airway patency and secure as required ☐ Administer oxygen at FiO2 1.0 to maintain oxygen saturation ≥ 95% *(accept 'high flow oxygen')* ☐ Assess breathing: confirm bilateral air entry and assess tracheal position ☐ Assess circulatory volume and tissue perfusion (capillary refill/ blood pressure/distal pulses) ☐ Large bore IV access x 2 ☐ Start 1 L IV isotonic crystalloid or Start O negative blood if indicated ☐ Neurological examination: Glasgow Coma Scale, pupillary assessment, and assessment for distal neurological deficits ☐ **Left uterine displacement** *(2 points)* ☐ Full body exposure and check for abdominal tenderness and vaginal bleeding ☐ Log roll with spinal protection ☐ Active warming and prevention of hypothermia ☐ Focused Abdominal Sonography for Trauma (FAST) scan/Diagnostic Peritoneal Lavage (DPL) *(as patient is hemodynamically unstable)* ☐ Fetal FAST ☐ Portable imaging as indicated: *e.g.,* cervical spine/chest/pelvis ☐ Trauma laboratory panel *(detailed in Question 12)*	Max 14

Her chest X-ray is as follows:

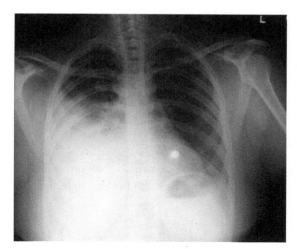

Figure 74.1

With permission: Figure 1 from Raju, V., Sadhasivam, S.K., Padmanabhan, C. et al. Pulmonary arteriovenous malformation with spontaneous haemothorax 2011. Indian J Thorac Cardiovasc Surg 27, 176–178.

There is no association between this case scenario and this patient's image. Image used for educational purposes only.

3. What is the most likely diagnosis?   1

☐ Right hemothorax

4-A. What procedure should be performed as the primary mode of treatment for this condition?   1

☐ Insertion of a chest drain

4-B. Indicate the required technical modifications specific to this patient, relative to the standard technique.   1

☐ Insertion in the third/fourth intercostal space as opposed to the fifth (due to pregnancy-induced upward displacement of the diaphragm)

5-A. What additional advanced intervention might be required to treat this condition?   1

☐ Thoracotomy

5-B. List two possible indications for this intervention in this patient. *(1 point each)*   Max 2

☐ Massive hemothorax on initial drainage (≥1500 mL)
☐ Ongoing bleeding (200 mL/hr for 2–4 hours)
☐ Refractory hypotension or hemodynamic decompensation after initial response to resuscitation

The patient's blood results reveal the following:

		Reference ranges *(not specific to pregnancy)*
Hemoglobin (g/L)	79	110–140
Hematocrit (%)	20	28-39
White cell count ($\times 10^9$/mm^3)	16.2	3.5–9.1
Platelet count ($\times 10^9$/L)	81	150–450
Blood type and screen	A-negative; atypical antibodies not detected	
Sodium (mmol/L)	141	130–140
Potassium (μmol/L)	4.9	3.2–5.1
Creatinine (μmol/L)	66	44–80
Estimated glomerular filtration rate (mL/min/1/.73m^2)	98	>70
International Normalized Ratio (INR)	1.7	0.9–1.0
Partial Thromboplastin Time, activated (s)	45	26.3–39.4
Fibrinogen (g/L)	1.9	2.0–4.0

6. Based on these laboratory results, what is the most likely diagnosis?   5

☐ DIC/consumptive coagulopathy

Special note:
Patient's score for overt DIC in pregnancy is '4' using the Modified International Society on Thrombosis and Hemostasis (ISTH) *(see Chapter 21, Suggested Reading 2 – Clark SL et al. Am J Obstet Gynecol 2016 Oct; 215(4):408–12)*

7. Indicate two pathophysiological mechanisms by which DIC/consumptive coagulopathy   Max 2
might develop in a trauma patient. *(1 point each)*

☐ Bleeding-induced depletion of coagulation factors and platelets and deposition into injuries
☐ Hyperfibrinolysis
☐ Diffuse endothelial cell injury
☐ Qualitative platelet defect *(more common with head injury)*

8. Delineate the necessary steps in the management of this abnormality. *(1 point each)* — Max 5

- ☐ Initiate the local massive hemorrhage (transfusion) protocol
- ☐ Transfuse packed red blood cells: fresh frozen plasma: platelets in a 1:1:1 ratio
- ☐ Transfuse cryoprecipitate/fibrinogen
- ☐ Tranexamic acid 1 g IV, then 1 g IV over eight hours if in hemorrhagic shock
- ☐ Point of care testing, *e.g.,* TEG (Thromboelastography) and ROTEM (Rotational Thromboelastometry) to guide blood component therapy
- ☐ Reassess for ongoing/concealed hemorrhage and ensure definitive control

9. Which other laboratory tests and diagnostic imaging should be performed in the ongoing management of this patient? *(1 point each, unless specified)* — Max 11

Imaging/other tests:
- ☐ CT head spine/chest/abdomen/pelvis *(3 points)*
- ☐ Arterial blood gas
- ☐ ECG
- ☐ Echocardiogram, *if indicated*

Serum:
- ☐ Lactate
- ☐ Troponin
- ☐ Amylase
- ☐ Glucose
- ☐ Feto-maternal haemorrhage screen (*e.g.,* Kleihauer-Betke test)

Urine:
- ☐ Urinalysis
- ☐ Toxicology screen

10. How is fetal well-being supported in this patient? *(1 point each)* — 6

- ☐ Initiation of continuous fetal monitoring with tocometry in the secondary survey
- ☐ Support of maternal blood pressure
- ☐ Maintenance of maternal oxygenation
- ☐ Avoidance of aortocaval compression
- ☐ Tocolysis, if appropriate and haemodynamic stability achieved
- ☐ Cesarean delivery, if indicated

11. List three factors associated with increased risk of fetal loss in maternal trauma. *(1 point each)*

    ☐ Maternal hypotension
    ☐ Injury severity score (ISS) >9 *(accept 'high ISS')*
    ☐ Abruptio placenta
    ☐ Uterine rupture
    ☐ Maternal tachycardia
    ☐ Maternal pelvic fracture
    ☐ Ejection from motor vehicle
    ☐ Abnormal fetal heart rate

Max 3

The patient suddenly becomes unresponsive. A rapid assessment reveals absence of central and peripheral pulses and respiratory effort. Her ECG is as follows.

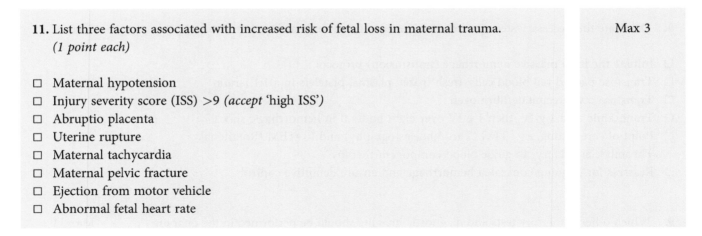

Figure 74.2

There is no association between this case scenario and this patient's ECG. The ECG used for educational purposes only.

12. Identify this rhythm.

    ☐ Pulseless electrical activity

4

13. List the steps required to treat this condition *(indicate correct rhythm is pulseless electrical activity in order to proceed). (1 point each, unless specified)*

    ☐ Start chest compressions and inflation breaths at a ratio of 30:2
    ☐ Establish definitive airway then asynchronous chest compressions
    ☐ Adrenaline 1 mg (10 ml of 1:10000) IV every 3–5 min
    ☐ Treat reversible causes simultaneously with resuscitation
    ☐ Reassess rhythm every 2 min
    ☐ Delivery by perimortem Cesarean section[†] at four minutes if no return of spontaneous circulation *(2 points)*

Max 7

Special note:

† At perimortem Cesarean section, a vertical skin scar may be considered to allow for exploratory surgery and intracardiac massage

14. What could be possible <u>reversible</u> causes of cardiac arrest in this patient? *(1 point each, unless specified)*

Max 12

☐ Hypovolemia[#]
☐ Hypoxia[#]
☐ Cardiac tamponade[#]
☐ Tension pneumothorax[#]
☐ Thromboembolism
☐ Hyper/hypokalaemia – hypo/hypermagnesemia – hypo/hypercalcemia (electrolyte imbalance)
☐ Toxins
☐ Eclampsia/intracranial haemorrhage
☐ Hypothermia

Special note:
[#] implies 2 points each

15. If hemodynamic stability of this patient is achieved and fetal well-being is assured, name three intramuscular injections you would then consider. *(1 point each)*

3

☐ Acellular pertussis vaccination
☐ Anti-D immunoglobulin
☐ Fetal pulmonary corticosteroids

TOTAL: **80**

CHAPTER 75

Substance Use in Pregnancy

Alexa Eberle and Amira El-Messidi

You are called to the A&E (E.R.) department of your tertiary center to assist in the care of your patient, a 22-year-old primigravida at 14^{+4} weeks' gestation who presents, accompanied by her partner, with a six-hour history of nausea, vomiting, and headache since her last consumed six-daily standard drinks of beer yesterday. At last week's baseline prenatal visit, you learned that medical history is only significant for an alcohol use disorder, for which she was motivated to enroll in a treatment program. Your medical notes indicate a normal body habitus and unremarkable physical exam. Prenatal investigations and first-trimester aneuploidy screening tests were normal. You had prescribed vitamins containing folic acid; the patient was not experiencing nausea or vomiting of pregnancy.

The urgent care physician informs you that mental status is normal, although she is anxious, tremulous, and diaphoretic. There is no evidence of trauma. Her blood pressure is 143/87 mmHg, pulse is 93 bpm, with normal temperature, oxygen saturation, and fetal cardiac activity. Urine toxicology screening performed with the patient's consent is negative, including her blood alcohol level.

Special note: *Although simultaneous polysubstance use may be more common than stepwise use of alcohol and other substance-related disorders, the case scenario is presented as such for academic purposes and to avoid overlap of content addressed in other chapters.*

LEARNING OBJECTIVES

1. Become familiar with validated brief alcohol screening questionnaires that may be used to detect patterns of maternal alcohol intake
2. Recognize various clinical syndromes of alcohol withdrawal, and collaborate with urgent care physicians to provide medical management of early withdrawal during pregnancy
3. Counsel on the importance of abstinence from alcohol and illicit substances during pregnancy and postpartum
4. Discuss potential maternal, fetal, and child risks of prenatal exposure to alcohol and marijuana
5. Understand that cocaine-induced hypertension may mimic preeclampsia, and appreciate an important difference in medical management

SUGGESTED READINGS

1. American College of Obstetricians and Gynecologists. Committee on Health Care for Underserved Women. Committee opinion no. 496: At-risk drinking and alcohol dependence: obstetric and gynecologic implications. *Obstet Gynecol.* 2011;118(2 Pt 1):383–388.

2. Committee on Obstetric Practice. Committee Opinion No. 722: marijuana use during pregnancy and lactation. *Obstet Gynecol.* 2017;130(4):e205–e209.

3. Department of Health. UK Chief Medical Officers' alcohol guidelines review: summary of the proposed new guidelines. 2016. Available at https://assets.publishing.service.gov.uk/government/uploads/system/uploads/attachment_data/file/489795/summary.pdf. Acessed April 22, 2022.

4. DeVido J, Bogunovic O, Weiss RD. Alcohol use disorders in pregnancy. *Harv Rev Psychiatry.* 2015;23(2):112–121.

5. Graves L, Carson G, Poole N, et al. Guideline No. 405: screening and counselling for alcohol consumption during pregnancy. *J Obstet Gynaecol Can.* 2020 Sep;42(9):1158–1173.

6. *Guidelines for the Identification and Management of Substance Use and Substance Use Disorders in Pregnancy.* Geneva: World Health Organization; 2014.

7. Dejong K, Olyaei A, Lo JO. Alcohol use in pregnancy. *Clin Obstet Gynecol.* 2019;62 (1):142–155.

8. Metz TD, Borgelt LM. Marijuana use in pregnancy and while breastfeeding. *Obstet Gynecol.* 2018;132(5):1198–1210.

9. Ordean A, Wong S, Graves L. No. 349 – substance use in pregnancy. *J Obstet Gynaecol Can.* 2017;39(10):922–937.

10. Thibaut F, Chagraoui A, Buckley L, et al. WFSBP* and IAWMH** Guidelines for the treatment of alcohol use disorders in pregnant women. *World J Biol Psychiatry.* 2019;20(1):17–50. [Correction in World J Biol Psychiatry. 2019 Apr 11]

POINTS

1. As your obstetric trainee accompanies you to attend to the patient, discuss <u>one</u> alcohol screening questionnaire[†] either developed for the obstetric population or which may assess prenatal risk drinking. *(1 point for any bullet)*

1

☐ T-ACE/T-ACER-3 *(Tolerance, Annoyed, Cut down, Eye-opener)*
☐ TWEAK *(Tolerance, Worry, Eye-Opener, Amnesia, K/Cut down)*
☐ SURP-P *(Substance Use Risk Profile – Pregnancy)*
☐ AUDIT-C *(a three-question tool)*
☐ NET *(Normal drinker, eye-opener, Tolerance)*
☐ The 4-Ps *(Pregnancy, Past, Partner, Parents)*

Special note:

† No one screening instrument is superior to another in identifying alcohol use disorders in pregnant women.

Refer to Question 1 in Chapter 76; framework of focused history may be applied to alcohol or substance use disorders in pregnancy

2. Outline to your trainee four syndromes of alcohol withdrawal appearing among problem drinkers. *(1 point per main bullet)*   4

☐ Minor withdrawal symptoms
  ○ *e.g anxiety, diaphoresis, tremors, palpitations, headache, nausea, vomiting*
☐ Tonic-clonic alcohol withdrawal seizures
  ○ *short duration with a brief post-ictal period*
☐ Alcoholic hallucinosis
  ○ *Visual (mostly) or auditory with autonomic stability*
☐ Delirium tremens *(more commonly in older population with prolonged drinking history, concurrent illness, and >48 hours after last drink)*

3. Serum investigations have been requested. In collaboration with the urgent care team, <u>detail</u> treatment and management of the patient at this time. *(1 point per main bullet unless specified)*   Max 6

☐ Hospitalization is recommended for management of alcohol withdrawal in pregnancy
  ○ Place the patient in a protected, quiet environment
☐ Peripheral IV access for hydration, electrolyte replacement, and medications
☐ If the patient cannot tolerate oral treatment, initiate IV treatment: Using the lowest dose for the shortest duration, may consider treatment with diazepam 5–10 mg IV every 5–10 minutes until symptomatic improvement *(2 points)*
  ○ *Benzodiazepines are first-line agents for all alcohol withdrawal syndromes*
  ○ *Diazepam or chlordiazepoxide should be considered first-line agents in early pregnancy*
☐ Thiamine (vitamin B1) 100 mg IV/IM once daily for three to five days, followed by oral treatment *(2 points)*
☐ Glucose replacement IV or orally (after thiamine)
☐ Supportive therapy including antiemetics, multivitamins
☐ Daily ascertainment of fetal viability during hospitalization
  ○ *Fetal monitoring should be considered at viable gestational ages*

During admission, symptomatic improvement from alcohol withdrawal is achieved and multi-disciplinary collaborations have been made. Although she recalls part of your brief intervention[†] discussion during the first prenatal visit,[‡] the patient requests repeat counseling of obstetric risks associated with alcohol use in pregnancy; she has also misplaced the patient information document on alcohol in pregnancy you had provided at the initial prenatal visit.[§]

Special notes:
† A brief intervention is patient-centered counseling to understand risks of alcohol and help change behavior or accept referral to treatment programs (raise awareness of risks, advise on strategies for reduction/elimination of drinking, and provide assistance)
‡ Universal screening for alcohol, tobacco, and illicit drug use is recommended at the first prenatal visit and subsequently throughout pregnancy; first prenatal visit screening based on risk factors only may miss problem drinkers and increase stereotyping
§ Resource sample: www.rcog.org.uk/en/patients/patient-leaflets/alcohol-and-pregnancy/

4. Counsel the patient on general recommendations for safe levels of alcohol intake, *if any*, and discuss prenatal and postnatal risks of consumption. *(1 point per main bullet, unless specified)*

    Max 7

☐ Safest approach is complete abstinence from alcohol intake during pregnancy, preconception and breastfeeding; there is no known safe amount of alcohol during pregnancy
   ○ *Alcohol cessation at any time during gestation may improve infant outcomes relative to continued antenatal exposure*

Maternal:
☐ Early pregnancy loss
☐ Preterm labor

Fetal/child:
☐ Teratogenicity; alcohol-related birth defects (ARBD)[†]
☐ Fetal growth restriction (FGR), low birthweight
☐ IUFD
☐ Fetal alcohol spectrum disorders (FASD), as a continuum of outcomes including: *(1 point per subbullet; max 2)*
   ○ Fetal alcohol syndrome (FAS)
   ○ Fetal alcohol effects (FAE)
   ○ Alcohol-related neurodevelopmental disorder (ARND)
   ○ Neurobehavioral disorder associated with prenatal alcohol exposure (ND-PAE)

Special note:
† *See Question 7*

5. Elicit socio-medical features associated with adversity from prenatal alcohol-use disorder, which may additionally increase risk of FAS. *(1 point per main bullet)*

    Max 7

Medical aspects:
☐ Type, amount, pattern, and timing of prenatal alcohol exposure *(especially prepregnancy alcohol consumption)*
   ○ *Heavy episodic drinking and/or binge drinking is associated with greater adversity to the fetus/neonate*
☐ Decreased maternal alcohol dehydrogenase metabolic capacity *(gene polymorphisms)*
☐ Concomitant use of substances, including cigarette smoking
☐ Concomitant mental health conditions or psychological stressors
☐ Advanced maternal age
☐ Multiparity

Social aspects:
☐ Prior physical, sexual abuse or neglect; low self-esteem
☐ Prior incarceration
☐ Nonmarried status
☐ Living alone
☐ Low socioeconomic status, unemployed
☐ Family history or partner use of alcohol, tobacco, or illicit drugs
☐ Ethnicity (e.g Native or African American)

Prior to discharge, the patient expresses continued optimism to modify her drinking behavior for the well-being of her unborn child and intends to adhere to prenatal care recommendations.

6. With focus on alcohol use disorder, discuss your <u>antenatal care</u> plan for this patient.   Max 5
    (1 point per main bullet)

☐ Frequent prenatal visits and/or telephone liaison for support and monitoring of maternal-fetal well-being
  ○ Include 'brief intervention' interviewing at each prenatal visit to maintain motivation for harm-reduction related to alcohol use
☐ Provide written or electronic materials on strategies for eliminating problematic drinking
☐ Referral for in-depth counseling and treatment of alcohol dependence (individual or group therapy)
☐ Nutritionist consultation and monitoring of gestational weight gain
  ○ Consideration for maintenance thiamine in heavy alcohol users; dietary supplementation of thiamine 1.4 mg/d is recommended antenatally and with breastfeeding *(no known adverse effects with high levels of thiamine)*
☐ Detailed second-trimester fetal morphology survey and consideration for fetal echocardiography, if required *(assess for alcohol-related fetal cardiac malformations)*
☐ Serial second- and third-trimester surveillance of fetal growth and well-being, particularly with continued alcohol intake or recurrent manifestations of withdrawal
☐ Neonatology/pediatric consultation

With simultaneous multidisciplinary psychosocial interventions, the patient decreased her intake of beer to one drink daily. She remains compliant with routine aspects of prenatal care and has not had obstetric complaints. She presents at 20 weeks' gestation for fetal morphology survey, performed in your center's maternal-fetal medicine unit.

7. Identify sonographic <u>fetal findings or malformations</u> that have been associated with   Max 3
    antenatal alcohol exposure, recognizing that none are pathognomonic. *(1 point each)*

☐ FGR
☐ Decreased head circumference
☐ Orofacial clefts *(through gene-environment interactions)*
☐ Congenital heart malformations *(e.g atrial or ventricular septal defects)*
☐ Renal malformations *(e.g aplasia/dysplasia/hypoplasia, horseshoe kidney)*
☐ Skeletal abnormalities *(e.g flexion contractures)*

Special note:
Characteristic craniofacial findings best appreciated postnatally include short palpebral fissures, a smooth or flat philtrum, and thin upper vermillion border

Fetal biometry, morphology, and placentation are normal. Although reassuring, the patient understands that postnatal surveillance for neurobehavioral manifestations, withdrawal and physical assessment of features associated with in utero alcohol exposure, remain necessary.

By 28 weeks' gestation, the patient manages to abstain from alcoholic beverages and remains compliant with prenatal care. She has not had obstetric complaints or complications; she is curious if she can resume *'some'* alcohol intake while breastfeeding.

8. Address principal elements of counseling on alcohol consumption during breastfeeding.   Max 7

Recommendations:
☐ Complete abstinence from alcohol is advised, although may not be practical *(5 points)*
  ○ *Do not consume immediately before feeding*
  ○ *Consider expressing breast milk in advance*
  ○ *Avoid breastfeeding for two to four hours after more than 2 drinks of alcohol*

Rationale: *(1 point each)*
☐ Alcohol does not accumulate in breast milk (unlike marijuana)
☐ Decreased lactation-induced milk ejection reflex, milk production and intake by infants
☐ Altered sleep-wake behavior pattern in infants
☐ Abnormal growth patterns
☐ Altered intellectual and psychomotor function

Special note:
Upper limits of alcohol intake for adult women (nonpregnant) varies among countries; United Kingdom (8 g pure alcohol/standard drink) advises two to three drinks per day, Unites States (13.7 g pure alcohol/standard drink) advises one drink per day, Canada (13.6 g alcohol/standard drink) advises two drinks per day

You maintain 'brief intervention' counseling at each prenatal visit, supporting her continued abstinence from alcohol. At 32 weeks' gestation, the patient indicates she started smoking cannabis (marijuana) for the past week to help with insomnia. She has not used other substances or resumed alcohol intake. Prior to discussing obstetric risks of marijuana, you provide her with safe and potentially effective sleep rituals.

9. Advise the patient on six recommendations to improve sleep health rather than marijuana consumption.   Max 7

Do's: *(1 point each; max 3)*
☐ Mindfulness, relaxation techniques, and yoga
☐ Reduce bedroom noise
☐ Regulate sleep time
☐ Use dim lights in the bathroom
☐ Exercise regularly, except where contraindicated in pregnancy and within four hours of bedtime

Don'ts: *(1 point each; max 4)*
☐ Drink/eat caffeinated products close to bedtime
☐ Drink large quantities of fluid close to bedtime
☐ Eat large, spicy, or fried meals in the evening
☐ Take daytime naps
☐ Use electronic devices in bed

10. With regard to her current marijuana intake, indicate important elements you would want
to know. *(1 point each)*   5

☐ Inquire about reasons for use, other than insomnia
☐ Access source, where and with whom she uses the drug
☐ Quantity, route, frequency, and verify duration of use
☐ Last use
☐ Symptoms of withdrawal *(e.g irritability, insomnia, anorexia, anxiety)*

11. Counsel the patient on perinatal recommendations regarding marijuana consumption,
including <u>possible</u> short-term and long-term risks from in utero exposure. *(1 point per
main bullet)*   7

☐ Complete abstinence from marijuana use in pregnancy and breastfeeding is advised
  ○ *No medicinal benefits justify fetal-neonatal risks of exposure*

Obstetric risks: *(Max 3)*
☐ FGR, low birthweight
☐ Preterm delivery
☐ Placental abruption
☐ IUFD *(likely confounded by smoking or multifactorial etiology)*
☐ Neonatal withdrawal syndrome
☐ NICU admission

<u>Long-term infant problems, including:</u> *(Max 3)*
☐ Evidence of neurodevelopmental delay, intellectual, memory and verbal dysfunction
☐ Dysfunction in abstract and visual reasoning
☐ Aggression, impulsivity, hyperactivity and inattention
☐ Mood disturbances, such as anxiety and depression
☐ Early substance use
☐ Abnormal sleep patterns
☐ Suboptimal height in childhood

12. Identify the <u>physiological</u> basis why the 'pump-and-dump' phenomenon during the
washout period after alcohol intake may not be adequate among marijuana users who wish
to breastfeed.   2

☐ Tetrahydrocannabinol (primary ingredient in marijuana) is highly lipophilic,
accumulating in breast milk, with a long half-life relative to alcohol

With modified behavioral practices and continued psychosocial therapy, sleep patterns improve
and the patient discontinues nightly marijuana by 35 weeks' gestation. Her obstetrical course is
otherwise unremarkable; fetal growth biometry and amniotic fluid volume have been normal.
Although universal vaginal-rectal GBS screening is recommended at 36^{+0} to 37^{+6} weeks' gestation,[†] you perform routine testing at this visit, in recognition of her antenatal risk factors for
prematurity. The test later reported to be negative.

The following week, she presents to the obstetric emergency assessment unit with spontaneous, acute abdominal pain and fresh vaginal bleeding that filled half a sanitary pad over 30 minutes. Her blood pressure is 160/108 mmHg, pulse is 105 bpm, and oxygen saturation is normal. Pupillary dilation is noticeable in room light. Her mood appears elated, and she is hyperalert to the surroundings. Fetal cardiotocography (CTG) shows a normal tracing with regular, palpable uterine contractions every three to five minutes. On examination, the cervix is 7 cm dilated with intact membranes; fetal presentation is cephalic. Serum laboratory investigations are unremarkable with absent proteinuria.

Special note:
† *Refer to* Prevention of Group B Streptococcal Early-Onset Disease in Newborns: ACOG Committee Opinion, No. 797 [published correction appears in Obstet Gynecol. 2020 Apr;135(4):978–979]. Obstet Gynecol. 2020;135(2):e51-e72.

---

13. Indicate the <u>most probable</u> causative agent accounting for the patient's presentation, assuming positive urine toxicology testing.   1

☐ Cocaine
  ○ *Urine testing assesses for the metabolite, benzoylecgonine, not cocaine*

---

14. Although mimicking preeclampsia, discuss an important caveat specific to treatment of cocaine-induced hypertension.   1

☐ Avoid labetalol
  ○ *β-blockade results in unopposed α-adrenergic stimulation, which may risk end-organ ischemia*

Special note:
Advise repeat blood pressure assessment prior to administering medication; cocaine-induced hypertension is often self-limited

---

Labor progresses rapidly with spontaneous delivery of a male newborn weighing 2780 grams with arterial pH of 7.20. The placenta delivers almost immediately, with gross evidence of abruption. Pathology evaluation of the placenta is requested.

On postpartum day 1, the patient admits to you that she smoked 150 mg of cocaine for the first time, shortly before delivery-hospitalization. She has minimal analgesic requirements, adequately controlled by paracetamol (acetaminophen) and nonsteroidal anti-inflammatory agents.

15. Discuss <u>postpartum</u> considerations most specific to this patient's antenatal course.

(1 point per main bullet)

Max 7

Mental health and addiction care:
☐ Screen for postpartum depression and continue to offer psychosocial counseling
☐ Refer to drug treatment programs (e.g cocaine, marijuana)
☐ Arrange for a clinic visit early in the postpartum period given significant antenatal stressors

Primary care:
☐ Communicate with her physician for ongoing care

Timing of discharge:
☐ Attempt accommodation of extended patient's hospital stay where neonate experiences withdrawal or other complications *(dependent on facility's capacity)*
☐ Arrange formal handover between hospital and community services for mother and neonate

Breastfeeding:
☐ Advise against breastfeeding with regular substance use
　○ After individual use of cocaine, discontinue breastfeeding for 24 hours

Contraception:
☐ Reassure the patient that contraceptive counseling serves to empower her to achieve the desired interpregnancy interval, rather than your judgement of her suitability for parenting
☐ Offer long-acting reversible contraception prior to hospital discharge
　○ *Encourage future preconception counseling*
☐ Encourage use of condoms for dual contraception to decrease risks of sexually transmitted infections

TOTAL:　　　**70**

CHAPTER 76

Opioid Use Disorders in Pregnancy

Tricia E. Wright and Amira El-Messidi

A 25-year-old primigravida at 21^{+5} weeks' gestation is sent by her primary care provider for urgent consultation and transfer of care to your tertiary center's high-risk obstetrics unit for increasing diaphoresis, body aches, and anxiousness since self-discontinuation of heroin upon recent knowledge of pregnancy.

Special note: *Although opioid use is often co-occurring with other substance-related disorders, including alcohol, recreational drugs, and psychiatric agents, the case scenario is presented as such for academic purposes and to ovoid content overlap; the reader is encouraged to complement subject matter with Chapter 75.*

LEARNING OBJECTIVES

1. Obtain a thorough prenatal history from a patient with opioid use disorder (OUD), and collaborate with addiction medicine experts to provide appropriate antenatal and long-term postpartum care to improve maternal-fetal and child outcomes
2. Recognize that OUD is a chronic relapsing condition requiring multidisciplinary and patient-centered care during pregnancy and beyond
3. Understand relevant aspects related to pharmacologic induction and maintenance treatment for OUD
4. Demonstrate the ability to plan intrapartum care of patients with OUD, and counsel on expectations related to neonatal withdrawal
5. Appreciate that cigarette smoking is common in patients with OUD and that pregnancy offers an optimal time to address smoking cessation interventions

SUGGESTED READINGS

1. Committee on Obstetric Practice. Committee Opinion No. 711: Opioid use and opioid use disorder in pregnancy. *Obstet Gynecol.* 2017;130(2):e81–e94.
2. Ecker J, Abuhamad A, Hill W, et al. Substance use disorders in pregnancy: clinical, ethical, and research imperatives of the opioid epidemic: a report of a joint workshop of the Society for Maternal-Fetal Medicine, American College of Obstetricians and Gynecologists, and American Society of Addiction Medicine. *Am J Obstet Gynecol.* 2019;221(1):B5–B28.
3. *Guidelines for the Identification and Management of Substance Use and Substance Use Disorders in Pregnancy.* Geneva: World Health Organization; 2014.

4.   Jones HE, Kaltenbach K, Heil SH, et al. Neonatal abstinence syndrome after methadone or buprenorphine exposure. *N Engl J Med.* 2010;363(24):2320–2331.

5.   Kampman K, Jarvis M. American Society of Addiction Medicine (ASAM) national practice guideline for the use of medications in the treatment of addiction involving opioid use. *J Addict Med.* 2015;9(5):358–367.

6.   Ordean A, Wong S, Graves L. No. 349 – substance use in pregnancy. *J Obstet Gynaecol Can.* 2017;39(10):922–937.

7.   Reddy UM, Davis JM, Ren Z, et al. Opioid use in pregnancy, neonatal abstinence syndrome, and childhood outcomes: executive summary of a joint workshop by the Eunice Kennedy Shriver National Institute of Child Health and Human Development, American College of Obstetricians and Gynecologists, American Academy of Pediatrics, Society for Maternal-Fetal Medicine, Centers for Disease Control and Prevention, and the March of Dimes Foundation. *Obstet Gynecol.* 2017;130(1):10–28.

8.   Substance Abuse and Mental Health Services Administration. Clinical guidance for treating pregnant and parenting women with opioid use disorder and their infants. HHS Publication No. (SMA) 18-5054. Rockville, MD: Substance Abuse and Mental Health Services Administration; 2018.

9.   The ASAM national practice guidelines for the use of medications to treat opioid use disorders 2015 with focused update 2020. Available at www.asam.org/docs/default-source/practice-support/guidelines-and-consensus-docs/asam-national-practice-guideline-supplement.pdf. Accessed December 8, 2020.

10. Wright TE, ed. *Opioid Use Disorders in Pregnancy, Management Guidelines for Improving Outcomes.* Cambridge: Cambridge University Press; 2018.

POINTS

1. With regard to OUD, what aspects of a focused history would you want to know? *(1 point per main bullet, unless specified)*	Max 35

History related to chronic opioid use:
☐   Name of the drug(s)
☐   Access source, where and with whom opioid(s) are used
☐   Last use
☐   Quantity, route, frequency and duration of use
 ○   *Route of use helps assess for potential complications*
☐   Previous treatment programs and longest period of abstinence *(if any)*

Symptoms of opioid withdrawal: *(in addition to her reported diaphoresis,[‡] aches,[‡] and anxiety[‡])*
☐   Cravings
☐   Palpitations
☐   Tremors
☐   Sleep disturbance, yawning
☐   Nasal congestion, rhinorrhea, lacrimation[‡]
☐   Gastrointestinal upset (cramps, nausea/vomiting, diarrhea)[‡]
 ○   Symptoms may overlap with pregnancy

Concomitant medications:
☐   *(particularly)* Benzodiazepines, selective serotonin reuptake inhibitors (SSRIs), antipsychotics
 ○   Consequences of alcohol and benzodiazepine withdrawal can result in fatality; vigilance in detection is advised

Social factors and routine health maintenance:
- ☐ Coercive sexual activity, physical abuse, or neglect
- ☐ Financial status, exchanging sex for money, occupation, housing situation
- ☐ Caffeine intake
- ☐ Cigarette smoking *(common in ~80%–90% of women with OUD)*
- ☐ Alcohol consumption or use of recreational drugs *(polysubstance use)*
- ☐ Prior incarceration
- ☐ Vaccination status *(e.g., influenza, hepatitis A and B, tetanus, Covid)*

Complications or comorbidities of substance use:
- ☐ Chronic pain syndromes, medical conditions
- ☐ *Psychiatric*: *e.g.*, mood, anxiety, eating disorders
  - ○ Determine presence of suicidal or homicidal ideation *(4 points)*
- ☐ *Oral:* e.g gum disease, abscesses
- ☐ *Musculoskeletal:* *e.g.*, substance-related amputations, burns, cellulitis, skin abscess
- ☐ *Hematologic*: e.g thromboembolic events, anemia
- ☐ *Cardio-respiratory*: *e.g.*, arrhythmias, endocarditis, asthma, chronic cough, hematemesis
- ☐ *Gastrointestinal*: *e.g.*, jaundice, hepatitis
- ☐ *Gynecologic*: *e.g.*, prior sexually transmitted infections (STIs), cervical dysplasia

Pregnancy:
- ☐ Establish whether dates were established by menstrual period or dating sonogram
- ☐ Assess her attitude toward pregnancy
- ☐ Involvement of partner, and assess for domestic violence/abuse
- ☐ Determine if patient had prior, *undisclosed*, spontaneous or therapeutic pregnancy losses

Family/partner history:
- ☐ Parental history of substance use
- ☐ Partner with an OUD or other substances

Special note:
‡ 5 of 11 components of the COWS (Clinical Opioid Withdrawal Scale)

You learn this is an unplanned, yet desired pregnancy, with her stable partner with whom she lives for two years. She started regular use of oxycodone four years ago after leaving her parents' home due to long-standing physical and emotional abuse. Last year, she switched to smoking heroin as oxycodone was costly. She smokes 1 g of heroin in two to six daily doses. Her last dose was two days ago after having a urine pregnancy test for suspected fetal activity. The patient also smokes at least 15 cigarettes per day, without alcohol or use of other substances. She does not have chronic pain, medical conditions, or prescribed medicinal agents. Her partner has been supportive, encouraging her to seek professional help for addiction.

With the willpower of providing safe care of her unborn child and given her partner's support, the patient decided to abstain from heroin during the remainder of pregnancy. However, six hours after her last heroin consumption, she became irritable with onset of body aches, progressively worsening over two days. With concomitant diaphoresis and anxiousness, she decided to seek medical care. She has no obstetric complaints.

Recognizing the urgent need to initiate treatment of OUD to optimize prenatal care, you call a colleague with expertise in addiction medicine.

2. Fundal height is at the umbilicus and fetal viability is ascertained. In collaboration with the addiction medicine expert, outline your <u>focused physical assessment</u> related to substance use. *(1 point each)*

Max 15

General findings and vital signs:
- ☐ Body habitus
- ☐ Slurred speech, yawning,‡ agitation, sedation, unsteady gait, tremor,‡ restlessness‡ *(i.e., signs of withdrawal)*
- ☐ Blood pressure, pulse,‡ respiratory rate, temperature, oxygen saturation

Integumentary:
- ☐ Jaundice (skin *or sclera*)
- ☐ Piloerection‡
- ☐ Needle tracks, scars, rashes, abscesses, cellulitis

Ocular:
- ☐ Pinpoint/dilated pupils,‡ conjunctivitis

Oral cavity:
- ☐ Poor dentition, gum disease

Oto-rhino-laryngeal *findings may include, but not limited to:*
- ☐ Hoarseness
- ☐ Perforation/excoriation of nasal septum
- ☐ Epistaxis, rhinorrhea
- ☐ Sinusitis
- ☐ Auricular discharge or otitis

Cardio-respiratory:
- ☐ Arrhythmias, murmurs
- ☐ Cough, crackles

Abdominal:
- ☐ Hepatomegaly *(physical examination may be difficult with advanced gestation)*

Pelvic:
- ☐ Ensure patient's permission prior to genital examination; consideration for offering presence of a support person (or witness). Be cognizant of likelihood of prior sexual abuse, and provide trauma-informed care, such as going slowly, asking permission at each stage of the exam, and allowing the patient to stop the exam at any time if needed
- ☐ Signs of infections *(e.g abnormal cervicovaginal discharge, ulcerations, vesicles)* and perform necessary testing

Special notes:
(a) ‡6 of 11 components of the COWS (Clinical Opioid Withdrawal Scale).
(b) Treatment of withdrawal is paramount and is practically initiated prior to completion of the physical exam; this structured approach is presented as such for academic purposes

Although she is restless, the patient is able to sit still with some difficulty and reports increasing anxiousness. She is of thin body habitus and appears flushed with observable facial moistness. Her resting pulse is 90 bpm, pupils appear larger than expected in room light, and you notice piloerection on her arms. Despite poor dentition, detailed physical examination is otherwise unremarkable; vaginal cultures have been obtained.

In discussion with the patient, the addiction expert discourages self-discontinuation of heroin and advises initiation of long-term medical treatment with concurrent psychosocial interventions to optimize maternal-fetal-child benefit. In response to your obstetric trainee's query, the addiction medicine expert indicates that '*medically assisted withdrawal, or detoxification therapy*' is a suboptimal regimen.

3-A. Outline what *medically assisted withdrawal* for OUD entails. 1

☐ Initiation of pharmacotherapy, followed by gradual weaning until discontinuation of medical treatment, with subsequent psychosocial interventions to prevent relapse

3-B. Identify the principal reason why *medically assisted withdrawal* is inferior to long-term pharmaco-psychosocial regimens for OUD. 1

☐ Increased opioid relapse rates, including risks of overdose and mortality
  ○ *Recent studies do not show increased rates of obstetric complications, as formerly considered (SOGC)*

---

4. In collaboration with the addiction medicine expert, outline your counseling of maternal-fetal-neonatal benefits of medication-assisted and psychosocial therapy compared with continued heroin use. *(1 point each)* Max 5

Maternal:[§]
☐ Improves perinatal outcome *(overlaps with fetal-neonatal benefits)*
☐ Improves adherence with multidisciplinary prenatal care and treatment plan for OUD
☐ Stabilizes daily serum drug levels, preventing opioid withdrawal symptoms
☐ Promotes social stability and potential for child custody
☐ Supports avoidance of drug-seeking environments or at-risk acts *(e.g., prostitution)*
☐ Decreases morbidity and mortality

Fetal/neonatal:
☐ No proven teratogenic effects of opioid agonist therapy
☐ Allows for preparation of postnatal management of infants whose mothers are in treatment programs for OUD

Special note:
§ Emphasize OUD is a chronic, relapsing condition requiring long-term treatment, similar to diabetes mellitus or hypertension; '*normalize*' therapy

5. Indicate potential <u>antenatal obstetric</u> complications if this patient were to continue illicit opioid use. *(1 point each)*   Max 6

☐ Low birthweight or FGR
☐ Third-trimester bleeding
☐ Placental abruption
☐ Preeclampsia
☐ Meconium aspiration
☐ Preterm labor and preterm rupture of membranes
☐ Malpresentation and Cesarean section
☐ IUFD

Special note:
Miscarriage is also associated with opioid use in pregnancy, although this patient presents in the second trimester

6. What are the two most common <u>opioid agonists</u> used for antepartum and postpartum management of opioid dependency? *(1 point each)*   2

☐ Buprenorphine
☐ Methadone

Special note:
Naltrexone (opioid antagonist) is not currently recommended for treatment of OUD in pregnant women, although studies are ongoing.

The addiction medicine expert explains that both buprenorphine and methadone are first-line agents with similar efficacy and safety for treatment of opioid-dependent pregnant women. During the decision-making discussion with the patient, the expert explains that buprenorphine can be started as the patient is in mild to moderate withdrawal (COWS score is 11); treatment initiation with buprenorphine where patients are not in withdrawal may otherwise precipitate symptoms. Induction will be initiated with sublingual combined buprenorphine with the opioid antagonist naloxone.[‡] The addiction medicine expert explains that although naloxone is not orally active, it serves to discourage product sharing or sale (*i.e.*, diversion) as severe withdrawal symptoms would occur with injection.

You sketch the benefits of the two opioid agonists, intending to teach your trainee after this consultation.

Special note:
‡ SOGC 2017 *(Suggested Reading 6)* recommends single agent buprenorphine during pregnancy

7. Discuss your sketched notes regarding maternal-neonatal <u>benefits of buprenorphine relative to methadone</u> in treatment of opioid-dependent pregnant women. *(1 point each)*

Max 7

Maternal:

☐ Discreet; possibility of dispensing medication in an office setting *(international policies may vary)*

☐ Improved side effect profile *(e.g.,* cardiovascular/arrhythmias)

☐ Decreased risk of overdose mortality,[§] unless combined with other central nervous system depressants

☐ Decreased sedative effect

☐ In the absence of sedation, switching from buprenorphine to methadone can be immediate, rather than the challenging reverse treatment

☐ Possibly decreased risk of preterm birth

Neonatal:

☐ Decreased incidence and severity of neonatal opioid withdrawal syndrome (NOWS)[†]

☐ Lower doses of morphine and shorter duration of treatment for NOWS

☐ Shorter hospitalization

☐ Possibly higher birthweight and larger head circumference

Special notes:

§ Due to its **mixed** opioid agonist/antagonist effects, whereas methadone is a **full** opioid agonist

† NOWS is not associated with long-term harm with adequate treatment; as such, severity of NOWS may not merit principal consideration for choice of pharmacotherapy

8. Discuss the maternal-neonatal <u>advantages of methadone relative to buprenorphine</u> as pharmacotherapy of opioid-dependent pregnant women. *(1 point each)*

Max 6

Maternal:

☐ Improves adherence to therapy with less dropout rates or relapse to opioid use

☐ Decreased diversion *(i.e., use of prescription medication by someone other than for whom it was intended)*

☐ Greater threshold limit for maximal equivalent dose *(i.e., absence of a 'ceiling effect')*

☐ Effective with failed buprenorphine treatment

☐ Decreased liver dysfunction or abnormal transaminases

☐ Generally, a simpler induction protocol with lower risk of precipitating withdrawal

☐ Lower cost *(international variations)*

Neonatal:

☐ Generally, more data available on long-term neurodevelopmental outcome

  ○ **Recently,** follow-up of children with in utero exposure to methadone compared with buprenorphine showed normal early childhood development of physical, cognitive, and language functions *(Kaltenbach K et al. Drug and alcohol dependence 2018;185:40–9)*

The patient complains of frequent perspirations, general myalgia and anxiousness. The addiction medicine expert proposes hospitalization[†] for induction and stabilization of pharmacotherapy, investigations, and coordination of care. Additional multidisciplinary consultations will be arranged with experts in nutrition, pediatrics, anesthesia, pain management, behavioral health, and social services.

Special note:

† Hospitalization may not be obligatory for induction of pharmacotherapy for prenatal OUD

9. Specific to this obstetric patient's chronic opioid dependency, outline your recommended investigations at hospitalization. *(1 point per main bullet)*   15

Imaging:[§]
☐ Dating sonography and detailed fetal morphology scan

Testing for infections:
☐ HIV antigen/antibody (*i.e.*, fourth generation testing)
☐ Covid testing
☐ Hepatitis A antibody *(plan vaccination if serology is negative)*
☐ HBV: HBsAg, HBsAb, HBcAb *(plan vaccination if serology is negative)*
☐ HCV antibody
☐ Syphilis testing (conventional or reverse algorithm screening)
☐ Toxoplasmosis IgG, IgM serology
☐ CMV IgG, IgM serology
☐ Tuberculosis (TB) testing (*e.g.,* purefied protein derivative or quantiferon)
☐ Urinalysis, culture, and testing for chlamydia/gonorrhea
☐ *Consideration* for Trichomonas vaginalis testing

General serum laboratory tests:
☐ CBC/FBC
☐ Ferritin
☐ Hepatic transaminases and function tests *(i.e., AST, ALT, GGT, bilirubin, INR)*
   ○ *May initiate pharmacotherapy prior to results*
   ○ *Buprenorphine is not contraindicated in liver disease, except with severe dysfunction*
☐ Creatinine and electrolytes

Special note:
§ Electrocardiogram (ECG) would be required to detect prolonged QT interval if methadone treatment was planned

10-A. Your obstetric trainee inquires why urine toxicology screening, and associated consent, have not been considered at the initial stage of investigations.   1

☐ Urine toxicology is unnecessary in the context of this patient's disclosure

10-B. Inform your trainee of four situations that *may or may not* apply to this patient, warranting consideration for biologic toxicology screening.[§] *(1 point each)*   Max 4

☐ Serially while on pharmacotherapy for OUD, to ensure no concurrent illicit use and compliance with prescribed pharmacotherapy
☐ At delivery-admission with history of illicit substance use at any time in pregnancy or on medication-assisted therapy for OUD *(depending on local and hospital policy)*
☐ Obtunded or unconscious patient
☐ Evidence of intoxication or patient falls asleep mid-sentences
☐ Recent physical evidence of injections (*e.g.*, 'track marks')
☐ Unexplained soft tissue infections or endocarditis
☐ Absence of prenatal care at the time of delivery
☐ Acute complications, such as fetal death, placental abruption, severe hypertension (*individualized assessment*)
☐ Unexpected reaction to buprenorphine (*may suggest fentanyl contamination*)

10-C. Discuss four characteristics of urine drug screening that justify why *universal* prenatal biologic testing is <u>not</u> recommended. *(1 point each)*   Max 4

☐ False-positive results may have legal and social repercussions, which are exacerbated by racial biases and have resulted in differential rates of loss of custody in communities of color
☐ Positive results are nondiagnostic of the incidence or severity of OUD, and may due to cross-reactivity with nonopioid drugs
☐ Negative results are common to inconsistent substance use, testing beyond the interval of drug detection, switching urine samples, and increasing water intake
☐ Biologic testing is limited by substances included in the panel
☐ Inability to detect alcohol use
☐ Cost

<u>Special note:</u>
§   Consent is required, unless the patient is unconscious

Sonography confirms a single viable male fetus with biometry consistent with 20^{+3} weeks' gestation, a nine-day difference from menstrual dating. Fetal morphology, placentation, amniotic fluid volume and cervical length are normal. Laboratory investigations reveal mild iron-deficiency anemia. All other serum and urine tests are unremarkable; she is immune to hepatitis B virus.

At admission, sublingual buprenorphine/naloxone 4 mg is given as a test dose. Without adverse reaction to the test dose, persistent physical manifestations of withdrawal 30 minutes later require dose escalation to 8 mg to achieve symptom resolution.[†] The following day, she receives 8 mg as given the day prior, and additional 4 mg daily increments are required until resolution of withdrawal symptoms is achieved on 8 mg twice daily. Recognizing antenatal repercussions of cigarette smoking and postnatal risks particular to opioid-dependent women, you counsel the patient and provide means for tobacco cessation.

The patient starts individual behavioral therapy and remains adherent to medical treatment. Her partner remains supportive and a social worker confirms a safe home environment.

Special note:
† Adequate dosing of buprenorphine/naloxone on the first day to achieve symptom resolution is advised to improve patient acceptance of treatment

---

11. Discuss your choice of gestational age estimate.   1

☐ Maintain menstrual dating given <10 days' difference between sonographic and menstrual dates at 16^{+0} to 21^{+6} weeks' gestation

Special note:
Refer to Committee Opinion No. 688: Management of Suboptimally Dated Pregnancies. Obstet Gynecol. 2017;129(3): e29-e32.

12-A. Indicate the principal risk of nicotine withdrawal particular to this patient with OUD.   1

☐ Increased opioid requirements due to loss of nicotine's analgesic properties

12-B. Discuss three principal interventions for smoking cessation you may offer this patient.   3
(1 point per main bullet)

☐ Psychosocial interventions, including:
  ○ Live or digital counseling with smoking health educators
  ○ Pregnancy-specific manuals
☐ Behavioral changes, including:
  ○ Disposing of ashtrays
  ○ Avoiding other smokers
☐ Pharmacotherapy: *(combined with psychosocial or behavioral interventions)*
  ○ Nicotine replacement therapy (transdermal patch, gum, nasal spray, lozenges)
  ○ Bupropion§

Special note:
§ No confirmed risk of fetal anomalies or adverse obstetric effects with use of bupropion; *refer to* ACOG Committee Opinion, No. 807. *Obstet Gynecol.* 2020;135(5): e221-e229, and Turner E, et al. *Nicotine Tob Res.* 2019;21(8):1001–1010.

Concerned about the effects of cigarette smoke on obstetric outcome, the patient agrees to start a nicotine patch, to be removed nightly. She prefers watching video-taped presentations by smoking educators, as she already attends regular psychosocial sessions for treatment of OUD.

13. Elicit this patient's <u>social factors</u> that support outpatient opioid agonist prescription. *(1 point each)*

3

☐ Safe home environment for storage of medication
☐ Discontinued illicit substance use
☐ Patient intent to adhere to clinical care plan involving combined pharmacotherapy and psychosocial interventions

14. Provide discharge counseling on *common* side effects of buprenorphine. *(1 point each)*

Max 2

☐ Fever, chills
☐ Insomnia, anxiety
☐ Nausea, vomiting, abdominal pain, change in bowel habits *(especially constipation)*

15. With focus on pharmaco-psychosocial therapy for OUD and related comorbidities, outline important aspects for her <u>outpatient antenatal</u> management. *(1 point per main bullet)*

Max 7

Maternal:
☐ Consideration for frequent clinic visits to decrease risks of buprenorphine diversion and improve adherence to care, particularly in the beginning of treatment *(individualized frequency)*
☐ Complete Covid vaccination series, if not previously done
☐ Monitoring of weight gain is of particular importance with OUD
☐ Correction of her iron-deficiency anemia with oral replacement therapy
　○ Treatment of anemia decreases maternal and perinatal adverse outcome[§]
　○ Anemia is common to patients with OUD
☐ Provide bowel regimen for constipation
☐ Consideration for repeat STI testing in the third trimester *(e.g., HIV, HCV, syphilis, chlamydia, gonorrhea)*
☐ Serial urine toxicology screening; consideration for monthly testing during buprenorphine maintenance treatment
☐ Continued multidisciplinary collaboration
☐ Advise the patient to present early in labor for analgesic care

Fetal:
☐ Consideration for fetal growth assessment in the later second or early third trimester
　○ *Lack of evidence for serial antenatal testing of patients who remain adherent to pharmacotherapy for OUD alone and have no other indication for testing (e.g., FGR)*

Special note:
§　Refer to Chapter 1 Question 11 for discussion of maternal-perinatal risks of iron-deficiency anemia

At 29 weeks' gestation, the patient complains of increased morning and afternoon cravings for heroin although she managed to resist consumption until contacting you. After recent neonatology consultation where risks and management of abstinence syndrome were discussed, the patient is ambivalent about increasing her pharmacotherapy. To date, serial urine toxicology screens are negative for illicit substances, and the patient is adherent to the management plan.

16-A. Address the patient's concern about the relationship between dosage of opioid agonists and neonatal opioid withdrawal syndrome (NOWS),[†] and discuss the management plan for her cravings, in collaboration with the addiction medicine expert. *(1 point each)*

2

☐ Reassure the patient that dose of opioid agonists is not correlated with severity of NOWS
☐ Increase buprenorphine/naloxone to 8 mg thrice daily sublingually *(max 32 mg/d sublingual)*

16-B. You take note to inform your trainee of factors that may affect the development and severity of NOWS. Identify four risk factors, which *may or may not* be related to this patient. *(1 point each)*

4

☐ Genetic, epigenetic, and environmental disposition
☐ Cigarette smoking
☐ Methadone treatment
☐ Concomitant medications *(see Question 1)*
☐ Insufficient rooming-in to promote skin-to-skin care, breastfeeding and family involvement
☐ Prematurity and low birthweight (decrease the risk of NOWS)

Special note:
† NOWS is used to describe opioid-only neonatal abstinence syndrome (NAS)

17. Although discussed with the neonatologist, the patient requests you outline the *general* method of assessment and treatment, should her newborn develop NOWS. *(1 point per main bullet)*

3

☐ Several[†] tools for assessment of NOWS exist, without an ideal screening index
  ○ *Tools do not apply well to preterm or polysubstance exposed infants*
☐ Nonpharmacological supportive therapy
  ○ *e.g.,* Recent development of the 'Eat, Sleep, Console model' [*Grossman MR et al. Hosp Pediatr 2018;8(1):1–6*]

☐ Pharmacologic treatment with opioids, most commonly morphine or methadone
   ○ *Individual nursery evidence-based treatment protocol is recommended*

Special note:
† 6 NOWS scoring systems have been published between the years 1975–2009

Reassured that increasing gestational requirements of opioid agonist is a normal phenomenon, without adversely affecting her child's risk of withdrawal, the patient agrees to the incremental dose adjustment; she has remained adherent to psychosocial sessions and is satisfied with the nicotine patch.

During this clinic visit at 29 weeks' gestation, you perform an obstetric sonogram, noting fundal height is at 25 cm. Reassuringly, fetal biometry on the 15th percentile for gestational age and amniotic fluid volume is normal.

18. What is the anticipated effect of buprenorphine on fetal biophysical parameters, *if any*, and what are potential differences with methadone treatment?

        Max 6

☐ Generally, buprenorphine may have little effect on fetal CTG or BPP parameters *(4 points)*
☐ Methadone may be associated with aberrations, such as: *(1 point per subbullet)*
   ○ Decreased variability
   ○ Decreased baseline fetal heart rate
   ○ Decreased breathing activity
   ○ Less frequent accelerations and movement

Special note:
Abnormalities may be less frequent with split-dosing of methadone and by delaying testing for four to six hours after ingestion

Routine aspects of prenatal care are unremarkable, and the remainder of pregnancy proceeds well with close multidisciplinary affiliations. The patient presents in spontaneous labor at 36^{+6} weeks' gestation; the fetus is in the cephalic presentation, CTG is normal, and her GBS swab was negative.

19. Outline essentials of <u>labor and delivery</u> management with regard to the patient's history of opioid use and antenatal buprenorphine pharmacotherapy. *(1 point per main bullet)*

Max 8

☐ Secure an IV line <u>early</u> in labor in case of obstetric emergency
  ○ *Anticipate risk of difficult venous access due to scars and sclerosed veins*
☐ Individualized consideration for biologic drug screening (*e.g.*, urine testing) upon admission
☐ Continue liaison with the addiction therapy team and request early intrapartum anesthesiology consultation
  ○ Neuraxial anesthesia (*e.g.*, epidural and combined spinal-epidural) is safe among patients with pharmacotherapy for OUD
  ○ Expect higher doses of opioids will be required to achieve analgesia
  ○ Alternatives for pain management include patient controlled analgesia (PCA) pump, mindfulness/relaxation training, gabapentin, ketamine
  ○ Doula may be helpful, if available
☐ Continue the patient's total daily buprenorphine dose, preferably in divided doses
  ○ Suggest verification of patient's self-administered agents
  ○ Do not rely on additional buprenorphine to achieve labor analgesia
☐ Reassure the patient that intrapartum opioids will not increase her relapse rate
☐ Use inhaled nitrous oxide in opioid-dependent women with caution *(risk of sedation)*
☐ Avoid intrapartum or postpartum use of opioid antagonists or agonist-antagonists, such as nalbuphine, naloxone, butorphanol, pentazocine *(precipitate withdrawal)*
☐ Continuous electronic CTG monitoring
☐ Neonatology assessment at delivery
☐ Pathology examination of the placenta and umbilical cord

Special note:
Where required, suggest ***standard dose*** protocol of magnesium sulfate for eclampsia prophylaxis or fetal neuroprotection; no evidence of additive neuro-cardio-respiratory depression with concomitant opioid agonist therapy

Early IV access and epidural analgesia are initiated in labor; the anesthesiologist notes a 30% higher dose of opioid compared to non–drug users. Intrapartum buprenorphine is continued in split doses and the addiction medicine expert concurrently follows the patient's labor analgesic needs.

She has an uncomplicated spontaneous vaginal delivery of a healthy neonate, as assessed by the neonatology team. Arrangements have been made to extend maternal hospitalization to five days, primarily for neonatal observation during the risk-period for NOWS.

20. What are important <u>postpartum</u> considerations and <u>discharge</u> recommendations, specific to this patient on medication-assisted treatment for OUD? *(1 point per main bullet)*

Max 18

Preferred **management of buprenorphine and analgesia:** *(in conjunction with respective experts)*

A. <u>Inpatient</u>:

☐ Continue her maintenance dose of buprenorphine
  ○ *Divided dosing may provide additional partial pain relief and lower risk of respiratory depression or sedation where concomitant opioids are needed*
☐ Nonopioids and nonpharmacologic analgesics on a scheduled basis rather than as needed treatment
☐ Judicious use of short-acting, low-dose opioids is generally reserved for post-Cesarean delivery, if needed

B. <u>Discharge</u>:

☐ Inform the patient that untreated pain can also trigger relapse of illicit opioid use
☐ Revision of her opioid requirements during hospitalization helps determine the need for outpatient opioid analgesia
  ○ Preferred avoidance of outpatient opioids after vaginal delivery, unless after extensive laceration repair or difficult delivery
  ○ Limit the dose and duration of outpatient opioids *(shared decision-making with the patient is advised)*
  ○ Suggest a reliable family member to dispense medication *when necessary*
☐ Continue combined buprenorphine/naloxone regimen used antenatally
☐ Encourage long-term opioid-agonist treatment for at least one year

<u>Mental health monitoring</u>:

☐ Screen for postpartum depression and continue to offer psychosocial support services
☐ Close postdischarge follow-up for risk of relapse/drug overdose

<u>Breastfeeding</u>:

☐ Provide lactation counseling or expert consultation
☐ Encourage breastfeeding with stable opioid agonist treatment, where no contraindication exists *(<1% and 1%–3% of maternal weight-adjusted dose of buprenorphine and methadone is present in breast milk, respectively)*
☐ Inform patient to suspend breastfeeding with relapse
☐ Continue breastfeeding as long as patient and infant desire; advise gradual weaning over approximately two weeks (once decision made to wean) to avoid infant withdrawal

<u>Contraception</u>:

☐ Reassure the patient that contraceptive counseling serves to empower her to achieve the desired interpregnancy interval, rather than your judgement of her suitability for parenting
☐ Offer long-acting reversible contraception immediately after delivery, if available
☐ Encourage use of condoms for dual contraception to decrease risks of STIs

Infant care:
☐ At discharge, educate the patient regarding signs and symptoms, and encourage early reporting of NOWS
☐ Arrange for local child welfare services to ensure safe care at home as required by law
   ○ Be aware of local requirements, while remaining mindful that loss of custody is more frequent in communities of color, and that many maternal-infant complications *(e.g., including overdose deaths, worse infant and child outcomes)* occur with loss of custody

Maternal outpatient follow-up:
☐ Arrange for a clinic visit at two weeks postpartum with addiction team and/or obstetrics
   ○ *Presence of significant stressors warrant very close follow-up; avoid gaps in care*
☐ Discourage future self-initiated discontinuation of pharmacotherapy with inadvertent pregnancy, and encourage preconception counseling, if possible

After the patient's discharge, your obstetric trainee indicates he or she appreciates the well-structured, comprehensive discharge plan; you find the trainee surfing the internet to learn of the benefits of breastfeeding, particular to women on opioid agonist therapy.

21. Discuss the maternal-neonatal benefits of breastfeeding, particular to women on opioid agonist therapy. *(1 point each)*	Max 5

Maternal:[†]
☐ Improved maternal-infant bonding
☐ Stress reduction and increased confidence
☐ Enhanced compliance with treatment of OUD, providing protection against relapse

Neonatal:
☐ Decreased severity of withdrawal syndrome
☐ Decreased need for, and doses of, opioid for treatment of withdrawal
☐ Shorter hospitalization

Special note:
† breastfeeding also reduces relapse to cigarette smoking

TOTAL:	**165**

CHAPTER 77

Acute Abdominal Pain in Pregnancy

Vincent Ponette and Amira El-Messidi

During your call duty, a 37-year-old obese G2P1 patient presents to your hospital center's obstetric emergency assessment unit at 33^{+3} weeks' gestation with pain and bruising in the lower aspect of the mid-abdomen. She holds her lower abdomen for support in between bouts of a residual dry cough after completion of antibiotic treatment for community-acquired pneumonia. Pregnancy has otherwise been unremarkable, and she has been compliant with prenatal care. She does not have vaginal bleeding or fluid loss. Two years ago, she had a Cesarean section for term breech presentation.

LEARNING OBJECTIVES

1. Appreciate the importance of maintaining a high index of clinical suspicion for less common causes of abdominal pain in late pregnancy and associated diagnostic challenges
2. Demonstrate awareness of particular signs on physical examination that may aid in distinguishing rectus sheath hematoma from other causes of acute intra-abdominal causes
3. Be familiar with clinical risk factors and pathophysiology for developing a rectus sheath hematoma
4. Recognize aspects of conservative management, with an understanding of the possible need for surgical intervention due to maternal-fetal morbidities risks associated with rectus sheath hematoma

SUGGESTED READINGS

1. Deb S, Hoo P, Chilaka V. Rectus sheath haematoma in pregnancy: a clinical challenge. *J Obstet Gynaecol.* 2006;26(8):822–823.
2. Eckhoff K, Wedel T, Both M, et al. Spontaneous rectus sheath hematoma in pregnancy and a systematic anatomical workup of rectus sheath hematoma: a case report. *J Med Case Rep.* 2016;10(1):292.
3. Gibbs J, Bridges F, Trivedi K, et al. Spontaneous rectus sheath hematoma in pregnancy complicated by the development of transfusion related acute lung injury: a case report and review of the literature. *AJP Rep.* 2016;6(3):e325–e328.
4. Machado-Gédéon A, Mitric C, Ponette V, et al. Spontaneous rectus sheath hematoma in pregnancy: a case report. *J Obstet Gynaecol Can.* 2020;42(11):1388–1390.

5. Tolcher MC, Nitsche JF, Arendt KW, et al. Spontaneous rectus sheath hematoma pregnancy: case report and review of the literature. *Obstet Gynecol Surv.* 2010;65(8):517–522.

6. Valsky DV, Daum H, Yagel S. Rectus sheath hematoma as a rare complication of genetic amniocentesis. *J Ultrasound Med.* 2007;26(3):371–372.

7. Wai C, Bhatia K, Clegg I. Rectus sheath haematoma: a rare cause of abdominal pain in pregnancy. *Int J Obstet Anesth.* 2015;24(2):194–195.

POINTS

1. What aspects of a <u>focused</u> history would you want to know? *(1 point each with section-specific max points)*   12

Details of abdominal pain: *(max 6)*
☐ Onset, duration, radiation, characteristics
☐ Presence of contractions
☐ Recent trauma
☐ Incisional pain at the Cesarean section site
☐ Aggravating factors apart from coughing
☐ Alleviating factors *(e.g., analgesics, maternal positioning)*
☐ Prior similar presentation

Associated symptoms, comorbidities, and surgical history: *(max 5)*
☐ Fever or chills
☐ Known or recent manifestations of preeclampsia/hypertensive syndromes
☐ Cardiorespiratory *(e.g., asthma, palpitations, [pleuritic] chest pain, shortness of breath)*
☐ Gastrointestinal symptoms *(e.g., nausea/vomiting, gastroesophageal reflux, constipation/diarrhea)*, or pain related to meals
☐ Renal *(e.g., dysuria, hematuria, back pain, abnormal urine color, known calculi)*
☐ Prior surgery apart from Cesarean section

Medications and social habits: *(max 1)*
☐ Prescribed anticoagulants or home-medicinals with anticoagulant effects
☐ Illicit substances *(e.g., cocaine)*

The patient informs you that the sharp pain is of spontaneous acute onset several hours ago, after an intense series of coughs from which she is recuperating. Also aggravated by fetal movements and touch, the pain remains superficial and well localized to the midline of the lower abdomen, where her husband noticed the bruised skin. There is no history of trauma, Cesarean incisional pain or uterine contractions. She is nauseous, without any other systemic complaints. Medications and social habits are noncontributory. She had a remote cholecystectomy.

2. Recognizing the extensive possibilities for abdominal pain in pregnancy, indicate four gynecological and nongynecological considerations, respectively, for this patient's presentation. *(1 point each)*

8

Gynecological:
☐ Placental abruption
☐ Labor
☐ Pedunculated or subserous degenerating fibroid
☐ Uterine rupture
☐ Ovarian mass

Nongynecological:
☐ Rectal sheath hematoma
☐ Evolving subcapsular liver hematoma
☐ Appendicitis
☐ Hernia
☐ Bowel obstruction
☐ Pancreatitis
☐ Gastroenteritis
☐ Hepatitis
☐ Urinary calculi/pyelonephritis

Special note:
The above list serves as a guide; other etiologies may be appropriate

3. Detail your <u>focused maternal</u> physical exam. *(1 point each with section-specific max points)*

14

Vital signs and cardiorespiratory: *(max 5)*
☐ Blood pressure
☐ Pulse
☐ Oxygen saturation
☐ Respiratory rate
☐ Temperature
☐ Pulmonary auscultation

Abdomen: *(max 8)*
☐ Evidence of trauma or abuse *(e.g., burns, cuts)*, distention
☐ Fundal height measurement
☐ Palpable contractions
☐ Palpable abdominal wall mass
☐ Palpable fetal parts
☐ Tenderness, guarding
☐ *Fothergill's sign* – mass does not cross midline; remains palpable with tensing of the rectus muscle
☐ *Carnett's sign* -exacerbation of pain by rectus muscle contraction while sitting up from supine position
☐ *Cullen's sign* – periumbilical ecchymosis
☐ *Grey Turner's sign* – ecchymoses in the flanks

Pelvic exam: *(1)*
☐ Cervical assessment

The patient is normotensive and afebrile; oxygenation is 98%, pulse is 105 bpm and respiratory rate is 18 breaths/minute. Slightly below one-third of the distance from the umbilicus to the symphysis pubis is a noticeable focal bruise, ~4 cm in diameter, without breaching of skin. At the region of pain, there is a localized, right-sided tender palpable mass, with no guarding or rebound tenderness elsewhere. Fothergill's and Carnett's signs are positive. Uterine size is appropriate for gestation without palpable contractions or scar tenderness. The cervix is long and closed with no bleeding on examination. Cardiotocography shows fetal baseline at 159 bpm, variability is ~6 bpm, with minimal accelerations that do not meet criteria for reactivity; there are no decelerations or sinusoidal waveforms. Uterine quiescence is maintained.

Results of comprehensive serum investigations are significant for a hemoglobin of 10.5 g/dL [105 g/L] *(normal 11.0–14.0)*, slightly elevated C-reactive protein at 8.5 mg/L *(normal 0.4–8.1)* and hepatic transaminases: ALT is 55 IU/L *(normal 6–45)* and AST is 45 IU/L *(normal 6–35)*. All other serum tests, including platelet concentration and coagulation profile, are unremarkable.

Report of her abdominal ultrasound indicates an intrauterine pregnancy in cephalic presentation with biometric measurements consistent for gestational age and normal amniotic fluid volume. The placenta is posterior. There is no suspicion of a hepatic subcapsular hematoma. At the region of her pain and skin bruising is a heterogeneous hypoechoic structure measuring 92 × 23 × 55 mm located anterior to, yet separate from, the uterine wall:

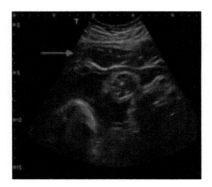

Figure 77.1

With permission: Figure [plate "a"] from J Obstet Gynaecol Can. 2020;42(11):1388–1390.

There is no association between this case scenario and this patient's image. Image used for educational purposes only.

4. Among your suspected etiologies for her abdominal pain, identify the <u>most probable</u> diagnosis.

☐ Rectus sheath hematoma

1

Max 4

5. While planning her current management, you highlight the patient's principal risk factors for rectus sheath hematoma. *(1 point each)*

☐ Abdominal straining *(e.g., her coughing; other mechanisms include sneezing, exercise, vomiting)*
☐ Pregnancy
☐ Multiparity
☐ Previous abdominal surgery
☐ Obesity

Special note:
Other risk factors for rectus sheath hematoma, though not specific to this patient, include anticoagulation, degenerative muscular disease, and amniocentesis

6. Outline essential aspects of your current management. *(1 point each)*

Max 8

Maternal:
☐ Hospitalization
☐ Oral, IV or IM analgesia
☐ Antiemetics and IV hydration
☐ Consideration for early anesthesiology consultation
☐ Serial testing of coagulation parameters and markers of inflammation
☐ Serial transaminase levels, and consideration for obstetric medicine consultation/ investigation of abnormal elevations
☐ Repeat abdominal sonography *(individualized interval)*
☐ Obtain blood group and antibody screening, if not recently available *(in case of need for blood product replacement)*

Fetal:
☐ Maintain continuous electronic monitoring until normalization of the tracing; serial monitoring thereafter
☐ Consideration for initiation of fetal pulmonary corticosteroids

Over the first 24 hours of admission, her abdominal pain subsides and laboratory markers remain stable. Investigations do not identify a cause for elevated hepatic transaminases. Fetal cardiotocographic (CTG) monitoring normalizes within 30 minutes of admission.

On day 2 of admission, the patient reports acute exacerbation of abdominal pain. Her vital signs remain stable. Hemoglobin concentration decreased to 8.9 g/dL [89 g/L], without evidence of coagulopathy. Fetal CTG is normal. She recalls abdominal probe tenderness upon presentation, declining repeat sonographic assessment. An MRI without contrast[†] is thereby initiated, revealing the following:

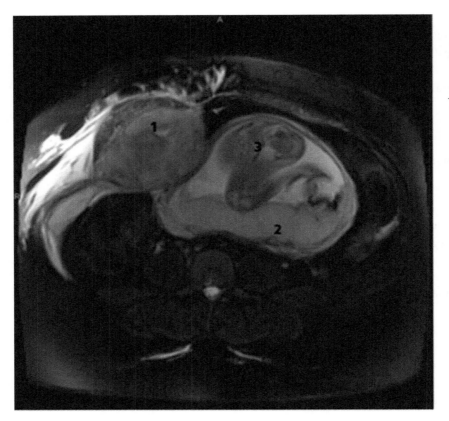

Figure 77.2

From J Med Case Rep. 2016;10(1):292. (suggested reading #2) 'Creative Commons-0': Permission for use of supplementary material is not required: There is no association between this case scenario and this patient's image. Image used for educational purposes only.

Type III‡ rectus sheath hematoma (1) measuring 11×12×20 cm, mainly right sided, starting to displace the uterine wall. The placenta (2) is posterior, without signs of abruption; the fetus is represented by (3)

Special notes:

† Refer to Chapter 42, Question 10 for discussion of MRI in pregnancy

‡ Patients with type III rectus sheath hematoma can present as hemodynamically stable or manifest signs of compromise

7. With focus on rectus sheath hematoma, provide a possible explanation for elevated hepatic transaminases.		1
☐ Release from trauma suffered by skeletal muscle		

8. Discuss the <u>pathophysiology</u> of spontaneous rectus sheath hematoma with your trainee.		1
☐ Shearing/tearing of the inferior epigastric artery or its branches, coursing deep to the posterior aspect of the right and left rectus abdominus muscles, causes blood to dissect along the rectus sheath		

You counsel the patient that given hemodynamic stability and fetal well-being, conservative management will continue with aim for delivery at term. She understands the possible need for blood replacement therapy, correction of developing coagulopathy, or emergent surgery and preterm delivery.

9. Identify a particular feature to consider if Cesarean delivery is required, assuming her rectus sheath hematoma remains of significant size.

1

☐ Consideration for midline vertical skin incision to avoid disruption of the rectus sheath hematoma

TOTAL: **50**

Index